Occupational, Industrial, AND Environmental Toxicology

Occupational, Industrial, *and* Environmental Toxicology

EDITOR-IN-CHIEF

MICHAEL I. GREENBERG, MD, MPH, FACEP, FAAEM

Associate Professor of Public Health, Allegheny University of the Health Sciences,
School of Public Health;
Associate Professor of Emergency Medicine,
Chief, Division of Occupational, Environmental, and Hyperbaric Emergency Medicine,
Allegheny University of the Health Sciences, School of Medicine;
Diplomate, American Board of Emergency Medicine;
Diplomate, American Board of Preventive Medicine (Occupational),
Consulting Toxicologist, Philadelphia Poison Control Center,
Philadelphia, Pennsylvania

EDITORS

RICHARD J. HAMILTON, MD

Instructor, Clinical Surgery/Emergency Medicine,
New York University School of Medicine;
Attending Physician, New York University/Bellevue Hospital;
Diplomate, American Board of Emergency Medicine;
Fellow, Medical Toxicology, New York City Poison Center,
New York University School of Medicine, New York, New York

SCOTT D. PHILLIPS, MD, FACP

Assistant Clinical Professor,
Department of Medicine, Division of Clinical Pharmacology and Toxicology,
Department of Surgery, Division of Emergency Medicine;
Diplomate, American College of Medical Toxicology;
Fellow, American College of Physicians,
Toxicology Associates, Prof LLC, Denver, Colorado

with 168 illustrations

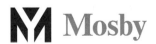

St. Louis   Baltimore   Boston   Carlsbad   Chicago   Naples   New York   Philadelphia   Portland
London   Madrid   Mexico City   Singapore   Sydney   Tokyo   Toronto   Wiesbaden

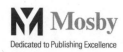
Mosby
Dedicated to Publishing Excellence

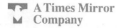
A Times Mirror Company

Vice President and Publisher: Anne S. Patterson
Editor: Laura DeYoung
Associate Developmental Editor: Jennifer Byington Geistler
Designer: Renee Duenow
Manufacturing Manager: David Graybill

Printed in the United States of America
Editing and production by Graphic World Publishing Services
Composition by Graphic World, Inc.
Printing/binding by Maple-Vail Book Mfg. Group

Mosby–Year Book, Inc.
11830 Westline Industrial Drive
St. Louis, Missouri 63146

Library of Congress Cataloging in Publication Data

Occupational, industrial, and environmental toxicology / [edited by]
  Michael I. Greenberg, Richard J. Hamilton, Scott D. Phillips. — 1st
  ed.
     p.   cm.
  Includes bibliographical references and index.
  ISBN 0-8151-3929-2
  1. Industrial toxicology. 2. Environmental toxicology.
I. Greenberg, Michael I. II. Hamilton, Richard J. (Richard Joseph)
III. Phillips, Scott D. (Scott David), 1955- .
  [DNLM: 1. Occupational Exposure—adverse effects. 2. Occupational
Diseases—etiology. 3. Environmental Pollution—adverse effects.
WA 400 0146 1997]
RA1229.0275 1997
615.9′02—dc20
DNLM/DLC
for Library of Congress   96-44661
                                    CIP

96 97 98 99 00 / 9 8 7 6 5 4 3 2 1

Contributors

José Eric Diáz Alcalá, MD, FAAEM
Assistant Professor of Clinical Surgery,
Emergency Medicine—Medical Toxicology,
Cooper Hospital/University Medical Center—RWJ,
Camden, New Jersey;
Assistant Professor,
Division of Medical Toxicology, Occupational and Emergency
  Medicine,
Department of Emergency Medicine,
Allegheny University of the Health Sciences,
Philadelphia, Pennsylvania

Franklin D. Aldrich, MD, PhD, FACP
Clinical Associate Professor of Medicine,
University of Colorado Health Sciences Center,
Denver, Colorado

Angela R. Babin, MS
Program Director,
Center for Safety in the Arts,
New York, New York

Amy J. Behrman, MD
Director, Occupational Medicine,
Department of Emergency Medicine,
Hospital of the University of Pennsylvania,
Philadelphia, Pennsylvania

Howard Blumstein, MD
Assistant Professor, Department of Emergency Medicine,
Allegheny University of the Health Sciences,
Philadelphia, Pennsylvania

Jeffrey Brent, MD, PhD
Associate Clinical Professor of Medicine, Surgery, and
  Pediatrics,
University of Colorado Health Sciences Center,
Denver, Colorado

Jeffrey R. Brubacher, MD, FRCP
Staff Physician, Department of Emergency Medicine,
Vancouver Hospital and Health Sciences Center,
Vancouver, British Columbia, Canada

Art Calise, MD
Department of Emergency Medicine,
Newark Beth Israel Medical Center,
Newark, New Jersey

William K. Chiang, MD
Research Director, Emergency Department;
Clinical Assistant Professor of Surgery/Emergency Medicine,
New York University School of Medicine,
New York, New York

Jeffery M. Cox, MD, FACEP
Assistant Clinical Instructor, Department of Surgery,
Brown University,
Providence, Rhode Island

Natalie M. Cullen, MD
Assistant Professor, Department of Emergency Medicine;
Fellow, Division of Toxicology,
Allegheny University of the Health Sciences,
Philadelphia, Pennsylvania

Francis J. DeRoos, MD
Assistant Professor, Department of Emergency Medicine,
University of Pennsylvania,
Philadelphia, Pennsylvania

Suzanne Doyon, MD, FAAEM
Assistant Professor, Department of Emergency Medicine,
New York Medical College,
Metropolitan Hospital Center,
New York, New York

Timothy Erickson, MD, FACEP
Toxicology Fellowship Director;
Associate Professor of Emergency Medicine,
University of Illinois,
Chicago, Illinois

Susan E. Farrell, MD, FAAEM
Assistant Professor, Department of Emergency Medicine,
Division of Toxicology,
Allegheny University of the Health Sciences,
Philadelphia, Pennsylvania

Swee-Cheng Foo, BSc, MSc, PhD
Associate Professor, Department of Community, Occupational,
  and Family Medicine,
National University of Singapore,
Republic of Singapore

Timothy R. Gablehouse
Managing Partner,
Gablehouse and Epel,
Denver, Colorado

Jeffrey C. Gershel, MD
Clinical Associate Professor of Pediatrics, Department of
    Pediatrics,
Westchester County Medical Center,
Valhalla, New York

Jerry V. Glowniak, MD
Fellow, Bioinformatics,
Biomedical Information Communications Center;
Associate Professor, Radiology and Internal Medicine,
Oregon Health Sciences University,
Portland, Oregon

Hernan F. Gomez, MD, FACP
Lecturer, Division of Emergency Medicine,
Department of Surgery,
University of Michigan Medical Center,
Ann Arbor, Michigan

Ronald E. Gots, MD, PhD
Principal, International Center for Toxicology and Medicine,
Rockville, Maryland

Tee Lamont Guidotti, MD, MPH
Professor of Occupational and Environmental Medicine;
Director of the Occupational Health Program,
Department of Public Health Sciences,
University of Alberta, Faculty of Medicine,
Edmonton, Alberta, Canada

Glendon C. Henry, MD
Assistant Director, Emergency Department;
Clinical Assistant Professor of Surgery/Emergency Medicine,
New York University School of Medicine,
New York, New York

Harold E. Hoffman, MD
Faculty, Occupational Health Program;
Attending Physician, Occupational Medicine Consultation
    Clinic,
University of Alberta Faculty of Medicine and Oral Health
    Sciences,
Edmonton, Alberta, Canada

Robert S. Hoffman, MD, FACEP
Director, New York City Poison Center;
Director, Fellowship in Medical Toxicology;
Clinical Assistant Professor of Surgery/Emergency Medicine,
New York University School of Medicine,
New York, New York

John P. Holland, MD, MPH
Occupational Medicine Consultant;
Clinical Assistant Professor,
Department of Environmental Health,
University of Washington,
Seattle, Washington

Mary Ann Howland, PharmD, ABAT
Clinical Professor of Pharmacy,
St. John's University College of Pharmacy;
Consultant, New York City Poison Center;
Consultant, Department of Emergency Medicine,
Bellevue Hospital Center,
New York, New York

Oliver L. Hung, MD
Fellow, Medical Toxicology,
New York City Poison Center,
New York University,
New York, New York

Raymond Iannacone, MD
Instructor, Department of Emergency Medicine,
Albert Einstein College of Medicine,
Bronx, New York

Lisandro Irizarry, MD
Assistant Professor of Emergency Medicine,
Allegheny University of the Health Sciences,
Philadelphia, Pennsylvania

Warren Jederberg, MSC, USN
LCDR, Naval Medical Research Institute Detachment
    (Toxicology),
Wright Patterson Air Force Base, Ohio

Peter T. Jezukaitis, MB, BS, AFOM (AACP)
Occupational Physician,
Adelaide, Australia

Christine Johnson, PhD
Henry Ford Health Sciences Center,
Detroit, Michigan

David Koh, MBBS, MSc, PhD, FFOM
Associate Professor, Department of Community, Occupational,
    and Family Medicine,
National University of Singapore,
Republic of Singapore

Wolfgang Köhnlein, PhD
University Professor;
Director, Institute of Strahlenbiologie,
Westfalische Wilhelms-Universitat Munster,
Munster, Germany

Lada Kokan, MD
Fellow, Medical Toxicology,
Rocky Mountain Poison and Drug Center,
Denver, Colorado

Edwin K. Kuffner, MD
Fellow, Medical Toxicology,
Rocky Mountain Poison and Drug Center,
Denver, Colorado

Ricky Lee Langley, MD, MPH
Clinical Assistant Professor, Occupational and Environmental
    Medicine,
Duke University,
Durham, North Carolina

David Lee, MD
Toxicology Fellowship Director,
Department of Emergency Medicine,
Allegheny University of the Health Sciences,
Philadelphia, Pennsylvania

Leon LeLeu
Senior Specialist (Director), Occupational Medical Services,
Senior Clinical Lecturer, Occupational Medicine (University
    of Sydney),
The Canberra Hospital,
Garran, Australia

Grace LeMasters, PhD
Professor of Epidemiology and Environmental Health,
University of Cincinnati,
Cincinnati, Ohio

Susan M. Lizarralde, PharmD
Assistant Director, Florida Poison Information Center,
Department of Pediatrics,
University of Miami School of Medicine,
Miami, Florida

Frank LoVecchio, DO
Fellow, Medical Toxicology,
Good Samaritan Regional Poison Center,
Phoenix, Arizona

Christine R. Medora, MD, MPH
Resident, Department of Internal Medicine,
The Cambridge Hospital,
Cambridge, Massachusetts

William J. Meggs, MD, PhD, FACEP
Associate Professor, Division of Clinical Toxicology,
Department of Emergency Medicine,
East Carolina University,
Greenville, North Carolina

Margaret P. Mueller, MD
Department of Emergency Medicine,
Rhode Island Hospital,
Providence, Rhode Island

Lewis Nelson, MD
Clinical Assistant Professor of Surgery/Emergency Medicine,
New York University School of Medicine,
New York, New York

Rudi H. Nussbaum, PhD
Professor Emeritus, Physics and Environmental Sciences
    and Resources,
Portland State University,
Portland, Oregon

Michael T. Parra, MD
Assistant Clinical Professor of Medicine,
University of Colorado Health Sciences Center,
Denver, Colorado

Jeanmarie Perrone, MD
Assistant Professor, Department of Emergency Medicine,
University of Pennsylvania,
Philadelphia, Pennsylvania

Dennis B. Phillips, DO, MPH
Assistant Professor, Department of Preventive Medicine,
Medical College of Wisconsin,
Milwaukee, Wisconsin

Liese O'Halloran Schwarz, MD
Resident, Department of Emergency Medicine,
Rhode Island Hospital;
Brown University,
Providence, Rhode Island

Richard D. Shih, MD
Associate Residency Director, Department of Emergency
    Medicine,
Morristown Memorial Hospital,
Morristown, New Jersey;
Attending Toxicologist, New Jersey Poison Center,
Newark Beth Israel Medical Center,
Newark, New Jersey

Susan Simpson, MS
Research Associate, Department of Environmental Health,
University of Cincinnati,
Cincinnati, Ohio

Dorsett D. Smith, MD
Clinical Professor, Department of Medicine,
Division of Respiratory Disease and Critical Care Medicine,
University of Washington,
Seattle, Washington

David Sonntag, MSPH, USAF, BSC
CAPT, University of Cincinnati,
Department of Environmental Health (AFIT/CIMI),
Cincinnati, Ohio

Kenneth Still, PhD, USN
Capt., Naval Medical Research Institute Detachment
    (Toxicology),
Wright Patterson Air Force Base, Ohio

Christine M. Stork, PharmD
Director, Central New York Poison Control Center;
Clinical Instructor, Emergency Medicine,
University Hospital,
Syracuse, New York

Surajit Suntornthan, MD
Pramongkutklao Hospital,
Bankok, Thailand

Anthony J. Suruda, MD
Director, Occupational Medicine,
Rocky Mountain Center for Occupational and Environmental
    Health,
University of Utah,
Salt Lake City, Utah

Valerie Thompson, MD
Assistant Professor of Pediatrics,
University of Miami School of Medicine;
Medical Director, Florida Poison Information Center,
Miami, Florida

Steven G. Turchen, BA, RN, DABAT
Hazardous Materials Toxicologist,
San Diego Regional Poison Center;
Instructor in Toxicology;
Adjunct Professor of Public Health,
San Diego State University,
Graduate School of Public Health,
San Diego, California

Mark J. Upfal, MD, MPH, FACOEM
Director, Division of Occupational and Environmental Medicine,
Department of Family Medicine,
Wayne State University,
Detroit, Michigan

Barry Wake, BSc, FGA, DGA, CHCM
University of London,
London, England

Richard Y. Wang, DO, FACEP, DACMT
Director, Medical Toxicology;
Assistant Professor of Emergency Medicine,
Department of Emergency Medicine,
Brown University;
Rhode Island Hospital,
Providence, Rhode Island

Paul M. Wax, MD
Assistant Professor of Emergency Medicine,
Department of Emergency Medicine,
University of Rochester School of Medicine,
Rochester, New York

Richard S. Weisman, PharmD, ABAT
Director, Florida Poison Information Center;
Research, Associate Professor of Pediatrics,
Department of Pcdiatrics,
University of Miami School of Medicine,
Miami, Florida

Michael A. Zaragoza, MD
Attending Physician,
Kent General Hospital,
Dover, Delaware

To James R. Roberts, MD, consummate
emergency physician, quintessential medical toxicologist, skilled
teacher, compassionate doctor. Without his mentoring influence this book
would never have been written because without his guidance and
friendship, I never would have become a toxicologist.

Michael I. Greenberg, MD

To my grandparents, who taught me the risks and rewards of work.
To my parents, chemists who sparked and flamed my interest in the natural world.
To my wife, Beth, the Copernican sun who warms and illuminates.
To my children, Richard, Catherine, and Aidan, fellow wanderers in the firmament.

Richard J. Hamilton, MD

To my loving wife, best friend, and eternal companion, Cyrel.
With love and thanks for your unwavering support and enthusiasm.
For protecting my time as if it were yours,
and for keeping the family going. You make the trip worthwhile.
To David and Daniel, who give me inspiration and life.
And to my parents, Ken and Marjorie, who showed me the way.

Scott D. Phillips, MD

Foreword

Occupational, Industrial, and Environmental Toxicology increases our potential to serve our patients. This effort further develops our understanding of environmental and occupational medicine and medical toxicology. The editors and authors have expanded our clinical perspectives. They enhance the traditional approach to the workplace setting by first focusing on the particular worker's occupation and then by emphasizing the potential toxins involved and their commonly associated clinical symptoms. By using this new structured approach to problem solving, the reader will have a better understanding of occupational epidemiology.

As the fields of medical toxicology and environmental and occupational medicine are developed and better understood, we are forced to be more creative in thinking about old and new problems. It is true that our data bases have been expanded, but our success remains based on meeting each patient's needs. Success can be achieved only when a fine and complete history and physical examination are accomplished. This allows the physician to think more clearly about the relationship between the worker's symptoms and his or her occupational site. The authors' enhancement of occupational and environmental epidemiology enriches our thinking about clinical dilemmas.

Medical toxicologists can expand this approach by considering the predisposing biologic makeup of the worker, the personal behavioral factors affecting health, the current medications used by the individual, and many other characteristics that make the clinician's tasks stimulating and provocative. Many of the chapters are based on an understanding of the biochemistry of toxicology. If clinicians improve their efforts in the investigation of an occupational exposure as developed in this text, the etiology and epidemiology of problems such as teratogenesis, carcinogenesis, and chronic diseases will be better understood.

The complex assessment of the worker, the workplace, and the environment necessitates a meticulous and comprehensive analysis. This text will allow physicians to think in a more systematic fashion about clinical problems and thus provide the stimulus necessary to improve the industrial environment and the health of workers. This enhanced understanding of the workplace and the environment will, I hope, allow us to increase our society's technology and creative potential without compromising the health and safety of the future worker.

Lewis R. Goldfrank, MD, FACP, FACEP
Director, Department of Emergency Medicine,
Bellevue Hospital Center and New York University
    Medical Center;
Associate Professor of Clinical Medicine,
New York University School of Medicine;
Medical Director, New York Poison Center,
New York, New York

Preface

Bernardino Ramazzini published the first edition of his *Discourse on the Diseases of Workers* in 1700. In the preface to that classic work, he admitted that his book was far from perfect, and he offered the hope that readers would be inspired by his work to investigate more completely the problems addressed in that book. Basically, he encouraged his readers to fill in the blanks.

Now, almost 300 years later, by this book, we have undertaken a task no less daunting than the one Ramazzini attempted. We have written our own "discourse" on the toxicologic diseases of workers. Despite the fact that our tools vastly surpassed those Ramazzini had at his disposal, the luxury of computer searches, word processors, laptop computers, E-mail, and the "Net" did not seem to adequately ease the burden of accomplishing what we set out to do.

The major task we set for ourselves was to take a fresh look at the body of knowledge relevant to occupational, industrial, and environmental toxicology and come up with a better way of delivering it to the reader. Realizing that all previous writers had chronicled the information in the traditional toxicologic model—by toxin or by the body system affected—we sought a new and different organization for the information, an approach that we hoped would be better suited to the clinician's daily use. After all, the clinician is the person who is actually called upon to sort out the complaints of the patient and whose task it is to formulate a diagnosis that takes into account, for example, the patient's occupational and environmental life history. With the relevant information organized by occupation and industry, we feel that a practical problem is solved. Those who treat patients regularly recognize that patients often tell the physician that they are firefighters, accountants, food handlers, or sandblasters rather than recalling that they have been exposed to one toxin or the other by name. They often tell the physician that their hobby is boatbuilding or ceramics but rarely say they think a particular toxin is causing a particular set of symptoms. This is the strength of our book. It allows the clinician to take simple, readily available, and generally accurate information about the patient and narrow the symptom complex and complaints offered to a set of toxins that are most commonly encountered in that given vocation or avocation. We have done so for vocations and avocations covering in excess of 50 million workers. However, just as our confrere Ramazzini confessed weakness in his written work, so do we. This text does not address every occupation or industry under the sun. Certainly, it does not contain the work-related toxic diseases of every occupation. However, an importantly large number of them are included. Just as Ramazzini asked for the indulgence of his readers, so do we. Despite the fact that our work covers the potential toxic insults to many millions of workers, others surely are, to some degree, left out. The service we feel we have performed, like Ramazzini some 300 years previously, will be fulfilled if our readers become inspired to fill in the blanks in their personal knowledge bases by digesting the material we present. We hope they fill in the blanks by answering the hundreds of review questions we have provided. Finally, we hope they fill in the blanks by telling us where we may have overlooked an important toxin or a fascinating profession, occupation, or avocation, so that subsequent editions of this work will become even more useful to readers.

Michael I. Greenberg, MD
Richard J. Hamilton, MD
Scott D. Phillips, MD

Acknowledgments

We would like to acknowledge Joan Saraceni and Diane Mueller for their hard work and support in completing this project. We would also like to thank Detective Jeffery S. McCabe of the Upper Merion Township Police Department, King of Prussia, Pennsylvania; Lieutenant Frank Bason of the Pennsylvania State Police; and Deputy Chief of Detectives Timothy Woodward of the Montgomery County District Attorney's Office, Norristown, Pennsylvania, for their technical help in writing the chapter on Police and Law Enforcement Personnel. We would also like to thank Laura DeYoung and Jennifer Byington Geistler of Mosby, whose vision for this book and dedication to the project made this work possible.

Michael I. Greenberg, MD
Richard J. Hamilton, MD
Scott D. Phillips, MD

Contents

Section Two

Industrial Toxicology

Section Editor: Michael I. Greenberg

Section Three

Environmental Toxicology

Section Editor: Scott D. Phillips

Occupational,
Industrial,
AND Environmental
Toxicology

1

A Brief History of Occupational, Industrial, and Environmental Toxicology

Michael I. Greenberg

Scott D. Phillips

There have been many mass exposures to natural and man-made toxins throughout history. A few important human exposures have been primarily environmental. Many more have been occupational or industrial in origin, which have subsequently resulted in environmental contamination. They have resulted in illness and death for a great many people. Often, they begin as industrial accidents and conclude with mass public injury. The Bhopal, India, episode is the best example. In other episodes, the environment poisons the worker. Uranium tunnel mine workers have excess lung cancer from radon exposure. Most episodes follow some type of industrial accident. More than 20 such episodes are reported in the United States every year.

The frequency of these episodes has been increasing with the industrialization of the world. Many disasters involving hazardous substances are never recorded, especially in less developed countries. The public has become more aware of the environment and its pollutants since the publication of the book *Silent Spring* in 1962.[6] Many organizations formed before and since that publication are dedicated to limiting environmental contamination, and public opinion has certainly changed over the last several decades. The following is a partial listing of well-known environmental and industrial toxicologic episodes..

79 AD Pompeii: Volcanic gas from the eruption of Mount Vesuvius caused thousands of deaths. Heat, particulates, and gases, especially oxides of nitrogen and sulfur, played a role in these deaths. It is estimated that more than 2000 died.

994 AD Aquitania, France: Ergot alkaloids are thought to be responsible for the deaths of 40,000.

1692 Salem, Massachusetts: Ergot alkaloids were believed to be the cause of bizarre behavior.[5]

1700 Italy: Cotton dust caused a significant outbreak of respiratory complaints (byssinosis) during the processing of cotton, flax, and soft hemp.

1767 Devonshire, England: Lead-contaminated cider caused colic; later, gout was associated with this same episode.[48]

1700s England: Polycyclic aromatic hydrocarbons caused excess scrotal cancer in men who were exposed as chimney sweeps.

1800s New Jersey: Mercurous nitrate used in the felting process of the hatting industry lead to mercurialism.[49]

1800s Europe: Yellow phosphorus used in the manufacture of matches led to "phossy jaw."[19]

1828 France: Bread and wine contaminated with arsenious acid caused an estimated 40,000 cases of polyneuropathy.[29]

1846 Canada: Lead from soldered cans contaminated foodstuffs in the Franklin expedition.

1900s Staffordshire, England: Arsenic-contaminated sugar was used in beer manufacturing.[32]

1900s United States and India: β-Naphthylamine use in the dye industry resulted in an increase of bladder cancers.

1910 Manchester, England: Polycyclic aromatic hydrocarbons (PAHs) were associated with scrotal cancer: 24 in active mulespinners (cotton textile factory workers), 5 in former mulespinners, 1 in a chimney sweep, and 22 in tar and paraffin workers. Shale oil was used to lubricate the spinning cotton spindles.[15,28]

1915 to 1918 Ypres, Belgium: Chlorine, phosphorus, and mustard gases resulted in 100,000 dead. Overall, there were 1.2 million deaths from chemical warfare in World War I.

1920s to 1990s Worldwide: Asbestos exposure resulted in a marked increase in asbestos-related disease and cancer.[36]

1928 Cleveland, Ohio, Cleveland Clinic: Nitrocellulose-containing x-ray film burned. Cyanide, nitrogen dioxide, and carbon monoxide were generated during pyrolysis. This resulted in 97 deaths immediately and 26 additional deaths during the next month.

1930 United States, Europe, and South Africa: Triorthocresylphosphate (TOCP) resulted in ginger jake paralysis, a neurotoxic disease affecting tens of thousands of people.[35]

1930 Meuse Valley, Belgium: Smog from a thermal inversion resulted in illness and death for many from photochemical smog.

1937 United States: Diethylene glycol used in elixir of sulfanilamide resulted in renal failure.[13]

1939 to 1954 Japan: Cadmium-contaminated water contributed to Itai-Itai disease.[4]

1939 to 1945 Europe, World War II: Cyanide and carbon monoxide exposure occurred; more than 1 million died from Zyklon B (HCN) gas exposure.

1942 Boston, Massachusetts: Carbon monoxide and cyanide from a fire at the Coconut Grove nightclub caused 498 deaths.[11]

1944 Salerno, Italy: Carbon monoxide from a stalled train resulted in more than 500 deaths.

1948 Donora, Pennsylvania: Smog developed from a thermal inversion of photochemical air pollution; 20 died and thousands were ill.

1950s Minimata Bay, Japan: Organic mercury poisoning resulted from the consumption of fish that had eaten plankton that had organified inorganic mercury.[40]

1950–1980s Rocky Flats, Colorado: Beryllium disease was detected in more than 200 workers in a ceramics plant that supported the nuclear weapons trigger plant.[37]

1951 Atlanta, Georgia: Methanol-contaminated whiskey in "moonshine" with ocular toxicity and acidosis.[3,44]

1952 London, England: Photochemical smog epidemic caused the deaths of 4000, with countless others ill.[30]

1953 New York City: Smog from photochemical air pollution resulted in an excess of 200 deaths.

1954 Marshall Islands: Ionizing radiation from fallout during the nuclear testing program developed thyroid cancer.[47]

1956 Turkey: Hexachlorobenzene (C_6Cl_6) caused an estimated 3000 cases of porphyria cutanea tarda in three epidemiologic studies. Though it was withdrawn from the market in 1959, cases continued to be reported until 1961. Those exposed suffered from other illnesses, including skin changes, hepatomegaly, hypertrichosis (causing "monkey children"), and death in 10% of cases. Infants of exposed mothers developed weight loss and a 95% mortality. It was referred to as *pema yara* or pink sore.[41]

1959 Meknes, Morocco: Cooking oil was contaminated with turbojet lubricant containing Triorthocresylphosphate (TOCP).[42]

1960 England and Germany: Thalidomide as an antiemetic in pregnancy resulted in 5000 cases of phocomelia.[33]

1960 to 1970 Louisville, Kentucky: Vinyl chloride use in PVC polymerization workers resulted in hepatic angiosarcomas.[10]

1962 London, England: Smog from photochemical air pollution resulted in an excess of 700 deaths, more than 3000 fewer than the episode in 1952.

1962 Osaka, Japan: Smog from photochemical air pollution resulted in an estimated 60 excess deaths.

1965 Epping, England: Foodstuffs contaminated with methylenedianiline resulted in liver injury in 84 people. Biopsies on 4 patients showed both parenchymal and biliary damage.[25]

1968 Japan: Rice cooking oil contaminated with polychlorinated biphenols caused sensory neuropathy.

1969 France: Copper sulfate neutralized with hydrated lime "Bordeaux mixture" resulted in a granulomatous disease among sprayers of this mixture.[39]

1971 Iraq: Grain contaminated with methylmercury caused the hospitalization of 6530 persons and 459 deaths. The grain was marked with a red dye to indicate it was to be used as seed. People washed off the red dye and consumed the grain for up to 2 months.[1]

1973 Michigan: Polybrominated biphenyl (PBB) instead of magnesium oxide was mistakenly sent as a livestock feed additive. The PBBs were fire retardants; Firemaster was put in Nutrimaster feed bags. More than 25,000 cattle, pigs, and chickens died or were killed to prevent human exposure.[7,52]

1973 to 1975 James River, Virginia: Chlordecone insecticide allegedly caused an increase in neurologic abnormalities among 148 workers.[45]

1970s California: 1,2 dibromo-3-chloropropane DBCP injected in soil as a nematocide resulted in increased infertility, bothazospermia, and oligospermia in a dose-dependent fashion.[50]

1975 El Paso, Texas: Children living within a 6.6-km radius of a smelter had lead levels of at least 60 µg/dl.

1975 Kellogg, Idaho: Lead levels in children who lived near a smelter were greater than 40 µg/dl in 98% of 1- to 9-year-olds.[26]

1975 Jamaica: Parathion-contaminated flour caused death to 17 and illness in 62 others.

1975 Ann Arbor, Michigan: Pancuronium administration resulted in an endemic of respiratory and cardiac arrests.[43]

1976 Seveso, Italy: Dioxin was released after an explosion in a chemical manufacturing plant, with increased incidence of chloracne of those in zone 1.[18]

1978 Jonestown, Guyana: Cyanide-laced beverage resulted in 911 deaths in a mass suicide-execution.[17]

1978 Youngstown, Florida: Chlorine leaked from a punctured tank car carrying 90 liquid tons. This resulted in 8 deaths with 130 total exposures.[22]

1978 Love Canal, New York: Toxic wastes placed in trenches resulted in increased public concern for practical or discernible health effects.[20,38]

1978 Bennington, Vermont: *Campylobacter jejuni* in the community water supply affected more than 3000 people with a typhoidlike illness.

1979 Jackson, Michigan: Methanol-contaminated moonshine was found in a prison.[44]

1979 Taiwan: Polychlorinated biphenyl–contaminated rice cooking oil resulted in sensory neuropathy.[21]

1981 United States: Benzyl alcohol caused a gasping syndrome in children.[14]

1981 Spain: Contaminated rapeseed oil caused an outbreak of pneumonitis in 19,828 cases, 59% of whom were hospitalized and 16% of whom died.[23,46]

1982 San Jose, California: MPTP (1-methyl-4-phenyl-1,2,3,6-tetrahydropyridine), a meperidine analog, injected intravenously resulted in acute parkinsonism.[27]

1982 United States: Cyanide-contaminated acetaminophen tampering incident resulted in 7 deaths.[8]

1982 Iraq and Iran: Mustard gas used in the Iraq-Iran war caused hundreds of casualties.

1983 Times Beach, Missouri: Hazardous waste contamination after application of roadways resulted in much public concern and no discernible health consequences.

1984 Pakistan: Sugar contaminated with endrin, a chlorinated hydrocarbon pesticide, caused seizures in 192 people and a 10% case-fatality rate.

1984 Bhopal, India: Methyl isocyanate release from the Union Carbide plant resulted in 2000 deaths and 200,000 injuries.[34]

1985 California and Oregon: Aldicarb found in watermelons resulted in cholinergic symptoms in many cases. In all, more than 1000 cases were reported to state health departments.[16]

1986 Lake Nyos, Cameroon: Carbon dioxide release from the lake caused more than 1700 deaths.[2]

1986 Chernobyl, Soviet Union: Ionizing radiation after a fire in a nuclear power plant resulted in 32 immediate deaths. The radioactive cloud covered an area of more than 10,000 square miles and affected 5 million people.

1987 Prince Edward Island, Canada: Domoic acid and excitatory amino acid caused 107 patients to develop gastrointestinal symptoms, headache, and memory loss and 12 patients to develop seizures. Four patients died with extensive neuronal loss in the basal ganglia.

1988 Pittsburgh, Pennsylvania: 3-Methylfentanyl (China White) epidemic in intravenous drug abusers.

1989 United States: L-tryptophan associated with eosinophilia-myalgia syndrome.[24]

1990 Texas: A hydrofluoric acid leak from a petrol plant caused 3000 people to be evacuated, more than 1000 to seek medical attention, mostly for irritation symptoms, and 100 to be hospitalized, but no deaths were reported.[51]

1990 Bronx, New York: Carbon monoxide and cyanide in the Happy Land Social Club caused 87 deaths from smoke inhalation.

1990 Worldwide: *Rotavirus* is responsible for more than 870,000 deaths a year in children from diarrhea-associated dehydration.

1991 New York City: Fentanyl injected by intravenous drug abusers resulted in the "Tango and Cash" epidemic.[12,31]

1993 Milwaukee, Wisconsin: Cryptosporidiosis from the water supply affected 350,000 persons, with a massive economic expense to the community.

Ecologic disasters that have not resulted in human adverse health effects, such as the Exxon Valdez oil spill, the oil pipeline rupture in northern Russia, the Persian Gulf oil well fires, and the Yellowstone wildfire, have been excluded.

This chronology is also one of errors or misjudgments or purposeful attempts to harm others. With proper safeguards, protocols, and scientific principles applied, the loss of millions may have been prevented over the last century alone. The greatest loss of life comes from infectious environmental hazards. Providing clean drinking water and education to those affected throughout the world could save more than a million lives annually. Many environmental hazard issues are international. As developing nations undergo their own "industrial revolution," these episodes will continue to increase. From these episodes, we must learn to better manage disasters, contain releases, provide public health and education, treat victims, and, most of all, prevent future episodes.

REFERENCES

1. Bakir F, et al: Methylmercury poisoning in Iraq, *Science* 181:230, 1973.
2. Baxter PJ, Kapila M, Mfonfu D: Lake Nyos disaster, Cameroon, 1986: the medical effects of large scale emissions of carbon dioxide? *BMJ* 298:1437, 1989.
3. Bennett LL, et al: Acute methyl alcohol poisoning: a review based on experiences in an outbreak of 323 cases, *Medicine (Baltimore)* 32:431, 1953.
4. Cadmium pollution and Itai-Itai disease, *Lancet* 2:382, 1971.
5. Caporael LR. Ergotism: the satan loosed in Salem, *Science* 192:21, 1976.
6. Carson R: *Silent Spring,* Cambridge, MA, 1962, Riverside Press.
7. Carter LJ: Michigan PBB incident: chemical mix-up leads to disaster, *Science* 192:240, 1976.
8. Dunea G: Death over the counter, *BMJ* 286:211, 1983.
9. Eckert WG: Mass deaths by gas or chemical poisoning: a historical perspective, *Am J Forensic Med Pathol* 12:119, 1991.
10. Falk H, et al: Hepatic disease among workers at a vinyl chloride polymerization plant, *JAMA* 230:59, 1974.
11. Faxon NW, Churchill ED: The Coconut Grove disaster in Boston, *JAMA* 120:1385, 1942.
12. Fernando D: Fentanyl-laced heroin, *JAMA* 265:2962, 1991.
13. Geiling EHK, Canon PR: Pathological effects of elixir of sulfanilamide (diethylene glycol) poisoning: a clinical and experimental correlation—final report, *JAMA* 111:919, 1938.
14. Gershanik J, et al: The gasping syndrome and benzyl alcohol poisoning, *N Engl J Med* 307:1384, 1982.
15. Goldblatt MW: Vesical tumours induced by chemical compounds, *Br J Indust Med* 6:65, 1949.
16. Green MA, et al. An outbreak of watermelon-borne pesticide toxicity, *Am J Public Health* 77:1431, 1987.
17. The Guyana tragedy: an international forensic problem, *INFORM Rep* 11:2, 1979.
18. Holmsted B: Prolegomena to Seveso, *Arch Toxicol* 44:211, 1980.
19. Hughes JP, et al: Phosphorus necrosis of the jaw: a present day study, *Br J Indust Med* 19:83, 1962.
20. Janerich DT, et al: Cancer incidence in the Love Canal area, *Science* 212:1404, 1981.
21. Jones GRN: Polychlorinated biphenyls: where do we stand now? *Lancet* 2:791, 1989.
22. Jones RN, et al: Lung function after acute chlorine exposure, *Am Rev Respir Dis* 134:1190, 1986.
23. Kilbourne EM, et al: Clinical epidemiology of toxic-oil syndrome: manifestations of a new illness, *N Engl J Med* 309:1408, 1983.
24. Kilbourne EM, et al: Toxic oil syndrome: a current clinical and epidemiologic summary, including comparisons with eosinophilia-myalgia syndrome, *J Am Coll Cardiol* 18:711, 1991.
25. Koppelman H, Robertson MH, Saunders PG: The Epping jaundice, *Br J Med* 1:514, 1966.
26. Landrigan PJ, et al: Epidemic lead absorption near an ore smelter: the role of particulate lead, *N Engl J Med* 292:123, 1975.
27. Langston JW, et al: Chronic Parkinsonism in humans due to a product of meperidine-analog synthesis, *Science* 219:979, 1983.
28. Lee WR, McCann JK: Mulespinners cancer and the wool industry, *Br J Indust Med* 24:148, 1967.
29. Leschke E: Clinical toxicology: modern methods. In *The diagnosis and treatment of poisoning,* Baltimore, William Wood and Co., 1934.
30. Logan WPD: Mortality in the London fog incident, 1952, *Lancet* 1:336, 1953.
31. Martin M, et al: China white epidemic: an eastern United States emergency department experience, *Ann Emerg Med* 20:158, 1991.
32. Massey EW, Wold D, Heyman A: Arsenic: homicidal intoxication, *South Med J* 77:848, 1984.
33. McFadyen RE: Thalidomide in America: a brush with tragedy, *Clin Med* 11:79, 1976.
34. Mehta PS, et al: Bhopal tragedy's health effects: a review of methyl isocyanate toxicity, *JAMA* 264:2781, 1990.
35. Morgan JP: The Jamaica ginger paralysis, *JAMA* 248:1864, 1982.
36. Murray R: Asbestos: a chronology of its origins and health effects, *Br J Indust Med* 47:361, 1990.
37. Newman LS, et al: Pathologic and immunologic alterations in early stages of berylium disease. Reexamination of disease definition and natural history, *Am Rev Respir Dis* 139:1479, 1989.
38. Paigen B: Controversy at Love Canal, *Hastings Center Rep* 12:29, 1982.
39. Pimentel JC, Marques F: Vineyard sprayer's lung, *Thorax* 24:415, 1969.
40. Powell PP: Minimata disease: a story of mercury's malevolence, *South Med J* 84:1352, 1991.
41. Schmid R: Cutaneous porphyria In Turkey, *N Engl J Med* 263:397, 1960.
42. Smith HV, Spalding JM: Outbreak of paralysis in Morocco due to ortho-cresyl phosphate poisoning, *Lancet* 2:1019, 1959.
43. Stross JK, Shasby M, Harlan WR: An epidemic of mysterious cardiopulmonary arrests, *N Engl J Med* 295:1107, 1976.
44. Swartz RD, et al: Epidemic methanol poisoning: clinical and biochemical analysis of a recent episode, *Medicine (Baltimore)* 60:373, 1981.

45. Taylor JR, et al: Chlordecone intoxication in man. *Neurology* 28:626, 1978.

46. Toxic Epidemic Syndrome Study Group: Toxic epidemic syndrome, Spain 1981, *Lancet* 2:697, 1982.

47. United Nations Scientific Committee on the Effects of Atomic Radiation (UNSAEAR): *Sources, effects and risks of ionizing radiation. Report to the General Assembly, with Annexes,* New York, 1988, United Nations.

48. Waldron HA: The Devonshire colic, *J Hist Med* 25:38, 1970.

49. Wedeen RP: Were the hatters of New Jersey "mad"? *Am J Indust Med* 16:225, 1989.

50. Whorton MD, et al: Infertility in male pesticide workers, *Lancet* 2:1259, 1977.

51. Wing JS, et al: Acute health effects in a community after a release of hydrofluoric acid, *Arch Environ Health* 46:155, 1991.

52. Wolff MS, Anderson HA, Selikoff IJ: Human tissue burdens of halogenated aromatic chemicals in Michigan, *JAMA* 247:2112, 1982.

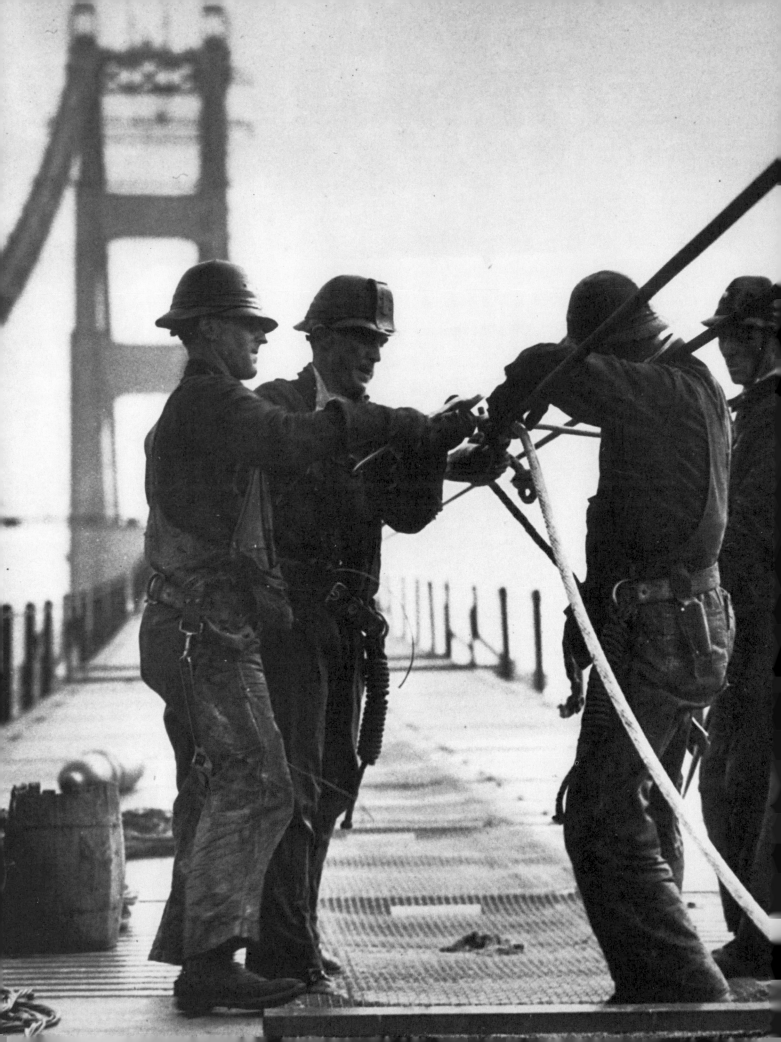

Section One

Occupational Toxicology

Section Editor

Richard J. Hamilton

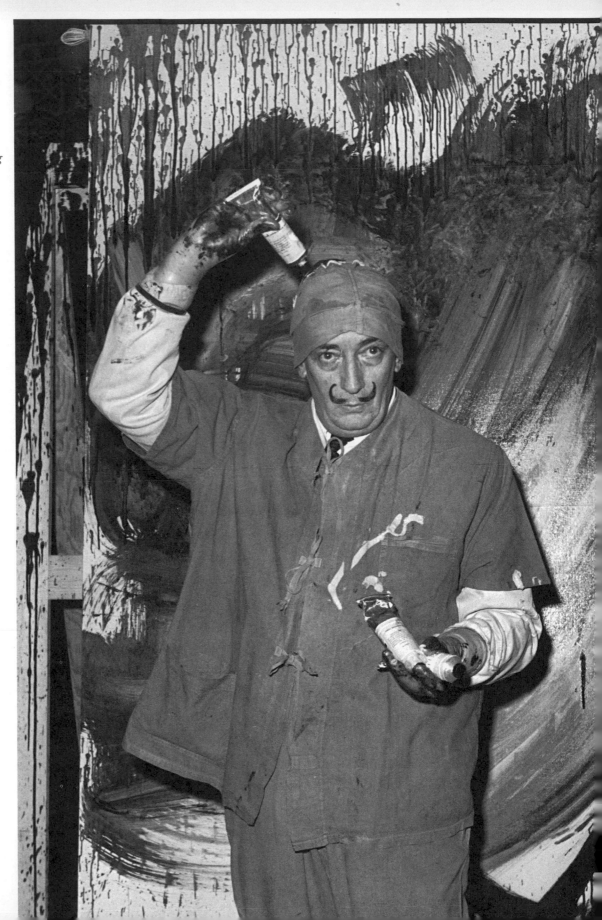

Famed painter, Salvador Dali, daubs paint on his head at the Berkshire Hotel while at work on his abstract impression of Bouguereau's "Nymphs and Satyr," a nineteenth century painting depicting four nude nymphs trying to lead a resisting satyr away. It took Dali ten minutes to finish the painting. Besides using a signpainter's brush, Dali applied paint to the canvas with his head, arm, and chest. He was able to keep the original Bouguereau in 1962 in return for his abstract version of the painting. March 23, 1960.
(Courtesy UPI/Corbis-Bettman)

2

Artists and Artisans

Richard D. Shih

Michael A. Zaragoza

Angela R. Babin

Cd   Hg   Pb

- Artists are exposed to many hazardous substances in a work environment that sometimes enhances the risk of acquiring toxicity

- Physicians who care for artists and artisans must obtain detailed occupational histories and understand the techniques employed by that artist

JOB DESCRIPTION

Artists and artisans, such as painters, sculptors, printmakers, potters, glassblowers, and dyers, are exposed to a variety of hazardous substances during their work. The Bureau of Labor 1992 Statistics identified 273,000 people working in the visual arts, 60% of whom were self-employed. Numerous case studies document heavy metal poisoning, carbon monoxide poisoning, dermatitis, silicosis, neuropathies, cancer, and other ailments.* Several important factors may increase artists' susceptibility to toxic exposures. First, education about prevention is inadequate in many art schools and textbooks.[37] Second, illnesses related to art hazards are uncommonly encountered by most physicians (such as manganism) or difficult to diagnose, in part because physicians are unfamiliar with the techniques employed in this trade.[19,38] Third, there are numerous materials with constituents with undefined toxicity. Lastly, the labeling of art materials is inadequate. Despite passage of the Labeling of Hazardous Art Materials Act in 1988, many products produced before this time and still available may not adequately document hazards. Imported art material is often lacking in appropriate hazard warnings, and some ingredients in art materials are considered trade secrets by the manufacturer and are not included on the list of ingredients.[22,30,51]

*References 11, 19, 22, 24, 32, 41, 48, 54, 59.

9

Table 2-1 Differences in work environment between industrial work setting and home art studios

Worker	Home art studio
Material safety data sheets available	Material safety data sheets may not be available
OSHA Hazcom protocols available	Toxic ingredients may not be known
Safety devices such as ventilation systems designed for task	Safety systems such as ventilation may be inadequate and often homemade
Shift schedule	Erratic work schedule (2–20 hr/day)
Personal protective equipment is often mandatory, available, and maintained	Personal protective equipment less available
Standard work protocols	Experimentation with materials and protocols

Awareness of art hazards dates back to the sixteenth century with Bernardini Ramazzini, who is considered the father of occupational medicine.[50] Published in 1713, Ramazzini's *De Morbis Artifacum (Disease of Workers)* describes silicosis in stone workers and lead poisoning in potters. Others have postulated that many of the masters, such as Rubens and Renoir, suffered from heavy metal poisoning due to pigment exposure.[47]

Artists are exposed to hazardous toxins via the many different media and the myriad of chemicals involved in their work. Exposure to art hazards usually occurs in one of three ways: (1) through inhalation, (2) by skin contact, and (3) via ingestions. Eating and sleeping in the workplace increases the risk of ingestion.[21,22] Prolonged inhalation and skin exposure are common since many artisans work long hours without proper protection, often in home studios (also exposing family members). These locations may be inadequately ventilated and probably lack material safety data sheets (Table 2-1). For further references on information about safety precautions, the reader is referred to the Center for Safety in the Arts, 155 6th Ave., 14th Floor, New York, NY 10013.

Information about toxicity from many of the agents used in this field are derived from occupational settings, and the Occupational Safety and Health Administration (OSHA) and the American Conference of Governmental Industrial Hygienists (ACGIH) safety standards are derived from data in industrial settings.[4,43] Time-weighted averages and permissible exposure limits are not applicable to artisans, who often work more than the traditional five, eight hour days in a week.[38] Finally, artistic experimentiveness creates new chemicals or materials with new possibilities for toxicity (Table 2-2).

TOXICOLOGIC EXPOSURES
Painting/Drawing

Toxicity to the artistic painter can occur through cutaneous exposure, inhalation, or ingestion. The artist's habit of "pointing" the paintbrush with the lips may result in inadvertent ingestion. Eating, drinking, or smoking in the workplace can lead to accidental ingestion and also increases the risk of exposure. Inhalation of powdered pigments or spray mist may occur while air brushing or using spray fixations.

Paint is made from pigments, vehicles, and binders. The two primary health hazards facing paint artists are exposure to the pigments in the paint and exposure to solvents used as thinners or in cleanup.[21,22,52,55] Paints can be water-based (watercolor, acrylic, gouache), solvent-based (alkyd, lacquer), or oil-based. Inorganic metal colors became used widely in the 19th and early 20th centuries. Organic synthetic pigments were utilized in the early 20th century. Inhalation of pigments can occur if the artist makes his or her own paint, uses pastels or sands, or torches the work in a finishing process.

The inorganic pigments have a wide range of potential toxicities. Lead, in the form of basic lead carbonate, lead antimonide, and lead chromate, is used to make a variety of whites and yellows. Most artists are aware of the hazards of lead pigments and avoid handling them in powder form because of the danger of inhaling the dust.[21,42] Even ready-to-use lead paints are dangerous to handle, and hand-washing precautions are crucial in preventing transfer to the oral cavity and subsequent ingestion. Lead toxicity, or plumbism, is well-described and may lead to peripheral neuropathy, hepatotoxicity, and hemolytic anemia, as well as reproductive abnormalities (see Chapter 36).[13]

Cadmium, a coloring agent in some yellow, red, and orange paints, can produce respiratory, dermatologic, or gastrointestinal symptoms with acute toxicity.[34] Inhalation may produce a febrile flulike syndrome, with laryngeal and facial edema resulting in progressive cough and dyspnea. With massive ingestion, pulmonary edema can occur. In cases of chronic exposure, genitourinary (decreased spermatocyte counts, testicular necrosis, hypercalciuria with nephrolithiasis, and proteinuria) and neurologic (vertigo, headache, and shivering) symptoms have been reported, as well as hypochromic anemia and pathologic fractures from bone resorption.[7] Both cadmium and chromate pigments are known or suspected carcinogens.[21,33]

The heavy metal manganese is present in blue, brown, and purple pigments. Toxic exposure may result in manganism, a disease with prominent psychiatric and neurologic manifestations.[30] Locura manganica, or manganese madness, is used to describe a complex of psychiatric symptoms including apathy, anxiety, insomnia, confusion, visual hallucinations, bizarre behavior, emotional lability, and decreased libido. Neurologic manifestations include nystagmus, disequilibrium, paresthesias, memory impairment,

Table 2-2 Art hazards

Technique	Material/process	Hazard
Airbrush	Pigments	Lead, cadmium, manganese, cobalt, mercury, and other metals
	Solvents	Mineral spirits, turpentine
Batik	Wax	Fire, wax fumes
	Dyes	Dyes
Ceramics	Clay dust	Silica
	Glazes	Silica, lead, cadmium, and other toxic metals
	Slip casting	Talc, asbestiform materials
	Kiln firing	Sulfur dioxide, carbon monoxide, fluorides, infrared radiation
Commercial art	Rubber cement	n-Hexane, n-heptane, fire
	Permanent markers	Xylene, propyl alcohol
	Spray adhesives	n-Hexane, 1,1,1-trichloroethane, fire
	Airbrushing	See *airbrush*
	Typography	See *photography*
	Photostats, proofs	Alkali, propyl alcohol
Computer art	Ergonomics	Carpal tunnel syndrome, poorly designed work stations
	Video display	Glare, extremely low frequency radiation
Drawing	Spray fixatives	n-Hexane, other solvents
Electroplating	Gold, silver, other metals	Cyanide salts, hydrogen cyanide, acids
Enameling	Enamels	Lead, cadmium, arsenic, cobalt, and other metals
	Kiln firing	Infrared radiation
Forging	Hammering	Noise
	Hot forge	Carbon monoxide
Glassblowing	Batch process	Lead, silica, arsenic
	Furnaces	Heat, infrared radiation
	Coloring	Metal fumes
	Etching	Hydrofluoric acid, fluoride salts
	Sandblasting	Silica
Holography	Lasers	Nonionizing radiation, electrical
	Developing	Bromine, pyrogallol; see also *photography*
Intaglio	Acid etching	Hydrochloric and nitric acids, nitrogen dioxide, chlorine gas
	Solvents	Alcohol, mineral spirits, kerosene
	Aquatint	Rosin dust, dust explosion
	Photoetching	Glycol ethers, xylene
Jewelry	Silver soldering	Cadmium fumes, fluoride fluxes
	Pickling baths	Acids, sulfur oxides
Lithography	Solvents	Mineral spirits, isophorone, cyclohexanone, kerosene, methylene chloride, and other solvents
	Acids	Nitric, phosphoric, hydrofluoric, hydrochloric, and others
	Talc	Asbestiform materials
	Photolithography	Dichromates
Lost wax casting	Investment	Cristobalite
	Wax burnout	Wax fumes, carbon monoxide
	Crucible furnace	Carbon monoxide, metal fumes
	Metal pouring	Metal fumes, infared radiation, molten metal
	Sandblasting	Silica
Painting	Pigments	Lead, cadmium, mercury, cobalt, manganese compounds, etc.
	Oil, alkyd	Mineral spirits, turpentine
	Acrylic	Trace amount of ammonia, formaldehyde
Pastels	Pigment dusts	Lead, cadmium, and mercury compounds
Photography	Developing bath	Hydroquinone, monomethyl-*p*-aminophenol sulfate, alkalis
	Stop bath	Acetic acid
	Fixing bath	Sulfur doxide
	Intensifier	Dichromates, hydrochloric acid
	Toning	Selenium compounds, hydrogen sulfide, uranium nitrate, sulfur dioxide, gold salts
	Color processes	Formaldehyde, solvents, color developers
	Platinum printing	Platinum salts, lead, acids, oxalates
Relief printing	Solvents	Mineral spirits
Sculpture, clay	See *ceramics*	See *ceramics*
Sculpture, lasers	Lasers	Nonionizing radiation, electrical
Sculpture, neon	Neon tubes	Mercury, electrical

From McCann M: *Artist beware*, ed 2, New York, 1992, Lyons and Buford, pp 11–13.

Continued.

Table 2-2 Art hazards—cont'd

Technique	Material/process	Hazard
Sculpture, plastics	Epoxy resin	Amines, diglycidyl ethers
	Polyester resin	Styrene, methyl methacrylate, methyl ethyl ketone peroxide
	Polyurethane resins	Isocyanates, organotin compounds, amines, mineral spirits
	Acrylic resins	Methyl methacrylate, benzoyl peroxide
	Plastic fabrication	Decomposition products (carbon monoxide, hydrogen chloride, hydrogen cyanide)
Sculpture, stone	Marble	Nuisance dust
	Soapstone	Silica, talc, asbestiform materials
	Granite, sandstone	Silica
	Pneumatic tools	Vibration, noise
Silk screen printing	Pigments	Lead, cadmium, manganese, and other compounds
	Solvents	Mineral spirits, toluene, xylene
	Photoemulsions	Ammonium dichromate
Stained glass	Lead	Lead
	Soldering	Lead, zinc chloride fumes
Weaving	Loom	Ergonomic problems
	Dyeing	Dyes, acids, dichromates
Welding	Oxyacetylene	Carbon monoxide
	Arc	Ozone, nitrogen dioxide, ultraviolet and infrared radiation, electrical hazards
	Metal fumes	Copper, zinc, lead, nickel, etc.
Woodworking	Machining	Wood dust, noise, fire
	Glues	Formaldehyde, epoxy
	Paint strippers	Methylene chloride, toluene, methyl alcohol, and other solvents
	Paints and finishes	Mineral spirits, toluene, turpentine, ethyl alcohol, etc.
	Preservatives	Chromated copper arsenate, pentachlorophenol, creosote

tremors, and lumbosacral pain.[21,33] In many respects, the neurologic syndrome can resemble Parkinson's disease. The most common respiratory complaint is dyspnea, which may result from a pneumonitis, pneumonia, or bronchitis caused by inhalation toxicity. Pathologic changes in the liver have also been described, although clinical hepatitis rarely develops.

Vermilion or vermilion mercury red pigments can cause mercury poisoning. Symptoms include behavioral changes, anorexia, weakness, peripheral neuritis, tremors, and renal impairment (see Chapter 8). Both barium and cobalt, which are used as pigments, are cardiotoxic heavy metals that can cause cardiomyopathy.

Other materials in paint include vehicles, preservatives, binders, and solvents. Most of the vehicles and binders (such as drying oils, egg yolk, gums, and casein) are essentially nontoxic except for quicklime, which is a skin and lung irritant. The most common vehicle in water-based media is acrylic emulsion. Although relatively safe, this emulsion contains a small amount of ammonia and formaldehyde, which may irritate the eyes, nose, and throat if used without proper ventilation.

Solvents are used as paint thinners and for cleanup of brushes and tools. Mineral spirits and turpentine are the most common, although a wide variety are available.

In general, turpentine is the most common solvent used in oil painting. Odorless paint thinner or terpenoid is recommended as a substitute because it is less flammable and less toxic. Solvents are also found in sprays that are used to fix drawings, and in spray-mounting adhesives used in graphic

arts. These sprays contain a wide variety of different aerosolized solvents, such as xylene, methylene chloride, and toluene (see box on p. 13).

Solvents cause dermatitis with sufficient contact. If ingested or inhaled in high enough concentrations, they can produce toxicity such as mental status obtundation, pneumonitis, hepatitis, cardiac sensitization to circulating catecholamines, and peripheral neuropathies. Chronic exposure to solvents has been associated with encephalopathy characterized by neuropsychologic abnormalities, memory impairment, and learning disabilities (see Chapters 21, 25, and 30).[27]

Sculpture

Sculpting is the art of representing figures and forms three-dimensionally. The materials used are most commonly stone, clay, marble, wood, and metals. Each material has its own specific toxicities associated with the material itself or the technique used.

Stone sculpting. Artists carve stone by chipping, grinding, and polishing. Traumatic injury is common and includes eye injuries due to flying debris, repetitive neurologic injuries, and vibration-induced injuries due to pneumatic or vibrational sanders.[27] Toxicologically, the predominant risk is associated with inhalation of dusts and powders during these processes. Many stones such as quartz, granite, and soapstone contain high quantities of silica. Silicosis in this endeavor is poorly documented and studied but is an exposure risk (for a more complete discussion of silicosis, see Chapter 32). Asbestos is a contaminant of stones such as

Past and Present Solvents Utilized by Artists	
Acetone	Isopropyl alcohol
Amyl acetate	Methanol
Amyl alcohol	Methyl acetate
Benzene	Methyl cellosolve
Benzine	Methyl chloroform
Butyl cellosolve	Methylene chloride
Carbon tetrachloride	Methyl ethyl ketone
Chloroform	Methyl isobutyl ketone
Cyclohexanol	Mineral spirits
Ethanol	Tetrachloroethylene
Ethyl acetate	Toluene
Gasoline	Trichloroethylene
Heptane	Turpentine
Hexane	Styrene
Isoamyl alcohol	Xylene
Isophorone	

soapstone and serpentine. The risk for asbestosis from stone sculpting is not known but remains a potential exposure risk (for a more complete discussion of asbestos, see Chapter 52).

Plaster sculpting. Plaster sculpting involves covering an internal wire support with plaster of paris. The plaster of paris is made of calcium sulfate and may be contaminated with lime. It is typically obtained as a powder and mixed with water. During this process, the powder is an exposure risk to the ophthalmologic and respiratory systems. Protective eye and respiratory equipment is recommended during this mixing process. Calcium sulfate is an eye irritant that can cause conjunctivitis. Treatment involves copious irrigation.

Respiratory exposure may cause minor upper respiratory symptoms, including cough and mucous membrane irritation. Lower respiratory effects are uncommon. Treatment involves removal from exposure and supportive measures.

Woodsculpting. Wood is carved, glued, and finished with varnishes and sealers.

Hardwoods such as the western red cedar (*Thuja plicata*), cocabolla (*Dolbergia retusa*), mahogany (*Shoreal sp.*), and California redwood (*Sequoia sempervirens*) are common sensitizers that can cause allergic dermatitis and asthma with exposure.[1] Hypersensitivity pneumonitis leading to fibrosis may occur on rare occasion. Chronic hardwood dust inhalation is also associated with nasal and nasal sinus adenocarcinoma.[60]

Softwoods such as pine can cause similar allergic and respiratory problems. These problems, however, are less frequent with softwood exposure than with hardwoods.[40]

Plywood and composition board are thin sheets of wood or wood chips and dust joined with a formaldehyde-containing glue. Heating and sanding these woods can release the formaldehyde. Exposure is associated with mucous membrane irritation and occasional allergic reactions.

A variety of glues are used to laminate and join wood. These include epoxy resins, cyanoacrylate, formaldehyde, casein, polyvinyl acetate, and contact adhesive glues.

Finishes, including varnishes, paints, and enamels, often contain a variety of solvents (previously discussed). Exposure occurs as the woodworker applies finish.

Wood preservatives may be used during harvesting and processing. Many chemicals used for this purpose are regulated in the United States, but fewer regulations abroad increase the risk of toxic exposure with imported woods. It is often not known (or difficult to find out) if wood has been treated with preservatives. The risk for exposure is higher with imported woods and wood treated for outdoor use. Toxins used for this purpose include chlorophenols, chromated copper arsenate (CCA), and creosols (see Chapter 5).

Metal sculpting. Metal sculpting involves a number of processes with potential toxic exposure: manufacturing (metal casting, forging, and/or welding), surface preparation (cleaning, grinding, and polishing), and finishing (etching, metal coloring, and electroplating).

Metals frequently used in this art form include iron, lead, bronze, brass, pewter, and aluminum. Precious metals such as gold, platinum, and silver are used in jewelry sculpting. Common methods for manufacturing metal are casting, forging, and welding.

Metal casting involves preparing a mold, heating metal to liquid form, and pouring the metal into the mold. Molds are hollow or have a core that melts when the liquid metal is poured. The core is often made of wax, polyurethane foam, polystyrene (Styrofoam), other plastics, silica, or organic material.[37] When the core is heated, a number of combustion products form that require proper ventilation. When wax is burned, by-products include acrolein, chlorinated phenyls, and formaldehyde. The polyurethanes can produce diisocyanate, polystyrene, cyanide, and methylene chloride. Other potential toxic inhalants include carbon monoxide, aldehydes, ammonia, chlorine, hydrogen chloride, hydrogen sulfide, sulfur oxide, and silica.[37]

Metals heated to extreme temperatures can produce toxic fumes. Oxides of zinc and other metals (copper, nickel, iron, and sulfur) can lead to metal fume fever (see Chapter 37). Lead from bronze can produce lead poisoning.

The use of junk metal is especially hazardous because it is frequently painted with paints containing lead, mercury, chromium, or cadmium that can be released during the heating process (see Chapter 12).[53]

Forging involves shaping the metal with different tools. Although this process can be done without heat, hot forging softens the metal and makes it more malleable. Toxic exposure occurs when the fumes of the molten metal are inhaled. Exposures are similar to the ones discussed in metal casting.

Metals are joined by soldering, brazing, and welding. These processes and related toxic risks are described in detail in Chapter 37. One process that is relatively rare in industry but common in jewelry sculpting is silver soldering. Silver solder can contain significant amounts of cadmium. Inhalation of cadmium fumes has led to serious toxicity in several reported cases.[9,34,52]

Welding processes included oxyacetylene and arc welding. Toxic exposures that can occur include infrared and ultraviolet radiation, unburned acetylene gas, nitrogen oxides of ozone, and metal fumes (see Chapter 37).

After forging, the metal surface is cleaned, filed, ground, and polished. The cleaning process involves the use of acids. Exposure to nitric, hydrochloric, hydrofluoric, and other acids can occur during this process.

High-powered grinding wheels produce respirable metal dusts. Sandblasting and polishing expose the artisan to high air concentrations of silica. Cases of pulmonary fibrosis have been reported in association with heavy exposure to metal dusts.[36]

Metal finishing includes chemical etching, painting, and electroplating. Etching involves the application of acids such as hydrofluoric acid. Metal painting may involve potential pigment exposures (previously discussed).

Electroplating is a process in which metal is electrically bound to another metal surface. Highly toxic gold and silver cyanate solutions are often used. Accidental cyanide toxicity has occurred during this process.[31] Other chemical and potential toxic exposures may exist, depending on the chemicals employed (see Chapter 12).

Plastics sculpting. Plastic sculpture involves working with plastic resins or working the finished plastics. Examples of material used in work with plastic resins include amino, phenolic, acrylic, epoxy, polyester, polyurethane, and silicone resins. They can be molded, cast, or foamed. Other additives are frequently used. Working finished plastics includes heating, bending, cutting, gluing, and other mechanical processes. These chemicals can include benzoyl peroxide, methyl methacrylate, formaldehydes, diglycidyl ethers, amines, vinyl toluene, styrene, Fiberglas, and isocyanates. (See Chapter 46 for a more detailed review of plastics toxicology.)

Printmaking

Several different techniques are used in printmaking. Traditionally, a flat surface of wood or linoleum is carved or etched to create a relief image. Different inks are applied to the surface and transferred to paper, cloth, or other materials by a press. Toxic exposures in this process involve the pigments or solvents in the ink and the solvents used during the cleanup process (discussed previously).[25]

The process of intaglio is similar. A copper, aluminum, or zinc background surface is used. Nitric acid, hydrochloric acid, or hydrofluoric acid is used to etch an image onto a plate. Ink is applied to the plate, filling the grooves of the etched portion. Excess ink from the background surface is removed with solvents. The ink is then transferred to paper by a high-pressure press. Toxic exposures are similar to those of relief printing, with the addition of acid exposure from the etching process. Nitric acid and hydrochloric acid are

corrosive agents that cause immediate skin burns. Further, in poorly ventilated surroundings, aerosolized particles can cause respiratory tract irritation. Treatment for these exposures is irrigation of exposed sites and wound care.

Hydrofluoric acid exposure is associated with symptoms of severe pain in exposed areas of skin. In closed spaces, high concentrations can cause respiratory tract irritation and symptoms. Pain is the most prominent early symptoms, with subsequent formation of burns. Treatment is application or injection of calcium and/or magnesium (for a more detailed discussion, see Chapter 41).

Lithography involves zinc or aluminum plates or stones as a background. Lithographic crayons (tuches) are used to draw an image on the surface. Lithographic etches, which typically contain dilute acids, are applied over this surface. A thin layer of metal or stone is removed by the acid except in the areas that are preserved by the tuches. Ink is applied to the surface and pressed onto paper or other material. Toxin exposures are similar to those in the intaglio process.

In screen printing, an image is cut into a stencil screen, and ink is forced through the stencil to create an image. Both solvent- and water-based inks are used. Solvent-based inks can contain up to 35% solvents, and high exposure can occur during this process. Further, solvents are often used to clean the screens. While pigment exposure from ink can occur, solvent exposure from the inks and cleaning fluids are the main exposure risk.[39,61]

Ceramics

Ceramics art uses clay for sculpting and pottery work. All the processes in producing a finished piece have potential for toxin exposure. The steps involved are selecting and preparing the clay, sculpting or molding the shape of the clay, firing the clay piece in a kiln to harden it (bisque firing), sanding and grinding the piece, applying glazes and colorants, and refiring of the piece in a kiln to fuse the glaze to the clay surface.

Clay is obtained in three manners. Ready-for-use, prepared clay can be purchased from potteries, kilns, or art supply stores, as can clay in the form of powder. When clay is dug directly from earth cleaning and drying yield clay dust.

The main toxicologic risk during this initial process comes from the mixing of the dry clay. Clay predominantly contains silicates as well as different amounts of free silica. It is also variably contaminated with kaolin (aluminum silicate), talc, and asbestos.

Inhalation of these materials can lead to toxicity. Bronchitis, bronchiolitis, and occupational asthma have been associated with ceramists, partly due to exposure to molds that grow on wet stored clay. Silicosis, asbestosis, and mesothelioma have been reported in association with this occupation.[23] However, the incidence and potential risk of these illnesses in artisans is not well studied.*

*References 14, 15, 18, 49, 57, 58.

After the clay has been sculpted, it is fired in a kiln to harden it (bisque firing) and fired a second time to color with glaze. During the firing process, toxic gases and fumes are produced. If these gases and fumes are not ventilated properly, then exposure can occur. Carbon monoxide gas from the incomplete combustion of organic material is produced, especially if a gas-fired kiln is employed. Fluorine, chlorine, nitrogen oxides, and sulfur dioxide can be released as the glazes are oxidized.[4,37] Heavy metal exposure such as lead, arsenic, antimony, barium, and cadmium can occur, especially during the glaze process.[6,17,46] All kilns need good ventilation systems to prevent inhalation of these gases and fumes. Another risk associated with the kiln firing process is infrared (IR) radiation exposure to eyes. Artisans looking through kiln peepholes can develop cataracts.

After the initial firing of the clay piece (bisque firing), the piece is prepared for the application of glazes or colorants. If the piece is sanded or grinding techniques are employed, clay dust exposure can again occur.

Glazes typically contain "frits"; metal colorants such as chromium, manganese, uranium, cadmium, antimony, and vanadium; zinc oxide; kaolin; and free silica.[37] The frits are made of fine ground glass that give the ceramic glossy finish after the final kiln firing. The frits contain silicon dioxide, lead, potassium, zinc, calcium, aluminum, boron, and other metals.[59]

Glazes come premixed or in powder form. Inhalation of glaze dust can occur during this mixing process when ventilation or protective clothing are not adequate. The glazes are applied either by brush or by spray painting. Aerosolized glaze is a serious potential exposure risk if safety equipment is not used properly.

Although ingestion of glazes among artisans is not common, this exposure associated with lead poisoning has been frequently reported in ceramic art programs at psychiatric facilities and nursing homes.[54,59]

Glass Art

Glassblowing. Glassblowing produces glass from raw materials. The most basic material involved is pure silica. Lead, silver, copper, cobalt, tin, selenium, barium, arsenic, manganese, zinc, and other metals are added to give the glass a particular color or strength.[11] These material mixes are called "batches." Although batches are available premixed, many artists prefer to make their own particular blend, which can pose an inhalational risk for silica and heavy metal.

The batch is heated in a gas furnace until molten and then removed at the end of a blowpipe. During this heating process, gases and fumes are emitted from the raw materials and furnace. The exposures are similar to the kiln firing process in ceramics. Exposure risks include carbon monoxide and heavy metal fumes.

Finished pieces can be sanded, ground, or abrasive blasted, posing the risk of inhalation of fine glass particles. Glass etching is often employed in this final stage, most commonly with hydrofluoric acid. Skin and inhalational exposure can cause toxicity (see Chapter 41).

Emphysema in glassblowers has been described.[44] Although not a common finding in this occupation, high rates of chronic cough, wheezing, and abnormal pulmonary function tests have been reported.[11,44] The cause for these nonspecific respiratory findings is not clear but may be due to the chronic low-level exposure to multiple inhalational toxins involved in this art process.[11]

Stained glass art. The production of stained glass requires cutting different colored glass and joining these pieces together between metal strips. The two most common techniques, *lead came* and *copper foil,* use lead or copper as the adjoining metal. Both techniques involve substantial amounts of soldering. The solder most commonly used contains lead and tin. Cases of lead poisoning are commonly reported in association with this process.[8,19,35] Soldering also involves the use of flux agents such as zinc chloride and hydrochloric acid. Both are caustic agents that can cause burns to skin and are respiratory irritants if inhaled (see Chapter 28).

Glass-finishing techniques are often employed in the final steps of this art form. These include glass coloring, decorating, and etching. Glass coloring utilizes such chemicals as copper sulfate (contact dermatitis), antimony, silver nitrate (skin corrosive, respiratory tract irritant), and selenium dioxide (skin irritant).

Glass etching typically uses hydrofluoric acid, which can cause painful burns to the skin and respiratory irritation when inhaled (see Chapter 41).

Textile Arts

The predominant toxin exposure risk in this art form is from the variety of dyes used for coloring different fabrics. They include acid, azoic, basic, direct, fiber reactive, mordant/ natural, and vat dyes.[28,37]

Acid dyes are used for wool, silk, and nylon. They are made of different color-imparting chemical groups, such as azo or anthraquinone chemicals that are bound to a sulfonic acid group. The sulfonic acid portion of the molecule has affinity to the basic amino groups found in these fabrics. During the process, the dye is made more acidic with sulfuric, acetic, or formic acid baths to increase the dye's affinity to fabric. The toxicity of the acid dyes is felt to be minimal, although long-term hazards are poorly studied. Exposure to the acids can cause skin and mucous membrane irritation and burns.

Azoic dyes, also known as *naphthol* dyes, are used to dye cotton, rayon, linen, silk, and polyester.[37] The dyes consist of two compounds, a diazonium and a naphthol compound, that are reacted together in fiber to produce the desired color. Contact dermatitis and hyperpigmentation has been associated with use of these dyes.[2] Little information is available about the long-term effects of these agents.

Basic dyes, cationic dyes, are used for fabrics with protein fibers (wool and silk) and cellulose fibers mordanted with tannic acid. Some of these dyes are associated with allergic skin reactions. Basic Orange 2 and Basic Violet 10 are suspected carcinogens. Little is known about long-term exposure.

Direct dyes have been used since the 1800s. Many of the dyes in this class were made from benzidine. Benzidine was an ideal agent that allowed bonding of the dye to a hydroxyl group in a cellulose molecule. Benzidine, however, is fairly well established as a bladder cancer carcinogen.* Although most direct dyes today are not benzidine containing, some continue to have benzidine derivatives.[37]

Direct dyes, used for linen, rayon, and especially cotton, are the ones commonly sold at grocery and hardware stores. The chronic health effects of nonbenzidine direct dyes are not well studied.

Fiber-reactive dyes react directly with fibers and are used for cotton and linen. The dye is applied in a warm bath over a short period of time (30 min). The dye is inactivated with water or sodium carbonate. These dyes are sensitizers and are associated with allergic respiratory problems. Sodium carbonate is a skin and mucous membrane irritant.

French dyes are solvent-based dyes that are usually bright colors that are used for painting on silk.[37] Most are ethyl alcohol based. Solvent exposure acutely and chronically is the toxicologic risk.

Mordant and natural dyes are synthetic or dyes derived from natural sources that use mordants to fix the dye to fabric. These dyes are used for dyeing wool and leather. The common mordants used are potassium aluminum sulfate (alum), ammonia, copper sulfate (blue vitriol), ferrous sulfate (copperas or green vitriol), potassium acid tartrate (cream of tartar), potassium dichromate (chrome), oxalic acid, tannic acid (tannin), stannous chloride (tin), and urea. The toxicity of these agents includes allergic sensitization, skin and mucous membrane irritation, causticity, and possible carcinogenesis. Little information is available on the long-term risks of most of these agents.

Vat dyes use air oxidation by the addition of chromic acid (potassium dichromate and sulfuric acid) to the dye bath.[28] These dyes are mildly irritative to skin and mucous membranes. The acids used are caustic agents with risk of severe burns. The long-term exposure risks are not well studied.

CLINICAL TOXICITY

The clinical toxicity of all these compounds are discussed elsewhere in this book.

CONCLUSION

The potential toxic exposures to artists and artisans are numerous. This chapter attempts to look at the most common art forms and their toxic risks. Many other art processes are not discussed and are beyond the scope of this chapter. For

additional information, readers are referred to the Center for the Safety in the Arts, 155 Sixth Avenue, Fourteenth Floor, New York City, NY 10013.

Accurate information about toxic exposure risk and disease in this field is hampered by a number of factors. Few studies have looked at the potential acute and chronic effects of the toxins in the setting of an artist's studio and work schedule. Multiple chemicals are often used together in art with the potential for synergistic effects. Government regulations do not adequately address the self-employed artisan. Diagnosis of toxicity is often missed by physicians who are unfamiliar with the toxins and the occupational risks.

Despite these problems, occupational exposures in this field are becoming better understood. Safety and art hazards are now standard curricula in most art schools. Understanding the specific processes employed and the potential toxic exposures can help in making proper diagnoses and instituting measures to prevent further exposure.

REFERENCES

1. Adams RM: Job descriptions with their irritants and allergens. In Adams RM, editor: *Occupational skin disease,* ed 2, Philadelphia, 1990, WB Saunders.
2. Alayon AA: Occupational pigmented contact dermatitis from Napthol AS, *Contact Dermatitis* 2:129, 1976.
3. Alexander WE: Ceramic toxicology, *Ceramic Potter* 2:8, 1974.
4. American Conference of Governmental Industrial Hygienists, *Threshold limit values for chemical substances and physical agents in the workroom environment,* Cincinnati, 1990, ACGIH.
5. Babin A: Proposed cadmium ban, *Art Hazards News* 12:1, 1989.
6. Bache CA, Lisk DJ: Epidemiologic study of cadmium and lead in the hair of ceramists and dental personnel, *J Tox Environ Health* 34:423, 1991.
7. Baker EL, et al: Subacute cadmium intoxication in jewelry workers: an evaluation of diagnostic procedures, *Arch Environ Health* 39:173, 1979.
8. Baxter PJ, Samuel AM, Holkham MPE: Lead hazards in British stained glass workers, *Br J Ind Med* 291:64, 1985.
9. Blejer HP, Caplan PE, Alcocer AE: Acute cadmium fume poisoning in welders: a fatal and a nonfatal case in California, *Calif Med* 105:290, 1966.
10. Bonser GM, Clayson DB, Jull JW: An experimental inquiry into the cause of industrial bladder cancer, *Lancet* 1:286, 1951.
11. Braun S, Tsiatis A: Pulmonary abnormalities in art glassblowers, *J Occup Med* 21:487, 1979.
12. Case RAM, et al: *Br J Ind Med* 11:75, 1954.
13. Cohen N: An esoteric occupational hazard for lead poisoning, *Clin Toxicol* 24:59, 1986.
14. Collins NA: The health and safety position in the ceramics industry— the record to date, *Ann Occup Hyg* 33:415, 1989.
15. Cone J: Silicosis in a ceramics technician. Paper presented at the first national conference on Health Risks in the Arts, Crafts, and Trades, Chicago, April 2, 1981.
16. Cook DG, Fahn S, Brait KA: Chronic manganese intoxication, *Arch Neurol* 30:59, 1974.
17. DeRosa E, et al: Lead exposure in the artistic ceramics industry, *Appl Occup Environ Hyg* 6:260, 1991.
18. Eichelmann A: Cancer in a ceramicist, *Art Hazards News* 3:2, 1980.
19. Feldman RG, Sedman T: Hobbyists working with lead, *N Engl J Med* 292, 1975.

*References 2, 3, 6, 8, 10, 12, 14, 15, 17, 18, 25, 28, 35, 36, 39, 44-46, 49, 56-58, 61.

20. Fishbein A, et al: Lead poisoning in an art conservator, *JAMA* 247:2007, 1982.
21. Fishbein A, et al: Increased lead absorption in a potter and her family members, *NY St J Med* 91:317, 1991.
22. Fishbein A, et al: Lead poisoning from art restoration and pottery work: unusual exposure source and household risk, *J Environ Pathol Toxicol Oncol* 11:7, 1992.
23. Fuortes LJ: Health hazards working with ceramics, *Postgrad Med* 85:133, 1989.
24. Goh C: Occupational dermatitis from gold plating, *Contact Dermatitis* 18:122, 1988.
25. Hart C: Art hazards: an overview for sanitarians and hygienists, *J Environ Health* 49:282, 1987.
26. Hine CH, Pasi A: Manganese intoxication, *West J Med* 123:101, 1975.
27. Hunter D, McLaughlin AIG, Perry KMA: Clinical effect of the use of pneumatic tools, *Br J Ind Med* 2:10, 1945.
28. Jenkins CL: Textile dyes are potential hazards, *J Environ Health* 40:279, 1978.
29. Kano K, et al: Lung cancer mortality among a cohort of male chromate pigment workers in Japan, *Int J Epidemiol* 22:16, 1993.
30. Lesser SH, Weiss SJ: Art hazards, *Am J Emerg Med* 13:451, 1995.
31. Letts N: Artist dies in basement cyanide accident, *Art Hazards News* 14:1, 1991.
32. Liden C: Occupational dermatoses in a film laboratory, *Contact Dermatitis* 10:77, 1984.
33. Linz DH, et al: Organic solvent induced encephalopathy in industrial painters, *J Occup Med* 28:119, 1986.
34. Lucas PA, et al: Fatal cadmium fume inhalation, *Lancet* 2:205, 1980.
35. Mapou RL, Kaplan E: Neuropsychological improvement from chelation after long-term exposure to lead: case study, *Neuropsychiatry, Neuropsychology, Behavioral Neurology* 4:224, 1991.
36. Mariano A, Sortorelli P, Innocenti A: Evolution of hard metal pulmonary fibrosis in two artisan grinders of woodworking tools, *Sci Total Environ* 150:219, 1994.
37. McCann M: *Artist beware*, ed 2, New York, 1992, Lyons & Buford.
38. McCann M: The impact of hazards in art on female workers, *Prev Med* 7:338, 1978.
39. McCann M: Silk screen printing hazards, *Art Hazards News* 2:7, 1979.
40. McCann M, Babin A: *Woodworking hazards*, 1995, Center for Safety in the Arts.
41. Miller AB, et al: Cancer risk among artistic painters, *Am J Ind Med* 9:281, 1986.
42. Murio T, et al: The analysis of metals contained in water colours and urinary Pb and Cd of children who practice painting in a private school, *Jpn Hyg* 31:399, 1976.
43. National Institute of Occupational Safety and Health: *Criteria for recommended standards: occupational exposure to*. Washington, DC, Government Printing Office.
44. Nauratil M, Fejsk K: Lung function in wind instrument players and glassblowers, *Ann NY Acad Sci* 155:276, 1968.
45. Neuman HG: The role of DNA damage in chemical carcinogenesis of aromatic amines, *J Cancer Res Clin Oncol* 112:100, 1986.
46. Ooi DS, Parkes M: A ceramic glazer presenting with extremely high lead levels, *Hum Toxicol* 7:171, 1988.
47. Pederson LM, Permin LT: Rheumatic disease, heavy-metal pigments, and the great masters, *Lancet* 1:1267, 1988.
48. Prockup L: Multifocal nervous system damage from inhalation of volatile hydrocarbons, *J Occup Med* 19:139, 1977.
49. Prowse K, Allen MB, Bradbury SP: Respiratory syndrome and pulmonary impairment in male and female subjects with pottery workers' silicosis, *Ann Occup Hyg* 33:375, 1989.
50. Ramazzini B: *De morbis artificum (Diseases of workers)*, ed 2, Chicago, 1940, University of Chicago Press (Translated by WC Wright; originally published in 1713).
51. Regulations [16CFR 1500.14(b)(8), 11500.135]. *Fed Reg* 1992, 46626–46674.
52. Siedlecki JT: Potential health hazards of materials used by artists and sculptors, *JAMA* 204:1176, 1968.
53. Sjogren BB, et al: Fever and respiratory symptoms after welding on painted steel, *Scand J Work Environ Health* 17:441, 1991.
54. Smith DC, et al: Lead ingestion associated with ceramic glaze—Alaska 1992, *MMWR Morb Mortal Wkly Rep* 41:781, 1992.
55. Stewart R, Hake C: Paint remover hazard, *JAMA* 235:398, 1976.
56. Swaen, GMH, Passier PECA, Van Attekum AMNG: Prevalence of silicosis in the Dutch fine-ceramic industry, *Int Arch Occup Environ Health* 60:71, 1988.
57. Trethowan WN, et al: Study of the respiratory health of employees in seven European plants that manufacture ceramic fibres, *Occup Environ Med* 32:97, 1995.
58. Valiante D, et al: Silicosis among pottery workers—New Jersey, *MMWR Morb Mortal Wkly Rep* 41:405, 1989.
59. Vance MV, et al: Acute lead poisoning in nursing home and psychiatric patients from the ingestion of lead-based ceramic glazes, *Arch Intern Med* 150:2085, 1990.
60. Wills JH: Nasal cancer in woodworkers: a review, *J Occup Med* 24:526, 1982.
61. Ziem G: Silk screen printing and heart attack, *Art Hazards News* 7:2, 1984 (letter).

3

Athletes

Edwin K. Kuffner

NO_x Cl_2
oxides of nitrogen   *chlorine*

- Athletes are often motivated to ingest potentially toxic substances that they perceive will enhance their performance

- Indoor ice-skating stadiums and swimming pools pose special problems to athletes because of the ambient gases peculiar to these arenas

OCCUPATIONAL DESCRIPTION

Although athleticism is often associated with good health, athletes are also susceptible to the effects of toxins and toxicants. The unique environments in which athletes compete and the dietary or medicinal supplementation some athletes use in an attempt to improve athletic performance are potential sources of toxic exposures.

The 1994 annual report of the American Association of Poison Control Centers (AAPCC) lists 819 exposures that are related to sporting equipment. There are no reported data on toxic exposures specifically in athletes.[41] According to the U.S. Bureau of Labor Statistics, there were approximately 81,000 professional athletes in the United States in 1994.[54] The number of U.S. athletes, defined as anyone who participates in a sporting activity at least weekly, is on the rise and estimated to be in the tens of millions. Clearly, a large number of Americans are at risk for sports-related toxicities, the diagnosis and management of which often extend beyond the practice settings of the toxicologist and the sports medicine specialist.

This chapter's discussion of sport-related toxicities is divided into two main sections: environment-related toxicities and supplementation-related toxicities. The former addresses the occupational risks associated with the settings in which athletes train or compete, and the latter examines common hazards associated with the nutritional and medicinal supplementation some athletes use in an attempt to improve their performance.

TOXIC EXPOSURES
Environment-Related Toxicities

Whether competing indoors or outdoors, athletes are at risk for toxicities related to air pollution. With the creation of domed stadiums and enclosed arenas, indoor air pollution has become a significant health risk. As compared with outdoor air pollutants, indoor air pollutants have the potential to produce greater toxicities because of the smaller dilution volumes of indoor air. Increased minute ventilations predispose exercising athletes more than coaches, spectators, and athletic support personnel to the effects of airborne toxicants. Deficient ventilation systems, inadequate regulations for monitoring indoor arena air quality, poor maintenance practices, and naive attitudes on the part of both athletes and physicians as to the magnitude of environmental health risks have contributed to the development of significant sports-related toxicities.

Indoor motor sports and race car drivers: carbon monoxide. Carbon monoxide (CO) exposures have occurred in formula one and stock car drivers, in motorcross and boat racers, and during indoor sporting events whenever there is incomplete combustion of fossil fuels. Elevated levels of CO have been measured in arena air after tractor pulls and monster truck competitions.[11] Many racing vehicles are outfitted with supercharged engines that require higher octane fuel, lack catalytic converters, and generate increased amounts of CO. Although the U.S. Environmental Protection Agency (EPA) has established national ambient air quality standards for CO in outdoor air and the Occupational Health and Safety Administration has limited an employee's exposure to CO to 50 ppm as an 8-hour time-weighted average, there are no specific nationally established air quality standards or monitoring procedures for CO in indoor arenas.[17]

Figure skaters, ice hockey players, and speed skaters: nitrogen dioxide and carbon monoxide. Indoor ice skaters, hockey players, spectators, and ice rink maintenance personnel are at risk for both carbon monoxide and nitrogen dioxide toxicity.[10,51] Mechanical ice resurfacers (nicknamed Zambonis after their inventor), ice edgers, and space heaters are commonly powered by gas engines that can emit both carbon dioxide and nitrogen dioxide. If these engines are serviced improperly and inappropriate fuel mixtures reach the carburetor, increased amounts of both carbon monoxide and nitrogen dioxide (NO_2) can be generated.

If indoor ice arenas are improperly ventilated, toxic amounts of both CO and NO_2 can accumulate. Ice arena ventilation is often complicated by a number of factors. In order to maintain constant near-freezing surface temperatures, most ice arenas are designed to minimize natural ventilation and limit the amount of warmer ventilated air that contacts the ice surface. This ventilation strategy has been shown to create a thermic inversion phenomenon whereby colder air and toxic gases, such as NO_2 and CO, can become trapped at ice level. The risks to skaters are further complicated by the fact that the emissions from ice-resurfacing equipment are discharged at the ice surface, that NO_2 is heavier than air, and that the Plexiglas hockey boards surrounding many indoor ice rinks can also act to impede air exchange at the ice surface.[5]

Table 3-1 Chemical structures of nitrogen oxides

Chemical structure	Name
NO	Nitric oxide
NO_2	Nitrogen dioxide
NO_3	Nitrogen trioxide
N_2O	Nitrous oxide
N_2O_2	Nitrogen peroxide
N_2O_3	Dinitrogen trioxide
N_2O_4	Dinitrogen tetraoxide
N_2O_5	Dinitrogen pentoxide

The liberation of toxic gases from the mechanical refrigeration systems used to maintain the ice is also a potential source of toxicity. The most commonly employed chemicals in the ice refrigeration process include ammonia, fluorocarbons, calcium chloride, and ethylene glycol. As the popularity of indoor ice skating and ice hockey increases, so will the risk of both CO and NO_2 toxicities.

Nitrogen oxides. Nitrogen oxides, designated as NO_x, can exist in many atmospheric forms (Table 3-1). Nitrogen dioxide accounts for the majority of sports-related human exposures. It is a yellow to reddish brown gas of intermediate water solubility and is heavier than air. Natural sources of NO_2 include decaying organic matter, volcanic emissions, atmospheric lightning, and forest fires. It is also formed when nitric oxide (NO), a product of the combustion of fossil fuels, is oxidized. Occupational exposures to nitrogen oxides frequently occur in firefighters, silo fillers and farmers, welders, missile site personnel, and those involved in the manufacturing of explosives, jet fuels, dyes, lacquers, and celluloid. The Occupational Safety and Health Administration (OSHA) has set a workplace ceiling value for nitrogen dioxide at 5 ppm.[17] Unfortunately, there are no federal regulations specifically outlining the testing of air in indoor ice arenas for NO_2.

Nitrogen dioxide exerts its toxicity through a number of mechanisms. The effects of any pulmonary toxicant are influenced by its water solubility, particle size, breathing zone concentration, temperature, and pH. Since NO_2 is of intermediate water solubility, it exerts its effects on both the upper airway (as do chemicals of high water solubility) and on the lower respiratory tract (as do chemicals of low water solubility). Nitrogen dioxide reacts with moisture present within the airway and on the respiratory mucosa and forms both nitrous acid (HNO_2) and nitric acid (HNO_3):

$$2NO_2 + H_2O \rightarrow HNO_2 + HNO_3$$

Following significant exposures, nitrous and nitric acid can cause a spectrum of irritant caustic mucosal injury and inflammatory reactions, both at the level of the upper airway and at the level of the terminal bronchioles and alveoli.[34] The NO_2-induced cellular injury results from lipid peroxidation, the generation of free radicals, and subsequent oxidative injury to proteins and nucleic acids.[42]

Pulmonary injury is often the direct result of damage to both alveolar type 1 and alveolar type 2 cells. Alveolar type 1 cells appear to be more susceptible to the effects of NO_2 than the surfactant secreting alveolar type 2 cells. Fortunately, permanent pulmonary damage is often limited by the ability of alveolar type 2 cells to proliferate and act as pneumocyte stem cells, eventually replacing and transforming into alveolar type 1 cells.[25] If repair by the type 2 pneumocytes is incomplete, persistent pulmonary fibrosis and diffusion abnormalities can occur. Alveolar cell injury can also initiate an inflammatory cascade, resulting in the transcapillary transudation of fluid and the development of noncardiogenic pulmonary edema.

Nitrogen dioxide and nitrous and nitric acid have been shown to cross pulmonary capillary membranes and induce systemic metabolic acidosis.[47] Nitrogen oxides are also chemical asphyxiants and interfere with the delivery of oxygen. By oxidizing hemoglobin's iron molecule from the ferrous (Fe^{+2}) to the ferric (Fe^{+3}) state, nitrogen oxides can produce methemoglobinemia (Met-Hb). The higher oxides of nitrogen, which chemically have greater oxidizing potential, have been shown, in vitro, to induce a greater percentage of Met-Hb.[35]

The clinical presentation of patients acutely exposed to NO_2 is highly variable but has traditionally been divided into two phases: an acute phase and a delayed phase. Although the severity of symptoms can be related to the duration of the exposure and to the concentrations of NO_2 within a given patient's breathing zone, victims at the extremes of age or with underlying pulmonary dysfunction often exhibit increased bronchial sensitivity to both lower concentrations and shorter exposures of NO_2.[44]

Following mild exposures, it is not uncommon for symptoms to be delayed. Patients present with mucous membrane irritation and complaints of conjunctivitis, rhinitis, sore throat, cough, dyspnea, and wheezing. Nausea, vomiting, headache, and dizziness are also common. Physical exam may reveal tachycardia, tachypnea, mucous membrane irritation, and bronchospasm with decreased oxygen saturations. The acute tracheobronchitis is often self-limited. Patients who initially exhibit only mild symptoms but have had a significant exposure warrant close observation because the delayed development of pulmonary edema has been reported.[34]

Although rare, severe NO_2 intoxications have caused immediate death from asphyxiation. Following severe exposures, patients often present with drooling, dysphonia, paroxysmal coughing, dyspnea at rest, and stridor. Acute airway obstruction secondary to both laryngospasm and progressive mucosal edema has been reported. The physical exam may reveal cyanosis secondary to either hypoxia or methemoglobinemia, hypotension related to either nitrate-induced vasodilatation or hypovolemia, and noncardiogenic pulmonary edema.[34]

Patients who survive the acute phase of NO_2 intoxication are at risk of developing bronchiolitis days to weeks following the exposure. Although this delayed phase has been more commonly reported to follow severe intoxications initially complicated by pulmonary edema, it has also been reported with mild acute intoxications.[42,48] All patients exposed to NO_2 need close follow-up during the weeks after exposure.

Since NO_2 poisoning in ice hockey players, skaters, or spectators is often less severe than in industrial settings, a high index of suspicion is needed to make the diagnosis. There is no specific antidote for NO_2 poisoning, and comprehensive supportive care is the mainstay of therapy. As in all poisonings, victims must be removed from the source of the exposure without placing rescue personnel or health care providers at risk.

Treatment of NO_2 toxicity should be initiated with the administration of 100% oxygen. Airway management is critical because increased secretions and necrotic mucosal sloughing can rapidly lead to life-threatening airway obstruction. Aggressive suctioning and pulmonary toilet are indicated. Endotracheal intubation may become necessary if hypoxia is refractory to 100% oxygen by nonrebreather mask, if secretions cannot be controlled effectively with suctioning, or if there is progressive upper airway edema and laryngospasm. Patients exhibiting wheezing should be treated with nebulized bronchodilators. Treatment of noncardiogenic pulmonary edema, characterized by a normal pulmonary capillary wedge pressure and a normal cardiac output, may require mechanical ventilation and positive end-expiratory pressure.

For managing severe NO_2 exposures, arterial blood gas analysis using a cooximeter in combination with serum electrolytes may be helpful in evaluating both the ventilatory and oxygenation status, as well as the presence of metabolic acidosis, either due to oxides of nitrogen within the systemic circulation or due to lactate. Mixed acid-base abnormalities are common. The cooximeter is critical in detecting methemoglobin that may be induced by the NO_2 or carboxyhemoglobin from a concomitant CO exposure. Methemoglobinemia induced by NO_2 rarely requires treatment with methylene blue.[47]

A chest x-ray is indicated in patients who exhibit signs of respiratory insufficiency, hypoxia, or pulmonary edema. Chest x-rays obtained shortly after NO_2 exposures can be misleading. Even following severe NO_2 exposures, the chest x-ray can initially appear normal. Chest x-ray findings consistent with pneumonia or pulmonary edema are common in the hours following exposure and have also been described as part of the delayed phase.[42] Although complete resolution of chest x-ray abnormalities usually occurs within 2 months, persistent interstitial infiltrates, consistent with bronchiolitis fibrosa obliterans and focal interstitial fibrosis, have been reported.[15,43]

Case reports suggest that corticosteroids may be beneficial, especially for treating delayed-phase pulmonary complications, but there are no well-designed human studies demonstrating efficacy.[15] Prophylactic antibiotics have not been shown to decrease morbidity or mortality. Nitrogen dioxide may account for chronic asthma in these athletes since it can act as a primary cause or exacerbate an underlying condition.

Swimmers, divers, and water polo: chlorine and chloroform. Swimmers and divers, especially those who train or compete in indoor pools, are at risk for toxicity from both chlorine (Cl_2) and chloroform ($CHCl_3$).

Chlorine, employed as a swimming pool disinfectant, is added to pool water in a number of ways. Although some larger public and commercial pools still add chlorine gas directly to the water, most pools are chlorinated with either sodium or calcium hypochlorite. Both chlorine gas and the liquid and solid forms of these hypochlorite bleaches have resulted in chlorine exposures to pool maintenance personnel and to athletes.[58]

Chlorine gas reacts with pool water to form hypochlorous acid (HOCl), the germicidal agent, and hydrochloric acid (HCl), an unwanted by-product[22]:

$$Cl_2 + H_2O \rightarrow HOCl + HCl$$

Pools that are not properly pH balanced may become too acidic when disinfected with chlorine gas. Pools chlorinated with inadequately neutralized hypochlorites have the potential to become too alkaline. Regardless of the method of chlorination, the pH of pool water should be maintained in the range of 7.2 to 8.[4]

Acidic pool water has been demonstrated to cause painful, disfiguring, and irreversible erosion of dental enamel, termed *swimmers' erosion*.[13] Despite fastidious testing, acidic pool water can go unrecognized if the pH falls below the range of the pH detection system, commonly 6.8 to 8.2 when phenol red is used. Wide-range pH indicator paper should be used, especially when the measured pH is at either end of the detection range.[56]

Even a properly chlorinated pool poses toxicologic risks to swimmers. The dermatologic effects of chlorine range from simple contact dermatitis to chloracne, a form of acne characterized by open comedones and most commonly associated with exposures to the chlorinated aromatic hydrocarbons such as dioxin.[27] Swimmers not wearing protective eyewear are also at risk for chlorine-induced chemical conjunctivitis. Before chlorine is implicated as the cause of a dermatitis or conjunctivitis, infectious etiologies must be excluded.

Chemical reactions between chlorine and organic substances in pool water can liberate halogenated compounds, including bromodichloromethane, dibromochloromethane,

bromoform, and chloroform (trichloromethane).[40] Chloroform, liberated from chlorinated pool water in higher concentrations than other halogenated compounds, is classified by the EPA as a B2 probable human carcinogen, based upon its demonstrated carcinogenic potential in animals. The OSHA workplace ceiling value for chloroform is 50 ppm.[17] Unfortunately, there are no federal regulations specifically outlining the testing of air in indoor swimming pools for chloroform.

Dermal absorption of chloroform from pool water has never been reported, but, like chlorine, chloroform can accumulate in indoor swimming pool air. The chloroform concentration of indoor swimming pool air has been correlated with the pool water chloroform concentration and the degree of water turbulence (the number of swimmers in the pool). Air chloroform concentrations are highest at the water surface, placing athletes at the greatest risk for exposure.[1] Chloroform in the alveolar air of swimmers and spectators has also been shown to correlate with the chloroform concentration in environmental air, the intensity of the sporting activity, the duration of time in the pool, and the type and pattern of swimming. With all other factors controlled, competitive swimmers had higher levels of chloroform detected in alveolar air than noncompetitive swimmers.[2] Although studies have documented elevated chloroform levels in athletes who were participating in indoor water sports, these studies have not addressed the acute or chronic effects of these exposures.

Irrespective of the method of chlorination, chlorine gas and chloroform can accumulate within indoor swimming facilities. Inappropriate chlorination and pool maintenance procedures, poor ventilation without adequate fresh air exchange, and inadequate regulations for monitoring of indoor chlorine and chloroform levels place both competitors and spectators at risk for toxicity.

Chlorine. At room temperature and atmospheric pressure, chlorine is a highly water-soluble, pungent, greenish yellow gas that is heavier than air. Under pressure or in combination with other chemicals, chlorine can exist both as a liquid and as a solid.

According to AAPCC data, the number of yearly chlorine exposures consistently ranks second to only carbon monoxide within the category of fumes, gases, and vapors. Occupational exposures to chlorine occur during the manufacturing of rubber and plastics, in the process of bleaching fabrics and paper, during the production of hydrochloric acid, during the process of water and sewage purification, and when cleaning personnel mix bleaches containing sodium hypochlorite with acidic cleansers. Chlorine, used for warfare in 1915 in World War I at Ypres, Belgium, has been replaced by other agents in modern military practice.[39] The OSHA workplace ceiling values for chlorine are 1 ppm, but there are no published national standards that outline monitoring procedures or acceptable levels of chlorine in indoor swimming pool air.[17]

Chlorine acts as an upper airway mucosal irritant. The mechanisms of chlorine's toxicity has not been fully established. In addition to the caustic mucosal injury that can occur when chlorine combines with water and liberates hypochlorous and hydrochloric acid, oxygen free radicals may also be generated[22]:

$$Cl_2 + H_2O \rightarrow 2\ HCl + [O]^*$$

Chlorine injury manifests as conjunctivitis, rhinitis, and laryngotracheobronchitis. Low-level chlorine exposures produce headaches, nausea, and vomiting. At higher concentrations, chlorine can cause pulmonary edema. Whether acute or chronic chlorine exposure can cause permanent lung damage remains controversial, although it appears that single acute exposures do not produce residual pulmonary abnormalities.[33,39]

After victims are removed from the source of chlorine exposure, treatment is largely symptomatic and supportive. Nebulized sodium bicarbonate, theorized to neutralize hypochlorous and hydrochloric acids generated on mucous membranes, is not recommended. Nebulized sodium bicarbonate has not been demonstrated in randomized controlled human studies to have a beneficial effect, and some animal evidence suggests that intrapulmonary sodium bicarbonate may produce a chemical pneumonitis.[8] Although hypoxia-induced lactic acidosis and hyperchloremic acidosis from systemic absorption of chlorine-derived acids have both been reported, the intravenous administration of sodium bicarbonate is also not recommended.[52] Case reports suggest that corticosteroids may be beneficial, but there are no well-designed human studies demonstrating efficacy. Prophylactic antibiotics have not been shown to decrease morbidity or mortality.[8,16]

Marathoners, triathletes, cyclists, and shooters: lead. Runners who train in urban areas have been shown to have elevated blood lead levels.[45] Marathoners, cyclists, triathletes, and those who exercise in urban environments, specifically in the vicinity of roadways, are potentially at risk. With the advent of unleaded gasoline and more stringent emissions laws, airborne lead levels have been reduced, thereby decreasing the risk of lead toxicity in these athletes. Unfortunately, the long-term effects of low-level lead exposures in athletes have not been studied.[31]

Lead toxicity has been reported in shooters, instructors, and firing range personnel training or working both at indoor firing ranges with insufficient ventilation and at covered outdoor firing ranges. Airborne lead particles are produced when conventional, nonjacketed lead bullets shear as they pass through the gun's chambers and barrel and when they fragment upon striking the target. Vaporized lead-containing primer has also been identified as a source of inhalational lead exposure. Lead exposures can be limited by using nylon-clad, zinc- and copper-jacketed bullets, by reducing the time shooters spend in the range, and by improving range ventilation. The long-term effects of low-level lead exposure in this population requires further study.[53]

Sport fishers. Sport fishers who consume fish caught in contaminated water are also at risk for toxicity. Many bodies of water and subsequently the fish they support are contaminated with DDT (1,1,1,-trichloro-2,2,-bis[p-chlorophenyl]ethane) and its metabolite DDE, dieldrin (1,2,3, 4,10,10-hexachloro-6,7-epoxy-1,4,4a,5,6,7,8,8a-octahydro-endo-exo-1,4,:5,8-dimethanonaphthalene), polychlorinated biphenyls, heavy metals, and other toxicants. When contaminated fish are ingested, there is the potential for both human carcinogenicity and toxicity. It has been suggested that current sport fish consumption advisories may be inadequate and that a standard risk assessment–based approach be adopted for the development of future fish consumption advisories.[28]

Supplementation-Related Toxicities

At all levels of athletic competition, outcomes are often determined by extremely small differences in athletic performance. To gain even the slightest advantage, athletes continually seek more effective and alternative training methods, improved equipment, better nutrition, and sometimes pharmacologic aids. Although self-administration of a toxicant may not fit the traditional definition of an *occupational exposure,* any discussion of athletic-related toxicology would be incomplete without addressing these potential sources of poisoning.

In today's sporting world, where winning can translate into million-dollar payoffs, many athletes and coaches believe that even one's health is a small price to pay for success. Although the true ergogenic potential of many pharmacologic and dietary supplements remains scientifically unproven and despite a lack of information regarding the safety of many of these products, many athletes are willing to risk personal injury in the hopes of becoming a champion.

Bodybuilders, weight lifters, football players, wrestlers, track and field throwers, and swimmers: anabolic steroids. Androgenic (referring to the masculinizing effect) and anabolic (referring to the muscle-building effect) characterize the synthetic derivatives of testosterone, commonly referred to as androgenic-anabolic steroids (AAS). Alkylation of testosterone at the 17-α position decreases first-pass hepatic catabolism and forms many of the oral AAS. The majority of the injectable AAS are formed by esterification of testosterone's 17-β hydroxyl position, thereby decreasing polarity and increasing fat solubility.

Since 1991, in accordance with the Anabolic Steroids Control Act of 1990, anabolic steroids in the United States have been regulated under Schedule 111 of the Controlled Substances Act under the auspices of the Drug Enforcement Administration (DEA). The DEA estimates that the majority of AAS used by U.S. athletes are smuggled from Mexico and subsequently purchased on the black market.[38] The AAS obtained from the black market are often of questionable quality and composition. Some athletes do obtain AAS with prescriptions written by unscrupulous physicians who choose to ignore both the FDA-approved medical indications for steroid use and product warning labels that clearly state that steroids have not been shown to be safe and effective for the enhancement of athletic performance and that there is a potential risk of serious adverse health effects from use in this setting.

Although a violation of U.S. federal law, the illegitimate use of AAS has been reported by American athletes at all skill levels. Use by nonathletes who are seeking to improve their physiques has also been reported. Studies have shown that 4% to 12% of high school males and 1% to 2% of high school females have used AAS at some time in their lives.[60] In 1991, it was reported that approximately 5% of Division 1, 4% of Division 2, and 2% of Division 3 athletes had used AAS, with the highest incidences being reported among college athletes participating in football (10%), track and field (4%), and baseball, tennis, and basketball (2%).[6] The pattern of AAS use at the professional and international levels of competition varies greatly by individual sport. Although AAS abuse has been reported across a wide range of sports, athletes competing in events that require strength as opposed to aerobic endurance are the most common abusers.

Despite a lack of evidence from well-designed human studies, many members of the athletic community believe that AAS are ergogenic and improve athletic performance by increasing lean body mass, augmenting strength, and decreasing muscle recovery time following workouts. A review of 16 well-designed studies involving the use of AAS concluded that only 7 demonstrated a clear increase in muscle strength.[57] The physiologic basis for improved performance and the specific factors influencing these gains remain poorly understood. Inconsistencies in human studies may be related to differences in the type, dosing, and length of AAS exposure, variable training regimens, nonstandardized methods of assessing improved performance, variable nutritional intake during study periods, and problems with true blinding of participants and investigators. Although it has been suggested that female and adolescent athletes may respond differently to AAS, there are insufficient published data to address this issue.

Since information from well-designed human trials is lacking, most dosing regimens used by athletes abusing AAS are not based upon pharmacokinetic data. Dosing practices vary widely in different sports and individual athletes. Typical dosing regimens include *cycling,* taking AAS for weeks with intervening drug holidays, and *stacking,* taking multiple different AAS at the same time during any one cycle.[22] It is not uncommon for athletes to use both oral and injectable AAS simultaneously.

Most studies documenting AAS-induced toxicity have been as flawed as those studies claiming to demonstrate ergogenicity. Adverse effects to the liver and the cardiovascular, reproductive, endocrinologic, and central nervous systems have been reported. Although most efficacy and toxicity studies have been seriously flawed, it is apparent to most health care providers that the adverse effects of AAS clearly outweigh any potential ergogenic effects. Unfortunately, many athletes and members of the athletic community have not critically analyzed the data and continue to base their decisions to use AAS on locker room hearsay.

The toxic endocrinologic and reproductive effects of AAS have been well documented. In males, exogenous AAS cause feedback inhibition–induced reductions in the levels of endogenous testosterone, luteinizing hormone, and follicle-stimulating hormone. Males abusing AAS develop testicular atrophy, prostatic enlargement, impotence, oligospermia, and abnormal sperm morphology and motility. Although hypogonadotropic hypogonadism usually resolves following cessation of AAS abuse, it has been reported to persist for up to 1 year following the discontinuation of AAS use.[37] Males can also undergo feminization with the development of gynecomastia and voice changes secondary to the aromatization of AAS to estrogens. It has been reported that some AAS abusers have unsuccessfully used nonaromatizable androgens, tamoxifen, and human chorionic gonadotropin in an attempt to reduce or prevent the sometimes permanent and disfiguring gynecomastia.[29] In women, AAS abuse induces virilization, often resulting in irreversible hirsutism, deepening of the voice, male pattern alopecia, breast atrophy, menstrual abnormalities, and clitoromegaly.[57] Both males and females may experience increased libido.

The cardiovascular effects of the AAS can be life-threatening. They alter lipid profiles, resulting in decreases in serum high-density lipoproteins (HDL) and increases in both low-density lipoproteins (LDL) and total serum cholesterol concentrations. Although the alterations in lipid profiles often are reversible following discontinuation of AAS use, they may increase the risk of atherosclerosis.[7,55] Based upon numerous case reports of myocardial infarction, cerebrovascular events, and deep venous thrombosis in otherwise healthy young athletes abusing AAS, it has been suggested that AAS are thrombogenic.[26,49] Unfortunately, a long-term follow-up study has never been conducted to address the cardiovascular risks of AAS abuse in athletes.

The AAS, especially those formulated for oral absorption and alkylated at the 17-α position, have been reported to cause altered hepatic structure and function. With discontinuation of AAS use, AAS-induced elevations of serum hepatic transaminases, bilirubin, and alkaline phosphatase appear to normalize. Unfortunately, hepatic hyperplasia and the development of hepatic nodules may not be reversible. The AAS have been reported to cause hepatic nodules and intraparenchymal blood-filled cysts (peliosis hepatis). Rupture of these cysts has caused life-threatening intraabdominal hemorrhage.[60] Deaths from cholestatic jaundice have also been reported. Based upon available data, the long-term risk of AAS-induced hepatic malignancy is difficult to assess. It has been suggested that hepatic adenomas and hepatocellular carcinoma can occur.[20] Physicians caring for athletes suspected of using AAS should regularly monitor their liver function tests.

Reported psychiatric manifestations of AAS abuse in athletes range from euphoria and heightened energy to irritability, hostility, paranoia, delusions, and hallucinations. Those factors that predispose certain athletes to developing aberrant psychiatric behavior while taking AAS remain to be elucidated. Depressive symptoms have also been described in athletes following the withdrawal of AAS.[46]

Other reported toxic effects of the AAS include acne, insulin resistance with impaired glucose tolerance, and abnormal thyroid function tests.[3,18] The mineralocorticoid properties of AAS can produce fluid and electrolyte abnormalities resulting in hypernatremia, hyperkalemia, hypercalcemia, and edema. The AAS have also been reported to cause premature closure of epiphyseal growth plates, resulting in shortened stature. By altering connective tissue tensile strength, AAS may also predispose athletes to ligament and tendon injuries.[59] Through needle-sharing practices, those athletes who inject AAS are also at risk for acquiring blood-borne infections such as hepatitis and the human immunodeficiency virus.

Most athletes' decisions to use AAS are influenced by their perceived rather than proven effectiveness. At the professional and international levels, when the difference between victory and defeat often pushes the limits of detection, a clinically immeasurable benefit of AAS may translate into millions of dollars or life-threatening toxicity.

Wrestlers, rowers, boxers, equestrians, bobsledders, and lugers: diuretics, laxatives, and emetics. Athletes who compete in sports in which weight class determines the level of competition or one's eligibility to participate have been known to employ pharmacologic agents in order to "make weight." Diuretics, emetics, and laxatives may cause life-threatening electrolyte imbalances and potentiate dehydration.

Boxers: mercury. The intramuscular and intravenous injection of mercury has been reported among boxers who believe that this heavy metal imparts strength. Intravenous injection has produced mercury embolization in the lungs and has also resulted in non-athletic-related suicide deaths.[9]

Nutritional supplementation. Good nutrition is clearly a component of athletic success. When athletes or physically active noncompetitive individuals adopt special diets, consume supplemental vitamins and minerals, or try to enhance their performance with herbal preparations, they may be at risk for toxicity. Hundreds of products, directly marketed toward athletes, claim to be ergogenic. The performance claims of many of these supplements remain scientifically unfounded.[32]

Vitamins

Vitamins—organic compounds that cannot be synthesized by the human body and whose intake is required to prevent a deficiency syndrome—are the most common athletic nutritional supplement. Athletes who ingest vitamins in doses exceeding the recommended daily allowance (RDA) may be at risk for toxicity.

Of the fat-soluble vitamins (A, D, E, K), both hypervitaminosis A and D are associated with significant toxicity. Vitamin A (retinol) toxicity has been reported to cause pseudotumor cerebri. This can occur after acute vitamin A toxicity from doses exceeding a few hundred thousand to a million international units (IU). It can present in conjunction with a desquamating erythematous rash. Chronic vitamin A toxicity occurs after ingestions greater than 25,000 IU/day and can often present with dry scaly skin, brittle nails, hair loss, perioral fissuring, hypercalcemia, and hepatotoxicity. Hypervitaminosis D, resulting from greater than 4 or 5 times the RDA of 400 IU/day of vitamin D, can cause hypercalcemia and the complications thereof.[14,46]

Of the water-soluble vitamins, vitamin C and vitamin B_6 are most commonly associated with toxicity. Vitamin C (ascorbic acid) in doses exceeding 4 g/day has been reported to increase the excretion of oxalic acid and theorized to potentiate renal calculi formation. In acute ingestions of greater than 12 g and in chronic doses exceeding 500 mg/day, vitamin B_6 (pyridoxine) can cause a sensory axonal neuropathy resulting in ataxia, decreased deep tendon reflexes, painful dysesthesias, and numbness.[14]

Minerals

Athletes also commonly ingest supplemental minerals, inorganic substances that cannot be synthesized by the human body and whose deficiency may lead to metabolic dysfunction. Chromium, vanadium, boron, manganese, zinc, and selenium are common constituents of sport supplements. Although toxicities from these substances are well described, specific toxicity in athletes secondary to supplementation has not been reported. The ergogenicity of these minerals remains scientifically unproven.[30]

Other nutritional supplements

The composition of athletically marketed nutritional supplements that claim to be ergogenic varies widely between specific products. Many contain protein and amino acid supplements, which have never been proven to enhance muscle mass in healthy subjects consuming a normal diet. The safety of excessive amounts of most amino acids has not been established. Athletes ingesting supplements containing tryptophan, which was banned by the U.S. Food and Drug Administration in 1990, are at risk for the eosinophilia myalgia syndrome. Although arginine and ornithine have been reported to increase pituitary secretion of human growth hormone, a beneficial effect on athletic performance has not been demonstrated.[36] Other common components of nutritional supplements include carnitine, creatine, lysine, choline dibencozide, inosine, γ-oryzanol, ferulic acid, yohimbine, and glandular extracts from animals. None of these compounds has been shown to enhance athletic performance.[32]

An analog of γ-aminobutyric acid (GABA), γ-hydroxybutyrate (GHB), is also believed by some athletes to stimulate endogenous growth hormone, enhance muscle mass, and aid in fat metabolism. Although there is a lack of evidence that GHB is ergogenic, experience in acute overdose has shown that GHB can cause somnolence, bradycardia, respiratory arrest, seizures, and coma.[23] Reportedly, GHB has been used by shooters in an attempt to reduce tremors.[30]

Herbal preparations claiming to increase athletic performance are also commonly marketed to athletes. Some athletes believe extracts from a group of plants of the genus *Smilax* and Mexican yam, which contains the plant sterol, diosgenin, used to synthesize oral contraceptives, have steroidogenic potential.[29] There is no research documenting ergogenic effects from these plant sterols. Bee pollen has also never been shown to have a beneficial effect on athletic performance. Unfortunately, the exact composition of herbal medications is unknown, and none has been shown to have an ergogenic effect.

"Soda doping" refers to the ingestion of alkaline salts, most commonly sodium bicarbonate (baking soda), just prior to high-intensity, short-duration exercise, such as sprinting, in an attempt to create an alkaline reserve capable of buffering lactic acid. The effectiveness of alkaline salts in boosting athletic performance remains a topic of scientific debate. They cause abdominal cramping, diarrhea, and dehydration, possibly secondary to the high sodium load.[30]

Banned and restricted pharmacologic agents. In an attempt to preserve the integrity of sports, to protect the health and safety of athletes, and to ensure the fairness of athletic competition, some of sport's governing bodies have banned athletes from taking certain pharmacologic agents both during training and during competition (see box). Although some potentially ergogenic pharmacologic agents have been universally banned, it is important for both athletes and their physicians to be aware of the specific substances whose use has been banned or restricted by the national or international athletic governing body under which the athlete is competing. In general, the United States Olympic Committee (USOC) and the National Collegiate Athletic Association (NCAA) observe the International Olympic Committee's (IOC) list of banned and restricted substances. This list is continually revised and updated. Some of the more common classes of banned and restricted pharmacologic agents are listed in the box. Unless exempted by the athletic governing body, no substance belonging to a banned or restricted class may be used by an athlete, even for medical treatment.

Before taking or prescribing any medication prior to competition, athletes and their physicians are respectively advised to consult either the athletic governing body under which the athlete is competing or the head physician responsible for a specific athletic event concerning the status of a particular medication. Athletes and their physicians need to understand that some over-the-counter medications, although obtainable without a prescription, may be banned or restricted. Some common components of over-the-counter cold, decongestant, and allergy medications that are banned include ephedrine, phenylpropanolamine, pseudoephedrine, desoxyephedrine, propylhexedrine, caffeine, and the ephedrine-like herbal preparation Ma Huang. In the United States, specific questions concerning athletic drug information can be directed to USOC via their toll-free confidential hotline at 1-800-233-0393 or to the NCAA at (913) 339-1906.

Unfortunately, education programs alone have been only minimally effective in curtailing the use of banned and restricted pharmacologic agents. Drug testing programs, in conjunction with strict penalties for offenders, have proven to be a more effective deterrent. Most athletic governing bodies subject their athletes to drug testing at any time, including during the off-season and when out of competition. Prior to most national and international competitions, athletes are required to declare all pharmacologic agents they have been taking and are also subject to testing, usually immediately following the competition. For specific drug testing procedures and policies, athletes and their physicians are advised to contact the athletic governing body under which the athlete is competing and the agency responsible for administering the tests.

Although *athletic doping* refers to the use of any foreign substance that could give an athlete an unfair competitive advantage, the term commonly is applied to the use of physiologic substances that are taken in an abnormal amount or by an abnormal route, with a specific ergogenic intent. Peptide and glycoprotein hormones and their analogs, such as erythropoietin and growth hormone, are two commonly abused doping agents that have been banned by most athletic governing bodies.

Although growth hormone has been documented to accelerate the growth of children, there are no data to support the claim that it has athletic ergogenic potential.

Classes of Commonly Banned or Restricted Pharmacologic Agents

Diuretics
β-blockers
Injectable anesthetics
β-2-agonists
Narcotic analgesics
Urine-manipulating agents
Androgenic anabolic steroids and corticosteroids
Recreational drugs
β-2-agonists
Sympathomimetics/stimulants
Narcotic analgesics
Peptide and glycoprotein hormones and analogs

Toxic effects of supplemental growth hormone include impaired glucose metabolism, irreversible acromegaly, myopathy, and skin changes.[19] The use of human growth hormone for nonmedical use is illegal in the United States. Athletes have been reported to induce erythrocythemia, termed *blood doping,* either with the administration of the hormone erythropoietin or by transfusion of red blood cells. These practices, which have been demonstrated to cause a physiologic increase in oxygen delivery to tissues and a subsequent increase in muscle exercise power, are banned by most athletic governing bodies. Life-threatening complications of erythropoietin are related to the increased vascular viscosity and the increased risks of thromboembolic events associated with hematocrits greater than 55%. Athletes, who during competition become dehydrated, thereby further increasing their already abnormally elevated hematocrits, may be at increased risk of toxicity.[50]

Although the emphasis of sports governing bodies has been on limiting ergogenic drugs, physicians should be aware of the more common ergolytic agents that may impair an athlete's performance. These include alcohol, marijuana, β-blockers, diuretics, sedating antihistamines, imipramine, phenytoin, and valproic acid.[24]

REFERENCES

1. Aggazzotti G et al: Plasma chloroform concentrations in swimmers using indoor swimming pools, *Arch Environ Health* 45:175, 1990.
2. Aggazzotti G et al: Chloroform in alveolar air of individuals attending indoor swimming pools, *Arch Environ Health,* 48:250, 1993.
3. Alen M et al: Androgenic-anabolic steroid effects on serum thyroid, pituitary and steroid hormones in athletes, *Am J Sports Med* 15:357, 1987.
4. American Public Health Association: *Public swimming pools: recommended regulations for design and construction, operation and maintenance,* Washington, DC, 1981, American Public Health Association.
5. Anderson DE: Problems created for ice arenas by engine exhaust, *Am Ind Hyg Assoc J* 32:790, 1971.
6. Anderson W et al: A national survey of alcohol and drug use by college athletes, *Phys Sports Med* 19:91, 1991.
7. Ansell JE et al: Coagulation abnormalities associated with the use of anabolic steroids, *Am Heart J* 125:367, 1993.
8. Bannister WK, Sattilaro AJ, Otis RD: Therapeutic aspects of aspiration pneumonitis in experimental animals, *Anesthesiology* 22:440, 1961.
9. Bartolome C, Khan MA: Mercury embolization of the lung, *N Engl J Med* 295:883, 1976.
10. Berglund M et al: Personal NO$_2$ exposure monitoring shows high exposure among ice-skating schoolchildren, *Arch Environ Health* 49:17, 1994.
11. Boudreau DR et al: Carbon monoxide levels during indoor sporting events—Cincinnati, 1992–1993, *MMWR Morb Mortal Wkly Rep* 43:22, 1994.
12. Burke LM, Read RSD: Dietary supplements in sport, *Sports Med* 15:43, 1993.
13. Centerwall BS et al: Erosion of dental enamel among competitive swimmers at a gas-chlorinated swimming pool, *Am J Epidemiol* 123:641, 1986.
14. Cetaruk EW, Aaron CK: Hazards of nonprescription medications, *Emerg Med Clin North Am (Concepts and controversies in toxicology)* 12:483, 1994.
15. Charnels EAR, Bootlace EH: Silo-Filler's disease, *Radiology* 74:232, 1960.
16. Chester EH et al: Pulmonary injury following exposure to chlorine gas: possible beneficial effects of steroid treatment, *Chest* 72:247, 1977.
17. *Code of Federal Regulations* 29 1910.1000, revised July 1, 1995.
18. Cohen JC, Hickman R: Insulin resistance and diminished glucose tolerance in powerlifters ingesting anabolic steroids, *J Clin Endocrinol Metab* 64:960, 1987.
19. Cowart VS: Human growth hormone: the latest ergogenic aid? *Phys Sports Med* 16:175, 1988.
20. Creagh TM, Rubin A, Evans DJ: Hepatic tumors induced by anabolic steroids in an athlete, *J Cain Pathos,* 41:441, 1988.
21. Deacon D: *Underground steroid handbook,* ed 2, Venice, Calif, 1989, HER Technical Books.
22. Decker WE, Koch HE: Chlorine poisoning at the swimming pool: an overlooked hazard, *Clin Toxicol* 13:377, 1978.
23. Dyer J: γ-Hydroxybutyrate: a health food product producing coma and seizure-like activity, *Am J Emerg Med* 9:321, 1991.
24. Eichner ER: Ergolytic drugs in medicine and sport, *Am J Med* 94:205, 1993.
25. Evans M et al: Transformation of alveolar type 2 cells to type 1 cells following exposure to NO$_2$, *Exp Mol Pathol* 22:142, 1975.
26. Ferenchick GS: Are androgenic steroids thrombogenic? *N Engl J Med* 322:476, 1990.
27. Fisher AA: Dermatitis from chlorine and certain chlorinated products, *Cutis,* 33, 20, 24, 1984.
28. Foran JA, Cox M, Croxton D: Sport fish consumption advisories and projected cancer risks in the Great Lakes basin, *Am J Public Health* 79:322, 1989.
29. Friedl KE, Yesalis CE: Self-treatment of gynecomastia in bodybuilders who use anabolic steroids, *Phys Sports Med* 17:67, 1989.
30. Fuentes RJ, Rosenberg JM, Davis A: *Athletic drug reference '94,* Durham, NC, 1994, Allen and Hanburys.
31. Grobler SR, Maresky LS, Kotze TJ: Lead reduction of petrol and blood lead concentrations of athletes, *Arch Environ Health* 47:139, 1992.
32. Grunewald KK, Bailey RS: Commercially marketed supplements for bodybuilding athletes, *Sports Med* 15:90, 1993.
33. Hasan FM, Gehshan A, Fuleihan FJ: Resolution of pulmonary dysfunction following acute chlorine exposure, *Arch Environ Health* 38:1983.
34. Horvath E et al: Nitrogen dioxide–induced pulmonary disease: five new cases and a review of the literature, *J Occup Med* 20:103, 1978.
35. Hugo C, Collier CR, Mohler J: In vitro methemoglobinemia formation in human blood exposed to NO$_2$, *Environ Res* 30:9, 1983.
36. Jacobson BH: Effect of amino acids on growth hormone release, *Phys Sports Med* 18:63, 1990.
37. Jarow J, Lipschultz L: Anabolic steroid-induced hypogonadotropic hypogonadism, *Am J Sports Med* 18:429, 1990.
38. Kenny J: *Extent and nature of illicit trafficking in anabolic steroids. Report of the International Conference on the Abuse and Trafficking of Anabolic Steroids,* Washington, DC, 1994, United States Drug Enforcement Administration.
39. Kowitz TA et al: Effects of chlorine gas upon respiratory function, *Arch Environ Health* 14:545, 1967.
40. Lahl U et al: Distribution and balance of volatile halogenated hydrocarbons in the water and air of covered swimming pools using chlorine for water disinfection, *Wat Res* 15:803, 1981.
41. Litovitz TL et al: 1994 annual report of the American Association of Poison Control Centers toxic exposure surveillance system, *Am J Emerg Med* 13:551, 1995.
42. Loury T, Schuman L: "Silo-filler's disease"—a syndrome caused by nitrogen dioxide, *JAMA* 162:153, 1956.
43. Morrissey W et al: Silo-filler's disease, *Respiration* 32:81, 1975.
44. Orhek J et al: Effect of short-term, low level NO$_2$ exposure on bronchial sensitivity of asthmatic patients, *J Clin Invest* 57:301, 1976.
45. Orlando P et al: Increased blood lead levels in runners training in urban areas, *Arch Environ Health* 49:200, 1994.

46. Pope HG, Katz DL: Affective and psychotic symptoms associated with anabolic steroid use, *Am J Psychiatry* 145:487, 1988.

47. Prys-Roberts C: Principles of treatment of poisoning by higher oxides of nitrogen, *Br J Anaesth* 39:432, 1967.

48. Ramirez J, Dowell AR: Silo-filler's disease: nitrogen dioxide–induced lung injury. Long-term follow-up and review of the literature, *Ann Intern Med* 74:569, 1971.

49. Rockhold R: Cardiovascular toxicity of anabolic steroids, *Annu Rev Pharmacol Toxicol* 33:497, 1993.

50. Simon TL: Induced erythrocythemia and athletic performance, *Semin Hematol* 31:128, 1994.

51. Smith W, Anderson T, Anderson HA: Nitrogen dioxide and carbon monoxide intoxication in an indoor ice arena—Wisconsin, 1992, *MMWR Morb Mortal Wkly Rep* 41:383, 1992.

52. Szerlip HM, Singer I: Hyperchloremic metabolic acidosis after chlorine inhalation, *Am J Med* 77:581, 1984.

53. Tripathi RK et al: Reducing exposures to airborne lead in a covered, outdoor firing range by using totally copper-jacketed bullets, *Am Ind Hyg Assoc J* 51:28, 1990.

54. U.S. Bureau of Labor Statistics: Personal communication.

55. Webb OL, Laskarzewski PM, Glueck CJ: Severe depression of high-density lipoprotein cholesterol levels in weight lifters and body-builders by self-administered exogenous testosterone and anabolic-androgenic steroids, *Metabolism* 33:971, 1984.

56. White GC: *Handbook of chlorination for potable water, wastewater, cooling water, industrial processes and swimming pools,* New York, 1972, Van Nostrand Reinhold.

57. Wilson JD: Androgen abuse by athletes, *Endocr Rev* 9:181, 1988.

58. Wood BR, Colombo JL, Benson BE: Chlorine inhalation toxicity from vapors generated by swimming pool chlorinator tablets, *Pediatrics* 79:427, 1987.

59. Wood TO et al: The effect of exercise and anabolic steroids on the mechanical properties and crimp morphology of the rat tendon, *Am J Sports Med* 16:153, 1988.

60. Yesalis CE, Bahrke MS: Anabolic-androgenic steroids current issues, *Sports Med* 19:326, 1995.

4

hexane

tri-ortho cresyl phosphate

- The inhalational toxicity associated with aviation fuels is primarily acute CNS intoxication, chronic psychomotor impairment, and peripheral neuropathy

- Hydraulic fluids still contain small quantities of tricresyl phosphate, of which tri-ortho cresyl phosphate is only a trace contaminant

Aviation Personnel

Richard J. Hamilton

OCCUPATIONAL DESCRIPTION

More than 1 million personnel work in the aerospace environment. Pilots, mechanics, ground crew, and aircrew constitute the main occupational groups. Each of these is associated with a unique aspect of the maintenance and operation of aircraft. The toxicologic profile of each profession varies with the type of aviation (military, civilian, or general) and the aircraft engine (turbine or piston).

It is of historic interest that the first airplanes presented toxicologic hazards that helped create the mystique of aviation and pilots. These simple engines had castor oil in the fuel as an engine lubricant. This caused a continuous mist of castor oil to be sprayed across the pilot. To counter this, aviators wore long scarves to wipe the mist from their goggles. In addition, the fine castor oil spray had a cathartic effect on the gastrointestinal tract. The reported antidote was a shot of brandy.

In our era, pilots operate aircraft and spacecraft. In 1993, there were 685,000 pilots in the United States. Of these, 283,720 were private pilots, and 117,000 were airline transport pilots. These pilots operate the 183,303 aircraft in this country, only 7297 of which are owned and operated by air carriers. The rest are owned and operated by general aviation pilots who fly everything from single-engine piston planes to turbine-driven props and jets. They are used for pleasure flying, transportation, and agricultural applications. General aviation pilots are the only pilots who commonly perform simple maintenance and repair of their aircraft. Corporate and commercial air pilots operate jet and propeller transports. They fly at higher sustained altitudes than general aviation pilots. Military pilots fly piston, turbine, propeller, and jet aircraft in high-intensity operations. Even when they are not flying, military pilots often live and work in the same area as the maintenance and refueling operations.[3]

Aircrew are essential to flight operations but do not fly the aircraft. They include navigators, flight engineers, flight attendants, weapons officers, and flight officers. They are frequently exposed to the same toxicologic hazards as pilots and are considered the same in this chapter.

Mechanics maintain the engine, environmental control, hydraulic, and electrical systems of propeller, turbine, jet, and rocket engines. In 1993, there were 401,080 aircraft mechanics in the United States.[3] They share many toxic exposures with automotive mechanics (see Chapter 20).

Ground crew refuel, de-ice, handle cargo, and move aircraft. The toxic materials they work with are directly related to the airport environment. Small civil airports, large commercial hubs, and aircraft carriers represent some of the diverse environments where numerous ground crew work.

TOXICOLOGIC EXPOSURES
Fuels

Aviation gasoline. Aviation gasoline (AVGAS) is quite similar to automotive gasoline except that (1) unique additives are formulated to increase performance, (2) it is leaded, and (3) it has a higher octane number. Octane number is a rating representing the antiknock properties of gasoline. It is determined by the percentage of isooctane that must be added to normal heptane to produce the knocking quality of the fuel being tested. Knocking occurs when combustion of the air-fuel mixture occurs before the maximum compression stroke of the piston. This combustion is heard as a knocking sound in the engine. It decreases the performance of a piston engine dramatically. The AVGAS is formulated in three grades and given four unique colors: 80 octane is colored red, 100LL (low lead) is colored blue, and 100 octane is colored green; turbine (jet) fuel is colorless and is not octane rated. Typically, AVGAS is 75% aliphatic hydrocarbons (C_4 to C_{12}), 24% toluene, 0.2% benzene, 0.1% antioxidant static disperser, 0.1% dye, and 0.1% icing inhibitor. It contains as much as 1.28 g/L of tetraethyl lead (compared to 0.5 g/L of leaded automotive gasoline).[1]

Exposure to AVGAS occurs during accidental spills, general maintenance, refueling operations, and sampling of fuel tanks for water contamination.

General aviation pilots and ground crew are both involved in fueling operations and fuel tank sampling. Refueling operations generally occur in the open air with fuel trucks or fixed ground pumps similar to automotive gasoline pumps. The tanks are filled without respiratory protection. Confirmation of the level of gasoline is performed by visual inspection or by putting a finger into the tank. This is essential because fuel gauges on these aircraft (usually light, single-piston-driven propeller aircraft) are not sensitive enough to determine the maximum amount of fuel in the tanks. Finally, during preflight, the pilot inspects the aircraft and withdraws a small fuel sample from each tank at gravity-dependent sample sites. Water is poorly soluble in AVGAS and appears as liquid at the bottom of the sample. This alerts the pilot of the possibility of water contamination in the fuel system. Small spills occur commonly during these procedures. Environmental Protection Agency (EPA) regulations require that these samples (often totaling 150 ml) be returned to the tanks. The common practice is to pour the sample onto the surrounding macadam or soil.

The significance of exposures during refueling operations is unknown. However, studies of automobile refueling stations demonstrate elevated levels of the alkanes (200 ppm) and less than 1 ppm of the aromatic hydrocarbons. This is consistent with the analysis of the liquid and vapor phase of gasoline. Although the aromatics compose 30% of the liquid phase (1% benzene, the remainder toluene and xylene), they are only 2% of the vapor phase. The vapor phase of gasoline is 90% C4 and C5 alkanes. Thus, the alkanes are the main source of inhalation hydrocarbon exposures to aviation personnel. In Europe, benzene accounts for up to 5% of the liquid phase of gasoline. Studies of gasoline station attendants in Italy revealed a mean time-weighted average (TWA) of 6.3 ppm (1.73 mg/m^3) when they were exposed to gasoline with 2.6% to 2.8% vol/vol benzene.[14] This exceeds the U.S. permissible exposure limit (PEL). Urine phenol is an inadequate monitoring parameter in this range. Urine phenylmercapturic acid and muconic acid concentrations at the end of the work shift may prove to be useful parameters for monitoring.[18] Table 4-1 details the exposures commonly encountered and their relationship to Occupational Safety and Health Administration limits.[10]

This vapor-liquid composition characteristic of gasoline accounts for the different toxicity profile that might be expected when groundwater is contaminated by gasoline. In

Table 4-1 Commonly encountered exposures to gasoline constituents and their relationship to exposure limits

Substance	Short-term exposure limit (15 min)	Typical one-time fueling operation at self-service station (2 min)	TWA	Service station attendants mean TWA[10]
Alkanes	500 ppm (1500 mg/m^3)	200 ppm	300 ppm (900 mg/m^3)	1.5 ppm
Benzene	5 ppm	1 ppm	1 ppm	0.1 ppm

the liquid phase, aromatic hydrocarbons constitute 30% to 50% of gasoline. In one study of a private residence that used gasoline-contaminated groundwater (approximately 300 μg/L benzene), maximum benzene concentrations occurred in the shower stall (758–1670 μg/m3) and bathroom (366–498 μg/m3) during and immediately after a shower was taken. The total benzene dose resulting from the shower was estimated to be approximately 281 μg, with 40% via inhalation and 60% via the dermal pathway. These results indicate that domestic use of gasoline-contaminated water can produce relatively high benzene exposures.[15]

If the extrapolation from automotive gasoline station attendants is valid, then mechanics involved in busy AVGAS refueling operations may be exposed to significant alkyl leads. However, 100LL AVGAS is the most common general aviation fuel, and this product is less than 0.1% tetraethyl lead.

Jet fuel. Jet fuel is designed for the performance needs of a turbine engine. It is a higher octane, higher energy, and lower freezing point blend of largely straight-chain and napthene hydrocarbons. While JP-4 is a mixture of 65% kerosene blends and 35% AVGAS, JP-5, JP-7, and JP-8 are essentially pure kerosene. The actual blends of these fuels are proprietary, and an exact molecular weight is unknown. The JP-4 was measured in the air of enclosed hangars at levels ranging from 533 mg/m^3 to 1160 mg/m^3 (130 to 282 ppm). Levels above 1000 mg/m^3 have been measured in the breathing zone of refueling personnel and in the cockpit of a U.S. F-4 fighter. The Air Force Occupational Safety and Health (AFOSH) PEL for JP-4 is an 8-hour TWA of 400 ppm and a 15-minute short-term exposure limit (STEL) of 500 ppm.[2]

Hydraulic Fluids

Hydraulic fluid is used in systems that operate controls and equipment on the airplane. Transport aircraft may have as much as 55 gallons of hydraulic fluid that is under 1500 to 3000 pounds per square inch (psi) of operating pressure. Damaged systems may spray fluid as a mist into the work environment of mechanics and pilots alike. These fluids come in quart or gallon containers and pose a hazard during refilling operations.

The most commonly encountered hydraulic fluid for piston operations is referred to as Mil Spec 5606.[19] It is 1% tricresyl phosphate; 4% 2,6-di-tert-butyl-p-cresol, butylate hydroxy toluene, and antioxidant; 6% methacrylic acid copolymer with methyl and lauryl esters; and 90% hydro-treated middle petroleum distillate and petroleum solvent.

The hydraulic fluid for high-performance jets is a phosphate ester mixture composed principally of dibutyl phenyl phosphate and tributyl phosphate (Skydrol, Monsanto Co.). Phosphate ester mixtures, such as tricresyl phosphate, have produced well-described organophosphate-induced delayed neurotoxicity. Tricresyl phosphate is a phosphate ester that is used in many industrial applications: commercial plasti-

cizers, nitrocellulose solvents, lubricants, gasoline additives, hydraulic fluid, flame retardants, and machine gun coolant. Triorthocresylphosphate (TOCP) is a contaminant of tricresyl phosphate (which predominantly contains meta- and para-isomers). Tricresyl phosphate hydraulic fluid was the TOCP-contaminated adulterant added to Jamaica ginger (jake) that caused the demyelinating neurotoxicity responsible for the "jake walk" of the prohibition era.[16]

Like TOCP, organophosphate esters are capable of producing peripheral neurotoxicity without antecedent cholinesterase toxicity.[6] Animal studies and case reports support the notion that significant exposures can result in toxicity.[7,8,17] The principal route of exposure is through the skin and respiratory tract during spills or leaks. No association has been identified between typical occupational exposures to hydraulic fluids and neurotoxicity. Contact dermatitis is well described and constitutes the main manifestation of toxicity for all hydraulic fluids.[21]

Pesticides

Agricultural application of organophosphate insecticides is done by small airplanes and helicopters. Spills can occur to aviation personnel during loading, unloading, and cleanup operations. The hazards of insecticide application are discussed in Chapter 13.

Aircraft disinsection (spraying airplanes to kill potential insect vectors) was discontinued approximately 15 years ago. Up to that time, aircraft cabins, baggage holds, and cockpits that arrived from overseas were commonly sprayed with DDT or organophosphates. Since the practice was thought to be ineffectual and placed crew members and passengers at risk, the Center for Disease Control (CDC) and the United States Department of Agriculture (USDA) discontinued the practice and sought reciprocal agreements with other countries. At present, several countries still require disinsection but permit either direct (aerosol) or residual. D-phenothrin (a pyrethroid) is most commonly used, and it represents a toxic risk for patients who have been sensitized to it or have an allergy to the chrysanthemum plants that produce the natural pyrethrums.[9]

Carbon Monoxide

Piston engines produce carbon monoxide (CO), depending on the type of engine and throttle setting. Carbon monoxide is 8.5% of a piston engine at takeoff power and 3% at cruise power. These fumes may enter the cockpit through heating mechanisms or breaks in the engine exhaust stack. In-flight fires also produce CO and combustion products such as CN. The relative hypoxia of altitude exposure magnifies a small exposure to CO. A 5% COHgB level is the hypoxia equivalent of 4000 feet. This accounts for the detrimental effect cigarette smoking has on oxygen-sensitive senses such as color differentiation and night vision.

General aviation pilots often employ simple "spot" indicators to identify CO toxicity before symptoms become apparent. The obvious toxic effects of these compounds exacerbate an already dangerous situation.

Jet engine exhaust contains less than 1% CO due to its efficient burn and is of no consequence.[20]

De-icing Fluids

These compounds contain methanol, isopropanol, and ethylene glycol and are sprayed on control surfaces and wings prior to departure. Many general aviation pilots carry small cans of methanol spray as a deicer. These generally do not cause toxicity unless massive inhalation occurs, which is possible in accidental spills.

CLINICAL TOXICOLOGY
Fuels

Aviation fuels such as AVGAS or JP-4 are primarily central nervous system (CNS) toxins when inhaled. The effect of acute in-flight exposure has been documented in one military jet when fuel vapors entered the cockpit during flight. The pilot experienced somnolence, incoordination, and slurred speech but was able to switch to 100% oxygen, recover the jet, and land. His neurologic symptoms resolved after he was removed from the cockpit. It was estimated that the level of JP-4 fumes were 3000 to 7000 ppm.[5]

Chronic exposure may cause CNS toxicity and peripheral neuropathy. A series of investigations of aircraft factory workers who were repeatedly exposed to jet fuel demonstrated psychomotor impairment as well as peripheral neuropathy. This relationship seemed strongest for workers with the greatest number of "heavy" exposures.[11,13] The statistical validity of this data is not robust. In addition, it appears that the truly affected workers probably suffered from an ongoing series of significant acute exposures with concentrations ranging from 500 to 3000 ppm or more. A later study more firmly links neurasthenic symptoms with chronic jet fuel exposure at a level consistent with the current National Institute for Occupational Safety and Health recommended exposure limit.[12] It is difficult to determine the true threshold for peripheral neurotoxicity from chronic low-level exposures. It may relate to the amount of n-hexane, a well-known neurotoxin (see Chapter 35).

Dermatitis

Dermal exposure causes a defatting dermatitis that can progress to chronic eczematous dermatitis. The practice of degreasing hands with gasoline often leads to this condition.

Hydraulic Fluids

Contact dermatitis is the most common manifestation of exposure to hydraulic fluids.[21] Peripheral neurotoxicity from triaryl phosphate compounds is a recognized concern, but case reports are few and relate to exposures not normally encountered in most maintenance operations.[7] Some animal studies support the notion that high-dose inhalational exposure can result in a decrease in cholinesterases,[6] but this is not without controversy.[17] Neurotoxic esterase, a similar enzyme, is decreased by organophosphates and TOCP and is the currently accepted theory for why these molecules cause peripheral neuropathy.[4]

REFERENCES

1. Agency for Toxic Substances and Disease Registry: *Gasoline toxicity. Case studies in environmental medicine,* Atlanta, 1993, US Dept of Health and Human Services.
2. Agency for Toxic Substances and Disease Registry: *Jet fuel toxicity. Case studies in environmental medicine 32,* Atlanta, 1993, US Dept of Health and Human Services.
3. Airline Owners and Pilots Association (AOPA): *1993 Fact sheet,* Frederick, Maryland.
4. Barret DS, Oehme FW: A review of organophosphorous ester induced delayed neurotoxicity, *Vet Hum Toxicol* 27:22, 1985.
5. Davies NE: Jet fuel intoxication, *Aerospace Med* 35:481, 1964.
6. Healy CE, et al: Subchronic rat inhalational study with Skydrol 500B-4 fire resistant hydraulic fluid, *Am Ind Hyg Assoc J* 53:175, 1992.
7. Jarvholm B, et al: Exposure to triaryl phosphate and polyneuropathy: a case report, *Am J Ind Med* 9(6):561, 1986.
8. Johannsen FR, et al: Evaluation of delayed neurotoxicity and dose response relationships of phosphate esters in the adult hen, *Toxicol Appl Pharmacol* 41:291, 1977.
9. Jordan JL: FAA major initiatives continue advancing, *US Medicine,* January: 39, 1996.
10. Kearney C, Dunham D: Gasoline vapor at a high volume service station, *Am Ind Hyg Assoc J* 47:535, 1986.
11. Knave B, et al: Long-term exposure to jet fuel: part II. A cross-sectional epidemiologic investigation of occupationally exposed industrial workers with special reference to the nervous system, *Scand J Work Environ Health* 4:19, 1978.
12. Knave B, Mindus P, Struwe G: Neurasthenic symptoms in workers occupationally exposed to jet fuel, *Acta Psychiatr Scand* 60:39, 1979.
13. Knave B, et al: Long term exposure to jet fuel: an investigation of occupationally exposed workers with special reference to the nervous system, *Scan J Work Environ Health* 3:152, 1976.
14. Lagorio S: Exposure to benzene of service station employees and composition of benzene, *Med Lav* 85:412, 1994.
15. Lindstrom AB: Gasoline-contaminated ground water as a source of residential benzene exposure: a case study, *J Expo Anal Environ Epidemiol* 4:183, 1994.
16. Morgan JP: The Jamaican ginger paralysis, *JAMA* 248:1864, 1982.
17. Mortensen A, Ladefoged O: Delayed neurotoxicity of trixylenyl phosphate and a trialkyl/aryl phosphate mixture, and the modulating effect of atropine on tri-o-tolyl phosphate-induced neurotoxicity, *Neurotoxicology* 13:347, 1992.
18. Popp W: Concentrations of benzene in blood and S-phenyl mercapturic and t,t-muconic acid in urine car mechanics, *Int Arch Occup Environ Health* 66:1, 1994.
19. Texaco. 01537 Aircraft Hydraulic oil 15. mil-H-5606E. Material Safety Data Sheet. 20 March 1987, Beacon, NY.
20. *US naval flight surgeon's manual,* ed 3, Pensacola, 1993, Naval Aerospace Medical Institute.
21. Wolf R, Movshowitz M, Brenner S: Contact dermatitis in Israeli soldiers, *J Toxicol Environ Health* 43:7, 1994.

5

$$\underset{H}{\overset{H}{\diagdown}}C{=}O$$

formaldehyde

H_2S
hydrogen sulfide

Cl_2
chlorine

SO_2
sulfur dioxide

- Hypersensitivity pneumonitis and asthma are two common toxic manifestations of pulmonary disease in these occupations

- Nasal carcinomas in woodworkers have been linked to a variety of toxic exposures

- Woods, preservatives, fungicides, and equipment account for most dermatitis

Carpenters and Loggers

Lada Kokan

OCCUPATIONAL DESCRIPTION

Carpenters and loggers work with wood and various wood-related products, including solvents, adhesives, preservatives, strippers, and finishes, that may cause illness. Carpenters may be exposed to sawdust during sawing and sanding and to preservatives and solvents used in finishing. Loggers are exposed to the adverse health effects of the woods they work with and additionally such toxins as chlorine, hydrogen sulfide, methyl mercaptan, and sulfur dioxide in the pulp and paper industry. Many types of wood are known to cause occupational asthma and dermatitis in those employed in wood-related industries. However, separating the health effects of the wood itself from the effects of chemicals used in production is difficult.

In 1994, there were 1,265,000 people employed as carpenters and 86,000 loggers in the United States. These numbers reflect the number of people currently employed in these wood-related industries. However, many more individuals are exposed to a similar group of toxins during such nonprofessional activities as home remodeling and hobbies such as carpentry and model making. Further, there was recently much public interest in formaldehyde as a cause of illness in homes with insulation and particleboard that contained formaldehyde. The use of these compounds in homes is widespread.

This chapter examines the various adverse health effects that have been reported in woodworkers. Hypersensitivity pneumonitis affects individuals exposed to many different antigens. Carpenters and loggers who are occupationally exposed to antigens found in wood constitute only a small portion of the affected individuals. Following this is a discussion of other diseases and specific toxins that physicians who care for woodworkers should be familiar with.

POTENTIAL TOXIC EXPOSURES
Hypersensitivity Pneumonitis

History. Hypersensitivity pneumonitis (extrinsic allergic alveolitis) is a syndrome of respiratory and systemic symptoms that develops in a predisposed host after repeated exposure to a specific antigen.[35] Early descriptions of hyper-

sensitivity pneumonitis outline the development of "farmer's lung" after exposure to grains and hay.[2,10] Since Campbell's classic description in 1932, a broad variety of antigens that induce hypersensitivity pneumonitis in susceptible individuals have been identified. These include various fungi, animal proteins, other organic dust, and chemicals found in wood and in industrial and medical settings[35] (Table 5-1). Because these antigens are readily encountered in many environments, many people are at risk for developing this

Table 5-1 Causes of hypersensitivity pneumonitis

Disease	Occupation	Source of antigen	Major antigen
Thermophilic bacteria and bacterial products			
Bagassosis	Bagass workers	Moldy sugarcane	*Thermoactinomyces sacchari*
Coffee worker's lung	Coffee workers	Coffee bean dust	*Thermoactinomyces* spp.
Detergent worker's lung	Detergent workers	Detergent beads, wood dust	*Bacillus subtilis*
Farmer's lung	Agricultural workers	Moldy hay or grain	*Micropolyspora faeni*
Fertilizer worker's lung	Fertilizer workers	Dirt	*Streptomyces albus*, Endotoxin
Humidifier lung	Office workers and others	Water reservoir, ventilation	*T. vulgaris, T. candidus, M. faeri*
Sisal worker's lung	Bag and rope makers	Rope dust	*Thermoactinomyces* spp.
Fungi			
Cheese worker's lung	Cheese workers	Cheese mold	*Penicillium caseei, P. roqueforti*
Dry rot disease	European old house occupants	Old wood	*Merulius lacrymans*
Horseback rider's lung	Horsepeople	Moldy barn straw	*Sprobolomyces* spp.
Malt worker's lung	Malt workers	Moldy malt and barley	*Aspergillus clavatus*
Suberosis	Cork workers	Moldy cork dust	*P. frequentans*
Summer-type hypersensitivity pneumonitis	Japanese wood house occupants	Wood dust	*Trichoderma cutaneum*
Sequoiosis	Redwood workers	Moldy redwood	*Aureobasidium, Pullaria, Graphium* spp.
Papermill worker's lung	Papermill workers	Moldy wood chips	*Alternaria* spp.
Wood pulp worker's lung	Loggers	Wood dust	*Alternaria tenius* *Saccharomonospora viridis*
Woodworker's lung	Maple bark strippers	Moldy bark dust	*Cryptostroma corticale*
Animal proteins			
Avian protein diseases	Bird handlers	Chicken, ducks, parakeets, pigeons, turkeys	Avian proteins from excretia, feather bloom, and serum
Furrier's lung	Furrier's	Fox fur	Animal hair protein
Rodent handler's disease	Animal lab workers	Rats, gerbils	Serum, urine proteins
Chemicals			
Bathtub refinisher's lung	Tub refinishers	Vapors	Diisocyanates
Chromatographer's lung	Pauli's reagent	Chromatography spray	Sodium diazobenzene, sulfonic acid
Chronic berylium disease	Berylium workers	Berylium particulate	Berylium dust or fume
Insecticide worker's hypersensitivity pneumonitis	Insecticide sprayers	Insecticides	Pyrethrum
Thesaurosis	Beauticians	Hair spray	Dimethylhydration, formaldehyde resin, polyvinyl pyrrolidone (povidone)
Medications			
Acebutolol-induced hypersensitivity pneumonitis	Heart patients	Beta blockers	Acebutolol
Amiodarone-induced hypersensitivity pneumonitis	Amiodarone	Amiodarone	Amiodarone

Modified from Zenz C, editor: *Occupational toxicology,* ed 3, St Louis, 1994, Mosby.

syndrome in occupational settings and during other activities that offer an opportunity for repeated exposure to the antigens.

Clinical course. Patients may present with acute, subacute, or chronic disease, all of which have a respiratory component and a varying severity of systemic symptoms. The acute presentation of hypersensitivity pneumonitis consists of cough, dyspnea, and fever associated with myalgias, nausea, headache, and malaise. The onset of illness typically occurs 4 to 6 hours following exposure to the inciting agent. These flulike symptoms may persist for days or resolve spontaneously within hours. They also typically recur following reexposure. Symptoms may commence months or even years after initial exposure to the inciting agent. Host factors and the degree of exposure play a role in the severity of a given episode.

The subacute presentation of hypersensitivity pneumonitis follows repeated exposure to the offending agent. Patients present with progressive dyspnea and productive cough, sometimes accompanied by weight loss and lethargy. These symptoms often resemble chronic bronchitis associated with an occupational setting. Typically, in these cases, the exposure is low grade and repetitive, and the symptoms develop gradually. These subacute symptoms characteristically resolve over a period of weeks following avoidance of the antigen and symptom-based treatment.

Still fewer patients present with chronic disease. This insidious process is characterized by progressive dyspnea, chronic cough, and weight loss. In the case of the chronic syndrome, the illness is permanent, and symptoms persist despite withdrawal of the inciting agent and appropriate treatment.

Signs of hypersensitivity pneumonitis vary with the stage of presentation. The patient with an acute presentation may appear quite ill, with marked dyspnea, hypoxemia, fever as high as 41° C, and fine basilar rales. Rhonchi are rarely heard. Cyanosis is seen only in severe cases. Leukocytosis and eosinophilia are common, though IgE levels are normal. A similar, though attenuated, presentation is expected in the subacute stage of disease. In both groups, the chest x-ray may show a fine reticulonodular pattern, sparing the apices, or, in severe cases, diffuse infiltration in a whiteout pattern may occur. These resolve over the course of weeks to months if reexposure and the consolidation of chronic disease are not allowed to occur. Chronic disease is characterized by features of interstitial fibrosis with high-pitched rales on examination and interstitial lung disease with diffuse fibrosis and honeycombing on chest x-ray. Death has occurred at all stages of disease.

On pulmonary function testing, restrictive changes typically occur 4 to 6 hours following exposure. A decreased forced vital capacity (FVC) and forced expiratory capacity in 1 second (FEV_1) occur, which may also be accompanied by early obstructive changes. In chronic disease, the restrictive pattern typically becomes fixed, though some individuals exhibit obstructive signs. Diffusion abnormalities and decreased arterial oxygenation are also found.

Differentiating hypersensitivity pneumonitis from other respiratory illnesses can be difficult. For example, an entity labeled *organic dust toxic syndrome* or *inhalation fever*,[30] which develops after inhalation of organic dusts 1 to 5 microns in size, appears very similar to the acute phase of hypersensitivity pneumonitis. However, organic dust syndrome occurs after the first exposure to antigen, whereas repeated exposure is required for the development of hypersensitivity pneumonitis. Once chronic disease is established, hypersensitivity pneumonitis cannot be differentiated from other causes of combined diffuse interstitial fibrosis with obstruction. Methacholine challenge demonstrates bronchial hyperactivity similar to that found in the late phase of asthmatic disease.

The course of this disease varies with the stage of presentation. If exposure can be terminated at the acute or subacute stages, complete resolution is expected. A patient who presents with acute or subacute disease and continues to be exposed to the offending antigen will go on to develop chronic disease. Once established, the symptoms of chronic hypersensitivity pneumonitis may be only ameliorated with treatment.

Pathophysiology. Granulomatous interstitial pneumonitis is the characteristic lung biopsy. Alveolitis with predominantly lymphocytic interstitial infiltration is present in most cases. Interstitial fibrosis with scattered lymphocytic infiltrates is also common. Capillary inflammation and macrophage infiltration filling the alveoli may occur early in the course of hypersensitivity pneumonitis. Later changes include a chest x-ray with "honeycombing" appearance from alveolar destruction. Bronchiolitis obliterans may also occur at this chronic stage.

Bronchiole washings of patients with hypersensitivity pneumonitis show increases in T lymphocyte populations that are largely of the suppressor type. Functional impairment of suppressor T cells and macrophages may be central to the development of hypersensitivity pneumonitis.[11,35] In support of this theory, monkeys can develop hypersensitivity pneumonitis when they are exposed to avian antigens and then subject to radiation-induced defects of suppressor T cells.[17]

It has also been proposed that endotoxin from gram-negative bacteria plays a role in the development of respiratory symptoms from exposure to cotton and grain dusts.[3,7] However, endotoxin alone does not account for all of the observed symptomatology in these studies.

There is also some evidence to support the causative role of both pulmonary infection and concurrent exposure to toxins. An example of a toxin that may potentiate the development of hypersensitivity pneumonitis is inhalation of hexachlorobenzene. This compound was used for cleaning barns (a natural pigeon roost) and has been implicated in the development of pigeon breeder's disease.

Treatment. As with any patient in respiratory distress, supplemental oxygen, monitoring, and general supportive care in severely ill patients are key to the initial management on emergency presentation. The administration of steroids (prednisone 0.3 to 1 mg/kg) initially and for several weeks may hasten disease resolution in the acute and subacute situation.[10,33] Computed axial tomography (CAT) scan of the chest and lung biopsy are helpful diagnostic tests.

The cornerstone of treatment of hypersensitivity pneumonitis is avoidance of the inciting agent. Consultation with occupational medicine specialists, pulmonologists, and a worksite representative should aid in the long-term management, diagnosis, and treatment of these patients.

In situations where removal from the job site is not feasible, sodium cromolyn inhalers may be useful if there is an asthmatic component to the disease,[33] and dust respirators should be used but cannot be considered to be entirely protective. Engineering measures that reduce dust production or enhance dust removal can also create a much more favorable working environment.

MALIGNANCY
Nasopharyngeal Carcinoma

Since an increased incidence of paranasal cancer was first identified in English furniture makers,[21] many authors in various countries have verified that woodworkers have an increased risk of nasal and paranasal sinus malignancy. Sinonasal adenocarcinoma is particularly common, although an increase in squamous cell carcinoma has also been found.[20,29] These malignancies are associated with such woodworking occupations as furniture makers, sanders, and wood machinists and increases with the number of years of exposure.

The agent causing nasal adenocarcinoma in woodworkers is not clearly defined. Both hard and soft woods have been associated with the risk of nasal carcinoma, although hardwoods such as oak, beech, and ash may pose a greater risk.[27,29] The role of wood preservatives, adhesives, pesticides, and other added substances (as opposed to the natural constituents of the wood dust) has not yet been defined. Similarly, the effect of particle size and the exposure threshold for carcinogenesis have not been clearly elucidated.

Tannins are complex polyphenols that are found in the dust of hard and soft woods and are carcinogenic in animals. The concentrations in hardwoods are an order of magnitude higher than softwoods.[24] Shoemakers are also exposed to tannins and, like woodworkers, have an increased risk of sinonasal cancer.

Other Malignancies

The data linking woodworking occupations to an increased incidence of lymphatic,[24,28] hematopoietic,[7,28] gastrointestinal,[31] and respiratory[16,25] cancers are inconclusive, with several authors reporting disparate results. Various substances found in wood products may play a role in carcinogenesis and confound attempts to identify the true toxins. A study that identified an increased risk of death from leukemia and non-Hodgkin's lymphoma in American furniture makers also frequently sampled toluene and xylene in the furniture plants studied.[24] Toulene and xylene are solvents commonly found in lacquers and paints. Similarly, an excess of respiratory cancer found in Finnish woodworkers was associated with the use of phenol and with pesticides. These workers were also exposed to other agents, and a phenol-cancer dose-response relationship could not be established.[16] These data were not completely reproduced by subsequent investigations of these workers because only the subset of sawmill workers was found to have a significantly increased number of cells with chromatid-type breaks.[28] Another study of American pattern and model makers utilized a cancer screening program to identify an increased risk for developing lymphocytopenia associated with exposure to both epoxy resins and wood dusts.[19] Finally, coal tar pitch volatiles are classified by the International Agency for Research on Cancer (IARC) as human carcinogens. These substances are polycyclic hydrocarbons that may be released from wood as well as from coal, petroleum, and other organic matter during preparation.[35] A large number of these volatiles are released with heating and inhaled and are certain to confound investigations into occupational cancers.

Asthma

Many types of wood induce various idiosyncratic reactions in individual hosts (Table 5-2). Perhaps the best described is the occupational asthma resulting from exposure to western red cedar *(Thuja plicata)*. This disease had an approximate prevalence of 5% in exposed British Columbian sawmill workers working with western red cedar.[4] Airway hyperresponsiveness develops after occupational exposure in affected individuals and persists even years after removal from exposure.[4] Unlike allergic asthma, the bronchospasm that is induced by exposure to western red cedar is not

Table 5-2 Woods that cause asthma

Wood	Industry
Beech	Carpenters
Cabreuva	Carpenters
Cocobolo	Carpenters
Ebony	Violin and other instrument makers
Iroko	Carpenters
Mahogany	Carpenters
Mansonia	Carpenters
Oak	Carpenters
Obeche (African maple, whitewood)	Sauna builders
Pau marfan	Carpenters
Rosewood	Carpenters
Teak	Carpenters
Western red cedar	Sawmill workers, carpenters

associated with atopy or high serum IgE levels, and non-specific bronchial hyperresponsiveness was not a predisposing host factor.[6] Nonspecific bronchial hyperresponsiveness did, however, develop in affected individuals, in parallel with the development of asthma. The same study suggested that the nasal symptoms that precede pulmonary symptoms may be an early disease marker and that jobs with higher dust concentrations were associated with the initiation of asthma symptoms.

Plicatic acid is a substance found in western red cedar that has been implicated in this condition. Inhalation challenge with plicatic acid (Fig. 5-1) induces histamine release. However, plicatic acid–specific IgE does not appear to be the mechanism by which histamine release occurs.[14] Lymphocytes also appear to play a role, although the exact mechanism is not yet clear.[5]

An increase in pulmonary symptoms such as cough have been shown in workers exposed to wood dust. A decrease in FVC has also been found that is inversely related to years of employment.[32] Acute changes in FEV_1 that develop across a workweek have also been correlated with long-term declines in FEV_1 values over a period of 27 months.[9]

Exposures in the Pulp and Paper Mills

Aberrations on pulmonary function testing have been found in pulp and papermill workers. The FEV and FVC have been found to be lower in exposed pulp and papermill workers than in controls.[13] In one study, lung function and the number of years of pulp mill employment were found to be inversely related. Exposures to chlorine, methyl mercaptan, and hydrogen sulfide may contribute to these respiratory function abnormalities. Self-reported chlorine "gassing" incidents correlate with decreased FEV : FVC ratios and decreased midmaximal flow rates in pulpmill workers.[18]

Chlorine gas exposure can result in significant respiratory symptoms. Severe exposures can result in delayed pulmonary edema and fatality. In less concentrated form, chlorine can cause irritative symptoms such as burning and itching of the mucous membranes, cough, chest tightness, and wheezing.

Methyl mercaptan is another toxic gas to which pulpmill workers may be exposed. It can cause delayed onset pulmonary edema as well as central nervous system depression and seizures. A characteristic rotten egg smell may give warning of exposure to methyl mercaptan.

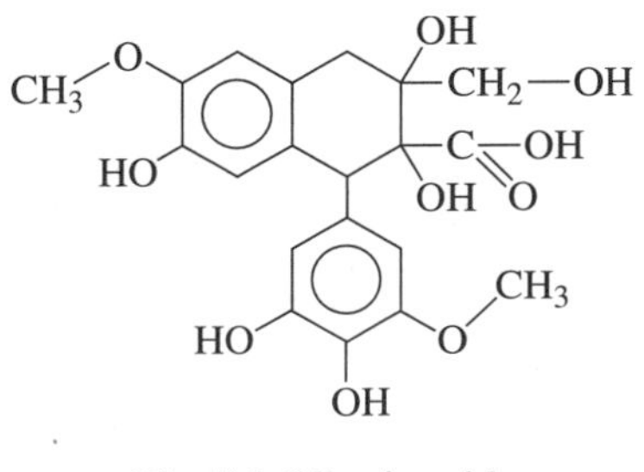

Another toxic gas with a rotten egg odor that pulpmill workers may encounter in the mill is hydrogen sulfide. This smell is noted at hydrogen sulfide (H_2S) concentrations lower than 100 to 150 ppm. Above this concentration, olfactory paralysis occurs. Once the odor is extinguished, workers may be fooled into thinking that the exposure is terminated when they have, in fact, encountered an even higher gas concentration. Headache, nausea and vomiting, dizziness, and an altered mental status may also warn of exposure to hydrogen sulfide. Marked respiratory irritation, CNS depression, seizures, and pulmonary edema occur at high levels of exposure. Above 600 ppm, H_2S may be rapidly fatal due to cardiovascular collapse and respiratory arrest.

Sulfur dioxide (SO_2) is another colorless gas that may be released during wood pulping. Like chlorine, it is a water-soluble irritant. This causes it to be readily deposited in the upper airways, where it reacts with water to create sulfurous acid on contact with mucous membranes. However, severe exposures may result in a significant enough load to also affect the lower airways, resulting in chemical pneumonitis and pulmonary edema. Irritation of the throat, nose, and eyes also occurs at lower levels of exposure. Wheezing may occur and is more likely in asthmatics. Sulfmethemoglobinemia has been reported from SO_2 exposure.

Fiberboard Toxicity

Medium-density fiber (MDF) board consists of wood fibers and carbamide resin glue, which contains formaldehyde. Woodworkers exposed to the MDF have been shown to have an increased number of airway and nasal complaints, an impaired sense of smell, and less mucociliary activity than a group handling traditional fiberboard.[14] However, no histologic changes of the nasal mucosa have been demonstrated.[14] Woodworkers using oriented strand board have also been demonstrated to have a decreased FVC : FEV_1 ratio compared with controls. This effect was more notable in smokers and changed significantly over the course of a work shift.[15] Self-reports of respiratory symptoms correlated with results of objective pulmonary function testing.

Due to the widespread use of urea formaldehyde insulation and furniture made of particleboard, there has been considerable public concern over formaldehyde exposure in homes. Formaldehyde is a gas at room temperature that has a characteristic odor that is detectable at low concentrations. At concentrations above 1 ppm, formaldehyde can cause mucous membrane irritation. The use of urea formaldehyde polymers has additionally been associated with complaints of headaches, nausea, and skin rashes. Formaldehyde is a sensitizer in immune-mediated bronchospasm and skin, by which it may mediate some of these effects. Its causative role in human carcinogenesis has not been established, although some studies show an increased incidence of nasopharyngeal cancer.

Fig. 5-1 Plicatic acid.

Fungi and Fungicides

Fungi may be found in significant concentrations in wood products. Immunocompromised individuals may be at an increased risk, as demonstrated in a case report of acute fatal microgranulomatous aspergillosis in a patient with chronic granulomatous disease who briefly shoveled moldy cedar chips.[10] As noted in an earlier section, various fungi have been implicated in the development of hypersensitivity pneumonitis from such agents as moldy hay and woods in which these fungi have been found.

The fungicides that control fungal growth in wood products may themselves be toxic. Pentachlorophenol (PCP) is a chlorinated phenol herbicide that enjoyed widespread use until reports appeared of its toxicity. Sawmill workers have died from this exposure in mills where PCP was used as a wood preservative.[23] The mechanism by which this occurs is interference with oxidative phosphorylation. Affected workers initially experienced profuse sweating with excessive release of heat, weight loss, and gastrointestinal complaints that led eventually to coma and death. This toxicity is likely to be exacerbated in a hot environment, where the body's ability to reduce heat may be overwhelmed. The PCP may also cause chronic effects on the immune system. This mechanism has been implicated in the development of non-Hodgkin's lymphoma in residents of log homes where PCP was used as a preservative.

In an attempt to curtail the use of chlorophenol fungicides such as PCP due to their toxicity, some sawmills use other agents. Dry, pruritic, and peeling skin, rashes, and nose bleeds have been reported after the use of 2-(thiocyanomethylthio) benzothiazole (TCMTB) as a fungicide in sawmills.[34] Chromium is also used as a fungicide despite the potential for carcinogenesis due to hexavalent chromium. Arsenic, too, is a fungicide with known toxicity. However, analysis for these latter compounds in a wood joinery shop showed that their levels were not elevated.[26] Copper and nickel are also found in wood preservatives. However, their potential for toxicity appears to be low.

Solvents

Solvents are often found in substances, such as paints and paint strippers, that carpenters use. Benzene, toluene, and xylene are the most common solvents. Benzene has been associated with the development of aplastic anemia and leukemia in chronic exposures. Toluene is commonly used as a substance of abuse by paint sniffers, who may have more severe exposures than do workers using toluene as a solvent. In severe exposures, it may cause renal tubular acidosis associated with metabolic acidosis, hematuria, and proteinuria, as well as an inability to acidify the urine below a pH of 5.5. Hypokalemia and hypophosphatemia severe enough to cause profound weakness can also occur. In addition, central nervous system dysfunction, including cognitive impairment, ataxia, tremor, and deafness, have been well described and are common in toluene abusers. Brain-imaging studies after chronic exposure may show cerebral,

Table 5-3 Woods that cause dermatitis

Wood	Active substance
Acacia	
Beech	
Boxwood	(?) Quebrachamine
Ebony	Quinones
Iroko	Stilbene
Mahogany	Anthothecol
Mansonia	Quinones and glycosides
Obeche	
Rosewood	Dalbergiones
Satinwood	(?) Alkaloids and (?) furocoumarins
Sequoia	
Teak	Desoxylapachol
Walnut	
Western red cedar	Tropolones

cerebellar, and brainstem atrophy, loss of gray and white matter differentiation, and increased periventricular white matter. Microcephaly and craniofacial and limb abnormalities similar to the fetal alcohol syndrome have been described in children whose mothers abused toluene during pregnancy. Concomitant alcoholism was also present in some of these cases.

Dermatitis

Dermatitis occurs in woodworkers after exposure to a variety of substances. Certain woods themselves can cause dermatoses. Allergic dermatitis may cause a pruritic rash of the exposed body parts that typically occurs during work with the offending wood and is relieved when this exposure stops. However, encounters with the same wood in other settings may result in similar symptoms. For example, there is a case report of a cabinetmaker who had allergic dermatitis to white pine wood (*Pinus monticola*) and who noted the same symptoms while camping near some pine trees on vacation.[22] Patch testing with an extract of the wood in question may reveal sensitivity to this wood. Other woods that can cause similar reactions are listed in Table 5-3.

Many compounds other than wood may cause dermal irritation to carpenters and loggers. These include the nickel found in carpenters' tools, hydroxyquinone in wood preservatives, rosin, adhesives, solvents, wet cement, oils, finishes, detergents, potassium dichromate in preservatives, the various mercapto compounds in rubber gloves, and itching from contact with rock wool.[1,35] Compounds such as creosote and pitch that may be encountered by carpenters and woodworkers may cause phototoxic or photoallergic reactions.[35] Hydroxyquinone may also cause toxic vitiligo.[35] Pentachlorophenol in wood preservatives has been well described to cause chloracne, thought to be caused by a dioxin contaminant. It has already been mentioned that TCMBT, another preservative, can also cause a dermatitis characterized by dry skin.

CONCLUSION

There are many toxic substances that carpenters and loggers may encounter. The woods themselves and some of their natural components are sometimes at fault. Additionally, multiple chemicals that are added to the wood or used in production to create a finished product are also toxic. The known toxicity of some of these compounds has resulted in either curtailed use of these compounds or in industry standards that limit workers' exposure to them. The information gained from studying the toxicity of wood and its related products in occupational settings is widely applicable to the many other individuals who are exposed to the same compounds in their homes and during leisure activities.

REFERENCES

1. Adams RM, ed: *Occupational skin disease,* New York, 1983, Grune & Stratton.
2. Campbell EJM: Acute symptoms following work with hay, *BMJ* 2:1143, 1932.
3. Castellan RM et al: Inhaled endotoxin and decreased spirometric values. An exposure-response relation for cotton dust, *N Engl J Med* 317:605, 1987.
4. Chan-Yeung M: Occupational asthma, *Chest* 98(suppl):148, 1990.
5. Chan-Yeung M: Mechanism of occupational asthma due to western red cedar *(Thuja plicata), Am J Ind Med* 25:13, 1994.
6. Chan-Yeung M, Desjardins A: Bronchial hyperresponsiveness and level of exposure in occupational asthma due to western red cedar *(Thuja plicata):* serial observation before and after development of symptoms, *Am Rev Respir Dis* 146:1606, 1992.
7. Clapp WD et al: The effects of inhalation of grain dust extract and endotoxin on upper and lower airways, *Chest* 104:825, 1993.
8. Conrad DJ et al: Microgranulomatous aspergillosis after shoveling wood chips: report of fatal outcome in a patient with chronic granulomatous disease, *Am J Ind Med* 22:411, 1992.
9. Dahlqvist M, Ulfvarson U: Acute effects on forced expiratory volume in one second and longitudinal change in pulmonary function among wood trimmers, *Am J Ind Med* 25:551, 1994.
10. Dickie HA, Rankin J: Farmer's lung: acute granulomatous interstitial pneumonitis occurring in agricultural workers, *JAMA* 167:1069, 1958.
11. Fink JN: Hypersensitivity pneumonitis, *Clin Chest Med* 13:303, 1992.
12. Frew A et al: Immunologic studies of the mechanisms of occupational asthma caused by western red cedar, *J Allergy Clin Immunol* 92:466, 1993.
13. Henneberger PK, Eisen EA, Ferris BG: Pulmonary function among pulp and paper workers in Berlin, New Hampshire, *Br J Ind Med* 46:765, 1989.
14. Herbert FA et al: Respiratory consequences of exposure to wood dust and formaldehyde of workers manufacturing oriented strand board, *Arch Environ Health* 49:465, 1994.
15. Holmstrom M, Rosen G, Wilhelmsson B: Symptoms, airway physiology and histology of workers exposed to medium-density fiber board, *Scand J Work Environ Health* 17:409, 1991.
16. Kauppinen TP et al: Chemical exposures and respiratory cancer among Finnish woodworkers, *Br J Ind Med* 50:143, 1993.
17. Keller RH et al: Immunoregulation in hypersensitivity pneumonitis. I. Differences in T-cell and macrophage suppressor activity in symptomatic and asymptomatic pigeon breeders, *J Clin Immunol* 2:46, 1982.
18. Kennedy SM et al: Lung health consequences of reported accidental chlorine gas exposures among pulpmill workers, *Am Rev Respir Dis* 143:74, 1991.
19. Kurttio P et al: Chromosome aberrations in peripheral lymphocytes of workers employed in the plywood industry, *Scand J Work Environ Health* 19:132, 1993.
20. Luce D et al: Occupational risk factors for sinonasal cancer: a case-control study in France, *Am J Ind Med* 21:163, 1992.
21. Macbeth R: Malignant diseases of the paranasal sinuses, *J Laryngol Otol* 79:592, 1965.
22. Mackey SA, Marks JG: Allergic contact dermatitis to white pine sawdust, *Arch Dermatol* 128:1660, 1992.
23. Menon JA: Tropical hazards associated with the use of pentachlorophenol, *BMJ* 12:1156, 1958.
24. Miller BA et al: Cancer and other mortality patterns among United States furniture workers, *Br J Ind Med* 46:508, 1989.
25. Miller BA, Blair A, Reed EJ: Extended mortality follow-up among men and women in a U.S. furniture workers union, *Am J Ind Med* 25:537, 1994.
26. Nygren O, Nilsson CA, Lindahl R: Occupational exposure to chromium, copper and arsenic during work with impregnated wood in joinery shops, *J Ind Hyg* 5:509, 1992.
27. Nylander LA, Dement JM: Carcinogenic effects of wood dust: review and discussion, *Am J Ind Med* 24:619, 1993.
28. Partanen T et al: Malignant lymphomas and leukemias, and exposures in the wood industry: and industry-based case-referent study, *Occup Environ Health* 41:593, 1993.
29. Perry GF: What is the association between nasal cancer and employment in the woodworking industry? *J Occup Med* 36:398, 1994.
30. Rask-Andersen A et al: Inhalation fever and respiratory symptoms in the trimming department of Swedish sawmills, *Am J Ind Med* 25:65, 1994.
31. Roscoe RJ et al: Colon and stomach cancer mortality among automotive wood model makers, *J Occup Med* 34:759, 1992.
32. Sharnssain MH: Pulmonary function and symptoms in workers exposed to wood dust, *Thorax* 47:84, 1992.
33. Terho EO: Extrinsic allergic alveolitis-management of established cases, *Eur J Respir Dis* 63(Suppl 123):101, 1982.
34. Teschke K et al: Recognizing acute health effects of substitute fungicides: are first-aid reports effective? *Am J Ind Med* 21:375, 1992.
35. Zenz C, Dickerson OB, Horvath EP, eds: *Occupational medicine,* St Louis, 1994, Mosby.

6

Concrete Workers and Masons

Frank LoVecchio

Richard J. Hamilton

Cr^{3+}
trivalent chromium

Cr^{6+}
hexavalent chromium

- Chromium is the main cause of dermatitis in cement workers

- Calcium hydroxide (Lime) is the source for the alkaline pH of cement and causes caustic burns

OCCUPATIONAL DESCRIPTION

To manage patients who work with concrete, physicians must familiarize themselves with the construction process and the components of cement. Large-scale construction projects in most developed countries use a prefabricated construction method, while on-site construction methods are often carried out for smaller buildings. The main substance used in construction today is cement. The conventional method of processing requires the complete fabrication process to be carried out on the construction site. The prefabrication method is carried out in a remote site and then transported to the construction site.

Most concrete today is premixed at a prefabrication factory and delivered to the site by a truck. Small jobs are mixed at the site with a machine or hoe. Most of this premix work is done by machines; therefore, exposure does not typically occur at this stage. Workers are exposed to concrete and its potential toxicologic effects during the pouring and cleaning process. After the concrete is poured into molds, cement workers (including cement pavers, cement masons, concrete floaters, and finishers) level and finish the surfaces. The concrete is spread to a desired consistency with a float. A float is simply a straightedge; it can be wooden blocks or more elaborate devices, depending on the job. Vertical surfaces are finished by moistening the surface and rubbing it with abrasive stones or by using a chisel or hammer. The hardened molds are sprayed with oil and cleaned, and defects in the concrete are repaired with epoxy resin.

POTENTIAL TOXIC EXPOSURES

The toxic work environment of concrete workers and masons is most often related to cements. As concrete is a mixture of cement and other additives that change its characteristics, it can be categorized with cement and cement's range of toxicity. Cement is a hydraulic bonding agent. It is a fine powder, obtained by grinding the clinker of a clay and limestone mixture at high temperatures. Adding water causes cement to reach a puree consistency, which gradually hardens at a rate that is dependent on the amount of water, the temperature, and the humidity. By varying the process or including additives, different types of cement may be obtained, such as waterproof, microporous, or asphalt tar.

There are two basic types of cement; natural cements and artificial cements. One of the sites of natural cement production is at the volcanic tuff. During the calcination process, the tuff may contain 70% to 80% amorphous free silica and 5% to 10% quartz. The natural cements, which are obtained from natural materials, need only to be calcined and ground. The artificial cements go through an intense manufacturing process and are by far the most common. The most commonly used construction cement is portland cement, so named by its inventor, Joseph Aspdin, in 1824, as it reminded him of a limestone used in England (Table 6-1).

Concrete is an admixture of cement with varying amounts of additives, usually sand, chemicals, and gravel. The addition of sand and gravel in concrete increases the irritant properties by increasing the likelihood of skin and ocular microtrauma. The addition of rubber epoxy resins and other additives to cement can also increase the allergen and irritant character (Table 6-2).

Cement is by far the most common cause of contact dermatitis among construction workers, primarily because of

hexavalent chromate. Other impurities, such as cobalt and nickel, have been implicated. In addition, rubber chemicals and epoxy resin may cause allergic dermatitis or act as skin sensitizers. Lead poisoning has been reported in bricklayers using mortar with a lead additive.[31]

Another potential exposure route is the respiratory tract. Chromate has been suggested as an irritant that may be responsible for chronic cough, bronchitis, and a multitude of pulmonary symptoms. Patients may have also been exposed to asbestos and silica.

Chromium

Chromium is a metal whose harmful effects are dependent on valence. Metallic chromium has a valence of 0, and other valences are the +2, +3, +4, +5, and +6 states. The trivalent state and hexavalent states are the only compounds known to cause human pathology. The hexavalent form most easily penetrates the skin.[13,20,26] It freely crosses the cell membrane but has a half-life of 2 to 4 hours. It reduces to the only form of chromium that is carcinogenic—the trivalent state. If the reduction occurs close to the DNA, in proximity to the nucleus, then the mutagenic potential is increased.

The total amount of chromium in portland cement ranges from 70 to 100 ppm or between 0.002% and 0.1%. This is variable among different countries.[8] In the United States, the amount of chromium varies among manufacturers. One study of 42 different manufacturers identified only 18 with measurable amounts of soluble chromate, ranging from 0.1 to 5.4/gms.[24] Other studies have shown a wide range of chromium content, from 0 to 0.2%.[8] On the average, 20% of the chromium content is found to be the soluble hexavalent chromium type. The origin of the chromium is unclear but hypothesized to be either the bricks of the furnaces, steel grinding balls, or the raw materials. Allergic reactions, most notably contact dermatitis, almost always arise from the hexavalent chromium. The National Institute for Occupational Safety and Health (NIOSH) lists 104 occupations in which more than 175,000 workers are exposed to chromium[22] (Table 6-3). During the construction of the England Channel tunnel, of the 5900 underground employees, 1138 were seen for occupational dermatitis. Although only a small number of the subset had formal patch testing, the majority showed allergies to chromate.[14]

Table 6-1 Summary of toxicologic hazards from cement

Hazard	Comments
Dermatitis	Often induced by chromium, less commonly by cobalt, nickel, and various additives or cleaners
Ocular irritation	Chronic conjunctivitis, blepharitis, and alkaline burns
Respiratory symptoms	Chronic bronchitis, cough, expectoration, rhinitis
Possible malignancy predisposition	Asbestosis (with asbestos-containing cements)
	Silicosis (with silica-containing cements)
	Gastrointestinal malignancies?
	Laryngeal malignancies

Table 6-2 Summary of allergens and irritants for the mason and cement workers

Allergens from rubber (gloves and additives)	Irritants in cement	Additional irritants and allergens
Potassium dichromate	Chromium	Cleaning solutions
2-Mercaptobenzothiazole	Cobalt	Phenylmercuric
Epoxy resin	Nickel	nitrate
Thiuram mix	Calcium chloride	O-Phenylmercuric nitrate

1964, US Dept. of Health Education and Welfare, Public Health Service.

23. Morris GE: The primary irritant of cement, *Arch Environ Health* 1:301, 1960.

24. Perone VB et al: The chromium, cobalt, nickel, contents of American cement and their relationship to cement dermatitis. *Am Ind Hyg Assoc J* May (35):301, 1974.

25. Perry GT Jr.: What is the current treatment of asphalt skin burns? *J Occup Med* 35:354, 1993.

26. Polak L: Immunology of chromium. In Burrows D, editor: *Chromium: metabolism and toxicity,* Boca Raton, Fla, 1983, CRC Press.

27. Rowe RJ, Williams GH: Severe reaction to cement, *Arch Environ Health* 7:709, 1963.

28. Sanders OA: The nonfibrogenic (benign) pneumoconioses, *Semin Roetgenol* 2:213, 1967.

29. Saric M, Kalacic I, Holetic A: Follow-up of ventilatory lung function in a group of cement workers, *Br J Ind Med* 33:18, 1976.

Cobalt and Nickel

Cobalt and nickel are two insoluble salts that exist in cement in approximately the same concentration as chromium does, but they are not as readily absorbed into the skin.[8] Most workers who are sensitive to cobalt and nickel are also sensitive to many other elements.[9,12] In a study in the Netherlands,[3] 126 concrete workers with eczema were skin tested; 11% documented a response to chromate and 2.3% to cobalt. In the control group of patients without eczema, only 2.6% responded to chromate and 0.7% to cobalt. In a study of 272 prefabrication factory workers, the prevalence of contact allergy was 15% for chromate and 1.8% for nickel. Interestingly, among the 5 with a nickel allergy, 2 were asymptomatic, 2 were allergic to their personal watches, and only 1 had an allergy to chromate, nickel, and cobalt.

Calcium Hydroxide

Cement dust is irritating to exposed tissues, especially the eyes and respiratory tract. Calcium hydroxide, because of its alkalinity, is responsible for its tissue irritant character. Mortar, a variant of cement, contains more free calcium hydroxide (lime) than concrete and is more alkaline. Lime rapidly dissolves in the skin; hence, it has been a longtime favorite for distorting proper identification of assassinated mobsters.

Water freely applied to the blade or tool during cutting operations can significantly decrease airborne dust levels. Some masonry and concrete tools have a water applicator incorporated into the cutting mechanism. Water application during cutting does not control all the airborne dust, however, and other control methods and respirators should be used. Most recently, NIOSH has recommended the use of "the most protective respirator that is feasible and consistent with the tasks performed." Personal protective equipment should be based on periodic air sampling (Table 6-4).

The pH of a water and cement mixture is 13. Hence, severe alkali burning can result from contact with wet cement.[27] Trivial splashes of mortar may cause "lime burns." Burns and ulcerations can result from kneeling in cement and mortar for long periods of time or from spilling it into boots or gloves (Fig. 6-1).[23,27] Workers often delay rapid decontamination because time constraints force them to complete their task before the concrete hardens.

Table 6-4 Personal protective respiratory recommendations for cement dust exposure

Total dust	Recommended protective equipment
Up to 50 mg/m^3	Dust respiratory filter
Up to 100 mg/m^3	Any dust respiratory (except single use) or self-contained breathing apparatus
Up to 250 mg/m^3	Powered air-purifying respirator with a dust filter operated in continuous flow mode
Up to 500 mg/m^3	Self-contained breathing apparatus with a full facepiece, any supplied air respirator with a tight mask operated in a continuous mode
Up to 7500 mg/m^3	Supplied-air respirator with a half mask and operated in a pressure-demand or other positive pressure mode

Modified from OSHA/NIOSH: *Pocket guide to chemical hazards,* Pub 85-114, Washington, DC, 1987, Government Printing Office.

Table 6-3 Examples of skin problems associated with chromium and chromium compounds

Chromium-containing materials	Occupational exposure
Chromium ore	Industrial chromium production
Leather and artificial leather tanned with chromium	Leather and footwear industries
Textiles and furs	Textiles and fur industries
Lubricating oils and greases	Metal industry
Cement	Cement production and workers
Wood preservation (Wolman salts)	Wood impregnation, carpenters, furniture industry
Chrome baths	Electroplating industry, graphic trades, metal industry
Chromate colors and dyes	Painters and decorators, graphic trades, textiles, rubber
Anticorrosive agents in water systems and greases	Diesel locomotive workshops, central heating and air-conditioning
Cleaning materials, washing and bleaching materials	Homemakers, cleaners, laundries

Modified from Polak L: Immunology of chromium. In Burrows D: *Chromium: metabolism and toxicity,* Boca Raton, Fla, 1983, CRC Press.

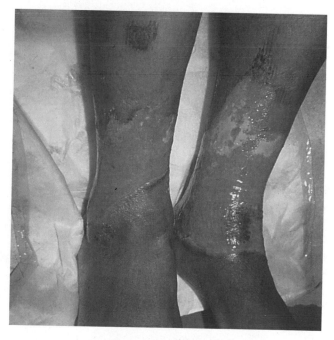

Fig. 6-1 Cement burns.

Silica

Free silica (SiO_2) or crystalline quartz is still a major occupational hazard. The number of potentially exposed workers range from 1.2 to 3 million, although the exact number of cement workers is not known. The major occupational exposures include sandblasting, road and building construction, mining, farming, stone cutting, and quarrying (particularly of granite).

Silica exposure in concrete and masonry workers is related to exposure quantity and protective measures. The lowest exposures are noted with those sawing concrete floors in a large room, with general ventilation. The highest exposures are noted during outdoor electric grinding of mortar. Exposure to quartz dust is present in excess of Occupational Safety and Health Administration (OSHA) standards and is probably common among concrete workers and masons.[32]

Are concrete workers at risk for silicosis? Some formal studies have shown a slight increase, approaching statistical significance.[33] Current concerns are based on anecdotal cases of concrete workers who had lung biopsies revealing silica particles.[2]

Asbestos

In the past, asbestos has been mixed with concrete to enhance heat resistance. Although this practice is no longer used, many modern-day concrete workers may have been exposed decades ago when the practice of pouring bags of asbestos powder into cement was common. Asbestos cement workers are at risk for chronic obstructive pulmonary disease (COPD) and various cancers, especially mesothelioma.[10] Radiographic evidence of asbestos is dose-dependent and continues well after exposure cessation.[17]

Miscellaneous

The oil that is spread on the molds is a known culprit in the development of folliculitis and contact dermatitis. The addition of rubber epoxy resins and other additives to cement can also increase the allergen and irritant character (see Table 6-2).

CLINICAL TOXICOLOGY

Chromium-Induced Skin Diseases

Jaeger and Pelloni were the first to associate chromate with cement eczema in 1950.[14] Skin disease is more frequent among cement users than among cement manufacturing plant workers, whose chromium exposure is minimal. However, overwhelming absorption has occurred from accidental immersion in hot chromium sulfate solution, leading to severe tissue damage and death.[19]

Workers from a variety of fields may come in contact with chromium and chromium-like products (see Table 6-3). Chromium dermatitis typically affects the backs of hands and distal forearms and may persist as eczema despite discontinuation of further cement contact.

Diagnosis. Diagnosis of skin-related dermatitis begins with a complete history and physical examination. Several factors facilitate chromium penetration of the skin: open sores, inflammation, alkaline pH, and traumatized skin. The incidence of chromium sensitivity in the general population is uncertain. However, the estimated U.S. range is 2% to 20%. In sensitized populations, the threshold for eliciting allergic contact dermatitis is about 10 ppm in solution.[7] Actual patch testing of cement is commonly negative because of the lack of reactivity of the chromates in the dry state. The recommended method for patch testing utilizes a 0.5% solution of potassium dichromate in either water or petroleum. The patch test may remain positive long after exposure, and patients should be forewarned.[4]

Prevention remains an important aspect in promoting dermatologic wellness. Protective gloves, clothing, and boots decrease the incidence of dermatitis. This, in conjunction with rapid decontamination after inadvertent contact, reduces the incidence to less than 1%. Other products added during the processing of cement may affect the incidence of chromium dermatitis. Ferrous sulfate significantly reduces the hexavalent chromium levels. The proposed mechanism for this is a reduction of the chromate by iron sulfate, with eventual precipitation of the trivalent chromium.[10] No side effects have been noted to be associated with this additive, although it is not currently used in the United States.

When pharmacologic intervention is required for chromium-induced dermatitis, topical steroids are the drug of choice. Superinfections are common and, when present, should be treated with a penicillinase-resistant antibiotic or first-generation cephalosporin. Hospital admission is rarely required; however, it should be considered for advanced disease or a poor response to outpatient therapy.

Removal of cement product from skin may pose a problem. The conventional method uses soap and water. If this fails, a 50:50 solution of povidone-iodine and mineral oil may be effective.[25] A report on the decontamination of asphalt cement exposure used the commercially available petroleum-based solvent De-Solv-It. It may be successful if conventional methods fail.[34]

Cement-Induced Pulmonary Disease

The prevalence of pulmonary disease among cement workers is unknown. Upper airway irritation, nasal septum perforation, and pulmonary sensitization have been reported in association with cement exposure. Historically, the pulmonary malignancies from cement exposure were associated with additives not used in cement today, such as silica and asbestos. Today, workers may become exposed to asbestos and silica when they work on older structures.

There are few well-controlled studies that address the issue of pure cement-induced pulmonary disease. Those that exist fail to adequately control for confounders such as smoking. When work habits are controlled, no significant statistical difference in respiratory symptoms exists between controls and cement workers.[6] Although one other study noted a trend for increased prevalence of pulmonary symptoms among cement workers, these data have not been reproduced elsewhere.[5] The National Institute of Health evaluated the overall mortality of U.S. portland cement and quarry workers. It followed a cohort of 5141 workers in 23 U.S. cement plants from 1950 to 1980.[1] A statistically significant decrease in mortality among white males was found for diseases of all causes. All malignant neoplasms, heart disease, respiratory disease including emphysema, chronic bronchitis, tuberculosis, and pneumonia were all found with decreased incident when compared with the control group. Also of note, death from stomach cancer increased after a 20-year latency. None of the groups in the subset evaluating gastrointestinal cancer approaches statistical significance. Hexavalent chromium is an established carcinogen; however, its exact role in pulmonary disease is not defined.

Chronic obstructive pulmonary disease (COPD) is the most common respiratory tract disease affecting cement workers and masons. Cement dust has been implicated as a cause of mucus hypersecretion and obstruction of the small airways. In some cases, IGE, direct broncoconstrictor substances, or directly irritating mechanisms have been proposed. The greatest prevalence of COPD was reported in one study as 63%,[35] although other studies put the range from 9.5% to 20%[6,18,21] among cement workers. Moreover, an increased incidence of chronic phlegm production is reported.

The calcium silicate and oxide in cement dust are a suggested toxin of the respiratory tract. Exposure is more common in workers who bag the finished product; however, radiographic evidence of disease is lacking even after 40 years of exposure.[28] Pulmonary function tests reveal an obstructive impairment[30] in this group, seemingly attributable to smoking.[29]

The mainstay of respiratory tract treatment remains proper prevention strategies. Chronic bronchitis can be treated in the traditional fashion with inhalational β-adrenergic agonists and anticholinergic agents (ipratropium bromide).

SUMMARY

Preventive measures concerning occupational dermatitis and respiratory protection are most effective. Routine screening for skin and pulmonary disease is recommended. Applicable chest radiographs and pulmonary function tests should be used only when prompted by the history and physical examination.

Cement workers and masons are exposed to a wide variety of airborne and dermatologic chemical hazards. When the overall mortality of the cement worker is compared with controls, however, the overall mortality is not increased.[16]

ACKNOWLEDGMENT

The author would like to thank Anu Bhatia for preparation of this manuscript.

REFERENCES

1. Amandus HE: *The mortality of U.S. Portland cement plant and quarry workers,* Washington, DC, 1985, National Institute of Occupational Safety and Health.
2. Bernadou JM et al: Silicosis in occupations handling concrete, *Arch Mal Prof* 31:617, 1970.
3. Coenraads PJ: Prevalence of eczema and other dermatoses of the hands and forearms in construction workers in the Netherlands, *Clin Exp Dermatol* 9:149, 1984.
4. Dooms-Goossens A et al: Follow-up study of patients with contact dermatitis caused by chromates, nickel, and cobalt, *Dermatologica* 4:249, 1980.
5. El-Sewefy AZ, Awad S: Chest symptomology in an Egyptian portland cement factory, *J Egypt Med Assoc* 54:457, 1971.
6. El-Sewefy AZ, Awad S, Abdel-Salem MS: Chest symptomology in an Egyptian cement-asbestos pipe factory, *J Egypt Med Ass* 53:84, 1970.
7. Foussereau J et al: Brick layers. In *Occupational clinical dermatitis, clinical and chemical aspects,* Philadelphia, 1982, WB Saunders Co.
8. Fregert S: Chromium valencies and cement dermatitis, *Br J Dermatol* 105(suppl):21:7, 1981.
9. Fregert S, Gruvberger B: Solubility of cobalt in cement, *Contact Dermatitis* 4:14, 1978.
10. Fregert S, Gruvberger B, Sandahl E: Reduction of chromate in cement by iron sulfate, *Contact Dermatitis* 5:39, 1979.
11. Giaroli C et al: Mortality study of asbestos cement workers, *Int Arch Occup Environ Health* 66:7, 1994.
12. Goh CL, Kwok SF, Gans SL: Cobalt and nickel content of Asian cement, *Contact Dermatitis* 15:169, 1986.
13. Gray S, Sterling K: The tagging of red cells and plasma proteins with radioactive chromium, *J Clin Invest* 29:1604, 1950.
14. Irvine C et al: Cement dermatitis in underground workers during construction of the Channel Tunnel, *Occup Med* 44:17, 1994.
15. Jaeger H, Pelloni E: Test epicutanees aux bichromates, positifs dans L'eczema au ciment, *Dermatologica* 100:200, 1950.
16. Jakobsson K, Horstmann V, Welinder H: Mortality and cancer morbidity among cement workers, *Br J Ind Med* 50:264, 1993.
17. Jakobsson K et al: Radiological changes in asbestos cement workers, *Occup Environ Med* 52:20, 1995.
18. Kalacic I: Chronic nonspecific lung disease in cement workers, *Arch Environ Health* 26:78, 1973.
19. Kelly WF et al: Cutaneous absorption of trivalent chromium: tissue levels and treatment by exchange transfusions, *Br J Ind Med* 39:397, 1982.
20. Korrallus U, Harsdorf C, Lewalter J: Experimental bases for ascorbic acid therapy of poisoning by hexavalent chromium compounds, *Int Arch Occup Environ Health* 539:247, 1984.
21. Mal'tseva LM, Tatanov YA: Respiratory diseases among workers occupied in the manufacture of cement, *Gig Tr Prof Zabol* 3:14, 1974.
22. Milby TH et al: Chemical hazards. In Gafafer WM (ed): *Occupational diseases: a guide to recognition,* PHS Publ 1097, Washington, DC,

30. Scansetti G et al: Cement, asbestos, and cement-asbestos pneumoconioses, *Arch Environ Health* 30:272, 1975.

31. Stockbridge H, Daniel W: Lead poisoning among bricklayers—Washington State, *MMWR Morb Mortal Wkly Rep* 40:169, 1991.

32. Tharr D: Silica exposure for concrete workers and masons, *Appl Occup Environ Hyg* 8:832, 1993.

33. Tornling G, Tollqvist J, Askergren A, et al. Does long term concrete work cause silicosis? *Scand J Work Environ Health* 18:97, 1992.

34. Tsou T et al: De-Solv-It for hot paving asphalt burn: case report, *Acad Emer Med* 3:88, 1996.

35. Vyskocil J: Long term follow up of chronic bronchitis in hydraulic cement workers, *Intern Med* 14:341, 1968.

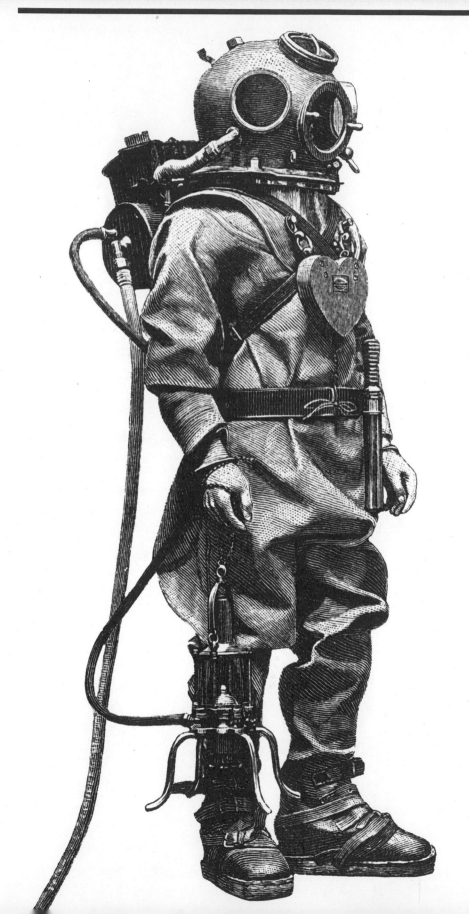

7

Divers

Raymond Iannacone

N₂   O₂
   CO₂

- Professional divers undertake the riskiest of dives, but have an excellent record of safety despite the toxicologic risk of compressed gases

- Nitrogen narcosis is the most common manifestation of diving toxicity

OCCUPATIONAL DESCRIPTION

Diving is a centuries-old practice that utilizes a variety of equipment and techniques. Alexander the Great used diving bells in the siege of Tyre around 332 BC, but not until Augustus Siebe's "open diving dress" in 1819 did the range and functionality of the diver become useful. This forerunner of the "classic" copper-helmeted diving suit tethered divers to the surface by only a lifeline and air hose. True freedom from the surface was achieved in the 1940s with the development of the self-contained underwater breathing apparatus (SCUBA). This advance also helped establish recreational diving.

In addition to these general advances in equipment, there were major advances in the understanding of diving physiology. Investigations into the effects of nitrogen led to the development of decompression schedules and treatment tables and an appreciation of the narcotic effect of this gas. An understanding of the benefits and risks of oxygen allowed an improvement in treatment tables and new types of diving that minimize decompression risk and extend bottom times (length of time at depth). In the last few decades, the use of helium and other inert gases has enabled divers to reach incredible depths, revealing previously unknown physiologic effects of high pressure.

It is difficult to say how many divers there are in the world. The vast majority are recreational divers. In the United States (where there are certification requirements), the Diver's Alert Network estimates there are 1 to 4 million recreational scuba divers. The number of commercial divers is in constant flux. There are roughly 3000 professional divers in the United States, fewer than 10% of whom are saturation qualified. The U.S. Navy employs the vast majority of military divers, including salvage, mine work, and combat swimming. There are approximately 3600 Navy divers, all of whom are qualified on at least one other diving apparatus besides scuba. This small number of commercial and military divers undertake the majority of dives beyond 30 msw,* and the majority of dives made with equipment and breathing gases other than the standard scuba-air combination. These specialists also continue to dive, using diving bells and surface-supplied "hard hat" diving.

POTENTIAL TOXIC EXPOSURES

Demand regulators, mixed gas (mostly helium), oxygen breathing rigs, and closed-circuit breathing systems (recirculate breathing gas by removing carbon dioxide) have markedly improved commercial and military diving. Saturation diving (divers stay at depth in a chamber between dives to avoid the lengthy compression and decompression) has made deep diving feasible. Much of this technology is now available to the recreational diving community. This has lead to "technical diving," in which high-tech equipment and "homemade" mixed gases combine to extend depth limits. This is much more dangerous than traditional scuba diving.

In spite of all this progress, the primary risks of diving have not changed: decompression sickness and arterial gas embolism. These conditions can be lethal or leave permanent sequelae. The toxicity of diving is less often encountered but nonetheless significant. Nitrogen narcosis is commonly encountered. Oxygen toxicity and the high-pressure neurologic syndrome (HPNS) are problems encountered during oxygen exposure and deep diving with mixed gas.

It is important to understand that the biologic effects of a gas are not determined by its relative concentration in the total breathing gas (that is, the percent of the total gas mixture). Instead, it is a result of the partial pressure, or total amount, of that gas. Thus, the biologic effect of 100% oxygen at 1 ATA is equivalent to 50% oxygen at 2 ATA because each represents a partial pressure of 1 ATA of oxygen. Also, the same innocuous 70% nitrogen of sea level air is converted into a deadly toxin at 300 feet.

CLINICAL TOXICOLOGY

Oxygen Toxicity

The toxic effects of elevated pressures of oxygen have been recognized for more than 100 years. Paul Bert first described the convulsive and eventually lethal effects of this vital gas in 1878. Lorrain Smith characterized the pulmonary toxicity of oxygen in 1899. Sporadic experiments and occupational experience ensued until the experiments of Albert R. Behnke in the 1930s elucidated some of the effects of hyperbaric oxygen (oxygen at an absolute pressure of greater than one atmosphere).[4] The modern era of oxygen toxicity research began with the hallmark experiments by Kenneth W. Donald

for the Royal Navy in 1942.[20] Many of the signs and symptoms of oxygen toxicity were first described or compiled in these efforts. At approximately the same time, aerospace research led to many experiments with hypobaric and hyperoxic exposure.[18] Mechanical ventilation with increased oxygen tensions provoked further research into the pulmonary effects of more prolonged exposures. Most recently, hyperbaric oxygen therapy has added a new facet to the oxygen toxicity experience.

Clinically, oxygen manifests its toxicity in the pulmonary or central nervous system. The lungs, as the organ of gas exchange, are exposed to a concentration many times higher than any other part of the body and are the primary site of toxicity. However, at oxygen pressures greater than 3 ATA (66 feet of seawater equivalent), acute central nervous system (CNS) toxicity usually develops before exposures are long enough to develop pulmonary symptoms. Overlap exists between these two ranges, and CNS symptoms including convulsions have been reported as shallow as 1.6 ATA.[13]

Many other organ systems, including the eye, liver, and erythrocytes, have been found to demonstrate toxic effects.

Oxygen is typically reduced to water in the mitochondria by cytochrome oxidase by the addition of four electrons. However, even under normal conditions a small percentage of oxygen undergoes a stepwise reduction to superoxide (O_2^-), hydrogen peroxide (H_2O_2), hydroxyl radical (OH), and finally water (Fig. 7-1).[14] This third step requires the presence of a transition metal (usually iron) and is described in the Fenton equation:

$$O_2^- + H_2O_2 \rightarrow O_2 + OH- + OH^{63}$$

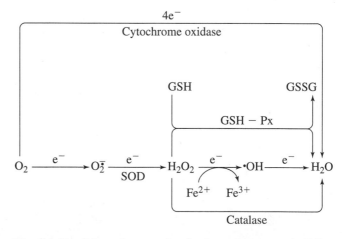

Fig. 7-1 Possible pathways of reduction of oxygen. Avoiding toxicity depends on minimizing production of hydroxyl radical (OH). *SOD,* Superoxide dismutase; *GSH,* reduced glutathione; *GSSG,* oxidized glutathione; *GSH-PX,* glutathione peroxidase. (From Clark IA: Tissue damage caused by free oxygen radicals, *Pathology* 18:181, 1986.)

---

*Thirty-three feet of seawater (fsw) = 10 meters of seawater (msw) = 1 atmosphere of pressure (atm) = 760 mm Hg = 1.013 bar. An ATA is atmospheres absolute, which simply adds the 1 atm of atmospheric pressure on the surface to the gauge reading, for example, 33 fsw = 2 ATA.

All these free radical species are highly reactive. They are known to react with and inactivate protein sulfhydryl groups.[65] They react with lipids to form lipid peroxides, hydroperoxides, and aldehydes that, in turn, can initiate free radical chain reactions.[14,42]

There are many sources of superoxide radical, such as hemoglobin, myoglobin, xanthine oxidase, aldehyde oxidase, and phagocytes.[49] These are increased in the presence of elevated partial pressures of oxygen.

The primary route of elimination of superoxide is through superoxide dismutases (SOD), a family of enzymes that catalyze the reduction of superoxide to peroxide. Typically, cytosolic SOD contains copper and zinc, mitochondrial SOD contains manganese, and others contain iron at the active site.[49] Hydrogen peroxide is metabolized principally by catalase (CAT), located primarily in peroxisomes of the liver and erythrocytes, and by the glutathione redox cycle. The CAT catalyzes the following reaction:

$$2\ H_2O_2 \rightarrow 2\ H_2O + O_2 \text{[63]}$$

This reaction, as well as the reduction of toxic lipid peroxides, is also catalyzed by glutathione peroxidase. This requires reduced glutathione produced by glutathione reductase and glucose 6-phosphate dehydrogenase.[40] In addition to these mechanisms, there are a host of antioxidants, including vitamins A, C, and E, that play key roles in protecting cells from the destructive effects of free radicals.[63]

Although the cause and effect have not been completely defined, there is evidence that the pathophysiology of oxygen toxicity is a result of excess free radicals.

In the lung, there are two phases of oxygen-induced damage: exudative and proliferative. Primate studies demonstrate that the exudative changes involve interstitial edema, which progresses to cellular infiltration and fibrin deposition. Subsequently, alveoli become obliterated by exudate. The initial site of injury is the capillary endothelium. In the exudative phase, there is initially destruction of type I epithelial cells, which leads to a proliferation of type II epithelial cells (which have a greater capacity for division). This thickens the air-blood tissue barrier, as does further proliferation of the interstitium. During this later phase, the exudative changes tend to resolve. Recovery from these exposures, which ranged from 4 to 13 days at pressures of 600 to 760 mm Hg, is complete in 2 to 3 months. However, examination of these lungs revealed that exposure long enough to produce proliferative changes resulted in residual scarring, despite clinical and functional normalcy.[45]

Ventilator patients demonstrate similar histologic changes, with more interstitial tissue, less prominent hyperplasia of the epithelium, and a pronounced endothelial injury.[44] Mechanisms for these pathologic changes are not completely elucidated, but evidence suggests that the primary derangement is endothelial cell injury. It is interesting that cultured human pulmonary artery endothelial cells lose their replicative function in 8 hours at 95% oxygen and in 48 hours at 60%.[48] These times parallel known limits for clinical oxygen toxicity and support the notion that there is a biologic basis for a threshold for oxygen toxicity.

There is no extensive body of research on pathologic or histologic changes in the CNS resulting from oxygen toxicity. However, there are significant studies on many different effects on CNS metabolic and chemical systems. Hyperbaric oxygen decreases cell metabolism, adenosine triphosphate (ATP) levels, and sodium-potassium gradients in cerebral cortex slices. Increased lipid peroxides may be causative.[43] Cell metabolism is more depressed in brain slices with higher baseline metabolic rates, and these latter tissues also develop oxygen toxic effects quicker.[47] This correlates well with the clinical findings that increases in metabolism by exercise[69] and hyperthyroidism[62] enhance sensitivity to oxygen toxicity and that decreases in metabolism by hypothermia, hibernation,[55] and hypophysectomy[62] diminish sensitivity. Finally, hyperbaric oxygen (HBO)-induced decreases in CNS γ-aminobutyric acid (GABA) levels have been demonstrated to correlate with decreased time to onset of seizures.[68]

There are three main histologic changes in the eye in response to elevated oxygen. Corneal endothelial cells thin, and their cytoplasm condenses. Lens epithelial cells exhibit pyknosis and nuclei loss. Finally, retinal edema, particularly of the inner nuclear and inner plexiform layers,[54] also occurs after exposure to HBO.

In spite of the incomplete understanding of the basis for oxygen toxicity, there is a relatively clear and consistent body of clinical experience in the area. The classic signs and symptoms of pulmonary oxygen toxicity were observed by Comroe and colleagues in an exposure to 1 ATA for 24 hours. The chief symptom was progressive substernal chest pain, exacerbated by inspiration, as well as cough, sore throat, and nasal congestion.[18] In studies at higher pressures for shorter durations, similar symptoms, in addition to fatigue, nausea, vomiting, and a tickling sensation in the trachea, have been described.[16,21]

Objective measurement of pulmonary oxygen toxicity has been a source of controversy. Vital capacity (VC) has remained the standard test since it is easy to perform and it correlates relatively well with clinical toxicity.[16,57] Figure 7-2 shows the results of some of the human exposure studies mentioned, plotting symptoms and VC changes versus time for a series of different exposure pressures. It is important to realize that VC can continue to decrease in the early postexposure period.[57] In the special situation of saturation diving, it has been shown that diffusing capacity actually is better than VC as an index of oxygen effect.[39]

The diagnosis of oxygen toxicity is based on clinical evidence. Characteristic symptoms in a person exposed to elevated pressures of oxygen should prompt the diagnosis. Decreases in VC can be roughly predicted, based on the

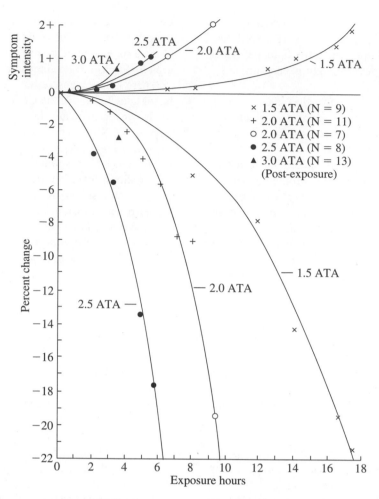

Fig. 7-2 Pulmonary symptoms and VC changes in humans during oxygen exposure at 3.0, 2.5, 2.0, and 1.5 ATA. (From Clark JM et al: Pulmonary tolerance in man to continuous oxygen exposure at 3.0, 2.5, 2.0, and 1.5 ATA in predictive study V. In Bachrach AJ, Bove AA, Greenbaum LJ Jr, editors: *9th International symposium on underwater and hyperbaric physiology,* Bethesda, Md, 1987, Undersea and Hyperbaric Medical Society.)

severity of exposure (see later in this chapter). Multiple studies have shown that vital signs (including respiratory rate), lung auscultation, radiography, and blood analysis, including alveolar-arterial oxygen gradient, do not correlate with the extent of oxygen toxicity.[16,18,21,57] The patient is removed from the source of oxygen if possible. Ancillary studies can help exclude other diagnoses, and pulmonary function tests may help confirm the diagnosis.

A similar approach is taken in diagnosing CNS oxygen toxicity. Proper symptoms (Table 7-1) in the proper exposure range are enough to make a presumptive diagnosis. Unlike pulmonary toxicity, there are no confirmatory tests. There is immense interindividual and intraindividual variability in onset and type of symptoms.[12,20]

Electroencephalographic (EEG) monitoring is not useful for predicting CNS toxicity because changes (increased delta wave activity) occur only seconds before the onset of seizures. In addition, a significant number of subjects have these changes and do not progress to seizures.[66]

There are no consistent warning signs, even for those having seizures.[20] Interestingly, all symptoms, including seizures, were increased or initially seen when the patient was taken off oxygen. This is also know as the "off effect." Decompression is also a convulsive stimulus during these times.[12]

The CNS toxicity may also lead to visual disturbances. Most classically, this is "tunnel vision" or contraction of the visual fields. Three ATA for 4 hours causes this contraction in the fourth hour of exposure, eventually to 10 degrees of central vision and impairment of visual acuity. These symptoms resolved within an hour of air breathing.[4] Patients treated with HBO have developed myopia over the course of 40 or more treatments, but it resolves within 10 weeks.[2]

The diagnosis of oxygen toxicity relies on a determination of the degree of risk from a particular exposure. Through pooled human exposure studies, the unit pulmonary toxic dose (UPTD) formula has been developed for the predicted change in VC based on the exposure pressure and time.

Table 7-1 Symptoms of O_2 toxicity and their frequency of occurrence

Private signs and symptoms	Toxicity episodes in which symptoms were observed	Percent of total symptoms	Percent of toxicity episodes in which symptoms were observed
Nausea	16	24.6	48.5
Muscle twitching	9	13.9	27.3
Dizziness	9	13.9	27.3
Tinnitus	5	7.7	15.2
Dysphoria	4	6.2	12.1
Confusion	3	4.6	9.1
Convulsion	2	3.1	6.1
Less auditory acuity	2	3.1	6.1
Aphasia	2	3.1	6.1
Tingling	2	3.1	6.1
Numbness	2	3.1	6.1
Choking sensation	2	3.1	6.1
Amnesia	1	1.5	3.0
Muscular rigidity	1	1.5	3.0
Lightheadedness	1	1.5	3.0
Poor concentration	1	1.5	3.0
Visual disturbances	1	1.5	3.0
Less mental alertness	1	1.5	3.0
Lower respiratory rate	1	1.5	3.0
Total symptoms 65	100		
Total toxicity episodes	33		

From Butler FK Jr, Thalmann ED: Central nervous system oxygen toxicity in closed circuit scuba divers II, *Undersea Biomed Res* 13:193, 1986.

Table 7-2 Proposed single-depth dive oxygen exposure limits

Depth (fsw)	Depth (msw)	Time (min)
20	6.1	240
25	7.6	240
30	9.1	80
35	10.7	25
40	12.2	15
50	15.2	10

Modified from: Butler FK Jr, Thalmann ED: Central nervous system oxygen toxicity in closed circuit scuba divers II, *Undersea Biomed Res* 13:193, 1986.

Recent modifications of this formula led to the following formula to roughly estimate the change in VC:

$$\% \ VC = 0.011 \ (Po_2 \ 0.5) \ time$$

where Po_2 is in ATA and time in minutes.[34]

A similar formula has not been developed for CNS limits; however, safe exposure limits have been suggested (Table 7-2). The preceding formula, the UPTD charts, and tables are only guidelines; individual responses are markedly varied. Toxicity may develop at times and depths severalfold less than these limits.

Numerous factors may increase or decrease the risk of developing oxygen toxicity. Hypothermia,[55] altitude acclimatization,[11] and pretreatment with progressive hypoxia,[10] 85% oxygen, or NO_2[19] may have a protective effect, based on animal experiments. Many studies, including human, have shown that both pulmonary and CNS toxicity are more common with work or exercise and in the wet environment.[20,69] These effects could be due to increased circulation or to the demonstrated fact that hypercapnia decreases time to seizure.[17] Hypercapnia is a common occurrence when a diver ventilates more than his breathing source supplies or when the carbon dioxide adsorbent is exhausted. All these features must be included in the composite assessment of exposure risk used in the decision algorithm.

Once symptoms develop and a diagnosis is made, treatment is simple: Remove the patient from the source, or minimize the exposure. The tracheobronchitis of pulmonary toxicity rarely requires bronchodilators or antibiotics and resolves in 1 to 3 days, depending on the exposure (Fig. 7-3).[15] Longer exposures may require several weeks.[39] Patients who are seizing should be switched immediately to air breathing. The CNS symptoms, including seizures, are short-lived, and patients recover rapidly if they have not suffered injury or death from trauma or drowning.

The real goal is prevention. The U.S. Navy formerly conducted an oxygen tolerance test (OTT) on all diver candidates. Studies showed, however, that interdiver and intradiver variability was so great that the test was not truly predictive, and it was abandoned.[20]

The most important technique for reducing the risk of oxygen toxicity is the scheduled use of intermittent air breathing or "air breaks." Animal data confirm increased survival times with the interspersed breathing of air at depth. A profile of 20 minutes of oxygen and 5 minutes of air has

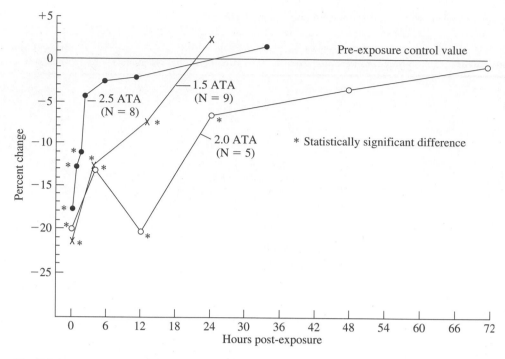

Fig. 7-3 Recovery of VC after oxygen exposure at 2.5, 2.0, and 1.5 ATA. Average percent changes in VC relative to preexposure control values are shown. (From Clark JM et al: Pulmonary tolerance in man to continuous oxygen exposure at 3.0, 2.5, 2.0, and 1.5 ATA in Predictive Study V. In Bachrach AJ, Bove AA, Greenbaum LJ Jr, editors: *9th international symposium on underwater and hyperbaric physiology,* Bethesda, Md, 1987, Undersea and Hyperbaric Medical Society.)

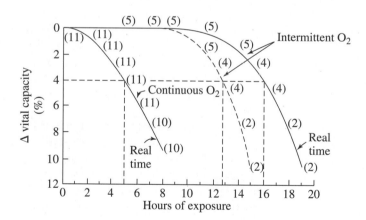

Fig. 7-4 Rate of onset of vital capacity change in continuous versus intermittent oxygen exposure at 2 ATA. First and second curves are in oxygen hours (second does not include air breaks). The third curve includes air break time. (Modified from: Hendricks PL et al: Extension of pulmonary O_2 tolerance in man at 2 ATA by intermittent O_2 exposure, *J Appl Physiol: Respir Environ Exercise Physiol* 42:593, 1977.)

been used in humans to nearly double the actual oxygen breathing time (Fig. 7-4) over that of controls.[36]

The dive plan is the key to avoiding potentially dangerous and even life-threatening toxicity. Air breaks, oxygen partial pressures, exposure times, and work load should all be controlled by the plan. In situations where the risk is still high, there should be contingency plans, such as buddy lines,

different breathing rigs, or more divers. The dive plan for elective HBO treatments is conservative enough that there are only rare instances of oxygen toxicity, and many of those are the myopia cases previously mentioned. Commercial and military diving plans may allow more exposure, yet oxygen toxicity is still a rare event. "Technical diving" is much less controlled, untethered, and increasing in popularity, which is leading to more common cases of oxygen poisoning. In spite of this, the prognosis is excellent if confounding circumstances (i.e., drowning, trauma) do not overtake the primary toxicity, and there appear to be no long-term effects of hyperoxic exposure.[53]

Nitrogen Narcosis

Divers have known for some time of the intoxicating effect of breathing air at elevated pressures. This "narcosis" was first elucidated by Albert Behnke in 1935 and characterized as "alterations of behavior, slowed mental activity, and impaired neuromuscular coordination."[5] Nitrogen was correctly postulated as the causative component. Since then, much research has more clearly defined the deficits induced by nitrogen at increased pressure as slowed reaction time, slowed movement time, amnesia, euphoria, and increased errors in performing tasks.[24]

Behnke observed a state of stimulation, alertness, and euphoria. He noted that, with effort, the divers could suppress the laughter and loquacity and that perception was preserved while response was slowed. Decreased recollec-

Table 7-3 Effects of repeated exposure to narcosis on symptomatology

Adjectives sensitive to narcosis	Adjectives that adapt to narcosis
Able to concentrate	Able to think clearly
Able to work hard	Dizzy
Alert	Elated
Businesslike	Hazy
Carefree	Light-headed
Cautious	Numb
Defiant	Tingling
Dependable	Uninhibited
Detached	
Dreamy	
Efficient	
Fuzzy	
Indifferent	
Intoxicated	
Reckless	
Self-confident	

Modified from Hamilton K, Laliberte MF, Heslegrave R: Subjective and behavioral effects associated with repeated exposure to narcosis, *Aviat Space Environ Med* 63:865, 1992.

tion, concentration, and arithmetical errors were also seen. Fine motor deficits were noted, but with greater concentration and slower movements these could be avoided. Symptoms increased with depth but not with duration of exposure.[5] Table 7-3 shows a list of adjectives that showed statistically significant correlation with the narcotic state.[33]

The original studies showed early effects at 3 ATA and definite effects at 4 ATA. A single exposure of a diver to 10 ATA revealed numbness, partial stupefaction, and greatly impaired neuromuscular function.[5] It is generally accepted that 4 ATA is the threshold for significant intoxication.[38] There is significant variation in the degree and nature of intoxication between divers, but the onset of symptoms is rapid (less than 3 minutes).[5] Recovery occurs as rapidly upon return to normal atmospheric nitrogen pressures.

More recent research has quantified the effects of nitrogen. In arithmetic testing, the number of problems completed and the number of correct choices are both decreased. Tests of perceptual speed, decision making, and fine motor skill all showed statistically significant decreases.[22] Other studies have shown that decrements in complex motor skills are a result of cognitive impairment as simple motor skills are preserved.[9] Primate studies using visual discrimination as a marker for sensory information processing have shown a decreased speed of processing with increasing depth. These effects are heightened with more difficult tasks and shorter input times.[3] Decreased response times are due to a general slowing of information processing (without distortion) throughout the perceptual-motor system. Long-term memory is the only function that suffers from true disruption of processing.[25]

This slowed processing may be the result of a depression of arousal and activation mechanisms.[23] Recent research

has demonstrated slowing of both the event-related brain potential P300 (a sensitive marker for stimulus evaluation time) and response time (stimulus evaluation plus the time to formulate and execute a response).[26]

Other studies reveal a more pervasive neurologic effect of nitrogen narcosis on divers that may be related to slowed information processing. The visual ocular reflex, responsible for maintaining foveal fixation in response to head movement, is disrupted by a decrease in compensatory eye movement velocity and the lag between eye and head position. These changes correlated with subjective reports of blurred vision and inability to fix gaze during head movement.[32] In addition, cold perception was decreased, even with decreases in core body temperature.[50]

The mechanism of action of nitrogen is believed to be similar to that of other inert gases and anesthetics. These gases share the property of being biochemically inactive; their action is a biophysical one. The Myer-Overton theory explains this phenomenon by stating that anesthesia is achieved when a chemically inert substance reaches a critical molar concentration within cells. This critical concentration depends directly on the lipid solubility of the substance; the more soluble, the lower the concentration needed.[51] In comparison, the critical volume hypothesis theorizes that anesthesia is achieved when the volume of a particular hydrophobic region of the cell is increased a critical amount. This latter hypothesis explains why general anesthesia is reversed by an increase in hydrostatic pressure (in the range of 100 ATA). The decrease in membrane expansion calculated for this pressure is equivalent to the increase calculated for the anesthetic.[52]

In a practical sense, narcosis can quickly and unwittingly incapacitate a diver. For this reason, researchers and divers have sought mechanisms to counteract the toxic effects of nitrogen.

Common diving lore states that "tolerance" can be developed to narcosis as in alcohol intoxication. Many experiments have been performed; no objective evidence of tolerance has been found. However, many have documented subjective improvement[9,33,58] (see Table 7-2). This may involve learned compensatory behavior; the diver sacrifices accuracy in an attempt to maintain speed.[9,23]

Alcohol appears to have a similar and additive effect on reaction time and general arousal as nitrogen. Amphetamines seem to reverse nitrogen's effects but not in doses that would be clinically acceptable for a working diver.[27] Carbon dioxide actually has a synergistic effect on narcosis.[37] This can be exogenous in the breathing gas or endogenous from swimming, working, a poorly ventilated helmet, overbreathing a gas supply, depleted adsorbent, or pooling of carbon dioxide in a loose-fitting suit. In addition, given the same pressure of nitrogen, elevated oxygen pressures have an additive effect on narcosis.[28] Avoidance of hazards (in addition to alcohol) has been a cornerstone of prevention.

The treatment of nitrogen narcosis is simple: Decrease the pressure! Resolution is almost instant. In dives greater than

200 fsw, the breathing gas should be switched to helium.

The effects of nitrogen have placed a major limitation on human exposure to depth. Many diving accidents and fatalities can be traced to a judgment error that seems out of character for a professional diver who was not experiencing nitrogen narcosis. A diver may misinterpret the environment, perform complex motor tasks inefficiently or incorrectly, and remember details of the dive erroneously. These place the diver at considerable risk.

High Pressure Neurologic Syndrome

High pressure neurologic syndrome (HPNS) was first identified in the mid-1960s. It had been called *helium tremors* in the past but has since been shown to be related to pressure.[64] This syndrome can be quite incapacitating and, in the open water environment, life-threatening. It stands as one of the major limitations to human exposure to depth.

The symptoms of HPNS are headache, vertigo, nausea, fatigue, and euphoria. Neurologic findings include tremor, myoclonus, dysmetria, opsoclonus, hyperreflexia, sleep disorders, and seizures. Memory and intellectual impairment can also be seen. There are also typical EEG changes.[41]

The tremor seen in HPNS is a postural and an intention tremor. The postural tremor is in the 6- to 10-Hz range and can involve the hands, arms, or entire body.[6] It is an exaggeration of the normal resting tremor and can be seen as shallow as 20 to 30 ATA. Myoclonus is seen at 50 to 60 ATA, and sleep disturbance at slightly over half that depth.[41] Hyperlocomotor activity is seen in animals at roughly 38 ATA, and seizures occur near 100 ATA.[1] Symptoms generally remain constant at depth and improve on decompression. Most symptoms resolve within hours, but some of the more subjective complaints may persist for days to weeks.[41] There do not appear to be any long-term sequelae.

The EEG demonstrates increases in the theta activity (4 to 8 Hz). Decreases in the faster components and increases in activity are less commonly seen. These changes occur during compression. If compression is stopped, theta activity may continue to rise for another 6 hours and then slowly return to control levels over 12 hours. It will rise again if compression is continued.[8] In studies of cerebellar and cerebral EEGs in rats, a spike and slow wave pattern resembling absence seizures develops while animals exhibit tonic-clonic seizures.[46]

Our understanding of the biochemistry and pathology of HPNS is incomplete. Derangements of both excitatory and inhibitory pathways have been implicated. Certain studies suggest that pressure exerts its effect on neuronal exocytosis.[35] Synaptosomes under pressure have decreased calcium uptake and γ-aminobutyric acid (GABA) efflux.[30,31] Dopamine, 5-hydroxytryptamine (5-HT), and glycine have also been implicated.[29,56,67]

In spite of these limitations on our understanding of mechanisms, significant advances in the techniques of deep diving and HPNS avoidance have been made. In the Atlantis series of dives at Duke University, Peter Bennett was able to bring three divers to the depth of 2250 fsw (69 ATA) with minimal symptoms by manipulating compression rates and adding narcotic gases to the breathing mixture. Slow exponential compression with frequent stops increases the threshold and decreases the severity of symptoms. In addition, nitrogen narcosis relieves many of the symptoms of HPNS. The Atlantis dives found that 5% nitrogen ameliorated the symptoms of HPNS and minimized narcotic side effects. Finally, these divers stayed at 650 msw for 4.5 days before the excursion to 686 msw.[7] This technique of excursions allows a greater maximum depth with a minimum of HPNS symptoms.

French studies with baboons have used these techniques to attain a depth of 1100 msw (111 ATA).[60] They have also successfully used the narcotic properties of hydrogen at 54% to 56% in a trimix with helium and oxygen to offset HPNS.[61] This group also selects divers who are less susceptible to the effects of pressure. As with other areas of diving, there is a large interindividual variation in the type of symptoms, threshold of onset, and severity. By measuring psychomotor effects and EEG changes at shallower depths (180 msw), they are able to identify divers particularly sensitive to HPNS.[59]

The HPNS has not shown to result in long-term sequelae. In the controlled environment of deep diving with highly trained, professional divers and supervisors, there are frequently ample warning and remedial measures in place. The major impact of this condition is diver discomfort and the limitation of depth and time.

Carbon Dioxide

There are many other possible toxicities involved in diving. However, they are not specific to diving. Carbon dioxide exacerbates oxygen and nitrogen toxicity. It also has a deleterious effect of its own. The symptoms are similar to hypercapnia in nondivers: dyspnea, somnolence, headache. Divers, however, can experience a unique combination of hypercarbia and hyperoxia that may mask some of these early symptoms. With higher pressures, normally not available on the surface, more serious symptoms may ensue (Table 7-4). Recall that elevated CO_2 levels may have three general sources. Excess production may be the result of work or exercise, including shivering. Impaired removal may be from inadequate ventilation on the part of the diver, the air supply, or exhausted carbon dioxide absorbent. Finally, the air supply may be an exogenous source of CO_2. Carbon dioxide is 175 times more narcotic than nitrogen. In one study, it produced irritability, difficulty in concentrating, and slowed thinking but no decrement in accuracy.[22] The danger of elevated CO_2 is twofold: It is continuously being produced, and its effects are multiplied by depth.

Carbon dioxide is not the only gas that can contaminate the breathing supply. During surface-supplied diving with

Table 7-4 Signs and symptoms of acute hypercapnia in normal men

Percent CO_2 (sea-level equivalent)	Effect
0-4	No CNS derangement
4-6	Dyspnea, anxiety
6-10	Impaired mental capabilities
10-15	Severely impaired mental function
15-20	Loss of consciousness
>20	Uncoordinated muscular twitching, convulsions

From Bove AA, Davis JC, editors: *Diving medicine,* ed 2, Philadelphia, 1990, WB Saunders Company.

compressors, the air intake may entrain any gas or vapor, such as carbon monoxide from engine exhaust. Deciphering a possible gas contamination may be even more difficult if the gas was stored in tanks that were filled weeks earlier or are from a commercial source. The toxicity of these gases are similar to surface exposure except that the relative concentration need not be as high to poison.

Miscellaneous

The divers' toxic exposures do not end with the breathing gas. Diving is merely a technique to work in a hostile environment. Once there, the work begins, and the diver may be exposed to any toxins in the surroundings. Many heavy metals, creosote, pesticides, and other chemicals are detectable at toxic levels in the waters where commercial diving takes place. In addition, commercial diving often involves working in the sediment on the ocean floor. In coastal areas such as shipyards and river outlets, this sediment may harbor the accumulated toxins of decades of industrial activity. In addition, the diver is subject to any biologic toxins that may be in the water. Fortunately, the diving dress, designed to secure breathing and to protect the diver from thermal and physical harm, offers substantial chemical protection from the environment. It is not foolproof, though, and dermal exposure, ingestion, and aspiration of small amounts are still possible. Specific dress is designed for chemical and even radioactive protection.

The diver can be exposed to many toxins. The three main areas of diving-specific toxicity, treatment, and prevention have been discussed. With proper vigilance and attention to proven procedures, the toxic effect of gases and pressure can be avoided or minimized.

REFERENCES

1. Abraini JH, Tomei C, Rostain JC: Quantitative study of behavioral disturbances in rats exposed to high pressure, *Ann Physiol Anthropol* 10:183, 1991.

2. Anderson B Jr, Farmer JC Jr: Hyperoxic myopia, *Trans Am Ophthalmol Soc* 76:116, 1978.

3. Bartus RT: Impairments in primate information processing resulting from nitrogen narcosis, *Physiol Behav* 12:797, 1974.

4. Behnke AR, Forbes HS, Motley EP: Circulatory and visual effects of oxygen at 3 atmospheres pressure, *Am J Physiol* 114:436, 1936.

5. Behnke AR, Thomson RM, Motley EP: The physiologic effects from breathing air at 4 atmospheres pressure, *Am J Physiol* 112:554, 1935.

6. Bennett PB: Inert gas narcosis and HPNS. In Bove AA, Davis JC, editors: *Diving medicine,* Philadelphia, 1990, WB Saunders Company.

7. Bennett PB, Coggin R, McLeod M: Effect of compression rate on the use of trimix to ameliorate HPNS in man to 686m (2250 ft), *Undersea Biomed Res* 9:335, 1982.

8. Bennett PB, Towse EJ: The high pressure nervous syndrome during a simulated oxygen-helium dive to 1500 ft, *Electroencephalogr Clin Neurophysiol* 31:383, 1971.

9. Biersner RJ et al: Diving experience and emotional factors related to the psychomotor effects of nitrogen narcosis, *Aviat Space Environ Med* 49:959, 1978.

10. Brashear RE, Sharma HM, DeAtley RE: Prolonged survival breathing oxygen at ambient pressure, *Am Rev Respir Dis* 108:701, 1973.

11. Brauer RW et al: Protection by altitude acclimatization against lung damage from exposure to oxygen at 825 mm Hg, *J Appl Physiol* 28:474, 1970.

12. Butler FK Jr, Knafelc ME: Screening for oxygen intolerance in US Navy divers, *Undersea Biomed Res* 13:91, 1986.

13. Butler FK Jr, Thalmann ED: Central nervous system oxygen toxicity in closed circuit scuba divers II, *Undersea Biomed Res* 13:193, 1986.

14. Clark IA: Tissue damage caused by free oxygen radicals, *Pathology* 18:181, 1986.

15. Clark JM et al: Pulmonary tolerance in man to continuous oxygen exposure at 3.0, 2.5, 2.0, and 1.5 ATA in predictive studies V. In Bachrach AJ, Bove AA, Greenbaum LJ Jr, editors: *9th International Symposium on Underwater and Hyperbaric Physiology,* Bethesda, Md, 1987, Undersea and Hyperbaric Medical Society.

16. Clark JM, Lambertsen CJ: Rate of development of pulmonary oxygen toxicity in man during oxygen breathing at 2.0 ATA, *J Appl Physiol* 30:739, 1971.

17. Clark LM: Effects of acute and chronic hypercapnia on oxygen tolerance in rats, *J Appl Physiol: Respir Environ Exercise Physiol* 50:1036, 1981.

18. Comroe JH Jr et al: Oxygen toxicity: the effect of inhalation of high concentration of oxygen for twenty-four hours on normal men at sea level and a simulated altitude of 18,000 feet, *JAMA* 128:710, 1945.

19. Crapo JD, Sjostrom K, Drew RT: Tolerance and cross-tolerance using NO_2 and O_2 I. Toxicology and biochemistry, *J Appl Physiol: Respir Environ Exercise Physiol* 44:364, 1978.

20. Donald KW: Oxygen poisoning in man, *BMJ* 1:667, 712, 1947.

21. Fisher AB et al: Effect of oxygen at 2 atmospheres on the pulmonary mechanics of normal man, *J Appl Physiol* 24:529, 1968.

22. Fothergill DM, Hedges D, Morrison JB: Effects of CO_2 and N_2 partial pressures on cognitive and psychomotor performance, *Undersea Biomed Res* 18:1, 1991.

23. Fowler B, Ackles KN, Porlier G: Effects of inert gas narcosis on behavior—a critical review, *Undersea Biomed Res* 12:369, 1985.

24. Fowler B, Adams J: Dissociation of the effects of alcohol and amphetamine on inert gas narcosis using reaction time and P300 latency, *Aviat Space Environ Med* 64:493, 1993.

25. Fowler B et al: The effects of inert gas narcosis on certain aspects of serial response time, *Ergonomics* 26:1125, 1983.

26. Fowler B, Hamel R, Lindeis AE: Relationship between the event-related brain potential P300 and inert gas narcosis, *Undersea Hyperb Med* 20:49, 1993.

27. Fowler B, Hamilton K, Porlier G: Effects of ethanol and amphetamine on inert gas narcosis in humans, *Undersea Biomed Res* 13:345, 1986.

28. Frankenhaeuser M, Graff-Lonnevig V, Hesser CM: Effects on psychomotor functions of different nitrogen-oxygen gas mixtures at increased ambient pressure, *Acta Physiol Scand* 59:400, 1963.

29. Gilman SC, Colton JS, Dutka AJ: Effect of pressure on the release of radioactive glycine and -aminobutyric acid from spinal cord synaptosomes, *J Neurochem* 49:1571, 1987.

30. Gilman SC, Colton JS, Hallenbeck JM: Effect of pressure on [^{3}H]GABA release by synaptosomes isolated from cerebral cortex, *J Appl Physiol* 61:2067, 1986.

31. Gilman SC, Kumaroo KK, Hallenbeck JM: Effects of pressure on uptake and release of calcium by brain synaptosomes, *J Appl Physiol* 60:1446, 1986.

32. Hamilton K et al: Visual/vestibular effects of inert narcosis, *Ergonomics* 36:891, 1993.

33. Hamilton K, Laliberte MF, Heslegrave R: Subjective and behavioral effects associated with repeated exposure to narcosis, *Aviat Space Environ Med* 63:865, 1992.

34. Harabin AL et al: An analysis of decrements in vital capacity as an index of pulmonary oxygen toxicity, *J Appl Physiol* 63:1130, 1987.

35. Heinemann SH et al: Effects of hydrostatic pressure on membrane processes, *J Gen Physiol* 90:765, 1987.

36. Hendricks PL et al: Extension of pulmonary O_2 tolerance in man at 2 ATA by intermittent O_2 exposure, *J Appl Physiol: Respir Environ Exercise Physiol* 42:593, 1977.

37. Hesser CM, Adolfson J, Fagraeus L: Role of CO_2 in compressed-air narcosis, *Aerospace Med* 42:163, 1971.

38. Hills BA, Ray DE: Inert gas narcosis, *Pharmacol Ther* 3:99, 1977.

39. Hyacinthe R, Giry P, Broussolle B: Development of alterations in pulmonary diffusing capacity after deep saturation dive with high oxygen level during decompression. In Bachrach AJ, Matzen MM, editors: *Underwater Physiology VII. Proc Seventh Symposium on Underwater Physiology*, Bethesda, Md, 1981, Undersea Medical Society.

40. Jackson RM: Molecular, pharmacologic, and clinical aspects of oxygen-induced lung injury, *Clin Chest Med* 11:73, 1990.

41. Jain KK: High-pressure neurological syndrome (HPNS), *Acta Neurol Scand* 90:45, 1994.

42. Jerrett SA, Jefferson D, Mengel CE: Seizures, H202 formation and lipid peroxides in brain during exposure to oxygen under high pressure, *Aerospace Med* 44:40, 1973.

43. Joanny P, Corriol J, Brue F: Hyperbaric oxygen: effects on metabolism and ionic movement in cerebral cortex slices, *Science* 167:1508, 1970.

44. Kapanci Y et al: Oxygen pneumonitis in man, *Chest* 62:162, 1972.

45. Kaplan HP et al: Pathogenesis and reversibility of the pulmonary lesions of oxygen toxicity in monkeys I & II, *Lab Invest* 20:94, 1969.

46. Kaufmann PG, Bennett PB, Farmer JC Jr: Cerebellar and cerebral electroencephalogram during the high pressure nervous syndrome (HPNS) in rats, *Undersea Biomed Res* 4:391, 1977.

47. Kovachich GB: Depression of $^{14}CO_2$ production from [U-^{1}4C] glucose in brain slices under high-pressure oxygen: relationship between metabolic rate and tissue sensitivity to oxygen, *J Neurochem* 34:459, 1980.

48. Martin WJ, Kachel DL: Oxygen-mediated impairment of human pulmonary endothelial cell growth: evidence for a specific threshold of toxicity, *J Lab Clin Med* 113:413, 1989.

49. McCord JM, Fridovich I: The biology and pathology of oxygen radicals, *Ann Intern Med* 89:122, 1978.

50. Mekjavic IB et al: Perception of thermal comfort during narcosis, *Undersea Hyperb Med* 21:9, 1994.

51. Meyer KH: Contributions to the theory of narcosis, *Trans Faraday Soc* 33:1062, 1937.

52. Miller KW et al: The pressure reversal of general anesthesia and the critical volume hypothesis, *Mol Pharmacol* 9:131, 1973.

53. Mosheli M, Abdallah SM, Azab YM: Pulmonary function in men with intermittent long-term exposure to hyperbaric oxygen, *Undersea Biomed Res* 7:149, 1980.

54. Nichols CW et al: Histologic alterations produced in the eye by oxygen at high pressure, *Arch Ophthalmol* 87:417, 1972.

55. Popvic V, Gerschman R, Gilbert DL: Effect of high oxygen pressure on ground squirrels in hypothermia and hibernation, *Am J Physiol* 206:49, 1964.

56. Requin M, Risso JJ: Effects of high pressure on striatal dopamine release in freely moving rats: a microdialysis, *Neurosci Lett* 146:211, 1992.

57. Ricardo JMP et al: Alterations in the pulmonary capillary bed during early oxygen toxicity in man, *J Appl Physiol* 24:537, 1968.

58. Rogers WH, Moeller G: Effect of brief, repeated hyperbaric exposures on susceptibility to nitrogen narcosis, *Undersea Biomed Res* 16:227, 1989.

59. Rostain JC et al: Estimation of human susceptibility to the high pressure nervous syndrome, *J Appl Physiol: Respir Environ Exercise Physiol* 54:1063, 1983.

60. Rostain JC et al: HPNS of baboons during helium-nitrogen-oxygen slow exponential compressions, *J Appl Physiol: Respir Environ Exercise Physiol* 57:341, 1984.

61. Rostain JC et al: Effects of a H_2-He-O_2 mixture on the HPNS to 450 msw, *Undersea Biomed Res* 15:257, 1988.

62. Smith CW, Bean JW, Bauer R: Thyroid influence in reactions to O_2 at atmospheric pressure, *Am J Physiol* 199:883, 1960.

63. Stogner SW, Payne DK: Oxygen toxicity, *Ann Pharmacother* 26:1554, 1992.

64. Thorne DR, Findling A, Bachrach AJ: Muscle tremors under helium, neon, nitrogen, and nitrous oxide at 1 and 37 atm, *J Appl Physiol* 37:875, 1974.

65. Tjioe G, Haugaard N: Oxygen inhibition of crystalline glyceraldehyde phosphate dehydrogenase and disappearance of enzyme sulfhydryl groups, *Life Sci* 11:329, 1972.

66. Torbati D, Simon AJ, Ranade A: Frequency analysis of EEG in rats during the preconvulsive period of oxygen poisoning, *Aviat Space Environ Med* 52:598, 1981.

67. Wardley-Smith B et al: Exposure to high pressure may produce the 5-HT behavioral syndrome in rats, *Undersea Biomed Res* 17:272, 1990.

68. Wood JD, Watson WJ, Murray GW: Correlation between decreases in brain GABA levels and susceptibility to convulsions induced by hyperbaric oxygen, *J Neurochem* 16:281, 1969.

69. Young JM: Acute oxygen toxicity in working man. In Lambertsen CJ, editor: *Underwater physiology IV. Proceedings of the fourth symposium on underwater physiology,* Bethesda, Md, 1969, Undersea Medical Society.

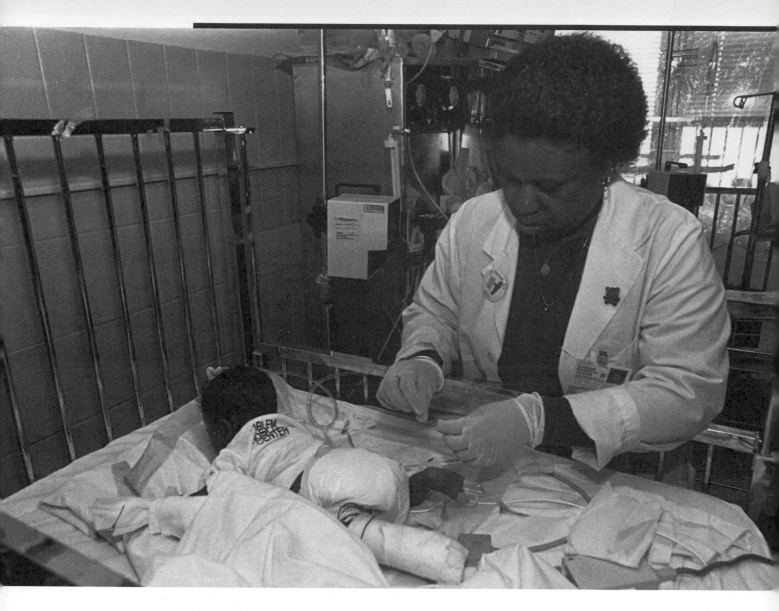

*A nurse at Harlem Hospital takes blood sample from a
baby with AIDS. March 1988.*

(Courtesy Reuters/Corbis-Bettmann)

Doctors, Nurses, and Dentists

Jeanmarie Perrone

Hg

ethylene oxide

- Mercury exposure occurs via inhalation of elemental mercury vapors in the preparation of dental amalgams

- Ethylene oxide is a known animal carcinogen and a probable human carcinogen

- Methyl methacrylate is commonly used as bone cement and can lead to dermal or pulmonary sensitization and irritation

- Waste anesthetic gas and antineoplastic agent exposures have consequential toxicity and exposure should be minimized via proper safety procedures and personal protective equipment

OCCUPATIONAL DESCRIPTION

Many health care professionals are exposed to a range of specialty-specific occupational toxins in the realm of daily patient care (Table 8-1). Although these exposures occur in diverse settings, they do share some similarities. All entail working indoors with low-level exposures that can often be prevented. The use of appropriate protective measures, worker education of health hazards, and increased ventilation or scavenger devices can minimize many encounters to insignificant levels.

The principal arenas of health care that raise concerns include operating room personnel (nurse anesthetists and anesthesiologists) administering volatile anesthetic gases, operating room technicians and other sterilant workers exposed to ethylene oxide, orthopedic surgeons and dentists utilizing methyl methacrylate as bone cement for fixation procedures and dental prostheses, dentists utilizing mercury in amalgams, oncology nurses and pharmacists involved in the preparation and administration of antineoplastic agents, and pathologists utilizing a variety of fixatives including formaldehyde in tissue preparations.

Epidemiology

Data from the Bureau of Labor Statistics for 1994 reveal that more than 5 million Americans are employed in hospitals. Of these, as many as 40% are physicians, nurses, pharmacists, dentists, and their assistants, with the various potential exposures described.[5] Many of these workers receive their occupational health care through a hospital-based employee health program that should be sensitive to the many sources of potential exposures. Of these 5 million health care workers, as many as 50% are women of childbearing age,

Table 8-1 Potential toxic exposures for health care workers

Exposure	Source	Route	Toxic effects	Permissible exposure limit
Mercury Elemental Mercury salts	Dental amalgams, tissue fixatives	Inhalation Dermal	Tremor, rash, gingivitis, asthma, CNS	0.1 mg/m^3 (ceiling)
Ethylene oxide	Used as cold sterilant for heat-sensitive equipment	Inhalation Dermal	Low levels: irritant High levels: pulmonary, edema, AMS	0.1 ppm (8-hr time weighted average [TWA])
Methyl methacrylate	Bone cement for fixation in orthopedic and dental prosthetics	Inhalation Probable dermal	Dermatitis Bronchospasm	100 ppm (8-hr TWA)
Antineoplastic agents	Prep and administration of chemotherapy	Inhalation Probable dermal	Mutagenicity, reproductive toxicity	
Waste anesthetic gases	Leaking gas delivery systems, scavenger system dysfunction	Inhalation	N$_2$O peripheral neuropathy; halothane, hepatitis	N$_2$O 25 ppm (TWA) 2 ppm ceiling (all others)
Formaldehyde	Tissue fixatives	Inhalation	Irritant, asthma, pulmonary edema; sensitizer	0.75 ppm (8-hr TWA)
Glutaraldehyde	Cold sterilant	Inhalation	Irritant, asthma, pulmonary edema; sensitizer	0.2 ppm (ceiling)

which must be considered in the assessment of exposures with potential reproductive toxicity.[5]

POTENTIAL TOXIC EXPOSURES
Mercury

Perhaps one of the most noteworthy exposures of occupational history is the now legendary toxicity of mercury in the "hatting" industry in the late nineteenth and early twentieth century. Since that time, mercury use in various settings, including dentistry, has been evaluated extensively. Mercury combines easily with metals such as gold, silver, and tin to form alloys called *amalgams*. These amalgams are routinely used in dental fillings. Exposure to mercury vapor or dust in a dental practice occurs commonly from various sources including instruments that mix amalgam (mechanical amalgamators), handling amalgam, sterilizing instruments contaminated with amalgam, and storing or cleaning mercury or amalgam. Elemental mercury is also used in Cantor tubes, thermometers, and sphygmomanometers, where exposure can occur following breakage or an incorrectly handled spill or repair. Mercury toxicity has been reported in these areas of hospital workers.[26]

Ethylene Oxide

Ethylene oxide has been used since the 1950s and is utilized daily in hospitals today for the gas sterilization of heat- or water-sensitive medical equipment. The National Institute of Occupational Safety and Health (NIOSH) estimates that approximately 96,000 hospital workers are exposed to ethylene oxide.

Methyl Methacrylate

Orthopedic surgeons utilize methyl methacrylate as bone cement for implantation of prosthetics or for fixation in the placement of stabilizing screws or devices. Methyl methacrylate is prepared by mixing liquid monomethyl methacrylate with polymethyl methacrylate powder. The plastic can be cured at room temperature or heated. Greatest exposures occur during the mixing process and can be significantly decreased with the use of a fume hood[28] or local ventilation.[4] Skin exposure can cause an allergic contact dermatitis that can be minimized with the use of gloves. A few case reports of nurses and dental technicians working with methacrylate for several years have demonstrated either immediate or late bronchospasm and asthma upon reexposure.[20,28] There are reports of local neurotoxic as well as central nervous system (CNS) effects, which have not been substantiated. Monitoring of workers exposed to methyl methacrylate should focus on examination of skin and respiratory symptoms. Air sampling of the workplace can be done. Mixing of the methacrylate should be done in a hood.[14] (See Chapter 16 for a complete discussion.)

Anesthetic Gases

According to NIOSH, an estimated 214,000 anesthesiologists, nurse anesthetists, and dentists, as well as other operating room personnel, are chronically exposed to trace anesthetic gases.[25] The potential effects of chronic exposure to these agents have raised concern regarding fertility, pregnancy outcome, malignancy risk, and possible CNS effects. Exposure occurs in the following situations: Anesthetic gas may seep under the mask, patients may exhale gas, scavenging systems may be neglected or operate inefficiently, or the delivery system may leak or be poorly assembled. Many studies have examined the toxicity of nitrous oxide and halothane. Trace concentrations of enflurane, isoflurane, and methoxyflurane are not clearly associated with toxicity.

Antineoplastic Drugs and Chemotherapeutics

The past 20 years of pharmacotherapy for malignancy have seen the production of increasingly cytotoxic drugs. The myriad of adverse effects in patients receiving these drugs have raised concerns over the potential toxicity via inhalation and dermal contact by pharmacists and nurses preparing and administering these agents. Initial concerns followed the demonstration that urine from nurses handling cytostatic drugs was mutagenic in the Ames assay.[6] Evidence of dermal or inhalational absorption of these drugs was demonstrated by Hirst and colleagues, who examined urine from nurses involved in cyclophosphamide administration and were able to demonstrate cyclophosphamide in a third of the urine samples obtained after preparation of drug.[11]

Formaldehyde

Formaldehyde is a naturally occurring compound that reacts with tissues and prevents their degradation. It is one of several available fixative agents widely used to prepare tissues in pathology laboratories. At low concentrations of aqueous formulation (0.1 to 2.5 ppm), nasal and ocular irritation occur, and the characteristic odor is detected.

Glutaraldehyde

Glutaraldehyde is also used as a tissue fixative and as a cold sterilizing agent (Cidex) like ethylene oxide for heat-sensitive medical equipment. It is volatile, and irritant skin and mucous membrane symptoms are common.[7,40] Glutaraldehyde is readily absorbed from skin; protective gloves such as vinyl, neoprene, or butyl rubber should be used when prolonged skin exposure is anticipated. Animal studies have not demonstrated carcinogenicity.[15]

CLINICAL TOXICOLOGY
Mercury

An overview of the forms and properties of mercury is necessary to comprehend the various potential toxicities of mercury compounds. Mercury toxicity, like that of most of the heavy metals, is related to its affinity to form covalent bonds with sulfhydryl groups diffusely disrupting enzyme systems in multiple organs. Toxicity can result from three different forms of mercury: elemental (Hg^0), mercuric (HG^{2+}), or organic mercury compounds such as methylmercury. Elemental or metallic mercury exists as a solid, liquid, or vapor. With increasing temperature, elemental mercury vaporizes, and with large inhalational exposure, acute pulmonary toxicity occurs. An erosive bronchitis or bronchiolitis with interstitial pneumonitis can result and usually develops within hours after exposure. Following low-level chronic exposure to elemental mercury or mercuric salts, a range of CNS effects may be seen. At the lowest levels, a syndrome of weakness, fatigue, anorexia, and gastrointestinal disturbances may be manifested, which is termed *micromercurialism*. Tremor, the hallmark of chronic mercury intoxication, is seen with increasing exposures and may be seen initially in the fingers, eyelids, and lips. Progression to generalized tremor accompanies more extensive CNS findings, including memory loss, insomnia, excitability, and depression. Subtle or explosive personality disturbances are classically described.

Mercuric salt (Hg^{2+}) exposure is less common than elemental exposures in the hospital. However, mercuric salts are used as tissue fixatives in the pathology laboratory. Inadvertent enteral exposure results in profound gastrointestinal toxicity and renal tubular dysfunction. Chronic exposure to mercuric salts may lead to a sensitization phenomenon with bronchospasm and dermatitis. Organic mercury in the form of methyl or alkylmercury compounds are principally encountered in dietary seafood and may confound attempts at biologic monitoring for elemental mercury in the workplace.

Route of exposure. Elemental mercury vapor is readily absorbed in the lungs and transported via red blood cells to the brain and other organs. Mercury is distributed to gray matter and accumulates in brainstem nuclei and in various parts of the cerebellum. Elemental mercury is not absorbed from the normal gastrointestinal tract, and, unlike inhalation, ingestion of mercury-contaminated dust is not a significant route of exposure.

Diagnosis. Physical examination to evaluate chronic mercury exposure includes a comprehensive neurologic exam and a focused neuropsychiatric assessment. Discussion with family members or co-workers may reveal subtle personality changes. Tremor, gingivitis, rash, or bronchospasm may be present. Environmental or biologic monitoring may be indicated. Methods of biologic monitoring must be directed at the acuity or chronicity of the likely exposure. Seafood ingestion as well as mercury-containing dental amalgams must be accounted for in the measurement of blood or urine mercury levels. Urine samples also reflect inorganic (elemental) mercury exposure without significant interference from seafood. Elevated urine mercury levels were recently demonstrated in dental personnel in an Israeli study but were all below the proposed occupational exposure limit.[35] Hair analysis, once thought to reflect total body burden of mercury without interference from dietary or dental amalgam sources, is confounded by elevation from mercury contamination in air. Currently, NIOSH recommends "periodic" urine mercury levels in workers who are routinely or accidentally exposed to mercury.[37] Environmental monitoring may be warranted and is especially important when a dentist takes over a long-standing practice site or in hospital areas where repair of mercury-containing instruments occurs to assess the residual mercury in floors, countertops, and other workspaces. Air sampling can be accomplished via several techniques, which vary in cost and accuracy.

Management. Management of significant acute elemental mercury inhalation would require treatment of the local pulmonary toxicity as well as chelation therapy with 2,3 dimercaptopropanol (British antilewisite or BAL) and dimercaptosuccinic acid (DMSA; succimer).[13] Any person with suspected chronic neurotoxicity from mercury exposure should be removed until an evaluation and a workup including mercury levels have been analyzed. Personnel without symptoms and 24-hour urine levels above 20 µg/L should be advised of protective measures in handling mercury, and an assessment of the source of exposure should be undertaken. In general, toxicity is first seen as levels approach 100 µg/L. Increased ventilation or local exhaust ventilation may be needed. Successful intervention requires an understanding of the work environment, surveillance for early, subtle symptoms, and an appreciation for the limitations of biologic markers.

Ethylene Oxide

In 1979, Hogstedt and colleagues reported three cases of leukemia in a small group of Swedish workers exposed to ethylene oxide.[12] Animal studies supporting carcinogenesis secondary to ethylene oxide exposure[21] have led to several cohort studies in ethylene oxide–exposed workers to examine cancer incidence and mortality trends.[34] Increasing concerns followed the demonstration of increased risk of lymphatic and hematopoietic neoplasms in a subgroup of this cohort after long-term exposure with a latency period.[33] Although individual studies have shown an increased risk for hematologic and gastric meta-analysis, a recent meta-analysis of 10 cohorts of ethylene oxide workers could not show an overall increased risk of leukemia by intensity or frequency.[32] However, the epidemiologic data were considered "inconclusive," and further studies were recommended. Not surprisingly, an increased incidence of spontaneous abortion was reported in Finnish sterilant workers exposed to ethylene oxide during pregnancy compared with a control nonexposed group.[10]

Pathophysiology. Ethylene oxide is a known alkylating agent and binds covalently to DNA. It is a highly reactive epoxide. Further evidence for human carcinogenesis is supported by the demonstration of cytogenetic mutations in the cells of workers exposed to ethylene oxide.[29]

Ethylene oxide acts as a sterilant and fumigant because of its ability to bind covalently to macromolecules, destroying all organisms. Acute high-level exposures occur when sterilizers or their exhaust systems malfunction. Most sterilizers are equipped with alarm systems to signal malfunction, as concentrations of ethylene oxide less than 700 ppm are below the odor threshold.

Diagnosis. Following an accidental discharge of ethylene oxide, mucous membrane irritation may result. Exposures to high concentrations may lead to marked dyspnea, vomiting, lethargy, seizures, and potential skin and conjunctival blistering and erosions. After supportive treatment for pulmonary symptoms is initiated, immediately decontaminate the skin and conjunctiva. Certain biologic markers as tools to monitor cumulative chronic exposure have been proposed. Mayer and colleagues demonstrated an increased frequency of ethylene oxide–hemoglobin adducts and sister chromatid exchanges in an ethylene oxide–exposed group compared with controls.[22] These techniques may play a role in workplace surveillance and prevention of carcinogenesis in the future. Currently, air sampling of sterilizer areas and frequent engineering checks of systems and alarms continue to diminish inadvertent exposure.

Toxicology of Anesthetic Gases

Nitrous oxide at varying levels and durations have been demonstrated to induce reproductive and teratogenic effects in rat and mice studies (reduction in litter size, skeletal anomalies). These studies were not representative of the trace levels found in anesthetic practice today. Rats exposed to low, intermittent nitrous oxide did not demonstrate an effect until nitrous oxide levels were in the 1000 to 5000 ppm range.[39] Several rat studies exposed at 10 ppm of halothane, simulating trace levels, induced fertility disorders and fetal CNS damage.[1] Human controlled and uncontrolled retrospective surveys have demonstrated an increased incidence of miscarriage and congenital malformations in the offspring of parents (anesthesiologists, nurse anesthetists) exposed to various anesthetic agents during pregnancy.[17,27] However, many of these studies were retrospective reviews potentially flawed by recall bias. When spontaneous abortion and malformation outcome was examined via a registry, no increased risks could be demonstrated.[9] Animal evidence supporting reduced fertility secondary to low-level nitrous oxide exposure prompted a study of dental assistants exposed to nitrous oxide.[30] Similar findings of reduced fertility in this group must be interpreted with caution due to selection bias and retrospective design; however, smoking, age, and previous history of pelvic inflammatory disease were factored. A suggestion of increased infertility at higher exposures was reported.

Other potential adverse effects of waste anesthetic gases include concerns of carcinogenicity, as well as hepatic and renal toxicity. Halothane-induced hepatotoxicity has been reported in occupationally exposed individuals.[2,16]

Nitrous oxide peripheral neuropathy. A peripheral neuropathy has been described in health care workers who abuse nitrous oxide.[19] A similar report by the same author included a neurologic syndrome with polyneuropathy in 13 nitrous oxide abusers and 2 dentists, whose chronic exposure in a poorly ventilated office was implicated.[18]

Management. Waste anesthetic gas exposure is largely minimized in the operating room today by the use of scavenging systems. Personnel outside formal operating rooms such as the labor and delivery suite[8] and small dental office operating rooms may be at increased risk because of less efficient or absent scavenging systems. Environmental monitoring of air samples remains the simplest technique for assessing exposures in the operating room setting.

Antineoplastic Agents and Chemotherapeutics

In 1985, a Finnish study demonstrated increased fetal loss in nurses occupationally exposed to antineoplastic drugs.[31] A more recent case control study in France demonstrated an odds ratio of 1:7 in risk of spontaneous abortion in nurses preparing chemotherapy after controlling for common confounders (smoking, age).[36] Specific individual adverse effects have been reported, including an acute urticarial reaction in one pharmacy technician who was preparing vincristine in a horizontally vented hood and a nurse who suffered gastroenterologic symptoms after prolonged dermal contact from a spill of carmustine.[23] Current recommendations by Occupational Safety and Health Administration (OSHA) are for the preparation of antineoplastic pharmaceuticals in one designated area with a vertical laminar flow hood (also referred to as a *biologic safety cabinet*) and the use of protective clothing and gloves. These techniques should diminish airborne and dermal exposure.

Formaldehyde

At increasing concentrations of formaldehyde, toxicity progresses from the upper to lower airways, and bronchospasm, pulmonary edema, and death have resulted. Formaldehyde can act as a sensitizer, inducing asthma or triggering bronchospasm in patients with asthma. Similarly, it can cause allergic contact dermatitis. Chronic low-level exposure in rats has demonstrated nasopharyngeal carcinomas, and formaldehyde is now classified by the Environmental Protective Agency as a probable human carcinogen. Human epidemiologic studies in varied categories of exposed workers have been deemed "inconclusive" due to limitations in study design and the very low incidence of nasal cancer overall.[3,24] In 1992, OSHA lowered the permissible exposure limit for an 8-hour time-weighted average from 1 ppm to 0.75 ppm.[38] Formaldehyde is covered in detail in Chapter 23.

REFERENCES

1. Baeder CH, Albrecht M: Embryotoxic/teratogenic potential of halothane, *Int Arch Occup Environ Health* 62:263, 1990.
2. Belfrage S, Ahlgren J, Axelson S: Halothane hepatitis in an anaesthetist, *Lancet* 2:1466, 1966.
3. Bernstein RS et al: Inhalation exposure to formaldehyde: an overview of its toxicology, epidemiology, monitoring and control, *Am Ind Hyg Assoc J* 45:778, 1984.
4. Brune D, Beltesbrekke H: Levels of methyl methacrylate, formaldehyde, and asbestos in dental workroom air, *Scand J Dent Res* 89:113, 1981.
5. Bureau of Labor Statistics: Current Population Survey, unpublished tabulations; personal communication: Randy Ilg.
6. Falck K et al: Mutagenicity in urine of nurses handling cytostatic drugs, *Lancet* 1:1250, 1979.
7. Fowler JF: Allergic contact dermatitis from glutaraldehyde exposure, *J Occup Med* 31:852, 1989.
8. Heath BJ et al: The effect of scavenging on nitrous oxide pollution in the delivery suite, *Aust N Z J Obstet Gynaecol* 34:484, 1994.
9. Hemminki K, Kyyronen P, Lindbohm ML: Spontaneous abortions and malformations in the offspring of nurses exposed to anaesthetic gases, cytostatic drugs and other potential hazards in hospitals based on registered information of outcome, *J Epidemiol Community Health* 39:141, 1985.
10. Hemminki K et al: Spontaneous abortions in hospital staff engaged in sterilising instruments with chemical agents, *BMJ* 285: 1461, 1982.
11. Hirst M et al: Occupational exposure to cyclophosphamide, *Lancet* 1:186, 1984.
12. Hogstedt C, Mamqvist N, Wadman B: Leukemia in workers exposed to ethylene oxide, *JAMA* 241:1132, 1979.
13. Houeto P et al: Elemental mercury vapour toxicity: treatment and levels in plasma and urine, *Hum Exp Toxicol* 13:848, 1994.
14. U.S. Department of Labor: Industrial exposure and control technologies for OSHA regulated hazardous substances, OSHA, Washington, DC, 1301, 1989.
15. Kari FW: *National toxicology program: technical report on toxicity studies of glutaraldehyde,* NIH Pub 93-3348, Washington, DC, 1993, National Institute of Health.
16. Klatsking G, Kimberg DW: Recurrent hepatitis attributable to halothane sensitization in an anesthetist, *N Engl J Med* 280:515, 1969.
17. Knill-Jones RP et al: Anaesthetic practice and pregnancy: controlled survey of women anaesthetists in the United Kingdom, *Lancet* 1:1326, 1972.
18. Layzer RB: Myeloneuropathy after prolonged exposure to nitrous oxide, *Lancet* 2:1227, 1978.
19. Layzer RB, Fishman RA, Schafer JA: Neuropathy following abuse of nitrous oxide, *Neurology* 28:504, 1978.
20. Lozewicz S et al: Occupational asthma due to methyl methacrylate and cyanoacrylates, *Thorax* 40:836, 1985.
21. Lynch D, Lewis T, Moorman W: Chronic inhalation study of ethylene oxide and propylene oxide in rats and monkeys, *Toxicologist* 2:11, 1982.
22. Mayer J et al: Biologic markers in ethylene oxide exposed workers and controls, *Mutat Res* 248:163, 1991.
23. McDiarmid M, Egan T: Acute occupational exposure to antineoplastic agents, *J Occup Med* 30:984, 1988.
24. McLaughlin JK: Formaldehyde and cancer: a critical review, *Int Arch Occup Environ Health* 66:295, 1994.
25. NIOSH: *A recommended standard for occupational exposure to waste anesthetic gases and vapors,* Washington, DC, 1994, National Institute of Occupational Safety and Health.
26. Notani-Sharm P: Little-known mercury hazards, *Hospitals* 54:76, 1980.
27. Pharoah POD, Alberman E, Doyle P: Outcome of pregnancy among women in anaesthetic practice, *Lancet* 1:34, 1977.
28. Pickering CAC et al: Occupational asthma due to methyl methacrylate in an orthopaedic theatre sister, *BMJ* 292:1362, 1986.
29. Richmond GW et al: An evaluation of possible effects on health following exposure to ethylene oxide, *Arch Environ Health* 40:20, 1985.
30. Rowland AS et al: Reduced fertility among women employed as dental assistants exposed to high levels of nitrous oxide, *N Engl J Med* 327:993, 1992.
31. Selevan SG: A study of occupational exposure to antineoplastic drugs and fetal loss in nurses, *N Engl J Med* 313:1173, 1985.
32. Shore RE, Gardner MJ, Pannett B: Ethylene oxide: an assessment of the epidemiological evidence on carcinogenicity, *Br J Ind Med* 50:971, 1993.
33. Stayner L et al: Exposure-response analysis of cancer mortality in a cohort of workers exposed to ethylene oxide, *Am J Epidemiol* 138:787, 1993.
34. Steenland K et al: Mortality among workers exposed to ethylene oxide, *N Engl J Med* 324:1402, 1991.

35. Steinberg D et al: Mercury levels among dental personnel in Israel: a preliminary study, *Isr J Med Sci* 31:418, 1995.

36. Stucker I et al: Risk of spontaneous abortion among nurses handling antineoplastic drugs, *Scand J Work Environ Health* 16:102, 1990.

37. United States Department of Health and Human Services: *Guidelines for protecting the safety and health of health care workers,* NIOSH 88-119, Washington, DC, 1988, National Institute of Occupational Safety and Health.

38. United States Department of Labor News: *OSHA issues amendments to regulation covering worker protection,* USDL 92-307, Washington, DC, 1992, US Dept of Labor.

39. Vieira E, Cleaton-Jones P, Moyes D: Effects of low intermittent concentrations of nitrous oxide on the developing rat fetus, *Br J Anaesth* 55:67, 1983.

40. Wiggins P, McCurdy SA, Zeidenber W: Epistaxis due to glutaraldehyde exposure, *J Occup Med* 31:854, 1989.

9

Domestic and Building Maintenance Workers

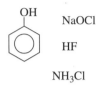

NaOCl

HF

NH₃Cl

- Mixing certain cleaning agents with bleach liberates chlorine, chloramine, and chlorine gas, which have pulmonary toxicity

- Detergents and disinfectants are common causes of irritant dermatitis

- Hydrofluoric acid burns demonstrate pain out of proportion to physical findings and are treated with calcium gluconate

Christine M. Stork

OCCUPATIONAL DESCRIPTION

Domestic and building maintenance workers have been in existence since the beginning of organized society. Many of the early poisonings and toxic exposures of domestic and building maintenance workers went unrecognized, but the Industrial Revolution and then the First and Second World Wars heightened our awareness of occupational toxins. In industrialized nations, there has been a concomitant increase in the number of laborers devoted to the tasks of building maintenance and domestic work.

Various studies conducted in the occupational setting have attempted to determine safe inhalational levels of toxins and to provide some degree of risk assessment for exposed building maintenance workers.[1,20] However, the vast array of toxins to which a domestic or building maintenance worker is exposed limits the reliability of these studies. For example, common passive exposure toxins (asbestos, radon, and carbon monoxide) may complicate the exposure to any chemical produced or emitted by the building itself.

The true number of exposures is difficult to estimate for building maintenance and domestic workers because exposures are undoubtedly underreported and occur in diverse settings. According to 1994 American Association of Poison Control Centers (AAPCC)-data, there were 151,871 reported exposures involving the toxins presented in this chapter.[26]

CLINICAL TOXICOLOGY
Chloramine

Pathophysiology, biochemistry, and management.
Chloramine exists in the gaseous state and forms when ammonia and sodium hypochlorite react. This typically occurs when household ammonia and bleach are mixed in a lavatory or other enclosed space. Another unique source of exposure is through the mixture of bleach, hydrochloric acid, and urine.[28] It is classified as an irritant gas and is highly water soluble.

Chloramine quickly produces a chemical pneumonitis. Symptoms consist of irritation of the upper airway, wheezing, and radiographic findings of pneumonitis.[38] The diagnosis of chloramine gas exposure is made through patient history and physical findings of pulmonary distress. Management is supportive. Bronchospasm is treated with bronchodilators and corticosteroids. Some of these patients may go on to develop chronic asthma.

Chlorine

Pathophysiology, biochemistry, and management.
Chlorine is a greenish yellow gas that is formed when strong chlorine-containing acids and bases react (e.g., HCl and sodium hypochlorite) or through the evaporative release of chlorine through concentrated chlorine solutions (e.g., swimming pools).[29] Historically, chlorine gas has been used in a very concentrated form as an agent of chemical warfare. It is classified as an irritant gas and has low water solubility, which allows it to bypass the upper airway and penetrate to the alveolar tissue level. Consequent to its low solubility in water, this agent can persist in the pulmonary tissue for prolonged periods prior to the manifestation of symptoms.

In the lungs, chlorine gas reunites with hydrogen and forms hydrochloric acid, a powerful chemical irritant. Exposure results in a chemical pneumonitis. Symptoms consist of irritation of the upper airway, wheezing, and respiratory distress, with radiographic findings typical of pneumonitis or pulmonary edema. In 100 patients acutely exposed to chlorine gas, 64 were admitted with a primary complaint of respiratory distress.[24] The authors of this study found that increasing air concentrations of chlorine correlated with the severity of clinical findings.[24] One ppm of chlorine was not considered dangerous, 30 ppm were associated with choking, and 40 to 60 ppm were associated with pneumonitis and pulmonary edema. Physical examination of these patients demonstrated increased airway resistance with normal tissue diffusion values.

Chlorine gas exposure is important to differentiate from other exposures because symptoms and radiographic findings may be delayed for as long as 6 hours after exposure.

Management of chlorine exposure is essentially supportive. Supplemental oxygen, bronchodilators, and corticosteroids are used to reverse hypoxia and to treat bronchospasm. Nebulized 2% sodium bicarbonate may alleviate symptoms, but it has not been conclusively demonstrated to improve patient outcome.[8] In this setting, sodium bicarbonate may act as a buffer-neutralizer, limiting parenchymal irritation. Pulmonary edema is treated in the same manner as other types of noncardiogenic pulmonary edema. Morphine was used successfully in a single case report of noncardiogenic pulmonary edema caused by chlorine gas exposure.[36] Fluid restriction, monitoring of arterial blood gases and hemodynamic parameters, and oxygen therapy are essential.

Several reports have documented the development of long-term asthma as a result of chronic exposure to chlorine gas.[15,30] Workers repeatedly exposed to chlorine gas complain of chronic respiratory symptoms as well as flulike symptoms.[5,12] One of the most highly reactive derivatives of chlorine gas is known as chloramine T. It is sometimes used as a disinfectant in foods. This agent has been reported to cause delayed asthma symptoms with fever and leukocytosis, which may be IgE mediated.[6,7]

Creosol and Phenol

Pathophysiology, biochemistry, and management.
Creosol and phenol are formed biochemically through substitutions of a benzene ring. These agents are known to be highly irritating to the skin and mucous membranes (Fig. 9-1).

Phenol (monohydroxy benzene) is commonly used as a surface disinfectant. It has the potential to be highly corrosive to intact skin because it interferes with the integrity of cellular membranes. In addition to being a topical corrosive, it is also well absorbed in the gastrointestinal tract. In a 5-year retrospective review, 96 cases of phenol exposure were identified.[42] There were 60 oral exposures, 11 of which developed rapid central nervous system depression accompanied by ventricular arrhythmias. Seventeen of the 60 patients developed gastrointestinal tract burns that were not well described. Isolated dermal burns developed in 19 of these patients.[42]

The treatment for acute exposure to phenol includes prompt decontamination, preferably with a polyethylene glycol–containing solution because phenol is not soluble in water. Meticulous supportive measures provide the mainstay of clinical care. Chronic exposure to inhaled phenol may produce symptoms such as anorexia, vertigo, headache, and salivation.[27] Dark, bilirubin-negative urine has also been reported. Substituted phenols such as hexachlorophene are also used as disinfectants, but these substituted phenols are not considered to be as "tissue toxic."

Creosol (dihydroxybenzene) is also corrosive to all tissues. It is a mixture of the ortho, meta, and para isomers of the parent compound. The documented effects from chronic exposure to creosol include skin decomposition, central nervous system depression, and possible renal and hepatic damage. The cumulative effects are thought to be similar to those expected for phenol.

Detergents

Pathophysiology, biochemistry, and management.
The biochemistry of detergents involves an anionic or cat-

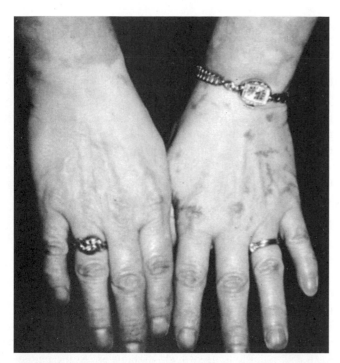

Fig. 9-1 Toxic vitiligo in a hospital custodial worker secondary to *p-tert*-amylphenol in a disinfectant cleaning solution. (From Zenz C, Dickerson OB, Horvath EP: *Occupational medicine,* ed 3, St Louis, 1994, Mosby.)

ionic surfactant that is able to permeate lipid membranes and to solubilize particles for removal from a surface. Some examples include sodium laurel sulfate, dodecyl trimethyl ammonium bromide, and potassium soap. Many detergents are available, and almost all domestic and building maintenance workers are routinely exposed to them. The most common occupational hazard incurred through prolonged exposure is a contact dermatitis.[19] In guinea pigs, exposure to different concentrations of various detergents caused epidermal erosion and a 40% to 60% increase in histamine content of the skin.[21]

The dermal irritant effects produced by surfactants is directly related to the concentration of the product, the duration of exposure, and the frequency of exposure. In addition, when detergents are mixed with water, increasing the water temperature tends to increase the irritant effects.[2] Chronic exposure to surfactant irritants often results in persistent effects with prolonged healing times.[43]

Finally, quaternary amine compounds have caused respiratory as well as dermal hypersensitivity.[4,10]

Hydrofluoric Acid

Pathophysiology, biochemistry, and management. Hydrofluoric acid (HF) is a liquid (volatile above a concentration of 40% to 48%) or gas that is used in occupational settings for glass etching, computer chip production, and removal of graffiti.

The most common route of exposure to HF is through the skin. Severity of symptoms depend on the concentration of HF, the duration of exposure, the type of skin exposed, and additives contained in the HF mixture. The typical hydrofluoric acid dermal burn involves the fingertip of a patient who was not adequately protected. It has been shown in a guinea pig model that skin depleted of epidermal lipids is injured to a greater extent by a given concentration of HF.[33]

Pain after HF exposure can be delayed up to 24 hours. However, the time to onset of pain may provide information about the seriousness of the burn and the concentration of the HF to which the person was exposed. The longer it takes for pain to appear, the less severe the burn and the lower the concentration of HF. The pain is usually characterized as a "hammerlike" pain unlike the sharp pain of other acid burns, and it may be resistant to conventional pain-control modalities.

Treatment of HF burns requires removal from exposure and decontamination of the skin with water. A complete discussion of the pathobiology and management of HF exposures is found in this book in Chapter 41.

Sodium Hypochlorite

Pathophysiology, biochemistry, and management. Sodium hypochlorite—household bleach—is ubiquitous in the domestic and building maintenance industry. It is most commonly found as a 5.25% solution that has a pH between 12 and 13. Sodium hypochlorite is also found in other cleaning products such as laundry bleach, hard-surface cleaning solutions, and toilet sanitizers.[37] It is commonly used to take color from fabric as well as to disinfect various areas. Recently, sodium hypochlorite was shown to inactivate the HIV-1 virus after 30 seconds of contact.[39]

Toxicity from sodium hypochlorite exposure generally results from prolonged dermal contact that causes a contact dermatitis. In a review of skin exposure data, a 4-hour exposure of undiluted bleach demonstrated weak irritation, a 2% solution resulted in similar findings after a 24-hour exposure, and a 1% solution resulted in no skin irritation after a 24-hour exposure.[37]

Enteral exposure to small amounts of sodium hypochlorite is generally thought to be nontoxic but may result in significant vomiting. In a case series of children who ingested sodium hypochlorite, there were 2 incidents of mucosal injury and 3 incidents of esophageal injury in 129 exposures.[35] These incidents happened from 1954 to 1962, the children were 1 to 7 years old, and 30 ml to 240 ml of an unknown percent of sodium hypochlorite solution had been ingested. There were no long-term complications in any of these children. In a reported death from sodium hypochlorite ingestion in a 1-year-old, 12 other household acids were found in the home, and the possibility of additional ingestants could not be excluded.[25] Large intentional ingestions of sodium hypochlorite, however, may result in protracted vomiting that requires medical attention.

Other routes of exposure to sodium hypochlorite have also been reported. Sodium hypochlorite injected intravenously has resulted in pain at the site of injection and left-sided chest pain that resolved spontaneously.[31] Another case of sodium hypochlorite injection into the maxillary sinus resulted in congestion and burning at the site, which resolved spontaneously after 1 day.[17]

LESS COMMON DOMESTIC AND BUILDING MAINTENANCE TOXINS

Glutaraldehyde

Glutaraldehyde is a disinfectant that is also used in leather tanning, radiopaque developing, and embalming. As a disinfectant, it is commonly used to clean medical and dental instruments and, as such, poses a hazard primarily to nurses, aides, technicians, and other hospital workers. Glutaraldehyde causes irritation and swelling of mucous membranes, headache, nausea and vomiting, pulmonary symptoms, and allergic contact dermatitis.[32] It also reportedly caused a keratopathy after it was inadvertently placed in an eye.[14]

Hydrogen Sulfide

Hydrogen sulfide is formed through the anaerobic metabolism of organic material. It is also a by-product in the petroleum industry, mining, leather tanning, and the production of synthetic fabrics. It is found commonly in sewers and in sulfur springs. It is colorless, odoriferous, irritating to mucous membranes, and flammable. Toxicity is related to its properties as a reversible chemical asphyxiant and irritant. (See Chapter 33.)

In a survey of workers exposed to unknown concentrations of hydrogen sulfide, headache, dizziness, chest pain, nausea, and vomiting were the most common complaints.[16] In the hospital setting, building maintenance workers are typically exposed to hydrogen sulfide when a clogged cast iron drain pipe is treated with 90% sulfuric acid.[34] First, inorganic calcium sulfide sludge is produced by degradation of plaster of paris under anaerobic conditions. When sulfuric acid is placed in the drain, hydrogen sulfide is produced when sulfuric acid reacts with the calcium sulfide. In one report, the worker became apneic and comatose and experienced seizures after this type of exposure.[34] With supportive care, full recovery occurred after 3 to 4 hours. In a retrospective case series conducted over 5 years, 221 cases of hydrogen sulfide exposure demonstrated a 6% mortality from coma, respiratory insufficiency, and pulmonary edema.[9]

Treatment for hydrogen sulfide poisoning is supportive, with removal from the source of exposure of primary importance. Hyperbaric oxygen therapy has also been tried when supportive measures were ineffective.[41]

Dettol

Dettol is a common household disinfectant comprised of 4.8% chlorxylenol, 9% pine oil, and 12% isopropyl alcohol. Complications associated with ingestion are nausea, vomiting, central nervous system depression, and respiratory depression. In a retrospective review of 67 patients who ingested 20 to 600 ml of dettol, the majority (84%) presented within 2 hours with primary complaints of nausea and vomiting (75%) and confusion or drowsiness (28%).[11] Five patients experienced aspiration complications deemed unrelated to their treatment with gastric lavage.

Mercury

Mercury is available in many forms, each with different toxicities. Mercurous compounds have been used as disinfectants by building maintenance and domestic workers. The most common route of exposure in these patients is dermal with a resultant contact dermatitis.[23] Mercury exposure in the workplace has also been reported to have adverse effects on reproductive function and humoral immunity.[18,40]

Hydrocarbons

Hydrocarbons are agents used by domestic workers and building maintenance workers for furniture and wood preservation. When applied topically for a prolonged period, hydrocarbons can dissolve and break down the lipid protective barrier of the skin (defat) to cause contact dermatitis. Hydrocarbons may also be absorbed through abraded tissue but are generally not absorbed through the gastrointestinal tract. The main toxicity of hydrocarbons are to the pulmonary vasculature and the central nervous system. Most hydrocarbons do not produce systemic toxicity unless they are aspirated. Once aspiration has occurred, the results can be devastating, with systemic effects of central nervous system depression, loss of pulmonary compliance, and possible late pneumatocele formation in survivors.[3,22]

In conclusion, domestic and building maintenance workers are routinely exposed to a multitude of toxic substances. Evaluation of these patients should include the identification of agents involved in their specific operation as well as the possible toxins that the workers may be passively exposed to in their work environment in general.

REFERENCES

1. Anderson HA et al: A radiographic survey of public school building maintenance and custodial employees, *Environ Res* 59:159, 1992.
2. Berardesca E et al: Effects of water temperature on surfactant-induced skin irritation, *Contact Dermatitis* 32:83, 1995.
3. Bergeson PS et al: Pneumatoceles following hydrocarbon ingestion, *Am J Dis Child* 129:49, 54, 1975.
4. Bernstein JA et al: A combined respiratory and cutaneous hypersensitivity syndrome induced by work exposure to quaternary amines, *J Allergy Clin Immunol* 94:257, 1993.
5. Bherer L et al: Survey of construction workers repeatedly exposed to chlorine over a three to six month period in a pulp mill: II. Follow up of affected workers by responsiveness 18-24 months after exposure ended, *Occup Environ Med* 51:225, 1994.
6. Blasco A et al: Bronchial asthma due to sensitization to chloramine T, *J Investig Allergol Clin Immunol* 2:167, 1992.
7. Blomqvist AM et al: Allergy to chloramine T and the demonstration of specific IgE antibodies by the radioallergosorbent test, *Int Arch Occup Environ Health* 63:363, 1991.
8. Bosse GM: Nebulized sodium bicarbonate in the treatment of chlorine gas inhalation, *J Toxicol Clin Toxicol* 32:233, 1994.
9. Burnett W et al: Hydrogen sulfide poisoning: review of 5 years' experience, *Can Med Assoc J* 117:1277, 1977.

10. Burge PS, Richardson MN: Occupational asthma due to indirect exposure to lauryl dimethyl benzym ammonium chloride used in a floor cleaner, *Thorax* 49:842, 1994.

11. Chan TYK, Lau MSW, Critchley JAJH: Serious complications associated with dettol poisoning, *Q J Med* 86:735, 1993.

12. Courteau JP, Cushman R, Bouchard F et al: Survey of construction workers repeatedly exposed to chlorine over a three to six month period: I. Exposure and symptomology, *Occup Environ Med* 51:219, 1994.

13. Cummings CC, McIvor ME: Fluoride-induced hyperkalemia. The role of Ca^{++} dependent K$^+$ channels, *Am J Emerg Med* 6:1, 1988.

14. Dailey JR, Parnes RE, Aminlan A: Glutaraldehyde keratopathy, *Am J Ophthalmol* 115:256, 1993.

15. Deschamps D et al: Persistent asthma after inhalation of a mixture of sodium hypochlorite and hydrochloric acid, *Chest* 105:1895, 1994.

16. Donham KS, et al: Acute toxic exposure to gasses from liquid manure, *J Occup Med* 24:142, 1982.

17. Ehrich DE, Brian JD, Walker WA: Sodium hypochlorite accident: inadvertent injection into the maxillary sinus, *J Endodontics* 19:180, 1993.

18. Ernst E, Lauritsen JG: Effect of organic and inorganic mercury on human sperm motility, *Pharmacol Toxicol* 69:440, 1991.

19. Flyvholm MA: Contact allergens in registered cleaning agents for industrial and household use, *Br J Indust Med* 50:1043, 1993.

20. Gage JC: The subacute inhalation toxicity of 109 industrial chemicals, *Br J Indust Med* 27:1, 1970.

21. Gupta BN et al: Dermal exposure to detergents, *Vet Hum Toxicol* 4:405, 1992.

22. Gurwitz D et al: Pulmonary function abnormalities in asymptomatic children after hydrocarbon pneumonitis, *Pediatrics* 62:789, 1978.

23. Handley J, Todd D, Burrows D: Mercury allergy in a contact dermatitis clinic in northern Ireland, *Contact Dermatitis* 29:258, 1993.

24. Hedges JR, Morrissey WL: Acute chlorine gas exposure, *JACEP* 8:59, 1979.

25. Jakobsson SW et al: Poisoning with sodium hypochlorite solution. Report of a fatal case, supplemented with an experimental and clinico-epidemiological study, *Am J Forensic Med Pathol* 12:320, 1991.

26. Litovitz TL et al: 1994 Annual report of the American Association of Poison Control Centers toxic exposure surveillance system, *Am J Emerg Med* 13:551, 1995.

27. Merliss RR: Phenol marasmus, *J Occup Med* 14:55, 1972.

28. Minami M et al: Dangerous mixture of household detergents in an old style toilet: a case report with simulation experiments of the working environment and warning of potential hazard relevant to the general environment, *Hum Exp Toxicol* 11:27, 1992.

29. MMWR 1991, Sep 13; 40(36)619-21, 627-9, Chlorine gas toxicity from mixture of bleach with other cleaning products.

30. Moore BB, Sherman M: Chronic reactive airway disease following acute chlorine gas exposure in an asymptomatic atopic patient, *Chest* 100:855, 1991.

31. Morgan DL: Intravenous injection of household bleach, *Ann Emerg Med* 21:1394, 1992.

32. Mwaniki DL, Guthua SW: Occupational exposure to glutaraldehyde in tropical climates, *Lancet* 340:1476, 1992.

33. Noonan T et al: Epidermal lipids and the natural history of hydrofluoric acid (HF) injury, *Burns* 20:202, 1994.

34. Peters JW: Hydrogen sulfide poisoning in a hospital setting, *JAMA* 246:1588, 1981.

35. Pike DG et al: A re-evaluation of the dangers of chlorox ingestion, *J Pediatr* 63:303, 1963.

36. Pino F et al: Effectiveness of morphine in non-cardiogenic pulmonary edema due to chlorine gas inhalation, *Vet Hum Toxicol* 35:36, 1993.

37. Recioppi F et al: Household bleaches based on sodium hypochlorite: review of acute toxicology and poison center experience, *Food Chem Toxicol* 32:845, 1994.

38. Reisz GR, Gammon RS: Toxic pneumonitis from mixing household cleaners, *Chest* 89:49, 1986.

39. Shapshank P et al: Preliminary laboratory studies of inactivation of HIV-1 in needles and syringes containing infected blood using undiluted household bleach, *J Acquir Immune Defic Syndr* 7:754, 1994.

40. Shenker BJ et al: Immunotoxic effects of mercuric compounds on human lymphocytes and monocytes. III: alterations in B-cell function and viability, *Immunol Immunotoxicol* 15:87, 1993.

41. Smilkstein MJ et al: Hyperbaric oxygen therapy for severe hydrogen sulfide poisoning.

42. Spiller HA, Quadrari-Kushner DA, Cleveland P: A five year evaluation of acute exposures to phenol disinfectants (26%), *J Toxicol Clin Toxicol* 31:307, 1993.

43. Wilhelm KP, Fretag G, Wolff HH: Surfactant-induced skin irritation and skin repair: evaluation of a cumulative human irritation model by non-invasive techniques, *J Am Acad Dermatol* 31:981, 1994.

10

Dry Cleaners

Paul M. Wax

$$Cl_2C=CCl_2$$
tetrachloroethylene

- Tetrachloroethylene, a chlorinated hydrocarbon, also known as *perchloroethylene* or *perc,* is the major solvent used in dry cleaning

- Acute toxicity from perc is mostly manifested by neurologic changes; cardiac and hepatic dysfunction is observed less commonly from perc exposure than from other chlorinated hydrocarbons, such as trichloroethylene or chloroform

- Chronic exposure to perc has been associated with a possible increase in prevalence of reproductive hazards and some types of cancer, although the definitive evidence for these adverse effects is lacking

OCCUPATIONAL DESCRIPTION
History

The first professional garment cleaners may have been the fullers of ancient Roman times. They were called *fullers* because they used fuller's earth (still used today in the treatment of paraquat poisoning) to adsorb greases and soils from garments thought to be too delicate for laundering. The use of lye and ammonia as laundering agents also dates back to this period.[37]

By the early eighteenth century, turpentine had become recognized as a good spotting agent for grease stains. A French manuscript from 1716 described the secret for stain removal from silk garments: "One rubs the spots on the silk with spirits of turpentine, this spirit evaporates and takes with it the oil in the spot."[9] In 1845 the first dry cleaning plant opened in Paris. The growth of the chemical industry during the nineteenth century led to the production of a variety of solvents that proved effective in nonaqueous cleaning. These early dry cleaning agents included benzene, camphene, naphtha, kerosene, and gasoline. Carbon tetrachloride was also introduced into dry cleaning because of its superior solvent properties.

The high flammability of gasoline and other similar petroleum distillates made dry cleaning a dangerous business. This stimulated a search for a safer solvent. In the 1920s, a less flammable petroleum distillate called *Stoddard solvent* was introduced.[9] Trichloroethylene was also used for a period of time. However, concerns about carbon tetrachloride and trichloroethylene toxicity contributed to the development of a less toxic solvent alternative.

Tetrachloroethylene, which had initially been developed as an antihelminthic, was introduced into the dry cleaning industry in the late 1930s. Tetrachloroethylene is also known as *perchloroethylene, perc,* or *PCE,* and for the remainder of this chapter is referred to as *perc.* At the time that perc was first used in dry cleaning, Stoddard solvent was the predominant dry cleaning solvent. By the late 1940s, perc replaced carbon tetrachloride because of the latter's potent hepatotoxic potential. Use of perc continued to increase through the 1950s, and by the early 1960s perc became the most commonly used solvent in the dry cleaning industry. These changes in dry cleaning solvents accompanied an exponential increase in the dry cleaning industry in the United States from a $55 million business in 1919 to a $5.3 billion business in the 1990s.[9]

Job Activity

Dry cleaning is one of the largest service industries in the United States. Approximately 48,000 dry cleaning plants are in operation across the country (about 3100 of which are located in New York state). Estimates of the number of employees working in dry cleaning in the United States range from 139,000 to 500,000.[1,46]

The main goal of dry cleaning is to remove soils (stains and dirt) from garments and other fabrics without adversely affecting garment integrity. To understand the chemicals used in dry cleaning, one must understand the different types of soil that commonly stain. Water-insoluble soils such as fats, greases, and oils solubilize in a variety of hydrocarbon-based solvents but not water. Water-soluble soils such as salt or sugar require some water for their removal. Solid soils such as sand, dust, or lint are insoluble in both solvents and water. Finally, some soils, such as nail polish, glues, inks, and paints, are known as chemically soluble soils because they often require a special solvent or other agent to assist in their removal.

Dry cleaning involves washing fabrics in specially designed machines with a variety of liquid solvents. The use of liquid solvents and small amounts of water in dry cleaning results in a cleaning process that is neither dry nor completely waterless. Certain fabrics such as wool or silk may become damaged in hot water through shrinking or leaching of dyes and are best cleaned by this mostly waterless dry cleaning method. Solvents are used for their ability to dissolve substances that are water insoluble without damaging the common textile fibers and dyes. Swelling of textile fibers, the bane of water cleansing, does not occur with the application of dry cleaning solvents. Dry cleaning also uses a variety of detergents that carry a small amount of water (about 1% of total cleaning solution concentration) to remove water-soluble substances such as sugars or salts. Solvents and detergents also help remove insoluble soils by suspending them, thereby enabling the dry cleaning machine to mechanically cleanse away the dirt.[37]

Most dry cleaning is performed in commercial dry cleaning plants. Coin-operated dry cleaning machines were introduced in the 1950s, but their use is not widespread. When garments first arrive at the dry cleaning store, they are tagged and sorted. Prespotting compounds may then be applied to facilitate the removal of spots. The clothes are then placed in the dry cleaning machine, where they are immersed in a nonaqueous solvent, usually perc. A water-based detergent is usually added to the solvent to facilitate the removal of water-soluble spots.

Two basic types of dry cleaning machines are currently in use. The dry-to-dry machine cleans, extracts, and dries in the same machine (Fig. 10-1). The wet-to-dry or transfer-type machine only cleans and extracts. Drying necessitates a hand transfer of the clothes to a separate drying machine. While the transfer machine includes a spin cycle that extracts much of the cleaning solvent, the clothes remain solvent-permeated during transfer. Residual solvent is eliminated only after the garment is transferred to the dryer and tumbled dry.

The elimination of the transfer step in the dry-to-dry machine is associated with less exposure to cleaning solvents. In plants with separate washers and dryers, machine operators who hand transferred solvent-permeated clothes were exposed to an average of 23 ppm perc. Using the dry-to-dry machine, average perc exposure was 16 ppm.[25] Despite the fact that the transfer type machine is considered antiquated, it continues to be used.[9] As of 1992, 27% of dry cleaners in New York state used transfer machines.

After laundering, difficult-to-remove stains are spot-cleaned with a variety of solvents and other cleaners (Fig. 10-2). These chemicals include trichloroethylene, ethylene glycol butyl ether, cyclohexanol, butyl acetate, sodium tripolyphosphate, hydrogen peroxide, and hydrofluoric acid. Finally, garments are sent to a finishing department, where they are steamed, ironed, and pressed to remove wrinkles and restore shape.

During and after the dry cleaning process, the solvents are filtered and reclaimed for reuse. Exhaust vapors from the dry cleaning machines are captured by large charcoal cartridges. Dry-to-dry machines recycle the great proportion of the solvent—up to 95% in well-maintained machines—and thereby reduce costs and indoor and outdoor environmental pollution. However, even among workers using dry-to-dry machines, needless exposure to the solvents may occur from improper use of the equipment, inadequate machine maintenance, or poor ventilation.

Job Categories

Although as many as 70% of dry cleaning outlets are "mom and pop" stores operating with as few as 1 to 4 workers, large dry cleaning establishments may employ 150 to 200 people.[9] Not all employees have the same occupational exposure to solvents. Dry cleaning machine operators load and remove garments from the machines and are often responsible for routine maintenance on the machines. Touch-up workers apply spotting solutions to stains and often double as machine operators. Dry cleaning machine operators may have four times as much exposure to solvents as other dry cleaning employees such as pressers, seamstresses, and counter personnel.[25]

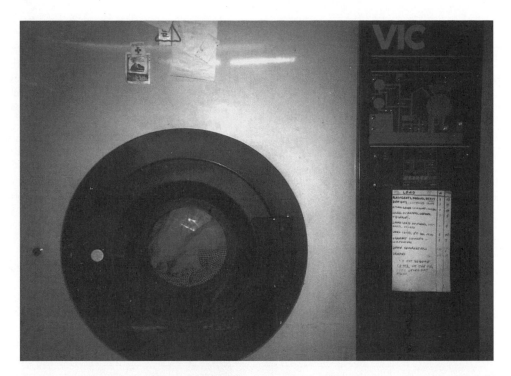

Fig. 10-1 The dry-to-dry machine is used by more than 75% of dry cleaning plants today. Usually the clothes are washed in perc, although Stoddard solvent is still used by some dry cleaners. Unlike the older transfer machines that require the machine operators to manually transfer the solvent permeated clothes into a dryer, the dry-to-dry machine cleans and dries in the same machine, thereby reducing solvent exposure.

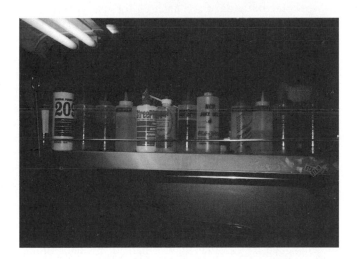

Fig. 10-2 Spotting tables in dry cleaning plants contain a number of toxic chemicals used to remove spots including trichloroethylene, hydrofluoric acid, butyl acetate, ethylene glycol butyl ether, cyclohexanol, methyl isobutyl ketone, and ammonia.

Another group at risk for exposure to dry cleaning solvents are the neighbors living above or in close proximity to dry cleaning stores. The indoor air of apartments above dry cleaners has perc levels considerably higher than levels found in control apartments not near dry cleaners. Recent evidence suggests that these upstairs neighbors may also have elevated blood concentrations of perc.[36]

POTENTIAL TOXIC EXPOSURES

A large number of solvents, detergents, caustics, and antiseptic agents are employed in the dry cleaning business (see box, top left, on p. 76). Currently, perc and Stoddard solvent are the two most commonly utilized solvents. Perc is used about 80% to 90% of the time, and Stoddard solvent is used about 10% to 20% of the time.[37] Much less commonly employed solvents include F-113, a fluorohydrocarbon used about 1% to 2% of the time, and 1,1,1-trichloroethane, a more toxic chlorinated hydrocarbon utilized less than 1% of the time.[37] Trichloroethylene, naphtha, and toluene may still be used by an occasional dry cleaning plant, but their role is largely obsolete.

Perc

Perc is *the* dry cleaning solvent. This unsaturated chlorinated hydrocarbon has the chemical structure $Cl_2 - C = C - Cl_2$. It is considered superior to other solvents used in the dry cleaning field because of its nonflammability and lower toxicity. Tetrachloroethylene should not be confused with its saturated cousin 1,1,2,2-tetrachloroethane, which is considerably more hepatotoxic.

Chemical properties. Perc is a colorless, volatile, nonflammable, poorly water-soluble liquid that gives off a chloroform or etherlike odor. Its odor threshold is 50 ppm, although it may be detectable at 5 ppm. Perc's molecular weight is 165.83 and specific gravity is 1.63, making it

Chemicals Used in Dry Cleaning	
SOLVENTS	**ANTISEPTICS**
Dichlorofluoroethane	Acetone
Fluorocarbon 113 (Valclene)	Ammonia
Naphtha	Ethyl alcohol
Stoddard solvent	Hydrogen peroxide
Tetrachloroethylene	Iodine
(perchloroethylene)	Potassium permanganate
Toluene	Sodium carbonate
1,1,1-Trichloroethane	Sodium hydrosulfite
Trichloroethylene	Sodium hypochlorite
	Sodium perborate
DETERGENTS	
Anionic detergents	**MISCELLANEOUS**
Cationic detergents	Amyl acetate
Nonionic detergents	Butyl acetate
	Butyl alcohol
CAUSTICS	Cyclohexanol
Ammonium bifluoride	Ethylene glycol butyl ether
Hydrofluoric acid	Formic acid
Phosphoric acid	Methanol
Potassium hydroxide	Methyl isobutyl ketone
Sodium hydroxide	4-Methyl-2-pentanone
Sodium triolyphosphate	Oxalic acid
Sulfuric acid	Ozone
Titanium sulfate	Sodium bisulfite
	Titanium dioxide

Uses of Perc	
Adhesives and glues	Printing inks
Antihelminthic	Resins
Chemical intermediate	Rubber coatings
Dry cleaning solvent	Sealants
Extractant in the	Semiconductor
pharmaceutical industry	manufacturing
Heat transfer medium	Silicones
Lubricants	Solvent soaps
Metal degreasing agent	Spot removers
Paint removers	Suede protectors
Pesticide intermediate	Textile processing
Polishes	Water repellents

considerably heavier than water. It has a relatively low vapor pressure at 14 mm Hg and a high boiling point at 121° C.

Impurities and stabilizers make up about 1% to 3% of technical and commercial grades of perc. The impurities predominantly consist of other chlorinated hydrocarbons such as carbon tetrachloride, chloroform, trichloroethylene, 1,1,1-trichloroethane, and 1,1,2-trichloroethane. Benzene may also be present as an impurity. Stabilizers include a variety of amines, epoxides, and esters; they are added to perc to prevent formation of hydrochloric acid.

Uses. In 1986, 600 million pounds of perc were used in the United States.[46] While dry cleaning consumes about 53% of the perc, a number of other industries also employ this solvent (see box, top right). Other important applications for perc include its uses as a chemical intermediate (including the production of 2-carbon chlorofluorocarbons [F-113]) and as a metal degreasing agent.[46] It is also used in textile processing, in semiconductor manufacturing, and as a heat transfer medium solvent serving as a nonflammable recyclable dielectric fluid for power transformers. Estimates of the total number of workers employed by industries using perc range from 500,000 to 1.6 million.

Until recently, perc was also used as an antihelminthic in the treatment of hookworm and some trematode infestations.[41] This medicinal use actually predates its use as a dry cleaning solvent. When first introduced in 1925, its relatively low toxicity made it preferable to carbon tetrachloride, another antihelminthic agent. Early animal studies showed that, while perc was more likely to cause sedation and respiratory depression, carbon tetrachloride was more likely to cause liver damage.[21] The recommended doses of perc for the treatment of hookworm infestation ranged from 0.5 to 8 ml. Side effects associated with this therapeutic use included giddiness, inebriation, and occasional vomiting or drowsiness.

Workplace standards. Standards for maximal acceptable perc exposure levels in the workplace have been lowered over the years (Table 10-1). The most recent Occupational Safety and Health Administration (OSHA) standard mandates that perc levels not exceed 25 ppm based on 8-hour time-weighted average (TWA). The National Institute of Occupational Safety and Health (NIOSH) has set a "no safe exposure limit" for perc because of this solvent's classification as a "suspected human carcinogen."

Stoddard Solvent

About 10% to 20% of dry cleaning plants use Stoddard solvent as their primary cleaning solvent. The Stoddard solvent was first manufactured in the 1920s and resulted from a desire to find a safer solvent than the older flammable solvents such as gasoline. It was named in honor of the National Institute of Dryers president W.J. Stoddard.[9]

Chemical properties. Stoddard solvent, also known as mineral spirits or white spirits, is a petroleum-based mixture of straight and branch-chain paraffins (30% to 50%), naphthalenes (30% to 40%), and alkyl aromatic hydrocarbons (10% to 20%). Benzene is not a constituent of this mixture. It is colorless and has a petroleum odor that is detected at 1 ppm. Unlike perc, it is lighter than water, with a specific gravity of 0.8. It is insoluble in water and readily soluble in most organic solvents. Pharmacologically and toxicologically, it resembles unleaded gasoline.

Table 10-1 Perc vapor concentrations, clinical effects, and workplace standards

Concentration	Clinical effects and workplace standards
1100 ppm	Coma after 30 min
400 ppm	Semicomatose state and mild liver injury after 3 hr
300 ppm	1976 OSHA standards: maximum ceiling (5 min in 3 hr)
200 ppm	1976 OSHA standards: acceptable maximum ceiling
	Headache, nausea, light-headedness, dizziness, tiredness, hangover and intoxication, eye irritation
100 ppm	1976 OSHA standards: threshold limit value for 8-hr TWA
	25% experienced mild headache; eyes, nose, throat irritation; slight light-headedness; some dysarthria after 7 hr; 40% slightly sleepy
50 ppm	Odor threshold
25 ppm	Current OSHA workplace standard
0 ppm	NIOSH recommends that since perc is classified as "suspected human carcinogen," no safe exposure limit should be set

---

Uses of Stoddard Solvent

Adhesives	Paint remover
Degreasing agent	Paint thinner
Dry cleaning	Photocopier toners
Herbicides	Printing inks
Metal cleaner	

Uses. Stoddard solvent also has a large number of industrial uses (see box above). It is used as a degreasing agent, metal cleaner, paint thinner, and paint remover. It may also serve as the solvent used in photocopier toners, printinginks, adhesives, and some herbicides.[27] About 1.7 million workers are potentially exposed to Stoddard solvent.[40]

Workplace standards. Workplace standards for Stoddard solvent include an 8-hour threshold limit value–time weighted average (TLV-TWA) not to exceed 100 ppm. According to NIOSH, the TLV-TWA should not exceed 67 ppm.

CLINICAL TOXICOLOGY: PERC
Toxicokinetics

Absorption. Perc is rapidly absorbed through the lungs and gastrointestinal tract and poorly absorbed through intact skin.[47] Occupationally, pulmonary absorption is the most important route of exposure. Ingestion of as little as 2 to 6 ml of perc can cause drowsiness. Inhalation of 5 ml of perc may cause significant central nervous system (CNS) depres-

sion. Dermal absorption is usually not great enough to cause toxicity. Following inhalation, peak blood levels occur as soon as exposure ceases. Peak levels occur 1 to 2 hours after ingestion.

Distribution. Due to its high lipophilicity, perc easily distributes to the brain.[26] Its lipophilicity may also lead to accumulation in the liver and kidneys. Its volume of distribution is 8.2 L/kg.[18] A two-compartment model describes the kinetics of perc.

Metabolism and elimination. Once absorbed, most of the perc (80% to 95%) is eliminated unchanged by exhalation through the lungs.[16] A much smaller amount is metabolized and excreted into the urine. Perc's predominant metabolite is trichloroacetic acid formed via the hepatic microsomal cytochrome P-450 mixed-function oxidase system. Tetrachloroethylene oxide and trichloroacetyl chloride are intermediates of trichloroacetic acid production.[22] A small amount of unchanged perc is also eliminated into the urine.[16] While earlier studies suggested that trichloroethanol (TCE) is also a metabolite of perc, TCE production in the setting of perc exposure is probably a result of the metabolism of trichloroethylene, a common impurity of perc production.[44] The extensive pulmonary elimination and limited metabolism of perc are characteristic and differentiate perc from other chlorinated hydrocarbons like trichloroethylene, which is predominantly metabolized to trichloroacetic acid and trichloroethanol.

Pulmonary elimination of perc may take some time. Although a high percentage is eliminated during the first 24 hours after exposure, the solvent's affinity for fat tissue contributes to a protracted period of pulmonary elimination that may last several weeks.[49] This prolonged exponential decay suggests that a brief acute inhalational exposure may result in sustained tissue exposure.

Pathophysiology

There are three general scenarios consistent with perc exposure. Acute exposure may occur as the result of a deliberate ingestion. While suicidal ingestions are quite uncommon, untoward effects from the oral use of perc in the treatment of parasites have also been reported. More commonly, acute exposure results from accidental (or deliberate) single inhalational exposure to high concentrations of perc. Chronic inhalational exposure to lower levels of perc may also result in toxicity.

Acute exposure. Acute exposure to perc is characterized by two stages of toxicity.[18] Initially, CNS disturbances are the predominant findings. Cardiac toxicity may also occur as a result of vasomotor collapse secondary to profound CNS depression or myocardial sensitization to catecholamines. Exposure to high concentrations of perc causes mucous membrane, eye, and dermal irritation. During the second stage of perc toxicity, hepatic and renal damage may ensue. These delayed insults most likely result from the metabolic activation of perc to highly reactive toxic intermediates.

Olfactory fatigue and extinction is characteristic of perc exposure. During the first 5 minutes of exposure to vapor at 100 ppm, subjects described the odor as moderately strong. After 7 hours of continuous exposure, only 40% were able to detect the solvent's odor.[49]

Several deaths from perc exposure have been reported.[23] In one report, a 33-year-old man who was attempting to clear a plugged line in a dry cleaning machine was found unresponsive next to the machine.[23] He was pronounced dead on arrival at the hospital. His blood perc level was 4.4 mg/dl, and his brain level was 36 mg/100 g. No perc was detected in the urine. In another report a 53-year-old dry cleaner who was cleaning and recycling perc was also overcome by the fumes and found dead at the scene.[24] He also had high levels of perc in the blood and tissues. In both these cases, the victims died from the anesthetic effects of the perc that caused CNS depression, respiratory depression, and cardiac arrest. Myocardial sensitization to catecholamines may have also played a role, although no electrocardiographic data are available to support or refute this hypothesis.

Neurologic. Perc's affinity for tissues with high lipid contents, such as the brain, explains the frequency of CNS symptoms seen with perc exposure. Perc's effects on the CNS is similar to anesthetic agents. The degree of depression is a function of the magnitude of exposure. The precise mechanism of perc's CNS effects remain unknown. As with other hydrocarbons, including ethanol, changes in lipid membrane fluidity resulting in altered neural transmission may partially explain its CNS effects.

Central nervous system findings range from light-headedness or drowsiness to obtundation and coma.[47] An initial excitation phase often precedes the depressive phase. Dizziness, inebriation, incoordination, mental dullness, and irresponsible behavior are common findings. Vertigo, agitation, and hallucination may also occur.[12,18] Abnormal Romberg testing has been observed with perc vapor pressures between 200 and 300 ppm.[47]

The major consequence of CNS sedation from perc is depression of the respiratory center and decreased ventilation. If left unattended, apnea and death may ensue. Once the exposure is terminated, resolution of CNS depression after exposures not associated with respiratory depression and hypoxemia is usually rapid and occurs within minutes.[47]

Cardiac. Exposures to certain chlorinated hydrocarbons have been associated with the development of arrhythmias. The proposed mechanism is a chlorinated hydrocarbon–induced sensitization of the myocardium to catecholamines that decreases the threshold to arrhythmogenic actions of catecholamines. Although an inhalational exposure study in dogs showed that chlorinated hydrocarbons such as 1,1,1-trichloroethane and trichloroethylene produced myocardial sensitization, arrhythmogenicity could not be demonstrated

with perc exposure.[39] In another animal study, however, intravenously administered perc did increase the vulnerability of the ventricles to arrhythmias.[17] Palpitations and premature ventricular beats have been reported in one case of perc exposure,[1] but little other clinical data are available linking perc use to arrhythmias. Sudden sniffing deaths have been associated with exposure to 1,1,1-trichloroethane, trichloroethylene, and chloroform, but not perc.

Profound CNS depression and peripheral vasodilation in the setting of perc exposure may result in hypotension and cardiovascular collapse. Respiratory failure and subsequent hypoxemia may lead to myocardial ischemia, further impairing myocardial function.[47]

Pulmonary. As with other hydrocarbons, the ingestion of perc may lead to aspiration and chemical pneumonitis. One report described a case of a 13-month-old boy who developed pneumonia and respiratory failure following ingestion of perc.[3]

Acute pulmonary edema has been reported in a man who had significant inhalational exposure to perc fumes.[35] Perc or its metabolites may have a direct or indirect adverse effect on capillary permeability. Since perc is heavier than air, hypoxia may also play a role.

Gastrointestinal. Ingestion of perc may cause significant gastrointestinal irritation. Nausea, vomiting, gastritis, and colitis may result.[18]

Hepatic. Compared with other halogenated hydrocarbons, particularly carbon tetrachloride and chloroform, perc has much less potential for causing consequential liver injury and is considered a weak hepatotoxin. Nonetheless, although reports of hepatotoxicity from perc exposure are rare, they do occur.[28] The pathogenesis of the hepatic injury is thought to be due to metabolic conversion of perc by the mixed-function oxidase system to a toxic epoxide intermediate. This toxic intermediate covalently binds to hepatocellular macromolecules and causes cell injury and death. The extent of hepatotoxicity is directly proportional to the amount of metabolism.[7] The development of hepatocellular tumors from perc is hypothesized to occur from repeated liver damage.[42]

Hepatic damage may occur from severe acute exposure or chronic lower-level exposure. Pathologic findings from perc exposure typically demonstrate centrilobular necrosis with fatty degeneration.

The time course of hepatic injury after high-level acute exposure may be similar to acetaminophen hepatotoxicity. In these cases, transaminases usually peak within 72 hours after the exposure, with AST and ALT elevation often above 1000 μ/L. Symptoms include nausea, vomiting, abdominal pain, and jaundice. At times, liver function test abnormalities may first become apparent only 2 to 3 weeks after exposure.[48] They may occur because, despite brief inhalational exposure to perc, protracted elimination may subject the liver to a more prolonged exposure. Chronic exposure to perc may also result in hepatitis.[15]

Renal. Glomerulonephritis and acute renal failure have been reported after oral ingestion of perc.[18] Renal injury may occur as a result of the hypotension produced by the peripheral vascular collapse secondary to CNS depression.[47] Renal injury from perc exposure has been manifested by moderate cloudy swelling of tubular epithelium. Proteinuria has also been reported.[13] These renal effects appear to have occurred at very high doses of perc.

Studies of dry cleaning workers exposed to chronic low levels of perc to determine whether such exposure causes renal dysfunction are inconclusive. In one study on 192 dry cleaning employees, no consistent relationship between perc exposure and abnormalities in renal function could be demonstrated as assessed by analyzing sensitive urinary indicators of renal dysfunction such as n-acetyl-glucos-aminidase.[45] However, in another study on 50 dry cleaning employees, subtle glomerular and tubular disturbances were found in the exposed group and not seen in matched controls.[31]

Hematologic. Coagulopathy has also been reported from acute oral ingestion of perc. Intravascular hemolysis may also occur from acute exposure.[3]

Skin. Direct skin contact with perc for 5 to 10 minutes may cause a mild to moderate burning sensation. Prolonged contact may cause erythema and blistering.[13] First- and second-degree burns may occur. One report described a "defatting" of the skin that occurred after a container of perc spilled on a dry cleaning worker and soaked his clothes.[30] Irritant contact dermatitis manifested by a pruritic rash and eczematous eruption has been associated with residual perc in dry-cleaned garments.[38] Corticosteroid treatment (systemic and topical) caused the lesions to regress over a 2-week period.

Chronic exposure. Certainly the most common type of perc exposure occurs chronically. Workplace employees of dry cleaning shops and other industries that manufacture or use perc are at greatest risk for long-term excessive perc exposure. Others at risk for chronic perc exposure include the neighbors of dry cleaning plants. Improperly configured ventilation systems may result in the venting of perc vapors into the outside air in proximity to, or into adjoining apartments and businesses. A recent investigation into indoor air contamination in residences above dry cleaners showed that apartments above dry cleaners using transfer-type dry cleaning machines had significantly elevated perc concentrations compared with apartments above dry cleaners using dry-dry machines.[33] Elevated levels of perc have also been found in food samples with high fat content (butter and margarine) obtained from retail stores located next to or near dry cleaning stores.[29] Another possible source of perc exposure is from the cleaned garments themselves. After garments are brought home from the cleaners, vapor emissions from freshly dry-cleaned clothing, drapes, or blankets may also elevate ambient air levels of perc to dangerous levels.

Neurologic. A moderate prenarcotic-like effect, headache, drowsiness, vertigo, nervousness, and fatigue have been observed during long-term exposure to perc in dry cleaning plants and semiconductor manufacturing plants.[43] Cross-sectional studies of dry cleaning workers describe symptoms of drunkenness, irritability, poor concentration, impaired short-term memory, and impaired psychomotor dexterity. One investigation showed that dry cleaning workers were more likely to have neurobehavioral impairments involving such functions as digit reproduction and perceptual speed compared with controls.[43] However, no differences in neurobehavioral function could be demonstrated between dry cleaning workers with high exposure and low exposure to perc.[43] Chronic long-lasting neurologic sequelae have not been described as a long-term consequence of perc exposure.

Reproductive. Since dry cleaning shops employ many women of reproductive age, significant concerns have arisen regarding reproductive hazards related to perc. Perc is thought to be mutagenic, and animal studies suggest that perc may be responsible for some reproductive failures.[34] However, human epidemiologic studies have not clearly shown that perc adversely effects reproductive outcome. Some studies have suggested that dry cleaning employees using perc were at increased risk for spontaneous abortions.[14,19] Other studies reported that perc exposure does not increase risk of adverse pregnancy outcome (spontaneous abortion, perinatal death, congenital malformations, or low birth weight).[2] In a study of male dry cleaner workers, semen analysis suggested that occupational exposures to perc may have subtle effects on sperm quality.[10] Perc is transmitted in breast milk, and its presence has been associated with a case of neonatal obstructive jaundice.[4]

Cancer. Perc is considered a suspected or possible human carcinogen. In animals, carcinogenicity has been demonstrated by mouse gavage and mouse and rat inhalational studies.[40] Hepatocellular carcinoma, renal cell adenoma, and leukemia have all been demonstrated in animal studies. Epidemiologic studies of dry cleaners have shown excess prevalence of total cancer as well as cancers of the urinary tract (kidney, bladder), cervix, skin, lung, pancreas, liver, colon, and esophagus.[5,6] Unfortunately, confounding variables such as smoking and ethanol use were not controlled for in many of these studies, and it could not be ascertained which specific solvent(s) each worker was exposed to. Furthermore, findings have not been consistent between studies. In a study of 1690 dry cleaning workers, a statistically significant excess in urinary tract (bladder and kidney) cancer was found without an excess of liver cancer.[6,26] Interestingly, the dry cleaning employees working in shops where perc was the predominant solvent did not show an excess mortality from urinary tract cancer. Studies on workers primarily exposed to Stoddard solvent and other petroleum solvents showed elevation in mortality rates for lung, pancreatic, and kidney cancers.[40] Another study showed an increase in liver cancer among women who worked in laundry and dry cleaning shops.[26] Again, many of these associations occurred in workers with the potential for mixed exposures to perc and other petroleum solvents.

CLINICAL TOXICOLOGY: STODDARD SOLVENT

Toxic exposure data are much more limited with Stoddard solvent than with perc. Expected toxicity from inhalational and oral exposure to Stoddard solvent is similar to other aliphatic hydrocarbon mixtures, such as gasoline and kerosene. The major problem with ingestion of these types of aliphatic hydrocarbon mixtures is pulmonary aspiration. Gastrointestinal (GI) absorption tends to be limited. Inhalational exposure may result in the typical biphasic excitatory-depression symptomatology associated with other hydrocarbon exposures (giddiness, agitation, light-headedness, somnolence, coma). Dermal exposure can result in a defatting dermatitis manifested by ulcerative and erythematous lesions.[32] Specific hepatic, renal, and hematologic toxicity has not been attributed to Stoddard solvent.[8] Studies on chronic long-term effects from Stoddard solvent exposure are also lacking, although some of the cancer studies suggest that Stoddard solvent may have some oncogenic potential.[40]

DIAGNOSIS
Examination

Diagnosis of perc poisoning is suggested by the occupational history or exposure to dry cleaning or other products that use perc. Symptomatology may include initial CNS excitation or depression. A chloroform-like odor may be detected up to several hours after exposure.[47] Hepatic and renal abnormalities may be present within several days of acute exposure. Examination of the skin and mucous membranes for evidence of dermatitis or mucosal inflammation should also be performed. Patients presenting after chronic perc exposure usually note nonspecific complaints such as light-headedness, fatigue, and malaise. A thorough occupational history is critical in correlating clinical presentation to a possible toxic etiology.

Recommended Lab Tests

Biologic indicators to evaluate occupational exposure to perc include alveolar air concentration, mixed expired air concentration, blood concentration, urinary perc, and urine and blood concentration of its metabolite trichloroacetic acid.[16] The most reliable indicator of perc absorption is blood perc or expired air perc.[44]

Definitive diagnosis of perc as the responsible etiologic agent for clinical presentation can be established by analyzing the patient's expired breath for perc with infrared spectrography or gas chromatography (GC). The breath concentration of perc in the most immediate postexposure period is correlative with the vapor concentration to which the person is exposed. A GC analysis of expired breath may detect perc days to weeks following overexposure. Measured breath perc levels are often useful for monitoring chronically exposed workers.

Blood concentration of perc may also be useful to establish the diagnosis of perc exposure, but these assays tend to be more difficult and are not readily available, certainly not in a timely manner. Blood analysis can be performed using GC and GC-electron impact mass spectrometry methods.[25] Since most perc is not metabolized, monitoring urinary concentration of chlorinated metabolites provides limited information. Urinary toxicology screens generally do not analyze for hydrocarbons.

Liver function tests (AST, ALT, alkaline phosphatase, bilirubin) are helpful in assessing for evidence of hepatotoxicity. Prothrombin time (PT) is an useful indicator of hepatic synthetic function and is particularly important in cases of significant hepatic injury. Urinary urobilinogen levels may also rise following hepatic injury from perc. This abnormality, also seen with hepatotoxicity from other industrial solvents, is noted 7 to 10 days following acute exposure.

Renal function tests (BUN, creatinine, urinalysis) may be abnormal in cases associated with significant renal dysfunction. When BUN and creatinine are normal, other renal markers such as n-acetyl-glucosaminidase and β-2-microglobulin may detect more subtle renal abnormalities.

Since perc is radiopaque in vitro, in cases of suspected perc ingestion, an abdominal radiograph may be helpful in demonstrating the presence of perc within the GI tract. Radiographic findings, if positive, may be useful in assessing efficacy of GI decontamination.

TREATMENT

Treatment of perc exposure is mainly supportive. No specific antidote exists. Since the most common route of absorption is inhalation, removal from the toxic environment should be performed immediately. In order to avoid becoming secondary victims, rescuers should use self-contained breathing apparatus if they are entering areas with potentially high concentrations of perc. During the initial acute resuscitation, an airway may need to be established and breathing assisted if respiratory depression is noted. The patient should immediately be placed on a cardiac monitor to check for arrhythmias and ventricular ectopy. Dermal and ocular decontamination should be performed as needed with copious amounts of water.

In cases of perc ingestion, gastric aspiration should be carefully performed. Unlike the GI decontamination approach in cases of aliphatic hydrocarbon ingestion (e.g., gasoline)—where the risks of pulmonary aspiration with syrup of ipecac, gastric tube placement, or activated charcoal administration are generally greater than the benefit of removing a substance that is poorly absorbed and causes minimal systemic toxicity—preventing absorption of chlorinated hydrocarbons such as perc requires more aggressive GI decontamination. The benefits of gastric removal of this toxic chemical most likely outweigh the risk of its removal. In patients who present with decreased mentation, gastric aspiration should be performed only after airway protection has been secured by endotracheal intubation. Actual instillation of fluid into the stomach for lavage is unnecessary. Syrup of ipecac should be avoided since perc can cause significant CNS depression. Although the binding capabilities of activated charcoal to perc are unknown, activated charcoal has been shown to decrease the blood levels of other solvents.[20] Furthermore, charcoal filters are used by dry cleaning stores to capture perc vapor emissions. Hence, oral instillation of activated charcoal may also be of some use in limiting absorption after ingestion of perc.

Enhancing the pulmonary elimination of perc with a trial of controlled hyperventilation has also been utilized in the treatment of perc toxicity.[18] Animal studies on hyperventilation in carbon tetrachloride–poisoned rats showed that this therapy was associated with significantly decreased transaminase elevations compared with controls. In addition, blood and tissue concentrations of carbon tetrachloride were also lower during this therapy.[11] Human experience with this approach after perc exposure is limited, but in one case hyperventilation therapy with a minute volume 3.3 times greater than normal resulted in a decreased half-life of perc and no evidence of hepatic or renal involvement, despite the initial comatose state.[18]

Perc-induced hypotension should be initially treated with fluids. Sympathomimetic pressor agents (e.g., catecholamines—dopamine, norepinephrine, epinephrine) should be avoided, if possible, because of the possibility of their inducing ventricular arrhythmias.

N-Acetylcysteine (NAC) may have a role in preventing hepatic toxicity either through its role in repleting glutathione stores or as an antioxidant, but clinical experience with NAC in the setting of perc hepatotoxicity is lacking.

CONSULTANT REFERRAL

Dry cleaning employees who develop any significant health changes while on the job should undergo toxicologic assessment to determine if a chemical exposure could be responsible for their illness. Any person with acute changes in mental status or sudden cardiopulmonary problems should immediately be sent to the emergency department for evaluation. Since perc-induced toxicity is an uncommon presentation, physicians should contact the poison control center for further assistance. Consultation with a medical toxicologist may greatly facilitate the evaluation of these patients.

REFERENCES

1. Abedin Z, Cook RC, Milberg RM: Cardiac toxicity of perchloroethylene (a dry cleaning agent), *South Med J* 73:1081, 1980.
2. Ahlborg G: Pregnancy outcome among women working in laundries and dry-cleaning shops using tetrachloroethylene, *Am J Ind Med* 17:567, 1990.
3. Algren JT, Rodgers GC: Intravascular hemolysis associated with hydrocarbon poisoning, *Pediatr Emerg Care* 8:34, 1992.
4. Bagnell PC, Ellenberger HA: Obstructive jaundice due to a chlorinated hydrocarbon in breast milk, *Can Med Ass J* 117:1047, 1977.
5. Blair A et al: Cancer and other causes of death among a cohort of dry cleaners, *Br J Ind Med* 47:162, 1990.
6. Brown DP, Kaplan SD: Retrospective cohort mortality study of dry cleaner workers using perchloroethylene, *J Occup Med* 29:535, 1987.
7. Buben JA, O'Flaherty EJ: Delineation of the role of metabolism in the hepatotoxicity of trichloroethylene and perchloroethylene: a dose-effect study, *Toxicol Appl Pharmacol* 78:105, 1985.
8. Carpenter CP et al: Petroleum hydrocarbon toxicity studies: iii. animal and human response to vapors of stoddard solvent, *Toxicol Appl Pharmacol* 32:282, 1975.
9. *Encyclopedia Americana*, vol 4, Danbury, Conn., 1994, Grolier.
10. Eskenazi B et al: A study of the effect of perchloroethylene exposure on the reproductive outcomes of wives of dry-cleaning workers, *Am J Ind Med* 20:593, 1991.
11. Gellert J, Goldermann L, Teschke R: Effect of CO_2-induced hyperventilation on carbon tetrachloride levels following acute CCl_4-poisoning, *Intensive Care Med* 9:333, 1983.
12. Haerer AF: Acute brain syndrome secondary to tetrachloroethylene ingestion, *Am J Psychiatry* 12:78, 1964.
13. Hake CL, Stewart RD: Human exposure to tetrachloroethylene: inhalation and skin contact, *Environ Health Perspect* 21:231, 1977.
14. Hemminki K, Franssila E, Vainio H: Spontaneous abortions among female chemical workers in Finland, *Int Arch Occup Environ Health* 45:123, 1980.
15. Hughes JP: Hazardous exposure to some so-called safe solvents, *JAMA* 156:234, 1954.
16. Imbriani M et al: Urinary excretion to tetrachloroethylene (perchloroethylene) in experimental and occupational exposure, *Arch Environ Health* 43:292, 1988.
17. Kobayashi S, Hutcheon DE, Regan J: Cardiopulmonary toxicity of tetrachloroethylene, *J Toxicol Environ Health* 10:23, 1982.
18. Köppel C et al: Acute tetrachloroethylene poisoning—blood elimination kinetics during hyperventilation therapy, *Clin Toxicol* 23:103, 1985.
19. Kyyrönen P et al: Spontaneous abortions and congenital malformations among women exposed to tetrachloroethylene in dry cleaning, *J Epidemiol Community Health* 43:346, 1989.
20. Laass W: Therapy of acute oral poisonings by organic solvents: treatment by activated charcoal in combination with laxatives, *Arch Toxicol* S4:406, 1980.
21. Lamson PD, Robbins BH, Ward CB: The pharmacology and toxicology of tetrachloroethylene, *Am J Ind Hyg* 9:430, 1929.
22. Leibman KC, Ortiz E: Metabolism of halogenated ethylenes, *Environ Health Perspect* 21:91, 1977.
23. Levine B et al: A tetrachloroethylene fatality, *J Forensic Sci* 26:206, 1981.
24. Ludwig HR et al: Worker exposure to perchloroethylene in the commercial dry-cleaning industry, *Am Ind Hyg Assoc J* 44:600, 1983.
25. Lukaszewski T: Acute tetrachloroethylene fatality, *Clin Toxicol* 15:411, 1979.
26. Lynge E, Thygesen L: Primary liver cancer among women in laundry and dry-cleaning work in Denmark, *Scand J Work Environ Health* 16:108, 1990.
27. McDermott HJ: Hygienic guide series: Stoddard solvent, *Am Ind Hyg Assoc J* 36:5553, 1975.
28. Meckler LC, Phelps DK: Liver disease secondary to tetrachloroethylene exposure, *JAMA* 197:662, 1966.
29. Miller L, Uhler A: Volatile halocarbons in butter: elevated tetrachloroethylene levels in samples obtained in close proximity to dry cleaning establishments, *Bull Environ Contam Toxicol* 41:469, 1988.

30. Morgan B: Dangers of perchloroethylene, *BMJ* 2:513, 1969.
31. Mutti A et al: Nephropathies and exposure to perchloroethylene in dry-cleaners, *Lancet* 340:189, 1992.
32. Nethercott JR: Genital ulceration due to Stoddard solvent, *J Occup Med* 22:549, 1980.
33. New York State Department of Health, Bureau of Toxic Substance Assessment: Investigation of indoor air contamination in residences above dry cleaners, Unpublished, October 1991.
34. Olsen J et al: Low birthweight, congenital malformations, and spontaneous abortions among dry-cleaning workers in Scandinavia, *Scand J Work Environ Health* 16:163, 1990.
35. Patel R, Janakiraman N, Towne WD: Pulmonary edema due to tetrachloroethylene, *Environ Health Perspect* 21:247, 1977.
36. Popp W et al: Concentrations of tetrachloroethene in blood and trichloroacetic acid in urine in workers and neighbors of dry-cleaning shops, *Int Arch Occup Environ Health* 63:393, 1992.
37. *Principles of Drycleaning,* International Fabricare Institute, Washington DC, 1995.
38. Redmond SF, Schappert KR: Occupational dermatitis associated with garments, *J Occup Med* 29:243, 1987.
39. Reinhardt CF, Mullin LS, Maxfield ME: Epinephrine-induced cardiac arrhythmia potential of some common industrial solvents, *J Occup Med* 15:953, 1973.
40. Ruder AM, Ward EM, Brown DP: Cancer mortality in female and male dry-cleaning workers, *J Occup Med* 36:867, 1994.
41. Sandground JH: Coma following medication with tetrachloroethylene, *JAMA* 117:440, 1941.
42. Schumann AM, Quast JF, Watanabe PG: The pharmacokinetics and macromolecular interactions of perchloroethylene in mice and rats as related to oncogenicity, *Toxicol Appl Pharmacol* 55:207, 1980.
43. Seeber A: Neurobehavioral toxicity of long-term exposure to tetrachloroethylene, *Neurotoxicol Teratol* 11:579, 1989.
44. Skender LJ, Karacic V, Prpic-Majic D: A comparative study of human levels of trichloroethylene and tetrachloroethylene after occupational exposure, *Arch Environ Health* 46:174, 1991.
45. Solet D, Robins TG: Renal function in dry cleaning workers exposed to perchloroethylene, *Am J Ind Med* 20:601, 1991.
46. Solet D, Robins TG, Sampaio C: Perchloroethylene exposure assessment among dry cleaning workers, *Am Ind Hyg Assoc J* 51:566, 1990.
47. Stewart RD: Acute tetrachloroethylene intoxication, *JAMA* 208:1490, 1969.
48. Stewart RD et al: Accidental vapor exposure to anesthetic concentrations of a solvent containing tetrachloroethylene, *Ind Med Surg* 30:327, 1961.
49. Stewart RD et al: Experimental human exposure to tetrachloroethylene, *Arch Environ Health* 20:224, 1970.

11

Electricians

Art Calise

Richard D. Shih

polychlorinated biphenyl

- Although it was originally thought that the polychlorinated biphenyls (PCBs) in dielectric fluids caused toxicity, it was later determined that the thermal degradation products polychlorinated dibenzofurans (furans), polychlorinated dibenzodioxins (dioxins), and polychlorinated quaterphenyls (PCQs) were responsible

- Chloracne and elevated liver transaminases are characteristic of PCB exposure

OCCUPATIONAL DESCRIPTION

At the beginning of the nineteenth century, Alessandro Volta manufactured the first electric pile—now more commonly known as a *battery*. Building on this work in 1808, Humphry Davy showed that electricity could produce light and heat when separated by two electrodes that carry a current. Following this in 1831, Michael Faraday demonstrated that a magnetic field can induce an electromotive force, a current, in conductors. He was thus able to produce the electric motor and the transformer. Shortly thereafter, Zenobe Gramme showed that electric current could be carried from one place to another by conductors, and Thomas Edison invented the first incandescent lamp. From that point on, electric power was rapidly implemented into factories and homes worldwide. With the advent of electric power came the occupation of the electrician.

The modern-day electrician invents, manufactures, installs, constructs, or repairs electrical devices. Aside from this concise definition of duties, the electrician's job description may include anything from digging trenches for the installation of pipe and wire to handling fluorescent lighting fixtures and air conditioners. Electricians work in a variety of settings, ranging from industrial and commercial complexes to private residences. Although occupational injuries among electricians are predominantly electrical burns or trauma, potential toxic exposures can occur from chemicals frequently used in electrical equipment (see box, top left, on p. 84).[34] Further, the myriad of chemicals that are related to any specific job site may also pose health risks.[13,36,45] The focus of this chapter is the toxins that are most commonly encountered in the daily practice of a general electrician and, in greater depth, the toxicity of polychlorinated biphenyl (PCB) exposure, the toxin historically most associated with electricians.

Potential Toxic Exposures for Electricians	
Asbestos	Mercury
Benzene	Nickel
Biphenylenes	Phenyl-xylyl-ethane
Chlorobenzenes	Polychlorinated biphenyl
Chromate	Polychlorinated dibenzo-
Chromium	furans
Dibenzodioxins	Polychlorinated quaterphe-
Dibenzofurans	nyls
Dioxin	Propyl diphenyl
Di(z-ethyl hexyl phthalate)	Solder
Electromagnetism	Solder flux
Epoxy resins	Solvents
Isopropyl biphenyl	Sulfur hexafluoride
Lead	Thallium
Man-made mineral fibers	Toluene
(MMMF)	Trichlorobenzene

Most Commonly Encountered Chemical Exposures Among Electricians	
Chlorinated biphenyls	Solder fluxes
Epoxy resins	Solvents
Lead	

Occupational Exposures

Electricians who are responsible for the maintenance and repair of major electrical equipment are often termed *linesmen.* Large electrical equipment such as transformers or capacitors are said to be *closed systems.* Fluctuations of temperature place stress on these systems and cause frequent leaks and need for maintenance.[39] Duties include sampling and testing of fluids for dielectric properties, adding fluids when levels are low, cleaning leaks, and repairing damaged equipment. It is not infrequent for linesmen to drain up to 200 gallons of PCB-containing fluid at a given time.[14] Workplace observations document frequent direct handling of contaminated equipment and frequent noncompliance with protective equipment.[39]

Exposure occurs by all routes, but dermal and inhalational routes are most important occupationally. Air samples document aerosolized PCBs, with the highest levels occurring during transformer repair and clean-up duties.[39] Wipe samples of skin, equipment, and work-related surfaces document high PCB concentrations and the dermal risk.[39,43]

POTENTIAL TOXIC EXPOSURES

Although the list of possible chemical exposures for electricians is quite vast, the toxins most commonly encountered by this group are listed in the box (top right). PCBs are the toxins historically linked with the electrical industry and the occupation of electricians. Because of their physical and chemical properties, PCBs are used in a variety of electrical equipment. Their exposure and clinical significance are described later in this chapter.

Epoxy resins are encountered frequently in this occupation. Electrical wire that is placed underground or in walls often requires housing in tubes for protection. Typically, the tubes used are made of polyvinyl chloride (PVC). They are joined together by resin "glues." Of the available resins, 90% require mixing epichlorohydrin with bisphenol A to produce monomers and polymers of diglycidyl ether of bisphenol A. This compound is associated with allergic contact and irritant dermatitis. Other compounds used as epoxy resins are also associated with similar dermatologic effects but cause these findings less frequently.

Lead is the predominant constituent in solder. Electricians frequently use soldering techniques to ensure good electrical contact. Exposure to lead can occur during this process (see Chapter 27). Another source of lead exposure for electricians is contained in the plastic coating of wires. Electricians have been known to chew the plastic coating throughout their workdays. Although lead poisoning from this source is uncommon, several cases have confirmed poisoning from this source of exposure (for a more detailed discussion on lead poisoning, see Chapter 35).[5]

Electricians often utilize solvents. To take apart PVC tubing, solvents are necessary to dissolve the epoxy resins holding the elbows together. Solvents are also frequently used for cleaning tools, other equipment, and hands and skin. Chronic long-term exposure to solvents such as toluene and other hydrocarbons have been associated with central and peripheral nervous system effects as well as other medical problems. For a more detailed discussion, see Chapters 24 and 29.[24]

CLINICAL TOXICOLOGY OF POLYCHLORINATED BIPHENYLS (PCBs)

Polychlorinated biphenyls (PCBs) are chlorinated aromatic hydrocarbon compounds that have chemical properties that make them useful in many electrical devices. They have a high dielectric constant, which make them excellent insulators, and their flame-resistant properties decrease the potential spread of electrical fires. These properties facilitated their introduction as dielectric fluids in transformers and capacitors in the 1930s. They quickly replaced mineral oil as the predominant dielectric fluid because of the decreased fire risk.[5] The main manufacturer of PCBs in the United States is Monsanto. Beginning in 1929, this company marketed different PCB-containing fluids under the tradename Aroclor. During peak production years, in the early 1970s, 85 million pounds of PCBs were produced annually in the United States.[12]

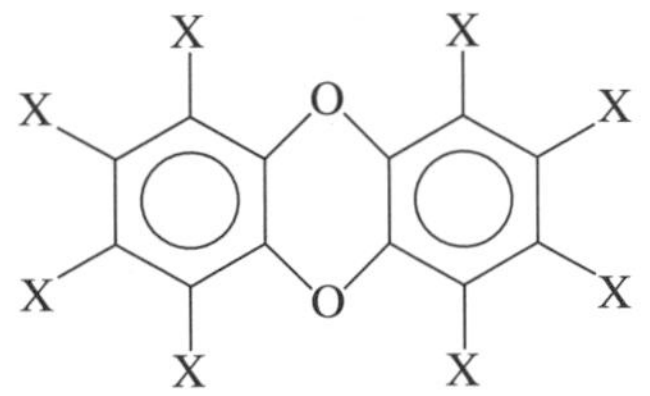

polychlorinated dibenzodioxins (dioxins)

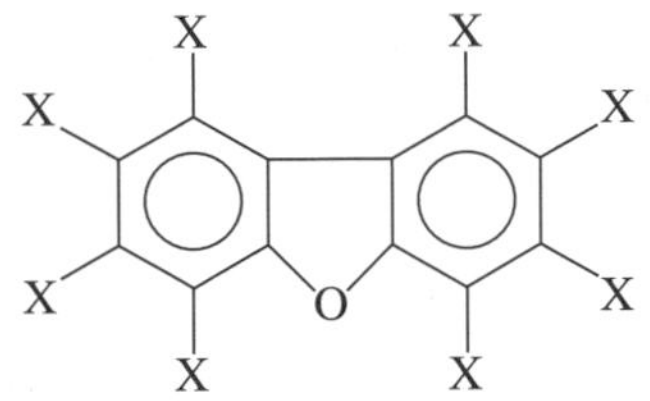

polychlorinated dibenzodifurans (furans)

Fig. 11-1 Thermal degradation products of PCBs (x = H or Cl).

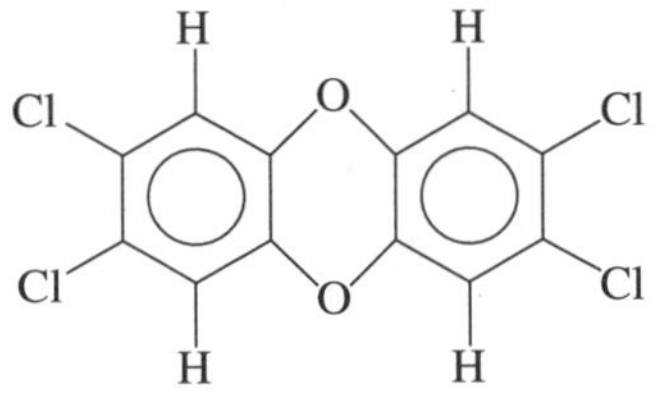

Fig. 11-2 Agent orange (2,3,7,8-tetrachlorodibenzo-p-dioxin [TCDD]).

dibenzo-p-dioxin (Fig. 11-2). This latter dioxin is the most toxic of the 75 dioxin isomers.[11]

Toxicity

The acute effects of PCBs are not well characterized. A clinical syndrome of "PCB poisoning" was described after two large epidemics involving contamination of rice cooking oils in Japan (1968, Yusho disease) and Taiwan (1969, Yucheng disease).[28,47] Patients ingesting the PCB-contaminated oils developed skin problems from itching dermatitis to severe chloracne, as well as clinical hepatitis. Nonspecific findings of fatigue, headaches, arthralgias, menstrual changes, and abdominal pain were also reported.[31,57]

Electrical fires that involve PCB fluids pose an exposure risk to furans. Several highly publicized PCB-related electrical fires document the production and potential toxicity from these thermal degradation products.[2,7,46,54,60] In addition to furans, dioxins, PCQs, and other thermally generated degradation products, such as biphenylenes, are produced. Soot from these fires can have high concentrations of these chemicals posing inhalational and dermal exposure risk.

The medical problems reported with electrical fires include complaints of nausea, eye irritation, sore throat, and headaches. Dermatitis and laboratory abnormalities in liver function tests and lipids are reported. These effects last hours to several days in most patients. Their clinical relevance and long-term effects are controversial, and studies are complicated by poor participant follow-up, often because of pending legal suits.[20,21] The sparse data available addressing chronic effects from this type of exposure do not find significant effects.[21]

The clinical effects due to acute exposure from PCBs unrelated to furans and PDQs are complicated by a number of factors. The PCB mixtures contain a number of different PCB cogeners, each with their own specific toxicity risks. Human studies are not able to look at individual cogeners, and it is not possible to identify the specific PCB cogeners that study participants were exposed to. Finally, most of the human data on PCB effects involve occupational studies in which other chemical exposures are frequent. These chemicals may have their own toxicities or synergistic effects with PCBs.

Pathophysiology

Animal toxicity. Animal experiments document a number of different organ system abnormalities.[25,27,56,58] Case re-

The PCBs are a group of chemical compounds that differ in the number and position of chlorine substitutions. They are entirely man-made, with no known natural sources. Two hundred nine different compounds, known as *cogeners,* exist in which 1 to 10 chlorine atoms are attached to the biphenyl backbone (Fig. 11-1). Further, commercial products contain a wide mixture of the differing PCB compounds, with the product identified by the number of carbon atoms and the percentage of total chlorine by weight (such as Arochlor 1254, 12 carbons and 54% chlorine; Arochlor 1260, 12 carbons and 60% chlorine).

The PCBs biodegrade very slowly, accumulating in soil and water systems.[17] Because of their ubiquitous presence in the environment and lipophilic nature, they can accumulate in the fatty tissues of animals and humans.[29] Although the acute and chronic health effects are poorly substantiated, the production of PCBs was banned by the U.S. Environmental Protection Agency in 1979 because of the potential health risks and their persistence in the ecologic and biologic systems.[29] Despite this ban, many older electrical devices continue to contain or be contaminated with PCB-containing fluids.[60]

Although toxicity of these compounds was initially attributed to PCBs, it was the polychlorinated dibenzofurans (furans), polychlorinated dibenzodioxins (dioxins), and polychlorinated quaterphenyls (PCQs) contaminating the oil that are now recognized as the main etiologic toxins (see Fig. 11-1).[9,23,35,41] These compounds are degradation products that are produced when PCBs are heated at high temperatures.[7] Those PCB fluids produced prior to 1970 and foreign-manufactured PCB fluids have had higher reported concentrations of furans.[10]

Agent Orange is a defoliant that contains a mixture of 2,4,5-trichlorophenoxyacetic acid and 2,4-dichlorophenoxyacetic acid, which is contaminated with 2,3,7,8-tetrachloro-

ports also attribute many medical problems to PCBs, including respiratory tract symptoms, elevated systolic and diastolic blood pressures, anorexia, weight loss, nausea, vomiting, abdominal pain, hepatitis, chloracne, dermatitis, pruritus, conjunctivitis, headaches, memory problems, sleeping abnormalities, and many types of cancer.* Abnormal laboratory values that have been reported include decreased polymorphonuclear cells, elevated liver function tests, decreased thyroxine levels, elevated 17-hydroxy corticosteroids, and elevated triglycerides and cholesterol levels.[8,16,19,38]

Hepatotoxicity. The PCBs are well-established potent inducers of the cytochrome P-450 enzyme systems.[49] They typically cause elevation in transaminitis. This effect may increase toxicity of commonly used solvents, drugs, and other chemicals.[4,33,38,43,50] Asymptomatic hepatomegaly and jaundice may occur.

Dermal toxicity. Chloracne is the most common manifestation of toxic PCB exposure, although this may largely be from furan contamination.[42,52] Chloracne develops weeks to months after exposure and can be refractory. These acneform lesions most often develop on the chin, periorbital and malar areas but may be found elsewhere. More recent studies, which have documented lack of furan contamination, have shown this finding to be rare.[19]

Carcinogenesis. The potential carcinogenic risk from chronic exposure to PCBs has been well documented in animals.[32,44,51] Human studies, however, are not conclusive, and this topic remains controversial.[26,37,61] Nonetheless, PCBs are considered probable human carcinogens. Recent reports from the Department of Veteran Affairs indicate that there is "sufficient" evidence to support the link between the dioxin exposures from the defoliant Agent Orange in Vietnam and the development of soft-tissue sarcoma, non-Hodgkin's lymphoma, Hodgkin's disease, the development of spina bifida in offspring, and chloracne. There is "suggestive" evidence to support the link to porphyria cutanea tarda.[1]

Clinical evaluation. The evaluation of potential PCB exposures includes a thorough exposure history, physical examination, and laboratory testing. The duration and intensity of exposure should also be assessed. The work duties performed by the individual and any workplace PCB air or skin monitoring levels, if available, may help assess this.

Physical examination should focus on the dermatologic and hepatic systems. Chloracne with elevated aspartate aminotransferase (SGOT or AST) and γ-glutamyl transpeptidase (GGTP or GGT) is presumptive evidence of PCB toxicity. However, lack of these findings does not eliminate the diagnosis. The PCB levels in blood, adipose tissue, and milk can be assessed by gas chromatography. The levels are difficult to interpret because increased levels do not correlate with clinical disease. Because PCBs are ubiquitous and all persons have some level of PCB exposure, background population levels need to be compared with the measured levels. For example, a history of eating fish caught in PCB-contaminated waters or living in contaminated areas would confound the significance of this laboratory data. Further, since PCB mixtures are made up of different cogeners and no standard mixture of PCB fluid exists, it is not clear what PCB cogeners should be analyzed. There is no standardized procedure for reporting PCB levels.[6] However, levels that rise over time may indicate recent exposure.[40] Liver function tests, plasma triglycerides, and serum cholesterol can function as surrogate markers for exposure.[3]

Treatment for acute PCB exposure involves decontamination and prevention of further exposure, as no specific antidotal therapies are available for treating toxicity. If acute exposure to PCBs or PCB-related compounds occurs, thorough skin decontamination is necessary. Immediate washing with water and acetone in animal models was able to remove only 59% of dermally applied PCBs.[59] Repeated washing with soap and water after acute exposure is recommended.

CONCLUSION

Electricians are exposed to a number of different toxins. Toxin injury, however, in this profession is relatively uncommon. Historically, PCB exposure is the most important toxin. Because PCB production has been discontinued, the risk of exposure from this toxin is decreasing.

REFERENCES

1. Agent Orange, spina bifida link posited, *US Medicine* 32:7, 1996.
2. Aitio A et al: Management of PCB accidents, *Environ Health Perspec* 60:351, 1985.
3. Baker EL et al: Metabolic consequences of exposure to polychlorinated biphenyls (PCB) in sewage sludge, *Am J Epidemiol* 112:553, 1980.
4. Bertazzi PA et al: Cancer mortality of capacitor manufacturing workers, *Am J Ind Med* 11:165, 1987.
5. Boykin RF, Kazarians M, Freeman RA: Comparative fire risk study of PCB transformers, *Risk Anal* 6:477, 1986.
6. Burse VW et al: Gas chromatographic determination of polychlorinated biphenyls (as Aroclor 1254) in serum: collaborative study, *J Assoc Off Anal Chem* 72:649, 1989.
7. Buser HR, Bossbardt HP, Rappe C: Formation of polychlorinated dibenzofurans (furans) from the pyrolysis of PCBs, *Chemosphere* 7:109, 1978.
8. Chase KH et al: Clinical and metabolic abnormalities associated with occupational exposure to polychlorinated biphenyls (PCBs), *J Occup Med* 24:109, 1982.
9. Chen PHS et al: Polychlorinated biphenyls, dibenzofurans, and quarterphenyls in the toxic rice-bran oil and PCBs in the blood of patients with PCB poisoning in Taiwan, *Am J Ind Med* 5:133, 1984.
10. De Voogt P, Brinkman UA: Production properties and usage of polychlorinated biphenyls. In Kimbrough RD, Jensen AA, editors: *Halogenated biphenyls, terphenyls, naphthalenes, dibenzodioxins and related products,* ed 2, Amsterdam, 1989, Elsevier Science Publishers.
11. *Dioxin toxicity,* ATSDR case studies in environmental medicine, Atlanta, 1990, Public Health Service, Agency for Toxic Substances and Disease Registry.

*References 4, 15, 18, 26, 38, 42, 48, 52, 53, 61.

12. Durfee RL: Production and usage of PCBs in the United States. In *Proceedings of the national conference on polychlorinated biphenyls, Chicago, 1975,* EPA-560/6-75-004, Washington, DC, 1975, Environmental Protection Agency.

13. Egedahl R, Rice E: Cancer incidence at a hydrometallurgical nickel refinery. In *Nickel in the human environment,* IARC Scientific Publication No 53, 1984, International Agency for Research on Cancer.

14. Emmett EA: Polychlorinated biphenyl exposure and effects in transformer repair workers, *Environ Health Perspect* 60:185, 1985.

15. Emmett EA et al: Studies of transformer workers exposed to PCBs: I. Study design, PCB concentrations, questionnaire, and clinical examination results, *Am J Ind Med* 13:415, 1988.

16. Emmett EA et al: Studies of transformer repair workers exposed to PCBs: II. Results of clinical laboratory investigations, *Am J Ind Med* 14:47, 1988.

17. Eshenroeder AQ, Doyle CP, Faeder EJ: Health risks of PCB spills from electrical equipment, *Risk Anal* 6:213, 1986.

18. Fishbein A et al: Clinical findings among PCB-exposed capacitor manufacturing workers, *Ann N Y Acad Sci* 320:703, 1979.

19. Fishbein A et al: Oculodermatological findings in workers with occupational exposure to polychlorinated biphenyls (PCBs), *Br J Ind Med* 42:426, 1985.

20. Fitzgerald EF et al: Assessing the health effects of potential exposure to PCBs, dioxins, and furans from electrical transformer fires: the Binghamton state office building medical surveillance program, *Arch Environ Health* 41:368, 1986.

21. Fitzgerald EF et al: Health effects three years after potential exposure to the toxic contaminants of an electrical transformer fire, *Arch Environ Health* 44:214, 1989.

22. Franco G, Cottica D, Minoia C: Chewing electric wire coatings: an unusual source of lead poisoning, *Am J Ind Med* 25:291, 1994.

23. Fu YA: Ocular manifestation of polychlorinated biphenyls intoxication, *Am J Ind Med* 5:127, 1984.

24. Gamberale F: Critical issues in the study of the acute effects of solvent exposure, *Neurotoxicol Teratol* 11:565, 1989.

25. Garthoff H, Cerra FE, Marks EM: Blood chemistry alteration in rats after single and multiple gavage administration of polychlorinated biphenyls, *Toxicol Appl Pharmacol* 60:33, 1981.

26. Gustavsson P, Hogstedt C, Rappe C: Short-term mortality and cancer incidence in capacitor manufacturing workers exposed to polychlorinated biphenyls, *Am J Ind Med* 10:341, 1986.

27. Hansen LG, Wilson DW, Byerly CS: Effects on growing swine and sheep of two polychlorinated biphenyls, *Am J Vet Res* 37:1021, 1976.

28. Hsu ST, Ma CI, Hsu SKH: Discovery and epidemiology of PCB poisoning in Taiwan, *Am J Ind Med* 5:71, 1984.

29. Humphrey HEB: Chemical contaminants in the Great Lakes: the human health aspect. In Evan MS, editor: *PCBs: human and environmental hazards,* Boston, 1988, Butterworth.

30. Jolanki R, Estlander T, Kanerva L: Contact allergy to an epoxy reactive diluent: 1,4-butane dilo diglycidyl ether, *Contact Dermatitis,* 16:87, 1987.

31. Kikuchi M: Autopsy of patients with Yusho, *Am J Ind Med* 5:19, 1984.

32. Kimbrough RD et al: Induction of liver tumors in Sherman strain female rats by polychlorinated biphenyl Aroclor 1260, *J Natl Cancer Inst* 55:1453, 1975.

33. Kluwe WM, Herrmann CL, Hook JB: Effects of dietary polychlorinated biphenyls and polybrominated biphenyls on the renal and hepatic toxicities of several chlorinated hydrocarbon solvents in mice, *J Toxicol Environ Health* 5:605, 1979.

34. Kobernick M: Electrical injuries: pathophysiology and emergency management, *Ann Emerg Med* 11:633, 1982.

35. Kunita N et al: Causal agents of Yusho, *Am J Ind Med* 5:45, 1984.

36. Kraut A, Lilis R: Pulmonary effects of acute exposure to degradation products of sulphur hexafluoride during electrical cable repair work, *Br J Ind Med* 47:829, 1990.

37. Lawrence C: PCB? and melanoma, *N Engl J Med* 296:108, 1977.

38. Lawton RW et al: Effects of PCB exposure on biochemical and hematological findings in capacitor workers, *Environ Health Perspect* 60:165, 1985.

39. Lees PSJ, Corn M, Breysee PN: Evidence for dermal absorption as the major route of body entry during exposure of transformer maintenance and repairmen to PCBs, *Am Ind Hyg Assoc J* 48:257, 1987.

40. Luotamo M, Iarvisalo J, Aitio A: Analysis of polychlorinated biphenyls (PCBs) in human serum, *Environ Health Perspect* 60:327, 1985.

41. Masuda Y, Yoshimura H: Polychlorinated biphenyls and dibenzofurans in patients with Yusho and their toxicological significance: a review, *Am J Ind Med* 5:31, 1985.

42. Meigs JW, Albom JJ, Kartin BL: Chloracne from an unusual exposure to Aroclor, *JAMA* 154:1417, 1954.

43. Moroni M et al: Occupational exposure to polychlorinated biphenyls in electrical workers: II. Health effects, *Br J Ind Med* 38:55, 1981.

44. Norback DH, Weltman RH: Polychlorinated biphenyl induction of hepatocellular carcinoma in the Sprague-Dawley rat, *Environ Health Perspect* 60:97, 1985.

45. Nordlinder R, Ramnas O: Exposure to benzene at different work places in Sweden, *Ann Occup Hyg* 31:345, 1987.

46. O'Keefe PW et al: Chemical and biological investigations of a transformer accident at Binghamton, NY, *Environ Health Perspect* 60:201, 1985.

47. Okumura M: Past and current medical states of Yusho patients, *Am J Ind Med* 5:13, 1984.

48. Ouw HK, Simpson GR, Silyali DS: Use and health effects of Aroclor 1242, a polychlorinated biphenyl in an electrical industry, *Arch Environ Health* 31:189, 1976.

49. Parkinson A et al: Polychlorinated biphenyls as inducers of hepatic microsomal enzymes: structure-activity rules, *Chem Biol Interact* 30:271, 1980.

50. Sahl JD et al: Polychlorinated biphenyls in the blood of personnel from an electric utility, *J Occup Med* 27:639, 1985.

51. Schaeffer E, Brein H, Goessner W: Pathology of chronic polychlorinated biphenyl (PCB) feeding in rats, *Toxicol Appl Pharmacol* 75:278, 1984.

52. Schwartz L: An outbreak of halowax acne ("cable rash") among electricians, *JAMA* 122:158, 1943.

53. Shalat SL et al: Kidney cancer in utility workers exposed to polychlorinated biphenyls (PCBs), *Br J Ind Med* 46:823, 1989.

54. Sherrell K et al: Polychlorinated biphenyl transformer incident—New Mexico, *MMWR Morb Mortal Wkly Rep* 34:557, 1985.

55. Smith AB et al: Metabolic and health consequences of occupational exposure to polychlorinated biphenyls, *Br J Ind Med* 39:361, 1982.

56. Treon JF et al: The toxicity of the vapours of Aroclor 1242 and Aroclor 1254, *Am J Hyg Assoc Q* 17:204, 1956.

57. Urabe K, Koda H, Asahi M: Present state of Yusho patients, *Ann N Y Acad Sci* 320:273, 1979.

58. Welsch F: Effects of acute or chronic polychlorinated biphenyl ingestion of maternal metabolic homeostasis and on the manifestations of embryotoxicity caused by cyclophosphamide in mice, *Arch Toxicol* 57:104, 1985.

59. Wester RC et al: Polychlorinated elimination, and dermal wash efficiency, *J Toxicol Environ Health* 12:511, 1983.

60. Wolff MS, Schecter A: Use of PCB blood levels to assess potential exposure following an electrical transformer explosion, *Occup Med* 34:1079, 1992.

61. Yassi A, Tate R, Fish D: Cancer mortality in workers employed at a transformer manufacturing plant, *Am J Ind Med* 25:425, 1994.

12

Electroplaters

Margaret P. Mueller
Richard Y. Wang

Cd   Cr

- Electroplaters can be exposed to the following potential toxins: organic solvents, inorganic acid and alkaline solutions, cyanide, heavy metals, and electrical injury

- Environmental and nutritional factors contribute to cadmium exposure

- Chronic cadmium toxicity affects the lung, bone metabolism, and kidney

- The oxidation state of chromium determines toxicity; with hexavalent chromium being the most toxic

- Acute chromium skin exposures can cause contact dermatitis and chemical burns

- Chelation therapy is not indicated for either chromium or chronic cadmium toxicity

OCCUPATIONAL DESCRIPTION

Few industrial processes have as rich a history or as ubiquitous a presence as metal plating. This technique is used to enhance the appearance of jewelry, strengthen machined parts, and provide corrosive resistance to weathered objects. Workers in this profession are subject to the ill effects of many chemicals, most notably, heavy metals. Toxicity can occur from the salts, solutions, or fumes of the metals, and manifestations may be localized or systemic.

The field began in the early 1800s with the discoveries of electrolysis and electromagnetic induction. These led to the invention of the magnetoelectric generator, which has become a cornerstone in the process of modern-day electroplating. The first patents for this process were granted to Joseph Shore in 1840. These patents were specifically for the electrodeposition of copper and nickel onto metallic surfaces by the voltaic battery. John Wright, a surgeon and chemist, experimented with gold and silver salts of cyanide and discovered that these solutions resulted in a superior finish. Wright made other modifications to the early methods of electroplating that allowed for the industrial application of this technique.[5]

Electroplating has evolved with the rapidly changing tastes and socioeconomic shifts of the last century. The metals used and the procedures employed in the process have been determined by the availability and cost of labor and materials. The field has also been shaped by changing tastes in jewelry, varying demands in industry, and increasing awareness of potential hazards in the work environment. Examples of these trends in electroplating are seen with flatware and costume jewelry. Flatware was once commonly electroplated, and the majority of silver use was for this purpose. As stainless steel became increasingly available, the plating of flatware turned obsolete. After the Great Depres-

89

sion, tastes in costume jewelry changed, and items became bigger, shinier, and yellower in color.[53]

The practice of electroplating is still very much in use and varies by region. States involved in the production of aircraft equipment, such as Washington and California, consume the majority of this country's cadmium. Rhode Island and Massachusetts are home to a large part of the costume jewelry industry. Thus, exposures to gold, nickel, and silver are more of a concern in these areas. Tin-plating is used in the production of semiconductors, which predominates in the Asian countries.[51]

Electroforming, another method of metal coating, is very similar to electroplating. This process creates objects by the electrodeposition of metal onto a mold, thereby creating a hollow figure. Household objects were commonly made by this method. However, as less expensive materials and more practical methods became available, the demand for electroforming declined.[51] An example of this change is silver tea sets. Initially, electroforming was the exclusive means of their production. This quickly gave way when it was discovered that they could be manufactured more easily by other means, such as pressing from preformed molds.

Presently, only a few articles are fashioned by electroforming. These include the wave guide system in radar equipment, certain gold and silver jewelry, cowboy belt buckles, and the Wimbledon women's singles champion trophy. Electroforming has the advantage of imparting more details than other means of manufacturing. It also lends itself well to forming lightweight pieces of gold and silver—ideal for certain jewelry. Historically, one of the most intriguing electroformed objects was an entire bed formed in intricately detailed relief from pure silver. This was made in Paris in 1851 for a maharaja of India, and its whereabouts today are unknown.[51]

POTENTIAL TOXIC EXPOSURES

The application of the metallic coat on an object can be accomplished by either flame spraying, vapor plating (use of high vacuum), or electrolytic action. This last process is the most commonly used and the foundation for the practice of electroplating. Objects are plated by being immersed in an electrochemical bath that contains salts of the desired metal. The physical and chemical nature of the metal determine which quality of the object is enhanced (luster, strength, or corrosive resistance). More than 18 types of metals and alloys are available for use in electroplating (Table 12-1).

Nickel is a popular finish because of the luster it imparts. This feature can be enhanced by applying an initial layer of copper. The largest use of nickel plating was in the jewelry industry in the 1920s and 1930s, when the dark shine of the metal was fashionable. The most commonly encountered form of nickel toxicity is contact dermatitis. Systemic manifestations are rare and usually result from the ingestion

Table 12-1 Electroplaters

Plating metal	Application	Base metal
Brass	Ornamentation Industry Electroforming	Iron, lead, steel, nickel
Chromium (bright)	Ornamentation	Iron, steel
Chromium (hard)	Automotive parts Household appliances	Aluminum
Copper	Ornamentation Jewelry Electroforming	Iron, plastic, brass, zinc, aluminum, steel
Gold	Jewelry Ornamentation	Stainless steel, brass, copper, nickel, silver
Iron	Printing plates* Military equipment	Ferrous and nonferrous metals
Lead	Items subject to corrosion by sulfuric acid	Ferrous and nonferrous metals
Nickel	Jewelry Lamps* Typewriters*	Steel, copper, zinc, aluminum
Palladium	Jewelry	Nickel, silver, gold
Platinum	Silverware	
Rhodium	Scientific and electrical equipment	
Silver	Jewelry Ornamentation	Copper, brass, steel, zinc, phosphor bronze
Tin	Canning Semiconductors	Ferrous and nonferrous metals
Zinc	Industry	Iron, steel, cast iron

*Former use.

of nickel salts or inhalation of nickel carbonyl.[25] Currently, nickel is used primarily to protect objects from corrosion and for decorating jewelry.[51]

Zinc is also used to protect steel and other metals from the elements of the environment.[51] The canning industry has been using the zinc alloy, tin, to plate their products in an effort to impart corrosive resistance for many years. Tin-plating exposes workers to tin oxide dusts and fumes that can cause metal fume fever and chemical pneumonitis. This process is now being replaced by a less toxic method involving lacquer coating.

When cadmium plating first became commercially feasible, it was heralded as the ideal metal for electroplating. It combined the corrosive resistance of zinc with the luster of nickel. This type of metal plating initially seemed very promising, and its use quickly grew in the airline, automotive, and marine industries. However, the widespread application of cadmium electroplating was short-lived as the toxicity of this metal was realized, and restrictions and modifications were enforced. Almost all of the initial applications of cadmium plating have now been replaced by other metals or techniques. However, cadmium electroplating is still extensively used for aircraft landing gears. No other practical process can provide the hardness and corrosive resistance needed in this type of equipment. These qualities imparted by cadmium are specifically due to its resistance to the deleterious effects of hydrogen embrittlement. Other metal coatings allow for the incorporation of hydrogen into the underlying steel, which actually weakens the structure.[51]

Chromium plating brought to the industry a finish that was durable and had a low coefficient of friction. This property was very useful for machined parts. The process was first described in 1854 by Blunsen, but it was not until 1925 that the method was perfected for use on a large scale.[5] Initially, chromium was plated from a cold chromic acid solution to form a relatively thick and dull finish. The chromic acid baths exposed workers to the hazards of corrosive chromic acid mists.[5] Today, the only commercial use for pure chromium is electroplating. Although the process has been modified to produce a more desirable finish, the acid baths are still present. The two main methods of chromium plating are hard plating, which improves the surface durability of a metal and involves a thick (5 to 10 microns) layer of chromium, and bright plating, which involves a much thinner layer of chromium (0.5 to 1 micron) and is used to impart a shiny finish on a surface.[18]

Iron, platinum, and cobalt are other metals used primarily because of their strength. Iron was originally used in Russia for making and coating printing plates. It experienced increased use during World War I for reinforcing worn or undersized parts of military equipment. The role of iron in plating has diminished because stronger and more decorative metals are now available. Platinum and cobalt plating are used sparingly due to their expense.[51]

The electroplating process consists of several cleaning and degreasing steps before electrolytic deposition occurs (Figs. 12-1 to 12-4). Each step has its own potential occupational hazard. To minimize these risks, a variety of protective measures have been mandated in the workplace. Examples of these measures are ventilators to remove solvent vapors and the installation of the degreasing baths away from the breathing region of the worker.

The base metal of the object is first mechanically cleansed of oxides (e.g., rust, scale, tarnish) to ensure a good-quality coating. During this abrasive cleaning, metallic dust is liberated into the air and can be inhaled to produce the risk of pneumoconiosis. Suction devices are present to remove the dust from the area to minimize worker exposure. Aluminum dust, which is combustible, is collected in a wet trap to avoid possible explosions. The object is then degreased with organic solvents (e.g., chlorinated hydrocarbons).[4] The solvents are often heated, which increases the danger of inhalation toxicity by producing more vapors. (For information regarding the toxic effects of organic solvents, see Chapter 25.)

The next step removes any remaining oxides and impurities from the metal object by pickling it in a concentrated acid or alkali solution. This process presents hazards associated with dermal and mucosal burns from concentrated caustic solutions. To protect against these potential hazards, adequate ventilation and irrigation facilities are required at the work site. When the quantities of oxides and impurities are small, the cleaning and pickling processes are often combined. This usually involves cleansers containing phosphoric acid mixed with wetting and emulsifying agents.[4]

The final stage before electrodeposition uses a degreasing bath, which often contains cyanide. If the object is not completely washed clean of all the acid from the previous step, hydrocyanic acid can form. Exposure to this toxic acid can result in the immediate death of the worker. Toxic effects are also possible through skin contact, inhalation, or ingestion of the cyanide salts.[9] To prevent these potential mishaps, proper hygienic conditions are mandated in the workplace. These include the strict prohibition of eating and drinking in the vicinity of the baths and stringent protocols on cleaning and rinsing before the cyanide degreasing bath.

The actual plating process occurs in a solution of metal salts that is connected to an electrical source. The object is dipped into the bath, and bubbles of oxygen and hydrogen form, which burst violently at the surface and liberate harmful mists. The mists contain the metal salts and can cause both local and systemic manifestations of toxicity. Floating balls, surface ventilation, and surfactants are used to reduce the workers' exposure to them.[18]

The temperature, current, and concentration of the electrochemical bath can be regulated to adjust the luster and color of the plating process. As the bath is heated and the current raised, mist production increases, and the workers' exposure is heightened. This is an issue of great concern and pertains specifically to the risks of hard and bright chromium plating. Hard plating uses a bath with a higher temperature and greater current than does bright plating. It has been shown that concentrations of airborne chromium are higher in hard plating plants and that biologic uptake, as measured by urine, is also greater.[18] Although bright platers are exposed less to chromium mists, they are at risk for other chemical hazards (e.g., solvents, inorganic acids, and alkali) because of the longer handling time associated with the process.[4] Thus, which of these two processes is fraught with more hazards remains unclear.

The voltage commonly used in electroplating systems is low (6 to 10 volts) and poses no significant risk to the worker. Exceptions are in the processes of anodizing and electrophoretic deposition. Anodizing imparts an oxide coat onto an aluminum base and uses between 40 and 50 volts. This process is most frequently used in the aircraft industry and is more of a regional concern for the Pacific Northwest. Electrophoretic deposition is used for automobile body finishing and undercoating. This process deposits a layer of lacquer or paint onto a metallic surface and requires between 60 and 80 volts.[53] Because of the higher voltage

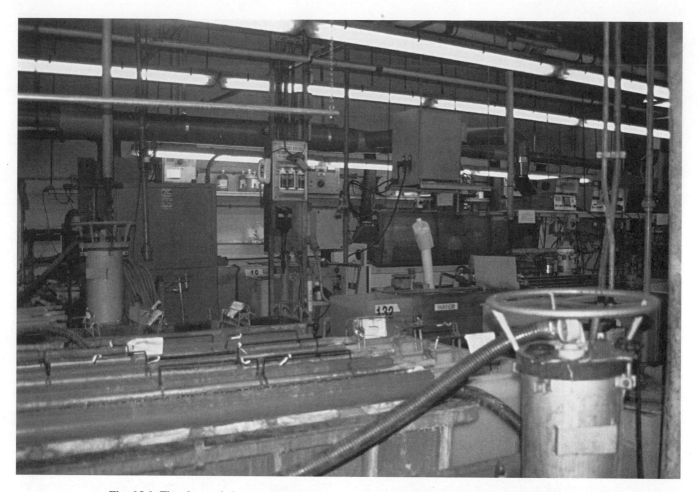

Fig. 12-1 The electroplating process involves several steps and is often contained in a large room.

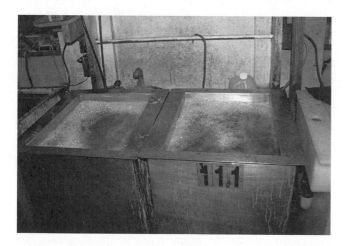

Fig. 12-2 Ultrasonic detergent cleansing baths are used to prepare certain items for electrolytic deposition.

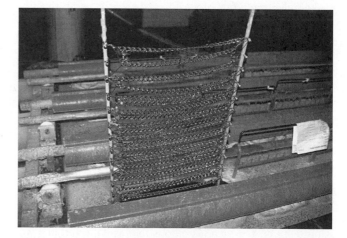

Fig. 12-3 Items being immersed in an electrolytic deposition bath to be nickel plated. These baths can be quite large so that many items can be processed at once.

involved with both of these processes, computer protocols are used to lessen human contact and risk of significant injury.

The most concerning and perhaps best studied hazardous exposure in the electrodeposition process is to the heavy metals. The electroplater can be exposed to a wide variety of heavy metals. Cadmium and chromium, however, are associated with more serious toxicities, and these exposures are discussed in the remaining portion of this chapter.

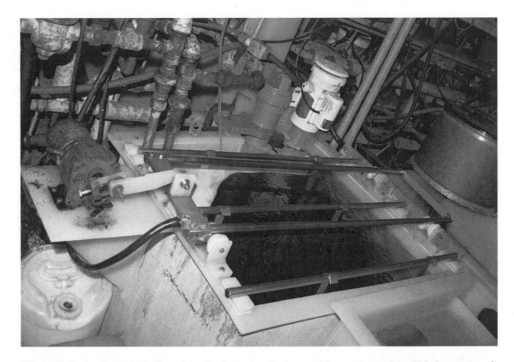

Fig. 12-4 Some electrolytic deposition baths are semiautomated for worker safety. This is an example of a gold-plating bath.

CLINICAL TOXICOLOGY
Cadmium

Pathophysiology and biochemistry. Cadmium is a ubiquitous metal that can be harmful to both workers and nonworkers. The nonoccupational sources of cadmium stem primarily from sources related to environmental contamination. Industrial by-products resulting from the production of plastic materials, batteries, and certain machined parts can enter the biologic food chain and are then eventually passed to humans. Seafood (especially shellfish), meat by-products, fruits, grain, drinking water, and vegetables all contain cadmium. Acidic beverages cause cadmium to leach out from certain containers. Fortunately, the amount of cadmium absorbed from the gastrointestinal tract is only about 5%. Nutritional deficient states (e.g., calcium, protein, and iron) tend to enhance gut absorption of cadmium.[17]

Some of the other nonoccupational sources of cadmium are tobacco and hobbies that involve welding, smelting, soldering, or grinding. Environmental cadmium is concentrated by production processes within the tobacco plants. So, cadmium is actually processed into cigarettes that, when smoked, expose the lungs to toxic cadmium oxide fumes. Each cigarette contains about 2 μg of cadmium, and the lungs absorb approximately 50% of exposed cadmium.[10] As a result, the body burden of cadmium in smokers is greater than that of nonsmokers.

Approximately 1.5 million workers are potentially exposed to cadmium in the United States today, and they are in industries that produce metal alloys, batteries, and plastic stabilizers, and those that involve electroplating.[35] Electroplaters commonly come in contact with cadmium oxide fumes, which can be inhaled to cause systemic toxicity.[17] Organ damage from absorbed cadmium is believed to result from the loss of homeostatic cellular function.[15] The mechanism responsible is unclear but may involve the disruption of enzymatic and regulatory protein activities.

Acute cadmium toxicity most commonly results from exposure via the oral or inhalational routes. Cadmium salts are caustic, and their ingestion results in nausea, vomiting, abdominal cramping, and diarrhea. Hypersalivation and choking may also occur. Increasing toxicity can cause gastrointestinal bleeding, hepatic and renal necrosis, cardiomyopathy, and metabolic acidosis.[15] This agent is a powerful emetic, and death has been reported following an ingestion of as little as 150 mg of cadmium.[11]

Inhalation of cadmium oxide fumes from heated metal can cause varying degrees of nasopharyngeal irritation, dyspnea, chest pain, vomiting, diarrhea, headache, dizziness, and weakness. The extent and time of onset of symptoms depend on the amount and duration of exposure. Exposures for as short a period of time as 1 hour can result in toxicity.[22] Because of the vague nature of these presenting symptoms, early toxicity is often mistaken for a viral illness. Prolonged hyperpyrexia has been reported and is associated with a poor prognosis.[11] Delayed chemical pneumonitis has been associated with cadmium fume exposure and can progress to noncardiogenic pulmonary edema and death.[11] Mortality from cadmium fume toxicity can be as high as 20%.[11] Pulmonary fibrosis is a long-term complication of acute lung injury from cadmium.

Chronic exposure to cadmium typically affects the lung, bone, and kidney. Long-term respiratory exposure to cadmium causes obstructive lung disease.[7] The onset of clinical symptoms usually occurs relatively late after exposure and can present initially as a chronic bronchitis. Progression of the disease leads to pulmonary fibrosis and emphysema. Pulmonary function testing demonstrates decreased vital capacity and increased residual capacity. The destruction of lung tissue is the result of lytic enzymes released by dying alveolar macrophages. Cadmium reduces α-1-antitrypsin activity in exposed workers; however, it is unclear whether this contributes to the development of obstructive lung disease.

The role of cadmium exposure in human lung carcinogenesis remains unresolved. Several human studies have suggested the association between cadmium exposure and lung carcinoma, but a definite link is yet to be established. A 1976 study of workers in a U.S. cadmium recovery plant demonstrated a statistically significant increase in deaths from respiratory cancer.[31] This finding was supported in a 5-year follow-up study.[47] Similar results were shown in nickel-cadmium battery workers.[44] The significance of these studies is limited by several issues. One is that these studies did not control for other cancer-causing agents (e.g., tobacco, arsenic, nickel). This design flaw limits the ability to make direct associations between cadmium and lung carcinogenesis. Also, the relevance of these findings to today's workers is weakened by the decreased amount of cadmium exposure in the current workplace. Finally, other epidemiologic studies of cadmium workers have failed to show a significant relationship between exposure and carcinogenesis.[35] The Environmental Protection Agency (EPA) and the International Agency for Research on Cancer (IARC) have classified cadmium as a probably human carcinogen when it is inhaled.[21]

Prostate carcinoma has also been a concern among cadmium-exposed workers. Animal studies have repeatedly demonstrated an association between cadmium exposure and prostatic cancer.[51] Epidemiologic investigations, however, have failed to uphold this relationship in cadmium-exposed workers.[47]

Bone disease occurs in late and severe cadmium exposures. Cadmium-induced bone disease is characterized by pathologic fractures, osteomalacia, and osteopenia. Patients often complain of pains in the back and extremities and difficulty in walking. The most noteworthy example of this manifestation is the well-documented outbreak of Itai-Itai disease in Japan (which translates to "ouch-ouch" disease).[48] This syndrome presented as severe renal tubular damage with osteomalacia and osteoporosis.[14] As a result of environmental contamination, 129 patients were afflicted by cadmium toxicity. The victims were mostly postmenopausal multiparous women. Their symptoms consisted of severe pain in the arms, legs, and back. As the disease progressed, pathologic fractures due to minor bone stress became more prevalent. These patients may have been more susceptible to bone pathology because of either preexisting malnutrition (i.e., calcium and vitamin D deficiencies) or their postmenopausal state.

Cadmium affects bone metabolism by several different mechanisms: increased urinary loss of calcium and phosphorus, inhibition of renal hydroxylation of vitamin D, and, possibly, inhibition of gut calcium absorption. Many of these physiologic findings are attributed to cadmium's specific toxicity to proximal renal tubule cells.[14] Diminished levels of 1-α-25(OH) vitamin D would cause decreased calcium absorption and demineralization of bone, as is observed in osteomalacia.

Renal dysfunction is another manifestation of chronic cadmium toxicity. It can result from oral or inhalational exposure. The onset is often delayed, about 2 to 10 years, and the extent of involvement is dependent on the toxic burden. Since it serves as the primary route of cadmium elimination from the body, the kidney is an important organ to recognize in the setting of cadmium toxicity. Cadmium elimination is a slow process (the biologic half-life of cadmium is 30 years) and accounts for the gradual accumulation of cadmium in the body over time. Nearly 50% of the body's burden of cadmium is stored in the kidney and liver.[14] In addition, certain renal functions can provide early indications of chronic cadmium toxicity. Such is the case with proteinuria.[38] Consequently, the urine of exposed workers should be analyzed on a regular basis.

Cadmium-induced proteinuria results from proximal renal tubule damage. Diminished resorption of low molecular proteins, amino acids, glucose, and phosphate allows their increased concentration in the urine. The low-molecular-weight proteins are β-2-microglobulin, lysozyme, and retinol binding protein.[38] These proteins play an important role in monitoring workers for cadmium exposure and toxicity and are discussed later in this chapter. Progressive exposure to cadmium can lead to glomerular damage, leakage of high-molecular-weight proteins (e.g., albumin, transferrin, and immune globulin) into the urine, and elevation of serum creatinine. Cadmium-induced renal injury is irreversible.[39] Once there is evidence of impaired function (e.g., proteinuria), work-related exposure should cease to limit further damage.

The specific mechanism of cadmium-induced renal disease is unclear; however, the accumulation of intracellular "free" or "unbound" cadmium is highly suspect. Once cadmium is absorbed into the bloodstream, it is bound by the carrier protein metallothionein and transported primarily to the liver and kidney. As long as cadmium remains bound to metallothionein, it is considered nontoxic. Hypotheses accounting for the presence of free or unbound cadmium involve the oversaturation of available protein-binding sites[34] and the dissociation of cadmium-metallothionein complexes upon proximal tubule resorption.[10] It has also been proposed that toxicity may result from cadmium's interference with essential trace metals.[37]

Laboratory. The measurement of cadmium concentration in body tissue samples is dependent on several factors, the most important of which is the proficiency of the laboratory with the technique. Cadmium levels should be measured from either whole blood or urine. Whole blood is a better indicator of the amount of exposure than serum because the majority of cadmium resides inside the red blood cell. Blood cadmium levels reflect only recent exposures and are not an accurate measure of the total body burden.[29] In normal adults without excessive exposure, the blood cadmium level is less than 0.1 µg/dl.[29] Smokers can be expected to have higher levels.

Urine cadmium levels can be useful in assessing long-term exposures because they are a better representation of body burden.[29] This is, however, dependent on renal function. Once renal dysfunction occurs, cadmium is spilled into the urine, and the level is no longer reflective of body burden. To account for diurnal variations in urinary cadmium elimination, a 24-hour urine collection is used for sample analysis. The urine cadmium level in nonexposed adults is less than 1 µg/L or 1 to 2 µg/g creatinine.[29] Smokers have elevated levels due to excessive exposure. A cadmium urine level higher than 10 µg/g creatinine suggests saturation of protein-binding sites and the likelihood of renal toxicity with proteinuria.[29]

Urine metallothionein levels can be used to assess urine cadmium levels and total body cadmium burden.[16] However, in the setting of renal damage, the level rises sharply and may be unreliable. This assessment is beneficial because there is no concern for external contamination of the specimen.[16] Excessive exposure to copper and zinc can also result in elevated urine metallothionein concentrations.[29] Urine levels for retinol-binding proteins can also be used to assess chronic cadmium exposure.[30] The advantage of this particular test is that it is not susceptible to variations in pH.

Hair analysis is not a reliable indicator for long-term exposure because of the possibility of external contamination.

Management. Treatment after a suspected inhalation exposure involves moving the patient to a clean and non-contaminated environment, administering 100% humidified oxygen, and assisting in ventilation if indicated. The patient needs to be monitored closely for signs of delayed pulmonary edema and treated with mechanical ventilation and positive end-expiratory pressure (PEEP) if necessary. Adequate hydration with intravenous fluids should be maintained.

Chelation therapy in the acutely exposed patient may be beneficial if administered early. Calcium disodium edetate (CaNa$_2$EDTA) has been demonstrated to increase urinary cadmium elimination when given before more metallothionein can be synthesized.[6] The body's metallothionein response to increased cadmium levels takes about 24 to 48 hours to occur. Once cadmium is complexed with this protein, chelating agents are not strong enough to free the metal and are ineffective as therapy. Also, with time, cadmium distributes to tissue stores that are inaccessible to certain chelating agents. Dimercaprol (BAL) therapy is not recommended because it can actually worsen

renal toxicity by increasing cadmium delivery to the kidneys.[16] Similarly, chelation therapy is not used for chronic cadmium exposures. Dithiocarbamate derivatives are being evaluated for use as chelating agents in this setting.[26]

The recommended regimen for CaNa$_2$EDTA is 75 mg/kg/day administered as a deep intramuscular injection (IM) or slow intravenous infusion, given in 3 to 6 divided doses for up to 5 days.[25] This may be repeated for a second therapeutic course after an interval of at least 2 days. Each course should not exceed 500 mg/kg body weight. Renal functions should be monitored during chelation therapy.

Patients with evidence of chronic cadmium toxicity should be removed from further exposure. Calcium and vitamin D supplementation is indicated if there is evidence of bone disease or calcium loss.[33] The vitamin D$_2$ regimen from the Itai-Itai experience was 100,00 IU/day administered orally for 10 days. After a 10-day holiday, this schedule can be repeated once. In addition, 300,00 IU of vitamin D$_2$ or D$_3$ can be administered IM up to 8 times a year to this population.

Prevention and monitoring. The protection of workers from occupational health hazards begins with proper personal hygiene and work habits. The addition of exhaust ventilators and personal protective devices has significantly reduced worker exposure. The Occupational Safety and Health Administration's (OSHA) permissible exposure limit (PEL) for cadmium fumes or cadmium oxide is 0.1 mg/m^3 and for cadmium dust is 0.2 mg/m^3 at the workplace.[36] The time-weighted average (TWA) according to the American Conference of Governmental Industrial Hygienists (ACGIH) for cadmium dust is 0.05 mg/m^3.[17]

Preemployment evaluations should include a detailed history of prior lung and kidney disease. Workers with these ailments should not be exposed to cadmium. Following a physical examination, laboratory values should be obtained for a complete blood count (CBC), serum renal and liver functions, whole blood and urine cadmium levels, urine analysis, and a baseline chest radiograph and pulmonary function test. The patient should be reassessed every 6 months with a complete physical exam and a urine evaluation.[17] This includes a routine urine analysis and urine quantitative levels for retinol-binding proteins (or β-2 microglobulin) and albumin. Abnormal urine protein levels need to be confirmed, and the patient should have further renal function studies. Pulmonary function tests are repeated annually and chest radiographs every 1 to 2 years.

Workers being evaluated for chronic cadmium exposure require all of these laboratory studies, and routine bone radiographs may be advisable. The use of such radiographs, however, should be guided by appropriate clinical judgment. Evidence of demineralization or pathologic fractures would support the diagnosis of cadmium toxicity. Blood cadmium levels are not helpful in the determination of chronic toxicity. When there is presence of end-organ disease (e.g., bone, kidney, lung), the worker should be removed from further exposure. Urine cadmium levels should not be allowed to rise above 5 µg/g creatinine.[50] The OSHA indicators for mandatory removal from work are urine cadmium higher than 15 µg/g creatinine, blood cadmium higher than 1.5 µg/dl, or urine β-2 microglobulin higher than 1500 µg/g creatinine.

Chromium

Pathophysiology and biochemistry. Chromium exists in several states of oxidation, which allows it to have many applications in industry. The hexavalent form (Cr^{+6}) is most commonly used in pigments and anticorrosive agents. The trivalent form (Cr^{+3}) is used in the production of alloys, such as stainless steel. Chromium electroplaters use chromic acid (Cr^{+6}) in their electrolytic baths. Understanding the oxidation state of chromium is essential because oxidation state specifically determines the nature of toxicity. In this regard, the trivalent (Cr^{+3}) and hexavalent (Cr^{+6}) forms are the only forms of any substantial clinical significance.

Exposure to hexavalent chromium is more hazardous than exposure to its reduced, trivalent form because of increased tissue solubility and cell membrane permeability. Once in the cell, hexavalent chromium is converted to the trivalent form, which binds to nucleic acids.[16] Trivalent chromium is the only form of chromium that is considered carcinogenic. It is important to note that trivalent chromium compounds, such as chromic oxide and sulfate, are not considered cancer risks because of their lack of tissue and cell permeability. However, hexavalent compounds (e.g., chromates, chromic acids) are a health risk because of their solubility and subsequent intracellular conversion to the trivalent form.[23]

Chromium exposures can present to the clinician with a variety of local and systemic clinical manifestations. One of the most interesting local reactions is the formation of "chrome holes" in the anterior portion of the nasal septum. The nasal septum is susceptible to damage from prolonged exposure to high concentrations of hexavalent chromium mist because of its somewhat limited vascular supply. Chromium deposits on the septum can lead to ulceration of the mucosa and subsequent necrosis of the cartilage. The resulting septal perforation absolutely will not heal, even upon discontinuation of exposure. Typically, this form of septal perforation does not cause disfigurement.[28]

Upon dermatologic contact, hexavalent chromium is capable of eroding the skin to form lesions known as *chrome ulcers*. These ulcers are more prone to develop over areas of broken skin and usually take many months to heal. Anatomic sites susceptible to chrome ulcer formation are the forearm, the dorsum of the hand, knuckles, finger webs, and nail root. Chrome ulcers tend to be painless and often penetrate deeply. Systemic absorption of hexavalent chromium can occur through open lesions and intact skin to cause significant toxicity and death.[28] It is important to remember that trivalent chromium is not corrosive and can be absorbed only through broken skin.

Allergic contact dermatitis is the most common local reaction to chromium. It has been widely described in cement workers, limestone workers, painters, leather workers, homemakers, and electroplaters.[28] The hexavalent form accounts for the majority of these cases because of its increased tissue permeability. Upon absorption by the cell, the chromium is reduced to the trivalent form, which covalently binds to proteins to form reactive allergens. After sensitization, workers with subsequent exposures to chromium can elicit an atopic reaction.

The ingestion of hexavalent chromium is an unusual occurrence and signifies either accidental or intentional (suicidal or homicidal) exposure. Gastric acid acts to reduce hexavalent chromium to its trivalent state, whereupon it is readily absorbed from the gut.[8] The amount of gut chromium absorption varies from 1% to 25%.[2] As little as 0.5 g of potassium dichromate can produce symptoms, and 1.5 g resulted in the death of a child.[24] The manifestations of toxicity can be dramatic and include both local and systemic derangements. The caustic nature of hexavalent chromium can lead to oropharyngeal and upper gastrointestinal distress. Significant ingestions can result in pronounced loss of fluid and blood from the gastrointestinal tract and has been reported to cause cardiovascular collapse and death. Esophageal and gastric burns are extremely concerning and warrant further evaluation. Manifestations of systemic toxicity include hepatic and renal failure, and red cell hemolysis.[42]

Chromic acid and chromate dust are irritating and can cause acute respiratory symptoms (e.g., dyspnea, chest pain, wheezing) upon inhalation. The onset of symptoms usually occurs between 4 and 8 hours following exposure. Delayed noncardiogenic pulmonary edema can result after an exposure to high concentrations of chromic acid mist.[11] In addition, these agents can sensitize workers to develop allergy-induced asthma.[11]

The organ most affected by chronic chromium exposure is the lung. Inhalation of chromium as large particles or poorly soluble forms (e.g., chromite ore) can lead to the development of a pneumoconiosis.[43] These particles deposit in the lower respiratory tree and can cause a reactive fibrosis. The chest radiograph in these cases shows fine nodules that are typically more radiopaque than those of coal miners' pneumoconiosis.

Early epidemiologic studies of workers demonstrated that long-term chromium exposure can be associated with lung carcinoma of almost all types.[4,19,41] Occupations involving chromates, dichromates, and chromium pigment production were shown to be at increased risk for the development of lung cancer. In addition, hard chromium platers have a higher incidence of lung cancer than bright platers.[13] These results must be interpreted cautiously because of certain issues, specifically, the lack of control for other carcinogens (e.g., tobacco, arsenic, nickel) within these studies, contrary results by other investigations,[20,46] and the lack of a supporting animal model. The EPA and the IARC have classified inhaled hexavalent chromium as a known human carcinogen. It is important to remember that the onset of carcinoma may be as late as 20 years, and the duration of exposure can be as short as 2 years.[23]

Laboratory. After systemic absorption, chromium becomes firmly bound to red blood cells and plasma proteins. The metal is transported to the liver, spleen, kidney, fat, and bone, where most of the body burden is stored. The lung, however, has the largest concentration of chromium because of the accumulation of inhaled insoluble particles.[45] Chromium elimination takes place predominantly via the kidney.

Whole blood and urine chromium levels can be used to evaluate exposures; however, certain issues need to be considered. Only laboratories experienced with the specific assays should be allowed to perform the analysis. Specimens are to be collected in acid-washed containers because certain plastics can leach chromium and cause spurious results. Confounding sources of chromium exposure need to be considered, including smoking and certain foods (e.g., meats, fish, fruits, alfalfa, and brewer's yeast). Urine samples should be collected over 24 hours because renal chromium elimination may be subject to diurnal variation. Hair and fingernail samples are not reliable indicators of exposure because of the potential for external contamination.[24]

Biologic fluid levels of chromium are higher in urban populations than among rural dwellers, primarily because of environmental contamination. Serum chromium levels in normal volunteers is in the range of 0.04 to 0.35 μg/L. The whole blood concentration is a better measure of acute exposure and is 20 to 30 μg/L in normal volunteers.[2] The normal range for urine chromium is between 0.1 and 0.5 μg/L or less than 10 μg/day.[1]

Management. The initial management of a patient ingesting hexavalent chromium centers around gastric decontamination and limiting local tissue damage. Inducing emesis is contraindicated, as the substance is corrosive and further damage may be incurred. A demulcent (e.g., 120 to 240 ml water) can be administered orally to the patient to dilute the caustic agent. Careful nasogastric tube lavage may be used to remove remaining gastric contents if the patient arrives to the hospital within about 1 hour after ingestion. If there is clinical evidence of a perforated viscus, then blind passage of a nasogastric tube is contraindicated. There is no role for activated charcoal, which binds poorly to heavy metals and can obscure the view of the endoscopist if an esophagogastroduodenoscopy becomes necessary in order to evaluate the resulting burns.

Gastric lavage with 10% ascorbic acid is recommended to limit local tissue toxicity by converting hexavalent chromium to the less caustic trivalent state.[27] Ascorbic acid may also have systemic benefits by reducing hexavalent chromium to the trivalent form, thus limiting cell permeability and toxicity. Oral administration of ascorbic acid following chromium ingestion has been shown to prevent chromium toxicity in rats.[40] Human data on the efficacy of ascorbic acid therapy for chromium ingestion are limited to the report of a 5-g sodium dichromate exposure in a 2-year-old.[52] This child was treated with 1 g of ascorbic acid daily and survived. Although the benefits of ascorbic acid therapy for systemic chromium exposures remain unclear, the agent is relatively benign and should be used if available. The initial dose of intravenous ascorbic acid in an adult is 3 g, given as 1-g boluses every 10 to 20 minutes.[27] Repeat doses may be necessary because ascorbic acid is eliminated quickly by the kidneys.

In an animal model poisoned with potassium dichromate, *N*-acetylcysteine (NAC) was shown to enhance urinary chromium elimination and reverse oliguria.[1] This agent was also used in a man who ingested a potentially lethal dose (16 g) of potassium dichromate.[49] The patient also was treated with hemodialysis and survived. The role of NAC in the treatment of chromium toxicity is unclear but should be considered in all significant acute exposures. The therapeutic dose of NAC is empiric and is the same as that used for acetaminophen toxicity (loading dose of 140 mg/kg followed by a maintenance dose of 70 mg/kg every 4 hours for a total of 17 doses).

Forced diuresis with IV fluid hydration is encouraged to enhance renal elimination of the heavy metal. If red cell hemolysis is evident, alkalinization of the urine to a pH of 7.5 may limit acute tubular necrosis. Hemodialysis has not been shown to offer any significant advantage in chromium clearance when renal function is adequate.[3] The onset of anuria is a poor prognostic indicator, and hemodialysis should be instituted to enhance chromium elimination. Chelation therapy with dimercaprol (BAL) and calcium disodium EDTA is not effective in removing chromium and is not indicated.[12]

Workers exposed to chromium fumes must be evacuated from the site and provided with oxygen and ventilatory support. Symptomatic patients should be observed for the delayed onset of noncardiogenic pulmonary edema and systemic toxicity. Continuous positive airway pressure or PEEP may be needed to maintain adequate oxygenation in the setting of pulmonary edema. Nebulized bronchodilator therapy is beneficial if bronchospasm is present. Steroids are of unproven benefit in preventing pulmonary edema, and their use should be individualized for each case.

Dermal exposures to hexavalent chromium must be washed immediately and thoroughly with soap and water. Topical application of 10% ascorbic acid solution may limit further damage by converting hexavalent chromium to the trivalent state. Chromium contact dermatitis can be prevented by repeated administration of a 10% ascorbic acid solution.[32] Daily washing of the nose and application of a protective layer of zinc or barium ointment to the nasal septum may help avoid local damage, necrosis, and perforation of the nasal septum. Chrome ulcers, should they occur, heal spontaneously over a period of weeks to months.

Prevention and monitoring. The health concerns for chromium electroplaters primarily involve chromic acid. Although this compound can cause burns and sensitization reactions, the issue of lung cancer risks is of greatest concern. The current workplace limit set by OSHA for chromic acid and chromates is an 8-hour TWA of 0.1 mg/m^3.[30] Despite the lack of evidence that exposures below this level will result in lung carcinoma, preventive measures and workplace monitoring are still necessary.

Proper personal hygiene and work habits are mandatory to limit chronic exposures. Smoking can increase the risk for lung cancer, and workers in this industry should be encouraged to immediately stop using tobacco. All workers using chromates or chromic acid must wear protective gloves. Any open wounds on the skin should be covered with a protective dressing to avoid the development of chrome ulcers. Workers with a history of atopy or a previous reaction to chromium should avoid all contact with chromium-containing compounds.

At the time of employment, a baseline evaluation should include a complete physical examination, whole blood and urine chromium levels, CBC, serum renal and liver functions, urine analysis, chest radiograph, and pulmonary function study. Annual reevaluations should be performed on a regular basis to monitor any changes. The risks for lung carcinoma are apparent only after lengthy exposures (i.e., more than 2 to 3 years) and is assessed by chest radiographs and sputum cytology.[24]

REFERENCES

1. Banner J et al: Experimental chelation therapy in chromium, lead, and boron intoxication with N-acetylcysteine and other compounds, *Toxicol Appl Pharmacol* 83:142, 1986.
2. Baselt RC, Cravey RH, editors: *Disposition of toxic drugs and chemicals in man,* ed 4, Chicago, 1995, Year Book Medical Publishers.
3. Behari JR, Tandon SK: Chelation in metal intoxication, VIII. Removal of chromium from organs of potassium chromate administered rats, *J Tox* 16:33, 1980.
4. Blum W, Hogaboom GB: *Principles of electroplating and electroforming,* New York, 1924, McGraw-Hill.
5. Burges DCL: Manufacturing processes electroplating, *J Soc Occ Med* 27:114, 1977.
6. Cantilena LR, Klaassen CD: Decreased effectiveness of chelation therapy for Cd poisoning with time, *Toxicol Appl Pharmacol* 63:173, 1982.
7. Davison AG et al: Cadmium fume inhalation and emphysema, *Lancet* 1:663, 1988.
8. DeFlora S et al: Circadian reduction of chromium in the gastric environment, *Mutat Res* 192:169, 1987.
9. Dodds C, McKnight C: Cyanide toxicity after immersion and the hazards of dicobalt edetate, *Br Med J Clin Res Ed* 291:785, 1985.
10. Dudley RE, Gammal LM, Klaassen CD: Cadmium induced hepatic and renal injury in chronically exposed rats: likely role of hepatic cadmium-metallothionein in nephrotoxicity, *Toxicol Appl Pharmacol* 77:414, 1985.
11. Dunphy B: Acute occupational cadmium poisoning: a critical review of the literature, *J Occup Med* 9:22, 1967.
12. Ellis EN et al: Effects of hemodialysis and dimercaprol in acute dichromate poisoning, *J Toxicol Clin Toxicol* 19:249, 1982.
13. Franchini I, Magnani F, Mutti A: Mortality experience among chromeplating workers: initial findings, *Scand J Work Environ Health* 9:247, 1983.
14. Friberg L, Kjellstrom T, Nordberg GF: Cadmium. In Friberg L, Nordberg GF, Vouk VB, editors: *Handbook on the toxicology of metals,* vol 2, Amsterdam, 1986, Elsevier Science Publishers.
15. Friberg L et al, editors: *Cadmium and health: a toxicological and epidemiological appraisal: effects and response,* vol 2, Boca Raton, Fla, 1986, CRC Press.
16. Goyer RA: Toxic effects of metals. In Doull J, Klaasen CD, Amdur MO, editors: *Casarett and Doull's toxicology: the basic science of poisons,* New York, 1986, Macmillan.
17. Grum EE, Bresnitz EA: *Case studies in environmental medicine. Cadmium toxicity,* Atlanta, 1990, Agency for Toxic Substances and Disease Registry, Dept of Health and Human Services.
18. Guillemin MP, Berode M: A study of the differences in chromium exposure in workers in two types of electroplating process, *Ann Occup Hyg* 21:105, 1978.
19. Hayes R, Lilienfeld AM, Snell LM: Mortality in chromium chemical production workers: a prospective study, *Int J Epidemiol* 8:365, 1979.
20. Horiguchi S, Morinaga K, Endo G: Epidemiological study of mortality from cancer among chromium platers, *Asia Pac J Public Health* 4:169, 1990.
21. International Agency for Research on Cancer: *Monograph on the evaluations of carcinogenicity: an update of IARC monographs,* vols 1-42, suppl 7, Geneva, Switzerland, 1987, World Health Organization, International Agency for Research on Cancer.
22. Johnson JS, Kilburn FH: Cadmium induced metal fume fever: results of inhalation challenge, *Am J Ind Med* 4:533, 1983.
23. Kapol V, Keogh J: *Case studies in environmental medicine. Chromium toxicity,* Atlanta, 1990, Agency for Toxic Substances and Disease Registry, Dept of Health and Human Services.
24. Kaufman DB, Di Nicola W, McIntosh R: Acute potassium-dichromate poisoning treated by peritoneal dialysis, *Am J Dis Child* 119:374, 1970.
25. Klaassen CD: Heavy metals and heavy metal antagonists. In Gilman AG et al, editors: *Goodman and Gilman's: The pharmacological basis of therapeutics,* ed 7, New York, 1986, Macmillan.
26. Kojima S et al: Effects of three dithiocarbamates on tissue distribution and excretion of cadmium in mice, *Chem Pharm Bull (Tokyo)* 38:3136, 1990.
27. Korallus U, Harzdorf C, Lewalter J: Experimental basis for ascorbic acid therapy of poisoning by hexavalent chromium compounds, *Int Arch Occup Environ Health* 53:247, 1984.
28. Langard S, Norseth T: Chromium. In Friberg L, Nordberg GF, Vouk VB, editors: *Handbook on the toxicology of metals,* vol 2, Amsterdam, 1986, Elsevier Science Publishers.
29. Lauwerys R et al: Significance of cadmium concentration in blood and in urine in workers exposed to cadmium, *Environ Res* 20:375, 1979.
30. Lauwerys R et al: Characterization of cadmium proteinuria in man and rat, *Environ Health Perspect* 54:147, 1984.
31. Lemen RA et al: Cancer mortality among cadmium production workers, *Ann N Y Acad Sci* 271:233, 1976.
32. Milner JE: Ascorbic acid in the prevention of chromium dermatitis, *J Occup Med* 22:51, 1980.
33. Nogawa K, Ishizaki A, Fukushima M: Studies on women with acquired Fanconi syndrome observed in the Ichi River Basin polluted by cadmium, *Environ Res* 10:280, 1975.
34. Nomiyama K, Nomiyama H: Critical concentration of "unbound" cadmium in the rabbit renal cortex, *Experientia* 42:149, 1986.
35. Oberdorster G: Airborne cadmium and carcinogenesis of the respiratory tract, *Scand J Work Environ Health* 12:523, 1986.
36. Occupational Safety and Health Administration, Department of Labor: *Air contaminants,* Final rule: 29 CRF Part 1910, *Fed Reg* 1989, 54(12):2322-2983.

37. Petering DH et al: Metabolism of cadmium, zinc, and copper in the rat kidney: the role of metallothionein and other binding sites, *Environ Health Perspect* 54:73, 1984.

38. Piscator M: Proteinuria in chronic cadmium poisoning. III. Electrophoretic and immunoelectrophoretic studies on urinary proteins from cadmium workers, with special reference to the excretion of low molecular weight proteins, *Arch Environ Health* 12:335, 1966.

39. Roels HA et al: Health significance of cadmium induced renal dysfunction at five year follow-up, *Br J Ind Med* 46:755, 1989.

40. Samitz MH, Epstein E, Katz S: Inactivation of hexavalent chromium. Studies of an antichrome agent, *Arch Dermatol* 85:595, 1962.

41. Satoh K et al: Epidemiologic study of workers engaged in the manufacture of chromium compounds, *J Occup Med* 23:835, 1981.

42. Sharma BK, Singhal PC, Chugh KS: Intravascular haemolysis and acute renal failure following potassium dichromate poisoning, *Postgrad Med* 54:514, 1978.

43. Sluis-Cremer GK, Du Troit RS: Pneumoconiosis in chromite miners in South Africa, *Br J Ind Med* 25:63, 1968.

44. Sorahan T, Waterhouse JAH: Mortality study of nickel-cadmium battery workers by the method of regression models in life tables, *Br J Ind Med* 4:293, 1983.

45. Sumino K et al: Heavy metals in normal Japanese tissues, *Arch Environ Health* 30:487, 1975.

46. Takahashi K, Okubo T: A prospective cohort study of chromium plating workers in Japan, *Arch Environ Health* 45:107, 1990.

47. Thun MJ et al: Mortality among a cohort of US cadmium production workers: an update, *J Natl Cancer Inst* 74:325, 1985.

48. Tsuchiya K: Epidemiological studies on cadmium in the environment in Japan: etiology of Itai-Itai disease, *Fed Proc* 35:2412, 1976.

49. Vasallo S, Howland MA: Severe dichromate poisoning: survival after therapy with intravenous N-acetylcysteine and hemodialysis. Paper presented at the annual meeting of the American Association of Poison Control Center, Baltimore, Maryland, October 1-4, 1988.

50. Verschoor M et al: Renal function of workers with low-level cadmium exposure, *Scand J Work Environ Health* 13:232, 1987.

51. Waalkes MP et al: Cadmium carcinogenesis in the male Wistar [Crl: (WI) BR] rats: dose-response analysis of tumor induction in the prostate and testes and at the injection site, *Cancer Res* 48:4656, 1988.

52. Walpole IR: Acute chromium poisoning in a 2 year old child, *Aust Ped J* 21:65, 1985.

53. Weissberg A (historian and first ex-president, Technic, Inc., Cranston, RI): personal correspondence, Oct 1995.

13

$$CH_3O \diagdown \ \ \ \ S$$
$$P$$
$$CH_3O \diagup \ \ \ O—\text{Leaving group}$$

Typical organophosphate

- Exterminators should have baseline and interval determinations of RBC cholinesterase to monitor for organophosphate toxicity

- Pyrethrums and pyrethroids may induce reactive upper airway and lower airway disease in individuals with pre-existing tendency for allergy

- Chronic organophosphate toxicity can occur without a significant acutely symptomatic episode

Exterminators

Glendon C. Henry

OCCUPATIONAL DESCRIPTION

Destruction of the insect population constitutes a large part of the work for exterminators. Today the two most widely used insecticides are the organophosphates (which include carbamates) and the chrysanthemum-derived pyrethrums and synthetic pyrethroids. There were 49,000 exterminators in 1992 according to the Department of Labor, Bureau of Labor Statistics. Exterminators apply pesticides as sprays, liquids, and solids. They frequently mix their pesticides from concentrates. Many exterminators are self-employed.

TOXIC EXPOSURES

Exposure to pesticides accounted for 61,182 (3.2%) of the 1,926,438 cases reported to the American Association of Poison Control Center Toxic Exposure Surveillance System in 1995. Although this number seems small, it was the seventh most frequent substance involved in human exposure and is an underestimation, since not all exposures are reported to poison centers. The U.S. Department of Labor, Bureau of Labor Statistics, reports 2621 case of injuries to exterminators. No deaths were listed, and there were only 65 cases of chemical exposures in pest controllers. The majority of these cases were minor and resulted in only 1 or 2 days of lost time at work. However, this type of work is frequently performed by migrant workers who avoid reporting exposures because they know they will lose their jobs. Organophosphates (OP) and carbamates account for 35% of the 61,182 pesticide exposures. Pyrethrins account for an additional 10% of the total exposures. Other agents include arsenic, piperonyl butoxide, and metaldehyde.

CLINICAL TOXICOLOGY
Organochlorines

Dichlorodiphenyltrichloroethane (DDT) belongs to the group of pesticides known as the organochlorines. These pesticides have been discontinued because of their harmful environmental toxicity.[46] Currently the only commonly used organochlorine is the scabicide lindane (Kwell). The organochlorines share some of the properties of the agents that replaced them. They are absorbed through the skin, mucous membranes, and pulmonary tree.[14] Toxicity is usually manifested by nausea, vomiting, headaches, and a change in mental status, seizures, lethargy, or coma.[23] The organochlorines, like other halogenated hydrocarbons, tend to sensitize the myocardium to catecholamines and may induce tachyarrhythmias.

Treatment of the toxicity induced by these agents includes decontamination of the area where absorption occurred, protection of the airway, termination of seizures with benzodiazepines, and treatment of tachyarrhythmias. The central nervous system (CNS) toxicity is usually transient and can be treated with supportive care until the agent is metabolized. Care should be taken not to induce vomiting with these hydrocarbon agents because of the added risk of aspiration.

Another commonly used insecticide that may cause toxicity if not handled properly is diethyltoluamide (DEET). Concentrations of 5% to 100% are sold over the counter. These agents cause toxicity when the higher concentrations are applied in excess on children, applied to damaged skin, or ingested.[44] Toxicity is manifested by central nervous system effects, but cardiopulmonary collapse can also be seen.[19,26]

Organophosphates

The group of agents referred to as organophosphates (OP) all contain at least one carbon associated with phosphoric acid or a derivative attached. Although these agents have been available for many years, they were initially employed as destructive agents against humans in time of war.

Pathophysiology. Organophosphates produce toxicity by interacting with the neurotransmitter acetylcholine. Acetylcholine is present at nicotinic and muscarinic receptors and in the central nervous system. Acetylcholinesterase is responsible for the degradation of the acetylcholine molecule into two inactive agents, choline and acetic acid. Organophosphates and carbamates bind to the acetylcholinesterase molecule and inactivate it, and allow acetylcholine to remain at its receptor site.[23,31]

Organophosphates can be absorbed from almost any site, such as the lungs, the gastrointestinal tract, the eyes, and the skin. The time of onset for symptoms is usually quickest via the pulmonary route (2 to 3 minutes) and slowest via the skin (30 minutes).

After absorption, the signs and symptoms of OP toxicity correspond to the receptors that are stimulated. When muscarinic receptors are stimulated, the patient experiences salivation, lacrimation, contraction of the bladder muscle with involuntary urination, diarrhea, nausea,

and vomiting. These constellation of signs and symptoms forms the mnemonic "SLUDGE" (salivation, lacrimation, urination, defecation, gastroenteritis, and emesis).[42] Other signs may include miosis, bradycardia, and hypotension.[42] Bronchorrhea-induced hypoxia may result in mydriasis. Nicotinic manifestations may predominate if the OP exposure occurs via the dermal route. Nicotinic stimulation causes sympathomimetic stimulation, can cause mydriasis, tachycardia, some bronchodilation, and increased blood pressure,[28] and leads to excessive muscle activity, fasciculation, weakness, and eventually flaccidity. Patients may complain of painful involuntary contractions of their muscles. Respiratory muscle fatigue can occur[20] and leads to respiratory arrest if bronchorrhea is severe.

Theoretically, carbamates do not cross the blood-brain barrier, but OP can alter the acetylcholinesterase in the CNS and lead to CNS depression, lethargy, coma, irritability, and seizures.[13,32] Survivors of OP poisoning do not suffer residual deficit in their cognitive function as a direct cause of the OP.[25]

The subacute form of OP toxicity (also called *intermediate syndrome*) usually presents 3 to 5 days after an exposure to an OP. The syndrome is characterized by proximal muscle weakness and cranial nerve abnormalities. The etiology is unknown, and total recovery is the norm.[41] It has been postulated that these patients may not have received enough 2-PAM during their initial therapy and that this syndrome represents ongoing toxicity.[3,21]

Chronic toxicity from OP presents as a mixed motor and sensory neuropathy without cranial nerve involvement. The patient usually demonstrates a lower-extremity polyneuropathy. The patient may complain of weakness, parasthesia, tingling, and burning.[29] This phenomenon can occur after severe, life-threatening acute exposure as well as after minimal exposures that required no treatment. Symptoms begin 1 to 2 weeks after an exposure. Treatment is symptomatic, and there is no role for atropine or protopam in any of these patients. The course is often protracted and may be permanent.[2] It is theorized that inhibition of neurotoxic esterase is the cause (see Chapter 4).

Laboratory diagnosis. Organophosphates inhibit all acetylcholinesterases, in particular, red blood cell (RBC) (true) cholinesterase and plasma (pseudo) cholinesterase. The RBCs, CNS, lungs, and spleen contain RBC (true) cholinesterase, while the liver, heart, pancreas, and some other parts of the nervous system contain plasma (pseudo) cholinesterase.[35] Depression of RBC cholinesterase is a more accurate determinant of OP exposure because it is not influenced by extrinsic factors such as liver or pancreatic disease. Unfortunately, the normal range is wide and variable, and interpretation is difficult without a baseline value. Serial levels may be very important in exterminators to monitor toxicity.

Obtaining a baseline level with monthly follow-up levels is a sufficient screening process for exterminators.[8,9] Exterminators with symptoms or a drop in enzyme activity should be removed from work until the enzyme activity has returned to normal or the symptoms abate.[8,9]

The RBC cholinesterase activity regenerates at about 1% per day. Plasma cholinesterase activity returns to normal in about 6 to 8 weeks but may be very variable because of other disease processes, malnutrition, or concurrent illness.[30] In either case, close monitoring of the level and attention to safety precautions in an effort to prevent toxicity is definitely warranted.

Therapy. Use a four-part treatment plan for these severely ill patients: (1) Protect your staff, (2) decontaminate the patient, (3) neutralize ongoing toxicity, and (4) prevent retoxicity.

All body fluids, including gastric contents and stool, may be contaminated with OP. Assume that the clothing, shoes, and undergarments may have become saturated with OP. Because of this, strict adherence to protecting all staff members and the health care team from accidental exposure to these agents is important. This may require wearing goggles, impenetrable clothing, gloves, and protective barriers for their shoes. Good ventilation in the area where decontamination will be taking place is also necessary. Hospital rubber gloves are permeable to organophosphates and should not be used in lieu of proper protection.

Remove and discard all clothing. Wipe down the patient with dry sterile dressings or dry rags to remove the remaining insecticide.

Atropine, a physiologic antagonist,[42] is the agent of choice for the immediate acute respiratory problems, and protopam (2-PAM), an oxime, is necessary for regeneration of the enzyme and treatment of the nicotinic dysfunction.[33,43]

Atropine, an anticholinergic agent, is effective in treating the muscarinic symptoms. It is capable of reversing all these symptoms but has no effect on the nicotinic symptoms.[40] Therefore, in patients who present with the SLUDGE syndrome, atropine is the agent of choice. Patients who exhibit respiratory compromise require immediate and potentially large amounts of atropine. In severe OP poisoning, treat bronchorrhea with 2 mg of atropine, and repeat this every 2 to 3 minutes until it resolves. The total dose of atropine administered may exceed 500 mg.[18] Watch for signs and symptoms of atropinization: tachycardia, altered mental status, mydriasis, spasm of accommodation, and red, dry, flushed skin.

Protopam has the majority of its effect on the nicotinic component of the toxicity and must be used with atropine.[11,38] Protopam binds to the OP while it sits on the serine site and removes it from the acetylcholinesterase enzyme.[34] It should be administered early in the exposure to prevent the OP from "aging"—or binding irreversibly—to the enzyme. If the protopam is not administered within 24 to 36 hours, its benefits may be negligible. However, since it is not clear when "aging" occurs and 2-PAM is rather benign, it may be beneficial to use it any time after the exposure in a seriously ill patient.[4,5,10] In addition, 2-PAM may be useful in fat-soluble OP that is released from tissue even days after the exposure.

Theoretically, carbamates do not "age" because they are bound to acetylcholinestrase in a reversible manner. Despite this, these patients should also be treated with protopam because of its atropine-enhancing effects. There is one case report of a patient who was exposed to carbaryl (a carbamate) who deteriorated after protopam administration without concomitant atropine administration. However, this has never been reported with any other carbamate.[9,42]

There are few side effects of protopam. If it is administered too quickly, the patient may exhibit dizziness, hypotension, and "intoxication."[24] Rarely, if given rapidly, cardiac or respiratory arrest may ensue.[37,39] The nonlethal side effects can be prevented or resolved by administering the agent slowly.

Pyrethrins. Along with organophosphates (and carbamates), pyrethrins constitute the other large group of agents employed by exterminators as insecticides. These highly effective insecticides are derived from the flower of the chrysanthemum cinerariaefolium plant and are nontoxic to the environment. Synthetic pyrethroids are more stable and also less toxic than pyrethrins.[47] Pipcronyl butoxide, which is added to enhance their effect, is not associated with human toxicity.

Unlike insects, humans have the ability to metabolize pyrethrins to nontoxic substances via the microsomal enzymes in the liver.[7] The mechanism of action of these agents is by alteration in sodium channel function and ATPase function, although these are not definitively proven.[12] Their rapid onset of action led to their use as "knock down" agents for stinging insects.

Human toxicity is dermatologic, neurologic, and pulmonary.[45] Dermatologic complications such as dermatitis, vesicular formation, facial itching, burning, and irritation of the eyes are the most common complaints.[15,27] The itching and burning may be relieved with topical vitamin E.[1,15,16]

Asthma usually is triggered in patients with preexisting allergy.[36] Exterminators with these conditions may be more likely to develop bronchospasm or rhinitis when exposed to a pyrethroid.[36] There is one case report of hypersensitivity pneumonitis.[6]

The neurologic complications of these agents includes hyperactivity, lethargy, confusion, coma, and seizures.[17] They may act as γ-aminobutyric acid (GABA) receptor antagonists.[22]

REFERENCES

1. Adamis Z et al: Occupational exposure to organophorous insecticides and pyrethroid, *Int Arch Occup Environ Health* 56:299, 1985.
2. Barret DS, Oehme FW: A review of organophosphate ester induced neurotoxicity, *Vet Hum Toxicol* 27:22, 1985.

3. Benson BJ, Tolo D, McIntire M: Is the intermediate syndrome in organophosphate poisoning the result of insufficient oxime therapy? *J Toxicol Clin Toxicol* 30:347, 1992.

4. Blaber LC, Creasy NH: The mode of recovery of cholinesterase activity in vivo after organophosphorous poisoning: 1. Erythrocyte cholinesterase, *Biochem J* 77:591, 1960.

5. Blaber LC, Creasy NH: The mode of recovery of cholinesterase activity in vivo after organophosphorous poisoning: 11. Brain cholinesterase, *Biochem J* 77:597, 1960.

6. Carlson JE, Villaveces JW: Hypersensitivity pneumonitis due to pyrethrins, *JAMA* 237:1718, 1977.

7. Casida JE: Oxidative metabolism of pyrethrins in mammals, *Nature* 230:326, 1971.

8. Coye MJ et al: Clinical confirmation of organophosphate poisoning by serial cholinesterase analysis, *Arch Intern Med* 147:438, 1987.

9. Coye MJ et al: Clinical confirmation of organophosphate poisoning of agricultural worker, *Am J Ind Med* 10:399, 1986.

10. Davies DR, Green AL: The kinetics of reactivation, by oximes, of cholinesterase inhibited by organophorous compounds, *Biochemistry* 63:529, 1956.

11. Dikart WL, Kiestra SH, Sangster B: The use of atropine and oximes in organophosphate intoxication: a modified approach, *J Toxicol Clin Toxicol* 26:199, 1988.

12. Dorman DC, Beasley VR: Neurotoxicity of pyrethrin and pyrethroid insecticides, *Vet Hum Toxicol* 33:238, 1991.

13. Durham WF, Hayes WJ: Organic phosphorus poisoning and its therapy, *Arch Environ Health* 5:21, 1962.

14. Feldman RJ, Mailbach HI: Percutaneous penetration of some pesticides and herbicides in man, *Toxicol Appl Pharmacol* 28:126, 1974.

15. Flannigan SA, Tucker SB: Variations in cutaneous sensation between synthetic pyrethroid insecticides, *Contact Dermatitis* 13:140, 1985.

16. Flannigan SA et al: Synthetic pyrethroid insecticide. A dermatological evaluation, *Br J Ind Med* 43:363, 1985.

17. Goldfrank L, Flomenbaum N, Weisman R: Rodenticides, *Hospital Physician* 17:87, 1991.

18. Golsousidis H, Kokas V: Use of 19590 mg of atropine during 24 days of treatment after a case of unusually severe parathion poisoning, *Human Toxicol*, 4:339, 1985.

19. Gryboski J, Weinstein D, Ordway NK: Toxic encephalopathy related to the use of an insect repellent, *N Engl J Med* 264:289, 1961.

20. Gutman L, Besser R: Organophosphate intoxication: pharmacologic, neurophysiologic, clinical and therapeutic considerations, *Semin Neurol* 10:46, 1990.

21. Haddad LM: Organophosphate poisoning: intermediate syndrome? *J Toxicol Clin Toxicol* 30:331, 1992.

22. He F et al: Clinical manifestations and diagnosis of acute pyrethroid poisoning, *Arch Toxicol* 63:54, 1989.

23. Holmstedt B: Pharmacology of organophosphorus cholinesterase inhibitors, *Pharmacol Rev* 11:567, 1959.

24. Jager BV, Staff GN: Toxicity of diacetyl monoxime and of 2 pyridine-2-aldoxime methiodide in man, *Bull John Hopkins Hosp* 102:203, 1958.

25. Joubert J, Joubert PH, Von Graan E: Acute organophosphate poisoning presenting with choreoathetosis, *Clin Toxicol* 22:187, 1984.

26. Lamberg SI, Mulrennan JA: Bullous reaction to diethyltolumide, *Arch Dermatol* 100:582, 1969.

27. Le Quesne PM, Maxwell IC, Butterworth STG: Transient facial sensory symptoms following exposure to synthetic pyrethroids: a clinical and electrophysiological assessment, *Neurotoxicology* 2:1, 1980.

28. Lerman Y, Hirschberg A, Shteger Z: Organophosphate and carbamate pesticide poisoning, *Am J Ind Med* 6:17, 1984.

29. Metcalf RL, Swift TR, Sikes RK: Neurological findings among workers exposed to fenion in a veterinary hospital, Georgia, *MMWR Morb Mortal Wkly Rep* 34:402, 1985.

30. Midtling JE et al: Clinical management of field worker organophosphate poisoning, *West J Med* 42:514, 1985.

31. Milby T: Prevention and management of organophosphate poisoning, *JAMA* 216:2131, 1971.

32. Minton NA, Murray SG: A review of organophosphate poisoning, *Med Toxicol* 3:350, 1988.

33. Namba T, Hiraki K: PAM (pyridine-2-aldoxime methiodide) therapy for alkyl-phosphate poisoning, *JAMA* 166:1834, 1958.

34. Namba T et al: Poisoning due to organophosphate insecticides: acute and chronic manifestations, *Am J Med* 50:475, 1971.

35. Nelson TC, Buritt MF: Pesticide poisoning, succinylcholine induced apnea and pseudocholinesterase, *Mayo Clin Proc* 61:750, 1986.

36. Paton DL, Walker JS: Pyrethrin poisoning from commercial strength flea and tick spray, *Am J Emerg Med* 6:232, 1988.

37. Pickering EN: Organic phosphate insecticide poisoning, *Can J Med Technol* 28:174, 1966.

38. Quimby GE: Further therapeutic experience with pralidoxime in organic phosphorous pesticide poisoning, *JAMA* 187:114, 1964.

39. Scott RJ: Repeated asystole following PAM in organophosphate self poisoning, *Anaesth Intensive Care* 4:458, 1986.

40. Selden BS, Curry SC: Prolonged succinycholine-induced paralysis in organophosphate insecticide poisoning, *Ann Emerg Med* 16:215, 1987.

41. Senanayake N, Karalliedde L: Neurotoxicity of organophosphorous insecticides, *N Engl J Med* 316:761, 1987.

42. Tafuri J, Robbers J: Organophosphate poisoning, *Ann Emerg Med* 16:193, 1987.

43. Taylor P: Anticholinesterase agents. In Gillman AG, Goodman LS, Gilman A, editors: *The pharmacologic basis of therapeutics*, ed 6, New York, 1980, Macmillan.

44. Tenenbein M: Severe toxic reactions and death following the ingestion of diethyltoluamide insect repellents, *JAMA* 258:1509, 1987.

45. Wax PM, Hoffman RS: Fatality associated with inhalation of a pyrethrin shampoo, *J Toxicol Clin Toxicol* 32:457, 1994.

46. Whorton D et al: Testicular function in DBCP exposed pesticide workers, *J Occup Med* 21:161, 1979.

47. Wouters W, Van den Berken J: Review: Action of pyrethroids, *Gen Pharmacol* 9:387, 1978.

Farmers and Farm Personnel

NO   NO$_2$

NH$_3$

CH$_4$

- Anhydrous ammonia is a caustic that causes severe respiratory and skin toxicity

- Silos produce complex gaseous hazards

- Confinement facilities are an ongoing source of toxic exposures

- Farming is one of the most hazardous of all occupations

Ricky Lee Langley

William J. Meggs

OCCUPATIONAL DESCRIPTION

Farmwork is one of the most hazardous occupations in the world. While the total number of farmworkers has declined in industrialized countries, the death rate remains higher than in other occupations.[18] The mortality rate in agriculture varies from 20.7 to 49 deaths per year per 100,000 farmworkers. By comparison, from 7.9 to 10 deaths per year per 100,000 workers are reported for the nonagricultural work force.[18]

A *farm* is defined as an establishment that in a normal year sells $1000 worth or more per year of agricultural products.[26] In 1992, there were an estimated 2,950,740 working farms in the United States. In 1991, 4,632,000 individuals (1.8% of the total U.S. population) lived on farms.[26] The number of workers on a farm varies with the season, with up to 3 million individuals working on farms during peak seasons. The majority of workers on farms are unpaid labor. Accidents and injuries vary with geography and with the type of animal or crop produced. Agricultural machinery is the major cause of death and disability on farms,[12,19,24] with tractor rollovers and runovers as the cause of the majority of machinery fatalities. Other common injuries on farms include animal attacks, falling objects, electric shock, fires, gas and chemical exposures, cave-ins, lightning, drowning, and asphyxiation.[12,21]

There are many other potential hazards on the farm, including zoonotic infections in farm animals, sun-related injuries, cold-related injuries, vibration, and noise. This chapter discusses the toxic hazards associated with farming.

POTENTIAL TOXIC EXPOSURES

Numerous chemicals are either produced or used on a farm. Some chemicals are purchased and have warnings and information about toxic potential. Failure to adhere to product use guidelines, inadvertent mishaps, and improper storage can lead to toxic exposures and poisonings. Toxic chemicals that are produced on the farm, such as hydrogen sulfide and methane from manure decomposition and nitrogen oxides from silage, can be deadly. Exposures to toxins resulting from fertilizer use, equipment use, the use of pesticides and fumigants, animal confinement facilities, and silos are discussed. Insecticide use is discussed in Chapter 13.

CLINICAL TOXICOLOGY
Fertilizers

Pathophysiology, biochemistry, management. Fertilizers are substances used to enhance and restore soil composition in order to increase crop yield. Fertilizer is generally a combination of nitrogen, phosphates, lime, and potash. A variety of forms and compositions exist, and fertilizer chemicals can be applied singly or in combination. Granular fertilizer is not as hazardous as gases and liquids.

Anhydrous ammonia fertilizer is a gas at atmospheric pressure; under pressure, it is a liquid. When dissolved in water, anhydrous ammonia forms an extremely alkaline solution that can cause severe burns of the eyes, skin, and mucous membranes.[3] Ocular exposure can result in severe corneal burns. First- and second-degree burns of the skin can occur as well. Exposure time and concentration are the primary determinants of the severity of these burns. The odor warning threshold for ammonia is 53 parts per million. This provides some margin of safety, as most severe effects related to ammonia occur at levels well in excess of this odor threshold. At the irritant threshold of 400 ppm, irritation of the eyes, nose, and throat occurs. Immediate eye injury occurs at exposures of 700 ppm. At 1700 ppm, laryngeal spasm and coughing can occur. Exposures of 2500 to 4500 ppm for 30 minutes can be lethal, while an exposure of 5000 ppm is rapidly fatal.[9,16] Upper airway edema can develop rapidly and leads to cyanosis and asphyxiation. Noncardiac pulmonary edema or adult respiratory distress syndrome has been reported after ammonia exposure. Chronic sequelae to an acute exposure can include bronchiolitis obliterans and chronic cystic bronchiectasis.[9,16]

After eye or skin exposure to ammonia, exposed areas should be decontaminated by copious flushing with water. Large amounts of water should be used, and irrigation should be prolonged. After eye exposures, several liters of water irrigation may be necessary, and irrigation should continue until after the pH of the tears has normalized (allow 10 minutes for equilibration after terminating lavage). The eye should be carefully examined with fluorescein to check for corneal damage, which should be treated using standard protocols for corneal injury due to alkali substances. Chemical burns to the skin should be treated like any other burn of similar size, location, and thickness.

Inhalation exposures to ammonia can be devastating. At the scene, victims should be removed to fresh air, and the emergency medical services system activated. Patency of the airway and adequacy of respirations and oxygenation should be verified. Endotracheal intubation and mechanical ventilation may need to be instituted. Since the onset of pulmonary edema may be delayed, a victim without initial pulmonary symptoms should be observed for at least 12 hours. A follow-up chest x-ray should be obtained before discharge from the emergency department.

Exposure to concentrated anhydrous ammonia most often occurs during the transfer from supply tanks to applicator tanks. Damaged hoses, leaking valves, and disconnected hoses are the main sources of exposure.[3]

Well water can become contaminated with nitrates from fertilizers, septic tanks, and animal manure. Infants of farm families who use well water are particularly at risk for developing methemoglobinemia from contaminated water. This increased susceptibility of infants is due to their relative absence of methemoglobin reductase, lower levels of reduced nicotinamide adenine dinucleotide phosphate (NADPH) in their red blood cells, and the sensitivity of fetal hemoglobin to oxidative stresses.

An in-depth discussion of the toxic hazards involved in fertilizer production and use is found in Chapter 40.

TOXINS ASSOCIATED WITH FARM EQUIPMENT

Farmers usually operate and repair a wide variety of farm machinery. In addition, they generally maintain and repair the buildings in which the machinery is housed. Solvents such as gasoline, diesel fuel, paint thinners and strippers, mineral spirits, kerosene, hydraulic fluids, and greases are used.[23] Many of these substances are flammable and potentially explosive. Farmers and farmworkers are exposed occupationally to solvents through skin contact, inhalation, and ingestion.

Solvents commonly act as upper respiratory and mucous membrane irritants. Central nervous system symptoms, such as dizziness, dysphagia, slurred speech, and mental confusion, can occur after systemic absorption. Seizure, coma, and death can occur in severe cases. Organic solvents can sensitize the myocardium to endogenous catecholamines, resulting in cardiac arrhythmias and sudden death.[20] Solvents defat the skin and cause dermatitis and, at high concentrations, severe burns.

Oral siphoning of gasoline with a rubber hose can lead to ingestion and aspiration. Severe lung injury can result from aspiration of hydrocarbons, including gasoline.[23]

Farmers occasionally solder or weld broken equipment, so welding hazards such as inhalation of metal fumes, ozone, nitrogen dioxide, or carbon dioxide are a toxicologic concern. Carbon monoxide toxicity associated with the use of high-pressure washing equipment has also been reported.[5] Metal fume fever, most commonly associated with zinc fumes and resulting from welding galvanized materials, is discussed in Chapter 36.

Gloves and protective clothing are essential when farmers work with chemical agents. Welding goggles and safety goggles can protect the eye from keratitis and chemical injuries. Chemicals on the skin should be removed immediately with water, and contaminated clothing should be removed. Children on farms present a special problem with regard to chemical exposures. Farm chemicals should be stored in sealed containers in secured areas, and children should be warned of chemical hazards.

TOXINS ASSOCIATED WITH ANIMAL CONFINEMENT

During the past 25 years, there has been increasing use of confinement facilities to raise cattle, pigs, and poultry. Almost a million workers are employed in these confinement facilities. These large buildings frequently house thousands of animals and generate large amounts of animal waste products. The waste usually drains through floor grates into a containment area. In other systems, the wastes are washed into gullies in the concrete floor and then into a storage pond or lagoon. Anaerobic degeneration of manure produces more than 150 different gases, most of which are toxic. Various alcohols, acids, amines, carbonyls, sulfides, nitrogen heterocycles, esters, mercaptans, and disulfides, as well as carbon monoxide, methane, ammonia, and hydrogen sulfide, are produced. Oxygen depletion may occur near the surface of the manure. Many deaths have been recorded when farmworkers are engaged in cleaning out manure pits. From 1982 to 1992, NIOSH recorded 104 fatalities in 68 such incidents in animal confinement facilities.[6] A manure pit should be entered only with self-contained breathing equipment and a partner located in immediate proximity, should an emergency arise.

Methane and carbon dioxide are simple asphyxiants. It is important to remember that death can occur from oxygen deprivation as well as exposure to these toxins. Methane can even accumulate to explosive levels. With ventilation system failure, carbon dioxide from animal pulmonary expiration can also rise to dangerous levels.

Hydrogen sulfide gas is a highly toxic metabolic poison similar to cyanide in its action. Cytochrome oxidase activity is blocked, so aerobic respiration ceases. The noxious rotten egg odor of hydrogen sulfide does not persist with continued exposure due to the effects of hydrogen sulfide on the olfactory apparatus. Above 150 ppm, the olfactory apparatus is quickly fatigued and paralyzed, and danger

may exist but not be recognized. Any exposure to a rotten egg odor should lead to evacuation of the area until risk can be determined. (See Chapter 32 for a complete discussion.)

Respiratory problems associated with confinement housing include the organic toxic dust syndrome, acute and chronic bronchitis, occupational asthma, chronic obstructive pulmonary disease, and hypersensitivity pneumonitis.[11]

TOXIC GASES IN SILOS

Silos are storage facilities for silage and animal feed. Silage is a fermented form of animal feed that is formed when bacteria digest a variety of crops, including corn, oats, and alfalfa. There are three basic types of silo structures on farms: oxygen-limited silos, conventional silos, and trench silos.[17] Trench silos have earth or concrete retaining walls with no structural component covering the top, and they hence have generally not been associated with respiratory hazards. Oxygen-limited silos have openings limited to the top of the silo and at the base for unloading the silage. As a result of limited ventilation, oxygen levels tend to be diminished, while carbon dioxide levels are high. Unprotected entry into an oxygen-limited silo can be immediately life-threatening from asphyxiation. Toxic levels of oxides of nitrogen can occur in oxygen-limited silos. Conventional silos have a series of small doors along the entire height of the silo. These doors provide access from which silage is unloaded. Conventional silos neither limit oxygen nor capture carbon dioxide. The danger of asphyxiation is much less in a conventional silo than in an oxygen-limited silo. The primary hazard associated with conventional silos results from the generation of oxides of nitrogen that are produced during the fermentation of silage.

Hazards from silos include becoming trapped in the grain and drowning, death from asphyxiation due to oxygen depletion, and the high levels of oxides of nitrogen within the silo.[4,12] Silo gases may seep out of the silo into nearby barns and affect both the animals and workers in the barn.

As the silage ferments, concentrations of carbon dioxide and oxides of nitrogen increase. Levels begin to rise within a few hours of loading the silo and reach peak concentrations in approximately 48 to 60 hours. High concentrations of these gases have been known to persist for several weeks. Nitrogen dioxide has an odor reminiscent of household bleach and may be visible as a slightly yellow or red-brown haze over silage. Inhaled nitrogen dioxide gas reacts with water in the airway to form acidic compounds that can result in severe pulmonary injury. This injury leads to the disorder known as *silo filler's disease*. Duration of exposure is one of the most essential determinants of clinical symptoms. Immediate upper airway irritation may occur after exposure, but it is important to remember that symptoms can be delayed for several hours. Cough, shortness of breath, light-headedness, choking, syncope, wheezing, chest pain, weakness, and eye and throat irritation may also occur. With increasing exposure, pulmonary edema or focal bronchial pneumonia may occur. After severe and prolonged exposures, symptoms may at first improve and then be followed by a clinical relapse 2 to 3 weeks later. The symptoms consistent with relapse include dyspnea, fever, and cough. This clinical relapse is due to the development of bronchiolitis obliterans, which represents a destruction of deep bronchial cells and subsequent sloughing of necrotic tissues. On occasion, an individual who develops bronchiolitis obliterans subsequently develops permanent pulmonary dysfunction.[11,14]

Concentrations of nitrogen dioxide greater than 200 ppm can be expected to produce immediate loss of consciousness. Sudden death can occur immediately upon entry into a silo structure because of high concentrations of nitrogen oxides. Acute laryngospasm, respiratory arrest, and asphyxiation are usually the clinical manifestations responsible for the sudden death in this setting. High levels of nitrogen dioxide are usually accompanied by oxygen depletion and high levels of carbon dioxide. It is important to remember that silo filler's disease must be differentiated from silo unloader's syndrome and farmer's lung disease.

Farmer's lung disease is a hypersensitivity pneumonitis related to inhalation of thermophilic actinomycetes and fungi. Acute farmer's lung presents with abrupt onset of high fever, chills, muscle aches, cough, and shortness of breath within 4 to 8 hours after exposure to dust from decomposing feed material from the top layer of silage. Chest radiography demonstrates diffuse ground-glass infiltrates, and pulmonary function testing shows restrictive lung disease. Subacute farmer's lung disease has a more gradual onset, with fever, night sweats, and weight loss accompanying productive cough and dyspnea. Permanent impairment of pulmonary function occurs in a few cases. Bronchoalveolar lavage in farmer's lung disease often identifies lymphocytosis in the airways. Lung biopsy reveals a mononuclear alveolitis with granuloma formation.

Silo unloader's syndrome is a form of organic dust toxic syndrome associated with a significant exposure to moldy elements at the top of a silo, generally when a silo is first opened or uncapped and moldy silage is handled. This syndrome is thought to be due to endotoxins, which are products from the cell wall of gram-negative bacteria. Mycotoxins, proteinases, and endogenous histamines may also play a role in this syndrome.[7] Silo unloader's syndrome is characterized by flulike symptoms, fever, malaise, muscle aches, headache, cough, chest tightness, wheezing, mild dyspnea, and nasal and throat irritation. Chest radiography and pulmonary function tests are usually normal. There may be a mild granulocytosis. Bronchoalveolar lavage and lung biopsy show neutrophil alveolitis and bronchitis with no granulomas. Organic dust toxic syndrome is not associated with long-term sequelae. Most individuals are able to return to work in a few days with symptomatic treatment.[11]

ANIMAL FEED, ADDITIVES, AND DISINFECTANTS

Numerous chemicals, including antibiotics and trace metals, are routinely added to animal feed as growth promoters and prophylaxis for disease. Handling animal feeds results in skin contact with a variety of chemicals. Ethylenediaminedihydroiodine, furazolidone, hydroquinone, and halquinol have all been implicated as causes of contact dermatitis. Ethyoxyquin (an antioxidant in animal feed) has been reported to cause contact dermatitis. The growth-promoting factor quindoxin can also cause photocontact dermatitis.

Other commonly used antibiotics causing dermatitis include neomycin, ethylenediamine, thiobendazole, sulfacetamide, sulfamethazine, tetracyclines, and bacitracin. Allergic reactions to nitrofurazone and tylosin in animal feed can occur. Manganese oxide is used as an additive in animal and poultry feed and can potentially cause central nervous system damage[25] (see Chapter 37).

Disinfectants used on animal farms can cause allergic or irritant reactions. Hypochlorite, iodine, and phenols are known to cause contact dermatitis. Allergic contact dermatitis can develop to rubberized clothing worn while working with animals. Chromate is used to preserve milk to be tested for quality control purposes, and there are documented cases of chromate allergy in milk testers.[1]

MYCOTOXINS

Mycotoxins are by-products of fungal metabolism that produce toxic effects when inhaled or ingested. Mycotoxins can contaminate foods and feeds such as nuts, corn, cotton seed, wheat, millet, sorghum, barley, peas, sesame, soybeans, cowpeas, Brazil nuts, pistachio nuts, almonds, beans, and sweet potatoes. Drought, high temperatures, insect infestation, and high humidity favor the growth of fungi and the production of mycotoxins in the fields.[8]

Of the numerous mycotoxins, aflatoxins, ochratoxins, trichothecenes, and zearalenones are the most troublesome.[22] Mycotoxins are responsible for numerous deaths among animals each year. The production of mycotoxins is lessened by proper food and feed cultivation and storage practices.

The most widely known mycotoxins are the aflatoxins. These substituted coumarin compounds are produced by *Aspergillus flavus* and *A. parasiticus*. Aflatoxins are known carcinogens and immune suppressers and have been associated with liver cancer. Reports of acute effects from aflatoxin ingestion are unusual in the United States. Reports of death due to hepatic failure and massive gastrointestinal hemorrhage among persons ingesting aflatoxin-contaminated grains have occurred in other countries.[8] In the United State, the federal Food and Drug Administration has responsibility to regulate aflatoxin levels in foods.

Suspended, Canceled, and Restricted Pesticides

Alar	Lead arsenate
Aldrin	Lindane
Amitraz	Mercury
Arsenic trioxide	Metaldehyde
Benomyl	Mirex
BHC	Monocrotophos
Bithionol	Ompa
Bromoxynil	10,10'-Oxybisphenoxarsine
Bromoxynil butyrate	Oxyfluorfen
Cadmium	Parathion (ethyl)
Calcium arsenate	PCNB
Captafol	Pentachlorophenol
Captan	Phenarsazine chloride
Carbon tetrachloride	Polychlorinated biphenyls
Chloranil	Polychlorinated terphenyls
Chlordane	Pronamide
Chlordimeform	Quaternary ammonium
Chlorobenzilate	compounds
Copper arsenate (basic)	Safrole
Creosote	Seed treatments
Cyanazine	Silvex/2,4,5-T
Cyhexatin	Sodium arsenate
DBCP	Sodium arsenite
Daminozide	Sodium cyanide
DDD (TDE)	Sodium fluoride
DDT	Sodium monofluoroacetate
2,4-D	Strobane
Dinoseb	Strychnine
Disinfectants	2,4,5-T
EBDCs	2,4,5-TCP
EDB	Thallium sulfate
Endrin	Toxaphene
EPN	Tributyltin (TBT)
Fluoroacetamide	Trifluralin
Heptachlor	Vinyl chloride
Kepone	

From Office of Compliance Monitoring, Office of Pesticides and Toxic Substances, U.S. Environmental Protection Agency (EPA), February 1990.

Pesticides Known to Cause Allergic Reactions

Allidochlor	Dichloropropene
Anilazine	Lindane
Antu	Maneb
Barban	Nitrofen
Benomyl	Propachlor
Captafol	Pyrethrum/pyrethroids
Captan	Rotenone
Dazomet	Thiram
Dichloropropane	Zineb

From *Allergy and pesticides,* North Carolina Cooperative Extension Service, January 1994.

TOXICITY OF PESTICIDES

Pesticides commonly used on farms include insecticides, herbicides, fungicides, and rodenticides (see Chapters 13 and 16 and boxes above).

Several classes of herbicides are in general use and can pose health hazards for farmers. Of the chlorphenoxy herbicides, 2,4-dichlorophenoxyacetic acid (2,4-D) is effective against broad-leaf plants and is commonly used as a weed killer on lawns and grain crops. Toxicity can result from ingestion, dermal contact, and inhalation, and multiple organ systems can be affected. Nausea, vomiting, diarrhea, pulmonary edema, cardiac arrythmias, bradycardia, muscle twitches, and myotonia have been reported. Dermal exposure to concentrated solutions can cause chemical burns. Peripheral neuropathy has been associated with chronic exposure. Painful paresthesias and muscle stiffness have been described.[13] Exposure of farmers has been shown to increase the risk of non-Hodgkin's lymphoma in a dose-dependent fashion.[27] The defoliating substance Agent Orange that was used extensively in Vietnam by U.S. forces was a mixture of 2,4-D and 2,4,5-trichlorophenoxyacetic acid (2,4,5-T), a herbicide that was banned in the United States in 1979 because of contamination with the by-product 2,3,7,8-tetrachlorodibenzo-p-dioxin (TCDD). The acute phase postexposure is characterized by gastrointestinal symptoms, hypotension, tachycardia, and coma. This may be followed by a transient peripheral neuropathy in the recovery phase.[15,19]

The urea substituted pesticides diuron, linuron, monolinuron, and monuron are inhibitors of photosynthesis. This class of herbicides presents only limited potential for systemic toxicity. These pesticides can be associated with the development of methemoglobinemia after ingestion. In cases of ingestion, the patient should be observed for cyanosis and monitored for elevated methemoglobin levels.

Endothall is a herbicide that is a mucous membrane and skin irritant. With ingestion, endothall has been reported to cause gastrointestinal hemorrhage, hypotension, disseminated intravascular coagulopathy, and death.[2,10]

Paraquat and diquat are herbicides of low toxicity from incidental inhalation exposure with field use, but ingestion can lead to devastating pulmonary toxicity.

REFERENCES

1. Abrams K, Hogan D, Maibach H: Pesticide related dermatoses in agricultural workers, *Occup Med* 6:463, 1991.
2. Allender WJ: Suicidal poisoning by endothall, *J Anal Toxicol* 7:79, 1983.
3. Centers for Disease Control: *Anhydrous ammonia safety,* NIOSH pub 93-131, 1993.
4. Centers for Disease Control: *NIOSH warns farmers of deadly risk of grain suffocation,* NIOSH update pub 93-116, April 28, 1993.
5. Centers for Disease Control: *NIOSH warns of carbon monoxide hazard using pressure washers indoors,* NIOSH update pub 93-117, May 10, 1993.

6. Centers for Disease Control: *NIOSH warns: manure pits continue to claim lives,* NIOSH update pub 93-114, July 6, 1993.

7. Centers for Disease Control: *Preventing organic dust toxic syndrome,* NIOSH alert, pub 94-102, April 1994.

8. Coulombe RA Jr: Aflatoxins in mycotoxins and phytoalexins. In CRC Handbook of Microbiology. Sharma RP, editor: Boca Raton, Fla, 1991, CRC Press.

9. Dalton M, Bricker D: Anhydrous burn of the respiratory tract, *Tex Med* 74:51, 1978.

10. Day LC: Delayed death by endothall, a herbicide, *Vet Hum Toxicol* 30:366, 1988.

11. Do Pico G: Hazardous exposure in lung disease among farm workers, *Clin Chest Med* 13:311, 1992.

12. Etherton J et al: Agricultural machine related deaths, *Am J Public Health* 198:766, 1991.

13. Goldstein NP, Jones PH, Brown JR: Peripheral neuropathy after exposure to an ester of dichlorophenoxyacetic acid, *JAMA* 171:1306, 1959.

14. Grover J, Ellwood P: Gasses in forage tower silos, *Ann Occup Hyg* 33:519, 1989.

15. Hayes WH Jr: *Pesticides studied in man,* Baltimore, 1982, Williams & Wilkins.

16. Millec T, Kucan J, Smoot CE III: Anhydrous injuries, *J Burn Care Rehabil* 10:448, 1989.

17. Murphy DJ: *Safety and health for production agriculture,* Washington DC 1992, American Society of Agricultural Engineers.

18. National Safety Council: *Accident facts,* 1993, Itasca, Ill, The Council.

19. O'Reilly JF: Prolonged coma and delayed peripheral neuropathy after ingestion of phenoxyacettic weed killers, *Postgrad Med J* 60:76, 1984.

20. Proctor N, Hughes J, Fischman M: Chemical hazards of the workplace, ed 2, Philadelphia, 1988, Lippincott Co.

21. Purschwitz M, Field W: Scope and magnitude of injuries in the agricultural workplace, *Am J Ind Med* 18:179, 1990.

22. Schneider E, Dickert K: Health costs and benefits of fungicide use in agriculture: a literature review, *J AgroMed* 1:19, 1994.

23. Shaver C, Tong T: Chemical hazards to agricultural workers, *Occup Med* 6:391, 1991.

24. Smith J, Rogers D, Sykes R: Farm tractor associated deaths—Georgia, *MMWR Morb Mortal Wkly Rep* 32:481, 1983.

25. Tanaka S: Manganese and its compounds. In Zena C, Dickerson OB, Horvath EP, editors: *Occupational Medicine,* St Louis, 1994, Mosby.

26. US Department of Agriculture: *Agriculture statistics 1992,* Washington, DC, 1992, US Government Printing Office.

27. Zahm SH et al: A case-control study of non-Hodgkin's lymphoma and the herbicide 2,4-dichlorophenoxyacetic acid (2,4-D) in eastern Nebraska, *Epidemiology* 1:349, 1990.

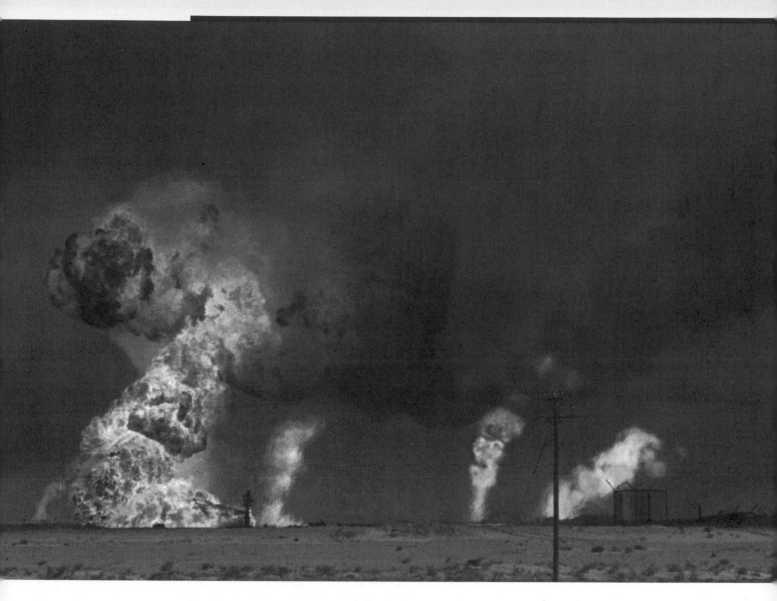

The oil fields of Kuwait continue to burn March 8. All 950 wells are either burning or in disrepair due to Iraqi sabotage. Some wells are expected to burn for more than a year. More than four million barrels of oil are burned daily. March 8, 1991.

(Courtesy Reuters/Corbis-Bettmann)

15

carbonyl fluoride

acrolein

Firefighters

Oliver L. Hung
Richard D. Shih

- Firefighters face toxins that range from pulmonary irritants to chemical and simple asphyxiants

- Solubility of pulmonary irritants determines the nature of clinical manifestations

- Hyperbaric oxygen remains the standard of care for carbon monoxide poisoning

- Sodium thiosulfate is the safe empiric treatment for presumed cyanide poisoning in fire victims

OCCUPATIONAL DESCRIPTION

Firefighters work in varied and complex environments that increase the risk of on-the-job death and injury. Each year, there are more than 100,000 firefighter injuries in the United States.[35] In 1993, there were 77 firefighter fatalities and an estimated 4850 firefighter injuries that required hospitalization.[35] Most injuries occur in the setting of fire emergencies or fireground operations. Of all injuries in 1993, 52,885 injuries (52.1%) occurred during fireground operations (Table 15-1).[35] Firefighters training during typical firefighting operations are shown in Figure 15-1. However, many firefighter injuries also occur during nonfire emergencies (e.g., rescue calls, hazardous materials calls, natural disasters), transport, training, or other on-duty settings (e.g., maintenance or inspection). This chapter focuses on the toxicologic manifestations of firefighter injuries, in particular, smoke inhalation injuries including carbon monoxide poisoning.

Smoke is the volatilized product of combustion. It varies according to the temperature, oxygen availability, and composition of the materials being burned.[52] The inhalational toxins contained in smoke are chemicals in the form of gases, vapors, aerosols, particulate, and fumes (see box on p. 115).[40] Some materials may produce many potentially toxic compounds. For example, polyvinyl chloride produces at least 75 potentially toxic agents, and wood produces as many as 200.[14,52] Temperature, oxygen availability, rate of burning, and ventilation affect the composition of smoke and the presence of inhalational toxins.

Injury from smoke is due to local pulmonary insult and systemic toxicity from the simple asphyxiant effects or systemic absorption of inhaled poisons. Local pulmonary insult results from thermal injury or chemical irritant injury

113

from gases or particulates. Simple asphyxiant effects occur when fire combustion consumes available oxygen or when inert inhalants displace the available oxygen of the environment. Systemic absorption of chemical asphyxiants such as cyanide further complicate toxicity.

Firefighting requires strenuous physical exertion, which increases oxygen demand and respiratory rate and thus in-

creases the risk of exposure to inhalational toxins and hypoxia.[66] Although all firefighters are equipped with respiratory protective equipment, they are not always used, particularly during the extinguishing or clean-up phases of firefighting, when smoke intensity and assumed exposure are thought to be low. The improper use of respiratory protective equipment at the scene of the fire is an important risk factor in the development of toxicity from smoke inhalation.[14,65]

TOXIC EXPOSURES
Physical Hazards

Thermal injuries. All building fires release a tremendous amount of heat into the air. The temperature of a top floor of a burning building may reach 900 to 1000° F. Fortunately, direct thermal lung parenchymal injury from smoke inhalation is rare. In general, inhaled smoke is composed of dry gases, which have a low heat capacity and a temperature of approximately 260° F.[40] The human respiratory tract has a

Table 15-1 Breakdown of fireground injuries, 1993[35]

Type of injury	Percentage
Strains, sprains, and muscle pains	35.6
Wounds, cuts, bleeding, and bruises	20.3
Burns	11.3
Smoke or gas inhalation	8.6

From Karter MJ, Lellane PR: US firefighter injuries in 1993, *NFPA Journal*, p. 57, Nov/Dec 1994.

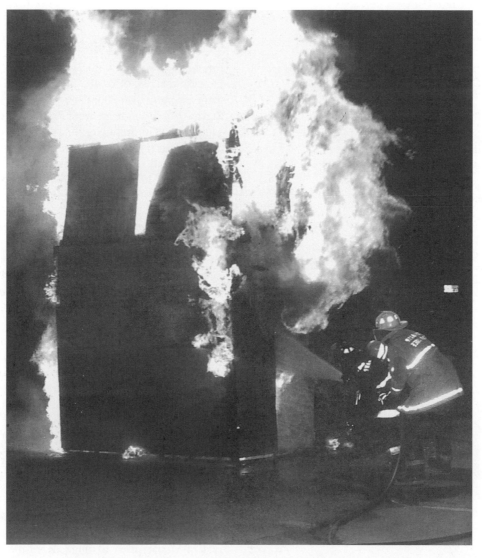

Fig. 15-1 Firefighters training during typical firefighting operations.

high heat-exchanging capacity that allows it to cool super-heated air before it passes the larynx.[8] In these situations, direct thermal injury is limited to the upper airway and rarely affects the pulmonary parenchyma. Pharyngeal edema, laryngeal edema, and laryngospasm are the classic signs of thermal injury to the upper airway, which can lead to life-threatening obstruction at the level of the vocal cords within the first 24 hours of presentation. In contrast, steam has 4000 times the heat-carrying capacity of hot air and may damage the entire respiratory system as far as the major bronchioles.[8] In conscious patients, the reflex closure of the larynx in response to heated gases may protect the distal airways from thermal injury. Patients with concomitant cutaneous burns and airway injuries have a high mortality. Smoke inhalation independently increases the mortality of cutaneous burns by 20%. If nosocomial pneumonia develops, burn mortality increases by 40%.[61]

Particulates. Soot particles (5 to 10 μm) are generally cleared by the respiratory tract. Occasionally, they may cause direct traumatic injury through nonspecific mechanical irritation of the upper respiratory tract or in massive exposures through anatomic obstruction of the airways.[27] Particulates such as hot cinders may also cause thermal injury to the respiratory tract. Particulates can also exacerbate airway injury caused by irritant gases. Irritant gases such as aldehydes and sulfur dioxide may adsorb to particulate matter, potentially increasing their contact with the mucosal surface of the tracheobronchial tree. This may result in increased damage to the affected airway. The site of injury depends on the size of the particulate. Particulates of 1- to 3-μm diameter are able to deposit in the alveoli. Those greater than 5 μm are unlikely to reach the alveoli.[48] At this

---

Definitions

Smoke. Volatilized product of combustion consisting of toxic gases and particulate matter.

Vapor. Gaseous phase of volatile liquid.

Gas. A substance is a gas if at standard conditions its normal physical state is gaseous.

Fume. Extremely fine, solid particulate formed by a process such as combustion or condensation. The term is generally applied to the condensation of metals from their gaseous state after volatilization and the subsequent formation of metal oxides. Fumes are usually 0.0001 to 1 μm in diameter.

Dust. Particulate formed from solid organic and inorganic material(s) reduced in size through a mechanical process such as crushing, drilling, grinding, blasting, or pulverization. Airborne dusts range from 0.1 to 25 μm in diameter.

Pyrolysis. Thermal degradation of organic material in oxygen-poor environment.

Combustion. Thermal degradation of organic material in oxygen-rich environment.

---

time, few studies have addressed the issue of toxicity related to particulate-toxin interaction.[38]

Chemical Irritants

Irritant inhalants have a direct cytotoxic effect on the epithelium of the oropharynx and respiratory tract and are capable of causing extensive damage to the airways and parenchyma. Highly water-soluble inhalants tend to remain in the upper airway because they dissolve in the mucous lining of the upper respiratory tract. Characteristic symptoms include irritation to the mucous membranes of the conjunctiva and upper airway, including the mouth, nose, throat, and bronchi. Highly water-soluble inhalants can also cause lower respiratory involvement if the patient is exposed to high levels of the irritant inhalant or has prolonged exposure. In these situations, the ability of the upper airway to "scrub out" the irritant inhalant from the inhaled air is overwhelmed, allowing penetration of the lower airways and possible consequent tissue damage.[40] Poorly water-soluble inhalants tend to affect the lower airway because they are less able to dissolve in the upper airway mucous lining. Exposed workers are often asymptomatic for hours or only mildly symptomatic. Bronchospasm and pulmonary edema continue to increase over the subsequent 24 hours.

Acrolein. Acrolein ($CH_2 = CHCHO$) is a highly water-soluble, three-carbon aldehyde that is the product of incomplete pyrolysis of organic materials (e.g., wood and cotton), tobacco, polymers, and plastics. It is the most common of the many aldehydes generated by fires.[36] It is also an intense irritant to the eyes and upper respiratory tract. At high concentrations, it can cause bronchitis and pulmonary edema.[2]

Although acrolein is toxic by all routes of exposure (dermal, oral, inhalational), it is primarily absorbed by inhalation. Consequently, the respiratory tract is the major site of injury. It has been shown to cause a reflex decrease in respiratory rate, ciliastasis, pulmonary hypersensitivity, and pulmonary edema. Although eye irritation is a common manifestation, eye injury has never been a reported clinical finding. Common symptoms of exposure include nasal irritation, cough, and dyspnea.

Exposure to 0.25 ppm can cause eye and skin irritation. The level immediately dangerous to life and health (IDLH) is 5 ppm. Exposure to 10 ppm may cause rapid pulmonary edema,[16,70] and 10-minute exposures have been fatal.[53] In a survey of 200 fires in Boston, 10% were noted to have acrolein levels exceeding 3 ppm.[70] Acrolein has been implicated as a major cause of fatalities due to smoke inhalation.[59]

Ammonia. Ammonia is a colorless, highly water-soluble alkaline gas that is highly irritating when in contact with the skin and mucous membranes. It easily dissolves in water to form the caustic solution ammonium hydroxide. In fires, it is liberated during combustion of nylon, silk, wood, and melamine.[59] Melamine is commonly used in office and household furnishings such as desks, bookshelves, and cupboards. In ordinary building fires, its concentrations in smoke is generally low.[66]

Symptoms of exposure include immediate irritation to the eyes, skin, and upper respiratory tract. Most will notice a pungent odor and burning to the affected areas after breathing even small amounts. With higher doses, coughing or choking may occur. Skin contact may result in burns, while eye exposure can cause corneal burns or blindness. Exposure to high levels of ammonia can cause death from laryngeal edema or from pulmonary pneumonitis. Because of its high water solubility, injuries are generally limited to the upper airway. The IDLH level of ammonia is 500 ppm.[45]

Halogen acid gases (HF, COF2, HBr). The halogen acid gases, including HF, COF2, and HBr, are products of combustion of fluorinated resins or films and fire-retardant materials containing bromine.[66] These gases are direct irritants to the mucosal surfaces, skin, and the pulmonary tract. Cutaneous manifestations vary from local irritation to deep penetrating necrotic lesions. Inhalation of these gases can result in a severe pneumonitis with dyspnea, chest tightness, and coughing. Hydrogen fluoride is particularly dangerous because the fluoride ion is a direct cellular poison, reacts with tissue proteins, and interferes with calcium metabolism.[11] The IDLH level of hydrogen fluoride is 30 ppm.[45]

Hydrogen chloride and chlorine. Hydrogen chloride, chlorine, and multiple other chemicals are produced when polyvinyl chloride (PVC) is burned in a process known as *thermal degradation.* The PVCs are found in many building and furniture fixtures. Typical symptoms after exposure to combustion products of PVCs include tachypnea, cough, hoarseness, dyspnea, chest tightness, and wheezing.[43]

Hydrogen chloride is a highly water-soluble gas with a sharp, irritating odor. It forms a dense white vapor when it comes in contact with air. When in contact with moist mucosal surfaces, it forms hydrochloric acid (HCl). Both are highly corrosive and may cause burns on contact. Most people can detect levels of 5 ppm. Brief exposure to 35 ppm causes throat irritation. Levels of 50 to 100 ppm are barely tolerable for 1 hour.[14] The IDLH is 100 ppm.[45] The greatest impact of exposure is on the upper respiratory tract. High-concentration exposures can rapidly lead to laryngeal edema and laryngospasm. Most seriously exposed persons have immediate onset of rapid breathing and narrowing of the bronchioles.[45] If escape from exposure is impossible, high levels (1000 ppm) may cause pulmonary edema.[16]

Chlorine is a yellow-green gas with a sharp or pungent odor and intermediate water solubility. In the presence of moisture, chlorine gas forms hypochlorous acid (HClO) and hydrochloric acid (HCl). The unstable HClO readily decomposes to form oxygen free radicals.[45] Chlorine gas is readily noticeable because of its olfactory and irritant properties. However, prolonged low-level exposures can lead to olfactory fatigue and tolerance to the irritant effects of the gas.[45] Chlorine gas is heavier than air and can cause asphyxiation

in poorly ventilated, enclosed, or low-lying areas.[45] Small exposures cause immediate burning of the eyes, nose, and throat, as well as coughing, wheezing, and tearing of the eyes. Since chlorine gas is of intermediate water solubility, it can affect both proximal and distal airways and cause damage to the entire respiratory tract.[40] Symptoms of mucous membrane irritation occur near the threshold limit value (TLV) of 0.5 ppm. The IDLH of chlorine is 30 ppm.[45]

Isocyanates. Isocyanates are produced by the pyrolysis of urethane isocyanate polymers or foams. The principal product is toluene diisocyanate (TDI). Isocyanates are intensely irritant gases and highly water soluble. They are believed to be the major irritants in the smoke of isocyanate-based urethanes.[66] Sites of toxicity include the eyes, gastrointestinal (GI) tract, and lungs.[15] Ocular manifestations include conjunctival irritation and inflammation. The GI findings include nausea, vomiting, and abdominal pain. Pulmonary irritation causes severe coughing, burning, and choking. Other pulmonary manifestations include chest pain, bronchospasm, and sometimes pulmonary edema. Chronic bronchitis can result from exposure to isocyanates. Occasional central nervous system (CNS) findings include headache, insomnia, euphoria, ataxia, anxiety neurosis, depression, and paranoia. At high concentrations, there is immediate cough and chest pain. At low concentrations, there may be no warning.[15] The TDI is also associated with allergic symptomology. In certain sensitized individuals, acute bronchospasm may occur.

Nitrogen oxides. Nitrogen oxides represent a mixture of gases designated by the formula NO_x. The mixture includes nitric oxide (NO), nitrogen dioxide (NO_2), nitrogen trioxide (NO_3), nitrogen tetroxide (N_2O_4), and nitrogen pentoxide (N_2O_5).[45] Nitrogen oxides are formed from the oxidation of nitrogen-containing compounds, such as celluloid, cellulose, nitrate, coal, diesel fuel, silage, and fabrics like wool. They are also formed during arc welding, electroplating, engraving, and dynamite blasting. The most hazardous of the nitrogen oxides are nitric oxide (NO) and nitrogen dioxide (NO_2). The nitrogen oxides are respiratory tract irritants that have relatively low water solubility. Nitrogen dioxide dissolves slowly in water to form nitric acid, a corrosive substance that dissociates into nitrites and nitrates. The nitrogen oxides have been shown to impair lung surfactant activity, increase sensitivity to bronchoconstrictors, and possibly initiate tissue destruction through lipid peroxidation.[13,21]

The primary site of toxicity is the lower respiratory tract. Because of poor water solubility, a person may be exposed to potentially hazardous levels of nitrogen oxides without clinical warning signs. Acute inhalation of low concentrations can cause mild dyspnea and cough. Higher concentrations may lead to pulmonary edema within 1 to 2 hours. Severe exposure can lead to bronchiolitis obliterans. It is unclear whether nitrogen oxides cause persistent severe respiratory impairment. The IDLH of NO is 100 ppm, and the IDLH of NO_2 is 50 ppm.[45] Inhalation of 20 ppm of NO in human volunteers has been shown to cause a rise in methemoglobin levels. Exposure to nitrogen oxides during fires may also result in methemoglobinemia.[31,60]

Phosgene. Phosgene ($COCl_2$) is a colorless, nonflammable gas above 47° F. It is produced by the combustion or decomposition of most volatile chlorinated organic compounds, such as solvents, paint removers, and dry cleaning fluids. It is also produced when carbon tetrachloride fire extinguishers are used in enclosed spaces.[15] At low concentrations, its odor is similar to that of green corn or freshly mowed hay. At high concentrations, its odor can be sharp and suffocating.[45] Phosgene is slowly hydrolyzed by moisture to form hydrochloric acid (HCl) and carbon dioxide.

At low levels, a single acute exposure is relatively nontoxic. Higher exposures can lead to pulmonary inflammation, which usually resolves in 2 to 3 weeks. At levels higher than 150 ppm, pulmonary edema may develop with a latency of up to 24 hours, although some authorities report a delay of up to 72 hours.[10] There are no reliable predictors of which patients exposed to phosgene will develop pulmonary edema. The IDLH level of phosgene is 2 ppm.

Sulfur dioxide. Sulfur dioxide is a gas produced when sulfur-containing natural or synthetic materials are exposed to heat or fire. It is a colorless, highly soluble gas with a pungent odor. When in contact with moisture, it produces the highly water-soluble sulfuric acid (H_2SO_4), which is intensely irritating to the eyes and respiratory tract. In one study, sulfur dioxide was detected in more than 50% of fires.[5] The concentrations ranged from 0.2 ppm to 42 ppm with 40% of these values greater than the TLV of 2 ppm. Exposures to 6 to 10 ppm cause immediate irritation. At low concentrations (1 to 50 ppm), most of the gas dissolves into the mucus of the nasopharynx and oropharynx. Involvement of the distal airways occurs only when exposures exceed this level. The IDLH level for sulfur dioxide is 100 ppm.[45]

Simple Asphyxiants

These gases produce hypoxia by displacing the available oxygen in the environment. Additionally, the fire itself contributes to a hypoxic environment by consuming available oxygen. It has been estimated that during the flashover phase of fire, when a room bursts into flames, the ambient oxygen content drops to 15% or lower. In general, a 17% inhaled-oxygen content is the safety limit for prolonged exposure. Oxygen content of 5% is the minimum compatible with life; 7% oxygen content produces stupor and memory loss; 10% produces dizziness, dyspnea, and tachypnea.[17]

Carbon dioxide and methane. Carbon dioxide is a ubiquitous by-product of the combustion of all organic products. It is chemically inert. Environments with high levels of carbon dioxide include carbohydrate fermentation sites (such as breweries, wineries, and silos), mine shafts, and dry ice storage facilities.[25] Methane can also act as a simple asphyxiant. It is produced in the combustion of polyvinyl chloride, wool, and wood and is commonly found in high concentrations in mine tunnels and enclosed organic decomposition sites (e.g., manure pits).[17]

Hydrocarbons. A variety of straight-chained and cyclic hydrocarbons have been measured in certain fire environments. In general, the straight-chained hydrocarbons can produce asphyxia in high concentrations. Medium-molecular-weight straight-chained hydrocarbons can also cause CNS depression.[17]

Chemical Asphyxiants

Carbon monoxide. Carbon monoxide (CO) is produced by the incomplete combustion of organic materials, which occurs in virtually every fire. Smoke from fires may contain from 0.1% to 10% carbon monoxide.[12] Poisoning from CO is the most common cause of death in fires.[30] Other sources of CO include faulty heaters, automobile exhaust systems, mine explosions, burning charcoal briquettes in confined spaces, and tobacco smoke. It has also been the cause of death for persons in homes with blocked chimneys.[24] Carbon monoxide is a colorless, odorless gas. Inhaled CO rapidly diffuses across the alveoli and binds to hemoglobin to form carboxyhemoglobin. Its rate of uptake depends on the percentage of inspired CO and oxygen, ventilatory rate, and duration of CO exposure.[11] The relative affinity of CO for hemoglobin is 210 times greater than that of oxygen. As a result, CO successfully competes with oxygen for the binding sites of hemoglobin, diminishes the oxygen-carrying capacity of blood, and increases tissue hypoxia. The binding of CO to hemoglobin also increases the bond strength of the remaining heme groups for oxygen, shifting the oxyhemoglobin dissociation curve to the left. Carbon monoxide also binds with other heme-containing proteins, such as the cytochromes, myoglobin, and peroxidases. At any given time, 10% to 15% of the total body burden of CO is bound to extravascular proteins.[7]

Acute clinical manifestations of CO poisoning result from carboxyhemoglobin-mediated tissue hypoxia and worsen as the blood carboxyhemoglobin (COHb) levels increase. However, there is a poor correlation between CoHb levels and clinical effects.[20,55] Initial manifestations of CO poisoning are varied and include nausea, vomiting, headache, malaise, weakness, fatigue, dyspnea, and dizziness. More ominous manifestations include seizures, syncope, myocardial ischemia, and coma. The classic cherry red coloration of the lips associated with CO poisoning is not usually apparent in patients with a carboxyhemoglobin concentration less than 40%, while cyanosis from respiratory depression is more often observed.[56] Acute mortality from CO poisoning usually results from ventricular arrhythmias precipitated by acute hypoxia from carboxyhemoglobin.[29]

Carbon monoxide poisoning has been associated with the development of delayed neuropsychiatric sequelae. Typically, there is a "lucid" period of 2 to 40 days after CO exposure before the development of abnormal neurologic effects. These include dementia, amnestic syndromes, psychosis, parkinsonism, paralysis, chorea, cortical blindness, apraxia and agnosias, peripheral neuropathy, and incontinence.[19] The incidence of development of neurologic sequelae in seriously poisoned patients has been reported in various studies to be between 12% and 40%.[6,23,63] Recent research with animal models suggest that delayed neurologic sequelae may be due to ischemia-reperfusion injury resulting from a hypoxic and hypotensive state. In serious poisonings, COHb causes tissue hypoxia and myocardial depression, resulting in hypotension and compromised cerebral blood flow. The cerebral ischemia leads to oxidative injury involving O_2 free radical formation and leukocyte-mediated lipid peroxidation.[67-69] Autopsy and magnetic resonance imaging studies suggest that CO-mediated injury involves areas of the brain with the poorest blood supply, including the globus pallidus, hippocampus, and cerebellum.[18,19,32,47,58] Delayed neurologic sequelae may resolve spontaneously; however, improvement may take as long as 2 years.[6,46]

The effects of frequent subclinical exposure to CO and the risk of neurologic sequelae remain poorly studied. However, the effects of long-term exposure to CO may be a very significant occupational health concern to firefighters.

The permissible exposure limit (PEL), an 8-hour time-weighted exposure limit established by the Occupational Safety and Health Administration, is 35 ppm. The human body can tolerate up to 100 ppm of CO for 8 hours. The IDLH of CO is 1500 ppm. Levels of 4000 ppm can be fatal in less than 1 hour.[16] At a level of 500 ppm, it takes 90 minutes for humans to attain a CoHb level of 20%. A CoHb level of 50% can be reached in 300 minutes at 500 ppm or in 60 minutes at 1000 ppm.[16] Of individuals who die from CO poisoning, 20% have CoHb levels lower than 50%.[52]

Hydrogen cyanide. Hydrogen cyanide is produced by the combustion of various nitrogen-containing products, such as wool, silk, polyacrylonitrile, nylon, polyurethane, synthetic rubber, asphalt, nitrocellulose, paper, polymers, and fire retardants.[3,62] Since these products are found in many commonplace materials such as plastic furnishing, upholstery, carpets, and fabrics, hydrogen cyanide is produced in most fires.[34] Hydrogen cyanide is rapidly absorbed by inhalation but can also be absorbed through the skin. It acts by binding to the ferric state (Fe^{3+}) of the cytochrome a-a_3 complex, inhibiting oxidative phosphorylation.[26] Hydrogen cyanide is a rapidly fatal cellular asphyxiant.

Unfortunately, cyanide has no reliable physical characteristic that indicates its presence in the cyanide-poisoned patient. One third of the population is unable to detect the characteristic odor of bitter almonds.[22] Initial symptoms include emesis, palpitations, confusion, anxiety, and vertigo. Elevated blood pressure and decreased pulse rate are followed by a decrease in blood pressure and a rise in pulse rate. Initial rapid respirations diminish to a slow and labored respiratory pattern, followed by coma and convulsions.[11] In one study of consecutive fire fatalities, 90% of victims had

been exposed to toxic levels of CO and 50% to toxic levels of cyanide.[41] The IDLH of hydrogen cyanide is 50 ppm. Hydrogen cyanide levels at various fire sites have been recorded between 0 and 75 ppm. Serum cyanide levels greater than 0.2 µg/ml are associated with toxicity. Levels greater than 2 to 3 µg/ml are usually fatal.[40]

Hydrogen sulfide. Hydrogen sulfide is produced from the burning and pyrolysis of hair, woolens, hides, and meats. It has a characteristic smell of rotten eggs and is highly water soluble.[11] It has the unique property of acting as both a chemical irritant and a chemical asphyxiant.

In contact with moisture, it forms a caustic, NaS_2, which is a direct irritant to the mucous membranes and respiratory tract. Hydrogen sulfide inhibits oxidative phosphorylation, which results in tissue hypoxia.[57] Additionally, hydrogen sulfide is detoxified to sulfmethemoglobin by red blood cells, further diminishing the oxygen-carrying capacity of blood.[24] The IDLH level of hydrogen sulfide is 300 ppm.

Miscellaneous Toxins

Depending on the fuel, a fire may produce additional inhalational toxins. Heavy metals such as antimony, bromine, cadmium, chromium, cobalt, gold, iron, lead, and zinc have been recovered in air samples from fires and in the soot recovered from the respiratory tract of fire victims.[4,9] Some of these metal fumes are associated with an acute, self-limited flulike illness after inhalation, while others may cause systemic toxicity in large doses. In addition, highly reactive free radicals are formed during combustion and may interact with tissues to cause lipid peroxidation and further respiratory damage.[71] At this time, these effects remain poorly understood.

CLINICAL TOXICOLOGY
Diagnosis

History. A careful history from the patient or witnesses may provide clues to the severity of potential injury from smoke inhalation. Important information concerning the circumstances of the injury are included in the box below.

The vast majority of smoke inhalation victims (90% to 95%) acutely complain of dyspnea, cough, or hoarse-

---

Historical Factors that Determine the Nature and Severity of Smoke Inhalation

Estimated duration of exposure
Open or closed space
Nature of the burning material
Presence of steam or explosion
Nature and function of respiratory protective equipment
Characteristics of the smoke (color, odor, amount)
History of fall or jump

From Goldstein IF et al: Acute respiratory effects of short-term exposures to nitrogen dioxide, *Arch Environ Health* 43:138, 1988.

ness.[44,54] Symptoms such as cough, sore throat, or hoarseness suggest upper airway injury and the potential for life-threatening airway obstruction. Dyspnea and wheezing suggest parenchymal injury. Headache, nausea, vomiting, dizziness, confusion, chest pain, palpitations, and syncope may suggest systemic poisoning or simple asphyxiant effects. It is also important to note if other firefighters, emergency response personnel, or medical units have similar symptoms.

The patient's age and past medical history are important risk factors for the development of injury. Patients with asthma or chronic lung disease may be more susceptible to the effects of irritant gas inhalation. Patients with coronary artery disease are at particular risk for increased myocardial ischemia from hypoxia due to bronchoconstriction, asphyxiant inhalants, and parenchymal injury.[42]

Physical examination. Initial assessment of all patients should begin with airway evaluation. Tachypnea, stridor, and cyanosis suggest impending respiratory failure or airway obstruction and the potential need for immediate airway intervention. Other typical signs and symptoms of airway injury include wheezing, rhonchi, rales, hoarseness, cough, singed nasal hairs, soot in the upper airways, carbonaceous sputum, hemoptysis, and facial and oropharyngeal burns.[8,28] Unfortunately, these suggestive findings have limited usefulness in the diagnosis of inhalation injury. In one report, only 67% of patients with facial burns had inhalation injuries, and 86% of patients with upper respiratory tract burns had no facial burns.[49] Most patients with inhalation injuries had no carbonaceous sputum at initial presentation, and only 50% later developed carbonaceous sputum or wheezing.[33,49] Wheezing, rales, and rhonchi may be found at presentation but are more common 24 to 36 hours after injury.[56] Singed nasal hairs were only 13% predictive of inhalation injuries.[33] Fewer than 25% of patients with upper respiratory tract burns requiring intubation developed hoarseness. Finally, lethal upper airway obstruction can occur acutely without the presence of facial burns.[49]

The presence of CNS signs and symptoms such as syncope, seizures, hallucinations, confusion, headache, and dizziness should alert the physician to asphyxiants, and systemic toxins, or both. Patients found unconscious in a fire probably have the highest risk of sustaining serious inhalational injuries.

Laboratory and diagnostic studies. Appropriate studies for all symptomatic victims of smoke inhalation and asymptomatic victims with significant risk factors (from history of exposure and past medical history) include pulse oximetry, arterial blood analyses, electrocardiogram and cardiac monitoring, and a carboxyhemoglobin level. Pulse oximetry is a simple and easy test to monitor oxygen saturation; however, it reads falsely normal in patients with carbon monoxide poisoning and errs toward a reading of 85% in patients with methemoglobinemia. Arterial blood gas analysis may indicate underlying hypoxemia or ventilatory failure. Although a single arterial blood gas may not be a sensitive marker for pulmonary dysfunction, serial arterial blood gases may be useful in detecting a declining respiratory pattern. An electrocardiogram is helpful in detecting myocardial ischemia. The presence of a myocardial infarct on the electrocardiogram may be the first sign that the patient has had significant smoke inhalation.

Finally, a carboxyhemoglobin level (which can be obtained from a venous or arterial blood gas) is extremely important because it is the only objective means to determine exposure to carboxyhemoglobin. An elevated carboxyhemoglobin level should raise concern for CO poisoning as well as potential exposure to other smoke inhalation toxins.

Direct laryngoscopy, preferably by fiberoptic laryngoscopy (or indirect laryngoscopy in the cooperative patient), should be performed to assess the upper airway of any patient with the potential for upper airway injury, such as those presenting with tachypnea, hoarseness, stridor, or orofacial burns. Laryngoscopy should be performed early during the emergency department evaluation because early endotracheal intubation may be required in selected patients to prevent the development of airway obstruction from progressing to upper airway edema.

Elevated methemoglobin levels have been reported in fire victims.[31] Fortunately, clinically significant methemoglobin toxicity from smoke inhalation is a rare occurrence. Methemoglobin analysis may be an appropriate test for smoke inhalation victims of fires with the potential for high levels of nitrogen oxides. In most hospital laboratories, a methemoglobin level is automatically measured by cooximetry when a blood sample request for a carboxyhemoglobin level is received.

Blood cyanide analysis is of little clinical use because of the delay of several hours in receiving cyanide levels from the laboratory. One study has suggested that an initial serum lactate greater than 10 mmol/L measured in the emergency department correlates strongly with cyanide poisoning in fires.[1] An elevated serum lactate level appears to be an important marker for cyanide poisoning. Unfortunately, even a delay of 30 minutes in obtaining a lactate level from the laboratory may limit its usefulness when therapeutic decisions must be made expeditiously.

For patients with abnormal chest examinations such as wheezing, rales, or asymmetric breath sounds, a chest radiograph may help determine the presence of pulmonary injury. Unfortunately, chest radiographs are commonly normal in the early course of smoke inhalation. Most often, abnormal chest radiograph findings such as local, patchy, or diffuse infiltrates are not evident until 24 to 36 hours after exposure.[64] Subtle findings such as perivascular haziness, peribronchial cuffing, bronchial wall thickening, and subglottic edema may be apparent within 24 hours of exposure.[39,64] Most patients with serious pulmonary injuries may have normal initial radiographs, while asymptomatic patients may present with markedly abnormal chest radiograph findings.

Nuclear pulmonary imaging, computed tomography of the chest, and pulmonary function tests have also been used to detect pulmonary injury. Unfortunately, these tests are of limited practical use, but they may detect early pulmonary abnormalities before chest radiograph or arterial blood gas abnormalities arise.

Treatment. All victims of smoke inhalation should begin treatment with high-flow supplemental oxygen (such as 100% oxygen by nonrebreather face mask at 12 L/minute), which should be adjusted based on arterial blood gas analysis, clinical history of chronic obstructive pulmonary disease, and suspicion of CO poisoning. In patients with severe respiratory distress (e.g., altered mental status, tachypnea, retractions, stridor), immediate endotracheal intubation with an adequate-size tube may be required. Increased positive end-expiratory pressure ventilation and frequent suctioning to remove debris and airway secretions may improve respiratory mechanics for a patient on artificial ventilation. Patients with evidence of upper airway edema by direct visualization through laryngoscopy should be intubated to prevent airway compromise by further airway swelling. Patients with upper airway erythema but without significant edema should be followed closely by serial evaluation.

The use of inhaled B_2 adrenergic agonists such as albuterol should be considered to reverse the bronchospasm induced by irritant gases. Although these agents are considered first-line therapy for the treatment of acute asthma or chronic obstructive pulmonary disease, their effectiveness among smoke inhalation victims remains unstudied. Corticosteroids are not recommended in inhalational injuries; however, they may be considered in selected patients with isolated inhalational injury and refractory bronchospasm. Corticosteroids have been shown to increase the risk of mortality and infection in the presence of burns and inhalational injury.[50] Antibiotics should not be administered unless a specific infection is documented by gram stain or culture.

Intravenous fluid therapy should be directed at replacing fluid losses from insensible losses and third spacing. In one study, patients with concomitant inhalational injuries and surface burns required greater fluid resuscitation per kilogram per % total body surface area burned than those patients with burns only.[37,51] Unfortunately, overhydration may exacerbate pulmonary injury caused by smoke inhalation. In the critically ill smoke inhalation patient, invasive cardiac monitoring should be used to better assess fluid requirements and optimize respiratory care for those patients requiring mechanical ventilation and high levels of positive end-expiratory pressure.

Patients with surface burns should receive dermal decontamination such as the removal of soot or chemical solvents from their skin. Extensive burns may require transfer to an appropriate burn facility after stabilization of the patient. Patients with ocular irritation should receive vigorous eye irrigation and appropriate care for corneal burns and other ophthalmologic injuries.

Carbon monoxide poisoning is initially treated with 100% oxygen by nonrebreathing face mask or endotracheal tube. Oxygen immediately enhances the dissociation of carboxyhemoglobin. At room air, the half-life of carboxyhemoglobin is 5 hours and 20 minutes. With 100% oxygen at 1 atmosphere absolute (ATA), the half-life of carboxyhemoglobin is reduced to 90 minutes. With hyperbaric oxygen, 100% at 3 ATA, the half-life is further reduced to 23 minutes. For those seriously poisoned by carbon monoxide, referral to an appropriate facility for hyperbaric oxygen treatment should be considered.

In a retrospective series, hyperbaric oxygen (HBO) therapy administered within 6 hours after discovery of the patient resulted in a decrease in mortality from 30% to 14%.[6] It may also diminish or prevent the effects of delayed neurologic sequelae, but this remains unproven. In animal models, HBO has been shown to prevent adherence of polymorphonuclear leukocytes to the microvascular endothelium, which causes endothelial injury, free radical production, and lipid peroxidation.[68] Generally accepted criteria for hyperbaric oxygen therapy are listed in the box below.

As mentioned previously, cyanide toxicity presents acutely without reliable early clinical or laboratory characteristics. Seriously ill smoke inhalation victims and those who are rapidly deteriorating despite supportive care should be considered for early empiric treatment with sodium thiosulfate. In a seriously ill patient, treatment should not wait for laboratory results such as lactate or cyanide levels. Amyl nitrite and sodium nitrite induce a methemoglobinemia that exacerbates concurrent CO poisoning. Nitrites should not be considered in the treatment of potential cyanide toxicity in the smoke inhalation victim without a measured methemoglobin and carboxyhemoglobin level. Chapter 19 includes additional discussion of cyanide poisoning and treatment.

Elevated methemoglobin levels are easily treated with oxygen in most cases. In those patients with levels greater

---

Criteria for Consideration of HBO

CoHb ≥ 25 in asymptomatic patients
Pregnancy in asymptomatic patients (especially if CoHb >15%)
Exposure to CO and any of the following:
- Syncope
- Neurologic impairment (e.g., coma, confusion, cognitive deficits, seizures, visual disturbance)
- Persistent neurologic findings despite oxygen therapy (e.g., headache, dizziness, ataxia)
- Myocardial ischemia or life-threatening arrhythmias
- Abnormal neuropsychiatric examination score

than 20% to 30% and serious symptoms, methylene blue may be appropriate treatment. Chapter 40 includes additional discussion of methemoglobin poisoning and treatment.

The observation period for asymptomatic patients without significant risk factors for chronic obstructive pulmonary disease or coronary artery disease is 4 to 6 hours. Those who remain asymptomatic during this observation can be discharged with appropriate follow-up and follow-up instructions. Asymptomatic patients with significant risk factors and symptomatic patients who rapidly improve should be observed for 12 to 24 hours. All other symptomatic patients should be admitted to the hospital.

REFERENCES

1. Baud FJ et al: Elevated blood cyanide concentrations in victims of smoke inhalation, *N Engl J Med* 325:1761, 1991.
2. Beauchamp RO: A critical review of the literature on acrolein toxicity, *Crit Rev Toxicol* 14:309, 1985.
3. Becker CE: The role of cyanide in fires, *Vet Hum Toxicol* 27:487, 1985.
4. Birky MM, Clarke FB: Inhalation of toxic products from fires, *Bull N Y Acad Med* 57:997-1013, 1981.
5. Brandt-Rauf PW et al: Health hazards of firefighters: exposure assessment, *Br J Ind Med* 45:606, 1988.
6. Choi IS: Delayed neurologic sequelae in carbon monoxide intoxication, *Arch Neurol* 40:433, 1983.
7. Coburn RF: The carbon monoxide body stores, *Ann N Y Acad Sci* 174:11, 1970.
8. Crapo RO: Smoke-inhalation injuries, *JAMA* 246:1694, 1981.
9. Davies JW: Toxic chemicals versus lung tissue: an aspect of inhalation injury revisited, *J Burn Care Rehabil* 7:213, 1986.
10. Diller WF: Medical phosgene problems and their possible solution, *J Occup Med* 20:189, 1978.
11. Dinerman N: Smoke (combustion) poisoning. In Arena JM, Drew RH, editors: *Poisoning: toxicology, symptoms, and treatment,* ed 5, Springfield, Ill, 1986, Charles C Thomas.
12. Dolan M: Carbon monoxide poisoning, *Can Med Assoc J* 133:329, 1985.
13. Dowell AR, Kilburn KH: Ultrastructural effects of nitrogen dioxide on the lung, *Am Rev Respir Dis* 101:197, 1979.
14. Dyer RF, Esch VH: Polyvinyl chloride toxicity in fires: hydrogen chloride toxicity in fire fighters, *JAMA* 235:393, 1976.
15. Eilers MA: Smoke inhalation. In Haddad LM, Winchester JF, editors: *Clinical management of poisoning and drug overdose,* ed 2, Philadelphia, 1990, WB Saunders.
16. Einhorn IN: Physiological and toxicological aspects of smoke produced during the combustion of polymeric materials, *Environ Health Perspect,* 11:163-189, 1975.
17. Ellenhorn MJ, Barceloux DG: Smoke inhalation. In Ellenhorn MJ, Barceloux DG, editors: *Medical toxicology, diagnosis and treatment of human poisoning,* New York, 1988, Elsevier.
18. Garland H, Pearce J: Neurological complications of carbon monoxide poisoning, *Q J Med* 36:445, 1967.
19. Ginsberg MD: Carbon monoxide intoxication: clinical features, neuropathology, and mechanisms of injury, *J Tox Clin Tox* 23:281, 1985.
20. Goldbaum LR, Ramirez RG, Absalon KB: What is the mechanism of carbon monoxide toxicity? *Aviat Space Environ Med* 46:1289, 1975.
21. Goldstein IF et al: Acute respiratory effects of short-term exposures to nitrogen dioxide, *Arch Environ Health* 43:138, 1988.
22. Gonzalez ER: Cyanide evades some noses, overpowers others, *JAMA* 248:2211, 1982.
23. Goulon M et al: Carbon monoxide poisoning and acute anoxia due to breathing coal gas and hydrocarbons. *Ann Med Interne (Paris)* 120:335, 1969; English translation, *J Hyperbar Med* 1:23, 1986.
24. Haggerty MA, Soto-Greene M, Reichman LB: Caring for toxic gas inhalation, *J Crit Illness* 2:77, 1987.
25. Hall AH: Simple asphyxiants, *Meditext (TM) Medical Management.* In Hall AH, Rumack BH, editors: *Tomes (R) Information System.* Denver, 1991, Micromedix.
26. Hall AH, Rumack BH: Clinical toxicology of cyanide, *Ann Emerg Med* 25:1067, 1986.
27. Haponik EF: Clinical smoke inhalation injury: pulmonary effects, *Occup Med* 8:431, 1993.
28. Haponik EF, Munster AM, editors: *Respiratory injury: smoke inhalation and burns,* New York, 1990, McGraw-Hill.
29. Hardy KR, Thom SR: Pathophysiology and treatment of carbon monoxide poisoning, *Clin Toxicol* 32:613-629, 1994.
30. Heimbach DM, Waeckerle JF: Inhalation injuries, *Ann Emerg Med* 17:1316, 1988.
31. Hoffman RS, Sauter D: Methemoglobinemia resulting from smoke inhalation, *Vet Hum Toxicol* 31:168, 1989.
32. Horowitz AL, Kaplan R, Sarpel G: Carbon monoxide toxicity: MR imaging in the brain, *Radiology* 162:787, 1987.
33. Hunt JR et al: Fiberoptic bronchoscopy in acute inhalation injury, *J Trauma* 15:641, 1975.
34. Jones J, McMullen J, Dougherty J: Toxic smoke inhalation: cyanide poisoning in fire victims, *Am J Emerg Med* 5:318, 1987.
35. Karter MJ, Lellane PR: US fire fighter injuries in 1993, *NFPA Journal* p 57, 1994.
36. Kirk M: Smoke inhalation. In Goldfrank LR, editor: *Toxicologic emergencies,* ed 5, Norwalk, Conn, 1994, Appleton & Lange.
37. Kirk MA, Gerace R, Kulig K: Cyanide and methemoglobin kinetics in smoke inhalation victims treated with the cyanide antidote kit, *Ann Emerg Med* 22:1413, 1993.
38. Kulle PJ et al: Pulmonary effects of sulfur dioxide and respirable carbon aerosol, *Environ Res* 41:239, 1986.
39. Lee MJ, O'Connell DJ: The plain chest radiograph after acute smoke inhalation, *Clin Radiol* 39:33, 1988.
40. Liu D, Olson KR: Smoke inhalation, *CMCC Crit Care Toxicol* 1:203-224, 1991.
41. Lundquist P, Rammer L, Sorbo B: The role of hydrogen cyanide and carbon monoxide in fire casualties: a prospective study, *Forensic Sci Int* 43:9, 1989.
42. Marius-Nunez AL: Myocardial infarction with normal coronary arteries after acute exposure to carbon monoxide, *Chest* 97:491, 1990.
43. Markowitz JS: Self-reported short- and long-term respiratory effects among PVC-exposed fire fighters, *Arch Environ Health* 44:30, 1989.
44. McGuigan MA: Smoke inhalation, *Clin Toxicol Rev* 7:1, 1985.
45. *Medical management guidelines for acute chemical exposures,* vol 3, Washington, DC, US Department of Health and Human Services.
46. Min SK: A brain syndrome associated with delayed neuropsychiatric sequelae following acute carbon monoxide intoxication, *Acta Psychiatr Scand* 73:80, 1986.
47. Miura T et al: CT of the brain in acute carbon monoxide intoxication: characteristic features and prognosis, *AJNR* 6:739, 1985.
48. Morgan WK: The respiratory effects of particles, vapours, and fumes, *Am Ind Hyg Assoc J* 47:670, 1986.
49. Moylan JA: Inhalation injury: a primary determination of survival, *Burn Care Rehabil* 3:78, 1981.
50. Moylan JA, Chan CK: Inhalation injury: an increasing problem, *Ann Surg* 188:34, 1978.
51. Navar PD, Affle JR, Warden GD: Effect of inhalational injury on fluid resuscitation requirements after thermal injury, *Am J Surg* 150:716-720, 1985.

52. Nelson GL: Regulatory aspects of fire toxicology, *Toxicology* 47:181, 1987.
53. Procter NH, Hughes JP, Fischman MI: *Chemical hazards of the workplace,* ed 2, Philadelphia, 1988, JB Lippincott.
54. Putman CE et al: Radiologic manifestations of acute smoke inhalations, *AJR Am J Roentgenol* 129:865, 1977.
55. Raphael JC et al: Trial of normobaric and hyperbaric oxygen for acute carbon monoxide intoxication, *Lancet* 2:414, 1989.
56. Robinson L, Miller RH: Smoke inhalation injuries, *Am J Otolaryngol* 7:375, 1986.
57. Rorison DG, McPherson SJ: Acute toxic inhalations. *Emerg Med Clin North Am* 10:409, 1992.
58. Sawada Y et al: Computerized tomography as an indication of long-term outcome after acute carbon monoxide poisoning, *Lancet* 1:783, 1980.
59. Schwartz DA: Acute inhalational injury, *Occup Med* 2:297, 1987.
60. Schwerd W, Schulz E: Carboxyhaemoglobin and methemoglobin findings in burnt bodies, *Forensic Sci Int* 12:233, 1978.
61. Shirani KZ, Pruitt BA, Mason AD: The influence of inhalation injury and pneumonia on burn mortality, *Ann Surg* 205:82, 1987.
62. Silverman SH et al: Cyanide toxicity in burned patients, *J Trauma* 28:171, 1988.
63. Smith JS, Brandon S: Morbidity from acute carbon monoxide poisoning at three year follow-up, *BMJ* 1:318, 1973.
64. Teixidor HS et al: Smoke inhalation: radiologic manifestations, *Radiology* 149:383, 1983.
65. Tepper A, Comstock GW, Levine M: A longitudinal study of pulmonary function in fire fighters, *Am J Ind Med* 20:307, 1991.
66. Terrill JB, Montgomery RR, Reinhardt CF: Toxic gases from fires, *Science* 200:1343, 1978.
67. Thom SR: Antagonism of carbon monoxide-mediated brain lipid peroxidation by hyperbaric oxygen, *Toxicol Appl Pharmacol* 105:340, 1990.
68. Thom SR: Carbon monoxide-mediated brain lipid peroxidation in the rat, *J Appl Physiol* 68:997, 1990.
69. Thom SR: Functional inhibition of leukocyte b2 integrins by hyperbaric oxygen in carbon monoxide-mediated brain injury in rats, *Toxicol Appl Pharmacol* 123:248, 1993.
70. Treitman RD, Burgess WA, Gold A: Air contaminants encountered by fire fighters, *Am Ind Hyg Assoc J* 41:796, 1980.
71. Youn Y, Lalonde C, Demling R: Oxidants and the pathophysiology of burn and smoke inhalation injury, *Free Radic Biol Med* 12:409, 1992.

Floor and Carpet Layers

Christine R. Medora

CH₃

methacrylic acid

- The diverse applications for the acrylic acids make them a commonly encountered workplace hazard

- Acrylic acids are potent sensitizers of the skin, mucous membranes, and lungs

- The carcinogenic potential is low

OCCUPATIONAL DESCRIPTION AND TOXIC EXPOSURE

This chapter discusses the occupationally related toxins that the following individuals may be exposed to: carpet layers, floor layers, paper hangers, and upholsterers.[5] Hispanic individuals are widely represented in the upholstery trade, accounting for nearly 25% of workers, while African-Americans make up only approximately 3% to 8% of persons employed in these four occupations (Table 16-1). Carpet layers, floor layers, paper hangers, and upholsterers are discussed together as they share a variety of potential occupational exposures, including specific musculoskeletal injuries associated with positional or repetitive motion trauma and contact dermatitis associated with the use of acrylate-containing adhesives.

Carpet layers install carpets or rugs in homes or other buildings.[6] According to the annual Current Population Survey conducted by the Bureau of Labor Statistics, there were 114,000 individuals employed as carpet installers in the United States in 1994 (see Table 16-1).[5] Carpet installation requires basic carpentry skills and physical strength. The installation of carpeting first requires preparation of the subfloor to eliminate imperfections. Often this involves the application of liquid underlayment and sealants that may contain gypsum and starch.[19] Staples may be used to secure carpet padding to the subfloor. A knee kicker, used to secure carpeting to the tackless strip placed around the perimeter of the floor, consists of a knee pad at one end and metal "teeth" embedded in a plate at the opposite end. Operation of the knee kicker requires repeated, powerful flexion of the knee while in the kneeling position, in order to allow the teeth to penetrate the carpeting. Use of the knee kicker has im-

Table 16-1 Craft employment in 1994

	Carpet layers	Floor layers	Paper hangers	Upholsterers
Total	114,000	56,000	543,000	61,000
Women	2.4%	3.0%	6.3%	24.3%
African-American	4.2%	3.6%	7.5%	7.6%
Hispanic	15.1%	11.1%	17.7%	24.6%

From Current Population Survey, Bureau of Labor Statistics, US Dept of Labor: *Employment and earnings* 42:175, 1995.

plications in the development of repetitive trauma. A power stretcher may be employed to stretch the carpeting, and a wall trimmer is utilized to finish carpet edges. For installation of cushion-backed carpeting and juxtaposition of seams, a coat of adhesive is applied with a trowel to the underlying floor. These adhesives may contain acrylic resins, styrene, butadiene, rubber latex, and halogenated hydrocarbons (Table 16-2). A plastic syringe may be used to inject contact adhesive into holes where "bubbles" develop in the carpeting. Wood baseboard or vinyl cove base is also installed with adhesives applied from a notched trowel or putty knife, although certain vinyl cove base is manufactured with a self-adhesive backing. The nature of carpet installation requires a carpet installer to spend a significant amount of time on either one or both knees. The performance of rigorous, repetitive motions using the knee kicker may predispose to repetitive motion injuries of the hip or knee joints. During a medical interview, the history and physical should be directed toward symptoms and signs of such trauma. In addition, the use of acrylate-based adhesives may predispose workers to the development of contact dermatitis, and close attention should be paid to complaints of rashes on the hands, forearms, and face. The effects of occupational exposure to acrylates and methacrylates is extensively discussed in this chapter.

In 1994, there were 56,000 floor layers in the United States (see Table 16-1).[5] This number includes both hard and soft tile setters. Hard tiles are ceramic or marble, and soft tiles are linoleum and other sheet floor coverings. Hard tile setters apply tile to walls, floors, ceilings, and roof decks, generally following specific design patterns.[6] Other floor layers apply blocks, strips, or sheets of decorative coverings to floors and cabinets.[6] The term *floor layers* excludes the installation of carpeting.

Floor installation requires preparation of concrete or wooden subfloors with floor levelers and sealants similar to those used in carpet laying. These liquid underlays are used to smooth, level, fill, patch, and moisture-proof subfloors. Floor-leveling compounds may contain gypsum and can result in eye and skin irritation; burns may result from an exothermic reaction of large quantities of material.[19] A variety of adhesives are used for the installa-

tion of flooring, depending upon both the flooring material and the nature of the subfloor. For example, latex adhesives are best used to apply vinyl composition tile to concrete or wood, whereas alcohol-resin adhesive is better suited for the application of vinyl, rubber, cork, or linoleum.[19] Table 16-2 lists some potential exposures of floor layers. In the case of hard tile setting, grout and mortar are used to apply decorative ceramic tiles to various surfaces. Often, these products contain acrylic copolymers, as well as ethylene glycol and limestone. Due to the precision required for the installation of hard tiles, it would not be surprising if workers are unlikely to wear protective gloves. Because of the substantial exposure to acrylate-containing adhesives, the floor layer who arrives for an office visit should be thoroughly questioned and examined regarding hand dermatitis and other symptoms that may be less frequently associated with long-term acrylic resin exposure.

Wallpaper hangers are commonly grouped together with painters, most likely because many workers are skilled in both trades, often being employed in "paint and paper" businesses. The Bureau of Labor Statistics groups the two occupations together and estimates that 543,000 individuals were employed as paper hangers and painters in 1994.[5] For the purpose of this discussion, paper hangers are discussed separately due to their common exposure to acrylate-containing adhesives. Paper hangers cover interior walls and ceilings of rooms with decorative wallpaper or fabric or attach advertising posters on surfaces such as walls or billboards.[6] Paper hangers are exposed to a variety of chemicals in the work environment (Table 16-3). Generally, wallpaper installation first requires the removal of preexisting paint or old wallpaper. Chemical wallpaper strippers containing halogenated hydrocarbon solvents, such as propylene glycol and dipropylene glycol methyl ether, are brushed or sprayed onto surfaces. The use of spray applicators is especially important to uncover in the occupational history, as this method of application may increase the likelihood of respiratory irritation and dermal and inhalational absorption of the solvent. Halogenated hydrocarbons are well known to affect the central nervous system. A second method of wallpaper removal uses a wallpaper steamer, in which steam from an electrically heated tank is pumped through a hose to a hand-held perforated plate.[53] The wallpaper is "steamed" off, and a putty knife can then be used to peel the softened wallcovering from the wall. Prior to hanging wallcovering, a primer is often used to promote the adhesion of the substrate, particularly for slick surfaces. These often contain nonvolatile acrylic copolymers and acrylic resins. Finally, installation of wallpaper requires the use of various adhesives, depending upon the nature and thickness of the wallcovering. Ethylene glycol and polyvinyl acetate may be in the adhesive. As is the case for carpet and floor layers, paper hangers' frequent exposure to acrylate-containing adhesives necessitates a well-directed history and physical

Table 16-2 Potential occupational exposures of carpet layers and floor layers

Product	Use	Contents	Toxicity
Latex carpet adhesive	Glue down carpet	Aromatic oil Kaolin clay Styrene butadiene rubber latex Hydrocarbon resin	Dermatitis Cancer
Multipurpose floor covering	Adheres sheet goods, adhesive tile	Heavy naphthenic distillate Styrene butadiene rubber latex Hydrocarbon resin	Eye injury Dermatitis CNS effects
Floor tile adhesive	Binds vinyl and asphalt tile	Toluene Heavy naphthenic distillate Petroleum hydrocarbon resin Styrene-butadiene polymer	Eye irritation Dermatitis CNS effects
Cove base adhesive	Binds rubber and vinyl cove base to walls	Oil resin Limestone Styrene butadiene latex mixture	Dermatitis
Floor leveler	Repairs surface imperfections	Gypsum Starch Wood floor	Eye irritation Dermatitis Burns
Tile repair mortar	Bonds tile	Polyvinyl copolymer Portland cement Silica quartz	Eye irritation Dermatitis
Marble cleanser	Cleans marble, seals, and polishes	Acrylic copolymer Ethylene glycol	Eye irritation Dermatitis
Ceramic tile adhesive	Bonds tile	Acrylic copolymer Ethylene glycol Limestone Triethanolamine	Dermatitis Eye irritation CNS effects
Tile grout	Repairs grout joints	Acrylic copolymer Limestone	Dermatitis

Table 16-3 Potential occupational exposures in wallpaper hangers and upholsterers

Product	Uses	Contents	Toxicity
Wallpaper hangers			
Wallpaper stripper	Dissolves wallpaper paste	Propylene glycol Surfactant Dipropylene glycol methyl ether	Eye irritant Dermatitis Asthma
Wallcovering adhesive	Adheres wallcovering	Polyvinyl acetate Ethylene glycol Starch	
Wallcovering primer	Promotes adhesion of wallcovering	Nonvolatile acrylic Copolymer Pigment	Dermatitis
Upholsterers			
Foam adhesive	Bonds flexible urethane or latex foam	Nonvolatiles Naphthol spirits Dimethyl ether	Eye irritation Dermatitis CNS effects

exam to identify symptoms and signs of contact dermatitis, respiratory compromise, and neurologic sequelae.

According to the Current Population Survey for 1994, there were 61,000 individuals employed as upholsterers, with women and Hispanics representing up to 50% of members.[5] Upholsterers make, repair, and replace upholstery of household furniture or automobiles, using knowledge of fabrics and upholstery methods. The trade includes workers in both manufacturing and nonmanufacturing industries but excludes workers who perform specialized operations such as sewing machine operators.[6] Upholsterers frequently utilize a hydraulic staple gun to apply fabrics to wood or synthetic furniture frameworks. They are exposed to acrylic resins through the use of rapid-drying fabric adhesives that bond materials such as foam together (see Table 16-3). The nature of their work requires that upholsterers be thoroughly questioned regarding symptoms of repetitive motion injuries. As is true of carpet layers, floor layers, and paper hangers, upholsterers should be examined for signs of contact dermatitis, particularly of the hands, arms, and face, as well as signs of respiratory distress that may be associated with the use of aerosolized adhesives.

CLINICAL TOXICOLOGY
Acrylic and Methacrylic Acids and Their Esters

Uses. Acrylic and methacrylic acids and their esters have a nearly unlimited number of uses in a variety of industries, including textiles, building materials, automotive, toy manufacturing, printing, medicine, and dentistry.[48] They are appropriate to discuss in the context of craftspeople in that acrylic resins are used extensively in the production of water-resistant and mineral-based floor coatings, floor topcoat paints, adhesives, glues, and anaerobic sealants.[25,59] Monomers of both ethyl acrylate and methyl methacrylate are primarily used in the production of acrylic and methacrylic polymers, respectively.[25] Methyl methacrylate is combined with acrylonitrile in the manufacture of acrylic fibers.[25,48] Hexanediol diacrylate and tripropylene glycol diacrylate monomers are used in ultraviolet (UV)-hardened acrylic primers, fillers, and varnishes.[59] Methyl methacrylate monomer is also used as a cross-linking agent in floor coatings[59] and as a component of prosthetic materials in dentistry and orthopedics.

Acrylic polymers and polymer mixtures are used extensively in lacquers, paints, glues, adhesives, floor coatings, and floor waxes.[59] They can be used in surface treatments for leather, fabric, and paper products.[25,59] Acrylic emulsion polymers, formed from the polymerization of the acrylic ester with water, are used in latex paints,[48] finishing agents,[59] and fabric coatings.[25] They are also used in the manufacture of paper, either as a coating to improve water resistance or as an ingredient in the pulp to provide resistance to oils.[48] They are added to leather to improve appearance and durability[48] and are used as metal, rubber, and plastics coatings.[59]

Perhaps the most widely employed acrylic resin polymer is polymethyl methacrylate. In 1909, the Rohm and Haas company began manufacturing "organic glass" and is still a leading producer worldwide.[48] Polymethyl methacrylate is used in sheets as Plexiglas or Lucite in such objects as bank teller windows, police cars, telephone booths, skylights, housewares, and industrial machinery guards, providing both transparency and durability.[25,48,59] It is also employed extensively in the health care industry. Originally used in denture bases in 1946,[48] polymethyl methacrylate is a component of dentures, orthopedic prostheses, surgical retractors, throat lights, hypodermic syringes, contact lenses, and bone cement.[25,48] The acrylic polymer 2-hydroxyethyl methacrylate (HEMA) is used in the production of soft contact lenses. The replacement of the polymethyl methacrylate methyl group with a hydroxyethyl group renders the polymer more hydrophilic and more comfortable to wear.[48]

Chemistry. Acrylic resins include both monomers and polymers. Of the monomers, the most common are acrylic acid, methacrylic acid, and cyanoacrylic acid.[59] Acrylic acid is also called *propenoic acid, acrolcic acid,* and *ethylene carboxylic acid.* Methacrylic acid is synonymous with 2-methyl propenoic acid and α-methacrylic acid.[28] These monomers are colorless liquids with a pungent odor. They readily evaporate and rapidly polymerize in the presence of light, heat, oxygen, and oxidizing agents.[25,48,59] At room temperature, they can present a major fire hazard.[59] Both compounds are soluble in water, ethyl alcohol, and ethyl ether.[25] By combining various monomers, a diverse group of polymers results, including rubbers and plastics.[48]

The term *acrylates* includes the derivatives of acrylic and methacrylic acids.[48] Acrylates can be classified as either monofunctional, difunctional, or multifunctional acrylates, depending on whether they contain one, two, or more than two acrylic groups, respectively.[28] Examples of each and their chemical structures are provided in Figure 16-1. In polymerization reactions, the physical characteristics of the resulting polymer are related to the ratio of monofunctional and multifunctional acrylates in the mixture. Adding multifunctional acrylates typically increases the number of reactive groups and decreases the viscosity of the polymer.[59]

Acrylic esters are formed by combining acrylic acid and alcohol, the resulting ester and its physical characteristics depending on which alcohol is employed in the reaction. Short-chain alcohols generally produce tougher, stronger, more transparent esters that are soluble in aromatic hydrocarbons, while longer-chain alcohols result in esters that are transparent but brittle and are soluble in aliphatic hydrocarbons.[25,48] Prepolymers are formed from the addition of two or more acrylic or methacrylic groups and include epoxies,

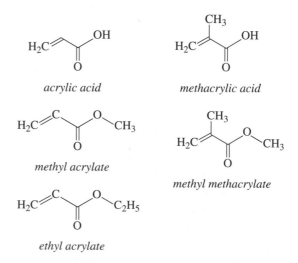

acrylic acid

methacrylic acid

methyl acrylate

methyl methacrylate

ethyl acrylate

Fig. 16-1 Acrylic acids and acrylic esters.

polyurethanes, polyesters, and polyethers.[59] The technical products that are the end result of polymerization processes can consist of a variety of acrylic compounds, including prepolymers, and monofunctional, difunctional, and multifunctional acrylates, in a multiplicity of combinations.

Production. Acrylic monomers are derived from petrochemicals.[48] The first process utilized in the production of acrylic acid involved the oxidation of propylene to acrolein and subsequently to acrylic acid.[25] Newer, more efficient techniques include the hydroxylation of acetylene and carbon monoxide to acrylic acid and acrylate, and the addition of ketene and formaldehyde to produce acrylate via the intermediate propriolactone.[25] Production of methacrylic acid involves oxidation of isobutylene via a catalyst to methacrylic acid, which can further be hydroxylated to form methacrylate. Generally, the ethyl and methyl acrylates are formed by using the same process as their acid moieties, but this is then followed by a reaction with ethanol or methanol, respectively. Methyl methacrylate production can also be accomplished with the addition of acetone and hydrocyanic acid to form acetone cyanohydrin. This is subsequently hydrolyzed with sulfuric acid in the presence of methanol to form the final product.[28]

Because acrylates polymerize readily when exposed to light, heat, or oxygen, their production requires the addition of stabilizers, typically hydroquinone or the monomethyl ether of hydroquinone.[59] Even with the addition of inhibitors, most products containing acrylate or methacrylate monomers have a shelf life of 1 year. In the case of adhesives sold for the purpose of do-it-yourself floor, carpet, or wallpaper installation, this date is generally indicated on the packaging.

The polymerization process can be accomplished with heat, cold, UV light, or electron bombardment. Polymerization can also be initiated by the addition of a catalyst such as peroxide.[59] Generally, UV light and electron bombardment are employed in the production of polymers that contain a prepolymer or a difunctional or multifunctional acrylate or methacrylate.[59] In order to produce sheets of polymethyl methacrylate, the monomer and a catalyst are mixed in a heated vessel to the desired thickness, cooled and poured into molds, and placed into an oven where polymerization takes place.[25] In order to manufacture a lower molecular weight polymethyl methacrylate, methyl methacrylate monomer and a second comonomer can be mixed to form a slurry, which dries to form a powder.[25] This powder polymer is used in combination with liquid monomer to form a "dough" that is used for molding prosthetics in dental and orthopedic settings.[48]

Metabolism. Exposure to acrylates and methacrylates occurs primarily through dermal and inhalation routes, for example, as tile setters spread acrylic copolymer-based adhesives and dental technicians mold methyl-methacrylate in denture material. The metabolism of monofunctional esters of acrylic and methacrylic acid has been studied primarily in animals, with studies focusing on dermal and inhalation routes.[59]

Many acrylates are readily absorbed through the skin and act as skin sensitizers.[59] In animal studies, the efficiency of acrylic acid absorption may depend upon the physical characteristics of the solvent. Absorption may occur rapidly from an acetone vehicle and may be enhanced at a more acidic pH.[58] In humans, preexisting dermatitis that may or may not be associated with the use of acrylates could predispose to more rapid absorption of these compounds. Although in vitro studies have shown acrylic acid to have a half-life of up to 10 hours in skin,[3] systemic absorption from dermal exposure in vivo may be limited by evaporative loss.[58] Acrylic acid is rapidly absorbed from the gastrointestinal (GI) tract of rats, although this route of exposure is unlikely in humans.

Acrylic compounds are also efficiently absorbed through the lungs.[59] Inhalation exposure to acrylates in the occupational setting has long been recognized, particularly in dentistry and orthopedic surgery, in which the mixing of denture materials or bone cements liberates volatile methyl methacrylate monomer into the breathing space.

The distribution of acrylic acid in major tissues is characterized by the highest tissue to blood concentration ratios in liver and kidney.[58] Administered to rats,[2,3-14] carbon-labeled ethyl acrylate becomes widely distributed throughout tissues, with highest concentrations in the GI tract, liver, and kidneys. It appears to bind to hepatic lipids and proteins, as well as to forestomach mucous membrane proteins; however, there is little evidence of binding to nucleic acids.[21] In animal studies, dermal exposure resulted in the highest level of radiolabeled compound being located in the dermis, with subsequent tissue damage and edema.[51]

Acrylic and methacrylic acid metabolism has been studied primarily in animals. The ester moiety of acrylates and methacrylates is hydrolyzed by carboxylesterases to acrylic acid and ethanol.[17,59] Administration of the carboxylase inhibitor triorthotolyl phosphate (TOTP) potentiates the toxicity of acrylates, supporting the role of carboxylesterases in their detoxification.[48] Metabolism of acrylic acid then occurs along a pathway of propionate catabolism, with carbon dioxide and acetyl CoA the end products of oxidation.[3] Subsequently, acetyl CoA is further oxidized to carbon dioxide via the tricarboxylic acid (TCA) cycle.[3] In mammals, propionic acid is formed from the β-oxidation of long-chain fatty acids and from the catabolism of branched-chain amino acids. There are several metabolic pathways for the oxidative metabolism of propionic acid. In mammals, the primary pathway involves the vitamin B_{12}–dependent metabolism of propionic acid to succinyl CoA via the enzyme methylmalonyl-CoA.[22] A secondary pathway that has also been reported involves conversion of propionic acid to acetate via acrylyl CoA, which is then hydrolyzed to 3-hydroxypropionate. This is further metabolized to acetate and carbon dioxide via malonic semialdehyde.[17] Although the vitamin B_{12}–dependent pathway is considered to be the major route of metabolism in mammals, evidence exists for the presence of the secondary non–vitamin B_{12}–dependent pathway. Acrylic acid is metabolized in vitro to carbon dioxide by the non–vitamin B_{12}–dependent pathway, as evidenced by detection of the intermediate 3-hydroxypropionate.[17] In addition, 3-hydroxypropionic acid has been detected in the urine of patients deficient in the vitamin B_{12}–dependent enzyme methylmalonyl-CoA,[1] and it may serve as a secondary pathway in humans with a defect in the major pathway of propionate metabolism.[58] Metabolism of acrylic acid is thought to be consistent with the non–vitamin B_{12}–dependent pathway and most likely occurs in the mitochondria.[17]

Metabolism of methyl methacrylate initially involves hydrolysis to methacrylic acid.[9] Methacrylic acid is a normal intermediate in the catabolism of valine,[48] as branched-chain methylmalonyl-CoA.[4] This is subsequently converted to succinyl-CoA by methylmalonyl-CoA mutase, after which the four carbon atoms enter the citric acid cycle and are oxidized to carbon dioxide. Exogenous methyl methacrylate may be metabolized along the same pathway, thereby explaining its rapid conversion and excretion in the form of carbon dioxide.

Elimination of acrylic acid occurs primarily in the form of carbon dioxide in expired air, with urinary excretion accounting for only 3% to 6% of the administered dose.[13] Rats exposed either orally or by gavage to acrylic acid were found to have metabolized 45% to 80% of the dose to carbon dioxide within 12 hours.[3] The rate of acrylic acid oxidation in the kidney is 15 times higher than that in the liver, which is twelvefold higher than the rate of oxidation in skin.[3] The high rate of metabolism observed in the kidney may be related to the high capacity for renal oxidative metabolism, rapid mitochondrial reactions, and higher levels of short-chain fatty-acyl CoA synthetase, which is necessary for the first step in acrylic acid metabolism.[3]

Teratogenicity. Some controversy has surrounded the question of whether acrylates and methacrylates and their esters pose embryotoxic or fetotoxic risk. Although one early study reported the development of fetal hemangiomas in rats after intraperitoneal injection of ethyl acrylate,[52] numerous subsequent studies have reported negative results. Authors have refuted the earlier findings, citing an inappropriate method of administration and a lack of histologic evidence.[29] When pregnant Sprague-Dawly rats were exposed to ethyl acrylate via oral and inhalation routes, maternal toxicity was observed at the highest dose level and was associated with a statistically insignificant increase in fetal malformations, including hypoplastic tails and missing vertebrae.[41] The oral median lethal concentration (LC_{50}) of ethyl acrylate in rats has been reported as 1020 mg/kg body weight, and the inhalation LC_{50} as 1000 to 2000 ppm over a 4-hour exposure.[43] No embryotoxic or teratogenic effects were observed in pregnant rats exposed to vapor concentrations of

between 40 and 360 ppm of acrylic acid, an end product of acrylic ester metabolism.[29] The majority of studies conducted to determine the embryotoxicity of acrylic resins show no substantial evidence that methyl methacrylate is teratogenic at levels that are not also maternally toxic.[54] When exposed to the monomer methyl methacrylate by inhalation during days 6 to 15 of gestation, mice embryos exhibited only a slight increase in fetal weight in the exposed study group.[36] In a subsequent study, pregnant rats exposed to the monomer via inhalation exhibited a decrease in maternal body weight overall when compared with controls. In addition, a significant increase in fetal skeletal abnormalities was reported at an intermediate dose; however, because these results were not reproduced at the highest dosing level, the changes were not considered exposure-related.[54] The majority of studies conducted to assess the developmental toxicity of ethyl acrylates and their esters point away from any significant teratogenicity.

Mutagenicity. Animal studies on the carcinogenic potential of acrylic acids and their esters have demonstrated conflicting results; however, the majority of in vitro and in vivo studies point to a lack of significant carcinogenic potential. In a study of rats dosed for 3 months with ethyl acrylate, study animals at the highest dose level demonstrated hyperemia and ulceration of the gastric mucosa, hyperemia and edema of lung alveoli, and necrotizing tubular nephroses. In a longer study, animals at the highest dose level developed changes in drinking and feeding habits. The authors concluded, however, that the incidence of tumors between study and control groups did not differ significantly and that no systemic toxicity or carcinogenic effects could be attributed to acrylic acid in the long-term drinking water study.[24] Chronic exposure of mice to acrylic acid via dermal application similarly did not produce an increased incidence of epidermal tumors.[14] In separate studies, acrylic acid has resulted in a negative AMES *Salmonella* mammalian activation assay,[2] leading to the conclusion that acrylic esters do not induce detectable gene mutations.[35] In the Chinese hamster ovary mutation assay, and the *Drosophila* sex-linked recessive lethal assay, mutation frequencies associated with acrylic acid exposure were below or within acceptable background levels.[35] Acrylic acid did not induce unscheduled DNA synthesis when tested in rat hepatocytes.[35] However, in Chinese hamster ovary cells in culture, acrylic acid did produce a dose-related increase in chromatid breaks and exchanges.[35] This in vitro clastogenic activity was explained by a number of mechanisms, including the production of a genotoxic moiety by acrylic acid that directly interacts with DNA, addition of acrylic acid to the nucleophilic center, or induction of genotoxicity indirectly by treatment conditions such as pH and ionic concentration.[35] Overall, however, evidence for the direct interaction of acrylic acid with DNA nucleophiles is weak, and other assays for mutagenicity such as those just mentioned have been negative.[35] Acrylic acid has been mutagenic in the in vitro mouse lymphoma assay, but the author explains this as a result of a predominance of small colony mutants and a clastogenic effect.[39] Ethyl acrylate has been shown to be both mutagenic[44] and nonmutagenic[56] and has been associated with the development of forestomach papillomas and carcinomas in rats.[21] The author attributed the mechanism of neoplasia to promotion by ethyl acrylate of spontaneously initiated cells, as there is no evidence to support mutagenic potential.[21] Rats exposed to methyl acrylate and *n*-butyl acrylate developed neoplastic changes of nasal mucosa and corneal epithelium, which were attributed to the irritant effect of acrylic esters.[46] Human exposure to either methyl acrylate or *n*-butyl acrylate does not seem to constitute a significant health risk as prolonged exposure to significant amounts of acrylic ester vapor would be too irritating to withstand.[46]

Data regarding human genotoxicity are still somewhat limited. In one study, authors examined chromosome aberration rates and sister chromatid exchange frequency in the peripheral lymphocytes of male workers exposed to methyl methacrylate vapor through organic glass production.[49] Results indicated an increased frequency of sister chromatid exchange in methyl methacrylate–exposed workers compared with the control group, even when smoking was controlled for, but no difference in chromosome aberration rates was observed.[49] A possible factor contributing to the observed difference was the higher average age of subjects in the study group.[49] In a separate study, men occupationally exposed to methyl methacrylate through manufacturing and processing were studied with regard to sister chromatid exchange frequency in peripheral lymphocytes. Overall, no significant difference in frequency was observed between exposed and unexposed groups; however, a significant difference was observed in workers who had been exposed to peak levels of methyl methacrylate.[32] Although methyl methacrylate did not appear to pose a significant mutagenic risk, high exposure levels for a protracted time may become more important. In support of this theory, a study that looked at prevalence of colorectal cancer in a cohort of workers with documented or probable exposure to methyl methacrylate found small increases in disease among exposed workers. These subjects were most likely to have been exposed to the highest levels of methyl methacrylate. Although no sound evidence exists to explain the mutagenic potential of methyl methacrylate, a connection between high levels, extended exposure, and colorectal cancer cannot be excluded.[57]

Dermatitis. Acrylates are the fourth most common cause of contact sensitization from resins.[55] The ability of an acrylic compound to produce contact allergy is dependent on its physical and chemical properties. While increasing the number of acrylic double bonds results in an increased irritant potential, α-methylation, as occurs in the methyl methacrylate monomer, results in a decreased sensitizing potential.[55] Therefore, compared with diacrylic and triacrylic monomers, dimethacrylic and trimethacrylic mono-

mers are weak sensitizers, whereas monoacrylates and methacrylates are weak sensitizers compared with their double bond–containing diacrylic and triacrylic analogs.[55] In general, the polymer end product of polymerization is inert and has little to no sensitizing potential, as in the case of polymethylmethacrylate. In cases where the polymer is suspected of causing a contact allergy, traces of residual monomer may actually be responsible. For example, the use of hearing aids has been associated in some patients with a long-standing contact dermatitis to the hearing aid ear molds.[37] Complaints included discomfort at the external auditory canal, including itching, redness, and swelling.[30] Materials commonly employed in the production of ear molds include methacrylic plastics polymerized from methyl methacrylate or other monomers, polyvinyl chloride, or silicone.[37] To produce methacrylic ear molds, methacrylate monomers are placed in a chamber for polymerization with UV light. Incomplete UV curing due to variable light penetration into the chamber may result in incomplete polymerization of the monomers. Residual monomer could act as a potent allergen if present in the final product.[30] When patch tested, patients developed a positive reaction to the monomers methyl methacrylate, triethyleneglycol dimethacrylate, and urethane dimethacrylate. The subjective symptoms of discomfort reported by patients resolved upon changing to a vinyl ear mold.[30] Similarly, cases of stomatitis associated with an intense burning sensation of the oral mucosa have been reported with the use of dental prostheses.[55] These reactions are considered the result of residual monomers left from the UV curing process.[55]

By far, one of the most common exposures to acrylic and methacrylic resins occurs in dental technicians and personnel who mix bone cement in orthopedic surgeries. Acrylic and methacrylic monomers are used in the production of dental and orthopedic prostheses. Polymerization occurs with the mixing of the polymethylmethacrylate polymer powder with methyl methacrylate liquid monomer, the latter of which is a strong sensitizer.[55] Dental personnel frequently mold the prosthetic material with their bare hands,[55] as wearing protective gloves presumably makes achieving the proper contours more difficult.[45] Even when protective gloves are worn, they are often not helpful due to permeability to the monomer.[45] Proper polymerization should result in little of the unreacted monomer remaining to cause sensitization. Processing of the polymerized product by filing or sawing may liberate residual monomer in the form of fine dust, increasing the likelihood of dermal irritation.[45] Examples of exposure include a 49-year-old woman who had worked for 20 years as a dental assistant. She had a long-standing history of eczema on her hands, forearms, upper eyelids, and perioral area. When she was away from work, her skin lesions improved, then relapsed a few days after her return. Physical exam revealed erythematous, scaly, fissured skin on the back of both her hands and forearms, as well as red and scaly skin on her face, and swelling of her upper eyelids.

Patch tests were positive to ethylene glycol dimethacrylate, and her symptoms improved with decreased exposure.[55]

Acrylic bone cement used in orthopedic surgery is responsible for multiple cases of contact sensitization in orthopedic surgeons, technicians, and nurses.[26] In two separate cases, female nurses who mixed bone cement during orthopedic procedures developed pruritis, redness, and eczema of the hands. In the first case, the patient presented with erythematous, infiltrated skin, with vesicles and exudative areas present on both the palmar and dorsal surfaces of both hands. The second patient presented with better-defined pustules covering several fingers.[26] Both women wore double-glove protection while mixing the bone cement. An orthopedic surgeon who mixed bone cement while wearing two pairs of gloves initially complained of pruritus of the fingers on evenings following surgery. This progressed to paresthesias, pruritus, swelling, and crythema of the index fingers on both hands. Symptoms improved within days following the exposure. Patch testing was positive only to methyl methacrylate.[20] Of 13 cases of dermatitis associated with handling bone cement, 7 patients developed a positive patch test reaction to methyl methacrylate monomer.[20]

Outside the health care industry, occupational exposure to acrylic resins is seen primarily in workers who handle acrylic sealants and adhesives. Dimethacrylate adhesives polymerize in the presence of metal, in an anaerobic environment, and are widely employed in the automotive industry.[18] A 43-year-old woman who had worked for 27 years assembling parts for automobile distributors developed a red, pruritic rash on the dorsa of her wrists and her left forearm. The dermatitis appeared 4 months after introduction of an adhesive containing dimethacrylate. Patch tests with dimethacrylate were positive.[18] A 25-year-old male packer who had been working with a UV-cured lacquer for 6 months developed eczema on his hands, arms, and face. The lacquer contained an amino-substituted diacrylate, bis-3-aminoethyl propanoate ester of tripropylene glycol (BAPETG).[7] Although there are few reported cases of dermatitis developing in craftspeople, including floor layers and carpet layers, acrylic copolymers are used extensively in the lacquers and adhesives used daily in these occupations.

Nonoccupational exposures to acrylic and methacrylic esters also occur. These substances may cause contact dermatitis in patients. Exposure occurs via the acrylate-containing adhesives found in medical tape and adhesive pads, such as those used in electrocardiographic monitoring. A case of contact dermatitis to the adhesive contained in a nicotine transdermal patch was reported in which the patient developed irritation and inflammation at the sites of application.[16] The adhesive contained methyl methacrylate and an ethyl acrylate copolymer; the patient had developed a contact sensitization to the former.[16] Two-hydroxyethyl methacrylate was identified as the cause of eczema that developed at the site of electrode pad application in a female patient;[34] the acrylate components of surgical tape caused eczematous lesions to develop in a male patient following surgery for malignant melanoma.[10]

Finally, the ubiquitous nature of acrylates and methacrylates in manufacturing makes domestic exposure likely. They are used extensively in products such as tapes, glues, and cosmetics, like adhesives for false nails.[10] A 52-year-old woman developed a positive patch test to methyl methacrylate and other acrylic compounds after she sought treatment for eczema that had developed in both hands after she used nail varnish hardener.[10] Generally, removal from exposure and avoidance of acrylate-containing products result in resolution of symptoms. However, with widespread industrial use of acrylates and the difficulty involved in accurately identifying the source of irritation, sensitization to acrylic and methacrylic esters is likely to continue to occur.[10]

Occupational asthma. Although the most commonly observed toxicity associated with exposure to acrylates is contact dermatitis, occupational asthma has also been reported. Acrylic compounds reported to cause airway reactivity include acrylates, methacrylates, and cyanoacrylates. The monomer methyl methacrylate is extensively employed throughout the automobile, furniture, and construction industries, as well as in health care.[32] Respiratory disorders, including cough, sore throat, irritation, and asthma, are reported in humans.[32] Marez and colleagues studied methyl methacrylate–exposed workers and found that functional signs were more common in these individuals than in unexposed control subjects. Complaints included morning cough, chronic cough, morning sputum production, chronic sputum production, dyspnea, wheezing, asthma, and previous episodes of bronchitis.[32] In a separate study, methyl methacrylate–exposed workers also complained of frequent cough and sputum production and throat irritation.[38] Differences persisted when tobacco use was controlled for. Pulmonary function testing revealed a decrease in performance following the work shift that was more pronounced in study subjects, with evidence of a mild obstructive pattern. Methyl methacrylate exposure could not be excluded as a cause for the increased cough and airway obstruction observed in the exposed group, although larger studies would be helpful in elucidating the connection.[32] In patients with methyl methacrylate exposure, respiratory sequelae may include sneezing, rhinorrhea, congestion, throat irritation, cough, chest tightness, rales, wheezing, and respiratory distress.[47] Occupational asthma has been reported among dental technicians and in a plate engraver using methyl methacrylate–containing glue.[47] Removal from exposure reduced but did not eliminate these patients' respiratory symptoms, and long-term medical treatment was required.[47] Similarly, two patients who were exposed to acrylates in printing inks and sealant paste, respectively, required long-term medical management due to persistence of respiratory symptoms after the patients' removal from the source.[47] Little work has been done to improve measurement of acrylate and methacrylate vapor concentrations in workplace air, and little is understood regarding the mechanism of respiratory compromise. Because acrylates are contact sensitizers, they may also act to produce pharyngitis and rhinitis via a Type IV delayed hypersensitivity reaction.[47] There is no evidence to support the role of an IgE-mediated allergic reaction.[47]

Neurotoxicity. Peripheral nerve toxicity associated with exposure to acrylic resins has been reported. As with contact dermatitis, symptoms have been most widespread in dental technicians and handlers of bone cement who tend to have the most prolonged and intense exposure to acrylic monomers. In one study, 25% of dental technicians surveyed reported having experienced digital and palmar paresthesias, as well as pain and whitening of the fingers.[45] Donaghy and colleagues described the case of a 55-year-old dental technician who began complaining of paresthesias in the tips of his right thumb and index finger with loss of manipulation and opposition strength, as well as leg weakness. Physical exam revealed atrophy and weakness of the small muscles of the hand, distal and proximal extremity weakness, and decreased deep tendon reflexes. The patient had been molding dental prostheses without the use of protective gloves for 30 years. He mixed the dental acrylate by hand, holding the mixing vessel against his chest. This created a significant inhalation and dermal exposure.[15] Nerve conduction studies were consistent with generalized neuropathy, demonstrating decreased amplitude. Nerve biopsy revealed a chronic axonopathy, with loss of large-diameter fibers and unmyelinated axons.[15] Similar neurophysiologic testing in 22 dental technicians who had experienced contact dermatitis revealed slowed conduction of the right median nerve and the radial aspects of the fingers.[50] The greatest degree of slowing was observed in the median nerve branches from digits with the most significant degree of exposure.[50] The mechanism of the observed axonopathy and neurotoxicity is unknown. One postulated mechanism invokes the reaction of methyl methacrylate with sulfhydryl groups that are essential to the function of enzymes involved in axonal transport.[50] Neurotoxicity associated with exposure to acrylamide monomer, which is structurally similar to acrylates, is well documented. It is not possible at this point to quantify the degree of exposure that is required before the development of neurologic sequelae.

Cardiovascular. Finally, methyl methacrylate has been shown to affect the myocardium. Patients who have undergone total hip replacements that involved the use of methyl methacrylate–containing bone cement have developed significant cardiovascular compromise, with hypotension and death resulting.[33] In a continuous electrocardiographic monitoring of exposed and unexposed workers, study subjects demonstrated a significantly increased number of supraventricular ectopic beats, as well as nonspecific repolarization changes.[33] In regard to this latter effect, the authors postulated a possible effect of methyl methacrylate on the autonomic nervous system, such as that seen with acrylamide.[32]

Such a mechanism might simultaneously help to explain the effects of methyl methacrylate exposure on peripheral nerves.[32]

Diagnosis. Accurate diagnosis of methyl methacrylate–induced toxicity requires a thorough occupational history to elucidate a history of exposure, including association of symptoms chronologically with work. Physical exam should include a thorough skin exam with particularly close attention to the pattern of dermatitis (particularly involvement of face, arms, and neck). It should also include a thorough chest exam to look for signs of asthma and a head and neck exam to look for upper respiratory irritation. If contact dermatitis to acrylates is suspected, referral of patients to a dermatologist capable of performing the required patch testing may be mandated. In regard to patch testing, monoacrylates should be tested at concentrations of 1% or less in petroleum.[55] Monomethyl acrylates can be tested at higher concentrations, as they are less sensitizing. The entire series of acrylates and methacrylates should be reserved only for patients who are strongly suspected of having allergic contact dermatitis to acrylates in order to avoid active sensitization. The patients' own products may be tested in 1% petroleum.[55] Finally, if a diagnosis of occupational asthma is suspected, an inhalational challenge test can be performed. Although removal of the patient from the exposure is the main treatment, it can also serve to elucidate the diagnosis if resolution of symptoms is noted.

Treatment. Treatment of toxicity associated with chronic exposure to acrylates and methacrylates is highly dependent on the route of exposure and the subsequent illness. However, the most apparent and effective treatment for any exposure is removal from the source. This may not be as simple as job relocation. Instead, the worker must start using personal protective equipment and safe handling methods, while the employer must provide a safe and clean work space, as free from exposure as possible.[47]

For health care workers who are exposed to acrylates through handling dental prosthetic material or bone cement, protection may not be as simple as wearing a pair of gloves. Several studies reveal the ineffectiveness of regular latex gloves.[40] Dental technicians have reported the dissolution of certain gloves in monomeric acrylate.[45] The rate of passage of acrylates and methacrylates through various glove materials depends upon both the molecular weight and the solubility of the monomer, as well as on the thickness of the glove.[20] Methyl methacrylate monomer has been demonstrated to diffuse directly through certain types of gloves.[20] Vinyl glove tips were heavily affected, and latex rubber gloves became wrinkled and brittle when exposed to acrylates in vitro.[20] Wearing multiple gloves may serve to increase the time over which diffusion occurs. Conversely, gloves may serve to keep the monomer close to the skin.[20] This increases the risk of sensitization, as otherwise the monomer would rapidly evaporate.[20] In a separate study, a patient who had developed contact dermatitis of the hands was able to return to work only with the use of 0.48-mm-thick butyl rubber gloves.[26] However, these gloves offer less tactile sensitivity than latex gloves. A second type of glove that is impervious to methyl methacrylate is the 0.07-mm-thick 4-H glove, consisting of an outer layer of polyethylene, an intermediate layer of ethylene vinyl alcohol copolymer, and an inner layer of polyethylene.[12]

Respiratory toxicity can be prevented by implementing personal protective measures, including the use of respirators. Fume hoods and extraction fans can reduce the level of acrylate vapor.[8] In the orthopedic surgical suit, use of a punctual field suction aggregate directly over the surgical field may substantially decrease the concentration of methyl methacrylate in the breathing space.[11] Improved monitoring of air levels is also needed. One sampling method for methyl methacrylate employs a sample tube that would allow for improved analytical sensitivity at lower vapor concentrations.[23] Finally, a yearly physical exam of workers exposed via inhalation to methyl methacrylate may help elucidate symptoms or detect changes in pulmonary function tests. This may help in the early identification of respiratory compromise. Early recommendation for work transfer may help to avoid a more prolonged exposure and severe pulmonary sequelae.[32]

Alternate mechanisms of monomer mixing have been proposed to decrease both dermal and inhalation exposure. In the dental setting, Clark and colleagues have proposed the use of a mixing envelope. This technique involves placing the polymer into a polyethylene pouch and adding the liquid monomer through a small opening with a syringe. The pouch is then sealed and kneaded to produce mixing. Because the envelope is thicker than gloves of the same material, monomer diffusion time is increased, rendering exposure less likely.[8] A similar closed-container approach is useful in the orthopedic setting. Mixing of the monomer with the polymer in one system occurs directly in a cartridge that is subsequently used for application of bone cement into the joint cavity.[11] A second system utilizes a closed mixing chamber in which the cement is mixed in a box inside a second container. Both systems result in decreased levels of aerosolized monomer than those seen in open mixing systems. A cement gun for placement of bone cement into the joint also serves to reduce the risk of exposure.[11]

In patients who develop sensitization to acrylates, treatment should include discontinuation of the offending substance and substitution with a nonsensitizing agent. In patients who develop inflammation of the ear canal secondary to wearing acrylate-containing ear molds, a new ear mold should be fashioned that contains decreased levels of monomer, or a vinyl or silicone ear mold should be substituted.[37] Patients with long-standing dermatitis of unknown origin should be questioned regarding occupational exposure history and sent to a dermatologist who specializes in occupational allergens if a source cannot be determined.

REFERENCES

1. Ando T et al: 3-hydroxypropionate: significance of beta-oxidation propionate in patients with propionic acidemia and methylmalonic acidemia, *Proc Natl Acad Sci U S A* 69:2807, 1972.
2. Andrews LS, Clary JJ: Review of the toxicity of multifunctional acrylates, *J Toxicol Environ Health* 19:149, 1986.
3. Black A, Finch L, Frederick CB: Metabolism of acrylic acid to carbon dioxide in mouse tissues, *Fundam Appl Toxicol* 21:97, 1993.
4. Bratt H, Hathway DE: Fate of methyl methacrylate in rats, *Br J Cancer* 36:114, 1977.
5. Bureau of Labor Statistics, United States Department of Labor, Office of Employment and Unemployment Statistics: Current population survey, *Employment and Earnings,* 42:175, 1995.
6. Bureau of Labor Statistics, Office of Employment and Unemployment Statistics, United States Department of Labor: *Occupational employment statistics dictionary of occupations 1988-1996,* 1995.
7. Carmichael AJ, Foulds IS: Allergic contact dermatitis due to an amino-substituted diacrylate in a UV-cured lacquer, *Contact Dermatitis* 28:45, 1993.
8. Clark BR, Brown JR, Matranga LF: Methylmethacrylate: managing the toxicity. *J New Jersey Dental Association,* Summer, 1993, 25-29.
9. Crout HG et al: Methylmethacrylate metabolism in man, *Clin Orthop* 141:90, 1979.
10. Daeke C, Schaller J, Goos M: Acrylates as potent allergens in occupational and domestic exposures, *Contact Dermatitis* 30:190, 1994.
11. Darre E, Holmich P, Jensen JS: The use and handling of acrylic bone cement in Danish orthopaedic departments, *Pharmacol Toxicol* 72:332, 1993.
12. Darre E, Vedel P, Jensen JS: Skin protection against methyl methacrylate, *Acta Orthop Scand* 58:236, 1987.
13. DeBethizy JD et al: The disposition and metabolism of acrylic acid and ethyl acrylate in male Sprague-Dawley rats, *Fundam Appl Toxicol* 8:549, 1987.
14. DePass LR et al: Dermal oncogenicity bioassay of acrylic acid, ethyl acrylate and butyl acrylate, *J Toxicol Environ Health* 14:115, 1984.
15. Donaghy M, Rushworth G, Jacobs JM: Generalized peripheral neuropathy in a dental technician exposed to methyl methacrylate monomer, *Neurology* 41:1112, 1991.
16. Dwyer CM, Forsyth A: Allergic contact dermatitis from methacrylates in a nicotine transdermal patch, *Contact Dermatitis* 30:309, 1994.
17. Finch L, Frederick CB: Rate and route of oxidation of acrylic acid to carbon dioxide in rat liver, *Fundam Appl Toxicol* 19:498, 1992.
18. Foulds IS, Koh D: Contact allergy to 1-acetyl-2-phenylhydrazine in a dimethacrylate adhesive, *Contact Dermatitis* 25:251, 1991.
19. Fox J, editor: *Floors and floor coverings,* San Ramon, Calif, 1986, Ortho Books.
20. Fries IB, Fisher A, Salvati E: Contact dermatitis in surgeons from methylmethacrylate bone cement, *J Bone Joint Surg Am* 57:547, 1975.
21. Ghanayem BL et al: Relationship between the time of sustained ethyl acrylate forestomach hyperplasia and carcinogenicity, *Environ Health Perspect* 101(suppl 5):277, 1993.
22. Halarnkar PP, Blomquist GJ: Comparative aspects of propionate metabolism, *Comp Biochem Physiol* [B] 92:227, 1988.
23. Harper M: A novel sampling method for methyl methacrylate in workplace air, *Am Ind Hyg Assoc J* 53:773, 1992.
24. Hellwig J, Deckardt K, Freisberg KO: Subchronic and chronic studies of the effects of oral administration of acrylic acid to rats, *Food Chem Toxicol* 31:1, 1993.
25. *International Labor Organization Encyclopedia of Health and Safety,* ed 3, Geneva, 1983, International Labor Organization.
26. Kassis V, Vedel P, Darre E: Contact dermatitis to methyl methacrylate, *Contact Dermatitis* 11:26, 1984.
27. Kivimaki J, Riihimaki H, Hanninen K: Knee disorders in carpet and floor layers and painters, *Scand J Work Environ Health* 18:310, 1992.

28. Kivimaki J, Riihimaki H, Hanninen K: Knee disorders in carpet and floor layers and painters, *Scand J Rehabil Med* 26:97, 1994.
29. Klimisch HJ, Hellwig J: The prenatal toxicity of acrylic acid in rats, *Fundam Appl Toxicol* 16:656, 1991.
30. Koefoed-Nielsen B, Pedersen B: Allergy caused by light-cured ear moulds, *Scand Audiol* 22:193, 1993.
31. Marez T et al: Increased frequency of sister chromatid exchange in workers exposed to high doses of methylmethacrylate, *Mutagenesis* 6:127, 1991.
32. Marez T et al: Bronchial symptoms and respiratory function in workers exposed to methylmethacrylate, *Br J Ind Med* 50:894, 1993.
33. Marez T, Shirali P, Haguanoer JM: Continuous ambulatory electrocardiography among workers exposed to methylmethacrylate, *Int Arch Occup Environ Health* 64:373, 1992.
34. Marren P, de Berker D, Powell S: Methacrylate sensitivity and transcutaneous electrical nerve stimulation (TENS), *Contact Dermatitis* 25:190, 1991.
35. McCarthy K et al: Genetic toxicology of acrylic acid, *Food Chem Toxicol* 30:505, 1992.
36. McGaughlin RE et al: Methylmethacrylate: a study of teratogenicity and fetal toxicity of the vapor in the mouse, *J Bone Joint Surg* 60:355, 1978.
37. Meding B, Ringdahl A: Allergic contact dermatitis from the earmolds of hearing aids, *Ear Hear* 13:122, 1992.
38. Mizunuma K et al: Biological monitoring and possible health effects in workers occupationally exposed to methyl methacrylate, *Int Arch Occup Environ Health* 65:227, 1993.
39. Moore MM et al: Genotoxicity of acrylic acid, methyl acrylate, ethyl acrylate, methyl methacrylate, and ethyl methacrylate in L5178Y mouse lymphoma cells, *Environ Mol Mutagen* 11:49, 1988.
40. Munksgaard EC: Permeability of protective gloves to (di)methacrylates in resinous dental materials, *Scand J Dent Res* 100:189, 1992.
41. Murray JS et al: Teratological evaluation of inhaled ethyl acrylate in rats, *Toxicol Appl Pharmacol* 60:106, 1981.
42. Myllymaki TT et al: Carpet-layers knee: an ultrasonographic study, *Acta Radiol* 34:496, 1993.
43. Pozzani UC, Weil CS, Carpenter C: Subacute vapor toxicity and range-finding data for ethyl acrylate, *J Ind Hyg Toxicol* 31:311, 1949.
44. Przybojewska B, Dziubaltowska E, Kowalski Z: Genotoxic effects of ethyl acrylate and methyl acrylate in the mouse evaluated by the micronucleu test, *Mutat Res* 135:189, 1984.
45. Rajaniemi R, Tola S: Subjective symptoms among dental technicians exposed to the monomer methyl methacrylate, *Scand J Work Environ Health* 11:281, 1985.
46. Reininghaus W, Koestner W, Klimisch HJ: Chronic toxicity and oncogenicity of inhaled methyl acrylate and *n*-butyl acrylate in Sprague-Dawley rats, *Food Chem Toxicol* 29:329, 1991.
47. Savonius B et al: Occupational respiratory disease caused by acrylates, *Clin Exp Allergy,* 23:416, 1993.
48. Scolnick B: Acrylates and methacrylates. In Sullivan JB Jr, Krieger GR, editors: *Hazardous materials toxicology: clinical principles of environmental health,* Baltimore, 1992, Williams & Wilkins.
49. Seiji K, et al: Absence of mutagenicity in peripheral lymphocytes of workers occupationally exposed to methyl methacrylate, *Ind Health* 32:97, 1994.
50. Seppalainen A, Rajaniemi R: Local neurotoxicity of methyl methacrylate among dental technicians, *Am J Ind Med* 5:471, 1984.
51. Seutter E, Rijntjes NVM: Whole-body autoradiography after systemic and topical administration of methyl acrylate in the guinea pig, *Arch Dermatol Res* 270:273, 1981.
52. Singh AR, Lawrence WH, Autian J: Embryonic fetal toxicity and teratogenic effects of a group of methylacrylate esters in rats, *J Dent Res* 51:1632, 1972.
53. Smith S: *Painting and wallpapering,* San Ramon, Calif, 1984, Ortho Books.
54. Solomon HM: Methyl methacrylate: inhalation developmental toxicity study in rats, *Teratology* 48:115, 1993.
55. Tosti A, Guerra L, Bardazzi F: Occupational contact dermatitis from exposure to epoxy resins and acrylates, *Clin Dermatol* 10:133, 1992.
56. Wagemakers THJM, Bensik MPM: Non-mutagenicity of 27 aliphatic acrylate esters in Salmonella-microsome test, *Mutat Res* 137:95, 1984.
57. Walker AM: Mortality from cancer of the colon or rectum among workers exposed to ethyl acrylate and methyl methacrylate, *Scand J Work Environ Health* 17:7, 1991.
58. Winter SM, Sipes IG: The disposition of acrylic acid in the male Sprague-Dawley rat following oral or topical administration, *Food Chem Toxicol* 31:615, 1993.
59. Zenz C, Dickerson OB, Horvath EP Jr, eds: *Occupational medicine,* ed 3, St Louis, 1994, Mosby–Year Book.

17

tetramethylthiuram disulfide

3-n-pentadecatrienylcatechol
(a urushiol constituent)

- Plant-induced dermatitis is a ubiquitous problem in these occupations

- A wide range of chemicals are in use as fungicides

- All dithiocarbamates interact with alcohol to produce a disulfuram-like reaction

Florists and Groundskeepers

Lewis Nelson

OCCUPATIONAL DESCRIPTION

Any person who handles plants, shrubs, or trees in their native or preserved state, including their flowers, leaves, roots, fruits, seeds, or cones, is at risk for exposure to phytotoxins. This category includes those who plant, grow, harvest, arrange, and sell these products. In addition, this same group is exposed to agents used to prevent fungal, bacterial, or parasitic invasion and to increase the yield and quality of the plants.

Major Job Categories

Florists, nursery workers, horticulturists, market workers, importers, botanists, groundskeepers, gardeners, landscapers, golf course workers, food handlers, and forest workers include most workers in this group.

Relevant Statistics

Nearly one third of 462 floral shops surveyed had one employee with job-related dermatitis.[22] Evaluation of workers at four floristry centers found that 25% of workers had dermatologic manifestations, with 5% confirmed to be allergic and the remainder related to chemicals and pesticides.[44]

A Swedish study comparing horticulturists and a reference population noted reduced total mortality and mortality due to malignancy, cardiovascular and respiratory causes in the horticulturists. Mortality was noted to be elevated in patients due to gastric, dermal, and central nervous system tumors.[27a] In addition, chronic mixed fungicide use is significantly associated with reduced peripheral and autonomic nerve function in Dutch bulb farmers.[43]

135

Epidemiology

Because of the diverse and widespread use of plants and flowers, the population at risk is not readily delineated. In the floral industry itself, approximately 45,000 workers have been estimated to be at risk in the United States.[43] Workers manually handling pesticide-treated plants appear to receive significantly higher exposures than those applying the pesticide.[1] Because of the nature of the industry, with potentially large numbers of undocumented workers, in addition to the prevalence of gardening as a pastime, the true at-risk population is much larger. Additionally, many workers may not report the lesions because of their commonness[30] and the existence of effective over-the-counter and folk remedies.

POTENTIAL TOXIC EXPOSURES
Fungicides

Fungicides are a large group of unrelated agents that have in common the ability to selectively interfere with the function or metabolism of fungi. They are used extensively for the protection of grains, seeds, crops, and flowers during storage and shipment. Fungicides are also used in the home as mildew suppressors for carpet and paint. The fungicides currently in use are considerably safer than those used historically for several reasons. A more thorough understanding of the inherent differences between fungi and mammals has allowed the design of agents that are selectively fungicidal. Inadvertent human exposure to older, nonspecific toxins, such as methylmercury, resulted in several large-scale tragedies.[41] Additionally, the formulation of fungicides as wettable powders or other solid forms reduces dermal exposure and permits skin decontamination before absorption occurs.

Acute human toxicity of all the fungicides tends to be limited to dermatotoxicity, particularly irritant dermatitis and allergic sensitization. Although uncommon, metabolic effects may occasionally be seen, especially after large, intentional poisoning. The different classes of agents vary widely in their ability to produce human toxicity, but those within a given family produce similar manifestations.

There are many classes of agents used as fungicides (see box). Although not all are available in the United States, they may occasionally be found on imported fruits and other plant products. Only those classes that are widely used are covered.

Dithiocarbamates. Of the many classes of fungicides available today, the dithiocarbamates are most commonly used. In addition, they have other industrial uses, most commonly as accelerators in the vulcanization of rubber. The dithiocarbamates may be divided into three general classes: thiurams (bisdithiocarbamates, e.g., thiram, disulfiram), dimethyldithiocarbamates (metallo-bisdithiocarbamates, e.g., ferbam, ziram), and ethylene-bisdithiocarbamates (e.g., maneb, nabam, zineb). Many of the dithio-

---

Fungicides	
Chlorinated hydrocarbon	**Anilide**
Chlorothalonil	Carboxin
Hexachlorobenzene	
Pentachlorophenol	**Dinitrophenol**
Quintozene	Dinocap
	Inorganic
Phthalimide	Copper sulfate
Captan	Sulfuryl fluoride
Benzimidazole	**Guanidine**
Benomyl	Dodine
Thiabendazole	
	Dicarboximide
Imidazole	Vinclozolin
Imazalil	Iprodion
Acylalanine	
Metalaxyl	
Dithiocarbamates	
Thiuram: thiram	
Dimethydithiocarbamates:	
ferbam, ziram	
Ethylenebisdithiocarbamates:	
maneb, zinab	

---

carbamates are complexed with a metal or similar moiety, and this is reflected in the chemical name (e.g., zineb has zinc, and ferbam has iron). Through use in the treatment of recurrent ethanol intoxication, disulfiram, a thiuram, has been the agent most widely studied in humans.

The dithiocarbamates as a group possess a low order of acute toxicity. The dithiocarbamates are generally considered mucosal irritants and skin sensitizers.[20] Although the ethylenebisdithiocarbamate compounds tend to be more potent sensitizers, recurrent exposures are still necessary to elicit an immune response. Acute poisoning in humans may occur from extensive dermal exposure or after intentional ingestion but is rare from inhalation.[26] Various gastrointestinal and neurologic symptoms have been seen. However, it is unclear whether the symptoms are related to the dithiocarbamate and not the other compounds present in the mixtures.[25] Metabolism of dithiocarbamates results in the liberation of carbon disulfide (CS_2).[8] Acute exposure to carbon disulfide may produce headache, delirium, and encephalopathy, which are similar to the manifestations noted in patients after large dithiocarbamate intoxications.[5] It is therefore likely that CS_2 is responsible for at least part of the acute toxic effects of dithiocarbamates. Unlike the *N*-methyl carbamate insecticides, the antifungal carbamate derivatives do not appear to inhibit cholinesterase.[29]

Several poorly described chronic sequelae have been reported. Chronic exposure to carbon disulfide has been associated with Parkinson's disease, retinopathy, hearing loss, and accelerated coronary artery disease.[49] Indeed, parkinsonism has been seen in patients exposed to disulfiram[21] and maneb.[13,32] In addition to CS_2 formation, maneb contains manganese, a toxin known to induce parkinsonism.[18] In most other cases, the metallic moiety is unlikely to be related to toxicity as similar toxicity is produced by each group despite disparate metals.

Disulfiram, like all of the dithiocarbamates, elevates the serum acetaldehyde concentration through inhibition of aldehyde dehydrogenase.[6] This is probably the effect of greatest clinical concern in humans occupationally exposed to dithiocarbamates. Ethanol consumption just before or for a variable time after exposure to dithiocarbamate results in abdominal pain, vomiting, tremor, hypotension, or seizure. It is unknown if the other enzyme-inhibiting properties of disulfiram (e.g., dopamine β-hydroxylase) are common to the group.[31] Another potential but uncommon acute toxic event is the formation of sulfhemoglobinemia in workers with glucose-6-phosphate dehydrogenase deficiency.[37]

Both acute and chronic exposure to dithiocarbamate is associated with alterations in thyroid function in animals. Decreased uptake of radioactive iodine and glandular hypertrophy (goiter) have been noted consistently.[8] Additionally, ethylene thiourea, a metabolite of the ethylenebisdithiocarbamates, has been noted to be a thyroid carcinogen in animals.[26] However, thyroid abnormalities have not been noted in dithiocarbamate-exposed workers.[53] While the mechanism remains unknown, involvement of carbon disulfide, thiourea, or free elemental sulfur has been suggested.

In animal trials, ingestion of mancozeb caused reproductive toxicity only at exceedingly high dosing. Reproductive toxicity has been demonstrated with maneb.[28] Ethylene thiourea is a known teratogen, which raises suspicions about their safety with chronic use.[8]

The physical examination should contain a thorough dermatologic evaluation for signs of irritation or eczema. The thyroid gland should be carefully palpated for size, firmness, and masses. Signs and symptoms of alcoholism should be carefully elicited to avoid an inevitable "disulfiram reaction." Careful evaluations for subtle neurologic abnormalities such as memory, concentration, and peripheral motor and sensory function is indicated.

There are no widely utilized or accepted methods to biologically monitor workers exposed to dithiocarbamates. Some have suggested monitoring metabolite levels such as carbon disulfide, xanthurenic acid, or ethylene thiourea.[26] In addition, baseline and as-needed (postoverexposure, goiter) thyroid function tests should be performed. Hepatic and renal function should be considered before exposure. A pregnancy test should be performed if appropriate.

Patients with dermatitis should be removed from exposure and observed for improvement. Thyroid abnormalities should be further evaluated as needed. There is no antidote for overexposure to dithiocarbamate, so prevention and supportive care are indicated. The disulfiram reaction may be treated with intravenous fluids, and pressor agents may be needed if it is severe.

Pentachlorophenol

Despite its long history as a wood preservative, especially for telephone poles, pentachlorophenol (PCP) use has been severely restricted. The presence of contaminants such as polychlorinated dibenzodioxin and dibenzofurans[35] makes the unpurified form of this compound too toxic for general use. Most occupational exposure to PCP occurs to carpenters, electrical line workers, and fungicide applicators. Inhalational exposure to PCP results in upper respiratory irritation. Dermal exposure produces erythema, pain, and exfoliation of the epidermal layer. Cases of chloracne have likely been related to the presence of dioxin contaminants in PCP.[54]

Systemic toxicity is primarily related to the ability of PCP to uncouple oxidative phosphorylation. Uncoupling of oxidative phosphorylation produces a hypermetabolic state, including sweating, hyperthermia, and altered mental status. Several cases of systemic toxicity resulting from dermal exposure have been reported, including an epidemic in a newborn nursery linked to PCP-treated diapers.[41] As with all chlorinated hydrocarbons, myocardial sensitization with tachyarrhythmia is possible, as are central nervous system depression and seizures. After prolonged exposures, hepatotoxicity and aplastic anemia have been noted.[40]

Immediate concerns to exposed patients should be directed toward skin or gastrointestinal decontamination and cooling, if the core temperature is significantly elevated. There is some evidence that cholestyramine may interrupt the enterohepatic circulation and enhance elimination.[42] The Occupational Safety and Health Administration (OSHA) permissible exposure limit is 0.5 mg/m^3; the National Institute for Occupational Safety and Health (NIOSH) level of immediate danger to life and health (IDLH) is 150 mg/m^3; and the American Conference of Governmental Industrial Hygienists (ACGIH) threshold limit value (TLV) is 0.5 mg/m^3.

Benomyl

Benomyl is a carbamate derivative of the anthelmintic thiabendazole fungicidal agent. Despite the drug's structure, it, like the dithiocarbamates, is unable to inhibit cholinesterase except at exceptionally high levels. Benomyl and thiabendazole produce their effect through a benzimidazole group. These agents inhibit tubulin formation.[29,50] The acute toxicity of these agents is considered low, especially compared with the insecticidal carbamates, although complete toxicologic data in humans is lacking. Contact dermatitis has been recognized and may be particularly common in Japanese women.[51]

Phthalimides

Phthalimide fungicides include captafol, folpet, and the structurally similar captan and are widely used in both home and professional settings. The most frequently observed adverse reaction with the group is reversible dermatitis.[2] The presence of the phthalimide nucleus has raised concern about teratogenicity since this same region is shared by the antinausea medication thalidomide, well known for adverse fetal effects. Studies in several animal species known to be susceptible to thalidomide teratogenicity have suggested that the antifungal agents are safe.[8] In addition, there appear to be no adverse effects on chromosomes, and teratogenicity has not been reported or adequately studied in humans.

Organotin Compounds

There are several alkyl and aromatic derivatives of tin, including trimethyltin, triethyltin, triphenyltin, and tributyltin, which are employed as fungicides. Triphenyltin is used as an agricultural fungicide, while the alkyl-substituted agents are preservatives in paint, paper, and textiles. These agents appear to function by inhibiting oxidative phosphorylation and enhancing the permeability of mitochondrial membranes.[12] Organotin compounds are mucosal irritants, producing conjunctival, airway, and gastrointestinal symptoms on contact. Some of these agents, such as tributyltin, can cause dermal burns upon contact. Triphenyltin is responsible for most occupational exposure to organotin compounds.[4] Headache, nausea, dizziness, seizures, and dermatitis may be seen, as can elevation of hepatic transaminases. Chronic exposure to organic tin compounds leads to lymphoid tissue depletion and altered T-lymphocyte function, probably through microtubule inhibition.[4] Although the alkyltins tend to have more neurotoxic effects, such as headache, muscle weakness, and paralysis, and the aromatic derivatives are more hepatotoxic, there is much overlap.

PLANT DERMATITIS

Plants have devised many methods to ward off intruders and to attract guests. Many plants contain chemicals that have profound pharmacologic effect on animals, including humans. Examples include anticholinergic agents (atropine, scopolamine), strychnine, and essential oils (pennyroyal, safrole). However, these are seldom of any significance in the workplace unless, of course, a plant or plant part is ingested. Still, skin exposure to plant parts (leaves, bark, flowers, roots, sap, fruits) continues to be a major occupational hazard. Approximately half of the workers' compensation claims filed in California are for poison oak dermatitis.[10,24] A survey of retail florists compiled by

OSHA noted that in approximately one third of floral shops at least one employee was affected by dermatitis.[22] Toxicity is often unpredictable and may vary with the season, maturity, cultivar and growing area, and individual sensitivity.

Plant dermatitis is classified by mechanism, which may be mechanical irritation, chemical irritation, allergic sensitization, photosensitization, or pseudophytodermatitis (see box on p. 139), which relates to conditions mistaken for plant induced that are, in reality, due to pests or applied chemical agents.

The irritant dermatoses produce skin that may be intensely pruritic, with edema, erythema, and papular or vesicular lesions. Those patients with severe dermatitis may present with bullae or ulceration. Chronically exposed workers may have dry, fissured skin.

Mechanical irritant dermatitis results from contact with rough or spiny plant parts, such as thorns, leaves, branches, and fruiting bodies, that produce a tear or puncture of the skin. Grasses and cereal grains, as well as prickly pear cactus (Sabra dermatitis), are well known to produce this type of lesion. In addition to the irritation, foreign objects or infectious agents can be introduced into the wound. For example, cactus needles can break off in the skin and cause infection and granuloma formation.[19] Spores of the fungus *Sporothrix schenckii* introduced through breaks in the dermal barrier may lead to granulomas along the route of lymphatic drainage characteristic of sporotrichosis. A recent outbreak affecting 17% of those handling evergreen tree seedlings highlights the relative ease of transmission of the disease. Sphagnum moss and rosebushes are commonly associated with sporotrichosis.[3]

Chemical irritant dermatitis is produced by substances that exert a toxic effect on tissue in a nonimmunologic manner. Therefore, unlike allergic manifestations, no prior contact is needed to elicit a skin response. Chemical irritation is most commonly caused by members of the spurge family (Euphorbiaceae) and is due to the presence of diterpenes, known as *phorbol esters,* in the sap. Poinsettia (*E. pulcherrima*) and candelabra cactus (*E. lactea*) are common examples in homes and nurseries. Phorbol esters are, in addition, thought to be cocarcinogens due to their ability to increase cell division in vitro. Other families commonly associated with chemical contact injury include *Brassica* and Ranunculaceae (buttercup).

In some plant species, a specialized apparatus has developed to allow transfer of the irritant substances. The leaves of plants in the Arum family, such as *Dieffenbachia,* harbor idioblasts, which are small pouches containing crystals of calcium oxalate. With pressure, especially upon chewing, the oxalate needles are released, penetrate the skin or mucous membranes, and cause pain and itching. Workers in the bulb industries may develop a scaling, erythematous dermatitis from the large amounts of calcium oxalate present in daffodil or hyacinth bulbs.[17]

Florist List

Plants (irritant)

Euphorbia (phorbol esters)
Arum (oxalate)
Daffodils, hyacinth bulbs (oxalate)
Pineapples (oxalate and bromelin)
Criciferae (mustard, radish, horseradish) isocyanates
Ranunculae (buttercup, protoanemonin)

Contact dermatitis (sensitizer)

Toxicodendron (urushiol)
Lichens (d-usnic acid)
Orchids (quinone)
Tulips (α-methylene-γ-butyrolactone)
Primrose (quinone)
Compositae *Ambrosia* [(ragweed), chrysanthemum, feverfew] sesquiterpene lactones
Liverworts (sesquiterpene lactones)

Plants containing urushiol or other catechols

T. radicans, poison ivy
T. toxicarium and *T. diversilobum,* poison oak
T. vernix, poison sumac
Mango
Cashew nut
Lacquer tree
Indian marking nut
Rengas tree
Gingko (related catechols)

Plants containing sesquiterpene lactone
Family compositae asteraceae

Dandelions (Taraxacum)
Asters
Daisies
Dahlias
Weeds: feverfew, tanzy
Chrysanthemums
Marigolds
Lettuce, artichokes
Other families containing SLs
Magnoliaceae *(Magnolia stelata)*
Lauraceae (bay tree)
Jubulaceae (liverwort)

Treatment of chemical irritant exposures includes copious irrigation of the affected area with water. Ocular involvement may be very distressing to the patient, and early irrigation is critical to limiting the complications, such as corneal injury. Oral injury, especially of the posterior oral cavity, may produce dramatic swelling that may require aggressive airway support.

Contact urticaria may have an immunologic or nonimmunologic basis. True allergic responses appear to be more common in atopic patients. Tulips and lillies have been noted to produce contact urticaria.[23] Stinging nettles (Urticaceae) introduce histamine into the skin with spines like hypodermic needles and cause a urticarial response without an immunologic basis. Cowhage *(Mucuna pruriens)* are fuzzy pods with hollow, fine hairs capable of penetrating intact skin and injecting a pruritogenic peptide, mucunain. This produces urticaria, erythema, and pruritis[46] and accounts for its use as "itch powder."[25]

Allergic contact dermatitis requires sensitization through prior exposure. Most plant-related allergic contact dermatitis (phytodermatitis) is the result of a cell-mediated immune response against a protein component of the skin altered by a hapten. Plants may either constitutively release toxin-containing resin onto the plant surface (e.g., chrysanthemum) or may do so only in response to injury (e.g., poison ivy), although this difference may have little clinical relevance. In general, it is the potency of the class of sensitizer that determines the extent of contact required for sensitization, although not every person is capable of being sensitized. Although virtually all plants contain substances capable of sensitizing somebody, several large groups of allergens are commonly implicated in cases of contact phytodermatitis: the urushiols, the sesquiterpene lactones, tuliposide A, and quinones.

As mentioned earlier, poison ivy dermatitis is the major occupational problem of outdoor workers.[10] Poison ivy dermatitis develops in sensitized persons 12 to 48 hours after contact with the various *Toxicodendron* species (*T. radicans,* poison ivy; *T. toxicarium,* poison oak; *T. vernix,* poison sumac) and may occur in unsensitized persons 9 to 14 days after exposure ("late reaction"). The toxic principle is urushiol, a mixture of catechols with long alkyl side chains, such as pentadecylcatechol in poison ivy. Urushiol is a potent sensitizer, producing sensitization in most people after a single contact.[9] The patient typically develops an erythematous, papular, or vesicular linear eruption, which is intensely pruritic and localized to the area of toxin contact. Toxin contained under the fingernail may produce dermatitis on any body part that the patient touches. Patch testing is generally not recommended, as the toxin is very potent, and sensitization may occur in unsensitized patients.

The Compositae family includes more than 25,000 species and is the second largest plant family worldwide. As such, interaction between humans and these plants is frequent and largely unavoidable. In addition, the same allergen may also be found in several other plant families. Dermatitis is frequent and appears to be a disease largely of men over the age of 40 years, an association likely due to increased outdoor work.[16] The sensitizing agents belong to the group of sesquiterpene lactones, 15 carbon ringed structures bearing a requisite methylene group on the lactone ring.[34] Ragweed *(Ambrosia)* and other Compositae, may either release pollen or dried debris as the plant withers, either of which is capable of initiating a dermatitis due to their content of sesquiterpene lactone. The diffuse eczematous dermatitis may resemble photodermatitis and is often misdiagnosed as it, but involvement of the triangle behind the ear and other non–sun-exposed areas is not seen in photodermatitis.[16] The eruption may be acute, including vesiculation, but more commonly appears as lichenification or erythroderma that is unresponsive to corticosteroids. The symptoms typically subside in the winter but may become year-round after several seasons of exposure. Patch testing produces a positive response if the proper allergen is selected. Cross-reactivity between different sesquiterpene lactone allergens is frequent and unpredictable. However, with more than 1350 sesquiterpene lactones (SLs) identified, selecting allergens for screening is difficult. For this reason a "sesquiterpene lactone mix" was created that incorporates several representative SLs. Although able to identify most sensitized patients, false negatives occur with regularity.[7,27] In addition, sensitization may occur during patch testing. Treatment is removal from exposure, which may be difficult due to their ubiquitous nature.

A well-described occupational dermatitis in the flower bulb industry is "tulip finger." Tulip bulbs contain tuliposide A, a glycoside that, when cleaved, forms tulipalin A (α-methylene-γ-butyrolactone). This allergen is responsible for the erythematous, painful hyperkeratosis and fissuring of the skin and nails.[52] Other Liliaceae such as *Alstroemeria* (Peruvian lily) are resulting in more cases of significant dermatitis due to their content of tuliposide A or similar, cross-reacting compounds.[22,48]

Naturally occurring quinones are potent sensitizers. Most are found within the wood of large trees, thus affecting timber workers more commonly than groundskeepers. The primrose *(Primula obconica)* is a leading cause of occupational dermatitis in England[33] due to its content of a quinone, primin.

As with most toxic exposures, avoidance is best. If this is not possible, barrier creams, while not infallible, may prove useful[15] against poison ivy. The general management of allergic phytodermatitis is supportive and should include antipruritics and analgesics as needed. Immediate treatment exposure should include thorough washing of the affected areas with soap and water. For poison ivy in particular, removal of antigen from under the fingernails is critical to avoid further contamination. The patient who has not already done so should change and thoroughly wash clothing. Topical corticosteroids may be beneficial, and systemic dosing may be needed for extensive exposure (see box above). Prevention through hyposensitization has met with limited success in humans.[30] Hyposensitization is a long and sometimes uncomfortable procedure that uses increasing doses of purified urushiol containing oleoresin.[10] Although not currently considered useful, it may have a role in highly sensitive individuals at high risk of exposure. In addition, work is progressing toward both pharmacotherapy and immunotherapy of poison ivy.[10]

Contact of moist skin with the furocoumarin psoralen, with subsequent exposure to sunlight, may result in phyto-

---

Treatment of Contact Dermatitis
Mild
Calamine lotion
Warm or cool baths
Avoid topical antihistamines and corticosteroids
Moderate
Open bullae
Cool Burow's solution topically
Zinc oxide
Petrolatum
Potassium permanganate
Oatmeal baths
Antihistamines
Severe
As for moderate
Systemic corticosteroids tapered over 3 weeks (to avoid rebound)

---

photodermatitis. Patients experience pruritus, intense erythema, and bullae formation, often with hyperpigmentation upon healing. Weeds such as wild carrot (Queen Anne's lace, Umbilliferae) and yarrow (Compositae) are frequently associated with occupational photodermatitis. Strimmer rash, also known as *weed wacker dermatitis,* is commonly noted in workers who, while gardening with the common handheld nylon-fiber cutting machine, inadvertently cut psoralen-containing weeds.[14,38] The photodermatitis may resemble poison ivy dermatitis, with linear vesicular streaking called *dermatitis bullosa striata pratensis.*

Insects on or around the plant and substances applied to the plant may also produce a dermatitis simulating phytodermatitis. Pseudophytodermatitis has been noted from mites, insecticides, herbicides, and carnauba wax.[47]

Phytodermatitis is often difficult to identify unless the patient's occupational exposures are considered in detail. Once suspected, Santucci and colleagues have suggested a regimen that involves standard and specific patch testing with known allergens.[44] In addition, screening may be performed with a "sesquiterpene lactone mix" that contains the most common antigens.[7]

OCCUPATIONAL PULMONARY PROBLEMS

Respiratory symptoms related to plants and flowers have been studied less than dermatologic manifestations. Although clinically a common problem, the literature on occupational asthma related to plants consists largely of case reports and small series. A recent allergologic investigation of four patients linked the respiratory symptoms with occupational exposure to decorative flowers.[36] Greenhouse workers have a higher prevalence of both acute and chronic respiratory symptoms than controls. In addition, there may be an association between the length of time worked in a greenhouse and a reduction in ventilatory capacity.[55] It is unclear whether the same antigens responsible for allergic dermatitis also cause a respiratory allergy.

REFERENCES

1. Brouwer DH et al: Pesticides in the cultivation of carnations in greenhouses: part I, exposure and concomitant health risk, *Am Ind Hyg Assoc J* 53:575, 1992.
2. Camarasa G: Difolatan dermatitis, *Contact Dermatitis* 1:127, 1975.
3. Coles FB et al: A multistate outbreak of sporotrichosis associated with sphagnum moss, *Am J Epidemiol* 136:475, 1992.
4. Colosio C et al: Occupational triphenyltin acetate poisoning: a case report, *Br J Ind Med* 48:136, 1991.
5. Dalvi R: Toxicology of thiram (tetramethylthiuram disulfide): a review, *Vet Hum Toxicol* 30:480, 1988.
6. DeTorres GG et al: Blood acetaldehyde level in alcohol-dosed rats after treatment with ANIT, ANTU, dithiocarbate derivatives or cyanamide, *Drug Chem Toxicol* 6:317-328, 1983.
7. Ducombs G et al: Patch testing with the "sesquiterpene lactone mix": a marker for contact allergy to Compositae and other sesquiterpene lactone-containing plants, *Contact Dermatitis* 22:249, 1990.
8. Edwards R, Ferry DG, Temple WA: Fungicides and related compounds. In Hayes WJ, Laws ER, editors: *Handbook of pesticide toxicology,* vol 3, San Diego, 1991, Academic Press.
9. Epstein WL: Contact-type delayed hypersensitivity in infants and children: induction of Rhus sensitivity, *Pediatrics* 27:51, 1961.
10. Epstein WL: Occupational poison ivy and oak dermatitis, *Dermat Clin* 12:511, 1994.
11. Fairbrothers D, Kirby E, Lester RM, et al: Mucuna pruriens associated pruritis-New Jersey, *JAMA* 255:313, 1986.
12. Fait A, Ferioli A, Barbieri F: Organotin compounds, *Toxicology* 91:77, 1994.
13. Ferraz HB et al: Chronic exposure to the fungicide maneb may produce symptoms and signs of CNS manganese intoxication, *Neurology* 38:550, 1988.
14. Freeman K, Hubbard HC, Warin AP: Strimmer rash, *Contact Dermatitis* 10:117, 1984.
15. Grevelink SA, Olsen EA: Efficacy of barrier creams in suppression of experimentally induced Rhus dermatitis, *Am J Contact Dermatitis* 2:69, 1991.
16. Hjorth N, Roed-Petersen J, Thomsen K: Airborne contact dermatitis from Compositae oleoresins simulating photodermatitis, *Br J Derm* 95:613, 1976.
17. Hjorth N, Wilkinson DS: Contact dermatitis IV, *Br J Dermatol* 80:696, 1968.
18. Huang CC et al: Chronic manganese intoxication, *Arch Neurol* 46:1104, 1989.
19. Karpman RR, Spark RP, Fried M: Cactus thorn injuries to the extremities: their management and etiology, *Arizona Med* 37:849, 1980.
20. Kligman AM: Sensitization testing by human assay, *Drug Cosmet Ind* 100:46, 1967.
21. Krauss JK et al: Dystonia and akinesia due to pallidoputaminal lesions after disulfiram intoxication, *Mov Disord* 6:166, 1991.
22. Kuack DL: Handle with care, *Greenhouse Grower* December: 86, 1987.
23. Lahati A: Contact urticaria and respiratory symptoms from tulips and lilies, *Contact Dermatitis* 5:317, 1986.
24. Lampe KF: Toxic effects of plant toxins. In Amdur MO, Doull J, Klaassen CD, editors: *Casaret and Doull's toxicology: the basic science of poisons,* ed 4, New York, 1991, McGraw Hill.
25. Lewis WH, Elvin-Lewis MPH: *Medical botany: plants affecting man's health,* New York, 1977, John Wiley and Sons.
26. Liesivuori J, Savolainen K: Dithiocarbamates, *Toxicology* 91:37, 1994.

27. Lovell CR, Rowan M: Dandelion dermatitis, *Contact Dermatitis* 25:185, 1991.
27a. Littorin M, Attewell R, Skerfving S, et al: Mortality and tumor morbidity among Swedish market gardeners and orchardists, *Int Arch Occup Environ Health* 65:163-169, 1993.
28. Lu MH, Kennedy GL: Teratogenic evaluation of mancozeb in the rat following inhalation exposure, *Toxicol Appl Pharmacol* 84:355, 1986.
29. Machemer LH, Pickel M: Carbamate herbicides and fungicides, *Toxicology* 91:105, 1994.
30. Marks JF, Trautlein JJ, Epstein WL, et al: Oral hyposensitization to poison ivy and poison oak, *Arch Dermatol* 123:476-478, 1987.
31. McKenna MJ, DiStefano V: A proposed mechanism for the action of carbon disulfide on dopamine beta-hydroxylase, *J Pharmacol Exp Ther* 202:254, 1977.
32. Meco G, Bonifate V, Vanacore N, Fabrizio E: Parkinsonism after chronic exposure to the fungicide maneb (manganese ethylene-bis-dithiocarbamate), *Scand J Work Environ Health* 20:301-305, 1994.
33. Merrick C et al: A survey of skin problems in floristry, *Contact Dermatitis* 24:306, 1991.
34. Mitchell JC et al: Allergic contact dermatitis from ragweeds (*Ambrosia* species): the role of sesquiterpene lactones, *Arch Dermatol* 104:73, 1971.
35. Nadig RJ: *Pentachlorophenol toxicity: case studies in environmental medicine,* Washington, DC, 1993, Agency for Toxic Substances and Disease Registry, US Department of Health and Human Services, Public Health Service.
36. Piirila P: Occupational asthma caused by decorative flowers: review and case reports, *Int Arch Occup Environ Health* 66:131, 1994.
37. Pinkhas J et al: Sulfhemoglobinemia and acute hemolytic anemia with Heinz bodies following contact with a fungicide—zinc ethylene bisdithiocarbamate—in a subject with glucose-6-phosphate dehydrogenase deficiency and hypocatalasemia, *Blood* 21:484, 1963.
38. Reynolds NJ et al: Weed wacker dermatitis, *Arch Dermatol* 127:1419, 1991.
39. Rietschel RL, Fowler JF, editors: *Fisher's contact dermatitis,* ed 4, Baltimore, 1995, Williams & Wilkens.
40. Roberts HJ: Aplastic anemia due to pentachlorophenol, *N Engl J Med* 305:1650, 1981.
41. Robson AN et al: Pentachlorophenol poisoning in a nursery for newborn infants: 1: clinical features and treatment, *J Pediatr* 75:309, 1969.
42. Rozman T et al: Effect of cholestyramine on the disposition of pentachlorophenol in rhesus monkeys, *J Toxicol Environ Health* 10:277, 1982.
43. Ruijten MWMM et al: Effect of chronic mixed pesticide exposure on peripheral and autonomic nerve function, *Arch Environ Health* 49:188, 1994.
44. Santucci B, Picardo M: Occupational contact dermatitis to plants, *Clinics in Dermatol* 10:157-165, 1992.
45. Schmid R: Cutaneous porphyria in Turkey, *N Engl J Med* 263:397, 1960.
46. Shelley WB, Arthur RP: Mucunain, the active pruritogenic proteinase of cowhage, *Science* 122:469, 1955.
47. Stoner, JG, Rasmussen JE: Plant dermatitis, *J Am Acad Dermatol* 9:1-15, 1983.
48. Thiboutot DM, Hamory BH, Marks JG: Dermatoses among floral shop workers, *J Am Acad Dermatol* 22:54, 1990.
49. Tiller Jr, Schilling RSF, Morris JW: Occupational toxic factor in mortality from coronary heart disease, *BMJ* 4:407, 1968.
50. Urani C et al: Benomyl affects the microtubule cytoskeleton and the glutathione level of mammalian primary cultured hepatocytes, *Toxicol Let* 76:135-144, 1995.
51. Van Joost T, Naafs B, van Ketel WG: Sensitization to benomyl and related pesticides, *Contact Dermatitis* 9:153, 1983.

52. Verspyck Mijnssen GAW: Pathogenesis and causative agent of "tulip finger," *Br J Dermatol* 81:737, 1969.

53. WHO: *Environmental health criteria 78. Dithiocarbamate pesticide, ethylenethiourea and propylenethiourea: a general introduction,* Geneva, 1988, World Health Organization.

54. Williams PL: Commercial PCP toxic impurities, *Occup Health Saf* 52:14, 1983.

55. Zuskin E, Schachter EN, Mustajbegovic J: Respiratory function in greenhouse workers, *Int Arch Occup Environ Health* 64:521, 1993.

18

H   Cl
| |
—C=C—
polyvinyl chloride

- Meat-wrapper's asthma consists of respiratory symptoms temporally related to plastic wrap's being cut with a heated wire and price labels' being attached subsequent to heat activation

- Phthalic anhydride from the heat-activated label adhesive is responsible for most of the consequential respiratory symptoms

Food Preparation Personnel

Mary Ann Howland

OCCUPATIONAL DESCRIPTION

Food preparation workers include bakers, brewers, sugar handlers, flour millers, food sanitizers, and fish, fruit, meat, milk and egg, poultry, and produce handlers. In addition to repetitive motion injuries and those secondary to falls or accidents, dermatitis, allergy, and asthma are responsible for most of the other occupationally related problems (Table 18-1).

Very little occupational disease is derived from chemical toxins per se in the food preparation occupations. Most of the toxicity is related to the often antigenic nature of food (e.g., baker's asthma) or toxins associated with the constant cleaning process. The major source for occupational toxins other than these is phytophotodermatitis from produce and bronchospasm from exposure to heated plastic wrap.

Phytophotodermatitis from plants that contain furocoumarins (psoralens) has been reported, especially after handling celery. The pertinent list of plants that can induce phytophotodermatitis includes celery, carrot, fennel, parsnip, and fig.

This chapter specifically examines meat-wrapper's asthma as a disease entity that is truly an occupational toxicity associated with the preparation of food. Meat-wrappers are unique in that heat-generated toxins emanating from a hot wire cutting process induce an irritant and allergic reaction in susceptible workers.

143

Table 18-1 Food preparation workers

Occupation	Toxin	Problem
Bakers	Flour	Asthma
	Candida	Finger web yeast infection
Fish handlers	*Erysipelothrix*	Erysipeloid from direct contact with fish slime layer
Flour millers	Aflatoxins	Allergies
	Flour	Asthma
		Chronic bronchitis
		Eosinophilic pulmonary infiltrates
	Parasites in flour	Pruritus ("Gran itch")
	Molds	Dermatosis
Fruit		
Ripeners	Ethylene gas	Simple asphyxiant
Handlers		Dermatitis, immediate hypersensitivity
Preservers	Sulfur dioxide	Irritant—concentration dependent; workplace standards available
		Direct contact with liquid can produce serious eye injury and frostbite
Meat handlers	Anthrax	Infections
		Dermatitis and allergies, virus warts
		Erysipeloid
Milk handlers	Antibiotic residues	Dermatitis, allergy
Poultry handlers	*Chlamydia psittaci*	Ornithosis
		Virus warts
Product handlers	Psoralens	Dermatitis from celery, limes, lemons
	Capsaicin	Irritant from chili peppers
		Delayed hypersensitivity, especially from garlic, onions

POTENTIAL TOXIC EXPOSURES
Phytophotodermatitis

The food handler may be exposed to psoralen-containing produce during processing. This hazard is of special concern for those who may handle diseased celery.[3] If the skin is then exposed to the sun, the worker at first assumes that a strong solar burn is causing the painful erythematous maculae. This may progress to papules and bullae in severe exposures. These lesions are often confused with *Rhus* dermatitis. The erythema progresses to hyperpigmentation, which persists for weeks. Both lesions respond to topical corticosteroids, but reexposure is inevitable if the cause is not correctly identified.

Meat-Wrapper's Asthma

The meat-wrapper unrolls the required amount of plastic wrap onto the work area and then cuts it with an electrically heated wire. The wire may reach temperatures of 180° F to 300° F.[4] The meat is then wrapped in the plastic, and the seam is sealed on a hot plate. A price label is also heated and then attached.

Meat-wrappers who use this process are at risk for developing respiratory symptoms. The first case report describing the onset of asthma in three meat-wrappers was published in 1973.[13] The patients and authors alike recognized the implementation of a new technique for cutting the plastic wrapping with a hot wire as being the probable cause. As part of this process and recognized later as a significant contributing cause, heat was also used to affix the price label.[15]

In response to this report, there were many letters from other authors reporting similar experiences.[1,14] Subsequent investigations of meat-wrappers in the Houston area,[7] Seattle area,[9] and Boston area[6] suggested that meat-wrappers who smoked (in the first two studies) or had a history of allergy or asthma (last study) tended to have more respiratory symptoms. When transferred to other areas or jobs, the patients were asymptomatic. Use of a cool rod usually alleviates the problem. Conversion to a more efficient mechanized cutting process with a self-adhesive label has eliminated the problem. Bigger modern stores and those that are unionized are more likely to have incorporated the mechanized process.

Any worker who uses a hot wire to cut plastic or uses heat to attach the price label is at risk. Primarily meat-wrappers fall into this category. Produce workers on occasion have also used this process, but there are no reports in the literature concerning this group. Since the trend has been to display fresh, unwrapped produce, this is unlikely to become a problem.

The United Food and Commercial Workers union represents about 1 million supermarket workers, about half of the estimated total number. Of these 2 million employees, about 2.5% to 7% (30,000 to 140,000) are meat-wrappers or work in produce.

Epidemiologic investigations carried out at the height of this new hot wire cutting technique revealed prevalence rates of 12% to 80% for respiratory symptoms, depending on the study design.[7,9] In both studies, smokers were about twice as likely as nonsmokers to report respiratory symptoms. More minor symptoms of eye and throat irritation occurred even more commonly.

CLINICAL TOXICOLOGY
Pathophysiology

Rubber, metal, and glass were the materials used before the advent of plastics in the mid-1940s.[8] Polyvinylchloride (PVC) then took over the marketplace because of its superior attributes and low cost. Not until the 1960s was the toxic potential of these PVC plastics or their heated by-products studied.[5,8,11,12] Additives are incorporated into the plastic to give it flexibility, transparency, and stability.[8] The toxicity is related to the different additives, alcohol solubility, and the temperature to which the plastic is heated.[8] The additive epoxidized soybean oil, a plasticizer and stabilizer in PVC, was first identified in 1980 as the agent responsible for causing a decrease in forced expiratory volume in 1 second (FEV_1) in three severely affected patients.[10] He also challenged these patients with the fumes given off by heating the price labels. Phthalic anhydride was identified as the decomposition product from the heated price label. Phthalic anhydride caused an even greater decrease in FEV_1 than the PVC fumes.[10] The current conceptualized model suggests that phthalic anhydride produces either rapidly occurring irritant effects (alone or with PVC pyrolysates) or delayed antibody-mediated allergic effects.[4] Smoking, chronic bronchitis, or both appear to modulate these effects.[4]

Diagnosis

The diagnosis of occupational asthma or work-related respiratory symptoms is dependent on obtaining an accurate and detailed description of the process: how the plastic wrap is severed, how the price labels are attached, and the temporal sequence for the development of clinical manifestations. Meat-wrappers surveyed in the Portland, Oregon area reported respiratory symptoms, including exertional dyspnea, productive and nonproductive cough, bronchospasm, and chest soreness; mucous membrane irritation, including rhinorrhea, conjunctivitis, nasal congestion, and throat irritation; and systemic symptoms, including irritability, myalgias, peripheral neuritis, headaches, and Raynaud's syndrome.[4] Challenge tests in a different study group revealed a pattern of an immediate onset of symptoms followed by a delayed reappearance in approximately one third of affected patients. Peripheral eosinophilia may be noted.[2,4] The most severely affected patients, often smokers or those with an allergic history, show the biggest drop in pulmonary function tests after exposure to the heated price label adhesive or the heated plastic wrap.[4] Symptoms usually abate with termination of the exposure. However, instances of the development of persistent asthma in patients with no prior history have been documented.[4,13,15]

Meat-wrapper's asthma may be confused with polymer fume fever. However, patients with meat-wrapper's asthma rarely exhibit the triad of fever, chills, and sore throat.[2] An episode of polymer fume fever generally persists for a longer period of time.

Management and Treatment

The first step is to eliminate exposure to the fumes from the hot wire cutting process and the heat-activated price label. Heat is a prerequisite. Changing to a cool rod and a self-adhesive price label solves the problem. Converting to an entirely mechanized system is ideal.

Inhaled β-2 agonists and corticosteroids are the mainstay of asthmatic symptoms. Patients without a prior history of asthma rarely require uninterrupted therapy in the absence of continued exposure.

REFERENCES

1. Aelony Y: Meat-wrappers' asthma, *JAMA* 236:1117, 1976.
2. Andrasch RH, Bardana EJ: Thermoactivated price-label fume intolerance: a cause of meat-wrapper's asthma, *JAMA* 235:937, 1976.
3. Ashwood-Smith MJ, Ceska O, Chaudhary SK: Mechanism of photosensitivity reaction to diseased celery, *BMJ* 290:1249, 1985.
4. Bardana EJ Jr, Anderson CJ, Andrasch RH: Meat-wrapper's asthma: clinical and pathogenic observations. In Frazier CA, editor: *Occupational asthma,* New York, 1980, Van Nostrand Reinhold.
5. Cornish HH, Abar EL: Toxicity of pyrolysis products of vinyl plastics, *Arch Environ Health* 19:15, 1969.
6. Eisen EA, Wegman DH, Smith TJ: Across-shift changes in the pulmonary function of meat-wrappers and other workers in the retail food industry, *Scand J Work Environ Health* 2:21, 1985.
7. Falk H, Portnoy B: Respiratory tract illness in meat-wrappers, *JAMA* 235:915, 1976.
8. Guess WL, Haberman S: Toxicity profiles of vinyl and polyolefinic plastics and their additives, *J Biomed Mater Res* 2:313, 1968.
9. Johnson CJ, Anderson HW: Meat-wrappers asthma: a case study, *J Occup Med* 18:102, 1976.
10. Pauli G et al: Meat-wrapper's asthma: identification of the causal agent, *Clin Allergy* 10:263, 1980.
11. Peterson JE: Toxic pyrolysis products of solvents, paints, and polymer films, *Occup Med* 8:533, 1993.
12. Polakoff PL, Lapp NL, Reger R: Polyvinyl chloride pyrolysis products, *Arch Environ Health* 30:269, 1975.
13. Sokol WN, Aelony Y, Beall GN: Meat-wrapper's asthma: a new syndrome? *JAMA* 226:639, 1973.
14. Stevens JJ: Meat-wrapper's asthma, *JAMA* 227:1005, 1974 (letter to the editor).
15. Wegman DH et al: Respiratory effects of work in retail food stores. 3: pulmonary function findings, *Scand J Work Environ Health* 13:213, 1987.

Hairdressers and Cosmetologists

Suzanne Doyon

S—C—OH with O double-bonded to C

thioglycolate

NH_3 (benzene ring) NH_3

p-phenylenediamine

- Hairdressers dermatitis is characteristic in distribution and is caused by the sensitizers present in many hair dyes

- The pathophysiology of thesaurosis is poorly understood

OCCUPATIONAL DESCRIPTION

The work of hairdressers includes washing, coloring, bleaching, permanent waving, conditioning, and cutting scalp hair and shaving beards. The work of cosmetologists includes facial skin care, application of makeup, and body waxing. For the sake of this discussion, the word *hairdresser* refers to hair stylists, hair technicians, and barbers, and the word *cosmetologist* refers to estheticians, cosmeticians, beauticians, and beauty technicians.

Hairdressers are subjected to a number of physical and toxicologic hazards. The physical hazards include exposure to sharp objects (cuts and abrasions) and hot electrical equipment (burns) and the prolonged hours spent in the standing position. The toxicologic hazards are those resulting from exposure to a wide range of chemicals and from exposure to chemically active processes.[37] The different chemicals are usually classified under the category of cosmetics. The Food, Drug, and Cosmetics Act (FDCA) defines cosmetics as materials that may be "rubbed, poured, sprinkled or sprayed on, introduced into or otherwise applied to the human body for cleansing, beautifying, promoting attractiveness or altering the appearance without affecting the body's structure or functions." Cosmetic labeling is regulated by the FDCA and must obey rigid nomenclature from a reference text *(CTFA Cosmetics Ingredient Dictionary).* The labeling, as mandated by the Fair Packaging and Labeling Act, stipulates that the listing of all active ingredients must appear first, regardless of amounts, followed by the listing of the major inert ingredients in decreasing order of quantity. The regulation allows the listing of minor ingredients (concentrations of 1% or less) and any coloring agents in no particular order. Trade secrets

147

O
‖
S   C
‹   ╲
C   OH

Fig. 19-1 Thioglycolate structure.

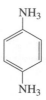

Fig. 19-2 *p*-Phenylenediamine.

(such as fragrance composition) are exempt from these regulations, but manufacturers must indicate their presence by adding "other ingredients" to the labeling.[50] This information on product composition is useful to both physician and consumer. Of note, professional products do not always adhere to these guidelines, and product labeling in Europe is not as stringent as in the United States.

Shampoos are composed mainly of surfactants that fall into one of three categories: anionic (e.g., ammonium lauryl sulfate or lauryl sulfates), which are the best cleansers; amphoteric, which are nonirritating to the eyes and are desirable for baby shampoos; and nonionic, which are adequate cleansers. Conditioning shampoos contain hydrolyzed animal proteins or polyvinylpyrrolidone (PVP). Medicated shampoos contain tar as an antiinflammatory agent, selenium as an antibacterial and antifungal agent, or salicylic acid as an antiinflammatory agent, which also aids scalp scale removal. Shampoo additives include thickeners, acidifiers, oiling agents, and formaldehyde. Formaldehyde is added to several less professional shampoos in order to prevent overgrowth of gram-negative bacteria. The need for hair conditioners arose from the fact that shampoos became too efficient at cleansing the hair and deprived it of its sebum. Hair conditioners can be film-forming and coat the hair shaft with polymers, cationic to counter the effect of anionic shampoos, or be protein-bound to restore hair protein. Protein-bound conditioners are the most popular.[13]

Permanent wave treatments are composed of a thioglycolate compound, ammonium hydroxide, a neutralizing agent (e.g., hydrogen peroxide, perborates, persulfates, bromates), and weak acid (e.g., citric acid, tartaric acid, acetic acid). The thioglycolate reduces and "breaks" the cysteine bonds in hair keratin. This bond is better disrupted by the addition of heat and water. The kerato-cysteine cross-linkages are reconstituted by oxidation with a neutralizing agent and a weak acid. Household permanent wave treatments (i.e., "cold" permanents) contain ammonium thioglycolate (ATG) and have been used extensively since 1943.[3] Professional permanent wave (i.e., "hot" permanents) usually contain glyceryl monothioglycolate (GMTG). (Figure 19-1 shows the basic thioglycolate structure.) In fact, GMTG-containing permanents, which were introduced in 1973, constitute 25% to 80% of the market.[5] Most professional permanent packages have three components: a small tube of GMTG in a concentration of up to 80%, a bottle of ammonium hydroxide, and a bottle of neutralizer and weak acid. The step-by-step procedure is as follows: washing the hair, applying a mix of thioglycolate and ammonium hydroxide in order to deliver an 18% to 20% solution to the hair, hot drying for 15 to 20

minutes, checking the test curl on the right index finger, washing out the thioglycolate solution with water for 8 to 12 minutes, applying the oxidizing agents, removing the rollers, applying the after-treatment cream, and styling.[13,53]

Hair-coloring products have evolved significantly over the last 80 years. The metallic salts traditionally used have been largely eliminated in light of the inherent toxicity of the heavy metals. Today, they can be found only in the progressive hair dyes, a descriptive term meaning that they color the hair shaft gradually after each application. They contain lead or silver sulfides. Hair-coloring products can be classified into three categories: temporary, semipermanent, and permanent. Temporary hair-coloring products contain large-molecular-weight acidic textile dyes that are deposited on the hair shaft but do not penetrate into it. They are easily washed away with one shampoo. Semipermanent hair-coloring products contain either natural vegetable dyes (e.g., henna) or low-molecular-weight dyes. They are removed after four to six shampoos. Permanent hair-coloring products are the most noxious class of hair dyes. The chemical reaction that colors the hair shaft requires that the *para* dye, usually *p*-phenylenediamine (PPD) (Fig. 19-2), be oxidized by hydrogen peroxide to form a reactive amine. Couplers react with this amine to form an indo dye that cannot diffuse out of the cuticle. An even hair cuticle is essential for even coloration, and pretreatment of the hair with conditioners is often required to smooth the cuticle surface before application of color.[13]

Hair bleaches contain a 20% to 30% solution of hydrogen peroxide in a vegetable or mineral base.[13]

Hair sprays contain polyvinylpyrrolidone (PVP) or polyvinyl acetate (PVA) copolymers, dimethylhydantoin, formaldehyde, lanolin, fragrances, and fluorohydrocarbons (Freon). The copolymers are polymerized plastic compounds used to stiffen the hair. The concentration of copolymer determines the amount of hold. Hair sprays that rely on shellac as a stiffening agent are no longer used. The environment-friendly and fluorohydrocarbon-free spritzer pump system is more widely used than the traditional aerosolized formulation. Hair gels and mousses contain the same copolymers found in cosmetic aerosols, but the delivery system is different. Brilliantine is an older hair gel containing *p*-dimethylaminoazobenzene, which was used in men's hair styling. Extremely high-hold hair gels, commonly referred to as *hair cement,* contain methylacrylate.[13]

Cosmetologists and pedicurists use a wide array of nail and skin care products including solvents (e.g., acetone, pentyl alcohol, benzyl alcohol), thinners (e.g., toluene, xylene, benzene), plasticizers (e.g., phthalates), resins (e.g., copal, urea formaldehyde, vinyl acrylic), and fragrances. Not surprisingly, the types of chemicals and practices vary widely around the world.[9,13,16,21,32]

CUTANEOUS DISORDERS

Cutaneous disorders remain the most important occupational hazards for hairdressers and cosmetologists. The overall prevalence of cutaneous lesions among hairdressers varies from 10% to 90%, with the highest prevalence among apprentices.[11,21,24,51,53] The average hairdresser's hands are exposed to water, detergents, dyes, bleaches, permanent wave treatments, metal equipment, heat, and frictional forces. It is believed that the dermatitis that results from the exposure to these chemicals actually starts off as an inflammatory skin reaction, irritant contact dermatitis (ICD). The persistent presence of the irritants results in the release of arachidonic acid and its metabolites, as well as vasoactive substances like histamine and kinins. The damaged skin is more easily penetrated by potential allergens.[11] Over a period of a few months to a year, continuous sensitization of the individual to the allergen results in an allergic contact dermatitis (ACD), which induces a cell-mediated immune response that forms the basis for patch testing. A predilection for the fingertips is, in fact, the hallmark feature of hairdresser's hand dermatitis.[49] Equally characteristic are lesions located on the distal part of the right index finger, where the test curl is typically unwound.[49] Some authors have suggested that the location of the dermatitis can be diagnostic, with finger webs more affected by shampoos and fingertips more affected by permanent wave treatments.[32] The physical hallmarks of contact dermatitis are the presence of (1) sharp margins that correspond to the areas of contact and (2) the presence of vesicles, papules, and bullae, lichenification of the epidermis, or both.[32]

There exists no standard way of testing for ICD. In ACD, however, the putative agent can be identified by patch testing. Therefore, ACD refers to a dermatitis with one or more positives on the patch test, and ICD refers to a dermatitis without a positive patch test but with a clear history of work-related exposure. Atopic dermatitis involves the hands as well as other distant body parts.[23] In order to assess the sensitivities of hairdressers, a hairdresser's series patch test (Hermal of Trolab, Germany) has been marketed. It commonly contains eight substances:

Glyceryl monothioglycolate	0.5 or 1% in petrolatum
Ammonium thioglycolate	1 or 2.5% in petrolatum
p-Toluenediamine sulfate	1% in petrolatum
o-Nitro-*p*-phenylenediamine	1% in petrolatum
Ammonium persulfate	2.5% in petrolatum
Resorcinol	2% in petrolatum
Pyrogallol	1% in petrolatum
Hydroquinone	1% in petrolatum

Some authors have modified the hairdresser's series to include 1% cocamidopropylbetaine or lavender oil.[6,54] Some

authors have used a series of 18 allergens.[49] Both a hairdresser's series and a North American Contact Dermatitis Group standard tray of allergens are applied as a patch to the skin of the subject after protocols established by the American Academy of Dermatology. Readings are performed as the patch is removed 48 hours after the application and then, again, in 96 hours. A positive reading can range anywhere from erythema to bullae formation.[32] The commonest sensitizers are, in decreasing order of frequency, PPD (19% to 24%), GMTG (19% to 58%), nickel (40%), ATG (36%), and even resin.* Past history of atopy does not impact the patch test results. Patch testing through different glove samples has demonstrated that all gloves, except neoprene, are inadequate physical barriers to these strong chemical agents. Patch testing is best done by experienced personnel.

Patients with ACD and a mild to moderate reaction to the patch test can be treated with the application of moisturizers, topical corticosteroid cream, and the occasional use of systemic antibiotics to treat suprainfection. Patients with severe reactions should be prescribed a short trial of systemic corticosteroids, although the response rate can be poor.[32] The nonmedicinal treatment of hairdresser's dermatitis involves reeducation on the correct use of these products, avoidance of the allergen as identified by patch testing, avoidance of nickel jewelry, constant thorough cleaning of all the working surfaces, washing hands with water only and drying only by towel, generous application of a water-resistant nonsticky hand cream (Atrix of Beiersdorf, Germany), and use of gloves. Vinyl gloves (Tru Touch Stretch; Beton, Dickinson and Company, Belgium) are believed to be better barrier protection than the readily available polypropylene gloves provided by the manufacturers, but they do allow some chemicals to seep through and reach the skin. Neoprene gloves (Super Etonette) and "4H" Danish gloves are the best choices. "Foam" gloves have never been scientifically tested and, despite their advertising, are not recommended. An 81% reduction in dermatitis was noted after implementation of these practices in a group of hairdressers.[54]

The GMTG-sensitized individuals should be instructed to avoid working on contaminated surfaces. The work surfaces can be spot tested for GMTG; however, surfaces wiped with regular household cleaners yielded undetectable levels. Hair treated with GMTG continues to release this allergen for up to 3 months.[35] It is recommended that GMTG-sensitized individuals avoid GMTG-treated hair for that period of time and avoid using this chemical on their own hair. Finally, although they both contain thiol groups, cross-reactivity between GMTG and ATG, the main active ingredient in household permanent wave treatments, is very unlikely. Sensitization to ATG is very rare; some authors believe that it may never occur.[11,49] Therefore, GMTG-sensitized individuals can safely work with ATG-treated hair.[15]

*References 10, 16, 19, 25, 49, 51, 53.

Certain precautions apply to individuals sensitized to PPD, a component of hair-coloring products. Avoidance of ester anesthetics (procaine and benzocaine), sulfonamides, and para-aminobenzoic acid (PABA)-containing products is recommended because of cross-reactivity. However, the PPD-sensitized individual need not avoid PPD-treated hair because this allergen, contrary to GMTG, does not persist in the hair over time.[15]

Finally, individuals with active atopic dermatitis, a history of severe atopic dermatitis, or severe nickel allergy (dermatitis extending beyond the ear lobes) should be discouraged from entering the hairdressing trade.[54]

RESPIRATORY DISORDERS

Hairdressers are exposed to a number of different inhalants in the workplace. Some are allergens, some are irritants, and some have been linked to a disease entity called *thesaurosis*. Lung diseases resulting from the exposure to organic particles have been, at best, difficult to study, and their etiology is difficult to prove.

In recent years, adult-onset asthma associated with exposure to chemicals in the workplace has received increasing attention in the medical literature. Inhaled persulfates, aerosol cosmetics, hair-coloring products, and henna have all been described as the cause of chronic asthma in hairdressers.[38,48] Some authors have even quantified the serum IgE antibodies to henna in symptomatic individuals.[48] The airway obstruction can be immediate or delayed and is usually easily reproduced in the laboratory. It can occasionally be blunted by the prophylactic administration of sodium cromolyn, suggesting that the mechanism of action may have to do with the release of mediators.[38,43,48] The airway obstruction did not warrant a hospital admission in any of the case reports. In all instances, subjects responded well to the administration of β-agonists, beclomethasone, or both. Hairdressing is a poor career choice for individuals with a history of severe asthma or steroid-dependent asthma.[32,54]

Little literature exists on exposure to irritants and development of allergic rhinitis in the workplace. It is important to remember that rhinitis can occur in the absence of asthma. One study linked rhinitis to exposure to inhaled permanent solution.[43] As previously mentioned, hair sprays essentially contain copolymers in an alcoholic or aqueous solution (PVP or PVA) and fluorochlorohydrocarbons as propellant. Aerosolized particles vary in size from 0.1 μm to 20 μm. They can be deposited anywhere in the respiratory tract but are predominantly deposited in the nasopharynx. They have been known to reduce mucociliary transport in this area after short-term exposure.[38] It is not clear from the literature which component of mucociliary transport—mucus composition or cilia action—is more affected by cosmetic aerosols. The noxious effect of hair spray on mucociliary transport may result from exposure to PVP, PVA, or the alcoholic solution but not from exposure to Freon.[5]

Thesaurosis is a lung storage disease ascribed to the chronic inhalation of hair spray and was first described by Bergmann in 1958.[2] *Thesaurosis* is derived from the Greek word *repository*. Bergmann and colleagues reported on two cases of household hair spray exposure. The patients had otherwise inexplicable signs and symptoms and chest x-ray findings of wide areas of homogeneously distributed spherical densities of 1 mm or less in diameter without marked reticular pattern. The differential diagnosis of such an x-ray includes alveolar microlithiasis, intravenous talcosis, berylliosis, farmer's lung, and bird fancier's lung.[7] More than 30 cases of thesaurosis followed Bergmann's original description.* Thesaurosis is thought to arise from the storage of nonbiodegradable macromolecules in the reticuloendothelial system. The macromolecules are believed to be PVP and PVA because these compounds cannot be metabolized by mammalian cells and are known to induce granulomata (with giant cells and epithelioid cells) when injected into laboratory animals.[14]

Authors remain skeptical and have argued that thesaurosis is a nondisease. Some have stated that Bergmann's findings could just as well be ascribed to sarcoidosis.[40] Total unexplained resolution of signs and symptoms, despite continued daily use of the aerosols, is true of many of the previously published case reports, including Bergmann's.[2,17,40,42] The skepticism from the medical community stems from the fact that no animal model has been able to reproduce this disease entity, and no single histologic lesion can be identified in the lungs of laboratory animals, and no epidemiologic study has supported the claims that thesaurosis is the result of exposure to hairspray.[40]

Multiple authors have attempted to reproduce this disease in the laboratory, looking at all the components of aerosol cosmetics, without much success. Laboratory animals exposed to inhaled hair spray do not develop definitive histologic changes in lung parenchyma or develop the same histologic changes reported in humans. No single histologic lesion can be linked to exposure to hair spray. When PVP is injected into the groin of laboratory animals, a subcutaneous granuloma may form; when PVP is inhaled by laboratory animals, however, granulomata may or may not develop in the lung parenchyma.[2,18,22,31] There is no consistency or dose-response relationship. Multiple human lung tissue biopsies have been examined, and pathologists describe lesions as harboring active chronic granulomatous inflammation with *p*-aminosalicylic acid (PAS)-positive cytoplasmic inclusions of interstitial and intraalveolar macrophages, as well as multinucleated giant cells.[17] Other authors have described granulomatous lesions in scalene lymph nodes and lung parenchyma.[2] Others have described lipoid pneumonia.[55] There is no consensus among authors. Furthermore, the presence of PAS-positive lesions cannot be used to support or disprove the diagnosis of thesaurosis because they

---

*References 3, 7, 8, 14, 36, 41.

are nonspecific. Infrared spectroscopy, spectrophotometry, thin-layer chromatography, electron microscopy studies, and animal inhalation models have all been inconclusive.[18,22,31,55]

Large epidemiologic studies involving hundreds of hairdressers have not uncovered a higher prevalence of pulmonary disease among this group of people.[12,40] Some authors have expanded the diagnosis of thesaurosis to include hairdressers with reduced forced vital capacity or reduced diffusion capacity, and, again, no link to hair spray exposure was found.[40] In light of the lack of a good animal model and lack of epidemiologic studies illustrating the relationship between exposure to inhaled aerosol hair spray and development of pulmonary disease, we have been unable to confirm the noxious nature of aerosol cosmetics. In the future, spritzer pumps will replace the traditional cosmetic aerosols. Spritzer pumps yield larger particles, and, therefore, upper respiratory tract problems are more likely to emerge.

NEOPLASTIC DISEASE

Of all the products used by hairdressers and cosmetologists, none has been more studied in relationship to potential carcinogenicity than the hair-coloring products. The International Agency for the Research in Cancer (IARC) found some hair dye components to be highly mutagenic in laboratory animals, particularly PPD and 2,4-diaminoptoluene, and the documentation was deemed sufficient to classify them as 2B.[27] This has been confirmed by other authors.[46] Endorsement by the IARC of PPD and diaminoptoluene as possible carcinogens has spawned a tremendous amount of research. Most of the available data originated from Scandinavian cancer registries. Cancer studies in the relationship between exposure to hair-coloring products and development of cancer fall into two categories: occupational exposure and household exposure.

A few studies demonstrated an increased incidence of hematopoietic cancers in hairdressers and cosmetologists. In female hairdressers, elevated risks of developing multiple myeloma, non-Hodgkin's lymphoma, and breast and ovarian cancer have been reported.* An even greater amount of literature, including studies from the IARC, has failed to demonstrate such an association.† In male hairdressers, elevated risks of bladder and lung cancers have been reported. A survey of the literature on the incidence of bladder cancer in hairdressers demonstrated that the majority of studies determined the risk estimate to be more than one. The potential carcinogen has been identified as *p*-dimethylaminoazobenzene (2B) a documented animal mutagen and component of brilliantine.[44,45] The literature on lung cancer is confusing mostly because of confounding variables, such as tobacco exposure, and no strong link to lung cancer has been established.

*References 4, 20, 26, 28, 30, 47, 52.
†References 1, 12, 27, 29, 34, 40, 52.

It seems fair to say that the human data are inconclusive concerning the exposure to hair-coloring products and the development of hematopoietic, ovarian, lung, or laryngeal tumors and that possibly a link between brilliantine (*p*-dimethylaminoazobenzene) and bladder tumors exists. Most cancers in these studies, however, are of the case-control type and suffer from small numbers, tremendous recall biases, and insufficient follow-up. Clearly, further research in this field is required.

Exposure to bromates (permanent wave neutralizer) has been linked to cases of renal failure and hearing loss. All of the cases occurred secondary to the ingestion of massive doses of potassium bromate. No similar data follow occupational exposures.[39,52]

REFERENCES

1. Alderson M: Cancer mortality in male hairdressers, *J Epidemiol Community Health* 34:182, 1980.
2. Bergmann M, Flance J, Blumenthal HT: Thesaurosis following inhalation of hair spray, *N Engl J Med* 258:471, 1958.
3. Bergmann M et al: Thesaurosis due to inhalation of hair spray, *N Engl J Med* 266:750, 1962.
4. Bofetta P et al: Employment as hairdresser and risk of ovarian cancer and non-Hodgkin's lymphomas among women, *J Occup Med* 36:61, 1994.
5. Borum P, Holten A, Loekkegaardn V: Depression of nasal mucociliary transport by an aerosol hair-spray, *Scand J Respir Dis* 60:253, 1979.
6. Brandao FM: Occupational allergy to lavender oil, *Contact Dermatitis* 15:249, 1986.
7. Caldwell DM, McQueeney AJ, Silipo SC: Pulmonary granulomatosis associated with the excessive use of cosmetic sprays, *Calif Med* 65:246, 1961.
8. Cares RM: Thesaurosis from inhaled hair spray? *Arch Environ Health* 11:80, 1965.
9. Clayton RP: Safety: hairdressing hazards, *Occup Health Saf* 35:212, 1983.
10. Conde-Salazar L et al: Contact dermatitis in hairdressers: patch test results in 379 hairdressers (1980-1993), *Am J Contact Dermatitis* 31:46, 1994.
11. Cronin E, Kullavanijaya P: Hand dermatitis in hair dressers, *Acta Derm Venereol Suppl (Stockh)* 59:47, 1979.
12. Discher DP, Hall CE: Prevalence of cardiorespiratory disease among cosmetologists. Paper presented at American Occupational Health Conference, New Orleans, 1978.
13. Draelos ZK: Hair cosmetics (review), *Dermatol Clin* 9:19, 1991.
14. Edelston BG: Thesaurosis following inhalation of hair spray, *Lancet* 2:112, 1959.
15. Fisher AA: Management of hairdressers sensitized to hair dyes or permanent wave solutions, *Cutis* 43:316, 1989.
16. Frosch PJ et al: Allergic reactions to a hairdressers series: results from 9 European centers. The European Environmental and Contact Dermatitis Research Group (EECDRG), *Contact Dermatitis* 28:180, 1993.
17. Gebbers JO, Tetzner C, Brukhardt A: Alveolitis due to hair-spray. Ultrastructural observations in two patients and the results of experimental investigations, *Virchows Archiv A, Pathol Anat Histol* 382:323, 1979.
18. Giovacchini RO et al: Pulmonary disease and hair spray polymers. Effects of long-term exposure of dogs, *JAMA* 193:118, 1965.
19. Guerra L et al: Contact dermatitis in hair dressers: the Italian experience, *Contact Dermatitis* 26:101, 1992.

20. Guidotti S, Wright WE, Peters JM: Multiple myeloma in cosmetologists, *Am J Ind Med* 3:169, 1982.

21. Guo YL et al: Occupational hand dermatoses in hairdressers in Tainan City, *Occup Environ Med* 51:689, 1994.

22. Gupta BN, Drew RT: The effect of aerosol hair spray inhalation in the hamster, *Am Ind Hyg Assoc J* 37:357, 1976.

23. Hanifin JM, Lobitz WC Jr: Newer concepts of atopic dermatitis, *Arch Dermatol* 113:663, 1977.

24. Hannuskela M, Hassi J: Hairdresser's Hand: Dermatosen in Beruf und Unwelt (Aulendorf, Federal Republic of Germany) 28/5:149-150, 1980.

25. Heine A, Laubstein B: Contact dermatitis from cyclohexanone-formaldehyde resin (L2 resin) in a hair lacquer spray, *Contact Dermatitis* 22:108, 1990.

26. Herrington LJ et al: Exposure to hair-coloring products and the risk of multiple myeloma, *Am J Public Health* 84:1142, 1994.

27. International Agency for Research in Cancer: *Some aromatic amines and related nitro compounds: hair dyes, colouring agents and miscellaneous industrial chemicals,* IARC monograph on the evaluation of the carcinogenicity risk of chemicals to humans No 16, Lyon, 1972, IARC.

28. International Agency for Research in Cancer. *Epidemiological evidence relating to the possible carcinogenic effects of hair dyes in hairdressers and users of hair dyes, IARC monograph on the evaluation of the carcinogenicity risk of chemicals to humans* No 27, Appendix 1, Lyon, 1982, IARC.

29. Kono S et al: Cancer and other causes of death among female beauticians, *J Natl Cancer Inst* 70:443, 1983.

30. La Vecchia C, Tavani A: Epidemiological evidence on hair dyes and the risk of cancer in humans, *Eur J Cancer Prev* 4:31, 1995.

31. Lowsma HB, Jones RA, Pendergast JA: Effects of respired polyvinyl-pyrrolidone aerosols in rats, *Toxicol Appl Pharmacol* 9:571, 1966.

32. Marks JG Jr: Occupational diseases in hairdressers (review), *Occup Med* 1:273, 1986.

33. Matsumotot I, Morizono T, Paparella M: Hearing loss following potassium bromate: two case reports, *Otolaryngol Head Neck Surg* 88:625, 1980.

34. Menck HR et al: Lung cancer risk among beauticians and other female workers, *J Natl Cancer Inst* 59:1423, 1977.

35. Morrison LH, Storrs FJ: Persistence of an allergen in hair after glyceryl monothioglycolate-containing permanent wave solutions, *J Am Acad Dermatol* 19:52, 1988.

36. Nevins MA et al: Pulmonary granulomatosis, *JAMA* 193:266, 1965.

37. Parmeggiani L: *Encyclopedia of Occupational Health and Safety,* vol 1, ed. 3, Geneva, Switzerland, 1983, International Labor Organization.

38. Pepys J, Hutchcroft J, Breslin BX: Asthma due to inhaled chemical agents—persulphate salts and henna in hairdressers, *Clin Allergy* 6/4:399, 1976.

39. Quick CA, Chole RA, Mauer M: Deafness and renal failure due to potassium bromate poisoning, *Arch Otolaryngol* 101:494, 1975.

40. Renzetti Jr AD et al: Thesaurosis—from hairspray exposure—a nondisease. Validation studies of an epidemiologic survey of cosmetologists, *Environ Res* 22:130, 1980.

41. Ripe E et al: Thesaurosis? Analysis of a case, *Scand J Respir Dis* 50:156, 1969.

42. Schraufnagel DE, Pare JA, Wang NS: Micronodular pulmonary pattern: association with inhaled aerosol, *AJR Am J Roentol* 137:57, 1981.

43. Schwartz HJ, Arnold JL, Strohl KP: Occupational allergic rhinitis in the hair care industry: reactions to permanent wave solutions, *J Occup Med* 32:473, 1990.

44. Skov T et al: Risk for cancer of the urinary bladder among hairdressers in the Nordic countries, *Am J Ind Med* 17:217, 1990.

45. Skov T, Lynge E: Cancer risk and exposure to carcinogens in hairdressers, *Skin Pharmacol* 7:94, 1994.

46. Sontag JM: Carcinogenicity of substituted-benzenediamine (phenylenediamine) in rats and mice, *J Natl Cancer Inst* 66:591, 1981.

47. Spinelli JJ et al: Multiple myeloma, leukemia and cancer of the ovary in cosmetologists and hairdressers, *Am J Ind Med* 6:97, 1984.

48. Starr JC, Yunginger J, Brasher GW: Immediate type I asthmatic response to henna following occupational exposure in hairdressers, *Ann Allergy* 48:98, 1982.

49. Storrs FJ: Permanent wave contact dermatitis: contact allergy to glyceryl monothioglycolate, *J Am Acad Dermatol* 11:74, 1985.

50. Stovall GK, Levin L, Oler J: Occupational dermatitis among hairdressers. A multifactor analysis, *J Occup Med* 25:871, 1983.

51. Sutthipisal N, McFadden JP, Cronin E: Sensitization in atopic and non-atopic hairdressers with hand eczema, *Contact Dermatitis* 29:206, 1993.

52. Teta MJ et al: Cancer incidence among cosmetologists, *J Natl Cancer Inst* 72:1051, 1984.

53. Van der Walle HB, Brunsveld VM: Dermatitis in hairdressers (I). The experience of the past 4 years, *Contact Dermatitis* 30:217, 1994.

54. Van der Walle HB: Dermatitis in hairdressers (II). Management and prevention, *Contact Dermatitis* 30:265, 1994.

55. Wright L, Crockcroft DW: Lung disease due to abuse of hairspray, *Arch Pathol Lab Med* 105:363, 1981.

20

Jewelers

Susan M. Lizarralde
Barry Wake
Valerie Thompson
Richard S. Weisman

CN Ag Au

- Jewelry manufacturing is often accomplished in small shops with simple equipment that when misused can result in toxic exposures

- Electroplating can result in cyanide exposure

- Nickel is a common component of ornamental jewelry

- Electroplating, lost wax casting, vacuum casting, investment heating, soldering, degreasing, and polishing are each associated with a substantial risk of toxicity

OCCUPATIONAL DESCRIPTION
History

"Empires have been built on gold; civilizations have been destroyed for it"[10]

Over the centuries, an amazing variety of materials have been valued and sought for their prized beauty. These desired objects are gemstones and precious metals hidden deep within the earth's rocky layers.

Gold is precious, partly because of its scarcity. The cumulative amount of gold secured in the world today, from the ancient Egyptian tombs to the rock obtained from modern large-scale strip mining, totals no more than 100,000 tons.[10]

Five thousand years ago, the Egyptians developed methods to fashion gold jewelry, and the same methods are still used today, only with modern equipment.

From the Byzantine era to the medieval times, crowns, pins, bangles, and bracelets adorned royal families, notorious conquerors, and clergy; jewels embellished objects of art like mosaics, paintings, murals, and sculptures. Cleopatra (69-30 BC) wore a pair of pearl earrings worth approximately $1 million by today's standards. Czar Ivan IV the Terrible (1530-1584) had built for himself a throne of gold garnished with rubies, sapphires, turquoise, and pearls. King Gustav III of Sweden (1746-1792) had a sword and scabbard studded with more than 1000 carats of precious gemstones. Peter Carl Fabergé (1846-1920) sculptured jeweled eggs and trimmed them with gold, enamel, and gemstones.[10]

Occupational Description

Jewelry is either valued subjectively and judged upon its decorative appearance or symbolic meaning or valued objectively, strictly upon physical characteristics. Industrial-quality jewels are graded by specific physical attributes, namely, the 4 Cs: clarity, color, cut, and carat weight. Figure 20-1 shows a Burmese ruby necklace.

The artistry of the jeweler must be tempered with working knowledge and an understanding of the potential hazards associated with each technical process a jeweler performs. In the jewelry manufacturing industry, the worker is likely to be confronted by a variety of toxic compounds that may exist in the solid, liquid, or gaseous state. Exposure to these toxins can occur primarily by inhalation or dermal contact.

Although the accident rate in this industry is low, recognized hazards include exposures to toxic substances, heat, noise, and vibration, in addition to physical injuries from production machinery.[11,22] The majority of toxic exposures are the result of dermal contact with caustics, molten metal, spilled solvents, flame torches, or heating elements or the inhalation of metal dusts, fumes, and solvent vapors.[11,39,44,52]

Illnesses and injuries are likely to present as acute dermal conditions (skin abrasions, burns, irritant and allergic dermatitis) and both acute and chronic pulmonary disorders (mucous membrane and upper airway irritation and allergic asthma.[39,44,52] Functional (restrictive) and benign pneumoconiosis has been described among industrial jewelry workers.[12,30] Serious chronic lung diseases such as allergic asthma and hypersensitivity pneumonitis can also occur from long-term metal fume and dust exposure.[39,44,52,56]

Precautionary measures should be incorporated into standard operating procedures to prevent toxic exposures to solvents, vapors, metal fumes and dusts, thermal heat injury, physical injuries, and noise pollution.

When the clinician is confronted by the ill or injured jeweler, the patient's work history becomes more meaningful if the clinician has a good understanding of the various processes and hazardous substances utilized in the jewelry

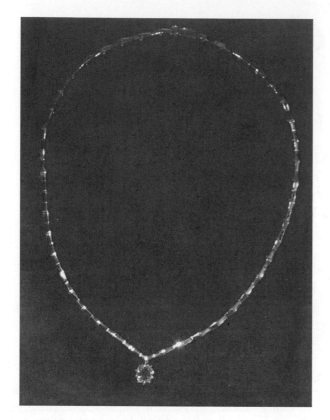

Fig. 20-1 Burmese ruby and diamond in 18-karat yellow gold necklace, valued at approximately $3250.

Table 20-1 Jewelry councils, societies, and associations

Council/association	Address	Telephone
American Craft Council (founded 1943)	72 Spring Street New York, NY 10012	(212) 274-0630
American Gem Society (founded 1934)	5901 W. Third Street Los Angeles, CA 90036	(213) 936-4367
Gemological Institute of America (GIA) (founded 1931)	1660 Stewart Street Santa Monica, CA 90404	(213) 829-2991
Jewelry Casters Association (founded 1951)	PO Box 1636 Grand Central Station New York, NY 10163	(212) 594-2714
Jewelry Manufacturers Association (founded 1919)	PO Box 46099 Los Angeles, CA 90046	(202) 725-5599
Manufacturing Jewelers and Silversmiths of America (founded 1903)	475 Fifth Street New York, NY 10017	(401) 274-3841
Society of North American Goldsmiths	5009 Londonderry Drive Tampa, FL 33647	(813) 977-5326

manufacturing industry. The jeweler's occupational history can provide information about chemical exposures that can assist the clinician in establishing both a diagnosis and a management plan.

Epidemiology

The U.S. Bureau of Labor Statistics summary report, *Survey of Occupational Injuries and Illnesses, 1993* noted approximately 133,800 jewelry workers in the industrial work force.[59]

Jewelry manufacturing is the largest industry in Rhode Island.[13] In the 1970s and 1980s, 20,000 to 30,000 jewelry workers resided in the state, accounting for approximately 20% of Rhode Island's total manufacturing employment.

Currently, there are 26,000 jewelry workers in Rhode Island.[13]

Technical training of jewelers. Jewelers learn their skills through apprenticeships. Most states have schools and associations that provide certificates and diplomas for jewelers, gemologists, artists, and designers. Table 20-1 lists jewelry councils, societies, and associations that provide information about schools and classes in the jewelry trade.

Jewelry Manufacturing Process

The procedures and materials discussed in this chapter comprise only a small segment of the processes employed routinely by large jewelry manufacturers and gold refineries.

Table 20-2 Basic jewelry manufacturing processes

	Function	Materials	Hazards
Drilling	To enlarge, shape, or texture metals and jewelry settings or frames	Twist drill bits, grinding wheels, cratex wheels (a mixture of emery powder and rubber) and shaped heads (burrs), metals	Respiratory effects from generated fumes and dusts
Electroplating	Restores the finish on items that have been soldered; coats jewelry with gold or silver finish	Silver cyanide salts, gold cyanide salts, and potassium/sodium cyanide; citric, phosphoric, and hydrochloric acids	Thermal burns from handheld propane gas torch or heated chemicals, *cyanide toxicity,* tooth erosion
Lost wax/plaster (investment) casting	For mass production of jewelry	Investment powder—may contain talc, asbestos, silica	Silica and metal alloy particles can cause irritant effects in upper airways; metal dust and fume inhalation, burns and itching, and irritation from direct skin contact from molten metal
Filing	Smooths sharp edges of gemstones and metals	Textured metal file/emery board or paper, metal, gemstones	Puncture wounds or scrapes from misdirected file; respiratory or dermal irritation from contact with metal dusts, sand, or chips
Soldering	To fuse or join together metal pieces	Solders (molten metal alloy mixtures); identified by melting point as: "easy," "medium," or "hard"; metal alloys: lead, tin, chromium, cadmium, copper, gold, silver, zinc; fluxes may contain fluoride, boric acid, zinc chloride, solvents	Thermal burns, exposure to lead (plumbism); metal fumes may cause upper respiratory tract irritation, metal fume fever, hypersensitivity pneumonitis, allergic asthma
Pickling	To remove tarnish and oxidation from metal bases	Phosphoric, sulfuric, nitric, and hydrochloric acids; sodium bicarbonate	Chemical burns, upper respiratory tract and ocular irritation from vapors or via direct acid contact; heating may produce phosgene or chlorine gas
Enameling	To fuse a colored, glasslike surface to a metal base	Silica, glass particles, solvents (toluene, xylene, acetone), gum tragacanth, hydrochloric acid	Simple asphyxiation from solvents, burns from hot materials and etching acids
Cleaning	Removes dirt and polishing compounds from jewelry	Ammonia, detergents	Skin irritation, upper respiratory irritation
Polishing	Removes smudges left on jewelry; gives a bright or matte finish to jewelry items	Polisher with rotary bristle brush and felt or muslin finishing mop; *polishes:* red rouge bar (iron oxides and fatty waxes), green rouge bar (chromium oxide), white rouge bar (fatty acids, glycerides, petroleum, silica dust 80%)	Dermal irritation from polishing materials and metal particles; abrasion of finger tips from aggressive polishing; oil mists from machinery can irritate upper airway and skin

Table 20-3 Bonding agents for metals and stones

Gold	Silver	Platinum	Stones
Phenolic epoxy	Epoxy polymide	Polyester + catalyst	Cyanoacrylate
Epoxy + polymine	Epoxy with methylene diamide catalyst	Epoxy polysulfide	
Epoxy/alkylester	Epoxy (bisphenol A based) + polyamide	Polyhydroxyether	
Polyhydroxyether	Polyamide/nylon based	Neoprene rubber	
Polyacrylic esters			
Vinyl chloride/vinyl acetate			
Polyurethane rubber			
RTV silicone			

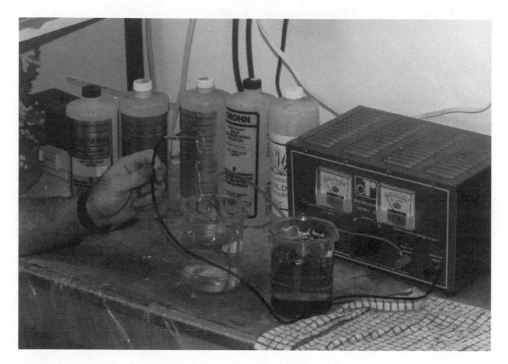

Fig. 20-2 Electroplating-stripping process: A gold ring is placed in stripping solution (sodium cyanide) prior to electroplating. The anode pole of the system is attached to the ring; the cathode pole is attached to a platinum plate, which is immersed in the stripping solution. The ring will be rhodium plated.

Industrial operations would most likely incorporate more complex manufacturing procedures.

Basic jewelry manufacturing processes are cutting and shaping precious, semiprecious, or synthetic stones, gemstone setting, gold and silver electroplating, lost wax or plastic casting, enameling, metal soldering, and shaping and finishing techniques.[11,25,44,52] Basic jewelry manufacturing processes are described in Table 20-2.

Hand drills are used to enlarge, shape, or texture metals and jewelry settings or frames.[25,47] Setter's shellac, a brittle wax softened with heat, is applied to protect and support delicate settings before gemstones are placed. After placement, the prongs or bezel edges of the metal settings are secured tightly over each gemstone. The setter's shellac is then removed from the jewelry by irrigating with a solution of warmed ethyl or isopropyl alcohol. Bonding agents

(epoxy resins) are also used to affix stones to metal plates or settings.[11,24] Bonding agents are listed in Table 20-3.

Metal chains and pendants are often coated with a metallic gold or silver layer by the process of electroplating. Electroplating requires two tanks, one containing a plating base (metal cyanide salts) and the other containing a metal stripping solution (sodium cyanide), each independently linked to an electrical power source. Both tanks have an anode (+) and cathode (−) pole; each pole is attached either to the voltage source or to the object to be plated. Before plating, the jewelry item is cleaned with detergent, rinsed under warm water, connected to the anode pole of the stripping tank, and then immersed in the solution. A stainless-steel plate is attached to the cathode pole and also placed into the stripping solution. Stripping removes the surface metal layer from the immersed jewelry piece. A

Table 20-4 Composition, melting point, and specific gravity of common metals

Common name	Composition (%)	Melting point (°C)	Specific gravity
Aluminum	100 Al	660	2.7
Antimony	100 Sb	631	6.7
Bismuth	100 Bi	271	9.7
Brass	67 Cu, 33 Zn	940	8.4
Bronze, commercial	90 Cu, 10 Zn	1050	8.8
Bronze, manganese	95 Cu, 5 Mn	1060	8.8
Cadmium	100 Cd	321	8.7
Chromium	100 Cr	1890	7.1
Copper	100 Cu	1083	8.9
Gold, fine	100 Au	1063	19.3
Gold, 22k (900)	91.66 Au, 4.16 Ag, 4.16 Cu	—	17.7
Gold, 18k (750)	75 Au, 15 Ag, 10 Cu	—	15.5
Gold, 14k (585)	58 Au, 25 Ag, 17 Cu	—	13.4
Gold, coinage	90 Au, 10 Cu	940	17.2
Gold, purple	79 Au, 21 Al	750	—
Iron	100 Fe	1535	7.9
Lead	100 Pb	327	11.4
Magnesium	100 Mg	651	1.7
Metal, monel	60 Ni, 33 Cu, 7 Fe	1360	8.9
Metal, white	75 Pb, 19 Sb, 5 Sn, 1 Cu	238	9.5
Nickel	100 Ni	1455	8.9
Nickel-silver	65 Cu, 18 Ni, 17 Zn	1110	8.8
Palladium	100 Pd	1549	12.2
Pewter	85 Sn, 7 Cu, 6 Bi, 2 Sb	—	7.7
Platinum	100 Pt	1774	21.4
Silver, fine	100 Ag	961	10.6
Silver, sterling (925)	92.5 Ag, 7.5 Cu	920	10.4
Silver, coinage (800)	80 Ag, 20 Cu (varies with nation)	890	10.3
Steel, ordinary	99 Fe, 1 C (some variation)	1430	7.8
Steel, stainless	90 Fe, 8 Cr, 0.4 Mn	1450	5.8
Tin	100 Sn	232	5.8
Titanium	100 Ti	1800	4.5
Zinc	100 Zn	419	7.1

Abbreviations for elements

Al	Aluminum	Mn	Manganese	Fe	Iron	Zn	Zinc
Ag	Silver	Ni	Nickel	Cu	Copper	Ti	Titanium
Au	Gold	Pb	Lead	Cr	Chromium	Sn	Tin
Bi	Bismuth	Pd	Palladium	Cd	Cadmium	Sb	Antimony
C	Carbon	Pt	Platinum	Mg	Magnesium		

selected contact metal (gold, platinum, copper, nickel) is then connected with the anode pole of the plating tank and suspended into a solution of warmed plating salts. The article to be plated is attached to the cathode pole and then immersed in the electrically charged plating bath (10 to 20 volts) for 30 seconds to several minutes.[47] Figure 20-2 shows the electroplating and stripping process.

Plating solutions contain metal cyanide complexes (e.g., cyanoaurate salts) and, occasionally, noncyanide salts such as silver succinimide or gold sulfite.[44] Gold-plating solutions often contain nickel, brass, or other metal cyanide complexes, potassium cyanide, potassium cyanaurate (gold potassium cyanide), potassium carbonate, and citric, phosphoric, or hydrochloric acid.[44,52] Silver-plating solutions

typically contain sodium cyanide, fine silver, lead (pewter), or antimony. Nickel-plating solutions are often prepared from nickel sulfate, boric acid, ammonium chloride, and sodium saccharin.[52] Copper-plating solutions may contain copper sulfate and sulfuric acid or copper cyanide, potassium cyanide, and potassium hydroxide.[52]

Stripping solutions contain sodium or potassium cyanide. In mass production, hydrogen peroxide 20% or 25% is sometimes added to cyanide stripping solution to hasten the removal of the top layer of gold from newly cast (raw) jewelry. This process is known as "the bombing procedure."

Charms and settings are mass produced by lost wax or lost plastic casting, referred to as *investment* casting, in which heated wax or plastic is first poured into a rubber mold and allowed to harden. The mold is removed, and the wax or plastic model or "tree" (3 inches × 6 inches) is encased in a flask containing investment paste.[11,52] Investment is composed of 45% cristabolite, 30% quartz, and hydrated calcium sulfate (gypsum or plaster of paris).[47] Until the last decade, some investment formulations contained asbestos.[30,44,52] The investment is mixed under vacuum to remove air bubbles and allowed to dry at room temperature. A hole is left in the bottom of the investment plaster block. The block is placed in a steam oven to allow the melted wax or plastic to drain from the bottom and then fired in a brick- or asbestos-lined oven at approximately 2000° C. When cooled to 1200° C, the block is filled with a casting metal. Casting metal mixtures are prepared from fine gold, platinum, or silver with the addition of one or more metal alloys.[44,52] Copper, antimony, pewter, aluminum, bronze, lead, brass, cadmium, tin, chromium, magnesium, zinc, and beryllium have been used as metal alloys.[44,47,52] Table 20-4 lists the composition, melting point, and specific gravity of common casting metals and alloys. In the industrial setting, casting metals are heated within a controlled environment of an inert gas to prevent the heated metal constituents from oxidizing.[44,52] Argon gas is commonly used for this purpose.[44,52] When molten, the alloy mix is injected into the hollow investment mold under a vacuum or by centrifugal force. After the metal has cooled, the investment plaster is dissolved with solutions of (1) ammonium carbonate, (2) hydrochloric acid and ammonium bifluoride, or (3) pressurized cold water.[44,52] The metal piece or tree is removed from the investment residue and then trimmed, bombed, filed, and polished (Figs. 20-3 through 20-5).

Jewelry and other ornamental pieces may be enameled. In this process, a mixture of silica and either glass particles or colored oxides are fused onto a base metal to form an enamel surface.[44,52] Prior to enameling, metals are prepared by the process of annealing (firing at temperatures 890° C to 1090° C) and "pickling." Pickling removes the firescale (oxidation) created from heating.[25,47] In this procedure, metals are pickled by immersion into dilute acid (usually nitric, hydrochloric, or sulfuric acid), followed by neutralization with a solution of sodium bicarbonate.[47] Gum tragacanth is then applied to the metal base to secure the enamel bond. Enamel is applied as a heavy paste or spray or as a powder that is dusted over the metal surface.[44,52] Metals are placed in a heated kiln (700° C to 900° C) and fired until the enamel melts. Hydrochloric acid is sometimes applied to the metal upon cooling to create a matte finish.[47] Excess enamel is removed with a mixture of ammonium bifluoride and hydrofluoric acid. Solvents such as toluene, xylene, and acetone are used to liquefy and clean enamel spray guns and equipment.[44,52]

The process of joining of two or more metal pieces together is called *soldering*. Soldering incorporates the appli-

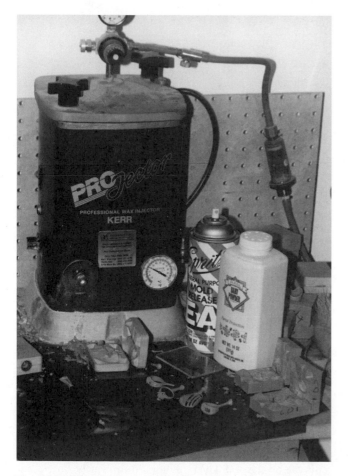

Fig. 20-3 Wax injection molding (lost wax casting): Pressurized melted wax (70°-85° F) is injected into a rubber casting mold. Before wax injection, talc is dusted over the mold to keep the rubber dry. Mold release spray (65% 1,1-dichloro-1-fluoroethane and 35% 1,1,1,2-tetrafluoroethane) prevents the cooled wax from adhering to the rubber mold.

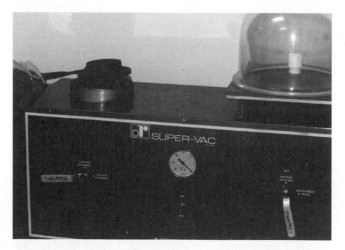

Fig. 20-4 Vacuum casting machine: Gold is melted in a crucible with other alloys before metal casting. The molten gold is then poured into the casting machine (flask) under vacuum. The gold fills the hollow spaces of the investment (plaster) block enclosed within the casting machine. The gold solidifies within seconds, is removed, and is allowed to cool at room temperature.

cation of a small amount of metal alloy (solder) selected to melt and flow at a temperature lower than the pieces to be joined.[44,52] Metal solders are selected by melting point, identified as "easy," "medium," or "hard."[25] Easy silver solder melts at approximately 715° C; medium and hard solders melt at 735° C and 750° C, respectively.[47] Table 20-5 lists the common components of silver and gold solders. Items to be soldered are placed on a heat-resistant asbestos board, charcoal block, or ceramic board. The metal ends of the jewelry are coated with "flux" prior to heating.[25,47] The flux prevents surface oxidation during the heating process and directs the flow of the melted solder. Flux formulations typically contain 10% to 20% boric acid or borax (sodium borate); ethyl alcohol, methanol, methylethylketone (MEK), or acetone; diammonium phosphate or sodium tripolyphosphate; and blue, green, or yellow dyes.[44,52] Zinc chloride fluxes are used for metals of extremely low melting points such as lead alloys[52] (Fig. 20-6).

Cleaning and degreasing remove flux and polishing compounds, respectively, from jewelry items.[25,47] Jewelry is cleaned with detergents and ammonia in an ultrasonic vibrating tub. Degreasing procedures involve either hot or cold (sodium hydroxide) mixtures and solvents. Sodium carbonate 45%, 20% sodium hydroxide, 30% disodium phosphate, 5% sodium metasilicate, and ammonia are chemicals commonly added to vibrating, degreasing tubs.[44,52] Trichloroethylene, perchloroethylene, or 1,1,1-trichloroethane are used for warm, nonvibrating, degreasing procedures[52] (Fig. 20-7).

The polishing process removes fine marks and yields a bright or matte finish to jewelry items. Felt or muslin polishing wheels and polishing compounds (rouges) are the materials involved in this procedure.[25] The selection of the polishing compound (red, yellow, black, green, and white) is dependent upon the type of metal or the hardness of the stone and the desired finish of the end product (i.e., bright or matte). Red rouge is used for gold and silver; black for white gold, platinum, and silver; green for high luster on chrome, stainless steel, and platinum; and white for stainless steel, chrome, and platinum[47] (Fig. 20-8).

Sources of Toxicity in the Work Environment

Much of the fine work in preparing and finishing jewelry is physically demanding. Jewelers, when faced with deadlines (like holidays or weddings) may work long hours, occasionally sleeping in their workplaces. Standard industrial limits

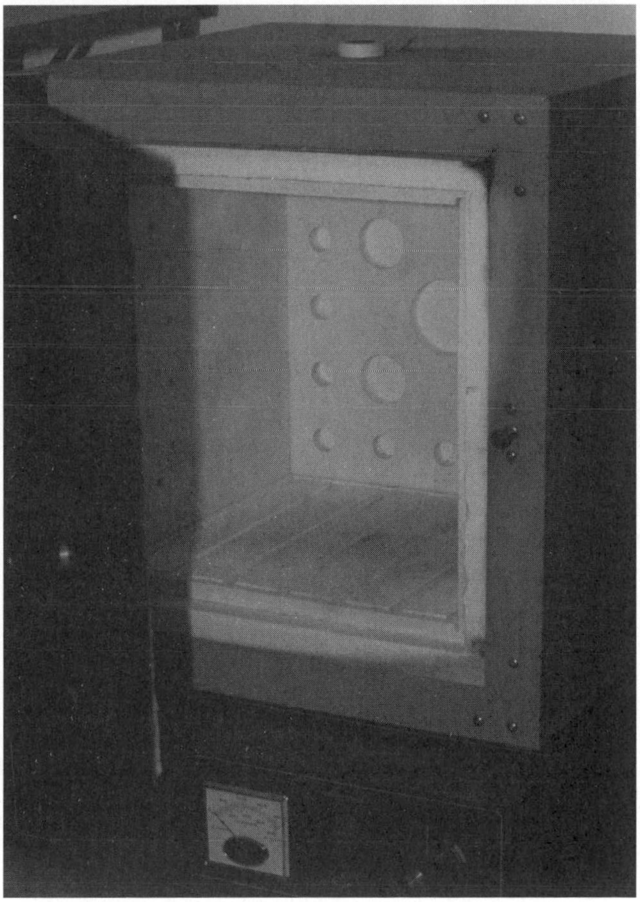

Fig. 20-5 Investment heating oven: Investment flasks or blocks are heated in ceramic, asbestos-lined ovens. This 24-inch × 30-inch oven is gas heated and holds up to 10 flasks of investment.

Table 20-5 Commonly used silver and gold solders

Solder type	Size	Composition
Hard solder		18 k (750) gold
	15 g	Fine silver
	6 g	Brass
Medium solder		
	15 g	Fine silver
	7.5 g	Brass
Easy solder		
	5.6 g	Fine silver
	2.2 g	Copper
	2.2 g	Zinc
Enameling silver solder		
	6 g	Fine silver
	1.5 g	Copper
	7.5 g	Fine gold
	0.3 g	Fine silver
	1 g	Copper
	1.2 g	Cadmium
14 k (585) hard solder		
	0.585 g	Fine gold
	0.18 g	Fine silver
	0.15 g	Copper
	0.085 g	Cadmium
14 k (585) medium solder		
	0.585 g	Fine gold
	0.115 g	Fine silver
	0.185 g	Copper
	0.115 g	Cadmium
Light-fusing gold solder		
	2 g	Fine gold
	9 g	Fine silver
	5 g	Copper
	1 g	Zinc

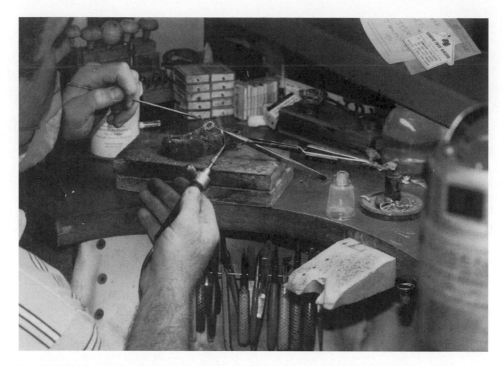

Fig. 20-6 Soldering: Jewelry is soldered on an asbestos board and charcoal block. A propane gas torch is used to heat the metal. The green liquid in the small bottle is a boric acid containing flux (Luxiflux) composed of 87% methanol, 12% boric acid, and a green dye.

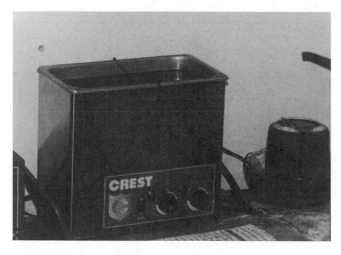

Fig. 20-7 This 3-gallon ultrasonic vibrating tank degreases jewelry and metals. Sodium carbonate, sodium hydroxide, disodium phosphate, sodium metasilicate, and ammonia are a common degreasing formulation for this type of tank.

for chemical exposures are predicated on an 8-hour workday, followed by 16 hours away from the work environment.[60] Many small jewelry shops employ fewer than 25 workers and therefore are less likely to incorporate a prospective medical surveillance program utilizing standard safety and manufacturing procedures. Potential problems in the work environment are summarized in the box on p. 161.

Ventilation systems found in jewelry production operations are frequently inadequate.[13,44,52] General ventilation systems, such as roof fans, merely push air around and give a false sense of security to employees. Local ventilation systems are more effective in eliminating airborne substances from the source of contamination.[52] Local ventilation consists of exhaust hoods, ducts that carry air away, and fans that push the air outside. Even when appropriate ventilation systems exist, air filter replacement and duct cleaning are neglected, ultimately reducing the effectiveness of the ventilation system.

Respirator masks and other protective equipment may be used or stored incorrectly (e.g., the wrong side of the mask is placed over the face), subsequently exposing the worker to the compound collected from the previous use!

Jewelry shops often exceed standards for heat exposure, especially during the summer. Industrial machinery, such as plating tanks, annealing ovens (a warming unit that makes a metal malleable), and casting furnaces, emit heat, and, if they are improperly vented, carbon monoxide gas accumulates.[52] The Occupational Safety and Health Administration (OSHA) recommends that work areas should be no warmer than 86° F where the work is considered "light" and the activities are continuous.[60]

Noise is a dangerous health and safety problem in the jewelry industry.[22,52] Poorly lubricated machinery, metal rollers and stampers, and high-speed drills contribute to factory noise.[52] The OSHA noise standard is 90 decibels per 8 hours to prevent loss of hearing.[60]

Privately owned jewelry shops may have limited space to perform all design and repair processes. Inadequate facilities

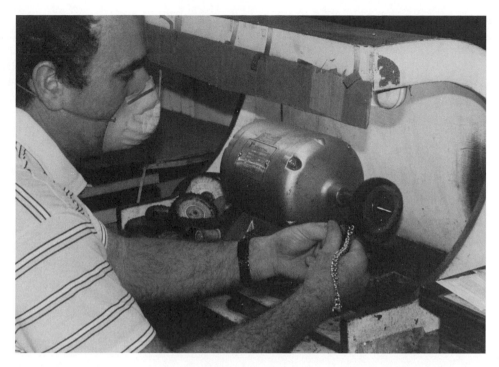

Fig. 20-8 Polishing: A motor-driven muslin wheel applies green rouge polish to a 14-karat gold bracelet. The vacuum beneath the pump pulls the gold dust downward and away from the worker.

for lunch and minimal time for rest breaks may encourage the jeweler to "eat on the job" and potentially expose food items to hazardous chemicals.

Jewelers may bring work clothing home and inadvertently expose family members to dusts and chemicals. Work shoes may contain dusts and materials that may contaminate household carpets and furniture. Some jewelers work in their homes and continuously expose themselves and family members to noxious vapors and dusts.

These potential problems place jewelry workers at a substantial risk for occupational illness and injury. Each activity performed by the jeweler is associated with a potential health hazard. Jewelers may be exposed to a variety of toxic chemicals and materials of different physical, pharmacologic, and pharmacodynamic properties.[24,44,52] Table 20-6 lists the potentially hazardous chemicals and materials that jewelers may be exposed to.

POTENTIAL TOXIC EXPOSURES
Organ System Toxicity

Toxicity from a hazardous materials exposure in the jewelry worker primarily involves the lung and dermal systems.[44,52] Less commonly, toxicity associated with other organ systems may be seen in this population. Although few accounts of occupational injury among jewelry workers have been published, the concerns for toxicity are predicated upon descriptions of organ system injuries associated with substances of established toxicity that are also utilized in jewelry manufacturing processes.

Potential Problems in the Work Environment

Old buildings with small work areas

Hot work area

"We don't need training" employee attitude

"We don't need education" management attitude

"Mystery mixture" unmarked bottles: chemicals, liquids, or acids

No chemical spill kits, outdated antidotes (i.e., cyanide kit)

First-aid boxes not checked or inadequate supplies

"Cutting corners"; slackened techniques due to seasonal rush (holidays and events; customer or boss waiting for jewelry to be finished)

Noise louder than 90 decibels

Inadequate exhaust and ventilation systems

Inadequate washing facilities

Contamination of chemicals due to poor measuring and cleaning techniques

No protective gloves, eye shields, or equipment

Incorrect mixtures—undiluted liquids, chemicals, and acids

Unapproved heating vessels used to heat acids

Improper acid and chemical disposal—usually down toilet or sink

Eating in the work area and exposing food to chemicals and vapors

Table 20-6 Potentially hazardous substances in the jeweler's workplace

Gases

Ammonia	Carbon monoxide	Hydrogen sulfide	Phosgene	Stibine
Argon	Chlorine	Nitrogen dioxide	Propane	Sulfur oxides
Arsine	Hydrogen cyanide			

Liquids

Acetone	Gum tragacanth	Mercury	Phenol	Toluene
Ammonium bifluoride	Hydrochloric acid	Methyl	Phosphoric acid	1,1,1-Trichloroethane
Benzene	(muriatic acid)	Methylethylketone	Potassium hydroxide	Trichloroethylene
Citric acid	Hydrofluoric acid	(MEK)	Sodium bisulfate	Turpentine
Diethyl ether	Hydrogen peroxide	Nitric acid	Sodium hydroxide	Xylene
Ethyl alcohol	Iodine	Oils, lubricants	Sulfuric acid	Zinc chloride
Epoxy resins	Isopropyl alcohol	Perchloroethylene		

Dusts

Aluminum	Borax (sodium borate)	Emery	Lead	Shell pearls
Antimony	Brass	Enamel	Marble	Silica (tridymite, pum-
Arsenic	Bronze	Epoxy resins	Nickel	ice quartz)
Asbestos (amosite, am-	Cadmium	Gold	Nuisance particulates	Silver
phibole, crocidolite,	Chromium	Graphite (carbon)	Plastics	Talc (soapstone, talcum)
serpentine)	Cobalt	Indium	Platinum	Tin
Beryllium	Copper	Iron	Precious stones	Zinc
Boric acid	Coral	Ivory	Rosin	

Fumes

Aluminum oxide	Beryllium oxide	Cyanide salts (gold,	Iron oxide	Nickel oxide
Ammonium fluoride	Cadmium oxide	nickel, silver, copper)	Lead oxide	Silver oxide
Ammonium chloride	Copper oxides	Divalent chromates	Manganese oxide	Stannic oxide (tin)
Ammonium carbonate	Cyanide (potassium or	Fluoride	Mercury	Zinc chloride
Antimony oxide	sodium)	Hydrofluoric acid	Nickel cyanide	Zinc oxide

Additional workplace exposures

Heat	Radiation
Noise	Vibratory insults

Pulmonary toxicity. Inhalation injuries are caused by three basic mechanisms: (1) deposition in the upper respiratory tract, lung parenchyma, or lymphatics with subsequent inflammatory or fibrotic reaction, (2) irritation of the lining of the tracheobronchial tree with inflammation, edema, or both, and (3) allergic or immunologic response.[40] Pathophysiologic pulmonary conditions resulting from metal and chemical exposures have been reported in the medical literature.*

Pulmonary toxicity in the jewelry worker may present as upper respiratory tract irritation, occupational asthma, functional or benign pneumoconioses, hypersensitivity pneumonitis, or oncologic disease.[1,28,40,56]

Upper respiratory tract irritation. Inhalation of metal dusts and fumes can produce both acute and chronic symptoms and signs. The severity of irritation depends upon several factors: the water solubility of a gas or vapor, the concentration, and the size and shape of the aerosol or particulate matter.[51] Metal dust-generating activities such as cutting, sawing, drilling, pounding, grinding, filing, scraping, and polishing can result in irritant effects on the eyes,

mucous membranes, and respiratory tract.[50] Liquid spillage, spraying, blowing, and pouring generate mists or fogs that may also irritate mucous membranes.[50] Sinus congestion, sore throat, coughing, chest pain, and dyspnea can be symptoms of metal and solvent exposure.[1,20,56] Table 20-7 lists mild and strong mucous membrane, ocular, and pulmonary irritants that jewelers may be exposed to. The following chemicals are particularly hazardous; exposure can be fatal.

Inhalation of elemental mercury vapors (quicksilver, Hg^0) can initially cause cough, chills, fever, and shortness of breath and may progress to pulmonary edema, respiratory failure, and death.[9,58] Acute interstitial pneumonitis, along with patchy atelectasis and emphysema, may be appreciated on chest radiograph.[9]

Inhalation of concentrated hydrofluoric acid for as little as 5 minutes can result in death within 2 to 10 hours due to a direct local toxic effect that produces hemorrhagic pulmonary edema or due to systemic toxicity.[26]

Occupational asthma. Asthma is a pulmonary disorder characterized by widespread partial obstruction of the airways that varies in severity, is reversible, and is not secondary to cardiovascular disease.[56] In occupational asthma, airway obstruction develops after workplace exposure to

*References 1, 5, 20, 23, 28, 41, 45.

Table 20-7 Mild and strong mucous membrane, ocular, and pulmonary irritants

Mild irritants	Strong irritants
Arsenic	Ammonia
Copper	Antimony
Fluoride	Beryllium
Silver	Cadmium
Tin	Chlorine
Acetone	Hexavalent chromium
Ethyl alcohol	Fluorine
Isopropyl alcohol	Hydrogen chloride
Diethyl ether	Hydrogen fluoride
Methylethylketone (MEK)	Hydrogen sulfide
Phosphoric acid	Iodine
Sodium hydroxide	Mercury
1,1,1-Trichloroethane	Nickel
Trichloroethylene	Nitric acid
Turpentine	Phosgene
Xylene	Sulfuric acid
	Zinc chloride

inhaled gases, dusts, fumes, or vapors.[56] Various etiologies have been suggested; an accepted pathogenesis of occupational asthma suggests that type I (immediate) and type III (immune-complex-mediated) reactions occur due to IgE and IgG antibodies, respectively.[56] The activation of complement via an alternative pathway, coupled with the nonimmunologic release of histamine, results in bronchoconstriction, inflammation, mucosal edema, and the accumulation of viscous secretions.[5,19,56] Low-molecular-weight metals such as cobalt,[2,21,48,57,61] chromium,[2,7,33,48,57] nickel,[7,42,48] platinum,[49] and zinc[43,62] have been reported to cause occupational asthma. In patients with asthma associated with nickel, cobalt, and chromium, IgE antibodies to these metals have been noted; however, the pathogenic mechanism of metal-induced asthma is not known.[2,42,48] Nickel exposure has been reported to cause both immediate and delayed allergy with allergic contact dermatitis, allergic contact urticaria, rhinitis, and asthma.[15]

Pneumoconiosis: functional and benign. Fibrogenic dusts, such as asbestos, cobalt, graphite (carbon), silica (pumice, quartz, tridymite), and talc (talcum, soapstone), are known to cause fibrotic pneumoconiosis with resultant restrictive disease.[14,63] Before 1970, investment powders used for molding and casting were often fortified with silica or asbestos for added firmness.[44,52] Oncologic disease can occur from chronic exposures to silica, asbestos, and talc.[56]

Asbestosis is an irreversible pulmonary condition caused by the deposition of asbestos fibers in the lower regions of the lung. *Asbestos* is a generic term for six fibrous minerals. The two major classes of asbestos are serpentine, which contains magnesium silicate (chrysotile), and amphibole, which includes crocidolite, amosite, anthophyllite, and tremolite fibers.[6] Chrysotile fibers account for 93% of the world's asbestos use. Asbestosis and lung cancer (often mesotheliomas) have been associated with chronic asbestos

exposure.[30,31] Although all asbestos fiber types can cause mesothelioma, several studies have suggested that the amphibole form may be more likely to induce this tumor than serpentine fibers.[6] Asbestos-related physiologic lung changes present after a latency period of 10 to 30 years. Lung cancers associated with asbestos exposure are discussed later in this chapter. Inhalation of asbestos fibers in the range of 5 to 10 microns in diameter can elicit a fibrogenic response, often involving the lower lung bases and pleura. Fibrosis results from the persistent release of inflammatory mediators such as lysoenzymes, interleukins, and fibroblast growth factors at the site of fiber penetration and deposition. Although most pleural plaques associated with asbestosis are benign, they can result in respiratory impairment. Lung fibrosis leads to restrictive lung disease and can increase pulmonary vascular resistance, which results in pulmonary hypertension and compensatory hypertrophy of the right heart.[6] Benign pneumoconiosis has resulted from iron and tin exposures because these radiopaque dusts deposit in the lung without eliciting fibrotic changes.[56] Tin-containing solders may produce tin oxide fumes. When inhaled, these fumes can result in a "benign" pneumoconiosis in which there is radiographic evidence of dust or fiber deposition in the lungs without measurable pulmonary function abnormalities.[45]

Silicosis is a form of pneumoconiosis associated with pulmonary exposure to silica. Intense exposure can result in a generalized systemic disease resembling a collagen vascular disease, such as systemic lupus erythematosus. Inhalation of silica may trigger an autoimmune disease.[1,5,40,56]

Diamond polishers in Belgium were reported to have developed diffuse interstitial lung disease after long-term exposure to cobalt dusts.[35] These dusts were generated from high-speed grinding disks coated with abrasive microdiamonds embedded in binding cobalt powder. The clinical, radiologic, and histologic findings in these workers were identical with those seen in hard-metal disease or cobalt allergy.

Hypersensitivity pneumonitis. Hypersensitivity pneumonitis (extrinsic alveolitis) is characterized by a granulomatous inflammatory reaction in the pulmonary alveolar and interstitial spaces. The condition is presumed to be immunologically mediated and typically requires repetitive exposures to a high concentration of an antigenic material such as copper and nickel sulfate.[5,15,40]

Lung cancers. Isolated reports of pulmonary cancers among jewelers have been published.[12,13,24,31] Exposures to silica,[11,29,56] chromium,[41,45,64] nickel,[23,38,41] and asbestos[1,6,12,30,31] have been associated with pulmonary cancers.

In 1989, the American College of Occupation Medicine Committee on Occupational Medical Practice reported that there was no known association between jewelry manufacturing and asbestos-related diseases[3]; however, isolated cases of mesothelioma in jewelers and others in similar trades have been published since that time. For example, a commercial jeweler developed biopsy-proven malignant mesothelioma secondary to investment powder exposure.[31] Amosite asbestos fibers were found in a lung specimen by scanning electron microscope (SEM) and energy-dispersive x-ray analysis (EDXA). The patient had manufactured asbestos soldering forms at a costume jewelry production facility and had been exposed to what was thought to be chrysotile asbestos during the first 25 years of his employment.

Another unusual asbestos exposure was identified in 5 cases of mesothelioma in a Native American pueblo of approximately 2000 people between 1970 and 1984.[12] All 5 people were exposed to asbestos during the manufacture of silver jewelry or during the preparation of leather leggings and moccasins. Workers used pounding boards (asbestos mats) to insulate worktables against the intense heat of brazing torches and molten metal. Aerosolization of the asbestos fibers occurred when these mats were slapped together for cleaning purposes. These findings underscore the dangers of asbestos exposure and represent the first reports of mesothelioma associated with jewelry manufacturing.

Occupational exposure to hexavalent chromium (CrVI) has been associated with increased lung cancer mortality.[7,37] The latency for chromium-induced lung cancer is greater than 20 years, and exposure duration may be as short as 2 years. Epidemiologic studies among stainless steel (SS) welders indicate a high risk of developing lung cancer if hexavalent chromium, zinc, and nickel are generated from the welding process.[38] Results suggest that these metals are capable of biologically altering several cellular defense mechanisms involved in the carcinogenic process.[38]

Metal fume fever. Metal fume fever is also known as *foundry ague, zinc shakes, Monday morning fever, welder's fever,* and *solderer's fever.*[39] It is called *Monday morning fever* because workers eventually develop a tolerance to the effects of the metal fumes from the repeated exposures. Tolerance may be lost over the weekend, but a flulike syndrome resumes on Monday evening, after the first day back at work. Substances associated with metal fume fever that a jeweler may be exposed to include copper, aluminum, antimony, iron, nickel, zinc, cadmium, and chromates.* Fever, fatigue, chills, cough, dyspnea, a metallic taste in the mouth, rhinitis, conjunctivitis, and muscle aches generally manifest the evening after the exposure to the metal fumes. Resolution occurs within 36 hours after fume exposure.[39]

Dermal toxicity. Jewelers are at risk for burns from hot surfaces (propane fuel torches, molten metals) and caustic chemicals and for the development of acute and chronic irritant dermatitis, allergic contact dermatitis, and contact urticaria. Many metals and solvents utilized in jewelry manufacturing and repair processes are known to cause dermal injury. Lipids and sweat act as a primary barrier to agents that contact the skin.[51] Alcohols and ketones break

down the skin's lipid barriers and promote enhanced contact with chemical agents. Skin that is abraded, inflamed, or denuded absorbs chemicals faster and to a greater extent than skin that is intact.[51] Caustics, such as hydrochloric (muriatic), hydrofluoric, sulfuric, phosphoric, and nitric acids, sodium or potassium hydroxide, ammonia, iodine, phenol, and zinc chloride, can produce serious burns.[18,26,27,46] Acid burns are characterized by immediate skin damage and early onset of resolution. Alkali burns tend to cause injury insidiously and are often more severe than acid burns.[18,46] A jeweler may use hydrofluoric acid to glaze pottery, etch glass, or remove rust.[39,44,52] Serious deep burns can occur initially without pain. Severe ocular and dermal injuries, as well as life-threatening systemic toxicity, have been reported from dermal exposure.[18] Hydrofluoric acid vapors can produce chronic bone and teeth damage (osteofluorosis).[26,34,52]

Most occupational dermatitis can be categorized as irritant or allergic. Clinically as well as histologically, both allergic contact and chronic irritant dermatitis are virtually indistinguishable.[46] However, chronic irritant contact dermatitis is characterized by erythema, scaling, fissuring, and pruritus. It may develop from long periods of exposure to a mildly irritating chemical. Allergic contact dermatitis is a cell-mediated reaction involving sensitized T cells. Sensitization occurs when substances penetrate the skin via epidermal cells, sebaceous and sweat glands, and hair follicles. Metals and epoxy resins can act as antigenic substances and cause sensitization after one or more dermal exposures. Nickel, cobalt, and chromium are known to cause skin sensitization.[5] Signs of allergic contact dermatitis include erythema and edema, which can progress to vesicle formation, rupture, and oozing dermatitis. The severity of the dermal response may increase for several days without further contact with the allergen; healing usually occurs within 2 to 4 weeks. Once developed, allergen sensitization persists long after healing. A subsequent exposure to even a small amount of the causative agent triggers another allergic reaction.[5] Patch testing may help to differentiate allergic contact and chronic irritant dermatitis.[4] However, patients should not be patch tested with known irritants, as the dermal reaction is inevitable and not based on sensitivity.

Metals. Metals such as gold,[53] chromium,[7,41,64] cobalt,[2] platinum salts,[46] and nickel[15,64] may produce acute contact dermatitis. Hexavalent chromium compounds (CrVI) are powerful oxidizing agents and tend to be irritating and corrosive. Argyria is a permanent, bluish black discoloration of eyes, nails, inner nose, mouth, throat, skin, and internal organs that develops from chronic inhalation of silver dust or fumes. Silver particles can become embedded in the skin and cause a permanent tattoo that appears identical to a malignant melanoma.[54]

Gold and silver electroplating solutions contain cyanide salts. Their metal cyanide complexes (e.g., cyanoaurate salts) release hydrogen cyanide when heated or treated with

---

*References 20, 23, 39, 41, 58, 64.

acid. Cyanide salts (sodium and potassium) are highly toxic by dermal contact, inhalation, or ingestion.[8,32] Chronic skin contact may cause skin rashes and promote dermal absorption of cyanide.

Chromium compounds can be sensitizers as well as irritants.[7,41] Lymphedema may be a complication of chronic allergic contact dermatitis attributed to both cobalt and chromium.[16] Hexavalent chromium compounds can cause persistent ulcers known as *chrome holes* on broken or denuded skin. These ulcers may penetrate into soft tissue and subsequently induce a secondary infection.[7] Repeated skin contact with chromium dust may lead to eczematous dermatitis with edema. Chronic inflammation of the skin and mucous membranes after prolonged exposure to high doses of hexavalent chromium is well known in the literature. Chromate dusts can irritate the conjunctiva and mucous membranes, as well as cause nasal ulcers and nasal septum perforation.[7]

Most of the reported cases of gold allergy have been allergic contact dermatitis caused by gold rings or other jewelry. Positive tests to patch testing with gold salts are difficult to interpret as the test material itself may cause dermal irritation and sensitization.[4] Oral contact hypersensitivity reactions to gold have been induced by gold crowns, bridges, and dentures.[4] Gingivitis caused by metallic gold has been reported. Black dermographism is a reaction to gold and gold alloys in which black lines appear immediately after the metal is rubbed on the skin.[53] The effect is the result of impregnation of the skin with black metallic particles produced when skin contaminants cause mechanical abrasion of the metal. Similarly, wearing gold jewelry has been known to cause blackening of the skin (smudge) beneath the metal. The mechanical abrasion of the gold jewelry, in addition to the corrosion of gold or gold alloys from components of sweat, may be the cause of the skin discoloration.[53]

Nickel allergy is the most common type of cutaneous hypersensitivity.[17] The prevalence of nickel allergy is lower in men than in women. As many as 10% of females are thought to have a nickel allergy. It has been suggested that exposure to nickel in metallic jewelry, especially earrings worn in pierced ears, may account for the female preponderance. Significant amounts of nickel can be released from stainless steel and other alloys even after silver or gold plating. Hand dermatitis has been reported to occur in up to 50% of nickel-sensitive women. Nickel sensitivity is also thought to result in atopic eczema.[17]

Epoxy resins. The primary dermal effect of epoxy resins is allergic contact dermatitis. The dermatitis is usually localized to the hands and forearms but occasionally appears on the face and neck.[18]

Gastrointestinal toxicity. A retrospective study of jewelry workers revealed a disproportionate number of deaths from gastrointestinal carcinomas.[24] Mortality was investigated for the years 1950 to 1980 among 1009 male members of a New York jewelry workers union and for the years 1984 to 1989 among 919 men and 605 women identified as jewelry workers on death certificates from 24 states. The author suggested that the wide variety of exposures in the jewelry industry, particularly to metals and solvents, could involve excess risk for malignancy of the gastrointestinal tract.

Cyanide. Cyanide salts, such as potassium cyanide and sodium cyanide, are used in the process of electroplating. The salts are colorless solids; when combined with acid, HCN (prussic acid), which is a colorless gas at room temperature, is released. Cyanide compounds have a faint, bitter almond odor, detectable at a threshold of 0.2 to 5 ppm. The ability to smell cyanide is a genetically determined trait that is absent in 20% to 40% of the population. Cyanide is absorbed through the lungs, gastrointestinal tract, and skin.[36,55]

CLINICAL TOXICOLOGY
Pathophysiology of Cyanide Toxicity

Mechanism of action. Cyanide binds to the cytochrome A_3 binding site within the cytochrome oxidase system, inhibiting cellular oxygen utilization. Blockade of the cytochrome oxidase system results in anaerobic metabolism with resultant lactate production and a severe metabolic acidosis. Cyanide also inhibits other enzymes and can combine with certain metabolic intermediates. Cyanide adversely affects the cardiovascular, respiratory, central nervous, and endocrine systems.

Exposure. Inhalation of 600 to 700 ppm HCN for 5 minutes or approximately 200 ppm for 30 minutes may be fatal. Symptoms can occur within seconds after inhalation or minutes after ingestion of cyanide salts. Symptom onset may be delayed up to 12 hours after the ingestion of cyanogenic compounds. Cyanide is absorbed via the mucous membranes and eyes; dermal burns have resulted from handling molten cyanide salts or from immersion in cyanide solutions. Gilders and silverplaters are at risk for potentially fatal cyanide toxicity, primarily from cutaneous or inhalational exposure to cyanide salts. Cyanide exposure can occur during the process of electroplating or stripping, as both processes require cyanide salts. Inhalational, dermal, and ocular exposures of cyanide may occur.

Clinical presentation. Acute cyanide exposure affects the central nervous system (CNS), initially producing stimulation, which may be followed quickly by depression.[8,32] Signs and symptoms of acute cyanide toxicity reflect cellular hypoxia. Fainting, flushing, anxiety, excitement, perspiration, vertigo, headache, drowsiness, prostration, opisthotonos, trismus, tremors, convulsions, stupor, paralysis, and coma may occur after exposure. Retinal veins and arteries may appear similarly red in color because cyanide blocks cellular utilization of oxygen and elevates venous Po_2. The brain is particularly susceptible to cyanide poisoning because of its high metabolic demands. A decrease

Table 20-8 Common toxicities and potential injuries in jewelers

Agent	System	Symptoms
Carbon monoxide	Neurologic	Headache, confusion, drowsiness (acute or chronic)
		Psychosis
		Peripheral neuropathy
		Dementia
		Amnestic syndromes
	Hematologic	Carboxyhemoglobin
Hydrogen cyanide	Neurologic	CNS stimulation, depression
		Headache
		Vertigo
		Tremors
		Convulsions
		Peripheral neuropathy
		Optic neuropathy, atrophy
		Visual failure
		Deafness
		Extrapyramidal signs
	Cardiovascular	Palpitations
		Myocardial depression drop
	Respiratory	Tachypnea (central-mediated)
		Pulmonary edema (? neurologic)
	Cutaneous	Cherry red color
		Cyanosis
	Ocular	Fundal vasculature with cherry red color
	Endocrinologic	Goiter
Heavy metals	Neurologic	Paresis or sensory disturbances of extremities and digits
		Ataxia
		Convulsions
		Extremity weakness (wrist drop)
		Headache
		Sleep disturbances
		Visual changes
		Confusion
		Personality changes
		Parkinson-like symptoms (tremor, rigidity, bradykinesia)
	Ocular	Excoriation due to metal particles
		Blue-black staining due to silver
	Renal	Proximal tubule injury
		Glomerular injury
	GI	Cancer
Halogenated hydrocarbons	GI/Hepatic	Hepatic necrosis, cirrhosis
	Neurologic	Cancer
		Trigeminal nerve anesthesia
Mechanical (due to excessive vibration)	Renal	Acute tubular necrosis
	Musculoskeletal	White finger disease (due to Raynaud's phenomenon)
		Degeneration of bone and cartilage

in the cellular ATP:ADP ratio occurs in cyanide poisoning because of the predominance of anaerobic metabolism. The electrical activity in the brain is altered secondarily to the disruption of calcium-dependent neurotransmitters; this factor appears to be important in the manifestation of cyanide-induced neurotoxic effects, such as tremors and convulsions. Delayed-onset Parkinson-like syndromes have been described after severe cyanide poisoning as well as after carbon monoxide poisoning. It has been suggested that the basal ganglia are sensitive to the neurotoxic effects of both agents.[8]

Diagnosis. In patients with suspected cyanide toxicity, whole-blood cyanide levels are not useful and should not be used. Red blood cell or serum cyanide levels can help to confirm the diagnosis. These levels take 4 to 6 hours and are not useful in acute poisonings. Indirect indicators of cyanide poisoning include lactic acidosis and a loss of the AVO_2 difference.[8,32]

Management. The management of cyanide poisoning deserves special mention, as cyanide toxicity is rapidly fatal unless expedient and appropriate therapy is begun. Emergency management for victims of cyanide poisoning initially

Table 20-9 Potential toxin-associated pathologies found on physical examination

System	Symptom
Lungs	Wheezing, prolonged expiration
	Decreased breath sounds
	Dullness to percussion
Neurologic/CNS	Altered mental status (e.g., agitation, depression)
	Tremors
	Altered position sense
	Cranial nerve impairment
	Fine-motor function disturbances
	Gait abnormalities
	Hearing impairment
Ocular	Diminished visual acuity
	Funduscopic evidence of optic nerve damage
	Excoriations of sclera or cornea
	Abnormal staining of sclera
Skin	Evidence of atopy
	Scars, old burns
Musculoskeletal	Joint swelling or contractures
	Muscle atrophy
	Fat pad wasting (especially fingertips)
Endocrinologic	Thyroid abnormality (enlargement)
	Diminished or elevated cue temperature
	Exophthalmos

involves basic life support. Airway management, ventilation, administration of 100% oxygen, and cardiovascular support with crystalloid and vasopressors should be initiated.[8,32] All contaminated garments should be removed, and the skin washed with soap and copious amounts of water. Cardiorespiratory monitoring should be instituted. Blood gas analysis, electrolytes, and serum lactate should be obtained to monitor the patient's oxygen and acid-base status. Metabolic acidosis with an elevated serum lactate level is indicative of cyanide poisoning.

The only approved antidote in the United States is the Lilly Antidote Kit. The kit contains amyl nitrite, sodium nitrite, and sodium thiosulfate. The nitrites reverse cyanide toxicity by inducing methemoglobinemia. Methemoglobinemia detoxifies cyanide by forming cyanomethemoglobin. The cyanomethemoglobin ultimately breaks down to cyanide and methemoglobin. Thiosulfate serves as a sulfur donor that is catalyzed by rhodanese to convert the cyanide to thiocyanate, which is less toxic and eliminated renally. Methemoglobin is then reduced to hemoglobin by methemoglobin reductase.

In severe cases, hyperbaric oxygen therapy, exchange transfusion, or both are instituted.

Experimental agents that may be future antidotes include 4-methylaminophenol (DMAP) and dicobalt ethylenediamine tetraacetic acid (cobalt EDTA), which are used in other countries.[32] These agents have not yet been approved by the Food and Drug Administration.

In cases of chronic poisonous exposure, the patient should avoid the source of cyanide. End-organ system injury should be treated symptomatically.

General Clinical Evaluation

The diagnosis of illnesses and injuries commonly encountered by jewelers can be difficult because of the wide variation in techniques, chemicals, materials, and machinery used in the industry—from meticulous handcrafting to the operation of large machinery. A review of potential toxicities and injuries in jewelers is presented in Table 20-8.

The physical examination of these patients should focus on the assessment of neuropsychiatric, ophthalmologic, cardiovascular, and thyroid functions. Table 20-9 provides a relevant guide to physical assessment.

INJURY PREVENTION

Injury prevention strategies are targeted at the prevention and control of both acute and chronic respiratory and dermal injuries.

Prevention of respiratory illness requires both sufficient ventilation and climate control of the work area. Employees should receive mandatory safety education and access to personal protective equipment and devices such as respirators, uniforms, gloves, boots, goggles, and face masks. Education should emphasize proper storage, cleaning, and repair of the equipment.

Decontamination stations for both dermal and ocular exposures should be accessible to all employees.

Detailed information regarding potential hazards in the workplace should be available to all employees; OSHA requires all employers to keep material safety data sheets (MSDS) on all industrial chemicals and materials.

Improvement and maintenance of personal habits and activities are also important in the prevention of illnesses and injuries. Jewelry workers who handle toxic agents such as acids and metal dust should have appropriate facilities for handwashing and showering. A specific area should be designated for eating and drinking to prevent food contamination by metal dusts, fumes, and other toxic substances.

Seasonal workload increases that occur before Christmas and Valentine's Day necessitate that employees receive adequate time for lunch or rest. Careless accidents are often the result of employee overload and fatigue.

REFERENCES

1. Abraham JL: Environmental pathology of the lung. In Rom WN, editor: *Environmental and occupational medicine,* ed 2, Boston, 1992, Little, Brown.
2. Allenby CF, Basketter DA: Minimum eliciting patch test concentrations of cobalt, *Contact Dermatitis* 20:185, 1989.
3. Andstadt GW: Genesis of mesothelioma, *J Occup Med* 31:643, 1989.
4. Aro T et al: Long-lasting allergic patch test reaction caused by gold, *Contact Dermatitis* 28:276, 1993.

5. Brooks BO, Sullivan JB: Immunotoxicology. In Sullivan JB, Krieger GR, editors: *Hazardous materials toxicology: clinical principles of environmental health,* Baltimore, 1992, Williams & Wilkins.

6. *Case studies in environmental medicine: asbestos toxicity,* ATSDR, Atlanta, 1990, US Department of Health and Human Services, Public Health Service.

7. *Case studies in environmental medicine: chromium toxicity,* ATSDR, Atlanta, 1990, US Department of Health and Human Services, Public Health Service.

8. *Case studies in environmental medicine: cyanide toxicity,* ATSDR, Atlanta, 1990, US Department of Health and Human Services, Public Health Service.

9. *Case studies in environmental medicine: mercury toxicity,* ATSDR, Atlanta, 1992, US Department of Health and Human Services, Public Health Service.

10. *Colored stones,* vol 15, series 2, Santa Monica, Calif, 1991, Gemological Institute of America.

11. Copplestone JF: Jewelry manufacture. In Parmeggiani L, editor: *Encyclopaedia of occupational health and safety,* ed 3, Geneva, 1983, International Labour Office.

12. Dricoll RJ et al: *Malignant mesothelioma: a cluster in a Native American pueblo, N Engl J Med* 318:1437, 1988.

13. Durbrow R, Gute D: Cause-specific mortality among Rhode Island jewelry workers, *Am J Ind Med* 12:579, 1987.

14. Dutoit RSJ: Tiger's eye pneumoconiosis, *Am J Ind Med* 22:605, 1992.

15. Estlander T et al: Immediate and delayed allergy to nickel with contact urticaria, rhinitis, asthma and contact dermatitis, *Clin Exp Allergy* 23:306, 1993.

16. Fitzgerald DA, English JS: Lymphoedema of the hands as a complication of chronic allergic contact dermatitis, *Contact Dermatitis* 30:310, 1994.

17. Gawkrodger DJ et al: Contact clinic survey of nickel sensitive subjects, *Contact Dermatitis* 14:165, 1986.

18. Geehr ED, Salluzzo RF: Dermal injuries and burns from hazardous materials. In Sullivan JB, Krieger GR, editors: *Hazardous materials toxicology: clinical principles of environmental health,* Baltimore, 1992, Williams & Wilkins.

19. German DF: Clinical immunology. In LaDou J, editor: *Occupational medicine,* Norwalk, Conn, 1990, Appleton & Lange.

20. Gerr F, Letz R: Solvents. In Rom WN, editor: *Environmental and occupational medicine,* ed 2, Boston, 1992, Little, Brown.

21. Gheysens B et al: Cobalt-induced bronchial asthma in diamond polishers, *Chest* 88:740, 1985.

22. Grant K et al: Case studies: biochemical hazards in a jewelry manufacturing facility, *Appl Occup Environ Hyg* 8:90, 1993.

23. Guidotti TL et al: Hazards of welding technologies. In Rom WN, editor: *Environmental and occupation medicine,* ed 2, Boston, 1992, Little, Brown.

24. Hayes RB et al: Cancer mortality among jewelry workers, *Am J Ind Med* 24:743, 1993.

25. Hickling JE: *Practical jewelry repair,* Ipswich, Suffolk (Great Britain), 1987, NAG Press.

26. Hoffman RS: Caustics and batteries. In Goldfrank LR et al, editors: *Goldfrank's toxicologic emergencies,* ed 5, Norwalk, Conn, 1994, Appleton & Lange.

27. Hughes JP, Letz G: Some clinical manifestations of occupational chemical exposure seen in emergency medical situations. In Hathaway GJ et al, editors: *Proctor and Hughes' chemical hazards of the workplace,* New York, 1991, Van Nostrand Reinhold.

28. Hughes JP, Letz G: Some physical clues to occupational poisoning. In Hathaway GJ et al, editors: *Proctor and Hughes' chemical hazards of the workplace,* New York, 1991, Van Nostrand Reinhold.

29. Kabir H, Bilgi C: Ontario gold miners with lung cancer: occupational exposure assessment in establishing work-relatedness, *JCM* 35:1203, 1993.

30. Kern DG: Asbestos-related disease in the jewelry industry: report of two cases, *Am J Ind Med* 13:407, 1988.

31. Kern DG et al: Malignant mesothelioma in the jewelry industry, *Am J Ind Med* 21:409, 1992.

32. Kerns WP, Kirk MA: Cyanide and hydrogen sulfide. In Goldfrank LR et al, editors: *Goldfrank's toxicologic emergencies,* ed 5, Norwalk, Conn, 1994, Appleton & Lange.

33. Keskinen H et al: Occupational asthma due to stainless steel welding fumes, *Clin Allergy* 10:151, 1980.

34. Krenzelok EP: Hydrofluoric acid. In Sullivan JB, Krieger GR, editors: *Hazardous materials toxicology: clinical principles of environmental health,* Baltimore, 1992, Williams & Wilkins.

35. Lahaye D et al: Lung disease among diamond polishers due to cobalt? *Lancet* 156:1984.

36. Landrigan PJ, Nicholson WJ: Benzene. In Rom WN, editor: *Environmental and occupation medicine,* ed 2, Boston, 1992, Little, Brown.

37. Langard S: Role of chemical species and exposure characteristics in cancer among occupationally exposed to chromium compounds, *Scand J Work, Environ, Health* 19(suppl 1):81, 1993.

38. Langard S: Nickel-related cancer in welders, *Sci Total Environ* 148:303, 1994.

39. Lesser SH, Weiss SJ: Art hazards, *Am J Emerg Med* 13:451-458, 1995.

40. Letz G: The diagnosis of occupational disease. In Hathaway GJ et al, editors: *Proctor and Hughes' chemical hazards of the workplace,* New York, 1991, Van Nostrand Reinhold.

41. Lewis R: Metals. In LaDou J, editor: *Occupational medicine,* Norwalk, Conn, 1990, Appleton & Lange.

42. Malo JL et al: Isolated late asthmatic reaction due to nickel sulphate without antibodies to nickel, *Clin Allergy* 15:95, 1985.

43. Malo JL et al: Occupational asthma due to zinc, *Eur Respir J* 6:447, 1993.

44. McCann M: *Artist beware,* ed 2, New York, 1992, Lyons & Burford.

45. Nadig RJ: Cadmium and other metals and metalloids. In Goldfrank LR et al, editors: *Goldfrank's toxicologic emergencies,* ed 5, Norwalk, Conn, 1994, Appleton & Lange.

46. Nethercott JR: Occupational skin disorders. In LaDou J, editor: *Occupational medicine,* Norwalk, Conn, 1990, Appleton & Lange.

47. O'Connor H: *The jeweler's bench reference,* ed 10, Crestone, Colo, 1993, Dunconor Books.

48. Park HS et al: Occupational asthma caused by chromium, *Clin Exp Allergy* 24:676, 1994.

49. Pepys J et al: Asthma due to inhaled chemical agents: complex salts of platinum, *Clin Allergy* 2:391, 1972.

50. Piantanida LG, Walker TJ: Industrial hygiene aspects of occupational chemical exposure. In Hathaway GJ et al, editors: *Proctor and Hughes' chemical hazards of the workplace,* New York, 1991, Van Nostrand Reinhold.

51. Proctor NH: Toxicological concepts-setting exposure limits. In Hathaway GJ et al, editors: *Proctor and Hughes' chemical hazards of the workplace,* New York, 1991, Van Nostrand Reinhold.

52. Quinn M et al, editors: *What you should know about health and safety in the jewelry industry,* Providence, RI, 1980, Jewelry Workers Health and Safety Research Group.

53. Rapson WS: Skin contact with gold and gold alloys, *Contact Dermatitis* 13:56, 1985.

54. Sarsfield P, White JE, Theaker JM: Silverworker's finger: an unusual hazard mimicking a melanocytic lesion, *Histopathology* 20:73, 1992.

55. Savitz DA et al: Review of epidemiologic studies of paternal occupational exposure and spontaneous abortion, *Am J Ind Med* 25:361, 1994.

56. Sheppard D et al: Occupational lung diseases. In LaDou J, editor: *Occupational medicine,* Norwalk, Conn, 1990, Appleton & Lange.

57. Shirakawa T et al: Occupational asthma from cobalt sensitivity in workers exposed to hard metal dust, *Chest* 95:29, 1989.

58. Sue YJ: Mercury. In Goldfrank LR et al, editors: *Goldfrank's toxicologic emergencies,* ed 5, Norwalk, Conn, 1994, Appleton & Lange.

59. *Survey of occupational injuries and illnesses, 1993,* USDL-95-5, Washington, DC, 1995, US Department of Labor.

60. *1995-1996 Threshold limit values for chemical substances and physical agents, and biological exposure indices,* Cincinnati, 1995, American Conference of Governmental Industrial Hygienists.

61. Van Cutsem E et al: Combined asthma and alveolitis induced by cobalt in a diamond polisher, *Eur J Respir Dis* 70:54, 1987.

62. Weir D et al: Occupational asthma due to soft corrosive soldering fluxes containing zinc chloride and ammonium chloride, *Thorax* 44:220, 1989.

63. White NW, Chetty R, Bateman ED: Silicosis among gemstone workers in South Africa: tiger's eye pneumonitis, *Am J Med* 19:205, 1991.

64. Wilkenfeld M: Metal compounds and rare earths. In Rom WN, editor: *Environmental and occupation medicine,* ed 2, Boston, 1992, Little, Brown.

21

Mechanics

$$\text{Cl}-\text{C}=\text{C}-\text{Cl}, \text{Cl}, \text{H}$$

trichloroethylene

- "Degreaser's Flush" occurs after chronic exposure to trichloroethylene and ethanol

- Hydrocarbon exposures in mechanics are associated with dermatologic, cardiovascular, neurologic, and renal abnormalities

Jeffrey M. Cox

Richard Y. Wang

OCCUPATIONAL DESCRIPTION

Mechanics perform a variety of services on motorized equipment that can include inspection, maintenance, and repair of these devices. In the past, mechanics learned their trade through apprenticeships; however, as technology became more sophisticated, vocational schools and specialized postsecondary training programs became necessary. These training programs are typically 1 to 2 years in duration, and there are approximately 117 U.S. community colleges that grant associate degrees in automotive mechanics. As such, the "general" mechanic is now harder to find. In the United States, there are about 1,286,000 mechanics,[50] of whom 900,000 work as automotive mechanics, 175,000 as diesel mechanics, and 130,000 as aircraft mechanics. These estimates underrepresent the true number of workers because many individuals perform these duties in an unofficial capacity.

The members of this profession can be categorized by the devices they service. This may be by either the type of engine (e.g., gasoline, diesel) or the function of the equipment (e.g., aircraft, automotive, motorcycle, and small engine). Some mechanics specialize in the service of a specific system. Brake system mechanics work specifically on drum, disk, and hydraulic braking systems. They inspect, adjust, repair, and replace brake shoes, disks, drums, hydraulic fluid lines, and master cylinders. Front-end mechanics evaluate the steering and suspension systems. They adjust, service, and replace suspension parts, such as tie rods, ball joints, and shock absorbers. Using special alignment equipment, they also align and balance wheels. Transmission mechanics adjust, repair, and replace clutch assemblies, gear trains, hydraulic pumps, and automatic transmission parts. Tune-up mechanics evaluate, adjust, and service electrical ignition and fuel economy systems. These mechanics specialize in the use of sophisticated devices and computerized diagnostic equipment to evaluate and repair malfunctions in fuel, ignition, and emission control systems. They also replace points, spark plugs, and electrical ignition triggering systems and adjust valve clearance and timing systems.

Many types of businesses employ mechanics. These workers may serve large national chains, dealerships, independent repair shops, gasoline service stations, leasing chains, or federal, state, or local governments. Most automotive mechanics work in small shops and perform several functions, including the refueling of cars. Some work in large shops that have the work area separated by the type of repairs being performed. Others work for shops that specialize in only one type of repair and service. Thus, working conditions and work hazards can vary tremendously from shop to shop.

Mechanics are subject to musculoskeletal injuries, as they may be required to lift heavy parts and equipment in awkward positions. Minor cuts, bruises, and burns are common. Specialization in the profession can affect the type of potential exposure they encounter. A brake specialist may have minor exposure to asbestos dust from the lining of clutch and brake pads (see Chapter 34). Radiator mechanics are subject to potential dermal injuries from working with the caustic alkaline solutions used to clean radiator ribbing. They also encounter ethylene glycol and methanol as they replace antifreeze fluid.

Chemical solutions of all types are located at the workplace, and they represent a significant concern to every mechanic. Many of these agents are flammable, and fires and explosions may result. The worker is at greatest risk for inhalational and dermal exposure to these agents, which can cause both acute and long-term manifestations of toxicity. The installation and proper use of contained working areas and specialized ventilation systems have limited such exposures.

POTENTIAL TOXIC EXPOSURES

The mechanic uses solutions for a variety of purposes, including as solvent degreasers, lubricants, and sources of fuel. All of these solutions contain chemicals that belong to a class of organic compounds known as hydrocarbons. For the purpose of this discussion, hydrocarbons are essentially liquids that contain carbon and hydrogen atoms. These agents can be further classified according to their structure and to whether they contain other atoms (e.g., oxygen and halogens). On the basis of structure, there are two classes: the aliphatics and the aromatics. The aromatic hydrocarbons are cyclic in structure and derived from benzene, the simplest compound in this series. The aliphatics are the alkanes, alkenes, alkynes, and their cyclic analogs. The oxygenated hydrocarbons include alcohols,

Table 21-1 Oxygenated hydrocarbons

Type	Example	Purpose
Alcohols	Ethyl alcohol (ethanol)	Octane enhancers, fuel,
	Isopropyl alcohol (isopropanol)	brake, and transmission system cleaners
	Isobutyl alcohol	Antifreeze
	Methyl alcohol (methanol)	Windshield washer fluid
Glycols	Ethylene glycol	Antifreeze
	Propylene glycol	Refrigerant
	Polyalkylene glycol	Refrigerant oil
Ketones	Acetone	Solvent
	Methyl *n*-butyl ketone (MnBK)	Octane enhancer
Ethers	Ethylene glycol monomethyl ether	Deicer
	Ethylene glycol monoethyl ether	Diluent in brake fluid
Esters	Alkyl polyglycol ether ester	Diluent in brake fluid

Table 21-2 Petroleum distillates

Fractions (synonyms)	Uses	Carbon number*
Petroleum ether (benzine)	Solvent	C5-6
Gasoline	Fuel	C4-14
VM & P naphtha	Paint thinner	C5-11
	Varnish thinner	
	Lighter fluid	
Mineral spirits (Stoddard)	Solvent	C10-16
	Degreaser	
	Paint thinner	
Kerosene	Fuel	C12-18
	Solvent	
Lubricating oil	Motor oil	C20-30

*Carbon number defines the distillate but also implies volatility and viscosity.

glycols, ketones, ethers, esters, and phenols (Table 21-1). The halogenated compounds, which usually contain either fluorine or chlorine, are found in cooling units and certain degreasing solutions. They have unique cardiovascular toxicity and more information can be obtained from the chapter on dry cleaners.

Petroleum distillates are a unique class of hydrocarbons because they are not just one agent but, rather, a collection of hydrocarbons. The distillates are extracted from crude oil by boiling it at high temperatures. As the temperature rises, individual distillates can be separated from the oil at varying points of vapor condensation. They can be collected in distinct fractions that contain varying amounts of aliphatic and aromatic hydrocarbons. Benzene, hexane, and toluene occur naturally in petroleum distillates. Table 21-2 contains a list of the common petroleum distillates.

Gasoline, for instance, contains at least 150 different compounds. The composition of these compounds varies between blends and the octane rating of the gasoline. The type of hydrocarbons also changes between the liquid and vapor phases.[38] The liquid phase contains of about 60% to 70% alkanes, 25% to 30% aromatics, and 6% to 9% alkenes; the vapor phase contains up to 90% alkanes and only about 2% aromatics. The percentage of benzene in different gasoline formulations varies from 1% to 5%.[41] The threshold limit value (TLV) recommended for occupational exposure to gasoline vapors is based on the benzene component of gasoline.

Mechanics are exposed to gases such as solvent vapors and exhaust fumes. Exhaust fumes result from servicing motorized equipment while the engine is running. Carbon monoxide poisoning may occur in poorly ventilated or enclosed areas. The chapter on firefighters discusses carbon monoxide toxicity.

Control measures are established to decrease gasoline vapor release at service stations. Stage one control devices collect and recover gasoline vapors released during bulk transfer. Stage two devices recover vapors being released during refueling. These devices help to decrease exposure and health hazards from gasoline vapors. When spills occur in poorly ventilated settings, significant toxicity from the vapor can occur.

Leaded gasoline contains tetraethyl and tetramethyl lead as octane enhancers. Organolead compounds are potent toxins to the nervous system. Leaded gasoline contains ethylene dichloride (EDE) and ethylene dibromide (EDB) as lead scavengers to prevent lead deposits on engine parts. Acute exposure to EDB can cause intractable acidosis, hepatorenal failure, and death.[30] Ethylene dibromide is also a carcinogen. These health concerns resulted in the phasing out of leaded gasoline. Unleaded gasoline contains only trace amounts of organolead compounds and their scavengers. The chapter on smelters discusses occupational lead exposure.

Increasing the concentration of benzene and adding other aromatic and branched-chain alkane compounds enhance the octane rating and antiknock properties of unleaded gasoline. Reformulated gasoline contains oxygenated hydrocarbons acting as octane enhancers and antiknock agents.[24] Ethyl alcohol, methyl alcohol, and methyl tert-butyl ether (MTBE) are common octane enhancers. The concentration of these agents in gasoline varies between 5% and 15%. There are many other additives in gasoline to perform various functions (see box). These are present in only small amounts and pose a risk for hypersensitivity reactions.

Chemicals used as degreasers and solvents are the most common type of exposure for mechanics. There are generally five categories of agents used to degrease machined parts: (1) flammable solvents (e.g., kerosene and mineral spirits), (2) nonflammable halogenated solvents (e.g., 1,1,1-

Gasoline Additives	
Antifoam	Emulsifiers
Antiicing	Lead scavengers
Antioxidants	Oxygenates
Detergents	Viscosity index improvers

trichloroethane, trichloroethylene, and dichloromethane), (3) alkaline solutions (e.g., sodium carbonate and trisodium phosphate), (4) emulsifying cleaners that contain soaps and detergents blended with flammable solvents and other agents, and (5) safety solvents, which are blends of flammable solvents and halogenated hydrocarbons to reduce the risk of combustion.

Mechanics have traditionally used flammable, nonflammable halogenated, and safety solvents to degrease engine parts. Because halogenated hydrocarbons have significant toxicities, mechanics are limiting their use to flammable solvents to degrease parts. Other commercially available degreasing solutions, such as Stoddard solutions, have various quantities of aromatic hydrocarbons added to a mineral spirit base. Benzene and toluene are typical examples. Some over-the-counter degreasing solutions use isobutane and propane as propellants.

The degreasing process may involve simply washing parts with brushes in a small container or using commercially available degreasing machines. These machines have removable baskets that automatically submerge and move through the degreasing solution. The process of degreasing represents a potential health hazard to the worker through dermal and inhalational exposure to these agents.

Mechanics also use solvents to clean braking, hydraulic, and fuel systems. Major constituents of these solvents are aliphatic, aromatic, and oxygenated hydrocarbons. Methylene chloride, a halogenated hydrocarbon, is sometimes added to these solutions.

Another common exposure to mechanics is lubricating oils. Although they are relatively nontoxic, they may cause various skin problems. Some lubricants may contain the same additives found in gasoline. Grease is a mixture of lubricating oils and soaps, and it is similar in toxicity to lubricating oils.

CLINICAL MANIFESTATIONS

Hydrocarbons, especially the petroleum distillates, are responsible for the majority of toxic exposures to mechanics. In 1994, there were 64,634 human exposures reported to the American Association of Poison Control Centers.[32] The medical outcome for these cases was minor in 21,719 and major in 161. Twenty-six exposures resulted in death, and 23 of these events were by the inhalational route. The other three deaths were due to the accidental ingestion and aspiration of petroleum distillates. Mechanics are exposed to these agents by similar routes. Inhalation and dermal contact are common, and ingestion usually results from using the mouth to siphon petroleum distillates from one container to another.

Toxicity to hydrocarbons depends on their physical properties and by-products of metabolism. The physical properties are surface tension, viscosity, and volatility. Surface tension describes the cohesiveness of molecules on a liquid surface. A lower surface tension allows the substance to spread more easily along a surface. Thus, a small amount of a low-surface-tension solution can cover a large surface area. Viscosity describes the resistance to flow of a liquid. Saybolt second universal (SSU) is the unit used to measure viscosity and can predict the risk of aspiration. Liquids with an SSU less than 60 carries a high risk of aspiration, and those with an SSU over 100 carry a low aspiration risk.[17] Volatility describes the ability of a substance to convert from a liquid into a gas. The ingestion or aspiration of highly volatile compounds may displace alveolar oxygen and act as an asphyxiant. Liquids that have high volatility and low viscosity pose the highest risk of pulmonary toxicity. Lipid-soluble agents are likely to manifest neurologic symptoms because of their permeability to the blood-brain barrier.

Gastrointestinal

The ingestion of hydrocarbons, accidentally or otherwise, produces oropharyngeal irritation and upper gastrointestinal symptoms. Nausea and vomiting may be pronounced and would put the patient at risk for an aspiration pneumonia. The petroleum distillates, gasoline, kerosene, and mineral spirits have low viscosities and may result in this complication if ingested. Aspiration of motor oil is less likely due to its higher viscosity. The gastrointestinal absorption of small-chained and aromatic hydrocarbons does occur; however, in accidental exposures, systemic toxicity is unlikely. Alcohol-containing solvents are readily absorbed from the gut and can produce additional toxicities. The irritating nature of isopropanol can result in a hemorrhagic gastritis. Alcohol dehydrogenase metabolizes ethylene glycol and methanol to toxic by-products that can lead to life-threatening metabolic acidosis, renal failure, and blindness. If such an oral exposure is recognized, regardless of the amount, immediate medical attention is necessary.

Hepatotoxicity can occur after chronic or significant acute exposures. Many of the hydrocarbons are metabolized in the liver by the cytochrome P-450 enzyme and may interact with medications. Chronic exposure can lead to the induction of this enzyme system. Halogenated hydrocarbons are the most notorious, and carbon tetrachlorohydrate is the representative agent in this class. Hepatic fatty infiltration and centrilobular necrosis are the histopathologic findings. The order of toxicity relates to the number of halogens and the atomic weight of the halogen. Metabolism of these

agents forms free radical products that cause hepatocellular damage. Acute toxicity is observed within 3 days after exposure, and resolution is over 2 weeks. Halogenated agents are radiopaque, and, if ingested, their toxic burden can be assessed with an abdominal radiograph.[11]

The halogenated hydrocarbons are also associated with an increased risk for hepatic carcinoma. Animal experiments with trichloroethylene support an increased risk for hepatocellular carcinoma.[2] The mechanisms of carcinogenicity may be due to the formation of reactive epoxide metabolites. Since epidemiologic studies failed to control for other environmental factors, however, the ability to infer the carcinogenicity of these agents is limited.[2]

Pulmonary

The presence of respiratory symptoms signifies the likelihood of pulmonary aspiration. The onset of clinical manifestations may be immediate or delayed by 6 hours.[13] Coughing, gasping, choking, and a burning sensation in the chest indicate tracheobronchial irritation. Patients with cyanosis may be suffering from severe bronchospasm, asphyxia (due to the displacement of oxygen by volatile agents), or methemoglobinemia. Liquids containing nitrates and aniline dyes can cause methemoglobinemia upon their systemic absorption.[22,28]

Hydrocarbons of low viscosity can travel to the distal airway to involve the alveoli. There is destruction of the surfactant layer and collapse of the air sac, which results in ventilation-perfusion mismatch.[13] Hydrocarbons can directly irritate bronchoalveolar tissue to cause a hemorrhagic pneumonitis and a clinical presentation of hemoptysis.[13] Symptoms may continue to progress over the next 24 hours to noncardiogenic pulmonary edema.[7] Resolution occurs in 2 to 5 days after the event.

Abnormalities of the chest radiograph may be seen within 30 minutes or up to 12 hours after aspiration, and they tend not to correlate with clinical symptoms.[13] Initial findings include bibasilar, right basilar, and perihilar infiltrates. Pleural effusions, pneumothorax, and pneumomediastinum have rarely been reported. Radiographic findings usually peak in 3 days and then slowly clear. Pneumatoceles may develop 3 to 15 days after aspiration.[5] Motor oil aspiration produces a lipoid pneumonia.[18] The pneumonia is more localized, causes less inflammation, and tends to form granulomas.

The inhalation of gasoline, kerosene, mineral spirits, and alcohol vapors does not usually cause pulmonary pathology. Workers with underlying reactive airway disease may develop bronchospasm.[52] Exposure to high concentrations and of prolonged duration can lead to systemic absorption and toxicity. The nonpolar and lipid-soluble properties of hydrocarbons allow them to pass through the alveolar-capillary membrane readily to achieve high blood concentrations. The heart and brain are most susceptible to the acute effects of these agents because of their high blood flow and lipid content.

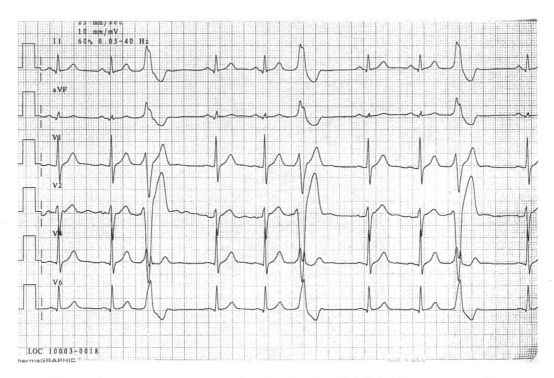

Fig. 21-1 Frequent PVCs in a truck driver after dermal and inhalational exposure to gasoline.

Cardiovascular

Cardiac arrhythmias and death can occur from exposure to hydrocarbons. This was originally observed and described as "sudden sniffing death" in individuals who died while being chased for inhalation abuse of solvents.[4] The several causes include hypoxia, acidosis, and hydrocarbon-induced myocardial sensitization to endogenous catecholamines. The synergistic effects of these factors can precipitate ventricular tachyarrhythmias and sudden death in the stressed individual. All hydrocarbons may cause cardiotoxicity; however, the halogenated compounds have the greatest risk. Gasoline, mineral spirits, and the aromatic hydrocarbons have also been reported to cause sudden death[37,39] (Fig. 21-1). Arrhythmias can develop in a delayed fashion from exposure because of either toxic metabolites or the redistribution of toxins from lipid stores.[47] Patients with evidence of cardiotoxicity or central nervous system (CNS) disturbance warrant prolonged observation.

Nervous System

Petroleum distillates are lipid-soluble agents, and they have both acute and chronic effects on the nervous system. Toxicity can occur by the inhalational, oral, or dermal route, and the severity depends on the duration and amount of exposure.[16] Acute CNS manifestations range from headaches and light-headedness to slurred speech, confusion, coma, and respiratory failure. The asphyxiant effects of the hydrocarbons and the presence of toxic metabolites (e.g., carbon monoxide) may contribute to these symptoms and should be evaluated. Dichloromethane (methylene chloride) is available in paint strippers and as a cleaning solvent for brake, hydraulic, and fuel systems. If absorbed, it is endogenously metabolized to carbon monoxide. Cranial nerve palsies can occur after inhalational exposure to trichloroethylene.[47] The trigeminal nerve is most commonly affected, and the neurotoxin is dichloroacetylene. Dichloroacetylene is a degradation product of industrial trichloroethylene.

Long-term exposure to hydrocarbons leads to neurobehavioral and intellectual impairment.[42] Toluene and hexane are two primary examples, and they can be found in petroleum distillates in varying amounts. Symptoms involve neurasthenia with fatigue, anxiety, insomnia, depression, and impairment of psychomotor skills. Encephalopathy, dementia, and cerebellar dysfunction have all been described in solvent abusers. Computed axial tomography and magnetic resonance imaging of the brain demonstrate abnormalities in the cerebral, cerebellar, and brainstem regions of these patients.[14,24] Patients with encephalopathy attributed to solvent exposure were noted to have elevated concentrations of albumin, immune globulin, and total protein.[35]

Disorders of the peripheral nervous system have been reported with chronic exposure to n-hexane, toluene, methyl n-butyl ketone, gasoline, and petroleum ether.[44] The pathology of n-hexane neuropathy is axonal degeneration and is well described. The metabolite of n-hexane, 2,5-hexadione, disrupts normal axonal function by inhibiting glutaraldehyde-3-phosphate dehydrogenase. Axonal nutrition becomes impaired, and the nerve fiber dies. Degeneration of the axon occurs first distally and then proximally, a process referred to as *dying back* neuropathy.

The neuropathy affects both motor and sensory long fibers and progresses in a symmetric and ascending pattern. Symptoms begin in the feet and advance proximally. At the time the knees are involved, the patient should begin to relate sensory disorders of the hand. A pure motor neuropathy has been described from the inhalation of a mixture of n-hexane and toluene.[41] If the axonal degeneration is not severe and the worker's exposure is discontinued, then complete recovery may be possible.

Dermatologic

A common complaint of mechanics is skin irritation because of their constant dermal exposure to hydrocarbons. These agents remove the protective lipid component of the stratum corneum, which allows the skin to become dry and cracked. Prolonged contact to these agents can result in partial- and full-thickness chemical burns.[21]

Marked erythema of the face, neck, and, at times, trunk can occur in the worker who drinks some ethanol. The "flushed" appearance is the result of vasodilatation of the superficial blood vessels of the skin and is known as *degreaser's flush.*[45] This reaction occurs in some individuals who consume ethanol after repeated vapor exposure to trichloroethylene (TCE). In daily alcohol drinkers, the flushing reaction does not occur until after 3 weeks of daily exposure to TCE vapor.[45] The reaction starts 30 minutes after a person starts to drink alcohol. The dermal response starts with the appearance of 5-mm red blotches on the malar eminences and nose. These lesions enlarge and become confluent, involving the skin of the face and neck. The flushing peaks within an hour, at which time small lesions can also be found on the upper chest and back. The dermal lesions gradually fade and completely disappear over the next hour. Alcohol ingestion 3 weeks after the last exposure to TCE vapors can still elicit this dermal response. Other solvents (e.g., xylene) may react in a similar fashion with ethanol.[36] The mechanism responsible for alcohol-induced flushing in individuals exposed to TCE and other solvents is unknown. No other physiologic derangements have been noted during flushing, and no specific treatment is needed except abstinence.

Chronic dermal exposure to hydrocarbons can lead to a variety of skin disorders. The most common is chronic dermatitis, which consists of drying and cracking of the skin. Acne vulgaris is also a problem among mechanics. Accidentally wiping oils on the face, back, chest, forearms, thighs, or neck blocks pilosebaceous follicles and causes impaction of keratin and lipids. These areas begin as a noninflammatory lesion and may later become inflamed and form erythematous papules, nodules, and cysts. Scarring can result from cystic formation and follicular rupture.

Exposure to halogenated aromatic hydrocarbons may cause a specific skin disorder, chloracne.[48] Chloracne is characterized by the presence of comedones in the malar crescent and postauricular areas. These lesions may be found in other areas, including the scrotum, axilla, neck, and buttock. Chronic inflammation and scarring may occur, as seen with acne vulgaris. Although cutting oils have been associated with squamous cell carcinoma in machinists, no similar findings have been linked with the hydrocarbons mechanics use.[49]

Hematologic

Hematologic abnormalities from exposure to petroleum distillates are uncommon. An exposure-dependent decrease in erythrocyte and hemoglobin concentrations was demonstrated in automotive workers who manually washed parts in kerosene.[51] The causes of anemia from these agents can be from either hemolysis, bone marrow suppression, or disseminated intravascular coagulation. Patients may present with weakness, fatigue, spontaneous bleeding, and serious infections. Red cell hemolysis is attributed to the direct damage of red cell membranes by hydrocarbons. Benzene is metabolized to hydroquinine and benzoquinone, which are toxic to the bone marrow.[26,33] The mechanisms of toxicity are the inhibition of protein synthesis and cell division.

Short-term exposure to benzene can cause leukopenia, thrombocytopenia, and anemia.[8] The initial marrow response may be hyperplastic. Longer durations of exposure can lead to irreversible aplastic anemia and leukemia. Early epidemiologic studies have shown associations between long-term exposure to benzene and leukemia.[25] The most common type is acute myeloblastic leukemia. The route of exposure does not affect the incidence of leukemia. The assertions made by these studies are limited by the lack of information on the amount and duration of exposure in relation to the incidence of leukemia, as well as the lack of control for other carcinogens (e.g., other solvents). The leukemic effects of benzene are further weakened by the lack of an in vivo model demonstrating the mechanism of mutagenesis and by corroboration by other studies.[9]

Ingestion of small amounts of aniline containing gasoline octane enhancers can induce significant methemoglobinemia, which would require antidotal therapy with methylene blue.[22,28]

Renal

Glomerulonephritis, distal renal tubular acidosis, and renal cell carcinoma are associated with chronic exposure to hydrocarbons.[6,16,27] Proteinuria and hematuria may be noted in the urine analysis. The exact mechanism by which these disorders occur is unknown. Gasoline, mineral spirits, toluene, degreasing agents, and glue vapors are implicated.

Reproduction

Hydrocarbons are associated with a variety of birth and gestational abnormalities.[12,31] Occupational exposure to these agents is associated with growth retardation and spontaneous abortions. In 15 pregnant women who were exposed to toxic levels of benzene, there were one still birth and seven spontaneous abortions.[43] Trichloroethylene in drinking water is associated with the development of congenital heart disease in children.[19] A retrospective study of 14 women occupationally exposed to mixed solvents, including toluene, suggested an increased risk of central nervous system anomalies and defects of neural tube closure in children exposed in utero.[23]

LABORATORY

The role of determining the concentration of hydrocarbons in biologic samples is to assess the degree of exposure in the worker. Blood samples have limited use in evaluating chronic exposures but may be useful to assess acute exposures. Urine samples are a better reflector of body burden and long-term exposure. Metabolites are measured when the compound is rapidly metabolized and no longer present for analysis. Certain considerations must be taken into account when interpreting the levels of these agents. The worker must be assessed for other sources of contamination, aside from the work site, including tobacco smoking, medications, and cosmetic products. The laboratory method of analysis must also be evaluated because certain techniques may yield false-positive results.[15] The workload of the worker must also be considered because labored activity increases the worker's minute ventilation and exposure to inhaled toxins. Finally, it should be emphasized that the measure of these agents in biologic samples is not used to aid in the management of the clinically apparent worker but rather is used to control for exposure.

Solvents and degreasing agents are commonly used by mechanics, and within these products are aromatic, halogenated, and oxygenated compounds. Benzene is a common aromatic agent that can be measured directly in whole blood and as its metabolite, phenol, in the urine of exposed workers.[26] The volatile nature of this agent requires head space sampling when whole blood is measured by gas chromatography. Improper storage of samples can result in significantly lower concentrations of benzene.[10] Blood levels are the best for evaluating systemic absorption after an acute exposure and are higher in smokers.[20] In volunteer nonsmokers, the average level is 0.2 μg/L. The next morning blood benzene level after an 8-hour exposure at 5 ppm (TWA) is about 20 nmol/L[1] (Table 21-3). Urine phenol is measured to assess for excessive routine work-related exposures. In a nonworker, the urine phenol is less than 10 mg/L.[40] After a TWA of 5 ppm, the urine phenol level should be less than 30 mg/L. Cosmetic and medication use can lead to elevations of phenol concentrations.[15] Muconic and phenylmercapturic acids are other urinary benzene metabolites that can be used to follow long-term exposures.

Trichloroethylene, once a popular degreasing agent, can be absorbed systemically by either inhalation, ingestion, dermal contact. It is rapidly metabolized to trichloroethanol and trichloroacetate, which can be measured in blood and urine.

The method of analysis can be performed either qualitatively in urine, by the Fujiwara test, or quantitatively by gas chromatography. The method of choice is gas chromatography because the Fujiwara can yield false positives if halogens are present in other forms (e.g., chlorine, bromine, fluorine).[3]

The metabolites of trichloroethylene have different rates of production and half-lives, which can assist in assessing the amount of exposure. Trichloroethanol has an early peak and a short half-life, making it useful in the assessment of recent exposures (e.g., at the end of the work day). Trichloroacetate is formed at a slower rate and has a longer half-life than trichloroethanol.[3] The American Conference of Industrial Hygienists Biological Exposure Index (ACGIH BEI) for whole blood trichloroethanol at the end of a shift at the end of a work week is 26.8 μmol/L.[1] The ACGIH BEI for urine trichloroacetate is 68 mmol/mol creatinine. Exposure to other agents can affect the levels of these metabolites.[3] Chloral hydrate is metabolized to similar by-products and can lead to elevated levels. Ethanol is metabolized by a similar pathway and can cause elevated levels and prolonged half-lives of these metabolites.

MANAGEMENT
General Management

Evaluating a mechanic with an acute exposure requires consideration of the variety of agents involved. The majority of these are hydrocarbons that have similar toxicities and treatment. The initial treatment of any exposed worker involves correcting any immediate life-threatening problems of the airway, breathing, and circulation. Once any immediate life-threatening problems have been stabilized, immediate decontamination measures should be taken to prevent further absorption of toxins. Usually removal from further exposure and supportive treatment are all that is needed.

All patients should be monitored with pulse oximetry, continuous cardiac monitoring, and a baseline 12-lead

Table 21-3 TWA of selected hydrocarbons

Agent	TWA (ppm)	Urine metabolite
n-Hexane	50	2,5-Hexanedione
Benzene	10	Phenol
Toluene	100	Hippuric acid
Gasoline	300	
Mineral spirits	100	
Kerosene	100	
Ethyl alcohol	1000	
Methyl alcohol	200-S	
Isopropyl alcohol	400	
Ethylene glycol	50	Oxalic acid
Methylene chloride	50	
Trichloroethane	350	Trichloroethanol Trichloroacetate
Trichloroethylene	50	Trichloroethanol Trichloroacetate

electrocardiogram (ECG). Supplemental humidified oxygen should be given for dyspnea and to maintain an arterial oxygen saturation (O_2sat) above 90%. Arterial blood gases are necessary in symptomatic patients and repeated as needed to assess worsening hypoxemia or hypercapnia. Because of the potential risk of carbon monoxide exposure in the workplace, any patient who presents with an altered mental status or exposure to methylene chloride should have a carboxyhemoglobin level drawn. Specific assessment for methemoglobinemia and for methanol and ethylene glycol toxicities is necessary as deemed appropriate.

Chest radiographs should be obtained on all patients who had or have respiratory symptoms to identify any acute pathologies and serve as a baseline. Chest radiographs abnormalities are usually seen within 30 minutes after aspiration, but abnormalities may be delayed up to 12 hours. It should be stressed that radiographic findings do not correlate with clinical symptoms.

Any exposed worker who presents with signs or symptoms of aspiration, respiratory dysfunction, cardiac arrhythmias or ECG changes, syncope, or central nervous system depression is to be admitted to a monitored bed for further observation. These patients should have a baseline CBC, electrolytes, renal and liver function panel, PT and PTT, and a urinalysis performed. Blood and urine hydrocarbon levels are needed only to confirm exposure; otherwise, they contribute little to management.

Cutaneous Exposure

Petroleum distillates, hydrocarbons, and oxygenated solvents are all local irritants. Skin contact can cause erythema and burns. Treatment consists of removing contaminated clothing, irrigating the skin with water, and then washing the skin with a mild soap. Topical steroids and emollients are standard treatment for both acute and chronic dermatitis. Topical antibiotic dressings (e.g., silver sulfadiazine) may be used for superficial and partial-thickness burns. Full-thickness burns should be referred to a burn care specialist. Significant exposure may result in systemic absorption and toxicity. These patients should be monitored and treated accordingly. Ocular exposure can produce a chemical conjunctivitis. After an ocular splash or vapor exposure, the eyes should be irrigated with normal saline and then pH tested. Alkali corneal burns require an immediate ophthalmology consultation.

Inhalational Exposure

Exposure to solvent vapors may induce or aggravate bronchospasm in susceptible people. Treatment with oxygen and nebulized bronchodilators is recommended. Epinephrine and isoproterenol may induce ventricular arrhythmias because of a sensitized myocardium. These agents must be avoided except for cardiac resuscitation. Parenteral steroids can be used for refractory bronchospasm.

Ingestions

The major risk from petroleum distillate ingestion is aspiration. Generally, these solutions pose a minimal risk for significant systemic toxicity after gastrointestinal absorption. Emesis and gastric lavage are not recommended unless the solution contains a highly toxic additive (e.g., halogens, heavy metals, methylene chloride, isopropyl alcohol, methyl alcohol, or ethylene glycol) or a large ingestion (greater than 1 ml/kg) has occurred. These compounds are rapidly absorbed from the gastrointestinal tract, which limits the usefulness of delayed gastric emptying. Otherwise, gastric lavage would be recommended for exposures within 1 hour and when no vomiting has occurred. If the patient is lethargic or comatose, the airway must be protected with a cuffed endotracheal tube before lavage.

Activated charcoal and cathartics are recommended as adjunctive therapies for toxic ingestions and may be effective in limiting absorption of these agents.[29] The recommended dose of activated charcoal is 1 to 2g/kg. One dose of a cathartic may be given with the charcoal if diarrhea is not present: sorbitol 1 to 2 g/kg in an adult with a maximum of 150 g per dose or magnesium citrate 4 ml/kg up to 300 ml per dose.

Patients who present with signs of aspiration require humidified oxygen, nebulized bronchodilator therapy, and hospital admission for close observation. Hypoxemia and hypoventilation can be assessed with an ABG and need to be monitored. Significant hypoxemia or hypercapnia requires mechanical ventilation. Positive end-expiratory pressure may assist oxygenation if significant distal airway and alveolar collapse are present. Prophylactic antibiotics and corticosteroids are not indicated in the treatment of chemical aspiration pneumonitis. If an infectious process can be demonstrated, antibiotic therapy is then administered. Extracorporeal membrane oxygenation and high-frequency jet ventilation have been utilized successfully in the management of severe cases of noncardiogenic pulmonary edema from chemical pneumonitis.[7,53]

PREVENTION AND MONITORING

Proper personal hygiene and work habits are always necessary to limit hazardous exposures at the workplace. At initial employment, a complete physical examination and history with special emphasis on renal, liver, and cardiac function need to be performed. Baseline laboratory values are to include complete blood count (CBC), serum renal and liver function panels, and urine analysis.

On an annual basis, the worker should be evaluated for hepatic, dermatologic, and, especially, neurologic disorders. Assessments can be made through neurophysiologic screening questionnaires and neuroradiologic studies. The questionnaires can ascertain disorders in affect, memory, and personality; however, they are highly sensitive and are subject to a high degree of false positives.[2]

The exposure monitoring can be performed by sampling either the air in the workplace or biologic specimens from the worker. The analysis of the air at the workplace is limited by the lack of correlation with what is truly absorbed by the worker and by difficulties in separating admixtures of solvents in the air.[34] Monitoring of biologic samples from workers is a better method of determining what is actually absorbed by the worker. This form of analysis is also affected by certain variables, including the workload of the worker and the physical properties of the solvent.[2] The amount absorbed by the worker can be assessed by measuring the concentrations of the parent compound or metabolites in the worker's urine or breath.[46] The amount measured in the exhaled breath within the first hour of exposure is usually an adequate representation of recent exposure. The amount measured in the exhaled breath the next morning (12 to 16 hours after work) represents the TWA.

The role of monitoring for the hematologic effects of benzene toxicity is limited by normal population variance and other factors that may affect the results (e.g., infections, medications). Other hematological parameters under consideration as biologic markers are cytogenetic abnormalities in the red blood cells and red blood cell distribution width (RDW).[2] Further studies are necessary to define the specificity and sensitivity of these parameters in workers exposed to benzene.

REFERENCES

1. Aitio A et al: Biological monitoring. In Zenz C, editor: *Occupational medicine: principles and practical applications,* Chicago, 1994, Year Book.
2. Axelson O, Hogstedt C: On the health effects of solvents. In Zenz C, editor: *Occupational medicine: principles and practical applications,* Chicago, 1994, Year Book.
3. Barceloux DG: Halogenated solvents. In Sullivan JB, Krieger GR, editors: *Hazardous materials toxicology,* Baltimore, 1992, Williams & Wilkins.
4. Bass M: Sudden sniffing death, *JAMA* 212:2075, 1970.
5. Bergeson PS et al: Pneumatoceles following hydrocarbon ingestion, *Am J Dis Child* 129:4954, 1975.
6. Bombassei GJ, Kaplan AA: The association between hydrocarbon exposure and antiglomerular basement membrane antibody-mediated disease (Goodpasture's syndrome), *Am J Ind Med* 21:141, 1992.
7. Bysani GK, Rucoba RJ, Noah ZL: Treatment of hydrocarbon pneumonitis, *Chest* 106:300, 1994.
8. Cody RP, Strawderman WW, Kipen HM: Hematologic effects of benzene, *J Occup Med* 35:776, 1993.
9. Collins JJ et al: A study of the hematologic effects of chronic low-level exposure to benzene, *J Occup Med* 33:619, 1991.
10. Collom WD, Winek CL: Detection of glue constituents in fatalities due to "glue sniffing," *Clin Tox* 3:125, 1970.
11. Dally S, Garnier R, Bismuth C: Diagnosis of chlorinated hydrocarbon poisoning by x ray examination, *Br J Ind Med* 44:424, 1987.
12. Daniell WE, Vaughan TL: Paternal employment in solvent related occupations and adverse pregnancy outcomes, *Br J Ind Med* 45:193, 1988.
13. Eade NR, Taussig LM, Marks MI: Hydrocarbon pneumonitis, *Dis Chest* 47:353, 1965.

14. Ellingsen DG et al: Patients with suspected solvent-induced encephalopathy examined with cerebral computed tomography, *J Occup Med* 35:155, 1993.
15. Fishbeck WA, Langner RR, Kochiba RJ: Elevated urinary phenol levels not related to benzene exposure, *Am Ind Hyg Assoc J* 36:820, 1975.
16. Flanagan RJ et al: An introduction to the clinical toxicology of volatile substances, *Drug Saf* 5:359, 1990.
17. Gerarde HW: Toxicological studies on hydrocarbons. IX. The aspiration hazard and toxicity of hydrocarbons and hydrocarbon mixtures, *Arch Environ Health* 6:329, 1963.
18. Glynn KP, Gale NA: Exogenous lipoid pneumonia due to inhalation of spray lubricant (WD-40 lung), *Chest* 97:1265, 1990.
19. Goldberg SJ et al: An association of human congenital cardiac malformations and drinking water contaminants, *J Am Coll Cardiol* 16:155, 1990.
20. Hajimiragha H et al: Levels of benzene and other volatile aromatic compounds in the blood of non-smokers, *Int Arch Occup Environ Health* 61:513, 1989.
21. Hansbrough JF et al: Hydrocarbon contact injuries, *J Trauma* 25:250, 1985.
22. Harvey JW, Keitt AS: Studies of the efficacy and potential hazards of methylene blue therapy in aniline-induced methaemoglobinaemia, *Br J Haematol* 54:29, 1983.
23. Holmberg PC: Central nervous system defects in children born to mothers exposed to organic solvents during pregnancy, *Lancet* 2:177, 1979.
24. Ikeda M, Tsukagoshi H: Encephalopathy due to toluene sniffing: report of a case with magnetic resonance imaging, *Eur Neurol* 30:347, 1990.
25. Infante PF et al: Leukaemia in benzene workers, *Lancet* 2:76, 1977.
26. Irons RD: Benzene and other hemotoxins. In Sullivan JB, Krieger GR, editors: *Hazardous materials toxicology,* Baltimore, 1992, Williams & Wilkins.
27. Kadamani S, Asal NR, Nelson RY: Occupational hydrocarbon exposure and risk of renal cell carcinoma, *Am J Ind Med* 15:131, 1989.
28. Kearney TE, Manoguerra AS, Dunford JV Jr: Chemically induced methemoglobinemia from aniline poisoning, *West J Med* 140:282, 1984.
29. Laass W: Therapy of acute oral poisonings by organic solvents: treatment by activated charcoal in combination with laxatives, *Arch Toxicol* 4:406, 1980.
30. Letz GA: Two fatalities after occupational exposure to ethylene dibromide, *JAMA* 252:2428, 1984.
31. Lindbohm ML et al: Spontaneous abortions among women exposed to organic solvents, *Am J Ind Med* 17:449, 1990.
32. Litovitz TL et al: 1994 Annual report of the American Association of Poison Control Centers toxic exposure surveillance system, *Am J Emerg Med* 13:551, 1995.
33. Macfarland HN: Toxicology of petroleum hydrocarbons, *Occup Med* 3:445, 1988.
34. McDermott HJ, Killiany SE: Quest for gasoline TLV, *Am Ind Hyg Assoc J* 39:110, 1978.
35. Moen BE et al: Cerebrospinal fluid proteins and free amino acids in patients with solvent induced chronic toxic encephalopathy and healthy controls, *Br J Ind Med* 47:277, 1990.
36. Mooney E: The flushing patient, *Int J Dermatol* 24:549, 1985.
37. Nierenberg DW et al: Mineral spirits inhalation associated with hemolysis, pulmonary edema, and ventricular fibrillation, *Arch Intern Med* 151:1437, 1991.
38. Page NP, Mehlman M: Health effects of gasoline refueling vapors and measured exposures at service stations, *Toxicol Ind Health* 5:869, 1989.
39. Reinhardt CF, Mullin LS, Maxfield ME: Epinephrine-induced cardiac arrhythmia potential of some common industrial solvents, *J Occup Med* 15:953, 1973.

40. Roush GJ, Ott MG: A study of benzene exposure versus urinary phenol levels, *Am Ind Hyg Assoc J* 38:67, 1977.

41. Runion HE: Benzene in gasoline, *Am Ind Hyg Assoc J* 36:338, 1975.

42. Scala RA: Hydrocarbon neuropathy, *Ann Occup Hyg* 19:293, 1976.

43. Schardein JL: *Chemically induced birth defects,* New York, 1985, Marcel Dekker.

44. Schaumburg HH, Spencer PS: The neurology and neuropathology of the occupational neuropathies, *J Occup Med* 18:739, 1976.

45. Steward RD, Hake CL, Peterson JE: "Degreasers' flush," *Arch Environ Health* 29:1, 1974.

46. Steward RD, et al: Diagnosis of solvent poisoning, *JAMA* 193:115, 1965.

47. Szlatenyi CS, Wang RY: Encephalopathy and cranial nerve palsies due to intentional trichloroethylene inhalation, *Vet Hum Toxicol* 36:348, 1994.

48. Tindall JP: Chloracne and chloracnegens, *J Am Acad Dermatol* 13:539, 1985.

49. Tsuji T et al: Multiple keratoses and squamous cell carcinoma from cutting oil, *J Am Acad Dermatol* 27:767, 1992.

50. United States Department of Labor: *Occupational outlook handbook,* Washington DC, 1994-1995, US Government Printing Office.

51. Upreti RK, Das M, Shanker R: Dermal exposure to kerosene, *Vet Hum Toxicol* 31:16, 1989.

52. Vega AR et al: Kerosene-induced asthma, *Ann Allergy* 64:362, 1990.

53. Weber TR et al: Prolonged extracorporeal support for nonneonatal respiratory failure, *J Pediatr Surg* 27:1100, 1992.

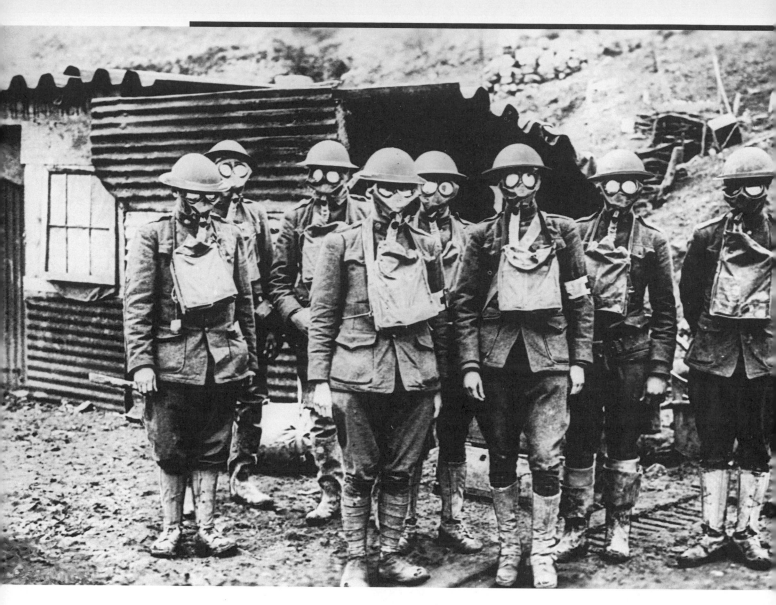

*Combating German frightfulness. The members of the
American Expeditionary forces in the first line trenches
at the Lorraine section, during WWI, were fully
prepared to fight in perfect safety despite gas attacks
of the enemy.*
(Courtesy Corbis-Bettmann)

22

2,3,7,8-tetrachlorodibenzo-p-dioxin
(TCDD)

halon 1301

- Military personnel frequently work and live in the same environment, thus complicating exposures
- The "healthy worker" effect frequently confounds studies of occupational risk factors

Military Personnel

David Sonntag

Warren Jederberg

Grace LeMasters

Susan Simpson

Kenneth Still

As a workforce, the U.S. Department of Defense (DoD) is formidable indeed, with a total active-duty strength of 1.5 million.[52] At a global level, the assorted governments of the world annually expend $868 billion to project forces of more than 27 million troops, with DoD's 1996 budget accounting for $270 billion.[16]

Recruiting propaganda for the armed services is typically aimed at the 17- to 18-year-old age bracket and touts the training that recruits can receive in more than 100 career specialties of their choice. Given the many professions represented in the military, describing the clinical toxicology associated with them all is obviously beyond the scope of this chapter and would repeat material covered in other chapters. Indeed, with minimal exceptions, most of the occupational toxins military members are exposed to are used in the civilian setting.

In a more pragmatic approach, this chapter considers how some of the qualitative differences in the military

The views expressed in this chapter are the personal opinions of the authors, and are not meant to represent official policy pronouncements for the University of Cincinnati, Department of Defense, or any of its component services.

workplace can affect traditional approaches to toxicologic risk assessments, discusses what occupational toxins are most commonly found in a military setting, and then reviews some of the lessons learned from previous military conflicts.

MILITARY HISTORY

While modern technology has changed much about warfare since the period surrounding the French Revolution, military historians trace many of the conceptual underpinnings of modern warfare to that era. The writings of Carl von Clausewitz and Henri de Jomini, still studied by military officers today, are relevant to understanding the differences between military and civilian exposure to toxins. Clausewitz's most commonly cited statement describes war as "nothing but a continuation of political intercourse with the admixture of different means."[20]

The planned violence and projection of force inherent in "different means" have mingled with them two elements that Clausewitz refers to as "fog" and "friction." These elements have a "pervasive atmosphere of uncertainty and opaqueness," which he describes more fully: "Everything in war is very simple, but the simplest thing is difficult. The difficulties accumulate and end by producing a kind of friction that is inconceivable unless one has experienced war . . . countless minor incidents—the kind you can never really foresee—combine to lower the general level of performance, so that one always falls far short of the intended goal."[20] The fog and friction of past wars have generated a large body of lessons learned in the preventive medicine community. It is well known, for instance, that during the Civil War, many more soldiers were disabled by chronic illness and infectious disease than by combat injury.[24]

The presence of fog and friction in the warfare environment makes evaluation of human exposure to occupational toxins particularly challenging, for a variety of reasons. The traditional epidemiologic triad of person, time and place, and agent becomes very obscure when fog and friction are introduced. Standard assumptions about toxin absorption, distribution, and elimination become questionable. It is thus important to recognize the relative merit of physiologically based pharmacokinetic (PBPK) models over classic pharmacokinetic models, which are flow-limited, and that PBPK models for military populations need to take into account wider variations in compartmental flow assumptions.

DEMOGRAPHICS

Another problem with application of traditional risk assessment models to military exposures has to do with demographics, including education level. Table 22-1 shows the demographic and military characteristics of personnel involved in the Persian Gulf war. The force tends to have high turnover rates among the youngest, least-educated troops, who account for the highest levels of hospitalizations and deaths attributable to occupational toxins. A survey of 1371 hospitalizations and 136 deaths attributable to occupational

exposures among U.S. Navy personnel showed strikingly high rates among the 17- to 19-year-old age group. The most frequent cause of toxin-associated death was from carbon monoxide poisoning (74%).[62]

Demographics of military populations are particularly important in epidemiologic studies because of the healthy worker effect. Since physical fitness is required for all active duty personnel and standards of fitness and body fat are maintained, the toxicologic consequences of exposure are expected to be somewhat different than for the normal population. The healthy worker effect is a common problem with proportionate mortality ratio (PMR) studies. Because of health criteria for active duty personnel, a low incidence of death from a particular cause, such as heart disease, can result in a proportionate excess of deaths from other causes. This effect shows up particularly in comparisons of proportionate incidence rates between workers from different populations. Selection criteria can also have subtle effects on epidemiologic studies. A study comparing health outcomes of Gulf War military personnel to civilian oil well firefighters in Kuwait was recently criticized because the authors ignored the self-selecting nature of the civilian firefighters.[22]

The assumptions used for routine risk assessment and the establishment of occupational exposure limits for Department of Navy personnel need to be interpreted with caution for operational personnel.[48] Among the issues raised is the fact that typical career patterns for military personnel are substantially different from their civilian counterparts, even though occupational specialties may be very similar. The typical military member does not spend 8 hours a day, 5 days a week, for 20 to 40 years doing the same thing. Soldiers, sailors, or airmen are much more likely than their civilian counterparts to experience significant periods of extended work hours with high-intensity tasking due to deployment, conflicts, or special operations. These activities lead to exposures for which routine assumptions would not apply.

In addition, confounding chemical (solvents, exhausts, etc.) and physical stressors (noise, temperature, fatigue) have unassessed impacts on critical performance parameters. The ability of occupational toxins to potentiate the effects of physical agents has been known for some time[30,40] but not evaluated to a great extent in the military environment. Because of this, a detailed description of seven navy subpopulations—basic underwater demolition students (BUDS), sea-air-land (SEALS), male aviators, female aviators, male fleet, female fleet, divers, and submariners—is being developed and will be used to model the differing effects of chemicals on duty performance for these populations.[23]

MEDICAL SURVEILLANCE

Routine industrial hygiene practices are enforced in all service branches, and professional hygienists provide workplace monitoring and surveys of military operations both at fixed bases[7,14,19,43] and afloat.[44] Due to various interagency agreements, the Occupational Safety and Health Adminis-

Table 22-1 Demographic characteristics of participants in Persian Gulf war

Characteristics	Active units (n = 580, 433) %	Reserve units (n = 72,348) %	National Guard (n = 43,781) %	Total (n = 696,562) %
Sex				
Male	93.7	84.9	89.1	92.5
Female	6.1	14.7	9.6	7.2
Unknown	0.2	0.4	1.3	0.3
Race				
White	69.6	73.4	77.7	70.5
Black	23.3	21.0	18.3	22.7
Other	7.0	5.7	3.9	6.7
Marital status				
Single	42.8	49.9	34.7	43.0
Married	54.3	44.8	57.8	53.5
Divorced	2.7	4.9	6.2	3.1
Unknown	0.2	0.4	1.4	0.3
Rank				
Enlisted	89.3	86.4	90.4	89.1
Officer	9.3	12.6	8.5	9.6
Warrant	1.4	1.0	1.0	1.9
Branch				
Air Force	12.2	7.6	14.7	11.9
Army	46.0	64.6	85.3	50.4
Marine	15.7	17.8		14.9
Navy	26.0	10.0		22.7
Coast Guard	0.1			0.1
Mean Age	27.4	30.4	32.6	28.0

From Lederberg J: *Report of the Defense Science Board (DSB) task force on Persian Gulf war health effects,* Washington, DC, 1995, http://www.dtic.dla.mil/gulflink/dsbrpt/index.html.

tration's Salt Lake City Analytic Laboratory (OSHA-SLCAL) has analyzed a large number of military industrial hygiene samples, and the results are stored on their OSHA computerized information system (OCIS).[46]

In addition, all services maintain medical surveillance systems that, to varying degrees, attempt to correlate person, time and place, and toxin exposure factors. Two of these comprise automated medical databases: the Army's OHMIS[14] and the Air Force's PHOENIX-Command Core.[10] For U.S. Navy personnel, a medical surveillance matrix is utilized and cross-matched to a specific hazard to determine appropriate medical surveillance. Routine medical surveillance for Navy personnel is conducted for 93 chemical, 9 physical, and 3 mixed stressors. Additionally, some 21 medical occupational certifications are required.[37]

MILITARY OPERATIONS
Pace and Setting

Military personnel are employed in all occupations normally seen in the industrial setting but are also exposed to unique

stress situations, including increased work tempos, and unusual work cycles. Because of this, many standard industrial hazards are juxtaposed with uniquely military stressors. These stressors may also contribute to increased severity of toxins normally considered to be of low risk. The pace and setting of military operations are best exemplified by looking at a number of naval operating environments.

Depending on the ship type, a sailor may be engaged in activities ranging from administrative watchstanding to nuclear power plant repair. Tenders, carriers, and other large platform ships are virtual floating industrial plants. In addition to the systems required to keep the ship itself operational, they may carry foundries, electric rewind capabilities, nuclear power plants, welding shops, oxygen generation shops, optical shops, weapons handling and repair areas, large storage areas, metal fabrication shops, electronic calibration and repair shops, electroplating and engraving shops, upholstery and carpenter shops, publication and duplication shops, photography shops, medical facilities, and hyperbaric chambers. Aircraft carriers have the capability to launch, store, refuel, and repair aircraft, from helicopters to jet planes. Consequently, carriers are floating airports. Conversely, submarines are self-contained vessels capable of full life-support and warfighting completely beneath the surface of the ocean, including repair and modification of the weapons systems, the boat, and certain activities exterior to the hull of the submarine. Submarines are also capable of search-and-rescue missions, including diving rescue. Navy divers operate from diverse Navy facilities, ship or shore.

When the mission of the ship is to support other fleet resources, it is not unusual for critical work to be conducted with around-the-clock efforts. In support of Operation Desert Shield/Desert Storm, divers from one repair ship (tender) spent extended hours underwater performing hull repairs on combatants. All of these occupational environments require full industrial hygiene support in the anticipation, recognition, evaluation, and control of exposure to toxins.

Under all operational circumstances, whether on a 5-person tugboat or a 5000-person aircraft carrier, shipboard personnel are exposed to various occupational hazards in the workplace and may continue to be exposed to the same agent away from the workplace. Onboard a surface vessel steaming the ocean, a sailor's home and workplace are almost indistinguishable. Sailors cannot escape the confines of the workplace by going home at the end of the workday, and the workday may extend well beyond the normal 8-hour workday as defined by OSHA. These extended work hours create unique workplace exposure situations that require special health standard development. Furthermore, the typical 40-hour workweek used in private industry to develop permissible exposure limits (PELs) or threshold limit values (TLVs) is nonexistent onboard ocean-going vessels. Twelve-hour days and 7-day workweeks are not uncommon under deployment conditions.

Special Forces

Unique occupational exposures are presented by the surface, aviation, submarine, and special warfighting operations (i.e., special forces) communities. Under these military platforms, peculiar combinations of stressors may yield potentially greater toxicities. Special forces personnel may encounter chemical, physical, and biologic agents in various concentrations and combinations that yield a greater toxic effect than ever encountered in private industry. When these stressor effects are added to the physical rigors demanded of these personnel and to a hostile environment, standards for health and well-being are extremely difficult to develop.

Submariners

Submarine sailors live and work in a world of their own. At work hundreds of feet below the ocean surface, they encounter occupational scenarios with no private industry counterpart. Even the air they breathe becomes a part of the routine atmospheric monitoring. Because of potential toxic combinations of certain chemicals, there is a whole class of prohibited materials onboard submarines. Relative humidity, dew point, oxygen concentration, barometric pressure, carbon dioxide concentration, and other factors must all be regularly monitored. The automatic monitoring systems used for this purpose must themselves be inspected routinely for malfunctions and alarm failures because, when the boat is transiting the polar icecaps, for example, the air supply cannot be replenished at a moment's notice. Some chemicals that are routinely used onboard a boat may yield by-products that are of some concern. For example, some submarine hydraulic fluid can produce 2,6-di-t-butyl-4-nitrophenols, a yellow residue that deposits on equipment and is potentially hepatotoxic.[66]

Aviation

The aviation community experiences many occupational stressors that are common in the private sector. Many of these hazardous conditions also can be encountered in the submarine community. The air that aircrews breathe becomes very important; airborne contaminants assume an increased hazardous role. Furthermore, because of the speed of many military aircraft, chronobiologic effects must be considered. The natural circadian rhythms that the human body experiences are disrupted drastically under some conditions. Do extant health standards apply equally under these conditions? Ground crews, whether ashore or onboard carriers, are potentially exposed to jet fuels, additives, noise, heat, and combinations of these agents not encountered elsewhere. Routinely used synthetic hydraulic fluids may contain chemicals that are neurotoxic, even at very low exposure concentrations, which cause performance decrements of concern. Trimethylpropane phosphate (TMPP) is one such chemical of concern.[51,65]

Surface Vessels

Surface vessels carry their own unique occupational circumstances. Consider the life of a boiler technician (BT). The BT's life exists well below the waterline of a ship under conditions of continuous high noise levels, high heat, high humidity, vibration, and use of numerous types of chemicals. Artificial light is all the "snipe" encounters for hours on end, day after day. When the workday has ended, these personnel leave one artificial environment for another. Shipboard noise is a fact of life, as is the constant low vibration of the engines and the scores of chemicals necessary to run the ship efficiently. Exposure from the occupational setting gradually blends into comparable exposures in the environmental setting and eventually into the living environment. Onboard a ship, it is difficult to escape from the hazards that are so rigorously controlled ashore.

Active duty populations may experience periods when exposures are similar to their civilian counterparts and significant periods when they are not (deployments, special operations, etc.). Shipboard life is physically and mentally demanding. The shipboard routine for the average sailor includes extended periods doing a primary job (e.g., welder, crane operator, supply clerk, radar station monitor, communications technician). Interspersed throughout the day, the sailor may be part of a damage control team, firefighting team, or other specialty group during drills. Thus the sailor could be preparing lunch one minute, then be in a full firefighting ensemble for 30 to 45 minutes, and then back to the galley for food preparations. Also, the sailor may stand any of numerous watches required to maintain the readiness of the ship. Any decrement in the mental or physical capabilities of the sailor has the potential to jeopardize the ship and crew.

POTENTIAL OCCUPATIONAL TOXINS
Fuels

Because of requirements to project force globally, one of the most common chemical exposures at all military bases is to petroleum, oils, and lubricants, often referred as POLs. At one point, the DoD consumed approximately 2.7% of the total petroleum production in the United States.[25] Specifically, jet fuel, gasoline, diesel fuels, and the products of their complete and incomplete combustion are among the sources of fuel exposure encountered. The U.S. Air Force reported the net amount of fuel issued for fiscal year 1995 on air force bases as approximately 64 million gallons of gasoline and diesel fuels; jet fuel usage totaled approximately 63 million gallons.[27] The National Occupational Exposure Survey (NOES), conducted by the National Institute of Occupational Safety and Health between 1981 and 1983, estimated that 4866 employees were exposed to JP-4 in the workplace.[41] Tables 22-2 and 22-3 presents a summary of the properties and uses of various POLs of military significance.

Gasoline. Gasoline is a complex chemical mixture that is potentially composed of more than 1000 substances.[39] Factors such as the source of crude oil, geographic region, octane rating, and blending of the stock all affect the composition of this fuel. Hydrocarbons are distributed in gasoline as 60% to 70% alkanes, such as paraffins; 25% to 30% aromatics; and 5% to 10% alkenes, including lead-scavenger agents and octane enhancers.[47] Some of the

Table 22-2 Properties and uses of important military fuels

Petroleum product	Principal carbon content	Important fractions	Use	Comments
JP-4	C_4-C_{14}	Benzene, 0.5% (wt/wt) Toluene, 1.33% Ethyl-benzene, 0.37% Total xylenes, 2.32%	Former DoD jet fuel; high vapor pressure (13 kPA)	Frequent contaminant found in groundwater and soil under and around military bases
JP-5	Kerosene coal oil		Fire-safe naval aviation turbine fuel; fuel oil no. 1	Neurotoxic
JP-7	Alkanes, cyclo-alkanes, alkyl-benzenes, naphthalenes		SR-71, U-2, and other supersonic high-altitude aircraft	
JP-8	Kerosene-based	n-Undecane, 8.88% n-Decane, 8.04% n-Dodecane, 6.73% n-Tridecane, 3.61% C_{13}-branched alkanes, 1.78% C_3-benzenes, 1.44% C_4-benzenes, 1.73% Naphthalene, 0.58% Methyl naphthalenes, 0.37%[25]	NATO countries, DoD replacement fuel for JP-4	Equivalent to commercial aviation turbine fuel
JP-10	Synthetic	exo-tetrahydro-bicyclopenta-diene (CAS 2825-82-3)	Cruise missile fuel	Carcinogenic, neurotoxic
Automotive gas	C_4-C_{11}	Benzene, toluene, ethylbenzene, xylenes (BTEX)	Civilian and military use	
Diesel fuel	C_{10}-C_{19}		Civilian and military use	
Stoddard solvent	C_7-C_{12}	Naphtha	Civilian and military use	
Purging fluid (Soltrol 2000)	C_{13}-C_{17}		To purge drained fuel tanks prior to maintenance work	Can accumulate volatile fractions from residual fuel; often recycled via on-site distillation.
Otto fuel II		Propylene glycol dinitrate Dibutyl sebacate 2-nitro-diphenylamine	Torpedo fuel	OSHA PEL for propylene glycol dinitrate is 0.05 ppm, 8-hr TWA

Table 22-3 Other fuel oils

Fuel product	Synonyms	Comments
Fuel oil no. 1-D	Diesel fuel, or diesel fuel no. 1	Nephrotoxic
Fuel oil no. 2	Home heating oil, gas oil, no. 2 burner oil	
Fuel oil no. 2-D	Diesel fuel oil no. 2, diesel oil no. 2, no. 2 diesel	Nephrotoxic
Fuel oil no. 4	Heavy residual fuel oil, marine diesel fuel, residual fuel oil no. 4	Dermal and hepatic carcinogen
Fuel oil UNSP		

Table 22-4 Selected fuel additives (percent volume at Hill Air Force Base, Ogden, Utah)

Function	Typical additive	Percent
Corrosion inhibitor	DuPont DCI-4A: Xylenes Ethyl benzene Benzene Fatty acid amines Sulfonates Alkyl carboxylates	0.005
Conductivity improver	DuPont Stadis 450: Toluene 50-60% Benzene, <0.06% Mixed aromatic solvents, 5-10% Isopropyl alcohol, 1-5% Dodecyl benzene sulfonic acid, 5-10% Polymeric alkyl sulfuric compound, 10-20% Polyamino polyol, 5-10%	0.0005
Antiicing	Ashland Glycol ether DM: Diethylene glycol monomethyl ether (EGME)	0.12

specific chemicals in gasoline include benzene and other substituted-aromatics, 1,3 butadiene, toluene, xylenes, ethylbenzene, n-hexane, and hexenes.[39] The American Conference of Governmental Industrial Hygienists (ACGIH) has established a TLV for gasoline of 300 ppm, with a short-term exposure limit (STEL) of 500 ppm.

Gasoline engine emission studies of 20 current fleet vehicles fueled with an industry average gasoline revealed that 89% of tailpipe exhaust included 44 different paraffin compounds, 20 aromatics, 18 olefins, and 9 oxygenates.[52,53] Unburned fuel has been shown to account for 50% to 65% of engine-out and tailpipe hydrocarbons.[53] Catalysts on current vehicles prevent the emission of about 90% of carbon monoxide (CO) and 95% of hydrocarbon (HC) and nitrogen oxides (NO_x).[28] Gasoline engine emissions reportedly contain 10 times fewer particles than emitted by diesel engines; with a catalytic converter, gasoline particles drop to 100 times fewer particles than diesel engine emissions.[67]

Jet Fuels and Jet Fuel Emissions

At least two thirds of the turbine fuels used by DoD are JP-8, a turbine engine fuel[37]; JP-8 is a kerosene-based distillate with a higher flashpoint, higher chain hydrocarbons, and no unsubstituted benzene. It is safer to use than JP-4, whose BTEX concentrations are shown in Table 22-2. Use of JP-8 was recently implemented at all U.S. bases, and it is used at most overseas installations.

As jet fuels are pumped to storage tanks, various additives are injected, as indicated in Table 22-4. Although the additives are in very low concentrations, the workers handle large volumes of fuel, increasing exposure opportunities. In such large quantities, the total of these small fractions may have substantial effects. Jet fuel also contains traces of metals, sulfur, oxygen, and nitrogen compounds. All metals through atomic number 42, except for rubidium and niobium, have been found in generally low concentrations, with the most prevalent metals being nickel and vanadium.[5] Studies of the chemical composition of emissions from various military and commercial aircraft engines have also been published.[59,60]

Both OSHA and Air Force Occupational Safety and Health (AFOSH) standards for jet fuel exposure are given in terms of "petroleum distillates" (naphtha). The PEL time-weighted average (TWA) is 400 ppm, and the STEL is 500 ppm. The AFOSH program has proposed guidelines for JP-8 exposure that are currently in the peer review process. The proposed guidelines set a TLV-TWA of 35 mg/m^3 and a 15-minute STEL of 1800 mg/m^3 and are currently under review by the Committee on Toxicology.

Studies of military personnel exposed in Kuwait to combustion by-products from oil well fires have shown clear evidence of mutagenic effect,[31] while in vitro studies have demonstrated the potential for similar effects from airborne particulates in a large metropolitan area.

Diesel Fuel

Diesel exhaust exposures are common in developed countries.[38] Rough estimates of population exposure to diesel exhausts are derived from the total suspended particulates (TSPs) or black smoke, consisting of particles less than 5 μm (primarily elemental carbon plus organics). The Environmental Protection Agency (EPA) estimated average U.S. diesel soot concentrations in 1986 to be 2.4 μg/m^3 in rural regions and slightly higher at 2.6 μg/m^3 in urban areas and nationwide.[12] The EPA projected soot concentrations in 1995 to be 1.5 μg/m^3 in rural areas and 1.4 μg/m^3 nationally.

Diesel exhaust is composed of more than 450 organic compounds. In its gas and vapor phases, it contains acrolein, ammonia, carbon dioxide, carbon monoxide, benzene,

1,3-butadiene, formaldehyde, formic acid, heterocycles, hydrocarbons (C_1-C_{18}) and their derivatives (acids, ketones, alcohols, nitriles, aldehydes, quinones, anhydrides, sulfonates, esters, halogenated and nitrated compounds), hydrogen cyanide, hydrogen sulfide, methane, methanol, nitric and nitrous acids, sulfur dioxide, toluene, and water. In its C_{14}-C_{35} fraction and derivatives (as previously), polycyclic aromatic hydrocarbons, inorganic sulfates, nitrates, and metals. Soot particles carry hydrocarbons, which are mutagenic.[38]

Other Toxins

Metals. Because of the corrosive environment in which many modern weapon systems must operate, large amounts of heavy metals are used in sealants, paints, and electroplated parts. Most prominent among these are hexavalent chromium, found in paint primers as strontium or zinc chromate. Cadmium plating is found on almost all steel components that come into contact with aluminum, and is used to prevent galvanically induced corrosion.

Alloys of metals commonly used in military weapon systems contain titanium, beryllium, boron, and magnesium-thorium. Beryllium's potential for producing granulomatous lung disease has long been known, with typical radiographic findings of diffuse nodular and linear infiltrates and bilateral hilar lymphadenopathy.[61,62]

Magnesium-thorium alloys are used on military aircraft because of their strength and light weight; F-4 gearboxes, F-16 gearboxes, and F-105 panels are examples of current uses. Any component containing less than 4% thorium by weight does not require a radioactive license. The air force does not permit decommissioned Boeing CIM-IOA Surface to Air Anti Aircraft missile from the Boeing and Michigan Aerospace Center (BOMARC), which have a high thorium content, to be used as practice targets because of the potential α-particle release when these alloys burn.

Depleted uranium (DU) is used as a ballast on almost all civilian and military aircraft, due to its density. It was also used extensively in the Persian Gulf war in armor-piercing rounds and is found in the plates of reactive armor. Although DU is an α- and β-emitter, its principal health hazard is its nature as a heavy metal.

Solvents and degreasers. The two most common types of contaminants found in the soil and water beneath and around military installations are POLs from leaking storage tanks or discarded solvents and degreasers. For almost 50 years, 1,1,1 trichloroethylene (TCE) and 1,1,1 trichloroethane (TCA) have been used as degreasers in the military, and a substantial proportion of the DoD's hazardous waste environmental remediation budget is spent for their cleanup each year.

Due to their environmental persistence, as well as concern about ozone depletion, their use has been curtailed, with most being replaced by d-limonene or similar monoterpene compounds. Common physical complaints from workers using d-limonene as a replacement for TCA include irritation and drying of the skin and mucous membranes.[32] While the odor of this citrus-based compound is pleasant at low levels, the high concentrations often found in poorly ventilated areas may require the use of an air-purifying respirator or accessory ventilation. Workers using TCA replacements often have to adapt to changes in amounts applied and to increased drying times. From a behavioral point of view, adaptation to TCA replacements can be very slow; TCA has been used as a military degreaser for almost three generations of workers. In fact, it is not uncommon to find workers hoarding or surreptitiously trading TCA, and the traditionally arcane military supply system has only facilitated this. Recent implementation of the hazardous material (HAZ MAT) pharmacy (single supply system with cradle-to-grave tracking and accountability) concept has made base-level control of these industrial chemicals much tighter, but the challenge will be to carry this level of control and accountability forward to the battlefield.

Other solvents commonly used include methyl ethyl ketone (MEK, or 2-butanone) and acetone. Stories of soldiers passing out from unprotected MEK use during the Persian Gulf war were not uncommon.[15]

Paints. Urethane-based paints are used extensively on military equipment, with the predominant toxicant exposure coming from associated isocyanates. In addition, a type of paint known as chemical agent resistant coating (CARC) has its own unique toxicologic properties.[62] Paint stripping involving methylene-chloride strippers can produce significant workplace exposures, and it has given way in fixed-base locations to bead-blasting, xenon-flash, and other abrasive or physical paint removal methods. However, these methods are not without their own inherent exposure problems. For example, while the change from a methylene-chloride and water-based paint removal method to plastic media bead-blasting (PMBB) is touted as being more "environmentally friendly," it has its own daunting industrial hygiene considerations. What was once a wet method, involving worker exposure to methylene chloride, is now a dry method with significant exposure to fine particulates produced by the blasting method, not to mention noise exposures on the order of 105 decibels, 8 hours TWA. Samples of this type of operation show high levels of cadmium, chromium, zinc, and lead.

Composites and resins. Because of their decreased weight and lower radar profile, advanced composites are found on a variety of weapon systems and are used in some smoke and dispersant agents. They are generally composed of carbon, Kevlar, or boron fibers reinforced in an epoxy or other type of resinous matrix. Carbon or graphite fibers are found in the Air Force F-15, F-16, and F-117 and the Navy F-15, F/A-18, AV-8B, B-2, F-22, C-17, ATF, V-12, and ATA (A-12). Boron fibers have also been used in the FB-111,

F-15, and B-1B.[55] The Air Force considers carbon and glass fiber as a nuisance dust and observes the ACGIH TLV of 10 mg/m^3; the Navy uses a PEL for carbon fibers of 3 fibers per cm^3.[45,55] A variety of other exposures, including epichlorohydrin, formaldehyde, and phenol, can occur during the prepreg and layout process.[11]

Asbestos. With the friction and fog of war comes heat and, consequently, the presence of asbestos. The effects of chronic exposure to asbestos were first observed in epidemiologic studies of shipyard workers in World War II.[56] Given the age of many weapon systems, asbestos is still found on military equipment, primarily in brake pads and gaskets. For example, the C-130 cargo aircraft has been in the inventory since 1958, and the Air Force plans to use it well into the next millennium. Although older-model aircraft usually end up being sold to foreign countries or transferred to Air National Guard units, depot-level maintenance of these aircraft is performed at active-duty military installations. Thus, it is still common to encounter asbestos-containing parts.

Hydrazines, hypergolic propellants. Hydrazines are used as propellants throughout the aerospace community. A mixture of 70% hydrazine and 30% water, H-70, is used by the F-16 fighter aircraft's emergency power unit (EPU). There are 1588 F-16 aircraft in the U.S. inventory, broken down as follows: Active Force, 804; Air National Guard, 634; Reserve, 150.[6] Each aircraft carries approximately 7 gallons of H-70. In wings flying the F-16 aircraft, EPU activation is a regular occurrence. Hill AFB, which has two active F-16 wings, has experienced about two to five EPU activations per month. Operational and periodic maintenance requirements of the F-16 also present a variety of potential exposure scenarios.

Unsymmetric di-methyl hydrazine (UDMH) is used in the fourth stage of the LGM118-A Peacekeeper missile, along with nitrogen tetroxide. The combination of these two produces a violent reaction and a characteristic red plume. There are 50 Peacekeepers in the U.S. inventory.[8] Hydrazines are also used as propellants on the space shuttle and several satellite systems, as oxygen scavengers in boiler systems, and in the coolants of nuclear reactors.

Halons. Given the high level of POL usage in the military, firefighting is an important consideration. Several halons (or halogenated methanes) are used in this capacity. Halons take their names from the number and nature of the elements contained in the compounds. Trifluorobromomethane, for instance, is simply referred to as halon 1301, with the numbers being derived as illustrated in the following table:

#C	#F	#Cl	#Br
1	3	0	1

Because of their potential as cardiac sensitizers and central nervous system depressants, as well as documented battle-field fatalities, use of halons has been curtailed in most military systems where confined spaces exist.[36,57] Additionally, exposure of halons to temperatures above 1800°F results in production of the hydrogen halides HCl, HF, and HBr, all of which are extremely irritating to the respiratory tract. It is also quite likely that phosgene (carbonyl dichloride, COCl$_2$) can form by the generation of free radicals found in high-heat fires.

Fire practice areas. Disposal of classified material can represent a significant problem, particularly in a wartime setting. Because of the need to practice fire-extinguishing techniques, most air force bases throughout the years constructed burn pits, or fire training areas, which were essentially open trenches or berms into which JP-4 was poured and ignited. Because the goal was to extinguish the fire, large amounts of unburned fuel have made their way into groundwater and soil, with potential to migrate into surrounding population areas.

In many cases, these burn pits were turned into convenient methods to dispose of classified materials. Open-pit burning of magnesium thorium components from the BOMARC missile was conducted by the Marquardt Corporation on a limited basis in the 1950s and 1960s, with the consent of the Atomic Energy Commission. More recently, civilian workers at a military base in Nevada alleged that large volumes of classified resins, solvents, and hardening agents used to coat Stealth aircraft were routinely dumped into open pits adjacent to populated areas of the base, soaked in jet fuel, and allowed to burn.[50] It is well known that incomplete combustion of plastics and resins can result in the production of highly toxic dioxins and dibenzofurans.[49] Such disposal would therefore be inadvisable under non-combatant conditions.

Riot control agents. Military organizations have recently been called upon to participate in numerous "peace-keeping" operations or other types of operations classified under the rubric military operations other than war (MOOT-WAs). One of the key features of a MOOTWA involves unique rules of engagement because of the need to counter extremist or factional groups in a domestic setting.

The use of riot-control agents, particularly CS gas (O-chlorobenzylidene malonitrile), can be deadly inside occupied buildings. As is the case with all nitriles, CS gas can break down in the presence of fire or heat to form hydrogen cyanide. Because of fatalities associated with their use in confined buildings in Israel and the United States, law enforcement officials have recommended that CS be used for crowd control only outside occupied buildings.

PROLIFERATION OF NBC

As scientific knowledge of toxicology, molecular genetics, and human biochemistry has grown, so, too, has the potential for propagation of nuclear, biologic, and chemical weapons. The production and use of the nerve agent Sarin in several attacks in Tokyo subway stations underscore the ease with which these types of weapons can be used by extremist groups as the "poor man's nuclear weapons." After the Oklahoma City bombing, President Clinton made reference in a news conference to a recent case in which the FBI, the Centers for Disease Control (CDC), and the Public Health Service had acted to narrowly avert a similar attack against U.S. interests. Although the CDC would investigate the use of a biologic agent and the FBI would investigate domestic terrorism, the true nature of this incident remains the subject of speculation.

The problems of proliferation of nuclear, chemical, and biologic weapons will be with us for some time.[58] As the Russian economy and political world continue in turmoil, concern is mounting about the security of their aging inventory of chemical weapons, as well as their violations of existing chemical weapons bans and treaties. In the early 1980s, Russian scientist Vil Mirzayanov renounced his membership in the Communist party and wrote a scathing report exposing Russia's violations of the chemical-warfare treaties, including development of several new agents, including those known as Novichok and FT.[33,63] According to Mirzayanov, Moscow's State Union Scientific Research Institute for Chemistry and Technology developed a chemical weapon comprised of three fluoroacetate derivatives that was similar in action to the rat poison sodium fluoroacetate, which affects critical metabolites of the tricarboxylic acid cycle. Reportedly, FT is hepatotoxic and leaves virtually no chemically identifiable residues. It was engineered specifically to wipe out large populations and leave no traces. Mirzayanov claims that a team of 10 scientists from the institute were conscripted by the KGB to field-test FT in Afghanistan, where they dumped it wholesale into domestic water supplies. The military leadership in Moscow, according to Mirzayanov, were thrilled with the results of the testing. Mirzayanov was later arrested for "betraying state secrets."

LESSONS LEARNED

Military debriefings of any large undertaking are never complete without a section to cover "lessons learned."

Herbicide Orange

Follow-up of a cohort of Air Force veterans exposed to dioxins (TCDD) from herbicides dispersed over 10% to 20% of South Vietnam between 1962 to 1971[29] is ongoing. Studies of serum dioxin have shown that of personnel who served in the Republic of Vietnam, the Ranch Hand group was the most highly exposed to herbicides. The CDC has also found that Ranch Hand personnel still show elevated levels of serum dioxin (TCDD), higher than U.S. Army ground troops stationed in Vietnam during the same period.[17,21]

More recently, the Air Force has found[9] the following significant findings associated with increased serum levels of TCDD in the Ranch Hand population:

- Negative correlation between TCDD and high-density lipoprotein cholesterol
- Increase in cardiovascular mortality in the most-exposed subgroup
- Glucose intolerance
- Elevated mean liver aspartate aminotransferase (AST), ALT, and GGT
- Increased IgA
- Decrease in serum testosterone
- Positive reactions to lupus and rheumatoid factor tests

Further follow-up examinations are planned for 1997 and 2002.

Gulf War

A telling lesson learned from the case of Herbicide Orange is that it can take years for the fog and friction of war to clear so that outcomes of wartime exposures can be discerned. The Pentagon recently declassified many documents from the Persian Gulf war and has also published the recommendations of several scientific review boards for research priorities.[20] These recommendations, along with a high political profile, should contribute to friction-lowering and fog-clearing so that veterans of this war see a speedier resolution of their complaints than their comrades from the Vietnam era experienced.

REFERENCES

1. Agency for Toxic Substances Disease Registry (ATSDR): *Toxicological profile for fuel oils,* Atlanta, 1993, The Agency.
2. Agency for Toxic Substances Disease Registry (ATSDR): *Toxicological profile for jet fuels JP-4 and JP-7,* Atlanta, 1993, The Agency.
3. Agency for Toxic Substances Disease Registry (ATSDR): *Toxicological profile for hydrazines,* Atlanta, 1994, The Agency.
4. Agency for Toxic Substances Disease Registry (ATSDR): *Toxicological profile for otto fuel II and its components,* Atlanta, 1995, The Agency.
5. Air Force (USAF): *The installation restoration program toxicology guide,* vol 4, Wright Patterson AFB, Ohio, 1989, Harry G. Armstrong Aerospace Medical Research Laboratory, Aerospace Medical Division, Air Force Systems Command.
6. Air Force (USAF): F-16 Fighting falcon fact sheet, Langley Air Force Base, Va, 1992, Air Combat Command, Public Affairs Office.
7. Air Force (USAF): *Occupational health,* Atlanta, 1992.
8. Air Force (USAF): *LGM-118A peacekeeper fact sheet,* Peterson Air Force Base, 1993, Air Force Space Command.
9. Air Force (USAF): *Air force health study,* Brooks AFB, Texas, 1995, Epidemiologic Research Division Armstrong Laboratory.
10. Air Force (USAF). (1995). *Command core selection summary,* Wright Patterson AFB, Ohio. Available e-mail: http://www.afmc.wpafb.af.mil:12000/organizations/HQ-AFMC/SG/ccs 12.htm: United States Air Force.
11. AAMRL: *Conference on occupational health aspects of advanced composite technology in the aerospace industry,* Wright Patterson AFB, Dayton, Ohio, 1989, Harry G. Armstrong Aerospace Medical Research Laboratory.
12. Akland GG: Exposure of the general population to gasoline, *Environ Health Perspect* 101(suppl 6):27, 1993.
13. Arias O, Friedman J, Rossiter C: Redirecting military spending worldwide to benefit humanity, *Christian Science Monitor,* Dec 26, 1995.
14. Army: *Preventive medicine. Army regulation 40-5, Chapters 5-11.*

Available e-mail: http://chppm-www.apgea.army.mil/Documents/Regulations/AR40-5/ar40-5   i.htm#C5.

15. Bauerlein M. (1995). *Collateral damage.* Available e-mail: http://www.citypages.com/articles/774/774cover.htm.

16. Blaisdell RA, Smallwood ME: *Evaluation of total petroleum hydrocarbon standard for cleanup of petroleum contaminated sites,* Wright Patterson AFB, Dayton, Ohio, 1993, Air Force Institute of Technology.

17. Centers for Disease Control (CDC), Serum 2,3,7,8-tetrachlorodibenzo-p-dioxin levels in Air Force Health study participants—preliminary report, *Morb Mortal Wk Rep* 37:309, 1988.

18. von Clausewitz K. In Howard M and Paret P, editors: *On war (Von Kriege),* Princeton, NJ, 1984, Princeton University Press.

19. Department of Defense (DoD): *Industrial hygiene and occupational health,* Washington DC, 1989, The Department.

20. Department of Defense (DoD). (1995). *Declassified military documents,* Washington DC. Available e-mail: www.dtic.dla.mil/gulflink.

21. DeStefano F et al: Serum 2,3,7,8-tetrachlorodibenzo-p-dioxin levels in U.S. Army Vietnam-era veterans, *JAMA* 260:1249, 1988.

22. Etzel RA, Ashley DL: Volatile organic compounds in the blood of persons in Kuwait during the oil fires, *Int Arch Occup Environ Health* 66:125, 1994.

23. Flemming CD, Little OM, Carpenter RL: Statistical description of physiological variables for seven naval populations. Unpublished manuscript, 1996.

24. Freemon FR: The medical challenge of military operations in the Mississippi Valley during the American Civil War, *Mil Med* 157:494, 1992.

25. Gleason CC, Martone JA: Pollutant emission characteristics of future aviation jet fuels, *J Air Pollut Control Assoc* 29:1243, 1979.

26. Gordon S: *Comparison of major organic species in JP-4 vs JP-8,* Seattle, WA, 1995, Batelle Laboratories.

27. Ground Fuels Stock Fund Manager: *Fuels usage,* Kelly AFB, San Antonio, Tex, 1996.

28. Hamerle R, Schuetzle D, Adams W: A perspective on the potential development of environmentally acceptable light-duty diesel vehicles, *Environ Health Perspect* 102(suppl 4):25, 1994.

29. Institute of Medicine (US) Committee to Review the Health Effects in Vietnam Veterans of Exposure to Herbicides: *Veterans and agent orange,* Washington, DC, 1994, National Academy Press.

30. Johnson AC et al: Effect of interaction between noise and toluene on auditory function in the rat, *Acta Otolaryngol (Stockh)* 105:56, 1988.

31. Kelsey KT et al: Genotoxicity to human cells induced by air particulates isolated during the Kuwait oil fires, *Environ Res* 64:18, 1994.

32. Kiefer M et al: Investigation of d-limonene use during aircraft maintenance degreasing operations, *Appl Occup Environ Hyg* 9:303, 1994.

33. Kincaid C: Russia's dirty chemical secret, *American Legion Magazine,* February, 1995.

34. Klassen CD: *Nonmetallic environmental toxins: air pollutants, solvents and vapors, and pesticides.* In Gilman AG et al, editors: *Goodman and Gilman's the pharmacological basis of therapeutics,* New York, 1990, McGraw Hill.

35. Lederberg J. (1995). *Report of the Defense Science Board (DSB) task force on Persian Gulf war health effects,* Washington, DC. Available e-mail: http://www.dtic.dla.mil/gulflink/dsbrpt/index.html.

36. Lerman Y et al: Fatal accidental inhalation of bromochlorodifluoromethane (Halon 1211), *Hum Exp Toxicol* 10:125, 1991.

37. MacNaughton MG, Uddin DE: *Toxicology of mixed distillate and high-energy synthetic fuels.* In Mehlman MA, et al, editors: *Advances in modern environmental toxicology. Volume VII. Renal effects of petroleum hydrocarbons,* Princeton, NJ, 1984, Princeton Scientific Publishers.

38. Mauderly JL: Diesel exhaust. In Lippman M, editor: *Environmental toxins—human exposures and their health effects,* New York, 1992, Van Nostrand Reinhold.

39. Mehlman MA: Dangerous and cancer causing properties of products and chemicals in the oil refining industry, *Environmental Research* 59:238, 1992.

40. Morata TC et al: Effects of occupational exposure to organic solvents and noise on hearing, *Scandinavian Journal of Work, Environment and Health* 19:245, 1993.

41. National Institute of Occupational Safety and Health: *National occupational exposure survey (1981-1983),* Cincinnati, 1990, National Institute for Occupational Safety and Health, US Department of Health and Human Services.

42. NEHC: *Medical surveillance procedures manual and medical matrix,* Norfolk, Va, 1991, Navy Environmental Health Center.

43. Navy: *Navy occupational safety and health (NAVOSH) program manual for forces afloat,* Oct, 1994.

44. Navy: *Navy occupational safety and health (NAVOSH) program manual for forces afloat,* Oct, 1994.

45. NEHC: *Advanced composite materials,* Norfolk, Va, Oct, 1991, Navy Environmental Health Center.

46. Occupational Safety and Health Administration. (1996). *OCIS Description.* Available e-mail: http://www.osha-slc.gov/OCIS/intro   ocis. html.

47. Page N, Mehlman MA: Health effects of gasoline refueling vapors and measured exposures at service stations, *Toxicol Ind Health* 5:869, 1989.

48. Risher JF, Jederberg WW, Carpenter RL: The assessment of health risk to occupationally exposed navy personnel: a consideration of issues, *Inhalational Toxicology* 7:983, 1995.

49. Rizzardini M et al: Toxicological evaluation of urban waste incinerator emissions, *Chemosphere* 12:559, 1983.

50. Rogers K: Groom Lake toxic burning alleged: a former worker at the secret Air Force base says poisonous substances were routinely ignited, *Las Vegas Review-Journal,* Mar 20, 1994, 1B.

51. Rossi J et al: An overview of the development, validation and application of neurobehavioral and neuro-molecular toxicity assessment batteries: specialized applications to combustion toxicology, *Toxicology* (in press).

52. Schuetzle D et al: Analytical chemistry and auto emissions, *Anal Chem* 63:1149A, 1991.

53. Schuetzle D et al: The relationship between gasoline composition and vehicle hydrocarbon emissions: a review of current studies and future research needs, *Environ Health Perspect* 102(suppl 4):3, 1994.

54. Secretary of Defense: *Military strength figures for October 31, 1995,* Washington, DC, 1995, Department of Defense.

55. Seibert JF: *Composite fiber hazards,* Brooks AFB, Tex, 1990, Air Force Occupational and Environmental Health Laboratory (AFSC).

56. Sinks T et al: A case-control study of mesothelioma and employment in the Hawaii sugarcane industry, *Epidemiology* 54:44(2)466, 1994.

57. Smith DG, Harris DJ: Human exposure to Halon 1301 (CBrF3) during simulated aircraft cabin fires, *Aerospace Medicine,* Feb 1, 1973, 198.

58. Smithson AE. (1995). *Alarm sounded about security of Russia's chemical weapons.* Available e-mail: http://www.stimson.org/pub/stimson/cwc/rusadv.htm.

59. Spicer CW et al: Chemical composition of exhaust from aircraft turbine engines, *Annales Geophysicae* 114:111, 1992.

60. Spicer CW et al: Chemical composition and photochemical reactivity of exhaust from aircraft turbine engines, *Annales Geophysicae* 12:944, 1994.

61. Sprince NL, Kazemi H: *Beryllium disease.* In Rom WN et al, editors: *Occupational and environmental medicine,* Boston, 1983, Little, Brown.

62. USAEHA. (1996). *USAEHA information paper: CARC.* Available e-mail: http://chppm-meis.apgea.army.mil/hmwp/infopapers/carc. html, US Army Environmental Hygiene Agency.

63. Waller JM: Russia's poisonous secret, *Reader's Digest,* October 1994, 128.

64. White MR, McNally MS: Morbidity and mortality in U.S. Navy personnel from exposures to hazardous materials, 1974-85, *Mil Med* 156:70, 1991.

65. Wyman JF et al: Evaluation of shipboard formation of a neurotoxicant (trimethylpropane phosphate) from thermal decomposition of synthetic aircraft engine lubricant, *Am Ind Hyg Assoc J* 54:584, 1993.

66. Wyman J et al: Comparative toxicity of 2,6-di-t-butyl-4-nitrophenols in human and rat hepatic tissue slices, *Toxicologist* 15:1532, 1995.

67. Zweidinger RA. In Lippman M, editor: *Environmental toxicants—human exposures and their health effects,* New York, 1982, Van Nostrand Reinhold.

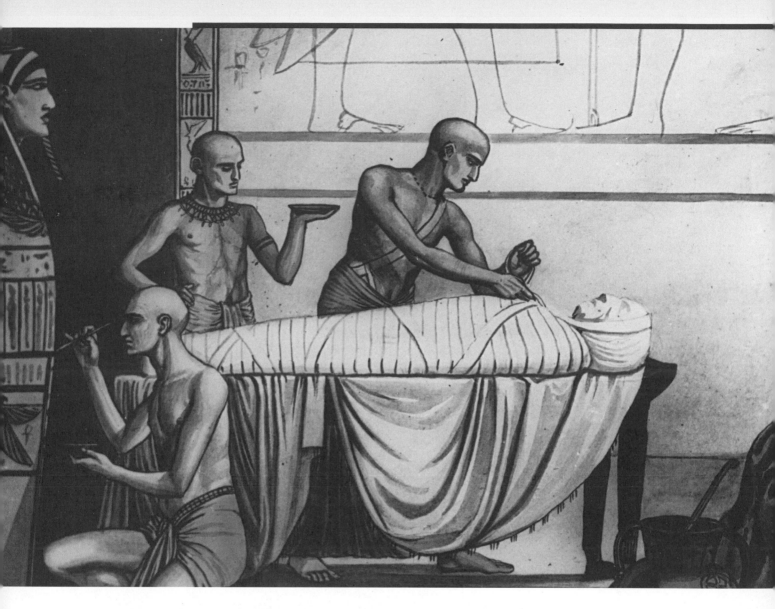

Embalmers bandaging mummy while assistant prepares
coffin. Colored wash drawing. Undated.
(Courtesy the Bettman Archive)

23

Morticians

Anthony J. Suruda

H
 \
  C=O
 /
H

- Formaldehyde is a potent respiratory and skin toxin as well as a sensitizer that causes bronchospastic disease and dermatitis

- Non–formaldehyde-containing embalming fluids are available

- Formaldehyde is suspect as a cause of nasopharyngeal cancer, but conclusive evidence is weak

OCCUPATIONAL DESCRIPTION

Morticians take custody of the dead and arrange funerals, cremations, and burials. The term *mortician* is synonymous with undertaker, funeral director, funeral service worker, and embalmer.[22] A mortician's work includes some or all of the following: collection of the dead body from the hospital or home, embalming, cosmetic restoration, provision of a casket, and arranging cremation, a funeral, and burial. In the United States most corpses are embalmed prior to cremation or burial. Embalming is a practice that is heavily influenced by religious, ethical, cultural, psychologic, and practical issues. Embalming and preservation of corpses have been practiced since before the time of the ancient Egyptians,[40] when embalming prepared the dead for the afterlife. In modern society, preserving dead bodies from decomposition is sometimes required for sanitary reasons such as to transport a body for long distances prior to burial.

Licensure requirements for morticians in the United States vary from state to state, and licensure is not required in all states.[22] Currently, there are approximately 14,400 U.S. funeral homes with a total of 71,000 employees.[44] In most cases, a funeral home employs at least one embalmer; however, at many homes all employees assist in the embalming, and thus are exposed to toxins.

Embalming can be accomplished by several methods. In general, chemical substances that are used coalesce and cross-link proteins and other organic molecules and so retard degradation. There are two physical methods for applying embalming products, which may be combined: (1) perfusion of the body or body area with embalming fluid by instillation into a vein, artery, or body cavity and (2) preservation by surface contact with chemicals in the form of gel, cream, or powder. Embalming solutions and powders may contain formaldehyde, phenol, glycerol, alcohol, glutaraldehyde, and coloring agents. Specialized creams and solutions are

195

Table 23-1 Potential toxic exposures for morticians

Toxic exposure	Source	Route of exposure	Toxic effects	Permissible limit
Infectious agents	Bodies and body fluids	Airborne, skin, needlestick, splash	Blood-borne diseases and tuberculosis	
Formaldehyde	Embalming fluids, disinfectants	Airborne, skin	Contact dermatitis, urticaria, asthma, suspected carcinogen	0.75 ppm avg 2.0 ppm short-term exposure limit (OSHA)
Glutaraldehyde	Embalming fluid	Airborne, skin	Contact dermatitis, asthma	0.2 ppm (NIOSH)
Methanol	Embalming fluid	Airborne, skin	Irritant, ocular damage	200 ppm (OSHA)
Isopropanol	Embalming fluid, disinfectants	Airborne, skin	Irritant	400 ppm (OSHA)
Phenol	Embalming fluid	Airborne, skin	Irritant, toxic to liver, kidney (CNS if ingested)	5 ppm (OSHA)
Dyes, perfumes, cosmetics	Cosmetic restoration	Skin	Contact dermatitis	
Floral arrangements		Skin	Contact dermatitis	

used on facial areas when public viewing is planned. Gels containing formaldehyde are applied to specific, difficult-to-penetrate areas, such as the hands and feet. Different procedures and solutions are used for normal, intact bodies, for bodies that have been altered by violence or by autopsy, and for bodies that are partly decomposed. Bodies donated to medical schools for anatomic research are given additional injections of fluids containing glycerin, phenol, methanol, and ethanol to maintain tissue flexibility for dissection.[8]

The body to be embalmed is placed on a metal table that is slightly inclined and equipped with a drain. The body is cleaned, shaved, and arranged in a natural position. A large needle is inserted into an artery, and embalming fluid is infused. Venous blood is allowed to drain out. Water is used to wash blood and any leaking embalming fluid from the table.[28,48] The viscera are embalmed by puncturing the abdominal wall with a trochar and introducing a more concentrated embalming solution. Several hours later, this fluid is drained and the hole sealed with a button. Gels and creams are applied to the face, feet, and hands. Cosmetic restoration may be done in addition to embalming.

In the case of autopsied bodies, viscera are embalmed separately. Embalming of autopsied bodies takes longer, requires larger volumes of embalming fluid, and results in higher exposures of airborne chemicals than embalming of intact bodies. Embalming of autopsied bodies or partly decomposed bodies commonly results in leaks and spills of embalming fluid onto the embalming table, which also tends to increase airborne exposure to formaldehyde.

POTENTIAL TOXIC EXPOSURES
Airborne

Commonly recognized potential toxic exposures of morticians are listed in Table 23-1. Exposure specifically to biologic hazards may occur through inhalation, skin contact,

or needlestick injury while injecting embalming fluids. Exposure to chemical substances may occur via inhalation or dermal absorption. It is common practice for embalmers to wear personal protective equipment such as gloves, aprons, and safety glasses to reduce the potential for toxic exposures. The primary means of controlling airborne exposures should be adequate ventilation of the embalming area, with the flow of air away from the breathing zone of the embalmer and the air exhausted from the building.[36] Ventilation systems in current use in embalming rooms may not be adequate to control airborne exposures such as from formaldehyde.[23,33] In one reported case, recirculated formaldehyde-containing air was inadvertently being drawn directly back into the building.[36]

Factors that increase airborne exposure are listed in the box on p. 197. The use of paraformaldehyde powder, a polymer that spontaneously decomposes to formaldehyde, can cause extremely high airborne concentrations of formaldehyde. When paraformaldehyde is used there is also the potential for inhalation of particulate matter containing formaldehyde.[23] The use of disinfectant sprays containing formaldehyde to spray down embalming tables and equipment also contributes to airborne formaldehyde exposure.[8]

Other components of embalming fluid with relatively high volatility that may be inhaled by embalmers include glutaraldehyde, methanol, isopropyl alcohol, and phenol. Air concentrations of these chemicals in embalming areas have been reported as low or below the limit of detection.[8,48]

The major airborne toxin in embalming rooms is formaldehyde. Average exposure levels to formaldehyde during embalming have been reported to range up to 3 ppm,[23,33,36,45,48] considerably more than the allowable U.S. Occupational Safety and Health Administration (OSHA) permissible exposure limit of 0.75 ppm as an 8-hour time-weighted average or the short-term exposure limit of

---

Factors that Increase Airborne Exposure to Formaldehyde Among Morticians

---

Embalming autopsied body
Use of paraformaldehyde powder
Spills or leaks of embalming fluid
Inadequate ventilation

---

2 ppm for a 15-minute period.[38] Average exposures of morticians to formaldehyde are comparable to those in manufacturing industries, but short-term or "peak" exposures are much higher.[6] Despite these exposures, the respiratory function of morticians as a group appears to be similar to control populations not occupationally exposed to formaldehyde.[28]

Mortality studies of morticians have not demonstrated excess deaths from nasal cancer or other respiratory cancers that might be related to formaldehyde exposure.[16,27,47] However, the statistical power of these studies to detect excess cancers was limited, and the largest study had 4046 deaths, with only 1.7 deaths expected from nasal cancer. There is one case report of nasal cancer in an embalmer with 24 years of experience.[10]

In one study, apprentice embalmers were noted to be more likely to complain of mucous membrane irritation from embalming chemicals than experienced embalmers.[20]

Skin

Embalming chemicals can be absorbed directly through the mortician's skin. This hazard can be limited by wearing gloves, aprons, and safety glasses. However, formaldehyde can be absorbed through the embalmer's skin even when gloves are worn. Common surgical gloves become permeable to formaldehyde solutions in 1 to 15 minutes after contact with concentrations in the 9% to 37% range, which are similar to concentrations used in pathology.[43] Fluids used for embalming are usually diluted to a formaldehyde concentration of 5% or less. Since glove permeability to chemicals is related to the concentration of the solution, the main hazard occurs secondary to spills of undiluted embalming fluid.

Contact dermatitis from embalming fluid is an occupational hazard of morticians. The prevalence of contact sensitivity to formaldehyde and glutaraldehyde is reported as 4% and 10%, respectively.[20] Observations during a field study[45] demonstrate that embalmers who are aware that formaldehyde is a suspect human carcinogen favored embalming fluids with lower formaldehyde content. Since the "low-formaldehyde" fluids had increased amounts of glutaraldehyde, their use might increase the possibility of contact dermatitis. Morticians who handle floral arrange-

ments are also at risk of contact dermatitis from plant sensitizers[13] (see Chapter 17).

CLINICAL TOXICOLOGY OF FORMALDEHYDE

Formaldehyde is a gas at room temperature. It has an irritating odor, polymerizes readily, and is very soluble in water. Gaseous formaldehyde is not available commercially per se, and pure formaldehyde can be obtained from spontaneous decomposition of paraformaldehyde. Formaldehyde is commonly available as formalin, a 37% to 50% aqueous solution that contains methanol to inhibit polymerization.

Formaldehyde is a necessary human metabolite for certain one-carbon reactions[34] and is normally present in the body in low concentrations.[29] More than 1 million U.S. workers are exposed to formaldehyde in manufacturing (see Chapter 49) and in health-related professions.[6] Individuals whose homes contain particleboard or urea-formaldehyde foam insulation are exposed by release of formaldehyde from these materials.

Formaldehyde is found in many consumer products. The Food and Drug Administration lists formaldehyde as present in more than 800 cosmetic preparations, and formaldehyde is present in products such as glossy papers, color photographs, and permanent-press clothing.[34] In Sweden and Japan, formaldehyde is forbidden in cosmetics.[13] Cigarette smoke contains up to 40 ppm formaldehyde.[19] All of us, even in wilderness areas, are exposed to small amounts of formaldehyde in air, which may originate from vehicle exhaust, industrial processes, or natural sources.[19]

Pathophysiology

Acute. Acute exposures to formaldehyde may occur from the gas or from contact with the liquid form as formalin. At air levels of 0.5 to 2 ppm, formaldehyde is an irritant and causes eye and mucous membrane irritation. Most individuals will not tolerate exposures above 5 ppm and will attempt to leave the area.[12] Acute pulmonary edema has been reported after inhalation of formaldehyde over several hours by workers who were preparing brain sections in a pathology laboratory.[41] The exposure level was not measured in this case, but the patient's wife smelled formaldehyde on his breath after he left the laboratory. Inhalation of more than 50 ppm formaldehyde may cause serious respiratory injury and death.[12] Eye damage does not normally occur from airborne formaldehyde because increased blinking rates and closure of the eyes protects the cornea.[34] Liquid formalin is extremely irritating to the eye, and splashes can lead to corneal opacities and loss of vision.[34]

Ingestion of a few drops of 40% formalin solution has caused death in a child,[35] and ingestions of 50 to 250 cc as overdoses by adults have also been fatal.[12,35] Postmortem findings of acute formaldehyde poisoning were gastric congestion and erosion, pulmonary edema, glottic and tracheal swelling, and discoloration of mucous membranes

Table 23-2 Acute effects of formaldehyde exposure

Area affected	Effects
Gaseous formaldehyde	
Eyes	Irritation, tearing
Upper respiratory tract	Irritation
Lungs	Irritation, bronchoconstriction, pulmonary edema (at high exposures)
Nose	Temporary reduction in ability to smell
Aqueous formaldehyde	
Blood	Hemolytic anemia in dialysis patients
Eyes	Corneal opacities and blindness
Mouth and esophagus	Coagulation of mucous membranes
Lungs	Mucosal and parenchymal edema
Gastrointestinal tract	Esophageal stricture; gastritis
Skin	Irritation, allergic contact dermatitis

in the mouth.[12,35] Exposure of hemodialysis patients to formaldehyde in contaminated dialysis water has caused hemolytic anemia[39] by depleting red blood cell adenosine triphosphate (ATP).

Acute exposure to formaldehyde reversibly diminishes the sense of smell.[34] Acute and chronic skin exposure can produce irritation, peeling, and an allergic contact dermatitis.[34] Ingestion of formaldehyde can produce urticaria and a skin eruption; in 1909, the U.S. Department of Agriculture evaluated formaldehyde as a food preservative and administered 100 mg of formaldehyde daily in milk to normal volunteers for 15 days. Four of the 15 subjects developed itching and a skin rash[35] (Table 23-2).

Chronic. Chronic skin exposure to formaldehyde causes contact dermatitis and occasionally urticaria. Formaldehyde has been reported as the tenth leading cause of contact dermatitis in patients who undergo patch testing.[34] The contact dermatitis from formaldehyde is sometimes more pronounced in sun-exposed areas of skin, raising the possibility of a photoallergic component.[30]

Currently, there is controversy concerning whether formaldehyde exposure can cause asthma.[5] A case report of two nurses exposed to formaldehyde in a dialysis unit describes their marked reductions in peak expiratory flow rates (PEF) when challenged with formaldehyde vapor.[17] The responses were of the delayed type. Bronchial provocation challenge with 2 ppm formaldehyde gas of 230 individuals with asthmalike symptoms who had previously been exposed to formaldehyde found 3 people who had immediate responses of a greater than 20% drop in PEF and 4 others with delayed responses characterized by PEF decreases of 20% or more.[37] Because high levels of formaldehyde were used for the provocation challenge (2 ppm), the observed effects were thought to have been due to nonspecific irritant reactions. However, studies of asthmatics exposed to formaldehyde

have not found decreases in airway flow such as those found with ozone. Bronchial provocation challenges of 9 asthmatics with 3 ppm formaldehyde for over 30 minutes and a similar challenge of 15 asthmatics with 2 ppm formaldehyde failed to show significant changes in expiratory flow.[42,49] Bronchial challenge with concentrations up to 3 ppm of 13 patients with suspected formaldehyde asthma failed to show significant decreases in expiratory flow.[14] A study of peak flow in medical students exposed to an average of 0.7 ppm formaldehyde in anatomy class found a small but significant decline during the course of the semester that reversed when the course was completed and exposure ceased.[25] Preshift and postshift spirometry in workers exposed to formaldehyde from particleboard or molding operations showed a small but significant decline in forced expiratory flow at 25% to 75% of forced vital capacity (FEF$_{25\%-75\%}$, a measure of small airway flow) in workers exposed to 0.5 to 1 ppm formaldehyde, compared with a control group.[21] No permanent reduction in flow was found. In summary, provocation challenges with formaldehyde in concentrations up to 3 ppm do not produce significant bronchoconstriction in small numbers of volunteer asthmatics, but studies of larger groups of presumably normal subjects have shown small airflow decreases that appear to be reversible.

One well-documented case of formaldehyde-related asthma in a nurse was confirmed by bronchial provocation challenge with 3 ppm formaldehyde for 5 minutes that produced a late asthmatic reaction with greater than 20% decrease in PEF.[18] Immunologic testing for antibodies to formaldehyde–human serum albumin has been suggested as a way to detect IgE and IgG antibody in persons allergic to formaldehyde,[15] but the clinical usefulness of this test in evaluating formaldehyde-induced asthma is unknown. To date, after consideration of all of the published evidence, it is safe to assume that true formaldehyde-induced asthma is rare.

Formaldehyde is a suspect human carcinogen based on findings that rats exposed to high doses (14 ppm) for several weeks developed nasal cancer.[1,24] The response was nonlinear, and excess nasal cancers did not develop at lower doses. Tissue concentrations of formaldehyde in the respiratory tract of rats sufficient to induce cancer are 6 to 8 orders of magnitude greater than naturally occurring tissue formaldehyde.[46] Formaldehyde is considered a rat carcinogen because at high concentrations it causes cell death and induces cell proliferation and mitogenesis,[32] which in themselves are tumor promoters.[2] Mice and hamsters do not develop cancers from formaldehyde.[26] Formaldehyde is unique as a suspect carcinogen in that it is present in normal tissue.

The epidemiologic evidence in humans for carcinogenicity of formaldehyde is weak, and the results of more than 30 studies have not been consistent.[6,31,46] Most studies have been of occupationally exposed groups, and findings in the various groups have differed. Excesses of nasal cancer have not been found in populations exposed to formaldehyde

Table 23-3 Chronic effects of formaldehyde exposure

Area affected	Effects
Skin	Sensitization and contact dermatitis
Nose	Dysplasia, squamous metaplasia
Lungs	Bronchospasm, pneumonitis

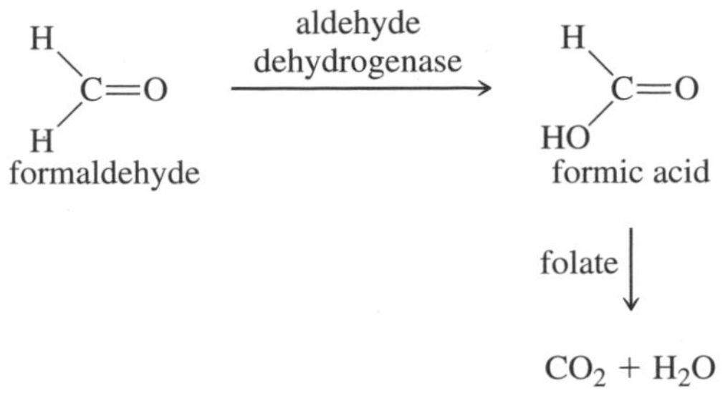

Fig. 23-1 Formaldehyde metabolism.

except in those exposed as well to wood dust, which is also associated with nasal cancer.[6,31] Nasopharyngeal cancer was associated with formaldehyde exposure[6] in one study of industrial workers. However, since major risk factors for nasopharyngeal cancer are tobacco and alcohol use, this finding could be from confounding factors. Lung cancer has not been found in excess in industrial workers or professionals exposed to formaldehyde.[6,31]

There is experimental evidence indicating formaldehyde gas can cause precancerous changes in humans. Chronic exposure to formaldehyde at levels of 0.5 to 2 ppm is associated with squamous metaplasia of human nasal epithelium,[9,11] with chromosomal alteration of nasal cells in the form of micronuclei,[3] and with chromosomal alteration expressed as micronucleus formation in blood lymphocytes[15] (Table 23-3). The significance of these changes and the potential for reversibility are unknown.

Multiple substance exposure. When formaldehyde is present together with other irritants, such as in smog, the smell threshold may be lowered to 0.01 ppm and irritant effects found at levels as low as 0.05 ppm. Formaldehyde in aerosols has more effect on airway resistance in guinea pigs than similar amounts of formaldehyde present as gas.[26]

Biochemistry

Formaldehyde is water soluble and readily absorbed through inhalation or ingestion. During nasal breathing, almost all inhaled formaldehyde is deposited on the mucous layer of the nasal mucosa; oral breathing allows it to deposit in the lower respiratory tract.[26] Formaldehyde is a normal metabolite and is involved in the transfer of methyl groups in dealkylation. Exogenous and endogenous formaldehyde are metabolized in a similar manner and are eliminated from the blood in 1 to 2 minutes.[34] Formaldehyde is oxidized to formic acid in erythrocytes and in the liver. The formic acid can then be oxidized to CO_2 or excreted in the urine. In humans and primates, metabolism of formaldehyde is decreased by folic acid deficiency,[34] causing the formic acid intermediate to increase (Fig. 23-1).

Formaldehyde is highly reactive and forms methylol adducts readily with the amines in nucleic acids and proteins. Formaldehyde also forms cross-links in proteins and nucleic acids by joining amines to its carbonyl group. In living organisms, these cross-links are unstable because of repair mechanisms such as aldehyde dehydrogenases and oxidases.[26]

Diagnosis

Adverse health effects can occur from ingestion, inhalation, or skin exposure. Because individuals vary in their reporting of irritant effects and because there may be individual variation in sensitivity to formaldehyde, it is difficult to set an exposure limit below which adverse effects are not seen.

Diagnosis of acute irritant reactions or overdoses may be made from the history of exposure. No peculiar physical features of skin or pulmonary disorders are due to formaldehyde exposure.

There are no laboratory tests specific for formaldehyde exposure. Because it is metabolized within a few minutes and because small quantities are present normally, formaldehyde levels in blood cannot be used to measure exposure. Some metabolized formaldehyde is excreted as urinary formate. Methanol, acetone, and substances that are metabolized to form one-carbon products, such as pectin in apples, are also metabolized to formate and contribute to urinary formate excretion. Because urinary formate excretion has multiple sources, it does not have value as a means for assessing formaldehyde exposure.[7] Exposure to formaldehyde by inhalation may be estimated from air sampling in the breathing zone of the individual.[7] There is no quantitative test to assess formaldehyde absorption through the skin or by ingestion.

Patch testing with nonirritating (less than 2%) solutions of formaldehyde can be used to test for delayed hypersensitivity.[4] The clinical usefulness of measuring IgE or IgG antibody to formaldehyde-protein complexes is unknown.[4,15]

Diagnostic dilemmas. Evaluation of the patient who develops asthma after exposure to an irritant such as formaldehyde presents the clinician with the dilemma of establishing whether the asthma arose de novo after the exposure or whether preexisting airway hyperresponsiveness had been quiescent until an attack was triggered by the irritant. Bronchial provocation challenge testing may be useful in establishing the degree of airway responsiveness. A drop in PEF or forced expiratory volume in 1 second (FEV_1) of 20% or more after challenge supports the diagnosis of formaldehyde asthma.

Patients may report irritant reactions to low levels of formaldehyde that do not bother other household members or workers. The complaints are usually subjective, and there is no diagnostic test to determine the presence of ocular irritation, headaches, and other "annoyance" reactions. Measurement of air levels of formaldehyde may be used to quantify exposure. Reduction of exposure by better ventilation, personal protective equipment, or assignment to another work area may alleviate symptoms.

Management and treatment. Irritant, allergic, and toxic reactions to formaldehyde should be managed by removal from exposure and symptomatic treatment. Topical steroid creams speed the resolution of dermatitis as long as exposure to formaldehyde stops. Bronchospasm should be treated with inhaled β-agonists, inhaled steroids, and parenteral steroids as indicated. Splash exposures to the eye should be treated immediately by washing with water and subsequently irrigated in the emergency department and examined for corneal abrasions.

Consultation, referral, and follow-up care. Consultation regarding formaldehyde contact dermatitis may be obtained from a dermatologist or allergist. Patients with possible formaldehyde asthma should be evaluated by an internal medicine or occupational medicine physician with experience in bronchial provocation testing.

There are no specific medications or therapies for formaldehyde toxicity, and follow-up care should be aimed at reducing or preventing future exposures.

REFERENCES

1. Albert RE et al: Gaseous formaldehyde and hydrogen chloride induction of nasal cancer in the rat, *J Natl Cancer Inst* 68:597, 1982.
2. Ames BN, Gold LW: Too many rodent carcinogens: mitogenesis increases mutagenesis, *Science* 249:970, 1990.
3. Ballarin C et al: Micronucleated cells in nasal mucosa of formal dehyde-exposed workers, *Mutat Res* 280:1, 1992.
4. Bardana EJ: Formaldehyde asthma. In Bardana EJ, Montanaro A, O'Hollaren MT, editors: *Occupational asthma,* Philadelphia, 1992, Hanley & Belfus.
5. Bardana EJ, Montanaro A: The formaldehyde fiasco: a review of the scientific data, *Immunol Allergy Prac* 9:11, 1987.
6. Blair A et al: Epidemiologic evidence on the relationship between formaldehyde exposure and cancer, *Scand J Work Environ Health* 16:381, 1990.
7. Boeniger MF: Formate in urine as a biological indicator of formaldehyde exposure: a review, *Am Ind Hyg Assoc J* 48:900, 1987.
8. Boeniger MF, Stewart P: *Biological markers for formaldehyde exposure in mortician students, report II: extent of exposure* (report 125.27), Cincinnati, 1992, National Institute for Occupational Safety and Health, Division of Surveillance, Hazard Evaluation, and Field Studies.
9. Boysen M et al: Nasal mucosa in workers exposed to formaldehyde: a pilot study, *Br J Ind Med* 47:116, 1990.
10. Brandwein M, Pervez N, Biller H: Nasal squamous carcinoma in an undertaker: does formaldehyde play a role? *Rhinology* 25:279, 1987.
11. Edling C, Hellquist H, Odkvist L: Occupational formaldehyde exposure and the nasal mucosa, *Rhinology* 25:181, 1987.
12. Feinman SE: *Formaldehyde sensitivity and toxicity,* Boca Raton, Fla, 1988, CRC Press.
13. Fisher AA: *Contact dermatitis,* Philadelphia, 1986, Lea & Febiger.
14. Frigas E, Filley WV, Reed CE: Bronchial challenge with formaldehyde gas: lack of bronchoconstriction in 13 patients suspected of having formaldehyde-induced asthma, *Mayo Clin Proc* 59:295, 1984.
15. Grammer LC et al: Evaluation of a worker with possible formaldehyde-induced asthma, *J Allergy Clin Immunol* 92:29, 1993.
16. Hayes RB et al: The mortality of U.S. embalmers and funeral directors, *Am J Ind Med* 18:641, 1990.
17. Hendrick DJ, Lane DJ: Occupational formalin asthma, *Br J Ind Med* 34:11, 1977.
18. Hendrick DJ et al: Formaldehyde asthma: challenge exposure levels and fate after five years, *J Occup Med* 24:893, 1982.
19. Hileman B: Formaldehyde: assessing the risk, *Environ Sci Technol* 18:216A, 1984.
20. Holness DL, Nethercott JR: Health status of funeral service workers exposed to formaldehyde, *Arch Environ Health* 44:222, 1994.
21. Horvath E et al: Effects of formaldehyde on the mucous membranes and lungs, *JAMA* 259:701, 1988.
22. Iserson K: *Death to dust: what happens to dead bodies?* Tucson, 1994, Galen Press.
23. Kerfoot EJ, Mooney TF: Formaldehyde and paraformaldehyde study in funeral homes, *Am Ind Hyg Assoc J* 36:533, 1975.
24. Kerns WD et al: Carcinogenicity of formaldehyde in rats and mice after long-term inhalation exposure, *Cancer Res* 43:4382, 1983.
25. Kriebel D, Sama SR, Cocanour B: Reversible pulmonary responses to formaldehyde, *Am Rev Respir Dis* 148:1509, 1993.
26. Leikauf GD: Formaldehyde and other aldehydes. In Lippman N, editor: *Environmental toxicants,* New York, 1993, Van Nostrand Reinhold.
27. Levine RJ, Andjelkovich DA, Shaw LK: The mortality of Ontario undertakers and a review of formaldehyde-related mortality studies, *J Occup Med* 26:740, 1984.
28. Levine RJ et al: The effects of occupational exposure on the respiratory health of West Virginia morticians, *J Occup Med* 26:91, 1984.
29. Lutz WK: Endogenous genotoxic agents and processes as a basis of spontaneous carcinogenesis, *Mutat Res* 238:287, 1990.
30. Maibach H: Effects of formaldehyde on skin. In Gibson J, editor: *Formaldehyde toxicity,* Washington, DC, 1983. Hemisphere Publishing.
31. McLaughlin JK: Formaldehyde and cancer: a critical review, *Int Arch Occup Environ Health* 66:295, 1994.
32. Monticello TM, Morgan KT: Cell proliferation and formaldehyde-induced respiratory carcinogenesis, *Risk Anal* 14:313, 1994.
33. Moore L, Ogrodnik E: Occupational exposure to formaldehyde in mortuaries, *J Environ Health* 49:32, 1986.
34. National Academy of Sciences, Committee on Aldehydes: *Formaldehyde and other aldehydes,* Washington, DC, 1981, National Academy Press.
35. National Institute for Occupational Safety and Health: *Criteria for a recommended standard. Occupational exposure to formaldehyde* (NIOSH publication 77-126), Cincinnati, 1977, Department of Health, Education, and Welfare.
36. National Institute for Occupational Safety and Health: *Health Hazard evaluation determination report, Cincinnati College of Mortuary Science Embalming Laboratory* (NIOSH report HE 79-146-670), Cincinnati, 1980, Department of Health and Human Services.
37. Nordman H, Keskinen H, Tuppurainen M: Formaldehyde asthma—rare or overlooked? *J Allergy Clin Immunol* 75:91, 1985.
38. Occupational Safety and Health Administration: Occupational exposure to formaldehyde, *Federal Register* 57:22290, 1992.
39. Orringer EP, Mattern WD: Formaldehyde-induced hemolysis during chronic hemodialysis, *N Engl J Med* 294:1416, 1976.
40. Palermo GB, Gumz EJ: The last invasion of human privacy and its psychological consequences on survivors: a critique of the practice of embalming, *Theor Med* 15:397, 1994.

41. Porter JAH: Acute respiratory distress following formalin inhalation, *Lancet* 2:603, 1975.

42. Sauder LR et al: Acute pulmonary response of asthmatics to 3.0 ppm formaldehyde, *Toxicol Ind Health* 3:569, 1987.

43. Schwope A et al: Gloves for protection from aqueous formaldehyde: permeation resistance and human factors analysis, *Appl Ind Hyg* 3:167, 1988.

44. *Statistical abstract of the United States 1990* (Table 1381), Washington, DC, 1990, Bureau of the Census.

45. Suruda A et al: Cytogenetic effects of formaldehyde exposure in students of mortuary science, *Cancer Epidemiol Biomarkers Prev* 2:453, 1993.

46. Universities Associated for Research and Education in Pathology, Inc: Epidemiology of chronic occupational exposure to formaldehyde: report of the ad hoc panel on health aspects of formaldehyde, *Toxicol Ind Health* 4:77, 1988.

47. Walrath J, Fraumeni JF: Mortality patterns among embalmers, *Int J Cancer* 31:407, 1983.

48. Williams TM, Levine RJ, Blunden PB: Exposure of embalmers to formaldehyde and other chemicals, *Am Ind Hyg Assoc J* 45:172, 1984.

49. Witek TJ et al: An evaluation of respiratory effects following exposure to 2.0 ppm formaldehyde in asthmatics: lung function, symptoms, and airway reactivity, *Arch Environ Health* 42:230, 1987.

24

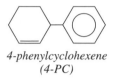

*4-phenylcyclohexene
(4-PC)*

- Buildings that create an isolated indoor environment are more likely to recirculate irritant and toxic substances found in the office

Office Personnel

William J. Meggs
Ricky Lee Langley

OCCUPATIONAL DESCRIPTION

Industrialized societies have increasingly large numbers of office workers. From 1983 to 1993, the number of managerial and professional specialty workers increased in the United States by 36%, from 23.6 million to 32.3 million workers. Administrative support personnel, which includes secretaries, receptionists, and file clerks, increased by 13%, from 16.4 million to 18.6 million. The total number of workers in occupations in which the majority of time is spent in offices or similar indoor environments increased 27%, from 50.57 million in 1983 to 64.62 million in 1993. During this same time, the number of workers in farming, forestry, and fishing decreased 11%, from 3.7 million to 3.3 million, and workers in manufacturing increased 6%, from 16.1 million to 17 million.

Office buildings are generally considered the safest of work environments. Certainly the job hazards of mining, farming, and factory work do not exist in office environments. Studies in occupational toxicology often use office workers as control groups because the specific toxins under investigation are not found in offices. In spite of this relative safety, the past decade has seen the emergence of health problems associated with office work.[40] Many of the problems are associated with the indoor air quality of office buildings rather than with exposures necessary or essential for the job.[46] Hence, many of the exposures of office workers are common to all workers in modern buildings, from schoolteachers and managers to clerks and professionals. Terms such as *sick building syndrome* and *multiple chemical sensitivity syndrome* have emerged as attempts to better define the illnesses associated with the contemporary indoor environment.[11]

Examples of toxicity associated with office workers include contact dermatitis associated with specific chemicals

203

handled in offices. Outbreaks of conjunctivitis in office buildings are often related to air quality. Specific contaminants of indoor air, such as radon, cigarette smoke, and asbestos, are carcinogenic. In addition, secondhand cigarette smoke has been associated with both lung cancer and coronary artery disease. Finally, solvents used in some office professions carry risks of solvent neurotoxicity.

POTENTIAL TOXIC EXPOSURES
Indoor Air Pollution

A number of pollutants are found in the indoor air of modern buildings, including offices, schools, and homes. The spectrum of toxicity associated with indoor air pollution range from carcinogenesis to minor irritant reactions. The box below lists air contaminants in modern buildings.

Carcinogens in the indoor air. Cancer-causing agents in the indoor air include radon, asbestos, environmental tobacco smoke, formaldehyde, and benzene.

Radon is a radioactive gas that is produced by the decay of nuclei in the earth's crust. Radon outgassing from the ground is trapped in buildings and can reach levels that cause health hazards. Approximately 10% of U.S. lung cancer deaths result from exposure to radon.[58] Exposure to radon is more likely in homes than in office buildings.

The health effects of cigarette smoking, with its increased risk of cancer, stroke, and heart disease, are well known. Recently, attention has been called to the health effects of environmental tobacco smoke on nonsmokers. Studies have shown an increased risk of coronary artery disease and cancer among those exposed to secondhand tobacco smoke.[28,83] Cigarette smoking has been banned in many offices, and addicted workers crowded around building entrances to smoke cigarettes have become a common sight.

Benzene and formaldehyde are known carcinogens. Airborne benzene is known to cause leukemia at levels as low as 1 ppm.[63] Formaldehyde has been associated with nasal cancer in rodents, but no data support a risk for office workers exposed to formaldehyde (see Chapter 23).

Volatile organic chemicals in the indoor air. A number of studies have demonstrated that the indoor air of modern offices, schools, and homes contains a complex mixture of volatile organic chemicals (VOCs). The total exposure methodology (TEAM) study measured VOCs in indoor air, outdoor air, drinking water, and exhaled air. This study documented that VOCs such as benzene, chloroform, trichloroethane, trichoroethylene, xylenes, styrene, carbon tetrachloride, and dichlorobenzene are exhaled by humans, and indoor air was identified as the source of this exposure.[82]

Emission rates of VOCs from different surfaces vary according to the surface, its chemical composition, and adhesives. The 1,1,1-trichloroethane emissions were determined to be 31 ± 15 mg/minute/m^2 from painted gypsum board (Sheetrock), 84 ± 48 mg/minute/m^2 from glued wallpaper, 180 ± 12 mg/minute/m^2 from glued carpet, and $37,000 \pm 15,000$ mg/minute/m^2 from a mixture of cleaning agents and pesticides. Emissions of *p*-xylene were found to be 26 ± 6.5 mg/minute/m^2 from glued wallpaper and 150 ± 24 mg/minute/m^2 from glued carpet.[68]

The VOCs in the air of office buildings are at levels below those associated with cancer. These compounds occur in a complex mixture of volatile organic chemicals, each component of which is thought to be below the level that is carcinogenic. However, the total burden of VOCs is above that which would cause cancer for some of the individual components. The carcinogenicity of these complex mixtures is not known at this time.

Pesticides in the indoor air. In many offices, schools, and private residences, it is the practice to spray with pesticides periodically. In one study, the airborne and surface concentrations of diazinon, chlorpyrifos, and bendiocarb (Ficam) were measured up to 10 days after broadcast spray application in offices. Diazinon and chlorpyrifos airborne concentrations peaked 4 hours after application; bendiocarb levels were at peak values during application. Airborne levels of diazinon persisted longer than those of chlorpyrifos or bendiocarb. Restriction of workers from their offices was recommended for 2 days after diazinon, chlorpyrifos, and bendiocarb application. Surface concentrations were found to be higher at 24 and 48 hours than at 1 hour. Thus, office workers are at continued risk for pesticide exposure after applications. Offices should be adequately ventilated, and surfaces should be cleaned before workers return to duty. Pyrethrins are frequently sprayed in offices, and sensitive individuals can develop pyrethrin-induced asthma.[61]

Neurotoxicity of pyrethrins and pyrethroids (synthetic derivatives of the naturally occurring pyrethrins) has been discussed,[30] but no cases of neurotoxicity among office workers have been reported. In a report of five cases concerning cypermethrin, a pyrethroid pesticide, contamination of air-conditioning ducts led to poisoning. Symptoms from this inhalation exposure were shortness of breath, nausea, headaches, and irritability. Diagnosis was delayed due to the treating physicians' lack of knowledge of pesticide toxicity, and these workers continued to enter the contamination area.[44]

Indoor Air Pollutants

Pesticides
Volatile organic chemicals
Asbestos
Radon
Environmental tobacco smoke

Organophosphate toxicity in office workers has been caused by spraying with chlorophyrifos (Dursban). In a report of five cases, the expected constant rate of recovery of the erythrocyte cholinesterase did not occur, which may be explained by ongoing release of organophosphates stored in a body compartment.[33]

Environmental tobacco smoke. Exposure to environmental tobacco smoke by nonsmokers has been linked to carotid atherosclerosis,[20] lung cancer,[25,56,85] nasal cancer,[89] breast cancer,[36] meningioma,[66] coronary artery disease,[28,77,83] inflammatory bowel disease,[42,75] and rheumatoid arthritis.[24] Nonsmoking women exposed to environmental tobacco smoke during pregnancy have an increased risk of spontaneous abortion[87] and infants of reduced birth weight.[47]

Exposure to passive cigarette smoke increases the incidence of chronic respiratory problems such as cough, phlegm, and bronchospasm.[59,64] Among nonsmokers, 86% believe that environmental tobacco smoke is harmful to their health, and 77% believe that smokers should not smoke in the presence of nonsmokers, according to a Gallup poll commissioned by the American Lung Association. Rhinitis patients with sensitivity to environmental tobacco smoke have increased nasal symptoms and measurable increases in nasal airway resistance when exposed to environmental tobacco smoke.[83] Exposure of sensitive nonsmokers to environmental tobacco smoke causes symptoms of headache, cough, nasal congestion, chest tightness, rhinorrhea, nose and throat irritation, and increases in nasal resistance.[4] Atopy and other respiratory diseases such as sinusitis are risk factors for intolerance of environmental tobacco smoke.[16] Nonsmokers exposed to workplace environmental tobacco smoke have increased serum carboxyhemoglobin levels and more cough, sputum production, eye irritation, chest colds, and days lost from work due to chest colds than unexposed workers.[76,86]

Groups at special risk for discomfort associated with indoor air pollutants may be those with asthma and rhinitis.[22] Surveys of patients with asthma and rhinitis indicate that chemical irritants common in indoor air, such as perfumes, environmental tobacco smoke, and pesticides, cause exacerbation of their disease.[52,69] Clinical challenges with perfume[69] and tobacco smoke[18,54] in asthma patients have verified that bronchospasm can be provoked by these substances in some asthmatics. Nasal inhalation studies with sidestream tobacco smoke have demonstrated that individuals giving a history of intolerance to tobacco smoke but not a control group have statistically significant changes in rhinitis symptoms, nasal airway resistance, and maximum inspiratory flow after a controlled exposure.[4,84] The fact that some but not all patients with asthma and rhinitis have disease provoked by chemical irritants suggests a susceptibility to chemical irritants in some subjects, and possible mechanisms have been reviewed.[3]

The prevalence of physician-diagnosed asthma with onset or exacerbation since building occupancy was 4.9 times greater in a sick building than in a control building.[35]

Photocopy Machines

Behenic acid, a fatty acid volatilized in photocopy machines, has been implicated as a cause of hypersensitivity angitis.[78] Thiourea in photocopy paper has been implicated as a cause of contact sensitivity.[39]

Carpets

Synthetic carpeting is known to emit a variety of VOCs. The styrene-butadiene rubber latex adhesive used in some carpeting emits 4-phenylcyclohexene (4-PC) and styrene. Carpeting with polyvinyl chlorine backing emits formaldehyde, vinyl acetate, isooctane, 1,2-propanediol, and 2-ethyl-1-hexanol. Carpeting with polyurethane backing emits hydroxytoluene.[33] Health complaints have been associated with the installation of new carpets in offices. Symptoms of burning eyes, chills, wheezing, rhinorrhea, sneezing, cough, chest tightness, hoarseness, sore throat, fatigue, memory difficulty, and difficulty in concentrating have been described. These symptoms are consistent with those of the sick building syndrome, with mucosal irritation and neurological symptoms. In one study, 4-PC was the single chemical found to correlate with new carpet installation.[31] Another study found 4-PC associated with odorous new carpeting.[14] Laboratory studies in rodents exposed to 4-PC found no evidence of eye, skin, nasal, or respiratory tract irritation over a 2-week period.[60] Groups of 5 and 10 animals were used in this study, and in human outbreaks the percentage of individuals affected is not high. For example, in the Hirzy study, 5000 people were exposed to the new carpeting, 122 individuals were adversely affected, 17 were unable to work at their normal duty stations, and 6 developed chronic chemical sensitivity.[31]

Carpeting is known to increase concentrations of indoor allergens relative to uncarpeted flooring[23] and may increase allergic symptoms to some indoor allergens. Carpet installers have an increased risk of oral and pharyngeal cancer, with an adjusted odds ratio of 7.7, relative to the population at large.[37]

Carbonless Copy Paper

Carbonless copy paper can cause contact dermatitis,[67] but more serious symptoms can result from exposure. Occupational exposure to carbonless copy paper can cause hoarseness, cough, rash, and flushing. The chemical alkylphenol novolac resin contained in carbonless copy paper gave a positive patch test result in susceptible individuals. Video endoscopy of the larynx verified the development of laryngeal edema with exposure, and plasma histamine was demonstrated to increase with exposure.[43] These findings suggest that immediate hypersensitivity is a factor in health problems associated with carbonless copy paper.

CLINICAL PROBLEMS ASSOCIATED WITH OFFICE WORK

Skin Diseases among Office Workers

Dryness and itching of the skin have been associated with low values of humidity in office buildings. A cross-over study in which two wings of an office building were maintained at relative humidities of 20% to 30% versus 30% to 40% found that symptom scores for dryness and itching increased significantly as the humidity was lowered.[62] Hence, adequate humidification of the air is essential for office workers' comfort.

Studies of contact dermatitis have found office workers to be in the four largest groups presenting with contact dermatitis[10] and that female office workers have an increased incidence of contact allergy to colophony (resins).[49] Some authors expect that the increasing complexity of the modern office environment has led to increased incidence of skin problems among office workers, with carbonless copy paper, duplicating machines, formaldehyde, video display terminals, and rubber bands being important etiologies of skin problems.[48] These authors stress that, though it is difficult to arrive at a correct diagnosis, the result is a complete cure.[67] Office workers have a lower rate of dermatitis of the hand than other occupational groups, such as nurses. In addition, the age-adjusted prevalence of dermatitis of the hand in office workers was not higher than that in the general population.[74]

The skin can convey toxins into the body and lead to systemic toxicity. Surface contamination with organophosphate pesticides, which are absorbed through skin contact, has been documented in office buildings that are routinely sprayed.[17]

Ophthamologic Problems among Office Workers

The name *office eye syndrome* was proposed for a syndrome of dry eyes and corneal staining found in 25% of office workers in four buildings in Copenhagen. There was a statistically significant relationship between reduced break-up time of the precorneal film and epithelial damage as measured by lissamere green stain. The correlation between eye irritation and different degrees of dry eyes was very significant, with a *p* value less than 0.00006.[27] Further investigations revealed that a thick, fatty layer may protect the eyes against development of dry eyes. The results indicate that deficiency in available meibomian oil is involved in the dry eye syndrome associated with eye irritation in the office environment. Diagnostic features that can be used to distinguish the office eye syndrome from other conditions with dry eyes include foam in the eye canthus, reduced break-up time of the precorneal film, clusters of epithelial damage on the bulbar conjunctiva, and a reduced fatty layer of the precorneal film.[26] Low humidity may be

one factor in this eye dryness.[62] The office eye syndrome is closely related to the sick building syndrome, as discussed later, in which mucosal irritation plays a prominent role. However, humidity alone cannot account for the sick building phenomena.

Hypersensitivity Pneumonitis

Fever, dyspnea, cough, infiltrates on chest x-ray, and precipitins to the causative agent are the hallmarks of hypersensitivity pneumonitis.[81] This acute illness occurs approximately 6 hours after exposure and is clinically similar to bacterial pneumonia. However, symptoms resolve within 24 hours if the causative agent is withdrawn. Subsequent exposures lead to recrudescence of disease. Office workers are at risk for hypersensitivity pneumonitis from contamination of air conditioning systems with agents such as *Thermoactinomyces vulgaris, Candida,* thermotolerant bacteria, protozoa, *Penicillium* species, and *Naegleria gruberi.*[15] Recurrent episodes have been associated with manipulations of the air conditioning system and in one instance led to vacating the building.[34]

Sick Building Syndrome

The *sick building syndrome* is defined as an outbreak of illness associated with a building. Symptoms are primarily irritation of mucous membranes (respiratory tract and eyes), headache, difficulty with concentration, lethargy, and irritability. Chest tightness and skin complaints have also been reported. No single etiology has been identified, but the illness is associated with modern buildings with sealed windows and recirculated air.[88] Early episodes of sick building syndrome were attributed to mass hysteria, but there are many differences between mass hysteria and the sick building syndrome. Mass hysteria tends to be acute and self-limited; sick building syndrome is chronic and ongoing. A number of investigations of sick buildings have been carried out, and little credence given to the mass hysteria hypothesis.[45]

Studies suggest that air quality is the dominant factor in sick building syndrome. A study in Sweden pumped air from a sick building into a booth on the sidewalk. Random subjects recruited on the street, blinded to the purpose of the study, were asked to sit in the booth and be interviewed by an examiner blinded to the exposure. Symptoms typical of sick building syndrome were demonstrated in subjects independent of their knowledge of exposure.[7]

A comparison of two buildings with similar occupants but different ventilation systems found that a number of symptoms were significantly increased among occupants of a tightly sealed building with air conditioning relative to the building with natural ventilation. Symptoms that were more common in the air-conditioned building were rhinitis (28% versus 5%), nasal blockage and dry throat (35% versus 9%), lethargy (36% versus 13%), and headache (31% versus 15%).[65]

A comparison of published studies of buildings with problems found that air-conditioned buildings were consistently associated with increased prevalence of work-related headache (prevalence odds ratio = 1.3-3.1), lethargy (POR = 1.4-5.1), and upper respiratory and mucous membrane symptoms (POR = 1.3-4.8).[1,2] Neither humidification nor mechanical ventilation without air conditioning was associated with higher symptom prevalence.[53]

A population study in Germany found that office workers have 50% more upper respiratory infections than a control group.[41] A meta-analysis of building surveys found a strong association between buildings with modern climate control and symptomatology, with a 50% increase in symptoms in modern buildings.[53] Those especially likely to be symptomatic are women and workers with a prior history of atopy and seborrheic dermatitis. Performing photocopying tasks, using carbonless copy paper, working in recently renovated buildings, and stressful work environments increase the likelihood of symptoms. Buildings with low outdoor air supply, strong sources of pollution, less frequent cleaning, and ultraviolet lights are more likely to be problems.[53] In one study, increasing airflow to 20 cubic feet per minute per occupant has been found to reduce symptoms, as has increasing relative humidity.[38]

Analysis of an outbreak of tuberculosis in a building with marginal air quality suggests that sick buildings put office workers at risk for communicable disease. In the building studied, 40% of office workers had skin test conversion after a 4-week exposure to a co-worker with active cavitary tuberculosis. Mathematical modeling suggests that infectivity rates decrease with increases of fresh air intake.[57]

There is a positive association between symptom prevalence rates and levels of airborne viable bacteria and fungi within groups of buildings with similar ventilation systems.[29] Whether these particles are a cause of sick building syndrome or a marker for inadequate ventilation has not been determined.

In conclusion, air quality represents a comprehensive cause of the sick building syndrome.[72,73] This quality is determined by adequate ventilation and humidity, the concentrations of volatile organic chemicals in the indoor air, and bioaerosols that contain irritants and allergens. Some individuals tolerate poor air quality better than others, so symptoms may be variable. In outbreaks of sick building syndrome, some individuals may progress to a generalized sensitivity to airborne chemicals, the multiple chemical sensitivity syndrome.[31]

Chemical Sensitivity

Chemical sensitivity is described as an intolerance of chemical inhalants, such as environmental tobacco smoke, perfumes, and pesticides. Chemical sensitivity is associated with rhinitis and asthma,[50-52,69] is often mild, and is different from the multiple chemical sensitivity syndrome (MCS). A number of definitions of MCS have been given.[55]

A prominent feature of these definitions is an acute or inducing chemical exposure, including organophosphate pesticide poisoning, a solvent exposure, or exposure to a chemical spill. In many patients, a single acute exposure cannot be identified at the onset of disease. Another feature of MCS is the involvement of more than one organ system. Like sick building syndrome, respiratory and neurologic symptoms are prominent, but gastrointestinal, dermal, and musculoskeletal symptoms have also been associated with exposures.

Mechanisms proposed for MCS include limbic kindling,[5] time-dependent sensitization, rhinitis with systemic manifestations of airway inflammation,[51,52] neurogenic inflammation,[3,52] classic conditioning,[9] and somatization disorder.[79] The extent that psychiatric phenomena are involved in MCS has been studied. Generally, studies using diagnostic questionnaires and structured interviews have found more psychopathology in this population than in a control group but also MCS patients with no psychopathology.[70,71]

Chemical sensitivity is a common complaint. A survey by the U.S. Environmental Protection Agency found that approximately one third of inhabitants of sealed buildings reported that they considered themselves especially sensitive to one or more common chemical exposures.[80] A general population study in Baltimore found that 25% of 60 respondents reported chemical sensitivity.[19] A survey of college students in Arizona found that 66% of 643 reported sensitivity to at least one of the five common chemicals surveyed.[6] A random-digit dial telephone survey of the general population found that 33% of 1027 respondents reported chemical sensitivity, although only 4.1% reported symptoms daily or almost daily.[52] The most commonly reported symptom was nausea, followed by headache and nasal symptoms. Specific syndromes such as the multiple chemical sensitivity syndrome may be less common.

Several studies have linked upper airway inflammation to chemical sensitivity. An elevated nasal resistance has been found in MCS patients relative to a control group.[21] A high incidence of sinusitis has been associated with an outbreak of environmental illness associated with poor ventilation in a high school.[13] Cigarette smoke increases nasal resistance in a sensitive population but not in controls.[3,4,84] Fiberoptic rhinoscopy has been used to document nasal inflammation in a chemically sensitive population,[51] and nasal biopsies have verified chronic inflammation.[52]

Patients with MCS are often disabled because they are unable to tolerate the poor indoor air quality of the modern environment. Sometimes the onset of illness is associated with exposures at work, such as overzealous pesticide use, installation of new carpeting, and solvent associated with remodeling.

SUMMARY

Traditionally, office work is one of the safest work environments. The health hazards workers have with machinery, equipment, and exposures to toxic fumes and heavy metals were not problems to the traditional office worker. Unfortunately, modern ventilation systems combined with outgassing from building materials, carpeting, and office equipment have created an unhealthy environment for office workers. As many as 30% of office workers suffer adverse health effects from the modern office environment. These difficulties are not innate to the work function of office workers. With proper choices in building materials, adequate ventilation and humidification, policies prohibiting the use of tobacco products and heavy perfumes, avoidance of routine spraying with pesticides, and scavenger systems to sweep emissions from point sources, the modern office can be the healthiest of places to work. It is no more expensive to construct a healthy office building than a sick building. Unfortunately, the cost of rehabilitating a sick building may be prohibitive. Since there are no regulations on indoor air quality, it is unlikely that volunteer measures will be undertaken. Hence, office workers will continue to endure an unhealthy environment, and a few percent will be unable to work in the "sick building" environment.

REFERENCES

1. Abbritti G et al: High prevalence of sick building syndrome in a new air-conditioned building in Italy, *Arch Environ Health* 47:16, 1992.
2. Bardana EJ Jr, Montanaro A, O'Hollaren MT: Building-related illness. A review of available scientific data, *Clin Rev Allergy* 6:61, 1988.
3. Bascom R: Differential susceptibility to tobacco smoke: possible mechanisms, *Pharmacogenetics* 1:102, 1991.
4. Bascom R et al: Upper respiratory tract environmental tobacco smoke sensitivity, *Am Rev Respir Dis* 143:1304, 1991.
5. Bell IR, Miller CS, Schwartz GE: An olfactory-limbic model of multiple chemical sensitivity syndrome: possible relationship to kindling and affective spectrum disorders, *Biol Psychol* 32:218, 1992.
6. Bell IR et al: Self-reported illness from chemical odors in young adults without clinical syndromes or occupational exposures, *Arch Environ Health* 48:6, 1993.
7. Berglund B et al: Mobile laboratory for sensory air quality studies in non-industrial environments. In Berglund B, Lindvall T, Sundell J, editors: Indoor air: proceedings of the 3rd International conference on indoor air quality and climate, vol 3, Stockholm, 1984, Swedish Council for Building Research.
8. Blood lead levels among office workers–New York City. *MMWR Morb Mortal Wkly Rep* 35:298, 1986.
9. Bolla-Wilson K, Wilson R, Bleecker ML: Conditioning of physical symptoms after neurotoxic exposure, *J Occup Med* 30:684, 1988.
10. Bruckner-Tuderman L, Konig A, Schnyder UW: Patch test results of the Dermatology Clinic Zurich in 1989: personal computer-aided statistical evaluation, *Dermatology* 184:29, 1992.
11. Burge S et al: Sick building syndrome: a study of 4373 office workers, *Ann Occup Hyg* 31:493, 1987.
12. Burge S, Robertson A: Asthma, humidifiers and "office worker's lung," *Occup Health* 38:82, 1986.
13. Chester AC: Environmental Illness, *JAMA* 265:2335, 1991.
14. Crabb CL: Odorous emissions from new carpeting: development of field monitoring and analytic techniques, master's thesis, 1984, University of Arizona.
15. Crystal RG: Interstitial lung disease. In Wyngaarden JB, Smith LH, editors: *Cecil textbook of medicine*, ed 18, Philadelphia, 1988, WB Saunders.

16. Cummings KM, Zaki A, Markello S: Variation in sensitivity to environmental tobacco smoke among adult non-smokers, *Int J Epidemiol* 20:121, 1991.
17. Currie KL et al: Concentrations of diazinon, chlorpyrifos, and bendiocarb after application in offices, *Am Ind Hyg Assoc J* 51:23, 1990.
18. Danuser B et al: Effects of bronchoprovocation challenge test with cigarette sidestream smoke on sensitive and healthy adults, *Chest* 103:353, 1993.
19. Davidoff AL, Key PM: Symptoms and health status in individuals with multiple chemical sensitivity syndrome from four different sensitizing exposures and a general population comparison group. Manuscript submitted for publication.
20. Diez-Roux AV et al: The relationship of active and passive smoking to carotid atherosclerosis 12-14 years later, *Prev Med* 24:48, 1995.
21. Doty R et al: Olfactory sensitivity, nasal resistance, and autonomic function in patients with multiple chemical sensitivities, *Arch Otolaryngol Head Neck Surg* 114:1422, 1988.
22. Dusse DJ et al: Cigarette smoke induces bronchoconstrictor hyperresponsiveness in substance P and inactivates airway neutral endopeptidases in the guinea pig. Possible role of free radicals, *J Clin Invest* 84:900, 1989.
23. Dybendal T, Elsayed S: Dust from carpeted and smooth floors. V. Cat (Fel l) and mite (Der p l and Der f l) allergen levels in school dust. Demonstration of the basophil histamine release induced by dust from classrooms, *Clin Exp Allergy* 22:1100, 1992.
24. Fischer KM: Hypothesis: tobacco use is a risk factor in rheumatoid arthritis, *Med Hypotheses* 34:116, 1991.
25. Fontham ET et al: Environmental tobacco smoke and lung cancer in nonsmoking women. A multicenter study, *JAMA* 271:1752, 1994.
26. Franck C: Fatty layer of the precorneal film in the "office eye syndrome," *Acta Ophthalmol (Copenh)* 69:737, 1991.
27. Franck C: Eye symptoms and signs in buildings with indoor climate problems ("office eye syndrome"), *Acta Ophthalmol (Copenh)* 64:306, 1986.
28. Glantz SA, Parmley WW: Passive smoking and heart disease. Mechanisms and risk, *JAMA* 273:1047, 1995.
29. Harrison J et al: An investigation of the relationship between microbial and particulate indoor air pollution and the sick building syndrome, *Respir Med* 86:225, 1992.
30. He F et al: Clinical manifestations and diagnosis of acute pyrethroid poisoning, *Arch Toxicol* 63:54, 1989.
31. Hirzy JW, Morison R: Carpet/4-phenylcyclohexene toxicity: the EPA headquarters case. In Garrick BJ, Gekler WC, editors: *The analysis, communication, and perception of risk,* New York, 1991, Plenum Press.
32. Hodgson AT, Wooley JD, Daisey JM: Emissions of volatile organic compounds from new carpets measured in a large-scale environmental chamber, *J Air Waste Manage Assoc* 43:316, 1993.
33. Hodgson MJ, Block GD, Parkinson DK: Organophosphate poisoning in office workers, *J Occup Med* 28:434, 1986.
34. Hodgson MJ et al: An outbreak of recurrent acute and chronic hypersensitivity pneumonitis in office workers, *Am J Epidemiol* 125:631, 1987.
35. Hoffman RE, Wood RC, Kreiss K: Building-related asthma in Denver office workers, *Am J Public Health* 83:89, 1993.
36. Horton AW: Epidemiologic evidence for the role of indoor tobacco smoke as an initiator of human breast carcinogenesis, *Cancer Detect Prev* 16:119, 1992.
37. Huebner WW et al: Oral and pharyngeal cancer and occupation: a case-control study, *Epidemiology* 3:300, 1992.
38. Jaakola J: Experimental studies in the assessment of the determinants of the SBS, *Proc Indoor Air* 1:719, 1993.
39. Kellett JK, Beck MH, Auckland G: Contact sensitivity to thiourea in photocopy paper, *Contact Dermatitis* 11:124, 1984.
40. Klitzman S, Stellman JM: The impact of the physical environment on the psychological well-being of office workers, *Soc Sci Med* 29:733, 1989.

41. Kroeling P: Untersuchungen zum "building-illness" syndrom in klimatisierten gebaeuden, *Gesundheits Ingenieur Haustechnik Bauphysik Umwelttechnik* 108:121, 1987.

42. Lashner BA et al: Passive smoking is associated with an increased risk of developing inflammatory bowel disease in children, *Am J Gastroenterol* 88:356, 1993.

43. LeMartre FP, Merchant JA, Casale TB: Acute systemic reactions to carbonless copy paper associated with histamine release, *JAMA* 260:242, 1988.

44. Lessenger JE: Five office workers inadvertently exposed to cypermethrin, *J Toxicol Environ Health* 35:261, 1992.

45. Letz GA: Sick building syndrome: acute illness among office workers—the role of building ventilation, airborne contaminants and work stress, *Allergy Proc* 11:109, 1990.

46. Macher JM, Hayward SB: Public inquiries about indoor air quality in California, *Environ Health Perspect* 92:175, 1991.

47. Mainous AG 3rd, Hueston WJ: Passive smoke and low birth weight. Evidence of a threshold effect, *Arch Fam Med* 3:875, 1994.

48. Marks JG Jr: Dermatologic problems of office workers, *Dermatol Clin* 6:75, 1988.

49. Meding B: Epidemiology of hand eczema in an industrial city, *Acta Derm Venereol Suppl (Stockh)* 153:1, 1990.

50. Meggs WJ et al: Prevalence of allergy and chemical sensitivity in a general population, *Arch Environ Health* (in press).

51. Meggs WJ et al: Reactive upper airways dysfunction syndrome (RUDS): a form of irritant rhinitis induced by a chemical exposure, *J Allergy Clin Immunol* 89:145, 1992.

52. Meggs WJ: Health effects of indoor air pollution, *N C Med J* 53:354, 1992.

53. Mendall M, Smith AB: Consistent pattern of elevated symptoms in air-conditioned office buildings: a reanalysis of epidemiological studies, *Am J Public Health* 80:1193, 1990.

54. Menon PK et al: Asthmatic responses to passive cigarette smoke: persistence of reactivity and effect of medications, *J Allergy Clin Immunol* 88:861, 1991.

55. Miller CS: White paper: chemical sensitivity: history and phenomenology, *Toxicol Ind Health* 10:253, 1994.

56. Morris PD: Lifetime excess risk of death from lung cancer for a U.S. female never-smoker exposed to environmental tobacco smoke, *Environ Res* 1995:68;3-9.

57. Nardell EA et al: Airborne infection. Theoretical limits of protection achievable by building ventilation, *Am Rev Respir Dis* 144:302, 1991.

58. Nero AV: Distribution of airborne radon-222 concentrations in U.S. homes, *Science* 234:992, 1986.

59. Ng TP, Hui KP, Tan WC: Respiratory symptoms and lung function effects of domestic exposure to tobacco smoke and cooking by gas in non-smoking women in Singapore, *J Epidemiol Community Health* 47:454, 1993.

60. Nitschke KD et al: Dermal sensitization potential and inhalation toxicological evaluation of 4-phenycyclohexene, *Am Ind Hyg Assoc J* 52:192, 1991.

61. Patton DL, Walker JS: Pyrethrin poisoning from commercial strength flea and tick spray, *Am J Emerg Med* 6:232, 1988.

62. Reinikainen LM, Jaakkola JJ, Seppanen O: The effect of air humidification on symptoms and perception of indoor air quality in office workers: a six-period cross-over trial, *Arch Environ Health* 47:8, 1992.

63. Rinsky RA et al: Benzene and leukemia. An epidemiologic risk assessment, *N Engl J Med* 316:1044, 1987.

64. Robbins AS, Abbey DE, Lebowitz MD: Passive smoking and chronic respiratory disease symptoms in non-smoking adults, *Int J Epidemiol* 22:809, 1993.

65. Robertson AS et al: Comparison of health problems related to work and environmental measurements in two office buildings with different ventilation systems, *Br Med J Clinical Research Ed* 291:373, 1985.

66. Ryan P: Risk factors for tumors of the brain and meninges: results from the Adelaide Adult Brain Tumor Study, *Int J Cancer* 51:20, 1992.

67. Rycroft RJ: Occupational dermatoses among office personnel, *Occup Med* 1:323, 1986.

68. Sheldon LS et al: *Project summary. Indoor air quality in public buildings,* vol 1, United States Environmental Protection Agency EPA/600/S6-88/009a, Springfield, Va, 1988, US National Technical Information Service.

69. Shim C, Williams MH Jr: Effect of odors in asthma, *Am J Med* 80:18, 1986.

70. Simon G: Psychiatric symptoms in multiple chemical sensitivity, *Toxicol Ind Health* 10:487, 1994.

71. Simon GE et al: Immunological, psychological, and neuropsychological factors in multiple chemical sensitivity, *Ann Intern Med* 19:97, 1993.

72. Skov P, Valbjorn O, Pedersen BV: Influence of indoor climate on the sick building syndrome in an office environment, *Scand J Work Environ Health* 16:363, 1990.

73. Skov P, Valbjorn O, Pedersen BV: Influence of personal characteristics, job-related factors and psychosocial factors on the sick building syndrome. Danish Indoor Climate Study Group, *Scand J Work Environ Health* 15:286, 1989.

74. Smit HA, Burdorf A, Coenraads PJ: Prevalence of hand dermatitis in different occupations, *Int J Epidemiol* 22:288, 1993.

75. Sonnenberg A: Occupational distribution of inflammatory bowel disease among German employees, *Gut* 31:1037, 1990.

76. Sterling TD, Collett CW, Sterling EM: Environmental tobacco smoke and indoor air quality in modern office work environments, *J Occup Med* 29:57, 1987.

77. Taylor AE, Johnson DC, Kazemi H: Environmental tobacco smoke and cardiovascular disease: a position paper from the Council on Cardiopulmonary and Critical Care, American Heart Association, *Circulation* 86:699, 1992.

78. Tencati JR, Novey HS: Hypersensitivity angitis caused by fumes from heat-activated photocopy paper, *Ann Intern Med* 98:320, 1983.

79. Terr A: Environmental illness: A review of 50 cases, *Arch Intern Med* 146:145, 1986.

80. United States Environmental Protection Agency: *Indoor air quality and work environment study,* vol 4, 21-M-3004, Washington, DC, 1991, U S Government Printing Office.

81. Utell MJ, Samet JM: Environmentally mediated disorders of the respiratory tract, *Med Clin North Am* 74:291, 1990.

82. Wallace LA et al: Personal exposures, indoor-outdoor relationships, and breath levels of toxic air pollutants measured for 355 persons in New Jersey, *Atmos Environ* 19:1651, 1985.

83. Wells AJ: Passive smoking as a cause of heart disease, *J Am Coll Cardiol* 24:54, 1994.

84. Willes SR, Fitzgerald TK, Bascom R: Nasal inhalation challenge studies with sidestream tobacco smoke, *Arch Environ Health* 47:223, 1992.

85. White F, Dingle J, Heyge E: Cancer incidence and mortality among office workers: an epidemiologic investigation, *Can J Public Health (Revue Canadienne de Sante Publique)* 79:31, 1988.

86. White JR, Froeb HF, Kulik JA: Respiratory illness in nonsmokers chronically exposed to tobacco smoke in the work place, *Chest* 100:39, 1991.

87. Windham GC, Swan SH, Fenster L: Parental cigarette smoking and the risk of spontaneous abortion, *Am J Epidemiol* 135:1394, 1992.

88. World Health Organization: The "sick" building syndrome. In *Indoor air pollutants: exposure and health effects,* EURO Report and Studies 78, Copenhagen, 1983, World Health Organization.

89. Zheng W et al: Risk factors for cancers of the nasal cavity and paranasal sinuses among white men in the United States, *Am J Epidemiol* 138:965, 1993.

25

CH₃
toluene diisocyanate

- The World Health Organization has described two different neurologic solvent syndromes: organic affective syndrome and chronic toxic encephalopathy

- Isocyanates are potent pulmonary toxins that can cause acute and chronic respiratory dysfunction

- Outdoor paints and paint removal continue to be a source of heavy metal toxicity

Painters and Furniture Refinishers

William K. Chiang

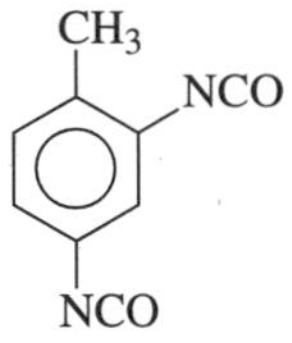

By the nature of their work, painters and furniture refinishers are exposed to the numerous chemicals contained in paints and paint removers, in particular, solvents such as tylene and oxyline. The effects of solvents on the lungs occur with relatively short exposures; however, the effects on the central nervous system may be acute or delayed by many years. Because of the long latency and the difficulty in estimating the amount and types of the exposure, studies to confirm these effects are difficult to perform and often have confounding variables.* Despite safe alternatives such as water-based paint and the removal of toxic compounds such as lead, cadmium, and mercury, there remain many potentially toxic compounds.[26]

PAINTERS
Paints and Varnishes

The use of paints for decorative and ritual purposes is an ancient and culturally diverse practice. The caves of Lascoux-Frand, the Egyptian burial sites, and the dwellings of ancient Rome were painted to enrich their attractiveness.

Currently, the United States produces more than 1 billion gallons of paints and varnishes per year. Paints consisted of three primary components: pigments, binders, and solvents. The pigments constitute 20% to 60% of the paint by weight, and the most commonly used pigments are from metallic ores, white titanium dioxide, carbon black, red lead, chrome yellow, molybdate orange, and zinc yellow. Many newer

*References 3, 7, 12, 18, 20, 24, 25, 28, 31, 32, 43, 45.

organic pigments are now available; they are generally more expensive but pose less acute toxicity than the inorganic pigments. The pigments are dispersed in binders (or resins), which allow the paint to adhere to the surface when the paint dries. The binders also serve to protect the paint surface and determine the gloss. The first binders were made from natural substances such as linseed and soybean oil, which are still present in some oil-based paints. Most of the binders today consist of polymeric materials: alkyd resins from acid, anhydrides, and alcohols, acrylic binders, vinyl, epoxy, and urethane resins. Polymers are formed with the help of an initiator (catalyst) such as benzoyl peroxide or by condensation reactions.[26]

The pigment-binder component is dispersed in a solvent. In the past, volatile organic solvents were most commonly used and posed significant health risks to painters. The important volatile organic solvents included xylene, toluene, and white spirit (mixture of aliphatic and aromatic hydrocarbons). Water-based paints have replaced much of the organic solvent-based paints. The water-based paints have significantly less volatile organic solvents; polar compounds such as plastic monomers (acrylates), glycols, and glycol ethers are most commonly used. While the glycols and glycol ethers are considered to be safer, they can cause respiratory irritations and myelotoxicity.[26,69] In a recent survey of available paints in Denmark, two thirds of the water-based paints still contained more than 20% volatile organic solvents.[63] Depending on the paint and its uses, the additives that may also be found in modern paints include thickening extenders, drying agents, insecticides, fungicides and other biocides, flattening agents, surfactants, deodorants, anticorrosive agents, and flame retardants. These additives may also contribute to toxicities.

Varnishes highlight and protect wooden and other decorative surfaces. They are divided into two different classes: oil and spirit. Oil varnish consists of drying oils such as linseed or tung oil, resins, and solvents. The most common solvents used are phenolics, coumarone, and different hydrocarbons. Spirit varnishes such as lacquer and shellac have resins dissolved in turpentine. They dry by evaporation rather than from a drying agent.

Methods of Application

Paints and varnishes can be applied by different methods, varying from manual hand applications with a brush or roller or spray to completely automated dipping and spraying processes. Automated processes have the potential to completely shield workers from any toxic exposure. Such automated processes are not possible for most circumstances because of cost or impracticality. The only possible means of limiting exposures for non–self-contained painting processes are through improved ventilation, proper personal respiratory protection, or safer paints or varnishes. Understanding of the different painting processes and painting systems is essential for the proper assessment of occupa-

Table 25-1 Painting processes

Method	Description
Hand	Objects are painted by using a brush, roller, or foam pad
Dipping	Usually the process is mechanically controlled in which an object is dipped and withdrawn from paint
Roller, curtain, veil-coating, and flow-coating	An even line of paint is applied by moving the object through a straight-line nozzle or line of paint jets
Spray painting	Air is used to apply pressure through a nozzle and produce an air-paint mist
Airless spraying	High pressure is directly applied to the paint through a nozzle producing a paint spray
Electrostatic spray guns	Charged nozzles can transfer a negative charge to the paint droplets, which are attracted to earthen objects; all spraying processes listed could be automated or applied manually
Electrocoating	The objects are charged and dipped into a water-based paint, thus attracting the paint[57]

tional paint exposures and toxicities. The types of painting processes are defined in Table 25-1.

In general, the highest risk of chemical exposures occurred in any of the aerosolization processes. Such processes are required by law in most states to be enclosed and with proper respiratory precautions for workers in the area.

HEALTH RISK ASSOCIATED WITH PAINTERS
Solvent Toxicity

Paints are aliphatic, alicyclic, aromatic, chlorinated, and oxygenated hydrocarbons. Systemic absorption of solvents predominantly takes place via the lungs because of the high vapor pressure of most organic solvents and the vast capillary networks in the lungs.[1] Dermal absorption is the other major route of solvent absorption.[14] Both acute and chronic toxicity are associated with solvent exposures. The acute narcotic effects of the oxygenated and chlorinated hydrocarbons have been used as inhalational anesthetic agents since the 1840s. Other classes of hydrocarbons have similar effects on the central nervous system (CNS) but not as potent as the oxygenated and chlorinated hydrocarbons. Acute solvent toxicity is characterized by dizziness, lightheadedness, incoordination, and transient psychomotor impairment.[2] These symptoms are reversible shortly after the termination of the exposure. The severity of the symptoms depends on the concentration, duration, and type of exposure. Unrecognized, these acute CNS symptoms may place the worker at risk for falls, slips, and other accidents at work.[30] For the chlorinated and aromatic hydrocarbons, concentrated exposure may sensitize the myocardium to endogenous and exogenous catecholamines, resulting in arrhythmias and potential deaths.[4] Methylene chloride, frequently found in paint and varnish removers, is metabolized by mixed function oxidase to carbon monoxide in the body.[38] The carbon monoxide level begins to rise in 2 to 3 hours. When the exposure is intense and prolonged (particularly when work is performed in an enclosed environment), the carboxyhemoglobin level may be significantly elevated (greater than 50% carboxyhemoglobin).[60]

The neurologic sequelae from chronic solvent exposure constitutes the single most important health risk to painters. It is sometimes called *painter's syndrome*.[2] The exact scope of the sequelae remains unclear. Despite some conflicting results in the literature,[23,67] the majority of the studies correlated solvent exposure to neurologic symptoms.* With the replacement of the oil-based paints, the incidence of solvent toxicity in painters is expected to decrease dramatically. The World Health Organization described two different syndromes: an organic affective syndrome and chronic toxic encephalopathy.[70] The organic affective syndrome is the mildest form of chronic solvent toxicity and is characterized by fatigue, irritability, depression, and apathy. The symptoms usually abate when the exposure is terminated. The second and most important syndrome is the largely irreversible chronic toxic encephalopathy. In the milder form, the symptoms include fatigue, mood disturbances, lack of concentration, short-term memory deficits, and psychomotor dysfunctions. Some of these symptoms may be reversible.[2] In the severer form, the mild symptoms may progress to impairment of judgment and abstract thinking, as well as other cortical functions. The memory deficits and personality changes become more pronounced. Corresponding structural abnormalities vary from normal to mild atrophy and have been identified by computed tomography, by magnetic resonance imaging, and at autopsy.[36,44,55] With cessation of further solvent exposure, patients with significant cognitive impairments improve or remain the same over the next several years.[17] The current phase out of oil-based paints should decrease the incident of solvent toxicity in painters.

Case controlled studies, cross-sectional studies, and isolated case reports have demonstrated significant association of these CNS abnormalities in house painters,[16,24] automobile painters,[31,32,43] shipyard painters,[62] paint manufacturer workers,[12,68] and other types of personnel with prolonged exposure to solvents.[3,20,37,45,51] Other convincing evidence for solvent-induced CNS toxicity originates in chronic solvent or paint abusers (usually toluene). Similar neurobehavioral changes were documented, along with histologic damages and atrophy in the cerebral cortex, cerebellum, and brainstem.[29,41]

Certain hydrocarbons such as n-hexane, methyl butyl ketone, and carbon disulfide are well-known causes of peripheral neurologic toxicities. These chemicals are not commonly used by painters and are only occasionally found in some mixed solvents. However, nerve conduction and electromyographic abnormalities and clinical peripheral neuropathy were reported in some painters exposed to solvent mixtures.[15,18,65] These results support some risk of peripheral nerve toxicity among certain painters. Symptoms suggestive of peripheral neuropathy such as numbness and paresthesia should be investigated.

There is no treatment available for the solvent-induced CNS toxicity. Prevention and regular monitoring of the at-risk individuals may be the most important goals. Regular worksite sampling of certain organic solvents may be helpful. However, neurologic symptoms may develop even at solvent concentrations substantially below permissible exposure limit values. Histories of memory difficulties and personality changes should be sought from the workers and their family members regularly. The most sensitive tool may be neuropsychiatric testing administered by an experienced health care provider. However, the precise neuropsychiatric test to be administered is debatable. A preemployment neuropsychiatric test and regular testing for cognitive deficits and personality changes may be the most sensitive method in screening for solvent-induced CNS toxicity. More simplified neuropsychiatric testing can also be performed on-site to assess acute toxicity at work.

Respiratory System

Numerous agents used by painters can elicit respiratory injuries by acting as nonspecific irritants, stimulating the parasympathetic nerves, and thus causing direct injuries or by stimulating immune-mediated mechanisms. Occupational respiratory dysfunctions occur by a number of mechanisms. All of these mechanisms result in respiratory distress with bronchospasm. Patients may experience an exacerbation of baseline RADs from irritants such as dust, volatile organic solvents, polar organic solvents (glycols and glycol ethers), biocides (tributyl tin oxide), and pigments. In addition, inflammatory reactions may occur to a patient exposed to ammonia, bleaching agents, and hydrochloric acid.

The mechanisms of irritant-induced occupational asthma remain unclear. Although no definitive studies confirm that nonspecific irritants may lead to permanent airway hyperresponsiveness, studies and case reports support the theory. It is also possible that these irritants may stimulate airway hyperresponsiveness in individuals with quiescent baseline reactive airway dysfunction syndrome (RADS).[34,35]

Occupational asthma is defined as airflow obstruction or airway hyperresponsiveness as a result of the work environment. It is estimated that 15% of the newly diagnosed asthma cases in adults are due to occupational asthma. More than 200 agents can cause occupational asthma, many of which are related to natural proteins from animals, insects, plants, bacteria, and fungi.[9,13] The most common cause of occupational asthma, however, is a family of relatively small chemicals, isocyanates.[9]

---

*References 3, 7, 12, 18, 20, 24, 25, 28, 31, 32, 43, 44.

Isocyanates (R-N = C = O) are highly reactive substances used in the manufacture of plastics, adhesives, insecticides, surface coatings, and polyurethane foam. Methyl isocyanate was the culprit in the Bhopal insecticide factory accident that resulted in numerous deaths and extensive acute respiratory distress. The following isocyanates may be found in polyurethane paint systems: toluene 2,4-diisocyanate (TDI), hexamethylene diisocyanate (HDI), diphenylmethane diisocyanate (MDI), and isophorone diisocyanate (IPDI). These chemicals are usually modified into prepolymers to minimize the volatility and thus the exposures to workers. However, if the paint is aerosolized, these isocyanate compounds may be inhaled and cause respiratory problems. Isocyanate exposure and toxicity have been widely reported in spray painters in the automobile and aerospace industries.[58,64]

The mechanisms of isocyanate-related pulmonary toxicity are not completely understood. Both immunologic and nonimmunologic mechanisms have been implicated. Isocyanates react with different biologic active groups in macromolecules, such as sulfhydryl, alkyl, amine, and carboxyl groups, and cause direct pulmonary epithelial damage and increased inflammatory reactions. Toluene 2,4-diisocyanate blocks the β-adrenergic receptors; it may also affect cAMP and then cause bronchospasm. In addition, isocyanates react with amino groups of proteins to form haptens, which results in a hypersensitivity reaction.[34] The IgE antibodies have been found in only 5% to 20% of symptomatic exposed workers.[8,34,58]

Originally, acute isocyanate exposure causes mucous membrane irritation of the eyes, nose, and throat, coughing, and shortness of breath. Hypersensitivity pneumonitis and bronchiolitis obliterans may also result, with fevers, chills, cough, dyspnea, and patchy infiltrates on the chest radiograph. Occupational asthma from isocyanate was first reported in 1951. The incidence has been determined to be from 5% to 30% of exposed workers.[58,64] Asthma most commonly develops in the first few months of exposures but may occur at any time. Many workers' symptoms persist even after removal from exposure.[9]

The proper diagnosis is important. The history of isocyanate exposure and work-related exacerbation of asthma and bronchospasm (i.e., relief during weekends and vacations) may be quite helpful in confirming the diagnosis. Symptoms such as cough or rhinitis should also be elicited since cough may be a symptom of asthma. Rhinitis may reflect reactive upper airway disease syndrome (RUDS). The IgE antibodies may be helpful in confirming the exposure but are nonspecific for isocyanate-induced occupational asthma. Methacholine and other pharmacologic challenges can confirm RUDS but they are also nonspecific and must be performed in a supervised medical setting because of potential adverse effects. A negative methacholine challenge makes the diagnosis of occupational asthma unlikely if the patient has returned to work for at least 2 weeks. The use of peak flow

monitoring at work for 2 weeks and away from work for 2 weeks may also help confirm the diagnosis. Finally, challenge testing with the specific suspected agent is of limited usefulness. A positive challenge test may confirm the diagnosis, but a negative test may not be helpful if the wrong agent is applied.[9] Because of the complexity associated with diagnosing occupational asthma and also the potential legal implications associated with the diagnosis, early and proper referral is important.

Once the diagnosis of occupational asthma with latency, such as isocyanate-induced asthma, is confirmed, the patient should be removed from her or his work or transferred to another job without the same exposure. Returning to the previous position, even with respiratory protection or improved ventilation, is usually not possible because even exposure with very low concentrations of the inciting agent can trigger the attack. Patients with occupational asthma may return to work when sufficient ventilation and respiratory protection are implemented.[9] The pharmacologic treatment of occupational asthma does not differ from standard asthma therapy (bronchodilator, inhaled steroids).

Dermatologic System

Most solvents that painters use cause a defatting dermatitis (Table 25-2). Others are sensitizers and irritants, such as chromates, isocyanates, epoxy resins, and sodium diocytl sulfosuccinate.

Hepatic System

Unlike some of the chlorinated hydrocarbons such as carbon tetrachloride and chloroform, aromatic and aliphatic hydrocarbons are considered unlikely to cause liver damage. However, acute liver necrosis and steatosis have been reported with large exposures to xylene.[52] The hepatorenal syndrome has been reported in toluene abusers (glue sniffers).[56] While most studies did not find significant correlation between normal occupational exposures and liver injuries,[39,46] others identify a cluster of painters with reversible focal liver necrosis and steatosis among a group of painters suspected of solvent intoxication and dementia and without significant alcohol consumption by history.[16] A more recent study also demonstrated mildly elevated liver

Table 25-2 The most common causes of dermatitis

Class of compound	Common examples
Solvents	Toluene, xylene, acetone, turpentine
Pigments	Zinc chromate, triglycidyl isocyanurate
Binders	Toluene 2,4-diisocyanates, hexamethylene diisocyanate
Biocides	Tributyl tin oxide, mercuric acetate
Binders	Linseed oil, epoxy resins, phenolic resins
Initiators	Methyl methacrylate, benzoyl peroxide
Hardeners	Aziridine[26]

function test with solvent exposures, but the interaction between solvent exposure and potentially hepatic toxic medications or solvents may be important.[47] Based on the current available evidence, painters are unlikely to be at risk for liver damages. There may be a higher risk in those with significant alcohol consumption or on potentially hepato-toxic medications.

Neoplasms

Some of the chemicals in paints are known carcinogens or mutagens. Benzo[*a*] pyrene, a polycyclic aromatic hydro-carbon contaminant found in carbon black pigments, is a known carcinogen responsible for causing scrotal cancer among the English chimney sweeps and mulespinners.[61] Studies of the carbon black identity have not demonstrated any increased cancer risk.[33] Solvents such as benzene and the chlorinated hydrocarbons (carbon tetrachloride, chloro-form, tetrachloroethylene, and trichloroethylene) are car-cinogens in animals (see the chapter about dry cleaners). The exposure to these hydrocarbons in painters is probably minimal. However, carcinogenic potential exists with sty-rene, xylene, and toluene because of their potentially toxic metabolites[66] (see the chapters on printers and the plastics industry).

Current evidence suggests an increased risk of certain malignancies among painters and paint manufacturers. Painters were found to have a higher risk for bladder and other urologic cancers, multiple myeloma, lung cancer, and stomach cancer.[5,19] Paint manufacturers were found to have an excess risk of acute leukemia and cancers of the lungs, esophagus, bladder, liver, skin, and colon.[5] Because of the complexity and the variety of the paint constituents, it is not possible to pinpoint the responsible agents.

Other Toxins

Painter's colic (lead). The advent of relatively inexpen-sive white-lead paint in the seventeenth century marks the expanded uses of paints. Lead toxicity was prevalent among painters at one time. In a review of occupational disease in Illinois in 1913, Alice Hamilton concluded that painters accounted for 30% of all occupational lead toxicity. *Painter's colic* denotes the common gastrointestinal symp-toms of lead toxicity, which were seen in more than 80% of the cases.[10] Painter's colic is an occupational disease of the past because most paints do not contain lead currently. Titanium dioxide and other pigments have supplanted lead. Currently, all interior paints are restricted by law to contain no more than 0.06% lead by weight, but some commercial paints still contain lead (up to 90% by weight). The other major factor in the reduction of lead exposure is related to the preparation of paints. In the past, by coloring their own paints with raw pigments, painters increased their exposure risk. Much of the paint today is premixed. Painters also risk lead exposure when they remove or prepare a surface containing leaded paint. Red lead (Pb_3O_4) remains an important weather-resistant coating for metals, particularly for bridges, ships, railways, and other iron or steel struc-tures.[11,40,42,53,59] The route of exposure may be secondary to inhalation of lead vapor or ingestion of the dust particles, resulting from mechanical abrasion of the paint (e.g., sand-blasting) and welding or torching of paint-coated steel structures. The use of heat guns is currently prohibited in the United States for removal of leaded paint. Lead vapor is particularly dangerous because it is readily absorbed through the alveoli and can penetrate the blood-brain barrier.[22] Acute encephalopathy may result from the lead vapor exposure (see the chapter on smelters).

Mercury. Phenylmercuric acetate was one of the most common biocides (for mold and mildew). Contact with it can cause a child to develop acrodynia, a childhood form of mercury toxicity that was last reported in 1990. This disease prompted the ultimate removal of mercury from interior paints.[49] Organic mercury affects the CNS system and causes tremors, shyness, emotional lability, nervousness, memory deficits, and diminution of psychomotor skills. Acrodynia symptoms are presence of erythematous rash and peeling of the hands, feet, and nose; fever; splenomegaly; irritability; insomnia; personality changes; and generalized weakness. These symptoms are quite similar to Kawasaki's disease except for acrodynia's lack of effects on the coronary arteries. Although mercury toxicity has not been reported in painters, indoor exposures and toxicity from recently applied mercury-containing paints have been reported.[27,50]

FURNITURE REFINISHERS

Since many of the chemicals used in varnishes and stripping fluids are similar to those used in other painting processes, furniture refinishers have similar exposures. However, there are some additional risks. Methylene chloride is a common agent for stripping old paints and varnishes from the furniture that is metabolized to carbon monoxide.[60] Because of the sanding process, wood dust poses additional problems for furniture refinishers. Wood dust may act as irritants and cause acute respiratory symptoms. Certain woods, such as western red cedar and eastern white cedar, are known causes of allergic reactions and reactive airway diseases[9,48] (see the chapter about carpenters). Tannins, which are polyphenols present in wood, are known animal carcinogens. The amount of tannin exposure correlates to the use of hard woods (e.g., oak, chestnut, mahogany) and the amount of wood dust exposure.[6] Epidemiologic studies have substantiated the increased risk of nasal cancer, particularly nasal adenocar-cinoma among woodworkers.[54] Although tannins are highly suspect as playing a significant role in carcinogenesis, the exact responsible agents have not been defined.

BATHTUB REFINISHERS

Bathtub refinishing is similar to other painting processes, with some variation in the technique and the chemicals applied. Initially, the porcelain surface is prepared by etching with hydrofluoric acid or ammonia bifluoride. The paint or porcelain used is then activated by a catalyst such as toluene 2,4-diisocyanate and applied by spraying. Because this procedure is often performed in a relatively enclosed environment in a home, the amount of the exposure could be significant. Hypersensitivity pneumonitis (bathtub refinisher's lung) secondary to diisocyanate has been reported with the bathtub refinishing process.[21]

REFERENCES

1. Astrand I: Uptake of solvents from the lungs, *Br J Ind Med* 42:217, 1985.
2. Baker EL, Fine LJ: Solvent neurotoxicity. The current evidence, *J Occup Med* 28:126, 1986.
3. Baker EL et al: Neurobehavioral effects of solvents in construction painters, *J Occup Med* 30:116, 1988.
4. Benowitz NL: Cardiotoxicity in the workplace, *Occup Med* 7:465, 1992.
5. Bethwaite PB, Pearce N, Fraser J: Cancer risk in painters: study based on the New Zealand cancer registry, *Br J Ind Med* 47:742, 1990.
6. Bianco MA, Savolainen H: Woodworker's exposure to tannins, *J Appl Toxicol* 14:293, 1994.
7. Brackbill RM, Maizlish N, Fischbach T: Risk of neuropsychiatric disability among painters in the United States, *Scand J Work Environ Health* 16:182, 1990.
8. Brugsch HG, Elkins HB: Toluene di-isocyanate (TDI) toxicity, *N Engl J Med* 268:353, 1963.
9. Chan-Yeung M, Malo JL: Occupational asthma, *N Engl J Med* 333:107, 1995.
10. Cherniack MG: Diseases of unusual occupations: an historical perspective, *Occup Med* 7:369, 1992.
11. Christophers AJ: Lead intoxication in paint removal workers, *Med J Aust* 146:559, 1987.
12. Colvin M et al: A cross-sectional survey of neurobehavioral effects of chronic solvent exposure on workers in a paint manufacturing plant, *Environ Res* 63:122, 1993.
13. Cullen MR, Cherniack MG, Rosenstock L: Occupational medicine, *N Engl J Med* 322:594, 1990.
14. Daniell W et al: The contributions to solvent uptake by skin and inhalation exposure, *Am Ind Hyg Assoc J* 53:124, 1992.
15. Demers RY, Markell BL, Wabeke R: Peripheral vibratory sense deficits in solvent-exposed painters, *J Occup Med* 33:1051, 1991.
16. Dossing M et al: Liver damage associated with occupational exposure to organic solvents in house painters, *Eur J Clin Invest* 13:151, 1983.
17. Edling C et al: Long term followup of workers exposed to solvents, *Br J Ind Med* 47:75, 1990.
18. Elofsson S et al: Exposure to organic solvents: a cross-sectional epidemiologic investigation on occupationally exposed car and industrial spray painters with special reference to the nervous system, *Scand J Work Environ Health* 6:239, 1980.
19. Engholm G, Englund A: Cancer incidence and mortality among Swedish painters. In Englund A, Ringen K, Mehlman M, editors: *Occupational health hazards of solvents,* Princeton, 1982, Princeton Scientific Publishing.
20. Fidler A, Baker EL, Letz RE: Neurobehavioral effects of occupational exposure to organic solvents among construction painters, *Br J Ind Med* 44:292, 1987.
21. Fink JN, Schlueter DP: Bathtub refinisher's lung: an unusual response to toluene diisocyanate, *Am Rev Respir Dis* 118:955, 1978.
22. Fischbein A et al: Lead poisoning from do it-yourself heat guns for removing lead-based paint: report of two cases, *Environ Res* 24:425, 1981.
23. Gade A, Mortensen EL, Bruhn P: Chronic painter's syndrome. A reanalysis of psychological test data in a group of diagnosed cases, based on comparisons with matched controls, *Acta Neurol Scand* 77:293, 1988.
24. Hane M et al: Psychological function changes among house painters, *Scand J Work Environ Health* 3:91, 1977.
25. Hanninen H et al: Behavioral effects of long-term exposure to a mixture of organic solvents, *Scand J Work Environ Health* 4:240, 1976.
26. Hansen MK, Larsen M, Cohr KH: Waterborne paints. A review of their chemistry and toxicology and the results of determinations made during their use, *Scand J Work Environ Health* 13:473, 1987.
27. Hirschman SZ, Feingold M, Boylen G: Mercury in house paint as a cause of acrodynia: effect of therapy with N-acetyl-D,L-penicillamine, *N Engl J Med* 269:889, 1963.
28. Hooisma J et al: Symptoms indicative of the effects of organic solvent exposure in Dutch painters, *Neurotoxicol Teratol* 16:613, 1994.
29. Hormes JT, Filley CM, Rosenberg NL: Neurologic sequelae of chronic solvent vapor abuse, *Neurology* 36:698, 1986.
30. Hunting KL, Matanoski GM, Barson M: Solvent exposure and the risk of slips, trips, and falls among painters, *Am J Ind Med* 20:353, 1996.
31. Husman K: Symptoms of car painters with long-term exposure to a mixture of organic solvents, *Scand J Work Environ Health* 6:19, 1980.
32. Husman K, Karli P: Clinical neurological findings among car painters exposed to a mixture of organic solvents, *Scand J Work Environ Health* 6:33, 1980.
33. Ingalls TH, Risques-Iribarren R: Periodic search for cancer in the carbon black industry, *Arch Environ Health* 2:249, 1961.
34. Kennedy AL, Brown WE: Isocyanates and lung disease: experimental approaches to molecular mechanisms, *Occup Med* 7:301, 1992.
35. Kennedy SM: Acquired airway hyperresponsiveness from nonimmunogenic irritant exposure, *Occup Med* 7:287, 1992.
36. Klinken L, Arlien-Soborg P: Brain autopsy in organic solvent syndrome, *Acta Neurol Scand* 87:371, 1993.
37. Knave B et al: Long-term exposure to jet fuel. II. A cross-sectional epidemiological investigation on occupationally-exposed industry workers with special reference to the nervous system, *Scand J Work Environ Health* 4:19, 1978.
38. Kubic VL, Anders MW: Metabolism of dichloromethane to carbon monoxide. III. Studies on the mechanism of the reaction, *Biochem Pharmacol* 27:2349, 1978.
39. Kurppa K, Husman K: Car painters exposure to a mixture of organic solvents. Serum activities of liver enzymes, *Scand J Work Environ Health* 8:137, 1982.
40. Landrigan PJ et al: Exposure to lead from the Mystic River bridge: the dilemma of deleading, *N Engl J Med* 306:673, 1982.
41. Lazar RB et al: Mutifocal central nervous system damage caused by toluene abuse, *Neurology* 33:1337, 1983.
42. Lead poisoning in bridge demolition worker—Massachusetts, 38:687, 1989.
43. Lee SH, Lee SH: A study on the neurobehavioral effects of occupational exposure to organic solvents in Korean workers, *Environ Res* 60:227, 1993.
44. Leira HL et al: Cerebral magnetic resonance imaging and cerebral computerized tomography for patients with solvent-induced encephalopathy, *Scand J Work Environ Health* 18:68, 1992.
45. Linz DH et al: Organic solvent-induced encephalopathy in industrial painters, *J Occup Med* 28:119, 1986.
46. Lundberg I, Hakansson M: Normal serum activities of liver enzymes in Swedish paint industry workers with heavy exposure to organic solvents, *Br J Ind Med* 42:596, 1985.
47. Lundberg I et al: Liver function tests and urinary albumin in house painters with previous heavy exposure to organic solvents, *Occup Environ Med* 51:347, 1994.
48. Malo JL et al: Prevalence of occupational asthma among workers exposed to eastern white cedar, *Am J Respir Crit Care Med* 150:1697, 1994.

49. Mercury exposure from interior latex paint—*MMWR Morb Mortal Wkly Rep* Michigan, 39:125, 1990.

50. Miller BA, Blair A, Reed EJ: Extended mortality follow-up among men and women in a U.S. furniture workers union, *Am J Ind Med* 25:537, 1994.

51. Moen BE et al: Reduced performance in tests of memory and visual abstraction in seamen exposed to industrial solvents, *Acta Psychiatr Scand* 81:114, 1990.

52. Morley R et al: Xylene poisoning: a report on one fatal case and two cases of recovery after prolonged unconsciousness, *BMJ* 2:442, 1970.

53. Muijser H et al: Lead exposure during demolition of a steel structure coated with lead-based paints. II. Reversible changes in the conduction velocity of the motor nerves in transiently exposed workers, *Scand J Work Environ Health* 13:56, 1987.

54. Nylander LA, Dement JM: Carcinogenic effects of wood dust, *Am J Ind Med* 24:619, 1993.

55. Obaek P et al: Computed tomography and psychometric test performances in patients with solvent induced chronic toxic encephalopathy and healthy controls, *Br J Ind Med* 44:175, 1987.

56. O'Brien ET, Yeoman WB, Hobby JAE: Hepatorenal damage from toluene in a "glue sniffer," *BMJ* 2:29, 1971.

57. Parmeggiani L: Painting and varnishing. In *Encyclopedia of occupational health safety,* Geneva, 1983, International Labour Organisation.

58. Phillips KK, Peters JM: Isocyanates. In Sullivan JB Jr, Krieger GR, editors: *Hazardous materials toxicology,* Baltimore, 1992, Williams & Wilkins.

59. Pollock CA, Ibels LS: Lead intoxication in Sydney harbour bridge workers, *Aust N Z J Med* 18:46, 1988.

60. Rioux JP, Myers RA: Methyene chloride poisoning: a paradigmatic review, *J Emerg Med* 6:227, 1988.

61. Rom WN: Polycyclic aromatic hydrocarbons. In Rom WN, editor: *Environmental and occupational medicine,* Boston, 1983, Little, Brown.

62. Seaton A, Jellinek EH, Kennedy P: Major neurological disease and occupational exposure to organic solvents, *Q J Med* 305:707, 1992.

63. Seedorff L, Olsen E: Exposure to organic solvents. I. A survey of the use of solvents, *Ann Occup Hyg* 34:371, 1990.

64. Seguin P et al: Prevalence of occupational asthma in spray painters exposed to several types of isocyanates, including polymethylene polyphenylisocyanate, *J Occup Med* 29:340, 1987.

65. Seppalaminen AM: Neurophysiological aspects of the toxicity of organic solvents, *Scand J Work Environ Health* 11:61, 1985.

66. Toftgaard R, Gustafsson J: Biotransformation of organic solvents. A review, *Scand J Work Environ Health* 6:1, 1980.

67. Triebig G et al: Cross-sectional epidemiological study on neurotoxicity of solvents in paints and lacquers, *Int Arch Occup Environ Health* 60:233, 1988.

68. Wang JD, Chen JD: Acute and chronic neurological symptoms among paint workers exposed to mixtures of organic solvents, *Environ Res* 61:107, 1993.

69. Wieslander G et al: Occupational exposure to water-based paints and self-reported asthma, lower airway symptoms, bronchial hyperresponsiveness, and lung function, *Int Arch Occup Environ Health* 66:261, 1994.

70. World Health Organization: *Organic solvents and the central nervous system and diagnostic criteria,* Environmental Health Series No. 5, Copenhagen, 1985, WHO Regional Office for Europe.

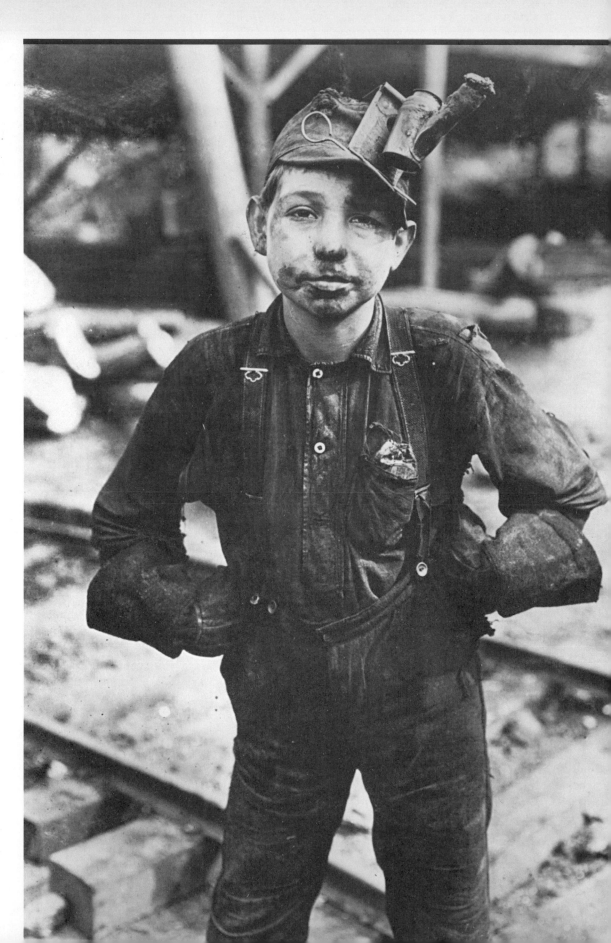

Mine "Tipple Boy,"
West Virginia Coal
Mine. Photograph by
Lewis Hine. 1908.
(Courtesy the Bettman
Archive)

26

Pediatric Laborers

Jeffrey C. Gershel

nicotine

- Illegal child labor continues to present a health hazard to children the world over

- Adolescents who are legally in the workplace may be at increased risk for occupational hazards

- Green tobacco sickness caused by nicotine represents one interesting occupational toxicity that particularly affects children

Childhood labor is defined as the paid employment of children younger than 16 years of age. Despite the fact that violations of appropriate child labor practices were thought to be a thing of the past, the numbers are definitely on the increase. The U.S. Department of Labor estimates that more than 4 million children under 16 years of age were employed in the United States in 1988. This number does not include those children who may be working off the books, in agriculture, in so-called street trades, or in sweatshops.[41]

Various significant socioeconomic factors have influenced the increasing number of working minors over the past decade. Among these factors, the following have been perhaps the most influential[35]:

1. A growing economy in the face of low unemployment has created an increasing need for unskilled workers.
2. More American children (20%) are now below the poverty line than 20 years ago. Consequently, the financial needs of these families represent a compelling reason to seek work.
3. Increasing illegal immigration to the United States has created a pool of children who are particularly vulnerable to exploitation because of their desperate financial needs and fear of discovery by immigration officials.
4. There has been an apparent relaxation of the enforcement of the federal child labor laws. In addition, with cutbacks in federal funding, there are fewer inspectors to ensure widespread compliance with the laws.

The situation with regard to child labor is substantially worse elsewhere in the world. According to the International Labor

Organization (ILO), at least 200 million children under 14 years of age are employed worldwide; in some countries, children comprise 20% to 50% of the workforce. Children are employed as rug weavers in the Middle East, underground tin miners in South America, and as metal workers, fireworks makers, textile weavers, and glass blowers in other countries. Particularly severe abuses occur in the so-called free enterprise zones, such as those that exist along the Mexico–United States border, where the labor and environmental laws are not generally strictly enforced.[30] The current ILO standards have designated 13 years as the minimum age at which children can undertake what has been termed "light work" and 15 years for other types of work.[46]

LEGISLATION IN THE UNITED STATES

In 1916, the first national child labor law, the Keating-Owen Act, established an 8-hour workday for children under 16 years of age and prohibited the interstate commerce of goods produced by children under 14 years of age. Nine months later, as a result of political pressure, this law was declared unconstitutional. In 1917, a second law imposed a 10% tax on the net profits of manufacturers who employed children younger than 14 years of age. Once again, this law was struck down, 5 years later in 1922. In the 1930s, the National Recovery Administration banned child labor in most industries for minors under 16 years of age; this standard was invalidated in 1935. Finally, in 1938, the Fair Labor Standards Act (FLSA) was passed. This act remains the major federal legislation that regulates the conditions under which children are employed. Its key provisions follow.[44]

Nonagricultural Jobs

1. No restrictions are imposed on youths who are at least 18 years old. Sixteen and 17-year-olds may perform any "nonhazardous" job, with no restrictions regarding hours. Fourteen and 15-year-olds may work during school hours, but there are limits on the number of hours a minor can work on a school day.
2. For persons under 18 years of age, employment is prohibited in any hazardous nonagricultural occupation. This includes jobs involved in mining, logging, brick and tile manufacture, roofing, and excavating. In addition, work involving meat processing, machinery, delicatessen slicers, and supermarket box crushers are specifically prohibited. There are no restrictions on newspaper delivery, media and theatrical productions, work performed for parents in solely owned businesses (except those involving manufacturing and/or hazardous jobs), and gathering evergreens and making wreaths.

Agricultural Jobs

In agriculture, hazardous work is prohibited for 12- to 15-year-olds. This includes handling category I or II pesticides and herbicides. However, all work on family farms is exempt (including if the child is under 12 years of age). There are no restrictions on the type or hours of work after the age of 16.

Recently, the ban on industrial piecework undertaken at home, also known as "industrial homework," has been repealed. This has resulted in children being exposed, at home, to solvents (electronic assembly) and to lead and cadmium (costume jewelry manufacture), among other toxins.[30] In addition, the School to Work Act of 1993 contains no specific provisions for occupational health and safety training of adolescents; these provisions, when addressed, are added on a state-by-state basis.[2]

MAGNITUDE OF THE PROBLEM

In September 1993, the entire issue of the *American Journal of Industrial Medicine* was devoted to the health hazards of children who work. However, virtually no data were presented concerning toxicologic exposures or injuries. There is little information available on the incidence or severity of work-related illnesses in children caused by toxic occupational exposures.[29] Since most of the hazardous exposure occurs in the context of illegal child labor, in small and difficult-to-access enterprises such as industrial homework, or in migrant populations,[28] it is difficult or even impossible to collect data or to effectively follow a cohort.

Similarly, specific information regarding childhood workplace injuries is limited, as these injuries may not be consistently reported or chronicled. Most injuries are underdiagnosed and, in fact, not reported. Often, adolescent minors do not seek medical attention or may not report that the injury even occurred at work for fear of loss of the job (especially if he or she is working illegally). In addition, physicians often neglect to obtain a complete history of occupational exposure in children.[30] What is known, at the very least, is that the number of American adolescents killed each year in work-related injuries is comparable to the number killed from falls, fires, and bicycles.[11] The risk of occupational injury is approximately 10 times greater for children employed under illegal conditions than for those working in compliance with the law.[27] It is reasonable to assume that toxic insults and exposures to working children would follow a similar pattern.

In New York, more than 1000 children and adolescents annually receive workers' compensation benefits.[7] This includes the categories of chemical burn, poisoning, and dermatitis. In Connecticut, a study of 16- and 17-year-olds found a work-related injury rate of 150 per 1000.[4] A review of trauma-related emergency room visits for 14- to 17-year-olds in Massachusetts showed that 7% to 13% of injuries requiring emergency care actually occurred in the workplace.[8] A survey of occupational injury deaths of 16- and 17-year-olds concluded that these workers are at greater risk than adults for death by electrocution, suffocation, drowning, poisoning, and natural and environmental factors.[9]

In the state of Texas, 30% of known child labor violations involve hazardous substances.[12] However, the entire magnitude of the problem is not clear as there are no reliable estimates of the number of working children, workers' compensation is voluntary in Texas (so many workers are not covered by the state surveillance system), and Texas does not require work permits for minors. In North Carolina, 86% of deaths of workers under age 18 involved circumstances that are reported to have violated the FLSA.[14]

INCREASED RISK FOR CHILDREN

It is not clear if the available adult data on toxicologic risks can be extrapolated to children. Children might be more susceptible to toxicologic exposure; almost no work has been done to explore this possibility. Some features that may increase the risk to children follow.

1. Physical differences, including an increased surface area (per kilogram of body weight) and a smaller size (increased dose in milligrams per kilogram; closer to the ground where toxins may settle). Also, children generally have more rapid respiratory rates (increased exposure of inhaled toxins) and different metabolism, so that detoxification mechanisms may not be fully developed.

2. Children exhibit significantly more hand-to-mouth activity than do adults.

3. Children are at greater risk for long-term accumulation and the effects of exposure after a long latency period. Some toxins (lead, polychlorinated biphenyls) can remain in body stores (bone, adipose) for many years, posing a long-term threat. The longer life expectancy of children (compared with adults) may translate into increased risk. Of particular concern are those substances noted to be possible carcinogens.

4. Children may also be more susceptible because of lack of experience in handling toxins, and the equipment used is generally designed for adult proportions.[44]

5. There is a concern that exposure in childhood may pose a reproductive risk later in life. Both lead and ethylene glycol ethers[38] fall into this category.

There are very few epidemiologic studies of the differences in susceptibility to toxins between children and adults. Research involving young workers and children exposed to lead reveals that at equal levels of exposure, children tend to absorb more lead and are more likely to develop irreversible neurologic complications than adults.[40] Children with blood lead levels above 120 mg per kilogram are reported to nearly always develop lead encephalopathy.[12] Workers in the slate pencil industry who develop silicosis have a higher mortality rate if they started work at younger ages.[43] Girls who began working at the age of 17 in spinning and weaving in a viscose fiber factory showed unfavorable changes in their cardiovascular and muscular systems by the end of the first year, as well as a higher general morbidity rate, when compared to those who started similar work at the age of 21. In an epidemiologic study on benzene exposure among 365 workers divided into three age groups, the youngest patients had not only the highest percentage of hematologic changes but also the worst. Higher rates of respiratory disease, as well as significant changes in hematological indices and physical development, occur in children from residential areas with excessively high concentrations of sulfur dioxide, nitrogen dioxide, carbon monoxide, and dust from nearby factories. Schoolchildren living in the vicinity of a cement plant have reduced mean values for forced expiratory volume.

SPECIFIC TOXINS

Despite the fact that few data regarding toxic hazards for child workers currently exist, it is possible that, for example, some cases of adolescent asthma might be related to occupational exposures to dust or sensitizing chemicals such as formaldehyde. Similarly, some cases of neurologic or behavioral dysfunction may be due to occupational exposure to solvents and pesticides, and some cases of leukemia and lymphomas may result from occupational exposure to benzene.[2]

Agricultural Industry

Agriculture is now considered to be one of the most dangerous industries. As mentioned before, child labor laws for agriculture are not as restrictive or protective as those for nonagricultural industries. Young children may work on family farms, minors as young as 12 can work on larger farms, and the handling of pesticides is prohibited only until 16 years of age.[48] In addition, child labor in agriculture often becomes a day care issue, as parents (especially migrant workers) often bring their young children into the fields because they lack accessible, affordable day care. Reliable data are lacking, but children account for a disproportionate share of farm fatalities and injuries.

Organophosphates

As mentioned previously, children may be at greater risk for exposure to pesticides because of their larger surface area–weight ratio, shorter height (closer to the leaves and ground), and increased hand-to-mouth behavior. The U.S. Department of Labor estimates that only 36% of farmworkers are covered by the Federal Sanitation Standard, which requires employers who hire more than 10 employees to provide in the field, free of charge, drinking water, toilets, and handwashing facilities.[34] Migrant workers may be housed in or near fields and be exposed to airborne pesticide drift, and irrigation water contaminated with pesticide runoff may be used for drinking and bathing. In a recent study, 48% of Mexican-American farmworkers reported working in fields while they were wet with pesticides, and 36% had been sprayed directly or indirectly by pesticide drift.[38] Although only a few states require mandatory reporting of pesticide-related illnesses, the EPA estimates as many as 300,000 cases a year.[46] There are possible associations between pesticide exposure and various types of cancer, including those involving lymphatic and hematopoietic systems, connective tissue, brain, prostate, skin, stomach, colon, and lip.[31] Also, there is increased risk of dermatitis. A review of 25 young patients with carbamate or organophospate intoxications reported that the most common presentation to the emergency department was central nervous system depression (coma, stupor, dyspnea, flaccidity).[42] Cholinergic symptoms were less common, and fasciculation and bradycardia were uncommon. In one study, children were found to suffer neuroophthalmologic impairments, including optic neuropathy, degeneration of the retina, and myopia, more frequently than adults.[24] These patients were sprayed with 3% malathion several times a year for 3 to 5 years. Also, some evidence suggests a link between acute organophosphate poisoning and chronic neurobehavioral changes.[39,41] A similar link has been observed with chronic organophosphate exposure.[26]

In addition, it is of great concern that DDT, lindane, chlordane, and heptachlor (organochlorine pesticides) are found in trace amounts in human breast milk despite the fact that, to date, no ill effects have been noted.[5] It is possible that the latency period is greater than the duration of any documented study, especially since pesticides are stored and tend to accumulate in adipose tissue.

Green Tobacco

Green tobacco sickness (GTS) was first reported in 1970[47] in a group of tobacco croppers, the youngest of whom was 9 years old. Age less than 30 was noted to be a significant risk factor,[10] and midadolescence represents the age when ability to work and susceptibility to toxicity result in peak incidence of disease.[20] This systemic illness results from absorption after dermal exposure to dissolved nicotine. Since nicotine is an alkaloid, it is soluble in water and can be drawn out of the leaf by rain, dew, or sweat.

GTS occurs most frequently in tobacco croppers who cut the tobacco leaves. During this process of cutting, a cropper's clothing can become saturated with dew and moisture from the plants after a few minutes of work. It is estimated that 100 ml of dew may contain as much as 9 mg of nicotine (equivalent to 6 cigarettes) and that croppers may be exposed to 600 ml of dew.[19] The disease is more common in Kentucky, where the burley tobacco is harvested by hand, than in North Carolina, South Carolina, and Virginia, where it is harvested by machine. In stringers, who place the leaves

on metal spikes, GTS is rare, as they wear aprons and gloves.[22]

Weakness, nausea, vomiting, dizziness, abdominal cramps, headache, and difficult breathing characterize GTS.[10] Some patients also demonstrate fluctuations in blood pressure or heart rate. The illness tends to have its onset about 10 hours after the patient began work, and it lasts for approximately 48 hours. Treatment is symptomatic, including antiemetics, fluids, rest, and thorough skin cleansing. In addition to the acute effects of nicotine exposure, there is a theoretical concern that nicotine can give rise to N-nitrosamines, which are proven carcinogens.[43] Rubberized nylon rainsuits[18] and rubber gloves[21] have both been shown to be effective in preventing GTS.

Service Sector Jobs

The service sector is currently the largest employer of adolescents, and the fast food industry is the single largest segment.[25] Teenagers are particularly attractive employees for the fast food industry because they do not generally command high wages, typically do not receive benefits, and are available to work during peak dinner hours. In this industry, minors are often subjected to physical as well as toxic hazards, with little or no training or supervision. Many minors work in this industry in violation of labor laws. A particular toxicologic concern for these workers is the effect of solvents and degreasers. Recent data regarding persons exposed to metal degreasers suggest a dose-response relation between cumulative solvent exposure and impaired psychometric test performance.[36]

Industry

Benzene. Unleaded gasoline contains 4% to 5% benzene, a known carcinogen. Adolescents are frequently employed at gasoline stations and may spend an entire day pumping gasoline with a significant risk of airborne and dermal exposure.[37] Benzene may also pose a reproductive risk. Results from a study evaluating maternal occupation in the year prior to a child's birth suggest an association between an increased risk of cancer and maternal exposure to benzene.[15] A similar finding comes from an English case-control study, which identified an association between paternal exposure to benzene and childhood leukemia.[33]

Formaldehyde and volatile organic compounds. Exposure to formaldehyde and volatile organic compounds occurs in many different industries and occupations. Formaldehyde exposure can occur in the garment industry. It is also found in new furniture, carpets, particleboard, and cigarette smoke. Exposure causes malaise, dizziness, eye irritation and tearing, and acute bronchospasm.[23,32] Specific data suggest that some cases of adolescent asthma may be related to occupational exposure to formaldehyde,[1] whereas chronic exposure has been linked to nasal malignancies.

Volatile organic compounds other than formaldehyde and benzene include propane, toluene, xylene, and halogenated compounds such as trichloroethane and trichloroethylene. These chemicals are found in paints, adhesives, cleansers, building materials and furnishings, dry-cleaned clothes, and gasoline.[17] Many are mucous membrane irritants that can cause gastrointestinal and respiratory symptoms. Some chlorinated solvents are suspected carcinogens.

Lead

Lead exposure can take place in many industries and employment sites, including brass and copper manufacturing, battery and aircraft manufacturing, painting, smelting, plumbing, firing ranges, and construction and bridge repair. While minor children are unlikely to be found employed at any of these sites or activities in the United States today, significant exposure does occur in other countries. One such situation arises in the cottage industry of lead reclamation from used lead-acid batteries. While most of this work is done on a rather extensive, high-volume scale by businesses whose goal is heavy metal reclamation and recycling, many home-based businesses perform the same function on a small scale. While the parents may be engaged in battery salvage in the basement, attic, or garage of the home, the children can be unknowingly exposed to volatilized lead in airborne dust in and around the house. In addition, it is well recognized that children are able to absorb a greater percentage of GI lead.[2] With lead dust from a home-based activity settling on food or eating utensils, children could suffer significant lead exposure. Since young children have a somewhat immature blood-brain barrier, small amounts of lead, when inhaled or ingested, can cause disastrous neurologic and neuropsychiatric consequences.[3] In fact, the most common presentation for acute lead intoxication in children is a toxic encephalopathy which may progress to coma, seizures, and sometimes death.

Another equally important and significant potential source for childhood lead exposure are parents engaged in lead industries or occupations who bring lead dust into the home on work clothes, shoes, and on hair and skin. Some specific parental occupations where lead exposure to children might be an issue are listed in the box at right.

An in depth discussion of the pathophysiology of lead is beyond the scope of this chapter. The reader is referred to other chapters in this text for more detailed information (see Chapter 36).

Asbestos. Minors can be exposed to asbestos during building abatement procedures. Asbestos exposure early in life is a risk factor for the later development of a mesothelioma. Asbestos may also be brought home by parents who may be exposed on the job.

Indoor air pollution. Workplace sources of sulfur dioxide, carbon monoxide, and nitrogen dioxide include improperly vented heaters and stoves and cigarette smoke.[48]

Parental Occupations that May Pose a Lead Exposure Threat to Children

Lead-acid battery industry
Home-based metal salvage
Painters
Bridge workers
Construction workers
Police officers, military personnel and others who might spend time on firing ranges
Home renovators (avocational or vocational)

There is a strong association between rates of chronic cough, bronchitis, and chest illnesses in preadolescents and measurements of particulate pollution, sulfur dioxide, and nitrogen dioxide. In addition, respiratory illness in childhood is a risk factor for respiratory illness later in life.

Working minors may smoke or be exposed to environmental tobacco smoke (ETS) from older co-workers. Among the known effects of ETS are wheezing and other respiratory illnesses, decreased lung function and FEV_1, decreased growth rate, increased rate of otitis media, hyperactivity, and a possibly increased risk of developing chronic obstructive pulmonary disease.[38]

OTHER CONCERNS

The possibility exists that birth defects and/or neurologic deficits may occur in the offspring of parents who experience occupational toxic exposures. The placenta may not be a barrier, as has been observed with lead, while polychlorinated biphenyls are excreted in breast milk. Also, the large number of rapidly dividing cells may increase the risk of carcinogens, such as diethylstilbestrol. There are some data associating paternal exposure to dyes and pigments, methyl ethyl ketone, and chlorinated hydrocarbon solvents with an increased risk of cancer.[39] Parental carbon monoxide exposure may cause reduced birth weight and delay postnatal growth. Recently, correlations were found between mental retardation in 10-year-olds and maternal occupation as a blue-collar worker in the textile and apparel industries. More of these mothers reported exposure to miscellaneous chemicals such as glue, ammonia, spray adhesives, and cleaning products.[13]

INTERNATIONAL CHILD LABOR

Even though the number of children at risk is prodigious in the United States, these numbers pale in comparison to the number of at-risk children, under the age of 15, reported from various countries around the world. The problem has not been characterized, although some world health bodies and various United Nations initiatives have at least begun to analyze the problem.

In 1959, the United Nations issued its "Declaration of Rights of the Child." This document stated, in part, that children "shall not be admitted to employment before an appropriate minimum age; in no case [shall children] be permitted to engage in any occupation or employment which would prejudice his/her health or education, or interfere with physical, mental, or moral development." Despite this strong admonition to protect working children, in 1987 the World Health Organization published its technical report 756, which reported that there is precious little compliance with these United Nations guidelines worldwide. Indeed, based upon WHO data for the developing nations of the world, the general health of working children is poor compared to the health of nonworking children. Their nutrition is poorer, their hemoglobin levels are lower, and they have a higher incidence of infectious diseases (including tuberculosis).

It is estimated that in developing nations at least 50 million children under the age of 15 are "economically active." In some countries such as Nepal and India, up to 50% of children under the age of 15 are reported to be employed full-time. The precise nature of the employment is unreported in almost all developing countries, and the potential for exposure to toxic hazards is, not surprisingly, almost completely unknown. These nations typically exert only weak legislative controls over child labor, especially where exposure to toxic hazards is concerned. Unfortunately, due to reluctance to confront and failure to report such abuses, we really know far too little about the nature, extent, and duration of toxic exposures to child workers in most developing nations. Much needs to be learned and even more needs to be corrected. It is up to organizations such as the United Nations, the World Health Organization, and the national governments of the more progressive nations of the world to begin to protect the world's children from toxic hazards in the workplace.

REFERENCES

1. American Academy of Pediatrics, Committee on Environmental Health: Ambient air pollution: Respiratory hazards to children, *Pediatrics* 91:1210, 1993.
2. American Academy of Pediatrics, *Committee on Environmental Health*: The hazards of child labor, *Pediatrics* 95 5:311, 1995.
3. American Academy of Pediatrics, Committee on Injury and Poisoning Prevention: Lead. In *Handbook of common poisonings in childhood* ed 3, Elk Grove Village, Ill, 1994, American Academy of Pediatrics.
4. Banco L, Lapidus G, Braddock M: Work-related injury among Connecticut minors, *Pediatrics* 89:957, 1992.
5. Baum C, Shannon M: Environmental toxins: cutting the risks, *Contemporary Pediatrics* 12:20, 1995.
6. Bellinger D et al: Low-level lead exposure and children's cognitive function in the preschool years, *Pediatrics* 87:219, 1991.
7. Belville R et al: Occupational injuries among working adolescents in New York State, *JAMA* 269:2754, 1993.
8. Brooks DR, Davis LK, Gallagher SS: Work-related injuries among Massachusetts children: a study based on emergency department data, *Am J Ind Med* 24:313, 1993.
9. Castillo D, Landen DD, Layne LA: Occupational injury deaths of 16- and 17-year-olds in the United States, *Am J Public Health* 84:646, 1994.
10. Centers for Disease Control: Green tobacco sickness in tobacco harvesters—Kentucky, 1992, *MMWR Morb Mortal Wkly Rep* 42:237, 1993.
11. Children's Safety Workplace: *A data book of child and adolescent injury,* Washington, DC, 1991, National Center for Education in Maternal and Child Health.
12. Cooper RP, Rothstein MA: Health hazards among working children in Texas, *South Med J* 88:550, 1995.
13. Decouflé P et al: Mental retardation in ten-year old children in relation to their mother's employment during pregnancy, *Am J Ind Med* 24:567, 1993.
14. Dunn KA, Runyan CW: Deaths at work among children and adolescents, *Am J Dis Child* 147:1044, 1993.
15. Feingold L, Savitz DA, John EM: Use of a job-exposure matrix to evaluate parental occupation and childhood cancer, *Cancer Causes Control* 3:161, 1992.
16. Fischbein A: Occupational and environmental lead exposure. In Rom WN, editor: *Environmental and occupational medicine,* ed 3, Boston, 1992, Little, Brown.
17. Flanagan RJ et al: An introduction to the clinical toxicology of volatile substances, *Drug Saf* 5:359, 1990.
18. Gehlbach SH, Williams WA, Freeman JI: Protective clothing as a means of reducing nicotine absorption in tobacco harvesters, *Arch Environ Health* 34:111, 1979.
19. Gehlbach SH, Williams WA, Perry LD: Nicotine absorption by workers harvesting green tobacco, *Lancet* 1:478, 1975.
20. Gehlbach SH et al: Green-tobacco sickness: an illness of tobacco harvesters, *JAMA* 229:1880, 1974.
21. Ghosh SK et al: Protection against "green symptoms" from tobacco in Indian harvesters: a preliminary intervention study, *Arch Environ Health* 42:121, 1987.
22. Hipke ME: Green tobacco sickness, *South Med J* 1993; 86: 989-992.
23. Horvath EP et al: Effects of formaldehyde on the mucous membranes and lungs: a study of an industrial population, *JAMA* 259:701, 1988.
24. Ishikawa S et al: Chronic intoxication of organophosphate pesticide and its treatment, *Folia Med Cracov* 34:139, 1993.
25. Kinney JA: Health hazards to children in the service industries, *Am J Ind Med* 24:291, 1993.
26. Korsak RJ, Sato MM: Effects of chronic organophosphate pesticide exposure on the central nervous system, *Clin Toxicol* 11:83, 1977.
27. Landrigan PJ, Belville R: The dangers of illegal child labor, *Am J Dis Child* 147:1029, 1993 (editorial).
28. Landrigan PJ, Pollack SH, Belville R: Child labor. In Rom WN, editor: *Environmental and occupational medicine,* ed 3, Boston, 1992, Little, Brown.
29. Landrigan PJ et al: Child labor in the United States: historical background and current crisis, *Mt Sinai J Med* 59:498, 1992.
30. Landrigan PJ et al: Child labor, *Pediatr Ann* 24:657, 1995.
31. Maroni M, Fait A: Health effects in man from long-term exposure to pesticides, *Toxicology* 78:1, 1993.
32. Martin DF: Chemical hazards in the home/workplace: plywood and phenol-formaldehyde resins, *Florida J Public Health* 3:19, 1991.
33. McKinney PA et al: Parental occupations of children with leukemia in west Cumbria, north Humberside, and Gateshead, *BMJ* 302:681, 1991.
34. Occupational Safety and Health Administration: 29 CFR Part 128: field sanitation; final rule, *Fed Reg* 52:16050, 1987.
35. Pollack SH, Landrigan PJ: Child labor in 1990: prevalence and health hazards, *Annu Rev Public Health* 11:359, 1990.

36. Rasmussen K, Jeppesen J, Sabroe S: Psychometric tests for assessment of brain function after solvent exposure, *Am J Ind Med* 24:553, 1993.

37. Rinsky RA et al: Benzene and leukemia: an epidemiologic assessment, *N Engl J Med* 316:104, 1987.

38. Rosenstock L, Cullen MR: *Textbook of clinical, occupational and environmental medicine,* Philadelphia, 1994, WB Saunders.

39. Rosenstock L et al: Chronic nervous system effects of acute organophosphate pesticide intoxication, *Lancet* 338:223, 1991.

40. Samuel HD: Regulation of child labor revisited, *Am J Ind Med* 24:269, 1993.

41. Savage EP et al: Chronic neurological sequelae of acute organophosphate pesticide poisoning, *Arch Environ Health* 43:38, 1988.

42. Sofer S, Tal A, Sahak E: Carbamate and organophosphate poisoning in early childhood, *Pediatr Emerg Care* 5:222, 1989.

43. Ulrich S: Haze still surrounds green tobacco sickness, *J Natl Cancer Inst* 86:419, 1994 (news).

44. United States Department of Labor, Employment Standards Administration, Wage and Hour Division: *Handy reference guide to the Fair Labor Standards Act,* WHD Publication 1282, Washington, DC, 1990, US Government Printing Office.

45. United States General Accounting Office: Hired farmworkers: health and well-being at risk, GAO/HRD-92-46, Washington, DC, 1992, US Government Printing Office.

46. Waldron HA: Danger: children at work, *Br J Ind Med* 45:73, 1988 (editorial).

47. Weizenecker R, Deal WB: Tobacco cropper's sickness, *J Florida* 57:13, 1970.

48. Wilk VA: Health hazards to children in agriculture, *Am J Ind Med* 24:283, 1993.

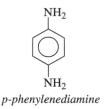

p-phenylenediamine

- Photographers can obtain many hazardous substances and frequently experiment to produce unusual photographic effects

- p-Phenylenediamine is a potent sensitizer and causes contact dermatitis that progresses to lichen planus

Photographers and Film Developers

Steven G. Turchen

Scott D. Phillips

OCCUPATIONAL EXPOSURES

Photographers work in a variety of situations. These conditions include darkrooms, locations, theatrical fogs, smokes, and a variety of outdoor conditions. In addition to chemical hazards, darkroom workers often work without adequate ventilation systems, particularly in smaller facilities. Contact with plants and animals is common, either on location or while they are subjects or props in the studio.

This group of workers might be exposed to new chemicals as processing techniques change. Developers might experiment with a variety of photographic processes in an effort to achieve a certain stylistic effect. Photographers try novel combinations of different processes empirically in an attempt to achieve a desired "look" for the final print. Recipes for processes utilizing gold, palladium, platinum, chromium, mercury, vanadium, and uranium salts are available in photography references.[1,3,4] The toxicity of many of these salts in nonphotographic occupations is discussed elsewhere in this text. Chemicals are surprisingly easy to obtain through retail outlets or mail order houses that cater to photographers.[1] Because this is a hobby, fume hoods, face shields, eye wash stations, and other safety measures common in larger laboratory settings are virtually nonexistent in smaller photographic labs.[12]

Safety materials are becoming more available. Concern for health does seem to be increasing for this trade, which is evident by the growing number of safety guides intended for photographers. Recent books on photographic laboratory techniques contain chapters on chemical safety issues. Those who work in larger laboratories are more likely to have access and knowledge on material safety data sheets (MSDSs). Photography journals have also been addressing safety issues, but the quality of safety information provided in articles is often incomplete. Recommendations to wear dust masks when mixing dry chemicals, to work with adequate ventilation, and to wear gloves when handling photochemistry are becoming common. However, advice on proper first aid is questionable.[1]

Technologic advances have done more to improve photographic safety than has education. Commercial photolabs using automated processors have substantially reduced chemical exposures for some workers. The amount of dermal contact with photochemistry is reduced by proper utilization of automated systems. Automated processing greatly reduces the incidence of occupational dermatitis in this branch of the industry.[11] Digital photography is evolving rapidly and in some instances has replaced film-based technology for capturing images. Printing of digitized images requires the use of photostatic and other processes that utilize a variety of dyes or toners in the work environment. A partial list of chemicals used in the photographic industry is in the box below.

TOXICOLOGIC EXPOSURES

It is useful for the clinician to have some understanding of the different processes photographers use. The familiar photograph is produced on films and papers coated with a gelatin emulsion containing light-sensitive grains of silver halide. Development selectively reduces light-exposed silver halide to metallic silver while leaving nonexposed silver halide in a soluble form. Developers are alkaline solutions that usually contain an aromatic developing agent. Hydroquinone and aminophenol are examples of black and white developing

agents.[8] Color developers are based on p-phenylenediamine or its congeners. Color developers act by oxidizing dye precursors, known as *couplers,* into visible dyes. The couplers may be present in the emulsion or in the developer. A typical coupler is α-naphthol. Development is halted by immersing the film or paper in an acidic solution (stop bath), almost always dilute acetic acid.[8] Immersing photographic film in wide, flat containers of developer and fixer solutions is an important vector of exposure. These tray characteristics lend to increased vaporization of the solutions because of their large surface areas. This, combined with poor ventilation systems, increases the risk of the individual to these hazards. Absorption in this environment is by dermal and inhalation routes.

Fixation is the stabilization of the developed image. Solutions of sodium or ammonium thiosulfate are used to dissolve away residual silver halides.[8] Prints and films are then washed, and black-and-white prints are often toned with selenium, gold, or a similar toner. Specific agents involved in the processing of images are shown in Table 27-1.

Major Toxins

Developers. Developers can cause a variety of toxic effects, depending on their formulation. Developers, at working strength, are generally alkaline. However, the concentrations typically used render them to be only irritants. Kits for mixing special purpose developers commonly contain alkaline corrosives. For example, potassium hydroxide pellets are an ingredient of Rodinal included in commercial kits. Many aromatic developers are skin or respiratory sensitizers.

Developers also often contain various sulfites used to stabilize prepared solutions that may contribute to sensitization. Contact dermatitis, lichen planus, and other dermatoses are well documented for many developers (see following section). Ingestion of developers is not uncommon in black-and-white labs. Many photographers who work in improvised labs acknowledge occasionally dipping a finger into a solution and then licking to distinguish developer from fixer; each has a characteristic taste.

Color labs require work in total darkness, and the author

Chemicals Used in the Photography Trade

Acetic acid	Mercuric chloride
α-naphthol	Metol
Aminophenol	p-Phenylenediamine
Ammonium thiosulfate	Platinum
Bromides	Palladium
Caustics	Potassium ferrocyanide
Chromic acid	Pyrogallic acid
Chromium	Selenium
Dyes	Silver nitrate
Formaldehyde	Silver halide
Gold salts	Sulfuric acid
Hydroquinone	Sulfur dioxide
Iodides	Uranium nitrate
Iron salts	Vanadium salts

Table 27-1 Photographic hazards by specific process

Process	Hazard
Process steps	Chemical agents
Developing baths	Hydroquinone, p-phenylenediamine, alkalis
Stop bath	Acetic acid
Fixing bath	Sulfur dioxide
Intensifier	Chromates, hydrochloric acids
Toning	Selenium compounds, hydrogen sulfide, uranium nitrate, sulfur dioxide
Color processing	Formaldehyde, solvents, p-phenylenediamine

has consulted on patients with severe gastritis as a consequence of confusing a glass of soft drink with a beaker of chemistry. Some developers contain solvents that are hazardous. Some liquid developers contain significant amounts of diethylene glycol, which in large quantities might cause central nervous system depression, high anion-gap metabolic acidosis, and renal failure.

Toning solutions. Toners are used in black-and-white photography to stabilize the image. Toners alter the color tone and contrast of the final image. Toners of greatest toxicologic concerns include selenium toner (probably the most widely used toner) and some rare formulations based on soluble heavy metal salts, including gold and uranium. Because of its ubiquitous nature, selenium toner would pose the greatest risk of toxic exposure. Despite its almost universal use by fine arts photographers, there have been no reports of acute or chronic toxicity from this product. Recognition of selenium toxicity is often difficult. Signs of chronic selenium toxicity include color changes or loss of hair or nails, elevated liver transaminases, gastrointestinal distress, and dermatitis. Acutely, inhalation of vapor can cause acute respiratory distress. The diagnosis of selenium toxicity is by appropriate history, clinical findings, and whole-blood selenium levels. Treatment of selenium poisoning is symptomatic and supportive. There is currently no effective chelating agent for selenium toxicity.[15] Bleaching (see later in this chapter) is required for some toning processes.

Stop bath. Dilute stop bath is acetic acid diluted with water to a pH of 4 to 5. At this dilution, it is not corrosive. Stock solutions of glacial acetic acid used by many photographers are extremely hazardous and often handled without adequate personal protective equipment.

Fixation solutions. Fixing solutions contain either sodium or ammonium thiosulfate. Both are of low toxicity. Old solutions of either can have a foul sulfur odor. Ammonium thiosulfate solutions can also have an ammonia odor. Either might produce respiratory irritation, especially in the poorly ventilated darkroom. Spent solutions are stored separately from other darkroom chemicals. They are disposed of as hazardous wastes or treated to remove dissolved silver in the spent fixer. The silver in the spent fixer is an environmental hazard, not an occupational hazard. The special handling given to fixer may cause some photography workers to become anxious about their exposure to spent fixer.

Cleaning agents. Film cleaner formulations vary, but almost all are based on aliphatic solvents. Heptane is a common ingredient. All too often, these volatile cleaners are used in poorly ventilated areas. The hazards of exposure to aliphatic solvents has been discussed elsewhere. Tray cleaners are typically acidic. Chromic acid based products are undoubtedly the most hazardous and produce both local and systemic symptoms from small body surface area burns. Chromates are discussed at length elsewhere.

Bleach. Potassium ferroyanide is used to bleach image silver. Although it is often feared by darkroom workers, the cyanide is tightly bound. Ferroyanide is an irritant and has low hazard potential.

Alternative processes. Alternative processes are techniques that use emulsions that are not based on gelatin silver to capture a latent image. The most popular alternative processes are platinum-palladium and gum bichromate. Both processes require the use of hexavalent chromium salts. Photography workers are seldom poisoned by the heavy metals. should be cautioned to use safer processes.

PATHOPHYSIOLOGY OF COLOR FILM DEVELOPERS
Dermal Effects of Photochemistry

Contact dermatitis, contact allergy, and a lichen planus (LP) as lesions occur as a consequence of exposure to color developers that are congeners of p-phenylenediamine[2,7,13] and less commonly from black-and-white developers.[13] There has been some controversy as to whether the lichen planus associated with color developers is a local effect or from the inhalation of vapors of the color developer solutions. The development of lichen planus associated with color developers has been described as following two courses: The first is a lesion of gradual onset that is clinically and histologically identical to lichen planus, with mucosal and sometimes glans and foreskin involvement. The second is a rapid-onset dermatitis that usually occurs in patients acutely and significantly exposed to the developer.[5] The dermatitis in the latter case was described as spreading rapidly and over several days to develop lichenoid characteristics. The existence of progressive LP from contact with developers has been challenged in more recent studies of the epidemiology and symptomatology of occupational exposure to these developers. Rashes are seen temporally related to exposure and resolved (over weeks) after exposure. Development of this rash has also been reported during the servicing of automatic self-photographing machines.[9] The LP symptoms returned upon reexposure and seemed be generally a consequence of direct skin contact with developer.[10] Three separate histopathologic pictures associated with color developer exposure are contact dermatitis, lichen planus, and a mixed lesion with features of both.[10] Cross-reactivity between different developer components has been reported.[7] Patients with occupational LP are usually patch test positive to developers, while LP patients without exposure to developers are typically patch test negative.[15] Treatment is symptomatic. Avoiding exposure is probably the most effective recommendation.

CONCLUSION

It is important to recognize that dental personnel, automated x-ray services, and hospital and office staff are also at increased risk from these agents. When in contact with these solutions, workers should always wear rubber gloves and eyewear protection. Accidental splashes from these agents might cause significant eye injury. Though contact lenses may block splashes from striking the cornea, vapors may absorb into them. The major risks are for sensitization to specific agents and caustic injury. The development of LP occurs, though infrequently, in this trade. Knowledge of the process chemicals and proper use of personal protective equipment will assist in limiting health complaints.

REFERENCES

1. Anchell SG: *The darkroom cookbook,* Boston, 1994, Focal Press.
2. Brandao FM: Colour developers and lichen planus, *Contact Dermatitis* 15:233, 1986.
3. Clerc LP: *Photography theory and practice,* New York, 1970, Focal Press.
4. Crawford W: *The keepers of light,* New York, 1979, Morgan & Morgan.
5. De Graciansky P, Boulle S: Skin disease from color developers, *Br J Dermatol* 78:297, 1966.
6. Eaton GT: *Photographic chemistry,* New York, 1986, Morgan & Morgan.
7. Goh CL, Kwok SF, Rajan VS: Cross sensitivity in colour developers, *Contact Dermatitis* 10:280, 1984.
8. James TH, Higgins GC: *Fundamentals of photographic theory,* New York, 1948, John Wiley & Sons.
9. Kersey PM, Stevenson CJ: Lichenoid eruption due to colour developer. A new occupational hazard of servicing automatic self-photographing machines, *Contact Dermatitis* 6:503, 1980.
10. Liden C: Occupational dermatoses at a film laboratory, *Contact Dermatitis* 10:77, 1984.
11. Liden C: Occupational dermatoses at a film laboratory. Follow-up after modernization, *Contact Dermatitis* 20:191, 1989.
12. Marlenga B, Parker-Conrad JE: Knowledge of occupational hazards in photography: a pilot study, *AAOHN J* 41:175, 1993.
13. Roed-Petersen J, Menne T: Allergic contact dermatitis and lichen planus from black-and-white photographic developing, *Cutis* 18:699, 1976.
14. Sollenberg J et al: Contact allergy to developing agents. Analysis of test preparations, bulk chemicals and tank solutions by HPLC, *Dermatosen in Beruf und Umwelt* 37:47, 1989.
15. Thomas DJ: Selenium. In Sullivan JB, Krieger GR, editors: *Hazardous materials toxicology,* Baltimore, 1992, Williams & Wilkins.

28

CFCl$_3$ CF$_2$Cl$_2$
freon 11   *freon 12*

- Asbestos and lead are important toxins that are less common exposures for plumbers

- Solder flux asthma is caused by colophony

- The increased use of plastic pipes will result in more solvent exposures

- Fluorocarbons are cardiac, CNS, and pulmonary toxins but rarely result in occupational toxicity

Plumbers

Richard J. Hamilton

OCCUPATIONAL DESCRIPTION

Plumbers and pipefitters install, maintain, and repair many different types of pipe systems. Steamfitters install pipe systems for liquids or gases under high pressure. Sprinklerfitters install automatic fire sprinkler systems. Plumbers and pipefitters held 351,000 jobs in 1992. Two thirds worked for mechanical and plumbing contractors engaged in new construction, repair, modernization, or maintenance work. One of six plumbers and pipefitters is self-employed.

TOXIC EXPOSURES
Soldering

Soldering utilizes a filler material that melts below 450° C (lead, zinc, or silver alloy) to join two metal surfaces. The effort to reduce lead exposure produced lead-free solders that are 4% silver and 96% tin. Some solders have a core of flux; others are solid. Fluxes are added to enhance the adherence of the solder to the surfaces and promote an even flow of solder when heated. Flux paste contains ZnCl and NH$_3$Cl in a petrolatum base. Flux paste is applied with a brush prior to joining and soldering the metals. Solder with a flux core is either corrosive (zinc chloride or hydrochloric acid) or noncorrosive (typically the highly allergenic pine resin, colophony). This material spreads with the melting solder. During this process, flux is heated and creates a flux vapor. If an acidic flux is used, respiratory irritant symptoms occur only after unusually high exposures. Colophony flux is a pine oil resin that acts as a sensitizer as well as an irritant. Thus, symptoms of bronchospasm occur on first exposure and at lower concentrations thereafter.

Solvents and Cements

Plastic pipes have revolutionized the plumbing industry. The ease of handling and the diverse applicability (pressure, heat, fluids) make them the first choice for many

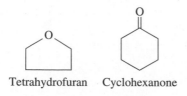

Fig. 28-1 Structure of tetrahydrofuran and cyclohexanone.

jobs. Rigid plastics include acrylonitrile-butadiene-styrene (ABS), polyvinyl chloride (PVC), and chlorinated polyvinyl chloride (CPVC). The most commonly used flexible plastic is polybutylene (PB). The ABS and PVC are used in drain systems. The PVC is a newer form of plastic that resists chemical damage and heat better than ABS. The CPVC and PB are used in water supply. Pipe is cut to fit with a saw. Each type of pipe can use a solvent-adhesive combination for that specific pipe or a general-purpose adhesive that works with many types of plastics. These solvents contain tetrahydrofuran, methyl ethyl ketone, and acetone and serve to clean the surface of dirt and oils that would prevent a good seal. The cement contains tetrahydrofuran and cyclohexanone. These agents (Fig. 28-1) produce typical hydrocarbon solvent symptom complexes: central nervous system (CNS) depression, mucous membrane irritation, and defatting dermatitis (see Chapters 10, 21, and 30).

Fluorocarbons

Exposure to fluorocarbons can occur during repair and installation of refrigeration devices. Two common fluorocarbons are dichlorodifluoromethane (Freon 12) and trichloromonofluoromethane (Freon 11).

Miscellaneous

Exposure to asbestos and lead is considered part of the toxic work environment of plumbers. However, asbestos-free construction and lead-free solders have reduced these exposures (see Chapter 52).

CLINICAL TOXICOLOGY
Fluorocarbons

Chemistry. Freon is a trade name for the class of fluorocarbons commonly used as propellants. Although fluorocarbons cause cardiac sensitization to catecholamines

in animal models, elimination is so rapid that only acute inhalation of high concentrations of fluorocarbons results in toxicity.[2] The distribution half-life of Freon 11 (CCl_3F) and Freon 12 (CCl_2F_2) is on the order of seconds, and elimination is complete in a few hours.[3] In addition, fluorocarbon leaks from a refrigeration unit into a closed space can result in asphyxiation by simple displacement of oxygen. Peak concentrations may reach anywhere from 1300 to 10,000 cm^3/m^3, well below the level that caused cardiac toxicity in animals.[1]

Clinical effects. Cardiac arrhythmias, pulmonary edema and fibrosis, and altered consciousness are produced to a greater or lesser extent by all fluorocarbons. Sudden death has been reported after inhalational abuse and after massive accidental exposures.[4,5,8]

Occupational exposures may produce cardiac arrhythmias. Dogs exposed to 25,000 to 100,000 cm^3/m^3 developed sinus bradycardia and asystole. This is half the inhaled concentration that a solvent abuser might achieve by using a plastic bag.[7] Occupational exposures may not achieve high enough concentrations to cause cardiac activity. A study of Freon 22 and 12 exposures during repairs with ambulatory electrocardiographic monitoring did not support a consistent cause and effect, although one subject did experience ventricular ectopic beats that corresponded to exposure.[1,6]

REFERENCES

1. Antti-Poika M, Heikkila J, Saarinen L: Cardiac arrhythmias during occupational exposure to fluorinated hydrocarbons, *Br J Ind Med* 47: 138, 1990.
2. Charlesworth FA: The fate of fluorocarbons inhaled and ingested, *Food Cosmet Toxicol* 13:572, 1975.
3. Chiou WL: Aerosol propellants: cardiac toxicity and lung biological half-life, *JAMA* 227:658, 1974.
4. Clark MA et al: Multiple deaths resulting from shipboard exposure to trichlorotrifluoroethane, *J Forensic Sci* 30:1256, 1985.
5. Crawford WV: Death due to fluorocarbon inhalation, *South Med J* 69:506, 1976.
6. Edling C et al: Cardiac arrhythmia in refrigerator repairmen exposed to fluorocarbons, *Br J Ind Med* 47:207, 1990.
7. Flowers NC, Hand C, Horan LG: Concentrations of fluoroalkanes associated with cardiac conduction system toxicity, *Arch Environ Health* 30:353, 1975.
8. Morita M et al: Case reports of deaths caused by freon gas, *Forensic Sci* 30:1256, 1985.

Police and Law Enforcement Personnel

Michael I. Greenberg

Se

- Selenosis is characterized by a garlic breath odor, gastrointestinal disturbances, metallic taste in the mouth, dermatitis, and upper airway irritation

- The gun blueing agent selenious acid is a potent caustic

- Exposures to lead, carbon monoxide, radar guns, and clandestine drug lab chemicals should be considered as occult sources of toxicity for police officers

OCCUPATIONAL DESCRIPTION

Law enforcement personnel at the turn of the 21st century can no longer simply be thought of as "the cop on the beat." Instead, modern law enforcement personnel work for dozens of different agencies and organizations on the local, state, federal, military, and international levels. The following agencies serve a law enforcement function in the United States today: local, municipal, and county police departments, state police departments, sheriffs' departments, state departments of public safety, law enforcement and investigative offices attached to state attorney generals' offices, local prosecutors' and district attorneys' offices, the U.S. attorneys' office, the U.S. Attorney General's office, the enforcement division of the Internal Revenue Service, the Federal Bureau of Investigation, the Bureau of Alcohol, Tobacco, and Firearms, the Financial Crimes Enforcement Network of the U.S. Treasury Department, the U.S. Coast Guard, the U.S. Secret Service, the U.S. Postal Inspection Service, military police (each branch of the military service has its own police and investigative units), the U.S. Drug Enforcement Agency, the U.S. Border Patrol, the U.S. Customs Service, the U.S. Immigration and Naturalization Service, the U.S. Marshals Service, the U.S. Bureau of Prisons, various state corrections departments, various local transit police, various local housing authority police units, the U.S. Fish and Wildlife Service, college and university campus police, city-based public school police forces, the U.S. Park Service Police, the U.S. Parole Commission, and

233

various units of the National Guard under appropriate federal or state direction. It is worth remembering that the Central Intelligence Agency is not a law enforcement organization and has as its only mission the development of intelligence resources for the U.S. government.

As the diversity of this list reflects, these agencies work in many different environments, often under a very wide variety of work conditions. In addition, specialization within the field of law enforcement has significantly complicated the characterization of the work environment for law enforcement personnel. Many law enforcement agencies have developed specific units tasked to be involved with specific aspects of law enforcement. Consequently, even small law enforcement agencies and police departments can be expected to have officers specifically assigned to duties in narcotics, homicide, traffic safety, special weapons and tactics, range officer duty, airborne patrol, motor patrol, hazardous materials, and other specialties. Given the "para-military" orientation of most law enforcement agencies, many of the jobs and duties within the profession mirror those found traditionally in the military setting. Previously male-dominated, the law enforcement occupations have increasingly come to include female members as well at all levels performing all descriptions of law enforcement activities.

All told, there are in excess of 1.7 million individuals engaged in law enforcement occupations today.[2] This is exclusive of individuals such as judges, district attorneys, assistant district attorneys, state and U.S. attorneys, and their respective office staffs. As a reflection of the vast manpower commitment for law enforcement in the United States today, in 1990 federal, state, and local governments spent approximately $74 billion for civil and criminal justice and law enforcement activities.[2]

Given the diversity of the various law enforcement agencies operating in the world today and given the diverse tasks they are expected to perform, it is not surprising to find an extremely wide spectrum of potentially toxic hazards that might impact on the personnel in various police agencies. While some toxic hazards may be common to many different law enforcement settings today, many of the specific hazards depend, in large part, on not only the tasks being performed but also the conditions under which they are being performed.

POTENTIAL TOXIC EXPOSURES

The potential toxic exposures for law enforcement personnel involve a wide range of substances (Table 29-1). Since virtually all personnel involved in law enforcement today carry and need to qualify with various weapons, the most ubiquitous hazards probably stem from the chemicals used to clean and maintain weapons as well as those toxic hazards (exclusive of direct injury) that result from use of the weapons. The use of hand gun cleaning agents poses a threat not only to the law enforcement officer but also poses a

Table 29-1 Major toxic hazards for law enforcement personnel

Hazardous toxin	Common locations of exposure for law enforcement	Agencies most commonly affected
Selenious acid	Firing ranges, barracks, headquarters, locker rooms, home	All; potential hazard for children of officers
Carbon monoxide	Tunnels, outdoor traffic control, fires	Local police, transit police
Radar (nonionizing radiation)	Speed enforcement	Local police, state police
Lead	Firing ranges, retained bullet/fragments	All
Clandestine laboratory chemicals	Clandestine drug laboratory sites	DEA, ATF, local police, state police
Cocaine, THC	Drug interdiction sites	All handling bulk, especially U.S. customs, DEA

hazard to members of their families if such agents are kept in and used in the home. Since many (if not most) law enforcement personnel also carry their weapons when off duty, gun-cleaning materials are frequently found in the homes, garages, and workshops of these individuals. Such gun-cleaning substances are discussed at great length as they pose a substantial toxic hazard.

Since all personnel are required to qualify on various ranges with various sorts of weapons, the toxic hazard of lead exposure due to simply spending time on firing ranges is discussed at some length. In addition, unfortunately an increasing number of law enforcement personnel are involved in incidents in which shots are exchanged with criminals. As a result, many officers are wounded annually. The lead hazard resultant from retained bullets and bullet fragments is also addressed as it represents a very specific occupationally related toxic hazard for law enforcement personnel.

Many law enforcement personnel work in areas that result in exposure to high levels of vehicular traffic. Consequently, these personnel may be subjected to dangerous levels of carbon monoxide. Depending on levels of ambient carbon monoxide, duration of exposure, and baseline levels of carboxyhemoglobin, significant elevations of carboxyhemoglobin can occur with resultant adverse health effects.

Certain law enforcement personnel work with radar devices used to ascertain speed limit violations by motorists. Speculation has arisen as to whether these devices are potentially causative of various types of cancer in these law enforcement personnel. The arguments surrounding this controversy are described and elucidated.

Drug enforcement and interdiction are major functions of many different law enforcement agencies from the federal to the local level. Many different potential toxic hazards can result from this drug enforcement function. The major hazards revolve around handling contraband substances. When law enforcement agencies raid and dismantle clandestine methamphetamine or "designer drug" laboratories, officers can be exposed to significant toxic hazards as well as the potential hazards of explosion of the various chemicals routinely used in such clandestine laboratory operations.

CLINICAL TOXICOLOGY
Selenious Acid

Pathophysiology. Gun blueing agents (such as the brand names Super Blue, Perma Blue, Herter's Belgian Blue, American Rust Blue, Brownell's Oxpho-Blue, Oxynate No. 7, Dicrophan IM, Nitre Blue, and 44/40) are colorless and are sold in the form of odorless liquid or pastelike agents. These materials are used by gun owners and gunsmiths to lubricate gun metal and to impart to it a bluish, metallic appearance. Blueing would also be applied to gun metal after use of the weapon or periodically to maintain the weapon's appearance. Typical gun blueing agents contain 4% to 6% selenious acid in conjunction with 2.5% cupric sulfate in hydrochloric acid. Other types of gun blueing compounds contain nitric acid and copper nitrate in conjunction with varying concentrations of selenious acid. Still other blueing agents contain primarily selenium dioxide.

In general, gun blueing agents are extremely caustic when ingested, and such ingestion often results in death. Specifically, the literature contains several case reports of death in children following ingestion of hydrogen selenide containing blueing compounds.[3,15] This is a special concern for law enforcement personnel, who often clean their service weapons (as well as other weapons) at home. The presence of gun blueing agents in and around the home represents a serious toxic hazard for the children of law enforcement officers as well as the officers themselves. Poisoning with gun blueing agent is decidedly uncommon.[1,10] Although most cases represent acute exposure episodes, chronic intoxication may occur as a result of chronic exposure. The toxicology of poisoning by gun blueing agents involves exposure to potentially several different substances. Depending upon the brand of blueing agent in question, exposures might include selenious acid, hydrogen selenide, copper, and nitric or other acids in varying combinations.

Selenium's potential as a toxic hazard to humans has been recognized since the early 1930s, when cases of selenosis were first reported.[14] The symptoms described in these early cases included garlicky breath odor, gastrointestinal disturbances, upper airway irritation, metallic taste in the mouth, and anosmia. In 1940, Lemly reported a rancher who developed selenosis secondary to exposure from natural sources.[9] He suffered severe pruritic dermatitis of the beard, pubic region, and hairy surface of the arms and thighs. His skin had a peculiar brownish-bronze tinge over its entire surface, and the affected areas were thickened, dry, and described as

"lichenoid with perifollicular pustules." The symptoms were noted to worsen following exposure to the sun.

Lemley later reported other cases of chronic selenosis in the South Dakota area.[8] Symptoms in these patients included dizziness, altered mental status, extreme fatigue, psychologic indifference, depression, emotional instability, epigastric pain, belching, and watery diarrhea. In addition, one patient was reported to have developed cirrhosis of the liver, as confirmed on biopsy.

Similar endemic selenium intoxication occurred in China, where hair loss and nail loss were reported as common features.[23] The nails were noted to have become brittle with white spots and longitudinal streaks on the surface. Sloughing of the nails followed a brief quiescent period. New nails that regrew were reported to be thickened and rough, with a marked increase in fragility. Repeated exposures were described as resulting in clinically apparent clubbing of the fingers. These manifestations are also associated with intensely pruritic rashes and gastrointestinal disturbances. Interestingly, an increased incidence of dental caries seems to be associated with these exposures as well. Central and peripheral nervous system abnormalities including peripheral anesthesia, paresthesia, hyperreflexia, and occasional hemiplegia were also reported.

The literature describes a woman who developed systemic selenium intoxication following the topical use of Selsun shampoo to treat an extensive and excoriated lesion of her scalp.[21] She developed a garlic odor to her breath, as well as gastrointestinal disturbances, lethargy, severe perspiration, and a generalized tremor. Laboratory evaluation revealed that her alkaline phosphatase was elevated, but other liver function tests were within normal limits. In addition, her urinary porphyrins were elevated.

Chronic granulomatous hypersensitivity reaction in the lungs has also been reported following long-term selenium exposure.[21] A case of chronic exposure to hydrogen selenide gas described facial eczema, asthenia, and bronchitis. Snodgrass reported two cases of children with cystic fibrosis who were treated with selenium on the advice of a veterinarian.[19] Both children developed electrolyte abnormalities, and one developed elevations of liver enzymes. Other reported effects of selenium toxicity include pallor, leukocytosis, microcytic hypochromic anemia, hemolytic anemia, urticaria, and teratogenesis.

Men exposed in an industrial accident that involved the inhalation of selenium oxide fumes developed bronchospasm associated with coughing and gagging.[14,15] In addition, some individuals also developed transient loss of consciousness. The exposed individuals complained of a bitter and acidic taste in their mouths and a burning sensation of the skin, conjunctivae, and mucous membranes. Following the acute phase, these individuals developed nausea, vomiting, diarrhea, malaise, dyspnea, headache, chills, and fever. Three of the exposed workers developed evidence of a chemical pneumonitis.

Sore throat and bronchitis with copious sputum production may develop after exposure to dogs injected with sodium selenite.[14] This reported exposure probably involved the dogs' respiratory excretion of dimethyl selenide. These symptoms are similar to the so-called "rose cold", which consisted of cough, sore throat, coryza, and bronchitis following dimethyl selenide exposure. A young girl who intentionally swallowed 400 ml of a 3 mg/ml sodium selenate solution developed a strong garlic odor of the breath; frequent loose, gray stools; T-wave flattening and Q-T interval prolongation on electrocardiogram; and elevations of alkaline phosphatase, bilirubin, and SGOT. A 3-year-old boy who ingested 1.8% selenious acid exhibited cyanotic extremities, bright red lips, excessive salivation, a strong garlic odor, carpal spasm, and coma.[3] He died shortly after admission despite resuscitative efforts. Autopsy revealed vascular engorgement and edema of the gastrointestinal tract, as well as pulmonary edema with congestion and focal hemorrhages in the lungs.

Acute exposure to hydrogen selenide gas in a 24-year-old man resulted in severe dyspnea with abnormal pulmonary function tests.[19] Subsequent testing revealed persistent pulmonary impairment consistent with obstructive disease. Selenium dioxide and selenious acid can penetrate intact skin and cause severe local irritation and inflammation, especially under the nails. Selenium oxychloride is a powerful vesicant capable of producing a third-degree burn. It is extremely toxic; one drop applied to the skin of a dog produced death within a few hours.

After acute ingestion of any selenium-containing substance, cardiorespiratory collapse can occur in hours. Marked hypotension may result from what is thought to be the combination of an extremely low peripheral vascular resistance and the primary cardiac effects of the toxin. In one case report, noncorrectable respiratory failure developed after ingestion of only a small amount of a hydrogen selenide containing a gun-blueing agent.[15] The patient was treated with extracorporeal membrane oxygenation and succumbed despite all efforts.

Biochemistry. Selenium is an essential trace element at lower concentrations and an extremely toxic substance at higher concentrations. Animals can metabolize both inorganic and organic forms of selenium by converting ingested selenium to mono-, di-, or trimethylated forms. Of all the methylated forms, the monomethylated are probably the most toxic.

The enzyme glutathione reductase converts selenoglutathione to hydrogen sulfide in the liver and red blood cells and is eventually excreted. Chronic selenosis occurs in animals who ingest plants containing 5 or more ppm of selenium. This amount of selenium would be equivalent to 2400 to 3000 μg/day in man. However, the lowest level of potentially dangerous intake in humans is estimated to be 500 μg/day of selenium. The acutely lethal dose of selenium is approximately 4 mg/kg of body weight for most animals.

Selenium exerts its toxic effects primarily by catalyzing the oxidation of sulfhydryl groups, which result in inactivation of the cellular oxidative processes. It can also inhibit the process of mitosis at metaphase. In addition, selenium causes abnormal bone and cartilage development and is teratogenic.

The highest levels of selenium can be found in the liver, where it is converted to trimethylselenium, which is then excreted in the urine. Smaller amounts are excreted in the bile and feces. At high doses or with chronic exposure, selenium is also converted to dimethylselenide, which is excreted by the lungs and causes the characteristic garlic breath odor. Most of a selenium load is excreted within 2 weeks; organic forms tend to be retained longer. In chronic selenosis, very high levels of selenium can be found in the nails. It is interesting to note that the thyroid also tends to accumulate selenium.

The specific systemic toxicity of selenium can be modified by a number of divergent factors. Various forms of selenium differ greatly in their toxicity. The box below lists the various forms of selenium and their relative toxicities. The relative toxicity of the selenium compounds expected to be found in gun blueing materials is quite high.

Selenium toxicity appears to be much greater in young, slender, fair-skinned people. The reason for this differentiation is unclear. A diet high in protein seems to reduce selenium toxicity in laboratory animals; however, the clinical utility for this information has yet to be clarified. Other compounds noted to be protective against selenium, at least in a laboratory setting, include arsenic, sulfate, linseed oil, methionine, silver, zinc, copper, and cadmium.

Tolerance seems to develop to selenium toxicity. This may explain the disparity often noted between urinary selenium levels and clinical symptoms. Mercuric salts increase the systemic toxicity of selenium. Increased selenium intake protects against the toxicity of dimethylmercury cadmium and methylated selenium compounds. Supplements of selenium do not decrease mercury levels in tissues of animals given methylmercury, but animals given selenium plus methylmercury may accumulate high levels of mercury without signs of toxicity. This apparent protective effect may be related to the prevention of oxidative damage at the

---

Relative Toxicity of Selenium-Containing Compounds in Decreasing Order

MOST TOXIC

Hydrogen selenide
Organic selenium compounds in grain
Selenites
Selenates
Selenides

LEAST TOXIC

Metallic selenium

cellular and subcellular level. The possible role of selenium in the defense against cellular and subcellular injury is well recognized, but the precise part selenium plays in immune system functions has yet to be specifically delineated.

Diagnosis. In the absence of a specific history describing exposure to selenium-containing compounds, the diagnosis should be suspected by the garlic odor of the breath. However, this odor disappears over the course of about a week unless the person is reexposed to the selenium source. In addition to selenium exposure, other substances, including phosphorus, lewisite, arsenic, pyridine, tellurium, dimethyl sulfoxide (DMSO), and garlic, produce a similar garlic odor to the breath. Perhaps the earliest symptom of selenium poisoning is a metallic taste in the mouth, but this finding is very nonspecific and somewhat variable.

Selenium is generally not detected on routine heavy metal screening; however, blood levels can be measured and do correlate with the selenium content of cells. Erythrocyte glutathione peroxidase enzyme activity correlates directly with blood selenium concentrations. Hair and nail samples may be useful in detecting past exposure and may be especially helpful in cases involving suspected homicide or suicide.

Urinary selenium levels of 0 to 150 μg/L are considered to be normal and reflect the normal dietary intake of selenium. Toxic concentrations of selenium range from 100 to 2000 μg/L. That being said, many investigators deny any significant clinical correlation between urinary selenium levels and the severity of symptoms. In one study, workers exposed to selenium with symptoms consistent with marked selenosis had urinary selenium levels less than 10% of the levels of people living in seleniferous geographic regions. Clinical symptoms have been reported at urinary concentrations as low as 10μg/L. Urinary selenium levels must be determined as soon as possible after sample collection because significant amounts of selenium may be lost from the sample due to volatilization.

Management and treatment. The treatment of acute ingestions of compounds containing selenious acid (e.g., gun blueing solution) has not been thoroughly investigated. Despite the fact that even very small amounts of this chemical are potentially lethal, no specific and effective treatment currently exists. All patients who ingest selenious acid should be evaluated by a physician who is knowledgeable in medical toxicology and hospitalized for observation.

Because gun blueing compounds containing selenious acid are highly corrosive and will produce esophageal burns, early consultation with appropriate specialists is mandatory. This acid is a serious systemic poison that is rapidly and efficiently absorbed. Consequently, the decision to employ decontamination measures is based on clinical judgment. Factors to consider in the decision to use decontamination procedures include the time since exposure, the amount of spontaneous emesis, the clinical condition of the patient, and the amount ingested. Because specific antidotes to selenious acid toxicity do not exist, treatment is generally expectant

(cardiopulmonary monitoring in an intensive care setting) and supportive (intravenous infusion, supplemental oxygen, and ventilation as needed). Poor outcomes are, unfortunately the rule rather than the exception.

The management of chronic selenium intoxication is generally supportive. Obviously, elimination of the selenium source is the most crucial step in the management of a patient suffering from chronic selenosis. It is important to remember that the indiscriminate use of BAL, CaNa$_2$EDTA, and D-penicillamine may enhance selenium toxicity. It is thought that this phenomenon is due to the formation of nephrotoxic complexes with selenium. Consequently, these particular chelating agents should not be used to treat intoxication due to selenium-containing compounds.

Bromobenzene has been demonstrated to increase the rate of excretion of selenium. Unfortunately, bromobenzene has an inherent toxicity of its own. In any event, bromobenzene has been recommended for use specifically in order to treat selenium-associated dermatitis.

Thiosulfate has also been suggested as a possible treatment agent in selenium toxicity.[21] Although thiosulfate is not usually considered to be effective against the systemic manifestations of selenium toxicity, it can be applied topically and acts specifically to relieve the pain produced by selenium dioxide, which may accumulate under the nails after such an exposure.

Several other treatment possibilities have been addressed in the literature. For example, vitamin C (ascorbic acid) has been reported to decrease blood selenium levels in one study.[21] However, in another similar study, it was determined that Vitamin C actually caused an increase in selenium levels as a result of decreasing the rate of selenium excretion.

Arsenical compounds can ameliorate some of the toxic effects of selenium and increase its excretion. However, this seems to be true only if it is administered within 20 days of the initial exposure to selenium.

Glutathione may act as a detoxifying agent, but this has not been demonstrated conclusively.

Carbon Monoxide

Pathophysiology. While the details of the pathophysiology of carbon monoxide (CO) exposure and poisoning are discussed elsewhere in this book (see Chapter 15), certain potential mechanisms of exposure to carbon monoxide are likely for law enforcement personnel in particular. In fact, the clinical diagnosis of CO poisoning is rarely made by the clinician who does not suspect the toxin in any person presenting with altered mental status. Consequently, it is, to some extent, more important to be able to recognize the potential for exposure than it is to understand the precise pathophysiology of the toxin (although that is, of course, of obvious interest and clinical importance).

Law enforcement personnel often spend long hours sitting inside vehicles that may not undergo proper and routine maintenance. It is not usual for police vehicles to be operated around the clock and taken out of service only for a mechanical failure. In this setting of constant use, holes in the manifold and exhaust system of the vehicle could easily go undetected. This could be especially hazardous in the winter when the windows would be closed. Officers who smoke can be expected to have minimally elevated carboxyhemoglobin levels (often up to about 10%). Small increases in ambient carbon monoxide could easily increase the blood CO level to ranges that would cause symptoms (see Firefighter). In addition to exposure due to sitting inside vehicles, personnel can be exposed due to prolonged work outdoors in high-traffic areas, or in toll lanes or tunnels.

Lead

Pathophysiology. Prior to the mid-1970s, when lead was finally eliminated from most gasoline products sold in the United States, police officers who directed traffic for long periods or who spent tours of duty in underground traffic tunnels often developed significantly elevated blood lead levels. To date, the chronic effects on these personnel have not been clearly documented. These exposures could potentially relate to any hypertension and/or renal disease which would be manifest long after the exposure terminated.

The lead hazard for law enforcement personnel today occurs on the firing range. All personnel are required to fire their weapons for qualification at least twice a year. Officers of the FBI, and the U.S. Secret Service, and special response teams are specifically required to qualify and practice with their respective weapons frequently. In addition, many officers spend long hours practicing on the range for either their own personal enjoyment or to increase their skills with small weapons.

Personnel who work on indoor ranges can easily develop elevated blood lead levels from respiratory exposure to lead-containing dust. Those individuals who clean the ranges are at highest risk for this type of exposure. The respiratory route is a very efficient way for lead to enter the body and be absorbed into the systemic circulation. Generally, personnel do not wear respiratory protection while firing on the range. In addition, if personnel consume food or beverages on the range or, after leaving the range, fail to wash their hands and change their clothes, significant gastrointestinal lead exposure can occur. The combination of inspired lead dust and ingested lead particles may result in serious lead exposures to personnel. In addition, these personnel may transport significant quantities of lead dust into their own home environments and thereby expose their spouses and children to lead.

It is an unfortunate occupational reality that many law enforcement personnel are wounded (and killed) in the line of duty. Often wounding bullets either are intentionally left in the body or cannot be surgically removed because of location. These retained missiles may rarely leach lead, in clinically significant amounts, into the systemic circulation.[11] When these bullets or fragments are in or near serosal or joint surfaces, the process of lead exuding from the bullet

or fragment is accelerated. The potential for systemic lead intoxication following one or more gunshot wounds is an indication for surgical exploration and bullet removal.[16] Failure to do so has resulted in significant systemic lead intoxication.

Latent periods between the lodging of a bullet or bullet fragment and the onset of clinical lead intoxication can be 6 months to many years. A 69-year-old male patient developed abdominal pain, generalized weakness, and other neurologic complications 19 years after he had been shot in the elbow.[22] At the time of presentation and evaluation for plumbism, this individual's blood lead level was 84 μg/dl per deciliter. Another report[7] documented the case of a child who suffered a gunshot wound to the head with retained intracranial lead pellets. This child did not demonstrate elevated blood lead levels until 12 months later. In another case, a patient, who was clearly asymptomatic for 9 years after sustaining a gunshot to the upper extremity, developed what classic symptoms of lead intoxication in conjunction with elevated blood lead levels.[22]

Elevated blood lead levels 7 years after a .22-caliber gunshot to the foot can be caused by minimal amounts of this small-caliber bullet's fragments and have been reported to result in lead poisoning.[6] This is unlikely unless the bullet, fragment, or pellet is retained within or in close proximity to a synovial cavity.[18] Vigorous degradation mediated by the synovial fluid is the mechanism of toxicity. In a dog model, lead disks implanted in the synovial spaces and various soft tissues of dogs demonstrated that lead in the synovial space is released quickly and peaks within 6 months, and lead within muscle is solubilized only very slowly.[12]

In summary, then, any law enforcement officer who has been wounded should be monitored for possible development of elevated blood lead levels. If the wounding missile is easily amenable to surgical removal, that should be carried out as soon as clinically advisable, especially if a synovial space or body cavity is involved. Any officer presenting with abdominal pain, vague neurologic symptoms, renal disease, or hypertension should be questioned closely to ascertain if they had ever been shot in the past. Long latent periods may intervene and blood lead screening is in order for such individuals, even if the shooting event occurred decades prior to presentation.

Radar Speed Timing Devices

Traffic radar is a type of nonionizing radiation at the same end of the electromagnetic spectrum as radio waves and microwaves. Nonionizing radiation is known to exert both thermal and nonthermal effects. The thermal effects have been investigated, but few studies have examined the nonthermal effects, particularly the long-term effects of low-level exposure.

There is very little specific knowledge regarding the etiology of testicular cancer in men. What is clear, however, is that rates of testicular cancer have risen steadily over the past 100 years, and the incidence among white men in the United States has increased significantly in the last 50 years.[4] The specific reasons for this increase are not certain.

Recently, a mortality study[4] of Washington state troopers revealed six cases of testicular cancer that occurred between 1979 and 1991 in two separate departments that served geographically contiguous areas. The affected officers were interviewed concerning work-related exposures; their past medical histories, work histories, and family histories were also reviewed.

The staffing of both police departments studied had remained constant for approximately 30 years. The total number of individuals participating in the study was 270 and 70 officers, from the two respective departments. All of the men diagnosed with testicular cancer were police officers as their primary lifetime occupations. In addition, all were noted to have been exposed to traffic radar regularly during their careers. None of the men diagnosed with testicular cancer had been born with undescended testes, none had experienced severe trauma to the testicles, and only one had previously had mumps orchitis. After careful analysis, it was concluded that the only exposure common to these men was that they all rested their radar guns, while in the "on" position, directly in their laps, "close to, pointing at, or directly adjacent to the testicles."[4]

Of the six reported cases, three were embryonal cell carcinomas, one was a mixed-cell carcinoma with an embryonal cell metastasis, and two were seminomas. The total number of expected cases of testicular cancer using the 1981 SEER registry rates were reported to be only 0.87 (observed/expected ratio = 6.9, $p < .001$, Poisson distribution).

Further support for an association between testicular cancer and radar gun exposure is the mean age at diagnosis of the affected officers, which was 39 years, clearly much older than the usually recognized mean age for testicular cancers. This in itself may be a reflection of the effect of this exposure in the workplace.

Radar lies within the microwave frequency of the electromagnetic spectrum. Electromagnetic fields (EMF) have been reported to be associated with the development of cancer in some studies, while in others there has been no association. None of the studies has shown a specific association between EMF exposures and testicular cancer.[4] Testicular cancer has previously been noted among microwave radar operators, but the significance of this report is uncertain.[13]

A larger cohort study is needed to more accurately ascertain whether an association truly exists and, if so, the size of the excess risk of testicular cancer from radar use.

Clandestine Drug Laboratories

Drug enforcement and interdiction are important functions for many law enforcement agencies in the United States and abroad. One of the most daunting challenges facing these

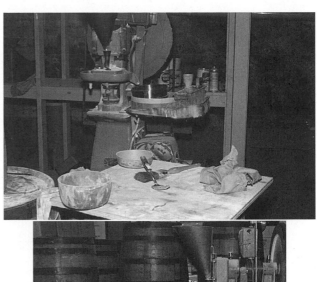
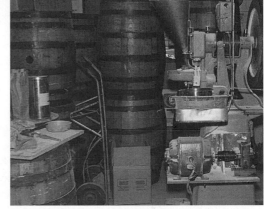

Fig. 29-1 Clandestine drug lab found during police raid.

law enforcement officers is locating and dismantling clandestine drug labs, the so-called "clan labs" (Fig. 29-1). These illicit laboratories are typically in a garage, basement, attic, or abandoned, isolated building structure in an out-of-the-way place. These labs are involved in the synthesis and manufacture of illicit drugs and serve as the first point of contact for the distribution of these substances as well. The illicit substances most commonly manufactured in these labs are listed in Table 29-2. The chemicals usually found on site in these clandestine labs are those used in the synthetic process for some of these illicit substances; they are listed in the box on p. 240. Officers who raid or dismantle these clandestine labs may come into contact with these hazardous substances and could suffer adverse health effects from any one of them or any combination. In addition, some of these substances, alone or in combination, represent significant explosive hazards to law enforcement personnel. For these and other reasons, many agencies have developed their own hazardous materials teams that dismantle and dispose of the hazardous materials found in these clandestine drug labs. In any event, the officers involved in this aspect of drug interdiction should be equipped with appropriate respiratory and other personal protective equipment and clothing. An extensive discussion of the biohazards and potential adverse health effects of each illicit substance listed is beyond the scope of this chapter, but the carcinogenic potential faced by

Table 29-2 Illicit substances commonly manufactured in clandestine drug labs

Common name	Chemical name
LSD	Lysergic acid diethylamide
Mescaline	3,4,5,trimethoxyphenethylamine
Amphetamine	
Methamphetamine	Methamphetamine HCl
STP	4-Methyl-2 dimethoxyamphetamine
THC	tetrahydrocannabinol
Methadone	
PCP	Phencyclidine HCl
Heroin	
Designer drugs	
DMT	N,N-Dimethyltryptamine

Chemicals Found on Site for the Production of Some Common Illicit Substances

LSD
Acetonitrile
Sodium sulfate
Alumina
Benzene
Chloroform
Diethylamine
Dimethylformamide
Ethanol
Ethyl ether
Methylene chloride
Isopropanol
Lithium hydroxide
Lysergic acid
Methanol
Sulfur trioxide
Sulfuric acid
Tartaric acid
Trifluoroacetic acid
Methanol
Methylamine
Palladium black
Phenylacetone
Potassium hydroxide
Sodium acetate
Zinc or aluminum foil

PCP
1-Phenyl-1-piperidinocyclo-
   hexane hydrobromide
1-Piperidinocyclohexane
   carbonitrile
Bromobenzene
Hydrobromic acid
Hydrogen chloride
Magnesium metal turnings
Phenyl magnesium bromide

METHAMPHETAMINE HYDROCHLORIDE
Ephedrine
Ethyl ether
Phenyl propylalamine
Hydrochloric acid
Hydrogen iodide
Lithium aluminum hydride

HEROIN
Morphine or opium
Acetic anhydride
Acetyl chloride
Acetone
Ether
Benzene
Hydrogen chloride gas
Sodium carbonate

---

officers who are repeatedly exposed to the substances found in clandestine drug labs is discussed.

Officers could be exposed to any of these or to a host of other potentially hazardous materials during work in and around clandestine drug laboratory operations. A given exposure must be clinically evaluated in light of the specific chemicals encountered. Consultation with a forensic chemist, forensic toxicologist, or other police officials may be warranted to define the scope and content of any single officer's exposure after involvement at a clandestine lab site.

No extensive scientific work has assessed the carcinogenic potential of the chemicals found in the typical clandestine lab. Perhaps the most significant threat is the inhalational exposure to benzene. This chemical is found in extremely large quantities in most clandestine lab operations. The pathophysiology of the development of such malignancies and their association with benzene exposure are discussed elsewhere in this book. The precise definition of the risk must await properly formulated epidemiologic studies of these at-risk populations.

An additional hazard for law enforcement personnel involved in drug interdiction involves handling large quantities of confiscated contraband drug substances, such as cocaine, heroin, and marijuana. When large amounts of these substances are confiscated, police officers collect, catalog, transport, and prepare for storage what can be, at times, tons of these materials. Typically these substances are found in plastic wraps or bags of varying degrees of strength and resilience. Significant quantities of drug-containing dust and particulate matter are in the atmosphere in and around sites where this work is taking place. In these settings, both inhalational and dermal exposures can result in systemic absorption of these (and other) drugs by the officers present. While the general systemic effects of absorption of these materials have been well described in toxicology texts, the very existence of these hazards for these personnel is often ignored. At the very least, such exposures could be expected

to result in positive urine screening, should these officers be tested within the ranges of time consistent with the half-lives of the drugs in question. One poorly controlled and statistically questionable investigation suggested that dermal absorption of cocaine and marijuana should not be detectable by a standard urine drug screen.[5] To the extent that systemic absorption does occur, the physician and, more specifically, the medical review officer (MRO) must be informed regarding the exposure potentials for these individuals in these venues. At the other end of the spectrum, systemic absorption in such uncontrolled settings could acutely threaten the health of officers on site. The potential for the development of, for example, an acute episode of chest pain reflective of coronary insufficiency in an officer during or after handling large quantities of cocaine is not beyond the realm of possibility. Other manifestations of acute toxicity reflective of the handling and exposure to other such illicit drugs should also be anticipated by physicians involved in the care of law enforcement personnel.

REFERENCES

1. Alderman LC, Bergin JJ: Hydrogen selenide poisoning: an illustrative case with review of the literature, *Arch Environ Health* 41:354, 1986.
2. Bureau of Justice Statistics Clearinghouse, 1995.
3. Carter RF: Acute selenium poisoning, *Med J Aust* 1:525, 1966.
4. Davis RL, Mostofi FK: Cluster of testicular cancer in police officers exposed to hand-held radar, *Am J Ind Med* 24:231, 1993.
5. ElSohly MA: Urinalysis and casual handling of marijuana and cocaine, *J Anal Toxicol* 15:31, 1991.
6. Fiorica V, Brinker JE: Increase lead absorption and lead poisoning from a retained bullet, *J Okla State Med Assoc* 82:63, 1989.
7. Kikano GE, Starge KC: Lead poisoning in a child after a gunshot injury, *J Fam Pract* 34:498, 1992.
8. Lemley AD: Subsurface agricultural irrigation drainage: the need for regulation, *Regul Toxicol Pharmacol* 17:157, 1993.
9. Lemly RE, Merryman MP: Selenium poisoning in the human, *Lancet* 61:435, 1941.
10. Mack RB: The fat lady enters stage left, acute selenium poisoning, *N C Med J* 51:636, 1990.
11. Magos L: Lead poisoning from retained lead projectiles: a critical review of cax reports, *Hum Exp Toxicol* 13:735, 1994.
12. Monton WI, Thal ER: Lead poisoning from retired missiles: an experimental study, *Ann Surg* 204:594, 1986.
13. Mostofi FK, Davis RC: Male reproductive system and prostate. In Kissane JM, editor: *Anderson's pathology,* St Louis, 1990, Mosby.
14. Motley HL, Ellis MM: Acute sore throat following exposure to selenium, *JAMA* 109:1718, 1937.
15. Nantel AJ et al: Acute poisoning by selenious acid, *Vet Hum Toxicol* 27:531, 1985.
16. Peh WE, Reinus WR: Lead arthropathy: a caux of delayed onset lead poisoning, *Skeletal Radiol* 24:357, 1995.
17. Pentel P, Fletcher D, Jentzen J: Fatal selenium toxicity, *J Forensic Sci* 30:556, 1985.
18. Roux P, Pocock F: Blood lead concentrates in children after gunshot injuries, *S Afr Med J* 73:580, 1988.
19. Snodgrass W, Rumack BN, Sullivan SB: Acute selenium poisoning: case report, *N Z Med J* 1:211, 1978.
20. Stromberg BV: Symptomatic lead toxicity secondary to retained shotgun pellets: case report, *J Trauma* 30:356, 1990.
21. Wilbur CG: Toxicology of selenium: a review, *Clin Tox* 7:171, 1980.
22. Wu PB, Kingery WS, Date ES: An EMG case report of lead neuropathy 19 years after a shotgun injury, *Muscle Nerve* 18:326, 1995.
23. Yang G et al: Endemic selenium intoxication of humans in China, *Am J Clin Nutr* 37:872, 1983.

30

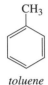

toluene

- Printers are exposed to aromatic and aliphatic solvents

- The type of printing job, the type of inks, and the cleaning methods determine the degree and severity of exposure

Printers

Richard J. Hamilton

OCCUPATIONAL DESCRIPTION

The printing process can be divided into three phases: prepress, press, and binding. Each phase employs a variety of specialty personnel. There were 167,000 jobs in the prepress phase, 240,000 jobs in the press phase, and 76,000 jobs in the binding phase according to 1992 Department of Labor statistics.[16] The prepress workers create the mechanicals (mockups of the actual final product) and plates (the metallic object that does the printing) by using a variety of photographic and computer-assisted techniques. The press operators monitor, maintain, and repair the printing operation. The bindery workers create the finished product from the printed pages.

Toxic exposures during prepress operations occur during the large-scale photographic process that makes metal printing plates from artwork. These toxins are no different than those encountered in photography (see Chapter 27).

Printing is the process that transfers the image from the metal plate to a substrate. Commercial printers use offset, thermography, flexography, and rotogravure techniques predominantly.

Offset lithography and offset printing are popular methods because the process can produce high-quality results quickly and inexpensively. Lithography is based on the immiscibility of oil and water. Lithographic plates have ink-receptive coating on the image area and a repellent coating such as water or silicone. The image is transferred from this inked plate to a rubber blanket on a drum. The rubber blanket ultimately contacts the paper and prints the image.

The offset printing press is a complex device with several components. The feeding unit delivers paper into the machine. Register units assure coordination of paper positioning and image. Ink units convey liquids to the plates. Printing units transfer the image to the paper. Inking units hold the ink in reservoirs called *fountains*. These are inverted plastic bottles or trough reservoirs. The press operator can control ink flow from the fountain onto rollers, which spread the ink evenly across the plate. Fountain solutions protect the image areas by applying fluids that contain acid, gum arabic, alcohol, and water to the plate via a system of rollers. The ink is applied mechanically in a thin layer from the ink fountain. The fountain solution must evaporate instantly from the plate and leave only the thin film of ink on the image area. If the paper becomes wet with fountain solution (such as multiple runs for color printing), it can stretch and each successive image is not properly centered. The quality of the print depends on the proper balance between ink and dampening solution. Press operators increase the concentration of the evaporative solvent in the fountain solution (most commonly isopropyl alcohol) to improve the speed of evaporation. Poorly ventilated print shops have large ambient air concentrations of isopropanol during these press runs.

Flexography is a process used for thick substrates such as labels and packaging. A raised image is inked with a water-based aniline dye by a special anilox roller.

Rotogravure or gravure printing is useful for production of large numbers or magazines or catalogs. It uses a plate cylinder, which is engraved with a diamond stylus guided by computer-controlled lasers. Gravure uses relatively thin ink that is wiped by a doctor blade before the impression is made on extremely smooth paper stocks. *National Geographic* magazine uses this technique for all its text and photographs, while the cover and advertisements are printed lithographically.

Thermography creates raised printing that is of similar quality to engraving. A slow-drying ink is offset onto the paper and then sprayed with thermography powder. Powder that does not adhere to the wet ink is vacuumed away. Heat is applied and fuses the powder and ink to create a raised image.

Engraving yields the sharpest images and is used to print detailed stock certificates, currency, invitations, and stationary. An etched plate is covered with thick ink, and the high-quality paper substrate is pressed onto the plate with high pressure, forcing the paper into the etched wells of ink.

Special ink blends provide special effects such as metallic colors, fade resistance, fluorescence, scents, and magnetic properties to the print. In order to comply with regulations to limit the environmental impact of solvents, many companies are using soy-based oil inks as well as water-based inks with hardeners that cure with ultraviolet light.

Most jobs require black ink. The presses must be thoroughly cleaned between ink changes to produce a high-quality product. First the pasty ink is troweled out of the fountain into a container for future use. The press is then

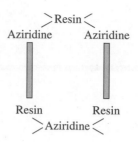

Fig. 30-1 Acrylic resin and aziridine cross-link to form hardened ink.

cleaned completely. It is during these cleanup operations that a great deal of solvent exposure occurs. In addition, "rubber-based" inks require frequent cleaning of the press to avoid damaging buildup. This maintenance prevents a costly drum replacement. The cleanup operations are most often done by hand. The drums are sprayed with solvents as the press runs and then wiped by hand with cotton rags. Inks that are not rubber-based can stay in the fountain and on the drum for many days without cleanup, which decreases maintenance costs and toxic exposures.

Protective coatings are applied either during the printing process or during the finishing and binding. For example, the glossy coating of a magazine is an acrylic mixture of polymer and water applied by a special coating unit. A complete discussion of printing techniques can be found in Mark Beach's *Getting It Printed* (Cincinnati, 1993, North Light Books).

TOXICOLOGIC EXPOSURES
Inks

Inks are oil- or water-based pigmented pastes. Their chemical composition is as varied as the effects the printers are attempting to achieve. Most black inks are carbon black with mineral oils. Many color pigments are azo compounds, which are characterized by the structures in R-N-N-R′ structure. The insoluble azos are free of any sulfonic acid or salt-forming groups in the R or R′ position. The soluble azo compounds have salt-forming groups in these positions that complex with the alkaline earth metals such as calcium, barium, strontium, and manganese. Simple inorganic pigments such as iron oxide and the metal silicates are also very common. The toxicity of these pigments is in the 5 to 10 g/kg range, with the exception of the aniline pigments, which are toxic at 0.3 mg/kg.

Hardeners are added to water-based acrylic inks to cross-link the acrylic resins without the use of volatile solvents (Fig. 30-1). Press operators, accustomed to the relative nontoxicity of other inks, may handle these inks without rubber gloves. A printing company experienced an outbreak of dermatitis when an aziridine hardener with trimethylpropane triacrylate replaced the usual volatile solvent-based ink.[8]

Rubber-based printing inks are typically composed of organic pigment, resin-rosin oil, light lube oil, wax, and vegetable oil in roughly equal proportions.

Newspaper inks are composed of carbon black (12%), mineral oil (85%), and indoline dye toner (3%). When the press runs, a mist of ink is created, which can be inhaled by those working in close proximity. Modernization has reduced exposures to this mist. However, higher press speeds produce greater amounts of mists. For instance, mineral oil mists in printers in the 1960s ranged from 2 to 16.6 mg/m^3. Twenty years later, the concentration ranges from 0.22 to 0.51 mg/m^3.[11] Nonetheless, more senior career press operators probably have a significant accumulated exposure to ink mist.

Carbon black is considered a carcinogen in mice.[10] This may relate to the absorption of polyaromatic hydrocarbons (such as benzo[*a*]pyrene) to the carbon black. Mean atmospheric concentrations of benzo[*a*]pyrene have been measured in the 4.1 to 75.6 μg/1000m^3. This is 10 times more than urban atmosphere concentrations, but 3 to 4 orders of magnitude below roof-tarring operations. Indeed, preliminary evidence links a long career in printing to development of lung cancer.[10]

Ultraviolet (UV) lamps are used to oxidize a printing surface and dry certain inks. A spark generated by a UV light coats the surface and enhances the subsequent adherence of ink. Since only modern presses utilize this technique, exposure is rare, and the presses are designed with proper ventilation and a high degree of mechanization.

Fountain Solution

The fountain solution contains isopropanol, butyl cellosolve, ethylene glycol, and water. The content of the isopropanol is increased to speed the drying process. This can produce a significant mist of isopropanol in the work area, and printers often avoid close proximity to the press during these operations to decrease exposure. Butyl cellosolve (ethylene glycol butyl ether) can cause delayed hemolytic anemia and renal failure. It has no dermal toxicity and produces little inhalational toxicity.

Solvents and Cleaning Solutions

The most important maintenance task for a press operator is cleanup, which is still done by hand at most commercial, modest-sized operations. The solvents used depend on the task. The water fountain is cleaned with 70% water, 10% isopropanol, 10% ethylene glycol butyl ether, and 8% ethylene. The press and ink fountain are typically cleaned with a solvent containing naphtha (for a discussion of aliphatic hydrocarbons, see Chapter 21), menthadiene, dipropylene glycol, and methyl ether. Toluene is the constituent of many of these solvents, although hexane may also be present in small amounts. The rags used for this process are left in a metal can and collected for cleaning by

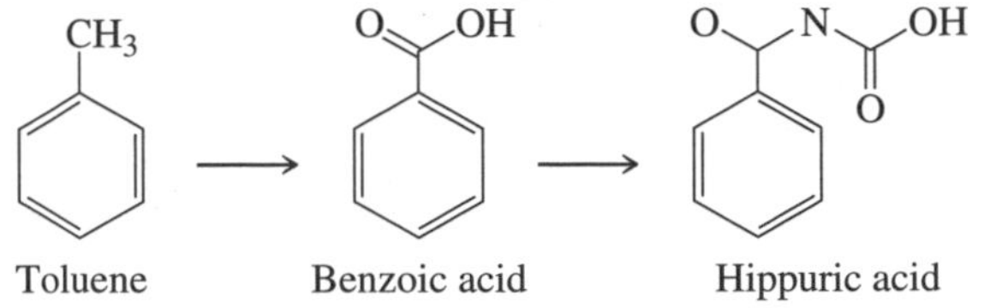

Fig. 30-2 Toluene metabolism.

a special laundry service that can handle the material properly.

In unregulated workplaces overseas, solvents with a large concentration of hexane are still prevalent. N-hexane is a solvent used to remove residual ink and clean the press. N-hexane exposures in the United States have been controlled by switching to hydrocarbon solvents, such as naphtha. N-hexane induces hepatic cytochrome P-450 and is metabolized to the neurotoxic 2,5-hexanedione. It is primarily absorbed from the respiratory tract but may also be absorbed through the skin (see Chapter 35).

In one Hong Kong print shop, an index case of peripheral neuropathy led to an investigation that identified symptomatic peripheral neuropathy in 20 (36%) workers and subclinical neuropathy in 26 (46%). Axonal degeneration and significant demyelination were confirmed by sural nerve biopsy. In addition, a subgroup of patients developed neuropathy, weight loss, headache, memory loss, vertigo, postural hypotension, and impotence.[5]

PATHOPHYSIOLOGY
Toluene

The National Occupational Hazards Survey identified 4 million workers who were potentially exposed to toluene in 271 different occupations. It is produced in cigarette smoke and is also prevalent as an indoor air contaminant.

Absorption and metabolism. Toluene (Fig. 30-2) is rapidly absorbed through during respiration and distributes into all tissues, particularly those with a high lipid content (brain, adipose tissue, and bone marrow).[1,7] Toluene accumulates in the marrow during the course of the exposure. It is 80% metabolized by the cytochrome P-450 system enzymes to hippuric acid, 19% expired unchanged, and less than 1% transformed into ortho, meta, and para cresols (see Fig. 30-2). Occupational exposures to toluene are not likely to result in clinically significant induction of cytochrome P-450 enzymes.[6]

Acute toxicity. Acute toxicity from inhalation is determined by the ambient concentration of toluene, the minute ventilation, and the activity of the affected individual. It is possible to develop central nervous system depression, headache, loss of concentration, staggering gait, and nausea at concentrations of toluene that are within the permissible exposure limit (threshold limit value, time weighted average is 100 ppm; short-term exposure limit is 150 ppm).[15]

Solvent abusers, who inhale or insufflate toluene-containing glues and paints for their intoxicating effects, generally must create an ambient concentration of 10,000 to 30,000 ppm. This is normally done by breathing from a closed bag ("baggers"), inhaling from a container ("sniffers"), or breathing from a soaked rag ("huffers"). At these concentrations, toluene sensitizes the myocardium to circulating catecholamines, which may result in fatal arrhythmias.[4] In addition, reversible metabolic acidosis, hypokalemia, hematuria, proteinuria, hepatotoxicity, and distal renal tubular acidosis develop.

Chronic. Symptoms of toluene exposure in the workplace are not as dramatic but involve the same organ systems as acute toxicity. Several studies demonstrate that printers working at a normal pace experience dizziness, nasal mucous membrane irritation, intoxication, and a sensation of altered temperature (hot or cold) at 75 to 200 ppm of toluene in the workplace. Thus, the current standards may need to be lowered to prevent symptoms. However, no decrement in performance of psychomotor tests can be reproducibly measured at levels below 300 ppm.[2,3]

Occupational exposure to toluene may cause cardiac autonomic dysfunction. Two small studies of the variation in electrocardiographic R-R intervals of rotogravure printers yielded conflicting results.[12,13] These printers had career toluene and mixed solvent exposures, with average workplace concentrations of 85 ppm. Further research is necessary to determine if toluene can affect autonomic control of the heart.

Hepatotoxicity in printers exposed to toluene is more likely to be from alcohol than from toluene.[14] Renal toxicity from hydrocarbons has been better characterized as early markers of renal dysfunction are identified. Serum laminin concentrations seem to correlate to basement membrane dysfunction. As basement membrane is destroyed, serum laminin levels rise. Hydrocarbon exposure and hypertension increased the serum laminin concentration. A subgroup of printers who had several years of hippuric acid concentrations recorded had a positive correlation with an acceleration of the age-related decline in creatinine clearance.[9]

Biologic Markers

A 24-hour urine collection for toluene metabolites can be obtained. The total hippuric acid correlates to the degree of exposure. Hippuric acid is a normal constituent in urine and rises when the diet contains canned food or fruit.

REFERENCES

1. Astrand I: Uptake of solvents in the blood and tissues of man. A review, *Scand J Work Environ Health* 1:199, 1975.
2. Baelum J, Andersen I, Molhave L: Acute and subacute symptoms among workers in the printing industry, *Br J Ind Med* 39:70, 1982.
3. Baelum J et al: Human response to varying concentrations of toluene, *Int Arch Occup Environ Health* 62:65, 1990.
4. Bass M: Sudden sniffing deaths, *JAMA* 212:2075, 1970.
5. Chang AM et al: N-hexane neuropathy in offset printer, *J Neurol Neurosurg Psychiatry* 56:538, 1993.
6. Dossing M, Baelum J, Lundquist GR: Antipyrine clearance during experimental and occupational exposure to toluene, *Br J Ind Med* 40:317, 1983.
7. Fiserova-Bergerova V, editor: *Modeling of inhalation exposures to vapors: uptake, distribution, and elimination,* Boca Raton, Fla, 1983, CRC Press.
8. Garabrant DH: Dermatitis from aziridine hardener in printing ink, *Contact Dermatitis* 12:209, 1985.
9. Hotz P et al: Serum laminin, hydrocarbon exposure, and glomerular damage, *Br J Ind Med* 50:1104, 1993.
10. Kay K: Toxicology and carcinogenic evaluation of chemical used in the graphics arts industry, *Clin Toxicol* 9:359, 1976.
11. Leon DA, Thomas P, Hutchings S: Lung cancer among newspaper printers exposed to ink mists: a study of trade union members in Manchester, England, *Occup Environ Med* 51:87, 1994.
12. Murata K et al: Autonomic and peripheral nervous system dysfunction in workers exposed to mixed organic solvents, *Int Arch Occup Environ Health* 63:335, 1991.
13. Murata K et al: Cardiac autonomic dysfunction in rotogravure printers exposed to toluene in relation to peripheral nerve conduction, *Ind Health* 31:79, 1993.
14. Nasterlack M, Triebig G, Stelzer O: Hepatotoxic effects of solvent exposure around permissible limits and alcohol consumption in printers over a 4-year period, *Int Arch Occup Environ Health* 66:161, 1994.
15. *Toluene toxicity: ATSDR case studies in environmental medicine,* Washington, DC, 1983, Agency for Toxic Substances and Disease Registry, US Department of Health and Human Services.
16. US Department of Labor, Bureau of Labor Statistics, *Bulletin 2450, 1992 Department of labor statistics* Washington, DC, 1994, US Government Printing Office.

Roofers and Roadbuilders

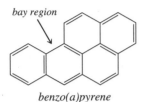

bay region

benzo(a)pyrene

- Coal tar increases the risk of skin, lung, gastric, and hematologic cancers

- Coal tar and asphalt fumes are skin and ocular irritants

- Tar warts

- "Bay regions" are tip-offs to carcinogenicity

Jeffrey R. Brubacher

OCCUPATIONAL DESCRIPTION
Background

The roofing and paving occupations are similar in that both use hot asphalt or coal tar pitch to provide a water- and weather-resistant surface. Vapors and dust from heated coal tar and asphalt products cause much of the occupational illness in these industries. According to U.S. government statistics, 239,000 people were employed in highway and street construction, and 187,000 people were employed in roofing, siding, and sheet metal work in 1987.[32] These figures may underestimate the actual number of persons employed as roofers or road builders.

Terminology: Asphalt, Coal Tar, Pitch, and Bitumens

Asphalt and coal tar pitch are both used to weatherproof and waterproof surfaces in the roofing and paving industries. These materials have similar physical properties; both are semisolids that become liquid when heated and harden when cooled. Both adhere to other materials (specifically to roofing felt and to road surfaces and fillers) and are waterproof. The two materials, however, come from different sources and contain different chemical constituents.

Bitumen is a generic term for a class of solid, semisolid, or viscous black or dark brown materials consisting primarily of high-molecular-weight hydrocarbons. Bitumen is produced during petroleum processing and also occurs naturally. *Asphalt* is the term given to solid or semisolid bitumens. Asphalt consists of very-high-molecular-weight hydrocarbons called *asphaltenes*. Today, most asphalt is derived from petroleum. Softer bitumens are referred to as *tars* or *pitches*. Tars and pitches derived from coal or wood are referred to, respectively, as *coal tar, coal pitch, wood tar,*

247

and *wood pitch.* About 80% of asphalt produced in the United States is used for road paving and repair. Roofing applications account for another 15% of asphalt use.

When organic material is pyrolized (heated in the absence of air), it yields dark viscous liquids referred to as *tars* and semisolids referred to as *pitch.* Coal is the largest source of industrial tars and pitches. Coal tar is a complex mixture of chemicals including benzene, toluene, phenol, styrene, cresol, naphthalene, and numerous polyaromatic hydrocarbons (PAHs), as well as tar bases and pitch. Compared to asphalt, coal tar has a much higher concentration of aromatic and polyaromatic hydrocarbons. Further processing separates coal tar pitch from the other constituents of coal tar. This pitch is used for aluminum smelting, and in the production of coal briquettes, as well as in the roofing and paving industries. In the United States, most roads (94%) are covered with asphalt, and only 6% are covered with coal tar pitch. In some parts of Europe, coal tar–derived road coatings are still prevalent.

Both coal tar pitch and asphalt are complex mixtures of aliphatic and aromatic hydrocarbons. The toxicity of bituminous materials is largely related to their content of PAHs. Asphalt contains primarily long-chain aliphatic hydrocarbons, whereas coal tar has more aromatic and polyaromatic hydrocarbons. When heated, both asphalt and coal tar pitch release significant amounts of hydrocarbon solvents. Other hydrocarbon solvents are added to roofing cement and cold applied roofing mixtures to improve their handling characteristics. Trucks carrying asphalt are sometimes cleaned with a spray of diesel oil, which exposes workers to another source of solvents.[6] Asphalt may also contain hydrogen sulfide, and there has been a report of roofers developing hydrogen sulfide toxicity from exposure to asphalt fumes.[15] Hydrogen sulfide is an irritant and a short-acting cellular asphyxiant similar in action to cyanide and exhibits a characteristic rotten egg odor (see Chapters 33 and 44).

Roofing

The specific tasks undertaken by roofers and the materials that they may be exposed to vary from job to job. In general, the most significant hazards are presented by exposure to fumes from asphalt and coal tar pitch. Additional hazards of the roofing industry include exposure to solvents, fiberglass, dust, solar ultraviolet radiation, and heat. There is also a significant potential for trauma (falls from a height).

The roofing process involves preparing the roof by removing preexisting surfaces. During these "tear-off" operations, roofers use power scratching machines that break up the old roofing material down to the roofing felt or insulation. The resulting debris is swept into rows and shoveled by hand into carts. The equipment used during the tear-off operation is cleaned by a power vacuum cleaner. All phases of the tear-off operation expose workers to dust from the old roof materials. Even when the new roof is made of roofing asphalt, roofers may be exposed to coal tar dust during the tear-off operation. Dust from old coal tar pitch roofs has been shown to be a potent inducer of skin cancer in a mouse model.[8] Applying water to the roof during the tear-off operation tends to decrease the amount of dust created. On occasion the old, underlying insulation may need to be removed and replaced. During these operations, roofers may come in contact with and need to handle fiberglass and various other insulation materials. Fiberglass can cause an intensely pruritic irritant dermatitis. After the insulation layer, a sheathing of plywood or boards is laid down to provide structural strength.

After these preparatory steps, an underlayment is applied. Underlayment consists of rolls of waterproof material that are made of fiberglass or felt saturated with asphalt or coal tar. Underlayment is held in place by nails and hot mopped asphalt, coal tar pitch, or cold applied roofing cement. During the underlayment process, areas where the roof is penetrated by vents or skylights are sealed with roofing cement. Roofing cements are mixtures of asphalt or tar with solvents added to improve handling characteristics. Fillers such as glass fibers, powdered aluminum, or rubber may also be added to these cements.

Industrial roofs are generally flat roofs made of built-up layers of asphalt or tar containing felts alternating with layers of asphalt or pitch. This is the so-called built-up roof (BUR). Both coal tar pitch and asphalt may be applied by a hot mop technique. Coal tar is softer than asphalt and melts at a lower temperature. Both products can be applied at temperatures near 200° C to 250° C but are often heated to much higher temperatures. Coal tar pitch is more water-resistant and is sometimes recommended on roofs where water pooling may occur. Asphalt is classified according to its melting point into four types: type I (dead level) asphalt has the lowest melting point and can be applied only to level roofs; type IV (special steep) has the highest melting point and can be applied to steep roofs in hot-weather areas. These products are heated in a kettle and applied by spray or by wheelbarrow. Exposure to fumes can be minimized by using the lowest possible temperature and by keeping the kettle covered. Some asphalt coatings are thinned with organic solvents so that they can be applied when cold. The entire structure is frequently covered with gravel.

Unlike industrial and commercial roofs, residential roofs are generally sloping and covered by shingles. As in industrial roofs, application of the underlayment may involve handling hot tar or asphalt. Shingles are most often made of roofing felt or fiberglass that has been saturated with asphalt. Because these materials are cold when roofers handle them, there is little exposure to asphalt or pitch fumes. Other shingle materials include wood, slate, and tile. Wooden shingles are made from various woods, of which western red cedar is the most popular. Cutting these shingles to size exposes roofers to dust from western red cedar (see Chapter 5).

Roadbuilding

The road is first formed with earthmoving equipment, and the base is stabilized by the addition of lime (calcium hydroxide) or cement. During this process, workers are exposed to significant amounts of cement, lime, and rock dust. Cement and lime are skin irritants. After the base is prepared, the road is paved to seal it. Paving involves the application of hot asphalt or coal tar pitch mixed with stone chips to the prepared surface. Stone chips are mixed with asphalt before application or applied after the asphalt has been laid down. Asphalt is usually applied from a truck, with one or more workers at the back of the truck to control asphalt flow. In hard-to-reach areas, asphalt may be applied manually with shovels and wheelbarrows. After asphalt application, other workers rake the asphalt into a uniform coating that is rolled by workers driving (or pushing) power rollers. After this, the surface is allowed to cool. The result is a waterproof and weather-resistant coating. All workers involved in this process are exposed to fumes from hot asphalt and to dust from the stone chips. Gang sprayers— workers who control the delivery of hot asphalt or coal tar pitch from the back of a truck—are exposed to the highest concentrations of asphalt or pitch fumes. Additional hazards include high temperatures, solar ultraviolet radiation, and fumes from combustion of diesel fuel. During the paving of tunnels or indoor surfaces or when road repair is performed in areas of heavy traffic, workers are frequently exposed to carbon monoxide.

POTENTIALLY TOXIC EXPOSURES
Coal Tar Fumes and Dust

Hot coal tar releases numerous volatile polyaromatic hydrocarbons (PAHs). Among the PAHs released are several compounds that are well-established animal carcinogens and mutagenic by the Ames test: chrysene, benzo(*c*)phenanthrene, benzo(*a*)pyrene, dibenzo(*a,j*)anthracene, dibenzo (*a,h*)anthracene, and indenol(1,2,3-*cd*)pyrene.[18] Of these compounds, benzo(*a*)pyrene and dibenzoanthracene are the most carcinogenic. Benzo(*a*)pyrene has been implicated as a human carcinogen.[10] Other compounds found in coal tar include benzene, toluene, xylene, styrene, phenol, cresol, and naphthalene. All of these compounds are irritants and play a role in the eye and skin irritation seen in roofers and pavers using coal tar–derived products. A newer variety of coal tar known as *coal tar bitumen* releases fewer volatiles on heating and may be less irritating to the skin.

The carcinogenicity of classic coal tar pitch, coal tar bitumen, asphalt, and dust released during the tear-off of a coal tar–covered roof was studied using a mouse bioassay. Dust from the tear-off operation, traditional coal tar pitch, and coal tar bitumen were all powerful carcinogens, although coal tar bitumen was significantly less potent than the other two. Roofing asphalt did not cause skin cancers in this model.[8]

The Occupational Safety and Health Administration (OSHA)-permissible exposure limit for coal tar volatiles is 0.2 mg/m^3, although some authors have recommended lowering this to 0.05 mg/m^3.[4] Instead of considering total coal tar volatiles, the National Institute of Occupational Safety and Health (NIOSH) considers PAHs and sets the recommended exposure limit for PAHs at 0.1 µg/m^3 (the lowest detectable concentration at the time of the recommendation).

Asphalt Fumes

Asphalt fumes have a much lower content of PAHs than do fumes from coal tar–derived products. Heated asphalt releases long-chain aliphatic hydrocarbons such as octanes, nonanes, decanes, and higher aliphatics. Toluene, xylene, other benzene derivatives, and higher aromatics are also found in small quantities.[6,24] Asphalt fumes cause skin and eye irritation and may be carcinogenic in humans, but this has not been definitively established. Asphalt is an animal carcinogen, although much less potent than coal tar.[5,25] Asphalt often contains added low-molecular-weight polyamines, which serve to increase adhesiveness and to act as emulsifiers. These chemicals are highly irritating and may account for some of the skin and eye irritation seen in road pavers.[20] The permissible exposure limit (PEL) for asphalt is 5 mg/m^3, although some authorities[4] suggest that this should be lowered to 0.5 mg/m^3.

Solvent Exposure

Asphalt and tar workers are exposed to organic solvents from heated asphalt and coal tar. Solvents may also be added to asphalt or to coal tar products to improve handling. Painters, printers, and other occupational groups exposed to high levels of organic solvents are at risk of developing a chronic toxic encephalopathy consisting of mood changes, short-term memory impairment, fatigue, attention deficits, and other cognitive deficits.[1] In contrast, asphalt and tar workers are exposed to relatively low levels of organic solvents, so severe solvent-induced toxic encephalopathy has not been described and is unlikely to occur in these workers under normal working conditions.[6,26] Nevertheless, asphalt workers do develop symptoms consistent with mild solvent exposure. A study comparing road repair and construction workers exposed to asphalt fumes to unexposed workers found that asphalt workers had a higher incidence of abnormal fatigue, reduced appetite, cough, and throat and eye irritation. These symptoms were more prevalent in workers using harder asphalt types and asphalt heated to higher temperatures and in those workers exposed to higher concentrations of asphalt fumes.[26]

Miscellaneous

Roofers may be required to handle fiberglass if a particular job involves the removal or placement of insulation. Fiberglass contains many sharp spicules that cause skin irritation. When wooden shingles are used, roofers may be exposed to wood dust from western red cedar, which can cause dermatitis and occupational asthma (see chapter on carpenters and woodworkers). Roadbuilders are exposed to particulate matter from the crushed stones used as fillers and from cement and lime added as stabilizers. Lime and cement are skin and eye irritants, and rock dust is a nuisance that may cause cough and throat irritation or ocular discomfort. The OSHA PEL for dust is 10 mg/m^3. This is often exceeded during roadbuilding operations.[6] There are no well-documented long-term sequelae from exposure to lime, cement, or rock dust.

The outdoor nature of roofing and paving results in high exposure to solar ultraviolet (UV) radiation. This plays a role in the skin and eye irritation caused by acute exposure to coal tar and asphalt vapors and may play a role in the development of skin cancer. Skin protection in the form of long sleeves, gloves, hats, and face coverings, as well as the use of sunblock, serves to decrease UV exposure. Heat exposure is another obvious hazard for both roofers and pavers in warm climates and especially in those workers directly handling heated tar or asphalt.

CLINICAL TOXICOLOGY
Oncologic

The association between exposure to tar and cancer was recognized in 1775 by the British surgeon Percival Pott, who noted the relationship between soot exposure and cancer of the scrotum in chimney sweeps. By 1907, the Workmen's Compensation Act in Britain recognized "epitheliomatous cancer or ulceration of the skin occurring in the handling or use of pitch, tar or tarry compounds" as occupational diseases. In 1920, these diseases became notifiable. In 1947, Henry analyzed 3753 cases of epitheliomata reported to the chief inspector of factories between 1920 and 1944. Road construction workers accounted for 22 of the cases. The vast majority of cases (3264) were caused by exposure to mineral oil in the cotton industry or to pitch and tar in the tar distilling, patent fuel, and coal gas industries.[13]

Several historical cohort studies have examined the incidence of cancer in asphalt workers and roofers. Comparison of medical records of members of the roofers union with records of the U.S. male population found an excess of cancer in the roofers. This increase was most marked for skin, head and neck, stomach, and bladder cancers and for leukemia.[10] This is caused by inhalation of benzo(a)pyrene and other agents found in the fumes of hot pitch. A 10-year historical cohort study compared Danish asphalt workers with unskilled workers employed outside the asphalt industry and demonstrated an increased incidence of cancer deaths in asphalt workers. This increase in cancer deaths reached statistical significance during the second 5-year follow-up period and was largely due to an increased incidence of respiratory, gastrointestinal, and bladder cancers.[12] In a similar study, a historical cohort of 679 mastic asphalt

workers was found to have a significant excess of lung and gastrointestinal cancers. Mastic asphalt is a mixture of sand, stone powder, powdered limestone, and hard asphalt used for roofing, flooring, and surfacing road. It is kept heated at approximately 250° C until application. The increased incidence of lung cancer was significant even in those workers who, because of their age, were unlikely to have worked with mastic asphalt during World War II, when coal tar was routinely added to it.[11]

Case-control studies found that roofers may be at increased risk for certain types of cancer. Of 2161 persons with lung cancer reported in Los Angeles County, roofers had a standard mortality ratio almost 5 times that of the general working population. Only asbestos and insulation workers had higher relative risks of developing lung cancer.[23] Another case-control study found that roofers have an increased risk of developing non-Hodgkin's lymphoma.[29]

These studies are confounded because they did not take into consideration the high prevalence of smoking in roofers. A recent U.S. government survey found that roofers have the highest smoking rate of all occupations surveyed: 59% of roofers smoked compared to 39% of all blue-collar workers and 24% of white-collar workers.[24]

A recent meta-analysis evaluated the cancer risk in roofers, highway maintenance and road workers, and miscellaneous bitumen and asphalt workers. Roofers had an increased risk for cancers of the lung, stomach, and skin (nonmelanoma) and for leukemia. Surprisingly, the increased relative risk for skin cancer in roofers did not quite reach statistical significance. Road workers had an increased relative risk for skin cancer.[27]

Since tar and asphalt are often mixed together and because a single worker usually is exposed to both agents during a career, the relative contribution of each agent to carcinogenesis is difficult to determine. A survey of 462 asphalt workers and 379 control workers concluded that there was no evidence that petroleum asphalt constituted a health hazard.[2] The meta-analysis discussed previously also addressed this issue but concluded that present studies were not able to answer this question. Others have measured volatilized and polyaromatic hydrocarbon exposures in pavers, using asphalt workers, and have concluded that they are occasionally exposed to harmful levels of potential carcinogens.[3,6] However, most authors conclude that coal tar poses a greater risk to the health than does asphalt.[6,17,18]

Dermatologic

Exposure to vapors and dust from coal tar or asphalt causes a variety of skin lesions: acneiform lesions, chronic dermatosis, benign skin neoplasms, and squamous cell carcinoma. Coal tar–induced photosensitivity reactions (also referred to as the *smarts* or *burns*) occur in more than half of coal tar workers. Symptoms consist of skin erythema, burning or pruritus, and blistering. Affected workers describe the burning as feeling as if they are exposed to a direct flame. The most commonly involved areas are the exposed skin of the face (nose, forehead, and central facial creases) and the forearms. Scaling may occur several days after initial symptoms even in the absence of erythema. Photosensitivity symptoms are described as different from a sunburn. Workers do not develop a tan after the burns, and symptoms tend to recur all summer long with little acquired protection. Burning starts within 1 hour of exposure to pitch and sunlight and persists for as long as the exposure continues. These symptoms are more prevalent in those with fair complexion and are worsened by exposure to UV radiation and to cold wind. Removal of the worker from the exposure results in resolution of symptoms over a period of several days to weeks. Some workers describe a benefit from showers and emollient creams used at the end of the day. Sunblock is likely to decrease symptoms, but this is rarely used by roofers. Protective clothing such as long-sleeved shirts, gloves, and face coverings decreases the incidence of the burns.[7]

Most tar workers develop acneiform lesions (more than 90% in one study),[15] including comedones on the face and shoulders, white or yellow sebaceous retention cysts on the face and neck, folliculitis on the head, body, and limbs, and true acne on the face and back. There appears to be no relation between development of acne and development of other tar-induced skin changes. Tar exposure may also result in a condition known as *chronic tar dermatosis,* which consists of skin thickening or atrophy, pigmentary changes (hyperpigmentation or hypopigmentation), and erythema or telangiectasia and most often occurs on the forearms, wrists, and hands.

Other benign skin lesions in tar workers include squamous keratosis and keratoacanthoma or tar warts. Squamous keratoses are dry, scaly, rough lesions that occur on the sun-exposed skin of the head and arms. Also known as *solar keratoses* and *senile keratoses,* these lesions are common in the general population but more prevalent in tar workers.[15] Keratoacanthomas are rapidly growing benign tumors that resemble squamous cell carcinomas. Keratoacanthomas are discrete, dome-shaped lesions that often have a central keratotic plug. They are found most commonly on the face around the eyes and nose but may be found elsewhere, including on the scrotum. These "tar warts" usually occur after decades of exposure to pitch but may occur after only a few years of exposure. They resolve spontaneously in about one quarter of cases and occasionally progress to squamous cell cancer; they are difficult to distinguish clinically from squamous cell cancer. Because of this, all "tar warts" should be biopsied and sent for pathologic examination. Finally, both roofers and road workers have a markedly increased incidence of nonmelanoma skin cancers.

Opthalmologic

Workers exposed to fumes from coal tar pitch and asphalt often complain of burning ocular discomfort, tearing, and conjunctival erythema. These symptoms are most marked on bright sunny and windy days and are more prominent in workers exposed to pitch than to those exposed to asphalt fumes. The cause appears to be keratoconjunctivitis related to photosensitization of the eye by coal tar volatiles. Experimental models in rabbits and anecdotal reports from roofers demonstrate that exposure to UV radiation is required in addition to fumes from heated coal tar or asphalt.[9] Persons with dark skin are not protected against ocular symptoms from tar exposure.[7] These ocular symptoms may impede a worker's vision and increase the risk of sustaining a work injury.

Pulmonary

Vapors from asphalt and coal tar products are irritating and may cause cough and pharyngeal irritation. Road workers handling asphalt developed these symptoms more frequently than other workers.[26] Roofers and pavers may be at increased risk of developing chronic obstructive pulmonary disease (COPD), and one study found an increased incidence of death from respiratory diseases in roofers. This conclusion must be interpreted in light of the extremely high incidence of smoking among roofers.[10] Exposure to dust from tear-off operations and from road preparation may also cause irritative respiratory symptoms. The most significant respiratory hazard in persons exposed to coal tar vapors is lung cancer.

Pathophysiology

Coal tar pitch is well described to be a human and animal carcinogen. Of the numerous constituents of coal tar, it is the polyaromatic hydrocarbons (especially benzo(*a*)pyrene) that are implicated as carcinogens. These compounds are absorbed through the skin and lungs of exposed workers.[31,33] Polyaromatic hydrocarbons (PAHs) are oxidized in the skin, liver, lungs, kidneys, and other organs to yield numerous metabolites. Certain pathways lead to the formation of reactive diol epoxides that are believed to mediate the carcinogenic activity of the PAHs. Not all PAHs have the same carcinogenic activity. The "bay region" theory states that diol epoxide metabolites of PAHs are carcinogenic if they occur in the bay region of a PAH (Fig. 31-1).[20] The potency of a PAH as a carcinogen thus depends on whether or not it contains a bay region, what percentage of its metabolites are bay region diol epoxides and the carcinogenic potency of the active metabolite(s). In vitro cell culture studies and in vivo mouse skin assays have shown that benzo(*a*)pyrene and dibenzoanthracene are potent carcinogens.[22] IARC considers benzo(a)pyrene and benzoanthracene to be animal carcinogens and probable human carcinogens.[27]

The PAH diol epoxides are highly reactive compounds that bind to molecules in the body to form adducts. When DNA-PAH adducts are formed, DNA is damaged, and there is a potential for malignancy. Organs with rapid cell turnover, such as skin and the gastrointestinal tract, seem to

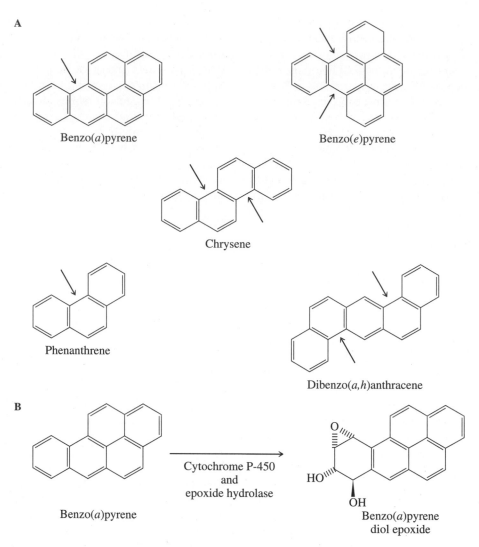

Fig. 31-1 A, Structures of common polyaromatic hydrocarbons. Arrows indicate the bay regions. **B,** Metabolism of benzo(a)pyrene to the carcinogenic metabolite benzo(a)pyrene diol epoxide. The highly reactive diol epoxide binds to DNA to form adducts that result in DNA damage.

be most affected by the formation of DNA-PAH adducts. The PAH diol epoxides also bind to the DNA of white blood cells or to albumin. Measurement of PAH-DNA adducts in white blood cells or of PAH-albumin adducts may provide noninvasive methods of biologic monitoring of exposed workers.[14,19]

Prevention

The most important preventative measures are steps taken at the worksite to minimize workers' exposure to harmful volatiles. Asphalt is safer than coal tar products and should be used whenever possible. The asphalt or coal tar mix should be heated at the lowest possible temperature. The softer types of asphalt or coal tar require lower temperatures and release less fumes and so are preferable. The kettles used to heat asphalt and coal tar should be kept covered, and there should be adequate ventilation whenever the work is indoors.

Personal measures to minimize exposure at work include protective clothing such as long-sleeved shirts, kerchiefs to cover the face, hats, and protective eyewear. Sunscreen may decrease irritative symptoms and lower the risk of skin cancer. Showering and changing clothes at the end of the workday and wearing clean clothes to work each day can decrease the duration of exposure to harmful dust that may have contaminated clothing and skin during the day. Because of the probable synergistic effect of smoking and exposure to PAHs in carcinogenesis, all persons handling coal tar or asphalt products should be counseled to stop smoking. Individuals who are particularly sensitive to coal tar or asphalt fumes may have to find alternate work.

Treatment and Screening

Most irritative skin and eye symptoms resolve in days to weeks following removal from exposure. Affected persons should be counseled regarding preventive measures. Specifically, protective clothing and eyewear, showers and clean clothes at the end of the workday, and use of emollient skin creams may minimize symptoms. The periodic health exam should include a search for suspicious skin lesions, and workers should be taught to recognize tar warts and other suspicious skin lesions and to report these to their physician. All such skin lesions should be removed and sent for pathologic examination. All workers should be counseled to stop smoking. Persons with respiratory symptoms should have chest radiographs to screen for cancer. Workers with weight loss, abdominal masses, or other suspicious signs or symptoms require appropriate investigations to rule out malignancy.

Exposure Monitoring

As mentioned in the pathophysiology section, PAHs are carcinogens by virtue of their binding to DNA to form PAH-DNA adducts. The PAHs also form adducts with albumin. Measurement of PAH-albumin adducts in blood or PAH-DNA adducts in white blood cells may give a measurement of exposure to PAHs. In patients with psoriasis treated with coal tar the measurement of PAH-DNA adducts in white blood cells by enzyme-linked immunosorbent assay (ELISA) is the most sensitive measure of exposure to PAHs.[28] Another biologic marker for PAH exposure is urinary excretion of 1:hydroxypyrene.[21] All these biologic markers for PAH exposure are relatively new and difficult to interpret because normal values are not well defined. Furthermore, numerous nonoccupational exposures to PAHs such as smoking, air pollution, psoriasis remedies, and consumption of PAH-containing foods like smoked or barbecued meats, roasted peanuts, coffee, and refined vegetable oil may all give positive results on these tests. The measurements of PAH adducts with protein or DNA must still be considered investigational.

The PAH exposure at the workplace may be approximated by measuring the total concentration of coal tar or asphalt volatiles in the ambient air. This is accomplished by passing a known volume of air through a filter and then extracting and measuring the coal tar or asphalt volatiles of the filtrate. The OSHA limit for coal tar volatiles is 0.2 mg/m^3, and that for asphalt volatiles is 5 mg/m^3. In these measurements, coal tar and asphalt volatiles are extracted with benzene or cyclohexane. For laboratory safety reasons, cyclohexane has generally replaced benzene. Some countries have set exposure limits for total PAHs or for benzo(a)pyrene and other specific PAHs. These can be measured by a similar method that is technically more difficult than measuring total volatiles. Personal exposure can be quantified by measuring PAHs and cyclohexane-soluble compounds in personal air filters to determine inhaled exposure and on dermally applied exposure pads to measure skin contamination. Monitoring personal exposure is expensive, requires worker cooperation, is not generally available, and has not been well standardized.

Measuring exposure is also complicated by the fact that, unlike the situation in a factory where the exposure is relatively constant from day to day, the exposure in the roofing and paving industries varies from job to job. Factors such as the type of coating used (asphalt or coal tar pitch), ventilation at a particular site (paving in a tunnel or another enclosed site), and the need for tear-off operations all contribute to the exposure involved with a particular job.

SUMMARY

Persons handling coal tar and asphalt products often suffer from irritative skin and eye symptoms that may be prevented by applying occupational hygiene measures and by appropriate use of skin and eye protection. Coal tar is a human carcinogen, and roofers and road workers have an increased risk of death from malignancy. Excess incidence of skin cancer, lung cancer, and gastrointestinal and hematologic malignancies are reported in these groups. Early detection may improve the outcome in persons developing these malignancies.

Although the risk of exposure to carcinogens from volatilized pitch and asphalt is very real, accidents cause more deaths than cancer in the roofing industry. In a recent New Jersey survey, roofers were second only to iron workers in fatal occupational accidents. The overall death rate from accidents in the construction industry was 14.5 per 100,000 persons per year. Roofers had an accidental death rate of 56.2 per 100,000 per year. Most of the deaths were caused by falls from a height.[30] These statistics emphasize the need to look at all aspects of workers' safety.

REFERENCES

1. Baker EL: A review of recent research on health effects of human occupational exposure to organic solvents, *J Occ Med* 36:1079, 1994.
2. Baylor CH, Weaver NK: A health survey of petroleum asphalt workers, *Arch Environ Health* 17:210, 1968.
3. Brandt HC, Molyneux MK: Sampling and analysis of bitumen fumes: part 2, field exposure measurements, *Ann Occup Hyg* 29:47, 1985.
4. Chong JP, Haines AT, Verma DK: A pragmatic approach to standard setting: the example of coal tar products and asphalt, *Ann Occup Hyg* 33:197, 1989.
5. Chong J et al: *Health effects of coal tar products and bitumens*, Ontario, 1986, Ontario Ministry of Labour.
6. Darby FW, Willis AF, Winchester RV: Occupational health hazards from road construction and sealing work, *Ann Occup Hyg* 30:445, 1986.
7. Emmett EA: Cutaneous and ocular hazards of roofers, *Occ Med* 1:307, 1986.
8. Emmett EA, Bingham EM, Barkley W: A carcinogenic bioassay of certain roofing materials, *Am J Ind Med* 2:59, 1981.
9. Emmett EA, Stetzer L, Taphorn B: Phototoxic keratoconjunctivitis from coal tar pitch volatiles, *Science* 198:841, 1977.
10. Hammond EC et al: Inhalation of benzpyrene and cancer in man, *Ann N Y Acad Sci* 271:116, 1976.
11. Hansen ES: Cancer incidence in an occupational cohort exposed to bitumen fumes, *Scand J Work Envir Health* 15:101, 1989.
12. Hansen ES: Cancer mortality in the asphalt industry: a ten year follow up of an occupational cohort, *Br J Ind Med* 46:582, 1989.
13. Henry SA: Occupational cutaneous cancer attributable to certain chemicals in industry, *BMJ* 4:389, 1947.

14. Herbert R et al: Detection of adducts of deoxyribonucleic acid in white blood cells of roofers by 32P-postlabeling. Relationship of adduct levels to measures of exposure to polycyclic aromatic hydrocarbons, *Scand J Work Environ Health* 16:135, 1990.

15. Hodgson GA, Whitely HJ: Personal susceptibility to pitch, *Br J Ind Med* 27:160, 1970.

16. Hoidal CR et al: Hydrogen sulfide poisoning from toxic inhalations of roofing asphalt fumes, *Ann Emerg Med* 15:826, 1986.

17. Jongeneelen FJ et al: Airborne concentrations, skin contamination, and urinary metabolite excretion of polycyclic aromatic hydrocarbons among paving workers exposed to coal tar derived road tars, *Am Ind Hyg Assoc J* 49:600, 1988.

18. Knecht U, Woitowitz HJ: Risk of cancer from the use of tar bitumen in road works, *Br J Ind Med* 46:24, 1989.

19. Lee BM et al: Immunologic measurement of polycyclic aromatic hydrocarbon-albumin adducts in foundry workers and roofers, *Scand J Work Environ Health* 17:190-94.

20. Levin JO, Andersson K, Hallgren C: Exposure to low molecular polyamines during road paving, *Ann Occ Hyg* 38:257, 1964.

21. Levin JO, Rhen M, Sikstrom E: Occupational PAH exposure: urinary 1-hydroxypyrene levels of coke oven workers, aluminum smelter pot-room workers, road pavers, and occupationally non-exposed persons in Sweden, *Sci Total Environ* 163:169, 1995.

22. Levin W et al: Oxidative metabolism of polycyclic aromatic hydrocarbons to ultimate carcinogens, *Drug Metab Rev* 13:555, 1982.

23. Menck HR, Henderson BE: Occupational differences in rates of lung cancer, *J Occ Med* 18:797, 1976.

24. Nelson DE et al: Cigarette smoking prevalence by occupation in the United States, *J Occ Med* 36:516, 1994.

25. Niemeier RW et al: A comparison of the skin carcinogenicity of condensed roofing asphalt and coal tar pitch fumes. In *Proceedings of the third NCI/EPA/NIOSH collaborative workshop: progress on joint environmental and occupational cancer studies,* Washington, DC 1984.

26. Norseth T, Waage J, Dale I: Acute effects and exposure to organic compounds in road maintenance workers exposed to asphalt, *Am J Ind Med* 20:737, 1991.

27. Partanen T, Boffetta P: Cancer risk in asphalt workers and roofers: review and meta-analysis of epidemiologic studies, *Am J Ind Med* 26:721, 1994.

28. Santella RM et al: Polycyclic aromatic hydrocarbon-DNA and protein adducts in coal tar treated patients and controls and their relationship to glutathione S-transferase genotype, *Mutat Res* 334:117, 1995.

29. Scherr PA, Hutchinson GB, Neiman RS: Non Hodgkin's lymphoma and occupational exposure, *Cancer Res* 52(suppl):5503s, 1992.

30. Sorok GS, Smith EO, Goldoft M: Fatal occupational injuries in the New Jersey construction industry, 1983 to 1989, *J Occup Med* 35:916, 1993.

31. Storer JS: Human absorption of crude coal tar products, *Arch Dermatol* 120:874, 1984.

32. US Bureau of the Census: *Statistical abstract of the United States,* (table 1192), ed 114, Washington, DC, 1994, US Government Printing Office.

33. VanRooij JGM et al: Absorption of polycyclic aromatic hydrocarbons through human skin: differences between anatomical sites and individuals, *J Toxicol Environ Health* 38:355, 1993.

Sandblasters

Liese O'Halloran Schwarz
Richard Y. Wang

Si

- Sandblasting generates crystalline silica particles that are associated with silicosis

- Silicosis is a fibrotic disease of the lungs; it can appear many years after toxic exposure ceases

- There is no known effective treatment for silicosis

- Prevention of silicosis consists of protection against inhaled crystalline silica particles, which is attempted by reducing the proportion of silica in the sandblasting abrasive, using wet abrasive technique, filtering the air, and ventilating the workplace

OCCUPATIONAL DESCRIPTION

Sandblasting is a method of industrial cleaning in which a stream of abrasive material is directed at a surface. The abrasive consists of tiny glass particles, metal spheres, wire fragments, walnut shells, pumice, or sand; it may be propelled by air, water, steam, or centrifugal force. Glass, freshly cast metal, and the sides of buildings or ships can all be cleaned by this method. Sandblasting was introduced at the beginning of the twentieth century and is most common in the construction industry, in shipbuilding, and in the iron and steel industries as a final step in metal casting.

Traditional metal casting has not changed significantly since antiquity. A model of the object to be cast is first created of wood or wax. A mold is constructed around the model by compressing sand against it. The sand mold maintains its shape with the aid of a binder (linseed oil, rosin, molasses, or glue). The cast is formed by pouring molten metal into the sand mold; the metal destroys the wooden or wax model but is constrained by the heat-resistant sand. After cooling, the cast item must be freed of the clinging sand in a sometimes arduous process.

Before mechanization, human workers accomplished every step of iron casting. The only skilled workers were the "molders," who pressed the sand against the molds. The other workers were unskilled, often immigrants, who mixed the sand and binder in large open vats, poured the metal, and performed the "shakeout." This last process freed sand from the castings with the use of sledgehammers and chisels. The cast metal surfaces were then finished with fine brushes or grinders. The air of the foundry twinkled with airborne sand, and all workers were exposed to it. After a workday, the workers turned sand out of the cuffs of their trousers and spit it from their mouths.

Mechanization came to the foundry in 1870 and paradoxically increased a foundry worker's exposure to inhaled sand. The mixing process was changed: 10 men with shovels and sieves were supplanted by 1 man operating a power mixer. Mixing became more efficient, enabling more sand to be mixed per work shift. The shake-out was also modernized: Sledgehammers and chisels gave way to pneumatic tools, which threw greater amounts of fine dust into the air. In the early 1900s, sandblasting replaced the wire brushes used in finishing work and filled the foundry's air with an enormous number of sand particles.

The famous Triangle Shirtwaist Factory fire of 1911 in New York City shed light on the abominable working conditions in that industry and spurred investigations of factory hazards. The New York State Factory Commission found immensely dusty foundries and was told by one public safety commissioner that "it would be practically impossible" to improve these conditions.[46] The Molder's Union sought in 1912 to confine the dusty processes of metal casting (the shakeout and the finishing work) to enclosed rooms so that not all workers were exposed to the same hazard. The union's attitude was that foundry work was inherently dusty, and while skilled workers ought to be protected, unskilled workers need not be.[46] In a minor measure to control exposure, the shakeout was restricted to the night shift. However, the sand lingered in the air to be breathed by the daytime workers, and no real improvement was achieved.

Sandblasting was one occupation felt to be particularly hazardous. In 1915, the Founder's Union published *Safety in the Foundry,* which detailed new industry protective measures.[2] The book stated that sandblasters were expected to wear special protective gear and work in separate, ventilated rooms. The book also lauded the tumbling mill, a device that cleaned small and hardy castings using agitated sand within a chamber. However, many foundries could not afford to adopt these changes, especially after the onset of the Great Depression.[1,15,47,54]

Concern for worker safety brought together many committees and investigative panels. However, by 1940, few changes had occurred. In the United States at that time, fewer than 15% of dusty industries had local exhaust ventilation, and only 3.2% of the operations were enclosed.[8] The proportion of workers wearing respiratory protection was also about 3%. Moreover, more than 96% of the operations that could have been done wet were being done dry, which increased airborne sand particles unnecessarily.[8] In the 1960s and 1970s in America, the creation of regulatory agencies such as the National Institute for Occupational Safety and Health (NIOSH) and the Occupational Safety and Health Administration (OSHA) paved the way for true reform of foundry working conditions.

Standard sandblasting today involves a compressed-air source, a stream of dry abrasive, and an enclosed blasting chamber. Other types of sandblasting use water or a spinning wheel to propel the abrasive material. The process can be performed in the open air, in a chamber, or in a tumbler. The number of Americans involved in sandblasting today is difficult to quantify because for many it is a part-time occupation; NIOSH estimated 100,000 sandblasters annually in America in 1992.[55] This number may be considerably greater in other countries.

SILICA

The major toxin associated with sandblasting is free crystalline silica, which after prolonged inhalation may cause silicosis, an interstitial fibrotic disease of the lungs. Silica dust is generated by the breakdown of the abrasive material or the surface being prepared into minute particles. In the early days of sandblasting, sand was the abrasive, and the exposure to silica dust was great. Currently, other abrasives are used; however, both these substances and the casting material being removed from a surface frequently contain some silica.

Silica is the most common mineral on earth. It composes about 90% of the earth's crust and exists in both amorphous and crystalline forms. The two amorphous forms are flint and diatomaceous earth, which is also known as *kieselguhr* or *tripolite.* The toxicity of diatomaceous earth is controversial; most amorphous silica is felt to be nontoxic. The crystalline form, most commonly encountered as quartz, occurs in a tetrahedral structure, with the silicon atom at the center and oxygen at the corners. Other forms of crystalline silica include tripoli, tridymite, and cristobalite. Different kinds of stones contain different proportions of silica: Sandstone is nearly 100%; granite is about 30%. Talc and asbestos are combined forms of silica, called *silicates,* and exposure to these can cause acute respiratory symptoms (cough, cyanosis, dyspnea) and cancer of the lung or pleura. The OSHA-permissible limit for occupational exposure to respirable silica is an 8-hour time-weighted average of 100 μm per cubic millimeter of air, which is double the maximal exposure recommended by NIOSH.[36,44,55] These numbers suppose a 10-hour/day exposure and a 40-hour workweek. In the United States, sandblasting abrasive should contain less than 1% free silica; in Great Britain, silica-containing abrasives have been abolished since 1950.

SILICOSIS
History

Disease caused by respirable crystalline silica is associated with many trades besides sandblasting. Hippocrates noted the breathlessness of metal miners. Lohneiss described mining in 1690: "the dust and stones fall upon the lungs, the men have lung disease, breathe with difficulty."[9] In 1700, Bernardo Ramazzini, the father of occupational medicine, wrote about miners' phthisis as a disease associated with dusty trades in his *De Morbis Artificum Diatriba.* Thomas Benson proposed in 1726 the wet grinding of flint for use in the pottery trade. He noted that "any person ever so healthful and strong working in that business cannot possibly survive above two years . . . the dust sucked into his body by the air he breathes . . . fixes there so closely that nothing will remove it."[9] The association between dust and disease was again observed among needle pointers. Those who used wet grindstones in their work lived into their 40s and 50s, while those who used dry grindstones died around the age of 30.[9] Throughout history, the affliction of these workers in dusty trades has been known by various names: "miners' phthisis," "dust consumption," "mason's disease," "grinders' asthma," "potters' rot," "sewer's disease," "stonecutters' disease," and "knappers' rot." Today, we know the disease as silicosis.

The emergence of the modern understanding of silicosis is a result of the work of statisticians around the turn of the century. Working for Metropolitan Life Insurance Company, Lee Frankl noted that foundry, quarry, and machine shop workers lost between 12 and 14 workdays to illness each year; clerks, bookkeepers, and butchers lost only 4 to 6 days.[46] Frederick L. Hoffman, a Prudential statistician, concluded in 1908 that "the dust-laden atmosphere of factories and workshops are a decidedly serious menace to health and life."[32] He added that there was, counter to public opinion at that time, "a paucity of bacteria in very dusty air" and that "dust in any form, when inhaled continuously and in considerable quantities, is prejudicial to health because of its inherent mechanical properties, destructive to the delicate membrane of the respiratory passages and the lungs."[32] Silica dust was identified in miners' lungs by Peacock and Greenhow in the 1860s.[35] Ten years later, Visconeti coined the name *silicosis* to mean the disease caused by silex or flint.[35]

Silicosis gained national attention in the 1930s in America, with the Gauley Bridge disaster.[13] The Hawk's Nest Tunnel, a hydroelectric power diversion over 16,000 feet long, was blasted into the rock near Gauley Bridge, West Virginia. An epidemic of acute silicosis followed, resulting in the death of 400 drillers and disability in the majority of the remaining workers. Federal hearings found that the tunneling had taken place through rock of greater than 90% pure silica. This event led many of the early giants of occupational disease to concentrate their efforts on silicosis. Victoria M. Trasko, who worked for the U.S. Public Health Service from 1937 to 1971, was the first to categorize silicosis by state, industry, and job description. Her investigations demonstrated that physicians did not reliably report cases of silicosis and led to the establishment of state-based surveillance of occupational diseases.[15]

Today, a multitude of occupations are associated with silica exposure: hard-rock mining, tunneling, quarrying, "flint-knapping" (an ancient, still-practiced British method of toolmaking), shipbuilding, stonecutting, and ceramic and glass manufacture. In 1980, the U.S. Department of Labor estimated that over 1 million American workers were exposed to silica dust and projected that 59,000 of those exposed would develop "silica-related pulmonary effects."[33] Silicosis has been associated with rubber processing, cosmetic and soap manufacture, and the jewelry industry. Finely ground silica (called *silica flour*) is used in the manufacture of numerous products and can be a source of "occult" toxicity. Two London women died from acute silicosis after having worked less than 5 years in a factory packing a scouring powder that contained silica flour.[39] The diagnosis was made only at autopsy.

Silica is not the only toxin associated with sandblasting. The cleaning of ferrous castings may produce iron oxide dust and cause siderosis, a benign pneumoconiosis. If the blasted surface contains hazardous metals such as lead, cadmium, or arsenic, the dust is accordingly toxic. Sandblasters may also be exposed to other hazardous substances associated with general foundry work, such as formaldehyde and products of combustion.

Pathology

During the seventeenth century, van Diemenbroeck, a professor of medicine in Utrecht, described cutting into a stonecutter's lungs at autopsy to be like cutting through sand. Indeed, silicotic lungs at postmortem examination are heavy and dark, with enlarged and fibrotic hilar and peribronchial nodes. Intraparenchymal nodules, variably calcified, are concentrated in the upper lobes and may range from 2 to 20 millimeters. Coalescent lesions (associated with progressive massive fibrosis, PMF) may cavitate, either from central necrosis or associated mycobacterial infection. On microscopic section, the early silicotic lung shows silica-containing macrophages and reticulin fibers. These areas organize as disease progresses and eventually form classic silicotic nodules. These nodules are like histologic tornadoes, with a quiet center of hyaline surrounded by whorls of collagen. The inflammatory periphery of macrophages and lymphocytes marches outward, causing a fibrous reaction in the normal structures of the lung (e.g., vessels, airways, pleura).[17,29] Polarized light may reveal crystalline silica as weak birefringence in the center of the nodule. Silicates are strongly birefringent, needle-shaped, and located at the active periphery of the nodule. These classic nodules are less common in steelworkers' lungs, which typically contain stellate lesions of reticulin and collagen.[37]

Acute silicosis presents with different pathologic findings than those of chronic silicosis, described previously. There is minimal fibrosis and an absence of nodules, and periodic acid-Schiff (PAS) stain–positive material fills the alveoli. This histologic appearance is known as *silicoproteinosis.*

Pathophysiology

Silica-induced lung damage begins with the entry of particles of crystalline silica, ranging in size from 0.5 to 3.0 microns, into the human alveolus. The exact mechanism that follows is unknown, but theories abound. The classic belief is that an alveolar macrophage ingests the silica particle and then dies, releasing proteolytic enzymes along with the silica particle, which is then ingested by another macrophage, and the cycle repeats itself. However, the process may be more complicated, involving fibrogenic factors such as interleukin 1(IL-1), leukotriene B-4, and tumor necrosis factor (TNF).[17,29,40,49] Another theory holds that alveolar macrophages are activated and not killed by silica ingestion. Electron microscopy of bronchoalveloar lavage (BAL) fluid taken from silica-exposed humans showed increased morphologic signs of activation (ruffling and filopodia) in the dust-containing macrophages.[53] The activation of pulmonary macrophages may lead to collagenase production and subsequent parenchymal lung destruction.[3]

Acute silicosis most likely has a very different pathologic mechanism. Electron microscopy of lungs affected by acute silicosis reveals hypertrophic type II pneumocytes lining the alveoli.[31] These cells are believed to produce exuberant amounts of proteinaceous material and surfactant protein, which fill the alveoli.

Free radicals may play a role in the evolution of silicotic lung injury. Freshly crushed silica contains a greater proportion of silicon free radicals than stored silica, and it has been shown to be more cytotoxic.[28] Sandblasting,[51] surface drilling,[6] and hard-rock drilling,[13] all of which produce freshly crushed silica particles, have each been associated with acute silicosis.

Clinical Presentation

The initial stages of silicosis are asymptomatic. Exertional dyspnea later develops and is typically the presenting complaint. The disease progresses to breathlessness at rest and increased cough and sputum production. Clinical syndromes of silicosis are distinguished historically, by time from toxic exposure to time of diagnosis.

The most common type of silicosis is chronic, also known as *classical*. It tends to occur after decades of moderate exposure to silica dust and is commonly diagnosed radiographically in the asymptomatic worker. Symptoms may take as long as 45 years from the time of last toxic exposure to develop.[52] On physical examination, patients may have stigmata of associated disease (emphysema, cor pulmonale), but they do not develop clubbing. They may become hypoxic with exercise. Chest radiograph reveals nodular lesions, predominantly in the upper lobes. Simple chronic silicosis is not usually disabling unless it is associated with mycobacterial infections or progresses to PMF, a disabling subset of chronic silicosis. It is marked on chest radiograph by large upper lobe opacities on a background of diffuse small nodular lesions, with basilar emphysematous changes. Patients who develop PMF are hypoxic at rest and predisposed to mycobacterial infections and spontaneous pneumothoraces. The disease progresses to cor pulmonale and respiratory failure.

Accelerated silicosis is a syndrome associated with greater silica exposure for less than a decade. One case report described 55 months of silica exposure in a 45-year-old South African foundry shotblaster, who presented with moderate dyspnea.[18] Two months later, cor pulmonale developed, and death came 10 months after that. Accelerated silicosis progresses despite removal from exposure, and it is frequently associated with autoimmune disorders, as discussed later in this chapter.

Acute silicosis is a striking syndrome and extremely uncommon.[10] It differs historically and pathologically from chronic silicosis and may develop by an entirely different mechanism. The patient with acute silicosis reports a large exposure over a relatively short period of time, perhaps as little as 1 year. Common symptoms are dyspnea, fatigue, weight loss, fever, and pleuritic pain. Silica flour exposure,[5,39] tombstone sandblasting,[51] and surface drilling[7] have all resulted in cases of acute silicosis. The Gauley Bridge tunneling disaster of 1931-1932 accounted for the largest American epidemic of acute silicosis.[13] The pathologic changes of acute silicosis consist of alveolar filling with proteinaceous material. The course of acute silicosis is dismal. The disease is relentlessly progressive and rapidly advances to respiratory failure after symptom onset.

Diagnosis

Diagnosis of silicosis requires a history of exposure to silica and a chest radiograph showing nodular opacities. Diseases with similar presentation need to be considered in the differential diagnosis; they include fungal infections, military tuberculosis, sarcoidosis, and idiopathic pulmonary fibrosis. Lung biopsy is rarely required for definitive diagnosis. Tissue can be examined with a nondestructive technique, energy dispersive x-ray analysis (EDAX),[20] which allows for scanning electron microscopy and elemental analysis.

Chest radiographs in chronic and accelerated silicosis reveal nodular opacities in the upper lung zones (Fig. 32-1). Lymph nodes calcify in a characteristic eggshell pattern, which is also seen in sarcoidosis, Hodgkin's disease after irradiation, blastomycosis, scleroderma, amyloidosis, and histoplasmosis. Progressive massive fibrosis is associated with large fibrotic masses and distortion of the lung architecture. There is upward displacement of mediastinal and hilar structures, due to volume loss in the upper zones. Lower lung zones become hyperventilated and emphysematous and may develop bullae.

Silicosis is classified by the International Labour Office (ILO) system, which incorporates degree of pleural involvement; size, shape, and profusion of opacities; and film quality.[52] Round nodules are called *p* if less than 1.5 mm, *q* if 1.5 mm to 3 mm, and *r* if 3 mm to 10 mm. If the nodules are irregular in shape, they are correspondingly called *s, t,* and *u.* Large nodules are named *A* if each one is greater than

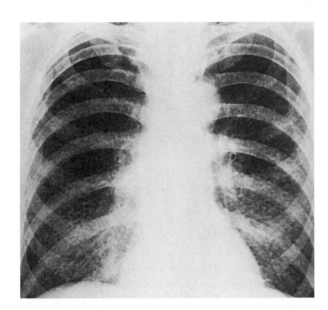

Fig. 32-1 Silicosis. Calcification in miliary nodules scattered throughout both lungs. (Eisenberg R: *Comprehensive radiographic pathology,* ed 2, St Louis, 1995, Mosby.)

1 cm and their summed diameters are less than 5 cm, *B* indicates nodules greater than 5 cm whose sum diameter is less than the right upper lobe, and *C* denotes nodules whose combined area is greater than the right upper lobe. Pleural involvement is graded by presence of calcification, thickening, or effusion.

Correlation between pathology and chest radiography is not always consistent.[57] Chest films of lungs with minimal changes have contained significant fibrosis on pathologic examination.[19] Chest computerized tomography (CT) may help to evaluate the presence of nodules and degree of emphysematous changes in complicated silicosis (Fig. 32-2). Chest CT may also reveal confluent lesions in what was previously graded simple silicosis by plain chest radiographs.[7] Emerging technologies for diagnosis include chest magnetic resonance imaging (MRI) and digitized radiography. These newer types of imaging have yet to be standardized for silicotic disease.

Acute silicosis, or silicoproteinosis, is radiographically different from chronic silicosis. The acute process has a ground-glass appearance, which is consistent with the pathologic alveolar filling. Linear opacities, signifying fibrosis, are usually present in the lower lobes. Hilar node enlargement may be impressive.

Pulmonary function tests in simple silicosis may be normal. As disease progresses, a restrictive pattern develops, with reduction in the volume of air exhaled in 1 second, forced vital capacity, total lung capacity, and lung compliance. Diffusion capacity also decreases. Obstruction of the airway due to fibrosis and distortion of lung architecture affects these flow parameters. Pulmonary function tests in acute silicosis also show a restrictive pattern.[7] Coexisting

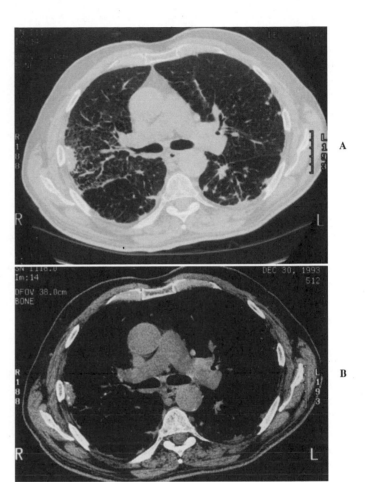

Fig. 32-2 A 73-year-old man with a history of employment in the granite industry in Vermont was evaluated for increased exercise dyspnea. Plain chest radiograph was nonspecific. **A,** High-resolution computed tomography, adjusted to optimize lung tissue density, demonstrates rounded opacities in low profusion. Multiple bilateral subpleural nodules are typical of silicosis. **B,** Calcification within the subpleural nodules, particularly at the right lateral chest, can be seen with the scan optimized for soft tissue density. (From Harber P, Schenker MB, Balmes JR: *Occupational and environmental respiratory disease,* St Louis, 1995, Mosby.)

factors, such as tobacco smoking and pulmonary infections, need to be considered when interpreting pulmonary function studies.

Bronchoalveolar lavage is not useful in diagnosing silicosis. Patients exposed to silica have silica and increased protein in their lung washings, regardless of the presence of disease.[5]

Treatment

Silicosis is a progressive disease, without any proven treatment. A variety of therapeutic modalities have attempted to decrease the inflammatory response to silica. Whole-lung lavage has led to symptomatic improvement but without changes in pulmonary function studies.[4] Pharmacologic approaches to the treatment of silicosis have included corticosteroids and aluminum citrate. One small controlled study showed improved pulmonary function tests and less inflammatory bronchoalveolar lavage fluid in symptomatic, silica-exposed patients treated with a 6-month course of corticosteroids.[51] Acute silicosis was reportedly reversed by corticosteroids in one case.[24] Despite these reports, corticosteroids are thought to be of little or no benefit in the treatment of silicosis. Inhalation of aluminum citrate powder (to coat the silica particles and render them less soluble) showed symptomatic improvement in controlled trials.[37] However, no change in objective disease or mortality was observed. The potential adverse effects of the aluminum citrate complex may limit its role in therapy.

Polyvinylpyridine-N-oxide (PVNO) concentrates silica particles intracellularly and has been shown to stabilize disease and improve patient functional ability.[12] The use of PVNO is limited by its hepatic and renal toxicity in animals. Further suggested therapies include alveolar macrophage inhibitors and monoclonal antibodies against IL-1.[11]

Although no therapy has proven beneficial in reducing mortality from silicosis, it is important to treat complicating conditions such as tuberculosis. Symptomatic patients with a chest radiograph suggesting silicosis should have a purified protein derivative (PPD) placed intradermally. A positive PPD should prompt a year of isoniazid therapy. Steroids should not be instituted until the absence of mycobacterial infection is confirmed. Some sources suggest treating empirically with isoniazid during steroid therapy, to prevent aggravation of undiagnosed mycobacterial disease.[25,50] Patients with silicosis should be removed from further silica exposure and treated with bronchodilators and supplemental oxygen as needed.

Prevention

Pliny the Elder commented in the first century that miners "envelop their faces with loose bladders, which enable them to see without inhaling the fatal dust."[9] The need for respiratory protection from the hazards of industrial dust has been recommended by all commentators since then. In the sixteenth century, Georgius Agricolus designed complex ventilation systems for mining.[34] By the beginning of the eighteenth century, mechanical ventilating devices were in place, and workers wore veils or scarves for protection.

True workplace reform was a sluggish process. In 1802, the Factory and Workshop Act made ventilation in British workplaces a requirement. However, factories remained dark and underventilated, because the window tax of 1696 was not revoked until 1851. The factory and workshop acts of 1864 and 1867 made more stringent requirements for ventilation and appointed an inspector, who could require fans or other devices be added to the workplace. In 1902, a Miner's Phthisis Commission was established to determine a "safe working level" of dust. Air sampling with a portable device measured dust levels that were correlated with medical findings. It was during this investigation that radiography was first used to diagnose silicosis.[54]

A variety of mechanisms protect today's sandblasting worker (Fig. 32-3). Blasting chambers are constructed to minimize human exposure to the large amounts of dust generated during the procedure. The chambers are sealed and vented and contain a series of baffles which allow the dust to be selectively extracted from the chamber. The venting system maintains a slight negative pressure within the chamber and pulls the exhausted air away from the worker's breathing zone. The air is filtered for abrasive, which is then recycled.

Sandblasters are provided with special personal equipment: overalls, apron, boots, and gauntlets. The fitted helmets are supplied with filtered air containing no more than 50 ppm of carbon monoxide and 1000 ppm of carbon dioxide. The blasting chamber and ventilation-filtration system are required to be inspected and tested at least monthly. A worker is not permitted to spend more than 40 continuous minutes inside the chamber, and a designated observer must monitor the process from outside the chamber. Open-air blasting is not as well controlled. It must occur a certain distance away from other workers and with appropriate ventilation. In addition, workers participating in open-air blasting must wear some respiratory protection. If the abrasive contains silica, the respirator must be a type CE, pressure-demand, abrasive blast SAR with an assigned protection factor of 2000 (Fig. 32-4, *A* and *B*).

Since OSHA and NIOSH came into being, worker safety has increased significantly. However, compliance with the regulations is difficult to monitor, and violations occur. Nearly half of surveyed U.S. foundries do not practice silica control, and one third of foundry workers are exposed to excessive amounts of airborne toxins.[43] According to NIOSH, cases of silicosis tend to occur in worksites where silica-containing abrasives are used, where ventilation or work practices are poor, where respiratory protection is inadequate, and where medical surveillance programs are not in effect.[55] In addition, many sandblasters are improperly trained and inadequately supervised. Continued efforts to promote worker safety are necessary.[56]

ILLNESSES ASSOCIATED WITH SILICOSIS
Silicosis and Tuberculosis

Silicosis and tuberculosis were poorly distinguished for some time. The diseases often presented together and appeared clinically similar. Patients seem to be consumed by their affliction, and the Greek term *phthisis*, meaning "wasting away," was applied to their disorder.

Koch's discovery of the tubercle bacillus in 1882 simultaneously advanced understanding of tuberculosis while it regressed understanding of silicosis. For several decades after Koch's discovery, all cases of phthisis were considered to be tubercular in origin and only peripherally associated with the inhalation of dust. Dusts were considered vehicles

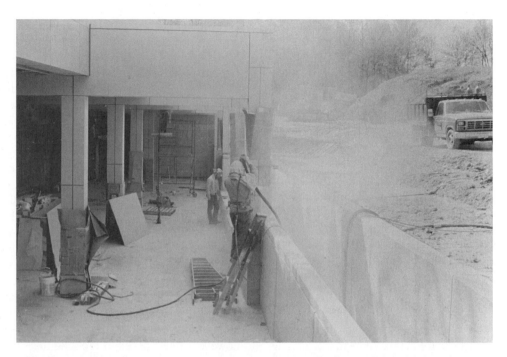

Fig. 32-3 Picture of a sandblaster in a cloud of dust. The blaster is using silica abrasive on a concrete structure to improve its appearance. The crystalline silica within the concrete poses additional risks of exposure to the worker. The worker is using a CE continuous-flow abrasive-blasting respirator. Note that the helper, who is standing 40 feet away, is not wearing any respiratory protection. (Courtesy Kenneth D. Linch, NIOSH.)

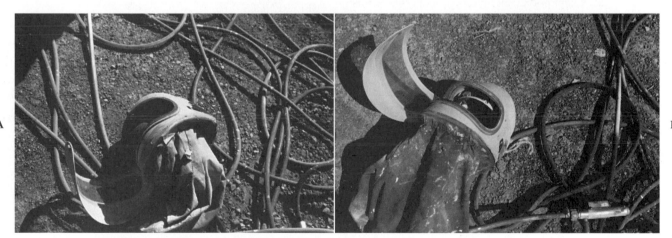

A   B

Fig. 32-4 Two type CE continuous-flow abrasive-blasting respirators that were used at a sandblasting site. The front glass portion of each respirator was removed to leave only the thin plastic liner in the doors (the doors are open). The purpose of the plastic liner is to protect the glass from being scratched by rebounding abrasive, not to protect the wearer. These respirators were not intended to be used in this fashion, thus violating the NIOSH certification. Note also the poor condition of these respirators: **A,** Duct tape used to hold the shroud to the helmet; **B,** several holes in the shroud. (Courtesy Kenneth D. Linch, NIOSH.)

of disease, carrying the tubercular germ, and not a cause of disease. This view was changing in 1902, when Thomas Oliver wrote that "the tendency of modern pathology is to look upon all pulmonary phthisis . . . as tuberculosis, but the fact remains that phthisis can be caused by dust."[41] Further progress was made when a group of British researchers described three separate types of phthisis: tuberculous, "fibroid," and a combination of the two.[32]

In 1915, Emery R. Hayhurst conducted a study of industrial hygiene, and his findings approximate the understanding of today. He concluded that dusts (i.e., cotton, coal, iron, and silica) resulted in pulmonary fibrosis, which ended "in a condition called phthisis, which is usually complicated by the presence of the bacillus tuberculosis."[26] The introduction of radiography, combined with the tuberculin test and sputum staining, allowed cases of pure silicosis to be distinguished from those mixed with tuberculosis.

Tuberculosis was a major cause of death at the turn of the century. In the 1920s, 80% of Vermont granite workers died from this illness. Today, the risk of tuberculosis is much less because of better dust protection, the evolution of antimycobacterial agents, and a decreased prevalence of the disease. However, mycobacterial infections still commonly complicate all forms of silicosis. Atypical mycobacteria such as *Mycobacterium avium intracellulare* and *M. kansasii* are increasingly seen. Thus, any sudden functional decline in a patient with silicosis warrants a prompt investigation for mycobacterial infection.

Silicosis and Cancer

The data regarding the carcinogenesis of silica are conflicting and unclear. No evidence for increased incidence of lung malignancy was shown in a group of South African gold miners.[24] However, among worker deaths in silica-exposed industries, an increased rate of lung cancer was found.[29] Further studies contradicted this latter finding.[22,36] The presence of other carcinogens (e.g., smoking tobacco, radioactive gases, and polycyclic hydrocarbons) makes this issue difficult to resolve. The International Agency for Research on Cancer commented in 1987 that, although there was "sufficient evidence" of silica's carcinogenicity to animals, "limited evidence" exists of its carcinogenic property in humans.[36]

Silicosis and Autoimmune Disease

Silicosis has been associated with various autoimmune diseases, such as rheumatoid arthritis, scleroderma, and progressive systemic sclerosis. Patients with silicosis tend to have serum antinuclear antibodies, rheumatoid factor, and high serum concentrations of immune complexes and immunoglobulins.[16]

Renal disease (e.g., nephrotic syndrome, renal failure) without pulmonary changes has been associated with silica exposure. Granite workers, Bedouins (exposed to dust storms), and Balkans who consume silica-contaminated water have increased incidence of end-stage renal disease.[21] Immune complexes in the glomerulus may be responsible for the observed damage.[42]

SUMMARY

Silicosis is an important occupational disease, both historically and at present. Many industries expose workers to free crystalline silica and to the potential for pulmonary fibrosis, autoimmune disease, and lung cancer. Sandblasting allows significant silica contamination and is common in the metalworking, shipbuilding, glass, and ceramic industries.

Chronic silicosis presents as dyspnea on exertion after decades of moderate silica exposure. Acute silicosis occurs less commonly and manifests symptoms within years after a large exposure. The acute process advances relentlessly to respiratory failure and death. The chest radiographs of these two forms of silicosis are dissimilar because of their different pathology. Chronic silicosis characteristically shows "eggshell" lymph node calcifications and small nodular opacities in the upper lung fields. This progresses to confluent areas of fibrosis and distortion of the normal lung architecture. Acute silicosis, an alveolar filling disease, is represented by a ground-glass appearance on the radiograph. Current therapies for silicosis are limited, and further investigations are necessary. Mycobacterial infection must always be sought and treated in the patient with silicosis.

Current practices for reducing industrial silica exposure include evaluating the amount and sources of exposure, replacing silica-containing materials, isolating and enclosing work processes, and using personal protective equipment and special ventilation. Despite such measures, however, rates of exposure continue to exceed OSHA recommendations.[56] Silica exposure in much of the Third World is even greater because of fewer regulations. Silicosis will be an occupational disease worldwide for many years to come.

REFERENCES

1. Abrams HK: Historical perspectives in occupational medicine. Diatomaceous earth silicosis, *Am J Ind Med* 18:591, 1990.
2. Alexander MW: *Safety in the foundry,* Chicago, 1915, National Founders' Association.
3. Bagchi N: What makes silica toxic? *Br J Ind Med* 49:163, 1992.
4. Banks DE: Strategies for the treatment of pneumoconiosis, *Occup Med* 8:203, 1993.
5. Banks DE et al: Silicosis in silica flour workers, *Am Rev Respir Dis* 124:445, 1981.
6. Banks DE et al: Silicosis in surface coalmine drillers, *Thorax* 38:275, 1983.
7. Begin R et al: CT assessment of silicosis in exposed workers, *Am J Radiol* 148:509, 1987.
8. Bloomfield J et al: *A preliminary survey of the industrial hygiene problem in the United States,* Public Health Service Bulletin 259, Washington, DC, 1940, US Department of Health, Education and Welfare.
9. Brown HV: The history of industrial hygiene: a review with special reference to silicosis, *Am Ind Hyg Assoc J* 26:212, 1965.
10. Buechner HA, Ansari A: Acute silicosis, *Dis Chest* 55:274, 1969.
11. Castranova V et al: Effects of bisbenzylisoquinoline alkaloids on alveolar macrophages: correlation between binding affinity, inhibitory potency, and antifibrotic potential, *Toxicol Appl Pharmacol* 108:242, 1991.
12. Chen SY, Lu XR: Clinical studies of the therapeutic effect of Kexiping on silicosis. In Institute of Occupational Medicine: *Proceedings of the therapeutic effect of Kexiping on silicosis,* Beijing, 1970, CAPM Press.
13. Cherniak M: *The Hawk's Nest incident: America's worst industrial disaster,* New Haven, Conn, 1986, Yale University Press.
14. Corn JK: Historical aspects of industrial hygiene, II. Silicosis, *Am Ind Hyg Assoc J* 41:125, 1980.
15. Costa C et al: Historical perspectives in occupational medicine: Victoria M. Trasko, *Am J Indust Med* 22:419, 1992.

16. Doll NJ et al: Immune complexes and autoantibodies in silicosis, *J Allergy Clin Immunol* 68:281, 1981.

17. Dubois CM, Bissonette E, Rola-Plescynski M: Asbestos fibers and silica particles stimulate rat alveolar macrophages to release tumor necrosis factor, *Am Rev Respir Dis* 139:1257, 1989.

18. Ehrlich RI, Gerston KF, Lalloo UG: Accelerated silicosis in a foundry shotblaster, *S Afr Med J* 73:128, 1988.

19. Fernie JM, Ruckley VA: Coalworkers' pneumoconiosis: correlation between opacity profusion and number and type of dust lesions with special reference to opacity type, *Br J Ind Med* 44:273, 1987.

20. Funahashi A, Siegesmund KA: Identification of foreign material in the lung by energy dispersive x-ray analysis—new approach to silicosis, *Arch Environ Health* 30:285, 1975.

21. Goldsmith DF, Winn DM, Shy CF: *Silica, silicosis, and cancer,* New York, 1986, Praeger.

22. Goldsmith GF, Guidotti TL, Johnston DR: Does occupational exposure to silica cause lung cancer? *Am J Ind Med* 3:423, 1982.

23. Goldsmith JR, Goldsmith DF: Fiberglass or silica exposure and increased nephritis or ESRD, *Am J Ind Med* 23:873, 1993.

24. Goodman GB et al: Acute silicosis responding to corticosteroid therapy, *Chest* 101:366, 1991.

25. Graham WG: Silicosis, *Clin Chest Med* 13:253, 1992.

26. Gross OB, Schneider H, Proto A: Eggshell calcification of lymph nodes: an update, *Am J Radiol* 135:1265, 1980.

27. Hayhurst ER: *Industrial health hazards and occupational diseases in Ohio,* Columbus, 1915, Ohio State Board of Health.

28. Heffner JE, Repine JE: Pulmonary strategies of oxidant defense—state of the art, *Am Rev Respir Dis* 140:531, 1989.

29. Heppleston AG: Silica pneumoconiosis and carcinoma of the lung, *Am J Ind Med* 7:285, 1985.

30. Heppleston AC, Styles JA: Activity of a macrophage factor in collagen formation by silica, *Nature* 214:521, 1967.

31. Hoffman EO et al: The ultrastructure of acute silicosis, *Arch Pathol* 96:104, 1973.

32. Hoffman F: *The mortality from consumption in dusty trades,* US Bureau of Labor Bulletin No 79, Washington, DC, 1908, Government Printing Office.

33. Holt PF: Silicosis. In Holt PF, editor: *Inhaled dust and disease,* New York, 1987, John Wiley.

34. Hoover H, Hoover L (translators): Agricola G: *De re metallica,* Book 6, London, 1912, Salisbury House.

35. Hunter D: *The diseases of occupations,* Boston, 1962, Little, Brown.

36. International Agency for Research on Cancer: *Monographs on the evaluation of the carcinogenic risk of chemicals to humans,* vol 42, Lyon, 1987, IARC.

37. Kennedy MCS: Aluminum powder in the treatment of silicosis of pottery workers and pneumoconiosis of coal-miners, *Br J Ind Med* 13:85, 1956.

38. Landrigan PJ: Silicosis. *Occup Med* 2:319, 1987.

39. McDonald G, Piggot AP, Gilder FW: Two cases of acute silicosis, *Lancet* 2:846, 1930.

40. Miller E et al: Induction of surfactant protein (SP-A) biosynthesis and SP-A mRNA in activated type II cells during acute silicosis in rats, *Am J Respir Cell Mol Biol* 3:217, 1990.

41. National Institute for Occupational Safety and Health: *Criteria for a recommended standard for occupational exposure to crystalline silica,* Publication No 75-120, Cincinnati, 1974, NIOSH.

42. Oghiso Y, Kubota Y: Enhanced interleukin 1 production by alveolar macrophages in Ia-positive lung cells in silica-exposed rats, *Microbiol Immunol* 30:1189, 1986.

43. Oliver T: *Dangerous trades,* London, 1902, EP Dutton.

44. Osorio AM et al: Silica and glomerulonephritis: case report and review of the literature, *Am J Kidney Dis* 9:224, 1987.

45. Oudiz J et al: A report on silica exposure levels in US foundries, *Am Ind Hyg Assoc J* 44:374, 1983.

46. Rossner D, Markowitz G: *Deadly dust: silicosis and politics of occupational disease in twentieth century America,* Princeton, NJ, 1991, Princeton University Press.

47. Russell AE et al: *Health of workers in dusty trades. II. Exposure to siliceous dust (granite industry),* Public Health Bulletin No 187, Washington, DC, 1929, US Public Health Service.

48. Schlueter DP: Silicosis and coal worker's pneumoconiosis. In Zenz C, Dickerson OB, Horvath EP, editors: *Occupational medicine,* ed 3, St Louis, 1994, Mosby.

49. Schmidt JA et al: Silica-stimulated monocytes release fibroblast-proliferation factors identical to interleukin 1, *J Clin Invest* 73:1462, 1984.

50. Sharma SK, Pane JN, Nerma K: Effect of prednisolone treatment in chronic silicosis, *Am Rev Respir Dis* 143:814, 1991.

51. Surrat PM, Winn WC, Brody AR: Acute silicosis in tombstone sandblasters, *Am Rev Respir Dis* 115:521, 1977.

52. Symanski H: Delayed onset sandstone pneumoconiosis: a case report, *Am J Ind Med* 2:101, 1981.

53. Takemura T et al: Morphologic characterization of alveolar macrophages from subjects with occupational exposure to inorganic particles, *Am Rev Respir Dis* 140:1674, 1989.

54. Teleky L: *History of factory and mine hygiene,* New York, 1948, Columbia University Press.

55. US Department of Health and Human Services: Request for assistance in preventing silicosis and deaths from sandblasting, *Alert,* NIOSH publication No 92-102, Washington, 1992, US Government Printing Office.

56. Valiante DJ, Rosenman KD: Does silicosis still occur? *JAMA* 262:3003, 1989.

57. Wagner GR: Chest radiography in dust-exposed miners: promise and problems, potential and imperfections, *Occup med* 8:127, 1993.

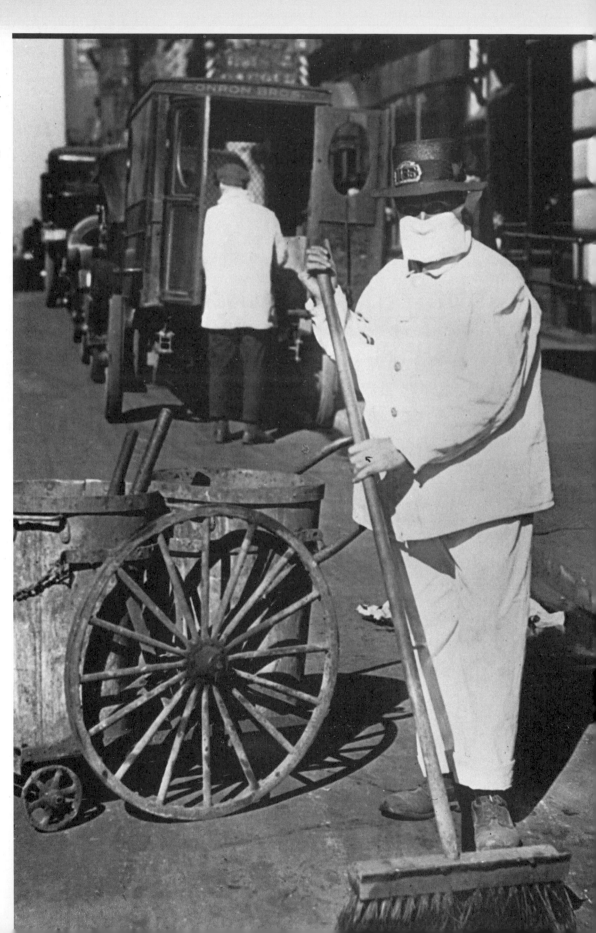

Influenza epidemic. Street cleaner with mask. The admonition of the New York Health Board to wear masks to check the spread of the influenza epidemic has been heeded. "Better be ridiculous than dead," is the view of one official. Undated. (Courtesy Corbis-Bettmann)

33

Sewer and Sanitation Personnel

Jeffrey R. Brubacher

H₂S

- Hydrogen sulfide is an irritant and chemical asphyxiant

- The TLV (10 ppm) for H₂S was designed to prevent ocular toxicity

- The "sewer workers' syndrome" is a self-limited illness that occurs after exposure to sewage sludge dust

BACKGROUND

Sewage systems are necessary for draining storm waters from city streets and for carrying human excreta outside the city for treatment and disposal. This must be done in such a way as to prevent the contamination of drinking water. Early sewers consisted of drains built to remove storm waters from city streets. The cloaca maxima, which drained the Roman forum into the Tiber River, is an example. Human waste was disposed of into cesspools or privies or carried in buckets to rivers. Garbage was often simply tossed into the street to be flushed away with the next storm. Many large cities had pigs and chickens that ate this garbage. Charles Dickens is said to have disliked New York City because of the estimated 20,000 pigs that ran loose in its streets.[18] These unsanitary conditions resulted in objectionable sights and odors and caused disease. This problem was solved in many European and North American cities by draining domestic wastes into the storm sewers. In 1842, Hamburg, Germany, became the first western city that built a separate system of pipes for carrying human wastes. These early sewage systems dumped untreated human waste into nearby fields or rivers, with resultant pollution of the surrounding waters. Sewage treatment plants were built to decrease the burden on the surrounding waterways.

Most sewer systems built today have large pipes draining waters from the streets and a separate smaller system of pipes for human waste. Sewage pipes draining buildings are generally about 6 inches in diameter; these pipes drain into

265

larger pipes that run 8 to 12 feet below city streets. The underground sewage pipes range in size from 12-inch-diameter street pipes to collecting sewers greater than 5 feet in diameter. That the pipes in storm sewers are generally larger than those in sanitary sewers reflects greater demand. Manholes give access to the sewage system at sites where pipes intersect, change direction, or change grade. In large cities such as New York, collecting sewers empty into large underground tunnels more than 10 feet in diameter called *interceptor sewers,* which carry sewage to centralized treatment plants. Sewage pipes slope downward so that sewage flows by gravity. When the sewage flows at a rate of at least 2 to 3 feet per second, sedimentation is less likely, and the sewer system is called *self-cleaning.*

The job of the sewer worker is to inspect and maintain the underground network of pipes that make up the sewer system. Storm drains have catch basins near their inlets that prevent solid garbage from entering the storm sewers. These catch basins must be periodically cleaned out. Where waste water contains high concentrations of grit or suspended particles or where sewage flow is slow, sewage pipes can become obstructed by sediment. Many of the pipes are too small for maintenance workers to enter and can be accessed only at certain points by manholes. These smaller pipes are cleaned with a water hose pulled from one manhole to the next. In this manner, silt is flushed out to a collection point, where it is carried to the surface. Sewer workers enter larger pipes to allow repair and removal of sediment. Sediment is shoveled into buckets, which are dragged to the nearest manhole and then raised to the surface with winches. All of this maintenance work occurs in poorly ventilated spaces so that sewer workers may be exposed to toxic gases volatilized from the sewage. Furthermore, skin contact with sewage may be unavoidable. Occasionally, sewage systems require emergency repair when a section of pipe becomes completely blocked or when a sewage leak has washed away the subsoil and allowed the floor of the sewer to collapse. In these situations, the damaged section of pipe is isolated by blocking each end, and a smaller pipe is used to temporarily bypass the damaged section, which is then pumped dry to allow repair to proceed. This repair work is particularly dangerous with a high risk of exposure to toxic gases, drowning, or becoming isolated if further structural damage to the sewage system occurs.

Biologic oxygen demand is a measurement of the oxygen requirement of the bacteria and other organisms as they decompose the organic material contained in sewage. Effluent with high biologic oxygen demand depletes oxygen in the receiving body of water and is harmful to aquatic life. Sewage treatment plants purify waste water by physical, biologic, and chemical means. These processes remove solid particles and reduce the biologic oxygen demand of the sewage. Objects such as rags, paper, and pieces of wood are removed by screens of various sizes. These screens may be cleaned automatically or manually. Alternately, grinders

known as *comminuters* reduce these objects to a manageable size. After screening or grinding, suspended materials such as sand, gravel, and ashes settle to the bottom of the slow-flowing sewage in basins known as *grit chambers.* Grit chambers are cleaned either manually or automatically. Smaller suspended solids are allowed to settle in sedimentation tanks known as *septic tanks.* This process occurs both before (primary sedimentation) and after (secondary sedimentation) aerobic oxidation. The sludge that settles to the bottom of these tanks undergoes anaerobic decomposition. Sewage is also digested by aerobic oxidation when it is exposed to oxygen in aeration basins or in trickling filters, where it is sprayed over stones. These biologic treatments reduce the biologic oxygen demand of the sewage. During the digestion process, methane, carbon dioxide, hydrogen sulfide, and other gases are released. Sewage may be chemically treated with a coagulant (usually ferric chloride) to cause formation of a floc, which can be removed by mechanical means. This process is expensive and generally reserved for the treatment of industrial wastes. Sewage sludge is often dried before being incinerated or otherwise disposed of.

Workers in sewage treatment plants are responsible for the operation and maintenance of treatment tanks and machines. Specific tasks include cleaning grit chambers and screens, emptying sedimentation tanks, cleaning sludge pipelines, operating aeration chambers, pump operation, operating dewatering and incineration equipment, and hauling and disposing of treated sludge. Workers in sewage treatment plants come into contact with gases volatilized from decomposing sewage and with dust and aerosolized bacteria from dried sewage sludge. In the sewage treatment plants, working in the pumping stations or near the sludge digestors is considered to be the most hazardous work because ventilation in these areas is generally poor. In the United States in 1992, there were 24,000 sanitation and sewer workers employed on the state and local level.[6]

HARMFUL AGENTS

Modern sewage is a complex mix of industrial chemicals, household waste, and human excrement. This mix contains numerous toxic substances, many of which are volatile. As it decomposes, sewage releases methane, hydrogen sulfide, and carbon dioxide. Since sewer maintenance and treatment plant personnel often work in confined spaces in intimate contact with raw or partially treated sewage, it is not surprising that they will frequently have inhalational exposure to the toxic gases, solvents, and aerosolized dust particles released from this sewage. Table 33-1 lists the volatilized chemicals and dusts to which sewage workers may be exposed.

Hydrogen Sulfide

Hydrogen sulfide is an irritant and a chemical asphyxiant. Because it is heavier than air, hydrogen sulfide gas collects

Table 33-1 Important inhalational exposures in sewage workers

Category	Examples	Clinical effects
Simple asphyxiants	Carbon dioxide Methane	Symptoms: Headache, altered mental status, coma, seizures, cardiopulmonary arrest. Treatment: Reversible on removal from exposure.
Chemical asphyxiants	Hydrogen sulfide Carbon monoxide *Hydrogen cyanide*	Symptoms: Headache, altered mental status, coma, seizures, cardiopulmonary arrest. Permanent or delayed neurologic sequelae in carbon monoxide exposure. Severe acidosis and continued deterioration in cyanide exposure. Rotten egg odor and irritant effects as well as hypoxic symptoms in hydrogen sulfide exposure. Treatment: Carbon monoxide and cyanide exposure require specific treatment. Hydrogen sulfide exposure may resolve entirely with removal from exposure and supportive care.
Irritants	Ammonia Chlorine	Symptoms: Burning eyes, cough, irritation of pharynx. High concentrations act as simple asphyxiants. Prolonged exposure may cause ARDS or delayed development of bronchiolitis obliterans.
Solvents	Benzene Toluene	Symptoms: Solvent exposure syndrome—headache, altered mental status, difficulty concentrating, nausea, malaise. Persistent neuropsychiatric sequelae may occur.
Dusts	Aerosolized bacteria Ashes from incineration of sewage sludge	Symptoms: Sewage worker's syndrome—headache, fatigue, fever, purulent-ocular discharge, skin irritation, diarrhea. Respiratory complaints: cough, purulent sputum, fever, sore throat, decreased pulmonary function.

in the bottom of tanks, in pits, and in enclosed spaces. Hydrogen sulfide is formed when sulfates are reduced under anoxic conditions and is released in significant quantities from sludge in sewage treatment plants. This occurs especially in primary sedimentation tanks, which fortunately are seldom entered. Hydrogen sulfide exposure can also occur during desludging operations in secondary sedimentation tanks, on the tops of sewage digestors, and during tanker loading and discharge.[16] Any situation in which sewage is allowed to decompose under anaerobic conditions can result in the release of hydrogen sulfide. These conditions occur in sewage treatment plants and in the underground sewage system when blockage or leakage of a pipe allows sewage to become stagnant. Similar conditions exist on farms where manure is collected in septic tanks. Entering septic tanks or damaged sewage lines without first ensuring adequate ventilation and measuring hydrogen sulfide levels is thus extremely dangerous.

Other Toxic Gases

Toxic gases are categorized according to clinical effect into simple asphyxiants, chemical asphyxiants, and irritants. The most prevalent gases released during sewage decomposition are the simple asphyxiants carbon dioxide and methane. Methane is frequently used as a fuel in sewage treatment plants. Simple asphyxiants act by displacing oxygen and creating an oxygen-poor atmosphere. Persons exposed to this environment suffer symptoms of hypoxia. Methane has a

characteristic unpleasant odor, but carbon dioxide and many other simple asphyxiants are odorless, so that the worker may be unaware of being exposed. All toxic gases act as simple asphyxiants when their concentration is high enough. Simple asphyxiants are immediately life-threatening when the fraction of inspired oxygen is less than 10%. Sewage workers may also be exposed to numerous other toxic gases. In the combined residential and industrial sewage of Zagreb, Croatia, investigators documented the presence of ammonia, carbon monoxide, carbon dioxide, hydrogen cyanide, hydrogen sulfide, and methane.[60] Ammonia is an irritant and is discussed in Chapter 9. Carbon monoxide and cyanide are chemical asphyxiants. Carbon monoxide and cyanide are discussed in detail in Chapters 15 and 20.

Solvents

Industrial wastes frequently contain volatile hydrocarbon solvents. The mixture of gases in Zagreb's sewage contained trichloroethylene, butane, propane, ethylene, and propylene.[60] Other workers have detected benzene and toluene in New York City sewage vapors.[27] Vapors from sewage in an industrial section of Cincinnati, Ohio, were found to contain numerous volatilized solvents including Stoddard solvent, trichloroethane, trichloroethylene, toluene, perchloroethylene, xylene, and chlorobenzene.[52] Sewer maintenance workers exposed to solvents have complained of eye and nose irritation, headache, and a metallic taste in their mouths.[52] Sewage treatment plant workers exposed to solvents have developed light-headedness, fatigue, and headache.[27] These symptoms are consistent with solvent exposure. Solvent toxicity is discussed in Chapter 25.

Aerosolized Bacteria and Endotoxin

Another special problem at sewage treatment plants is exposure to aerosolized bacteria and endotoxin. Gram-negative rods thrive in decomposing sewage and can become volatilized during various phases of sewage treatment. In sewage treatment plants in Sweden, concentrations of airborne bacteria ranged from 10 to 10^5 bacteria per cubic meter.[31] The highest concentrations occurred near areas where sewage was agitated. These bacteria may cause the sewer worker's syndrome, which is discussed later in this chapter. Endotoxin has also been measured in high concentrations (more than 100 ng/m^3) in wastewater treatment plants.[29] The mechanism of toxicity and the long-term effects after exposure to inhaled bacteria and endotoxin in this setting are incompletely understood. There is no accepted exposure limit for aerosolized bacteria or endotoxin, although a value of 30 ng/m^3 has been proposed for endotoxin.[44] At levels above 300 ng/m^3, endotoxin causes decreased FEV_1.[8]

Miscellaneous

Sewage workers may have skin or eye contact with liquid sewage or sewage dust. Many industries are required to pretreat their wastewater before disposal in the sewage system. Unfortunately, such regulations are not always followed, and sewage workers may be exposed to any number of toxic industrial chemicals, depending on local industry. In addition, household chemicals including paints and solvents may be disposed of into the sewage system. Pollutants found in sewage may include acids, alkalis, soaps, solvents, tars, phenol derivatives, heavy metals, and organic matter. Chloride, ammonia, sulfate, nitrites, cyanide, chromium, copper, nickel, lead, and cadmium were all detected in Zagreb sewage.[60] Compared to controls, workers exposed to this sewage had more chronic respiratory symptoms and decreased ventilatory capacity, as well as more complaints of headache and dizziness. Industrial sewage in Cincinnati, as well as containing numerous solvents, had a pH as low as 1.[52] In Kentucky, the industrial chemical hexachlorocyclopentadiene was dumped into a municipal sewage system. Sewage treatment workers exposed to this sewage developed higher rates of eye irritation, headache, and throat irritation. Several of the employees developed transient proteinuria and elevated lactate dehydrogenase after this exposure.[38] Sludge from a treatment plant in Toronto that was analyzed after an outbreak of irritant dermatitis was found to contain approximately 5% chromate by weight. Skin testing suggested that the chromate was not the cause of dermatitis in this instance.[39] Sewage sludge farmers in India were found to have higher urine cadmium levels than controls,

although no long-term effects of exposure to cadmium in this form have been documented.[57] The clinical effect of exposure to these industrial pollutants is poorly understood, which is not surprising because the chemicals that contaminate sewage vary from day to day and city to city. Perhaps these pollutants are responsible for the increased risk of some types of cancer in sewage workers that some authors have reported.[14,28] Pollutants may be responsible for the urinary mutagens detected in the urine of sewage workers[50] and for the finding that spouses of sewage workers have an increased incidence of fetal loss.[37]

CLINICAL EFFECTS
Sewer Worker's Syndrome

Compared to workers in other occupations, sewage treatment plant workers suffer more often from eye and skin irritation and nonspecific gastrointestinal, respiratory, and constitutional symptoms. Fever, chills, headache, fatigue, and malaise are commonly reported constitutional symptoms. Purulent ocular discharge and skin irritation are often reported, as are gastrointestinal symptoms including diarrhea. Cough, purulent sputum, and throat irritation are common respiratory symptoms. The term *sewer worker's syndrome* was coined in 1976 to describe the fevers, chills, fatigue, purulent ocular discharge, and skin irritation in Swedish sewage treatment plant workers.[48] In another Swedish study, 30% to 50% of sewage workers suffered from attacks of fever or purulent ocular discharge, and 13% reported episodes of diarrhea. All these symptoms were related to periods of heavy dust exposure at work.[34]

The agents responsible for the sewer worker's syndrome are unknown. Several authors have found an association between these symptoms and exposure to sewage sludge dust and specifically to aerosolized bacteria and endotoxin.[29,31,36] Some authors have suggested that workers with these symptoms have increased immunoglobulin levels,[49] but not all studies have duplicated these findings.[10,31] A New York study found that sewage workers had a higher incidence of headache, dizziness, sore throat, eye and skin irritation, and diarrhea than controls. This study found an association between eye and skin irritation and exposure to mutagens, as documented by the presence of urinary mutagens.[51]

Carcinogenesis

Sewage treatment workers may be at increased risk for developing cancer, but the data on this are inconclusive. A retrospective study of a cohort of sewer workers from Buffalo, New York, identified an increased risk of death from cancers of the larynx and liver. In this study, the overall cancer mortality rate in workers exposed to sewage effluent, sludge, or wastewater tended to be higher than that of the general population. Only the mortality rates from cancers of the larynx were identifiably work related and statistically significant.[28] A retrospective study of a cohort of Swedish

sewer workers found the mortality rate from cancer to be the same as the general population with a nonsignificant trend toward an increased incidence of brain, gastric, and renal cancers.[14] A proportional mortality study analyzing the death reports of 1026 sewage treatment workers showed more than expected deaths from benign malignancies and a nonsignificant trend toward increased deaths from gastric and esophageal cancer and from leukemia. The percentage of deaths from malignant cancers of all types was no different from that in the general population. The authors caution that an increased percentage of deaths from a given diagnosis in a proportional mortality study may reflect a true increased incidence of that disease or may reflect decreased deaths from other diagnoses.[5]

Although the data on deaths from cancer in sewage treatment workers are inconclusive, there is evidence that these workers are exposed to mutagens. Urine from sewage treatment plant workers in New York State was significantly more likely to contain mutagens as measured by the Ames test, which was performed both with and without hepatic microsomal activation. After correction for other factors, the adjusted odds ratio for the increase in urine mutagenicity was 2.2 (95% confidence interval 1.2-4.3) without activation and 12.9 (95% confidence interval 4.5-37.4) with activation. It was not determined which of the many potential chemicals in sewage sludge may be responsible for these urinary mutagens.[50]

Reproductive Effects

There is a concern that sewer workers may be exposed to pollutants that cause reproductive toxicity, although the data on this are inconclusive. In a California study that included 210 pregnancies, the wives of male employees at a waste water treatment plant were found to have an increased incidence of spontaneous abortions. In this study, the relative risk of a pregnancy terminating in a miscarriage was 2.86 (95% confidence interval 1.3-6.29) when the male partner had worked in the water treatment plant within the 4 months prior to conception compared with pregnancies where the male partner had not been exposed.[37] An Ohio group compared the fertility of 133 married male workers at a sewage treatment plant in an industrialized city with that of 86 controls who also worked for the city but were not exposed to sewage. To do this, they interviewed husbands and wives and determined pregnancy outcome data, history of infertility problems, contraceptive history, family history of infertility problems, and other pertinent information. From this information, they calculated a standardized fertility ratio (SFR) that compared actual live births with expected live births based on various risk factors. This study found no difference between the two groups, although there was a trend for the exposed group to have higher SFRs. In both groups, the SFRs were greater than one; that is, both groups of city workers had more live births than predicted.[30] This study differs from the previous one in that miscarriage rates were not documented.

Dermal Effects

Exposure to dust from dried sewage sludge causes an irritant dermatitis. This symptom is part of the sewer worker's syndrome.[31,49,51] An outbreak of irritant dermatitis in sewage treatment workers in Toronto was caused when the workplace became contaminated with dust from sewage sludge during the repair of a malfunctioning fan in a sludge incinerator. The workers suffered from an erythematous, scaly dermatitis on the exposed skin. Some workers also complained of eye irritation. These symptoms were successfully treated with cool saline compresses and topical steroids. The sludge was tested on rabbits and found to be very irritating. No further outbreaks of dermatitis occurred after an enclosure was built to hold the fan and measures were taken to remove dust from the workplace.[39]

Acute Inhalational Exposures

Because their work routinely involves entering closed spaces, sewer workers are at risk for inhalant exposure to volatilized toxins. The toxic gases most commonly encountered by this route are the chemical asphyxiants hydrogen sulfide and carbon monoxide and the simple asphyxiants methane and carbon dioxide. Of these, the most consequential is hydrogen sulfide.

Before entering any enclosed space, workers must follow proper procedures to ensure the presence of a safe atmosphere. Unlike other enclosed spaces, the atmosphere in a sewer may rapidly become hazardous as flammable or toxic gases are released from an ever-changing stream of sewage. Because of the constant danger involved, OSHA has specific recommendations for sewer entry.[43] The OSHA standards for sewer entry stipulate that only experienced persons well versed in proper procedure should enter the sewer system. These persons should be equipped with atmospheric monitoring equipment that has both a visible readout and an audible alarm that sounds when it detects hydrogen sulfide in concentrations greater than 10 ppm, carbon monoxide greater than 35 ppm, oxygen concentration less than 19.5%, or the presence of flammable gases. In certain situations, additional safety equipment may include use of an "escape" self-contained breathing apparatus, a device that gives a 10-minute supply of oxygen to allow escape, should atmospheric conditions deteriorate. Because these precautions are uniformly practiced, there are few reports of sewer workers overcome by toxic gases; nevertheless, failure to follow these procedures or unforeseen circumstances may place them at risk.

Entering an atmospheric containing toxic gases causes symptoms that depend on the type and concentration of toxic gases present. Toxic gases may be classified as simple asphyxiants, irritants, and chemical asphyxiants. Simple asphyxiants have no direct systemic toxicity and act simply

by displacing oxygen. Irritants and chemical asphyxiants, in addition to their other toxic properties, act as simple asphyxiants at high concentrations. As the ambient oxygen concentration decreases, exposed persons suffer from symptoms of progressive hypoxia. Headache, malaise, and exertional fatigue are common. An atmosphere with less than 10% oxygen is an immediate threat to life. Persons entering such an atmosphere rapidly lose consciousness and may suffer seizures or cardiopulmonary arrest. Methane and carbon dioxide are the simple asphyxiants most often found in sewers and septic tanks. Methane carries the additional hazard of being flammable.

Irritant gases are classified according to their water solubility. The highly water-soluble gases include ammonia, sulfur dioxide, and hydrogen chloride gas. Ammonia is often released from decomposing sewage and manure. These gases are highly irritating and cause immediate nose, throat, and eye irritation in exposed persons. Because of these uncomfortable symptoms, exposure is typically self-limited. Persons who are unable to escape may develop severe sequelae, such as upper airway obstruction or pulmonary edema. Ocular injury, including ulceration, may occur. The intermediate water-soluble gases such as chlorine cause less immediate irritation than the highly water-soluble gases but have the same overall clinical effect. The poorly water-soluble irritants, including phosgene and nitrogen dioxide, are uncommon constituents of the sewer atmosphere. These agents are less irritating than the highly water-soluble irritants and exposure tends to be prolonged. Pulmonary edema and bronchiolitis obliterans are common sequelae. Initial symptoms are often delayed for hours, and bronchiolitis obliterans typically occurs weeks after the original exposure.

Chemical asphyxiants cause systemic toxicity by interfering with oxygen delivery or utilization. Carbon monoxide (see Chapter 15) interferes with oxygen delivery by forming carboxyhemoglobin. In addition, carbon monoxide causes lipid peroxidation resulting in central nervous system injury. Hydrogen sulfide and cyanide interfere with mitochondrial utilization of oxygen. Cyanide is discussed in detail elsewhere (see Chapter 20). Agents that cause methemoglobin are also classified as chemical asphyxiants. Hydrogen sulfide, often referred to as *sewer gas,* is the most important toxic gas found in sewers. Because of modern safety precautions, sewer workers are now rarely exposed to this gas, although exposures have been reported in the past.[1,23] Persons in many other occupations are also at risk for hydrogen sulfide exposure. In a 5-year retrospective study in Alberta, Canada, 250 workers submitted claims to the provincial disability board for exposure to hydrogen sulfide. Of these exposures, 86% were associated with the oil and gas industry.[2] There are numerous reports of fatal hydrogen sulfide exposure in farmers and others working in and around septic tanks and manure waste pits.[13,32] Unfortunately, these often become multiple ca-

sualty situations as ill-equipped rescuers are overcome by the toxic gases.[42] Hydrogen sulfide exposure has also been reported in the pulp and paper industry,[2] shipyard workers,[58] construction workers,[56] roofers exposed to asphalt fumes,[22] workers cleaning hot spring reservoirs,[12] hospitals,[45] and numerous other industries.[56]

Hydrogen sulfide has a rotten egg odor that is detectable at concentrations as low as 0.02 ppm and becomes intense and unpleasant at 20 ppm. Exposure to hydrogen sulfide at concentrations above 50 ppm may cause keratoconjunctivitis. With continued exposure, reversible ulcers develop, a condition known as the *gas eye.* Corneal scarring and permanently impaired vision may occur with severe exposure. Levels above 50 or 100 ppm cause upper respiratory tract irritation with rhinitis and bronchitis. Prolonged exposure can cause lower respiratory damage and pulmonary edema. Even at low concentrations, hydrogen sulfide may cause increased airway reactivity in susceptible persons.[47] Respiratory symptoms in persons exposed to hydrogen sulfide include dyspnea, cough, sore throat, and chest pain. Cyanosis and hemoptysis may occur.[3,47] At concentrations between 100 and 200 ppm, olfactory fatigue, followed by olfactory paralysis, occurs. At high concentrations, hydrogen sulfide causes systemic toxicity by binding to and inhibiting cytochrome oxidase and other enzymes. Exposure to concentrations above 500 ppm results in rapid loss of consciousness ("knockdown"), and concentrations greater than 700 ppm cause immediate collapse with respiratory paralysis, cardiac arrhythmias, and death. The OSHA threshold limit values (TLV) for hydrogen sulfide is a time-weighted average of 10 ppm and a short-term exposure limit (STEL) of 15 ppm.

The brain and the lungs are the organ systems most affected by hydrogen sulfide exposure. Common clinical findings after exposure to hydrogen sulfide include syncope, headache, seizures, lethargy, dizziness, abnormal reflexes, sore throat, cough, dyspnea, cyanosis, pulmonary edema, hemoptysis, chest pain, eye irritation, weakness, nausea, vomiting, and malaise.[2,47] Of 250 workers reporting hydrogen sulfide exposure in Alberta, 138 (54%) lost consciousness, and there were seven (2.8%) deaths. After syncope, the next most common symptoms were headache (26%), nausea or vomiting (25%), dyspnea (23%), and disequilibrium (22%).[2]

Most persons who are exposed to hydrogen sulfide either die or recover completely. Of 243 survivors in one study, only 13 missed more than 2 weeks of work.[2] In another study of 221 workers exposed to hydrogen sulfide, the authors stated that there was no evidence of permanent neurologic sequelae in the survivors.[7] These studies were retrospective, with poor follow-up, and other authors have reported permanent sequelae after hydrogen sulfide exposure. Symptoms may include neuropsychiatric sequelae such as prolonged coma, dementia, incontinence, memory and learning

defects, and personality changes. Sensory abnormalities, including loss of hearing, loss of vision, and anosmia, and motor findings like ataxia, tremor, and muscle rigidity have also been reported. Neurologic sequelae may be delayed for several days after apparent improvement. Permanent brain damage usually does not occur in persons who were unconscious for less than 5 minutes. Cerebral computed tomography scans are often normal but may show cerebral atrophy, symmetric lucencies in the cerebral hemispheres, or basal ganglia lesions.[33,58,59]

Gastrointestinal Effects

Sewage treatment plant workers often suffer from diarrhea and other minor gastrointestinal complaints. Workers in New York sewage treatment plants were significantly more likely to have had diarrhea in the preceding month than drinking water treatment workers (odds ratio 2.4, 95% confidence interval 1.3 to 4.6).[51] Gastrointestinal symptoms are more common in newly employed workers. Symptoms tend to be minor and seldom result in time lost from work.[35] These symptoms are more common in workers with high exposure to sewage dust and are often related to specific jobs such as cleaning basins and servicing pumps. In these situations, the symptoms usually began a few hours after the work had started and had resolved by the following morning. Symptoms were also more likely to recur after return from a vacation period.[31]

Sewer workers are exposed to numerous bacteria, viruses, and parasites and may be at risk for infections from enteric pathogens. British sewage workers were found to have a 58% incidence of antihepatitis A IgG compared with a 34% incidence in controls (road workers).[46] Sewer workers in Singapore had an adjusted seroprevalence of antibodies to hepatitis A virus that was 2.2 times higher than nonexposed controls.[21] In another Singapore study, sewer workers and public cleansing workers (street and market cleaners) were found to be six times as likely to have high titres of leptospiral antibodies as control workers.[9] Egyptian sewage workers were more likely than nonexposed controls to have infections with intestinal parasites.[20] In contrast to the previous studies, American studies did not find an increased incidence of intestinal parasitic infections in sewage workers. This may be due to a lower prevalence of intestinal parasites in the American population or to a lower exposure to sewage in American sewage workers.[11]

Respiratory Effects

Sewage maintenance and sewage treatment plant workers have an increased incidence of respiratory complaints. Sewage treatment plant workers in Toronto were found to suffer more often than controls from cough, sputum production, wheezing, and sore throat. Those who worked near the sludge incinerator tended to have impaired lung function (decreased forced vital capacity and forced expiratory volume in 1 second), although this did not reach

statistical significance.[40] After controlling for incidence of smoking, sewer maintenance workers in Zagreb had a higher incidence of chronic cough, chronic sputum production, chest tightness, and throat irritation than control workers. Some measures of baseline ventilatory capacity in these Zagreb sewer workers were less than predicted, although not uniformly worse than in the control workers.[60] The agent or agents responsible for causing these respiratory complaints have not been determined.

In addition to the irritative complaints mentioned previously, sewer treatment workers may rarely develop occupational asthma caused by exposure to sewer flies. The seasonal asthma, rhinitis, and conjunctivitis of a sewer treatment plant worker in Michigan was attributed to sewer fly exposure. This patient's symptoms occurred during the warm months when sewer flies were abundant at his place of work. Bronchial challenge testing with sewer fly extract caused prolonged bronchospasm in this patient.[17] Several workers in a South African sewage treatment plant developed occupational asthma caused by exposure to sewer flies.[41] Hypersensitivity symptoms including bronchospasm are common in persons exposed to midges, which are closely related to the sewer fly.[15] Sewer flies rarely cause health problems but should be considered a possible cause of occupational asthma in sewer treatment plant workers.

PATHOPHYSIOLOGY

Hydrogen sulfide is both an irritant and a chemical asphyxiant. Tissues most affected by hydrogen sulfide toxicity are those with high oxygen requirements and those with exposed mucous membranes.[47] In the presence of water, hydrogen sulfide becomes a potent irritant that involves the eyes, nose, throat, upper airway, and, with continued exposure, the lower airway. Corneal epithelial cells swell, blister, and form vacuoles. Corneal vacuoles may progress to ulcers, which in severe cases may cause corneal scarring. The OSHA exposure limits (TLV-TWA 10 ppm) (STEL 15 ppm) for hydrogen sulfide are designed to prevent ocular injury. The effects of irritant exposure on the upper airway are well known. Hydrogen sulfide is relatively insoluble in water, which makes it less irritating than ammonia or chlorine, and exposed persons do not immediately suffer symptoms of upper airway or ocular irritation. Nevertheless, exposure to hydrogen sulfide is often self-limited because of the noxious odor. Because of its low water solubility, hydrogen sulfide tends to penetrate deeply into the respiratory tract to cause alveolar injury that results in pulmonary edema. Pulmonary edema requires inhalational exposure to sulfides and does not occur in experimental models with animals given lethal doses of sodium sulfide parenterally. In addition to this irritant effect on the respiratory tract, there is animal evidence that hydrogen sulfide may cause airway hyperresponsiveness. Prolonged exposure to low levels of hydrogen sulfide (1 to 100 ppm) caused increased sensitivity to a methacholine challenge test, and acute exposure to high levels of hydrogen sulfide increased both the sensitivity and maximal airway reactivity after methacholine challenge. Hydrogen sulfide causes a separation in tight junctions between mucosal cells, which increases airway permeability and allows metacholine better access to underlying bronchial smooth muscle. There is, however, little evidence that humans exposed to low levels of hydrogen sulfide develop reactive airways dysfunction syndrome.[19,25,47]

Inhaled hydrogen sulfide causes systemic toxicity identical to that of intravenous sodium sulfide. Like cyanide, sulfide interferes with mitochondrial respiration by inhibiting cytochrome a-a$_3$ activity.[26,53] Inhibition of cytochrome a-a$_3$ blocks the cytochrome oxidase system and thus interferes with oxidative phosphorylation and aerobic energy production. Energy production comes from less efficient anaerobic metabolism with resultant lactic acidosis. This results in markedly decreased ATP production and, with severe toxicity, inability to meet cellular energy requirements. Decreased oxygen extraction with increased venous po$_2$ is another marker of failure of oxidative phosphorylation.

Hydrogen sulfide is a well-known neurologic toxin. Hydrogen sulfide in concentrations greater than about 200 ppm paralyzes the olfactory nerves. Prolonged exposure or exposure to very high concentrations causes respiratory paralysis. At concentrations greater than 500 to 1000 ppm, rapid loss of consciousness ("knockdown") occurs.[19,47] Experimental animals dying of hydrogen sulfide poisoning have increased sulfide levels in the brain and particularly in the brainstem. It is unknown which site is responsible for neurologic toxicity. Part of the neurologic dysfunction may be due to cellular hypoxia from impaired mitochondrial respiration. Other effects of sulfide such as inhibition of sodium channels and of the sodium-potassium ATPase may also play a role. Sulfide also inhibits monoamine oxidase (MAO) and acetyl-cholinesterase. Inhibition of MAO results in increased levels of brain catecholamines and serotonin in experimental animals given sodium sulfide. Glutamate, glutamine, GABA, glycine, and other neurotransmitters are also increased in this experimental model.[47]

The effects of prolonged hydrogen sulfide exposure at the OSHA TLV (10 ppm) on organ systems other than the eye have not been extensively tested. Chronic low-level exposure causes respiratory dysfunction in animal models, but human data suggest that this effect is, at most, minimal.[47] In one study, Finnish pulp and paper workers chronically exposed to hydrogen sulfide had a trend toward increased mortality from cardiovascular causes.[24]

MANAGEMENT
Prevention

The skin and eye symptoms in sewage treatment plant workers is associated with sewage sludge or dust contact. The sewer worker's syndrome is associated with inhalation of bacterial aerosols. For this reason, workers' contact with these agents should be minimized. Occupational hygiene measures terminated an outbreak of irritant dermatitis in a Toronto plant.[39] Personal measures to minimize contact with the dust in the treatment plant are important. They include using boots, gloves, and masks, showering at the end of the workday, wearing clean clothes each day, and washing hands before meals and before smoking.

Preventing inhalational injury requires rigorous training and adherence to safety protocol for all persons who enter enclosed spaces. The OSHA guidelines for entering the sewerage system were described previously. Briefly, these guidelines include measuring concentrations of hazardous gases in the atmosphere and carrying a personal escape breathing apparatus to allow escape should conditions deteriorate. Because hydrogen sulfide is heavier than air and can accumulate in pits and depressions, persons can be overcome without actually entering an enclosed space. Perhaps the most important preventative measure is to keep rescuers from also becoming victims. When a worker collapses in an enclosed space, rescuers must obtain proper gear, including self-contained breathing apparatus, before entering that space. Having this gear readily available and training workers in its use prevent unnecessary exposures.

Treatment and Screening

Treating the nonspecific symptoms that comprise the sewer worker's syndrome involves first ensuring that contact with sewage dust is minimized, as previously described. Irritant dermatitis and ocular irritation have been successfully treated with topical steroids. Infectious diseases, specifically hepatitis A, leptospirosis, and giardiasis, may be screened for in workers with gastrointestinal symptoms. Although the long-term risks of exposure to pollutants in sewage are unclear, it is reasonable to periodically monitor renal and hepatic function. Similarly respiratory function tests should be obtained in those with respiratory symptoms. Persons who have lost consciousness following exposure to a toxic gas should be followed closely to detect any neuropsychiatric symptoms that may develop.

Collapse in an enclosed space is a true emergency, and the worker's life may depend on how quickly he can be extricated and resuscitated. After properly equipped rescuers remove the worker to a safe place, standard resuscitation measures should be instituted and the worker transported to the nearest hospital for definitive evaluation and treatment. The nonbreathing victim should receive mouth-to-mouth ventilation until more advanced care is possible. There is no evidence that mouth-to-mouth ventilation is dangerous for the rescuer of a victim of hydrogen sulfide inhalation. Medical personnel should institute advanced supportive care including intubation and mechanical ventilation as appropriate. The vast majority of exposures to simple asphyxiants and to hydrogen sulfide respond to simply removing the victim from the toxic atmosphere and perhaps assisting ventilation for a few minutes. Persons with respiratory distress after exposure to irritants should be treated supportively with humidified oxygen, bronchodilators and observation until symptoms have resolved. Exposure to low water-soluble irritants carries the risk of delayed development of adult respiratory distress syndrome (ARDS) and bronchiolitis obliterans. These persons should be observed in hospital for 24 hours. Persons who do not develop symptoms after this time can be discharged. Those who develop ARDS after such an exposure should be followed by a pulmonologist because of the risk of developing bronchiolitis obliterans.

The role for antidote therapy is undefined. Although nitrite-induced methemoglobin protects against sulfide poisoning in experimental models, this effect is seen only when methemoglobin is present before or shortly after sulfide exposure.[54,55] The protective effect of methemoglobin appears to be due to enhanced detoxification of sulfide by oxidation and not the formation of a sulfidemethemoglobin complex, as was previously thought.[4] However, sulfide is also rapidly oxidized in the presence of oxyhemoglobin and is essentially eliminated within minutes after exposure. Even in in vitro models with sulfide concentrations thousands of times higher than are seen clinically, oxyhemoglobin-catalyzed sulfide oxidation was 90% complete after 20 minutes.[4] Furthermore, inducing methemoglobin is dangerous in persons suffering from postanoxic encephalopathy or from carbon monoxide exposure. For these reasons, we do not recommend giving nitrites to persons overcome by a toxic inhalation unless there is reason to suspect cyanide exposure. There is no evidence that thiosulfate has any role in treating the victim of sulfide poisoning. Carbon monoxide levels should be obtained, and hyperbaric oxygen should be considered for victims of carbon monoxide exposure. The regional poison control center is often able to give valuable management guidelines. Persons who remain comatose after an inhalational injury should receive meticulous supportive care. It is also important to consider and search for potentially reversible causes, such as head trauma.

SUMMARY

Sewer and sanitation workers are exposed to the wide variety of toxic chemicals, microorganisms, and decaying organic matter that comprise sewage. These workers often suffer from a constellation of symptoms known as the *sewer worker's syndrome:* fever, chills, headache, fatigue, malaise, purulent ocular discharge, skin irritation, gastrointestinal symptoms including diarrhea, cough, purulent sputum, and throat irritation. Sewer workers appear to be exposed to mutagens and may be at an increased risk of developing cancers of the liver, larynx, brain, kidney, or stomach, although the data are inconclusive. Similarly, weak data suggest that spouses of sewer workers have an increased miscarriage rate. Proper occupational and personal hygiene measures should be taken to minimize exposure of workers to sewage sludge and dust.

Because they frequently enter enclosed spaces, sewer workers must be diligent to avoid exposure to toxic gases. Hydrogen sulfide is the most dangerous of these and in high concentrations causes rapid loss of consciousness and potentially death. Methane, carbon dioxide, and ammonia are also released from decaying sewage and may cause injury or death. Volatile solvents from industrial sewage and carbon monoxide pose additional hazards. Careful monitoring of atmospheric conditions inside the sewer before and during sewer entry minimizes the risk of inhalational exposure. Victims of inhalation exposure should be removed from the toxic atmosphere as quickly as possible but in a fashion that ensures the safety of the rescuer. Supportive care is the most important management step. Further management decisions may be made in consultation with the regional poison control center.

REFERENCES

1. Adelson L, Sunshine I: Fatal hydrogen sulfide intoxication: report of three cases occurring in a sewer, *Arch Pathol* 81:375-380.
2. Arnold IM et al: Health implication of occupational exposures to hydrogen sulfide, *J Occup Med* 27:373, 1985.
3. Beauchamp RO et al: A critical review of the literature on hydrogen sulfide toxicity, *Crit Rev Toxicol* 13:25, 1984.
4. Beck JF et al: Nitrite as an antidote for acute hydrogen sulfide intoxication? *Am Ind Hyg Assoc J* 42:805, 1981.
5. Betemps EJ, Buncher CR, Clark CS: Proportional mortality analysis of wastewater treatment system workers by birthplace with comments on amyotrophic lateral sclerosis, *J Occup Med* 36:31, 1994.
6. Bureau of the Census: *Statistical abstract of the United States* (table 494), ed 114, Washington, DC, 1994, Bureau of the Census.
7. Burnett WW et al: Hydrogen sulfide poisoning: review of 5 years experience, *Can Med Assoc J* 117:1277, 1977.
8. Castellan RM et al: Inhaled endotoxin and decreased spirometric values, *N Engl J Med* 317:605, 1987.
9. Chan OY et al: Leptospirosis risk in public cleansing and sewer workers, *Ann Acad Med* 16:586, 1987.
10. Clark CS et al: Sewage worker's syndrome, *Lancet* 1009, 1977.
11. Clark CS et al: Enteric parasites in workers occupationally exposed to sewage, *J Occup Med* 26:273, 1984.
12. Deng JG, Chang SC: Hydrogen sulfide poisonings in hot-spring reservoir cleaning: two case reports, *Am J Ind Med* 11:447, 1987.
13. Donham KJ et al: Acute toxic exposure to gases from liquid manure, *J Occup Med* 24:142, 1982.
14. Friis L, Edling C, Hagnar L: Mortality and incidence of cancer among sewage workers: a retrospective study, *Br J Ind Med* 50:653, 1993.
15. Gad ER, Kay AB: Widespread immunoglobulin E-mediated hypersensitivity in the Sudan to the "green nimitti" midge, *Cladotanytarsus lewisi* (Diptera: Chironomidae), *J Allergy Clin Immunol* 66:190, 1980.
16. Glass DC: An assessment of the exposure of water reclamation workers to hydrogen sulfide, *Ann Occup Hyg* 34:509, 1990.
17. Gold BL, Mathews KP, Burge HA: Occupational asthma caused by sewer flies, *Am Rev Respir Dis* 131:949, 1985.
18. Granick H: *Underneath New York,* New York, 1991, Fordham University Press.
19. Guidotti TL: Occupational exposure to hydrogen sulfide in the sour gas industry: some unresolved issues, *Int Arch Occup Environ Health* 66:153, 1994.
20. Hammouda NA, El-Gebali WM, Razek MK: Intestinal parasitic infection among sewage workers in Alexandria, Egypt, *J Egypt Soc Parasitol* 22:299, 1992.
21. Heng BH et al: Prevalence of hepatitis infection among sewer workers in Singapore, *Epidemiol Infect* 113:121, 1994.

22. Hoidal CR et al: Hydrogen sulfide poisoning from toxic inhalations of roofing asphalt fumes, *Ann Emerg Med* 15:826, 1986.

23. Hurwitz LJ, Taylor GI: Poisoning by sewer gas with unusual sequelae, *Lancet* 1:1110, 1954.

24. Jappinen P, Tola S: Cardiovascular mortality among pulp mill workers, *Br J Ind Med* 47:259, 1990.

25. Jappinen P et al: Exposure to hydrogen sulfide and respiratory function, *Br J Ind Med* 47:824, 1990.

26. Khan AA et al: Effects of hydrogen sulfide exposure on lung mitochondrial respiratory chain molecules in rats, *Toxicol Appl Pharmacol* 103:482, 1990.

27. Kraut A et al: Neurotoxic effects of solvent exposure on sewage workers, *Arch Environ Health* 43:263, 1988.

28. Lafleur J, Vena JE: Retrospective cohort mortality study of cancer among sewage plant workers, *Am J Ind Med* 19:75, 1991.

29. Laitinen S et al: Worker's exposure to airborne bacteria and endotoxins at industrial wastewater treatment plants, *Am Ind Hyg Assoc J* 55:1055, 1994.

30. Lemasters GK et al: Fertility of workers chronically exposed to chemically contaminated sewer wastes, *Reproduct Toxicol* 5:31, 1991.

31. Lundholm M, Rylander R: Work related symptoms among sewage workers, *Br J Ind Med* 40:325, 1983.

32. Madery G, Parker D, Shutske J: Fatalities attributed to entering manure waste pits—Minnesota, 1992, *MMWR Morb Mortal Wkly Rep* 42:325, 1993.

33. Matsuo F, Cummins JW, Anderson RE: Neurologic sequelae of massive hydrogen sulfide inhalation, *Arch Neurol* 36:451, 1979.

34. Mattsby I, Rylander R: Clinical and immunological findings in workers exposed to sewage dust, *J Occup Med* 20:690, 1978.

35. McCunney RJ: Health effects of work at waste water treatment plants: a review of the literature with guidelines for medical surveillance, *Am J Ind Med* 9:271, 1986.

36. Melbostatd E, Eduard W, Skogstad A: Exposure to bacterial aerosols and work related symptoms in sewage workers, *Am J Ind Med* 25:59, 1994.

37. Morgan RW et al: Fetal loss and work in a waste water treatment plant, *Am J Public Health* 74:499, 1984.

38. Morse DL et al: Occupational exposure to hexachlorocyclopentadiene. How safe is sewage? *JAMA* 241:2177, 1979.

39. Nethercott JR: Airborne irritant contact dermatitis due to sewage sludge, *J Occup Med* 23:771, 1981.

40. Nethercott JR, Holnes DL: Health status of a group of sewage treatment workers in Toronto, Canada, *Am Ind Hyg Assoc J* 49:346, 1988.

41. Ordman D: Sewage filter flies (psychoda) as a cause of bronchial asthma, *S Afr Med J* 20:32, 1946.

42. Osbern LN, Crapo RO: Dung lung: a report of toxic exposure to liquid manure, *Ann Intern Med* 95:312, 1981.

43. OSHA: *Sewer system entry,* Publication No 1910.146 App E, Washington, DC, 1994, US Government Printing Office.

44. Palchack RB et al: Airborne endotoxin associated with industrial scale production of protein products in gram negative bacteria, *Am Ind Hyg Assoc J* 49:420, 1988.

45. Peters JW: Hydrogen sulfide poisoning in a hospital setting, *JAMA* 246:1588, 1981.

46. Poole CJM, Shakespeare AT: Should sewage workers and carers for people with learning disabilities be vaccinated for hepatitis A? *BMJ* 306:1102, 1993.

47. Reiffenstein RJ et al: Toxicology of hydrogen sulfide, *Annu Rev Pharmacol Toxicol* 32:109, 1992.

48. Rylander R et al: Sewage worker's syndrome, *Lancet* 478, 1976.

49. Rylander R et al: Studies on humans exposed to airborne sewage sludge, *Schweiz Med Wochenschr* 107:182, 1977.

50. Scarlett-Kranz JM et al: Urinary mutagens in municipal sewage and water treatment workers, *Am J Epidemiol* 124:884, 1986.

51. Scarlett-Krantz JM et al: Health among municipal sewage and water treatment workers, *Toxicol Ind Health* 3:311, 19••.

52. Sewer collapse and toxic illness in sewer repairmen—Ohio, *MMWR Morb Mortal Wkly Rep* 30:89, 1981.

53. Smith L, Kruszyna H, Smith RP: The effect of methemoglobin on the inhibition of cytochrome c oxidase by cyanide, sulfide or azide, *Biochem Pharmacol* 26:2247, 1977.

54. Smith RP, Gosselin RE: On the mechanism of sulfide inactivation by methemoglobin, *Toxicol Appl Pharmacol* 8:159, 1977.

55. Smith RP, Kruszyna R, Kruszyna H: Management of acute hydrogen sulfide poisoning, *Arch Environ Health* 31:166, 1976.

56. Snyder JW et al: Occupational fatality and persistent neurologic sequelae after mass exposure to hydrogen sulfide, *Am J Emerg Med* 13:199, 1995.

57. Srikanth R, Khanam A, Rao V: Cadmium levels in the urine of male sewage sludge farmers of Hyberadad, India, *J Tox Environ Health* 43:1, 1994.

58. Tvedt B et al: Delayed neuropsychiatric sequelae after acute hydrogen sulfide poisoning, *Acta Neurol Scand* 84:348, 1991.

59. Tvedt B et al: Brain damage caused by hydrogen sulfide: a followup study of six patients, *Am J Ind Med* 20:91, 1991.

60. Zuskin E, Mustajbegovic J, Schachter EN: Respiratory function in sewage workers, *Am J Ind Med* 23:751, 1993.

Ship and Dockyard Personnel

Scott D. Phillips

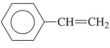

styrene

Pb$_3$O$_4$
lead oxide

Mg$_6$(Si$_4$O$_{10}$)(OH$_8$)
chrysotile asbestos

- Styrene is a potent neurotoxin and is the material often used in small craft construction

- Efforts to reduce asbestos exposure have been successful, but the long latency for this disease makes continued surveillance essential

- Lead oxide (red lead) is an important rust resistant paint that causes an ongoing lead exposure risk

Working in the dockyards is one of the oldest occupations. The construction of ships has changed dramatically over the last 50 years. Around 1940, both commercial and military vessels began using welded instead of riveted steel construction. The increased use of aluminum and other lighter-weight alloys has improved both productivity and performance of vessels. Over the years a massive amount of information has become available regarding these workers' exposures. In the United States, approximately 130,000 people are employed in building and repairing ships, roughly half in the private sector and half in the military sector.[24] This number omits those not directly involved in building or repair, such as administrators. Longshore, shipyard, dockyard workers perform a variety of tasks during the construction, repair, and breaking of ships. Loading and unloading cargo may expose workers to an unlimited number of chemicals and substances. Manual labor can result in ergonomic stress, vibration, and sun and thermal exposures. The modern-day shipyard is a production facility with multiple subassemblies working in concert toward a final product. The major job categories in this industry include welders, painters, pipefitters, shipwrights, sheet-metal workers, machinists, electricians, and other service workers. There are also material movers involved in the loading and off-loading of commerce and cargo from ships (Table 34-1). The most important exposure historically that has resulted in chronic illness is asbestos.

Cargo may include an almost endless array of potential hazards, from petroleum products to grains to ores. Fre-

Table 34-1 Various trades and their potential exposures, many of which have associated physical hazards

Trade	Potential exposures
Electricians	Solvents, metal fumes, fluxes, epoxy resins, naphthalenes, halogenated biphenyl, asbestos
Machinists	Synthetic cutting fluids, cutting oils, chromates, greases, lubricants, solvents, asbestos
Painters	Solvents, lead, chromium, cadmium, nickel, organotins, silica, asbestos
Pipefitters	Welding fumes, resins, asbestos, mineral fibers, plastic, magnesium
Riggers and material movers	Exposed to contents being moved
Sheet-metal workers	Welding fumes, asbestos, mineral fibers
Shipfitters	Welding fumes, asbestos, mineral fibers
Shipwrights	Solvents, wood dusts, glues, oils
Welders	Welding fumes, aluminum, arsenic, asbestos, beryllium, carbon monoxide, chromium, cobalt, copper, manganese, magnesium, ozone, phosgene, vanadium, zinc, dusts

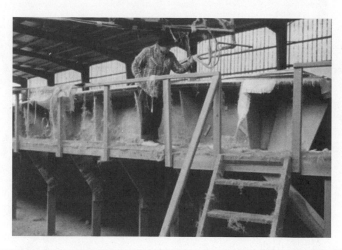

Fig. 34-1 Young woman building the hull of the trawler shown in Figure 34-2. (From Zenz C, Dickerson OB, Horvath EP: *Occupational medicine,* ed 3, St Louis, 1994, Mosby.)

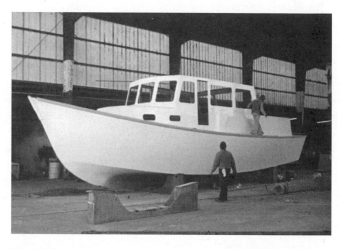

Fig. 34-2 A boat of the trawler type made almost entirely of fiberglass and polyester resins, with styrene as a major component. (From Zenz C, Dickerson OB, Horvath EP: *Occupational medicine,* ed 3, St Louis, 1994, Mosby.)

quently, substances such as crops require pesticide treatments to eliminate or prevent infestations. These fumigants may result in exposure to maritime workers.

For shipments of hazardous substances over water, a "dangerous cargo manifest" must be on the bridge of the vessel in a designated holder. It outlines the types and amounts of substances, the origin, destination, and loader's, captain's, and receiver's signatures. For barges, the tug must have the manifest in the pilot house.

Much more information is in the chapters dealing with those specific topics. As asbestos and lead are used prominently in this field, they are discussed in more detail.

POTENTIAL TOXIC EXPOSURES

Because of the nature of the building, remodeling, and day-to-day repair of ships, many different types of chemical and physical exposure are encountered. Potential toxic exposures classically include organic solvents, paints, oils, thinners, epoxy resins, inhalable dusts, asbestos, manufactured mineral fibers, lead and other metals from paint and ship rebuilding, diesel exhaust, styrene, and silica from sandblasting. The cargo onboard may also have toxic properties.

A common fumigant is aluminum phosphide. Phosphine is an insecticidal agent in ships carrying grain when applied as aluminum phosphide. Moisture onboard reacts with the aluminum phosphide to generate phosphine gas, leaving a harmless residue of aluminum hydroxide. The resulting gas may cause central nervous system (CNS) and gastrointestinal signs and pulmonary edema.

In shipbuilding, workers may be in confined spaces where toxic substances accumulate. Thus, not only are they in a potentially oxygen-deficient environment but also toxic fumes related to welding or flame-cutting may accumulate. Specific gases of concern are carbon dioxide, carbon monoxide, methane, hydrogen sulfide, hydrocarbon vapors, and more conventional vapors from welding (see Table 34-1). For example, shipyard welders who welded steel plates that were degreased with trichloroethylene have developed acute pulmonary edema from the generation of phosgene.

The vast majority of yachts of 150-foot length and some commercial fishing craft are constructed of fiberglass or glass reinforced plastic (GRP). Far less welding and pipefitting are involved. The exposures are mostly to

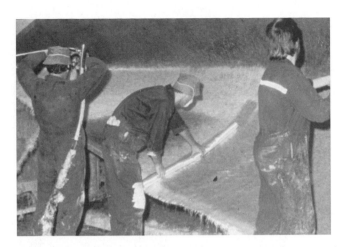

Fig. 34-3 Extensive hand work in applying the many layers of fiberglass in boat building; see Figure 34-4. (From Zenz C, Dickerson OB, Horvath EP: *Occupational medicine,* ed 3, St Louis, 1994, Mosby.)

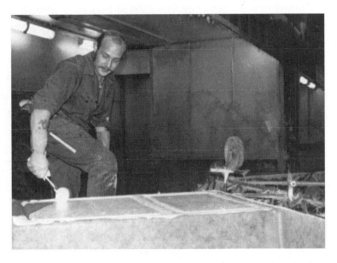

Fig. 34-4 Application of the many layers of fiberglass in boat building involves extensive hand work. (From Zenz C, Dickerson OB, Horvath EP: *Occupational medicine,* ed 3, St Louis, 1994, Mosby.)

epoxy resins and to solvents, including acetone and other highly aromatic compounds. Styrene is frequently used in nearly equal amounts to the resins in the production of plastics. During the assembly of these crafts, evaporation of styrene and other solvents may occur. Typically these crafts are constructed in environments with limited ventilation and exhaust. Further discussion on this topic can be found in Chapter 46 (Figs. 34-1 to 34-4).

Physical hazards include vibration, ergonomic stress, ionizing radiation, extreme temperatures, closed spaces, hypoxic environments, and noise. Epidemics of infectious diseases have also occurred. Epidemic keratoconjunctivitis—"shipyard eye"—has occurred from adenovirus infections. It results in corneal petechiae and infiltrates with visual impairment in about 50% of cases.

CLINICAL TOXICOLOGY
Asbestos

The leading health concerns involving shipyard workers have historically been asbestos exposure and lead poisoning. Asbestos is used for insulation of pipes and boilers. *Lagging* is the application of sheets of asbestos material for insulation purposes. Welders use asbestos sheeting for insulation against burning metal. Frequently, welders and painters have to move asbestos insulation to complete tasks. Prior to World War II, amosite was added to chrysotile. The crocidolite form has also been used. Asbestos has largely been replaced by manufactured mineral fibers, products that have their own risks. Although welders, painters, and pipefitters have the most exposure, virtually all other trades associated with shipbuilding and shipbreaking encounter asbestos. This exposure was most prominent before the mid-1970s. Asbestos-induced lung cancer is estimated to have a 20-year latency period.

Illnesses associated with asbestos include benign asbestos pleurisy, asbestosis, pleura plaques, mesothelioma, and lung cancer. The Occupational Safety and Health Administration (OSHA) has a specific shipyard standard covering workers in this industry due to the significant health risks. Specific exposure limits, medical surveillance requirements, and other programs are detailed in the Shipyard Standard (29 CFR 1915). The permissible exposure limit (PEL) time-weighted average (TWA) for asbestos is 0.1 fiber per cm^3 of air as an 8-hour TWA. Air samples taken in boiler rooms during the removal of lagging have found levels as high as 171 fibers per cc.[22]

Concern has risen over those living near shipyards. In order to better characterize this risk, The Small Area Health Statistics Unit (SAHFU) facility at the School of Hygiene and Tropical Medicine in London conducted a study of mortality from mesothelioma and asbestosis near the Plymouth Naval dockyards. Data were obtained between 1981 and 1987 within a 3-kilometer radius of the docks. The mortality rate for mesothelioma was higher than the national rate by a factor of 8.4, and that for asbestosis was higher by a factor of 13.6, findings that suggest that not only are those intimately involved with the repair and building of ships at risk but also the adjacent community may be at risk.[7]

The prevalence of asbestos-related health problems in this industry are well known. A study conducted during the 1970s among dockyard workers evaluated x-ray abnormalities related to asbestos. Of 1000 workers evaluated, the researchers found that 46% had evidence of either pleural or parenchymal chest x-ray abnormalities. If one breaks the prevalence down by job description, 74% of pipefitters, 40% of painters, and 36% of carpenters had radiographic abnormalities detected.[21]

The relative risk for developing lung cancer following asbestos exposure in dockyard workers is between 2 and 2.5.[6,8] Asbestos was common in vessels built prior to 1978. Appropriate medical surveillance should be done for those who served in their industry.[20] Not only is lung cancer elevated, a study evaluating the risk of mesothelioma at a naval dockyard in England found that occupational mesothelioma rates were similar to those recorded in London asbestos textile workers.[22]

The association between asbestos-related disease and fiber types or burden has been extensively studied. Recently, a study looking at asbestosis and fiber burden patterns in U.S. shipyard workers found that concentrations of amosite fibers correlated with airway fibrosis and asbestosis. Subjects with mesothelioma, lung cancer, pleura plaques, or no asbestos-related disease had about the same amosite concentrations. Analysis of fiber size measures (length, width, aspect ratio, surface, mass) showed pleura plaques strongly associated with high aspect ratio amosite fibers, and mesotheliomas were associated with low aspect ratio amosite.[5]

The relationship of asbestos and other diseases is poorly characterized. A recent study of the association of asbestos and ischemic heart disease found that those shipyard workers with asbestosis and impaired pulmonary function had an increased risk of death from ischemic heart disease. They found asbestosis independently associated with heart disease.[19] Other studies have not found an association in other occupational settings.[1,4,10,16]

Chest imaging of workers after asbestos exposure has traditionally been done with conventional radiography and International Labor Organization (ILO) criteria for interpretation. The utility of newer, more expensive techniques remains unvalidated. A study looking at the high resolution of computer tomography for early detection of asbestosis found that for asbestos-exposed workers with an ILO classification of less than 1/0 and functional impairment, a high-resolution cat scan (HRCT) examination should be considered.[15] Others examining the lung function in shipyard workers with pulmonary function tests as well as ILO chest x-ray readings, found no significant difference between workers without pleura plaques and those with visible plaques with respect to lung function values. With increase in length and width of the plaques, FVC FVV$_1$, FEF$_{25}$, and FEF$_{75}$ values tend to become lower. These results demonstrate that the changes detected on radiographs in lung pleura are the early indicators of possible asbestosis in shipyard workers.[25]

Radionucleotide studies have had some success in detecting asbestosis. Gallium scans as well as high-resolution computed tomography (HRCT) demonstrate that although only 21% of patients satisfy the common accepted criteria for diagnosis of asbestosis, 75% had evidence of disease by both HRCT and gallium scanning. This suggests that physical examination, pulmonary function tests, and chest x-rays are not useful early diagnostic indicators.[13]

The Finnish Institute of Occupational Health Asbestos Program (1987-1992) led to implementation of this study to prevent asbestos-related risks.[11] The goals were to minimize exposure to asbestos, identify those exposed, and improve the diagnostic studies, especially for cancers. Screening included 18,943 current and retired workers from the house-building, shipyard, and asbestos industries. Pleura and parenchymal changes were found in 22% (4133). In the Finnish population of 5 million, more than 150 mesotheliomas and lung cancers occur annually, and more than 2000 asbestos-induced cancer deaths are anticipated by the year 2010. Lung tissue was available for analysis of mineral fiber content in 94 cases.

Linear regression analysis showed a significant correlation between duration of exposure and asbestos bodies per gram of wet lung weight determined by scanning electron microscopy. Over the duration of exposure, shipyard workers had comparably higher asbestos contents than other workers (p <0.05). Mesotheliomas are associated with varying durations of exposure and asbestos burdens. There seems to be a rough correlation between duration of exposure and commercial amphibole content.[17]

Comparing the presence of asbestos bodies in bronchoalveolar lavage fluid to occupational history, asbestos bodies are found in concentrations equal or exceeding 1 asbestos body per ml in 85% of patients heavily exposed to asbestos and in only 7% of those who were not.

Others have sought to study possible predictors of mesothelioma in shipyard workers exposed to asbestos. In 3893 shipyard workers, medical monitoring, chest x-rays, spirometry, questionnaires, asbestos exposure, and respiratory symptoms were reviewed as possible predictors of mesothelioma. No strong association between different exposure parameters and the risk of mesothelioma could be identified. Impaired lung function and pleura plaques were not associated with increased risk of mesothelioma. Respiratory symptoms were of little value as predictors of mesothelioma. There are suggestions that traditional methods of surveillance are of limited value in identifying persons who are at increased risk of mesothelioma.[18]

Lead

During the process of shipbreaking or refurbishing ships, the grinding, burning, and chipping of paint have given workers significant exposures to airborne lead. Several layers of lead-based paint can occur in ships. The most important lead for use in paint is red lead (Pb_3O_4). Red lead is both a rust retardant and a primer coating. During the breaking process, oxyacetylene cutting torches vaporize the lead in the paint. Inhalation of lead fumes can result in significant pulmonary absorption. Chipping and grinding tend to create larger particles, which are inhaled or ingested. Lead concentrations found in the bulk lead paint samples range from 0.0037% to 11.5% by weight. In 1985, more than 441,000 metric tons of lead pigments were consumed.[23] In personnel conducting the paint removal process, 62% were exposed at or above the OSHA permissible exposure limit for lead, which is 50

Table 34-2 Summary of lowest observed effect levels for key lead-induced health effects in children

Lowest observed effect level (blood lead µg/dl)	Heme synthesis and hematologic effects	Neurologic effects	Renal effects	Gastrointestinal effects
80-100		Encephalopathic signs and symptoms	Chronic nephropathy (aminoaciduria, etc.)	Colic and other overt gastrointestinal symptoms
70	Anemia			
60		Peripheral neuropathies		
50				
40	Reduced hemoglobin synthesis Elevated coproporphyrin Increased urinary aminolevulinic acid	Peripheral nerve dysfunction (slowed NCVS) CNS cognitive effects		
30	Erythrocyte protoporphyrin elevation	Altered CNS electrophysiologic responses, effect on IQ	Vitamin D metabolism interference	
15	Aminolevulinic acid dehydrase inhibition Pyrimidine-5'-nucleotidase activity inhibition	MDI deficits, reduced gestational age, and birth weight (prenatal exposure)		
10				

From EPA 1986a (with updating).

µg/m². Correlations of airborne lead concentrations in bulk lead paint contents for chipping and grinding operations were found to be statistically significant, and blood lead levels were significantly higher in the follow-up blood tests than in the initial blood test taken prior to paint removal. However, blood lead levels were well below the OSHA allowable levels of 40 µg/dl.[26]

Other metals used in the shipbuilding industry include chromium, cadmium, beryllium, manganese, and aluminum. Metals are often colorants in paint: The addition of cadmium to paint results in a yellow coloration, and the use of chromates—typically lead chromates—results in a variety of colors including, green, yellow, and red. They may be used in the shipyard industry or in industrial equipment.

A study in southern Ontario looked at four different shipbreaking operations for lead toxicity. The air sampling results for lead were above the Ontario standard at all locations. Of 113 workers, 34 or 30% had at least one blood level above 3.4 µmols/L (70 µg/100 ml = 34 µmols/L). At one company, 50% of workers had results above 2.5 µmols/L.[14]

Lead exposure produces many health effects (Table 34-2). Programs must be in place to monitor air exposure levels, provide personal protective equipment, and ensure a regular medical surveillance program. Specific respirators are required depending on the ambient air lead levels (Table 34-3). As levels of lead increase in the body, certain biochemical changes appear. The earliest effect is on the inhibition of pyrimidine-5'-nucleotidase at blood levels over 10 µg/dl. Erythrocyte and protoporphyrin increase when the blood lead level approaches 30 µg/dl, with a reduction in the synthesis of hemoglobin at 40 µg/dl. Early effects on the nervous system may occur when blood lead levels reach a similar range. Frank encephalopathy occurs over 80 µg/dl.

The OSHA lead standard has created a blood-lead compliance plan. This scheme allows the physician or other medical provider to remove employees from exposure if they are at risk of material impairment from exposure to lead. The provider can remove an employee from exposures exceeding the action level (or less if needed) or can recommend special protective measures as necessary. Medical monitoring of workers during the medical removal period can be more stringent than that noted in Table 34-3 if the provider feels it is necessary. Workers may return to their previous jobs when the provider feels they are no longer at risk of impairment.

Proper personal protective equipment, frequent medical monitoring, and prompt removal from exposure are vital in preventing lead poisoning. The appropriate respirator type is dictated by airborne concentrations of lead (Table 34-4). Chelation may be indicated in certain individuals with marked exposures. Currently the drug of choice is DMSA (2,3-dimercaptosuccinic acid, Chemet). This is an oral, water-soluble analog of dimercaprol and a very effective

Table 34-3 OSHA blood-lead compliance scheme

A. Blood-lead level requiring employee medical removal (Level must be confirmed with second follow-up blood-lead level within 2 weeks of first report.)	>60 µg/dl or average of last 3 blood samples or all blood samples over previous 6 months (whichever is over a longer time period) is 50 µg/dl or greater unless last blood sample is 40 µg/dl or less
B. Frequency with which employees are exposed to action level of lead (30 µg/m³ TWA) must have blood-lead level checked (zinc protoporphyrin is also strongly recommended in each occasion that a blood lead is obtained):	
1. Last blood-lead level less than 40 µg/dl	Every 6 months
2. Last blood-lead level between 40 µg/dl and level requiring medical removal (see A above)	Every 2 months
3. Employees removed from exposure to lead because of an elevated blood-lead level	Every month
C. Permissible airborne exposure limit for workers removed from work due to an elevated blood-lead level (without regard to respirator protection)	30 µg/m³ 8 hr TWA
D. Blood-lead level confirmed with a second blood analysis, at which employee may return to work	<40 µg/dl

Modified from US Department of Labor, Occupational Safety and Health Administrator: *Lead standard,* 20 CFR 1910.1025, Washington, DC, 1990, US Government Printing Office.

chelator. There are still roles for dimercaprol (BAL), ethylenediaminetetraacetic acid (calcium disodium EDTA), and D-penicillamine in certain situations (see Chapter 36).

Aluminum is frequently used for its relative strength and light weight in the shipbuilding industry. Recent research suggests that serum and urine aluminum measurements can be elevated in many welders in this occupation.[9] Further studies are required to demonstrate causation in these workers.

Manganese is another metal frequently used in the manufacture of ships.[12] It is used in steel alloys. Manganese poisoning was first recognized more than 150 years ago. Inhalation of manganese, as dust or fumes, presents a potent neurotoxin. Symptoms are typical of parkinsonism. However, the brain lesions from manganese occur in the striatum and palladium in distinction to parkinsonism, in which the substantia nigra is damaged.[3]

Table 34-4 OSHA inorganic lead standard for respiratory protection

Airborne concentration of lead	Required respirator*
Not in excess of 0.5 mg/m³ (10 × PEL)	Half-mask, air-purifying respirator equipped with high-efficiency filters†‡
Not in excess of 2.5 mg/m³ (50 × PEL)	Full facepiece, air-purifying respirator with high-efficiency filters‡
Not in excess of 50 mg/m³ (1000 × PEL)	(1) Any powered, air-purifying respirator with high-efficiency filters;‡ or (2) half-mask supplied-air respirator operated in positive-pressure mode†
Not in excess of 100 mg/m³ (2000[Ts]PEL)	Supplied-air respirators with full facepiece, hood, helmet, or suit, operated in positive pressure mode
Greater than 100 mg/m³; unknown concentration or firefighting	Full facepiece, self-contained breathing apparatus operated sure mode

Modified from US Department of Labor, Occupational Safety and Health Administration: *Lead standard,* 20 CFR 1910.1025, Washington, DC, 1990, US Government Printing Office.
*Respirators specified for high concentrations can be used at lower concentrations of lead.
†Full facepiece is required if the lead aerosols cause eye or skin irritation at the use concentrations.
‡A high-efficiency particulate filter means 99.97% efficient against 0.3 µm size particles.

PHYSICAL HAZARDS

Working on ships frequently places workers in difficult positions in confined areas. Osteoarthritis occurs in skilled miners more often than in the unskilled. Because of similarities of confined working conditions, researchers looked at arthrosis in shipyard workers and found no difference between skilled and unskilled dockyard workers.[2]

Noise-induced hearing loss is typically in the high-frequency range. This is one of the most significant health-related issues in occupational health today (see Chapter 54).

Other physical hazards include ergonomic stress, ultraviolet light, radiation, vibration, electricity, and trauma (see box on p. 281).

CONCLUSION

The potential toxic exposures of those in the shipbuilding and shipbreaking industry are vast. These workers suffer the physical ills of other manual laborers. The confined spaces and heavy lifting places undue ergonomic stress on these workers. In addition, noise-induced hearing loss is prevalent in these occupations.

The most common toxicants encountered by these workers are lead and asbestos. Others include heavy metals, solvents, fumigants, diesel fumes, manufactured mineral

Physical Hazards that May Be Encountered in Shipyards

Ambient temperature	Vibration
Confined spaces	Ionizing radiation
Working at heights	Nonionizing radiation
Low oxygen	Electricity
concentrations	Trauma
Noise	Water hazards

fibers, and epoxy. The exposure of greatest concern and morbidity is asbestos. Many of the toxic risks associated with asbestos can be eliminated with proper protective equipment and medical monitoring.

REFERENCES

1. Albin M et al: Mortality and cancer morbidity in cohorts of asbestos cement workers and referents, *Br J Ind Med* 47:602, 1990.
2. Anderson JA: Arthrosis and relation to work, *Scand J Work Environ Health* 10:429, 1984.
3. Barbeau A, Inoue N, Cloutier T: Role of manganese in dystonia, *Adv Neurol* 14:339, 1976.
4. Beaumont JJ, Weiss NS: Mortality of welders, shipfitters, and other metal trades workers in boilermakers Local No. 104, AFL-CIO, *Am J Epidemiol* 112:775, 1980.
5. Churg A, Vedal S: Fiber burden and patterns of asbestos-related disease in workers with heavy mixed amosite and chrysotile exposure, *Am J Respir Crit Care Med* 150:663, 1994.
6. Edge JR: Incidence of bronchial carcinoma in shipyard workers with pleural plaques, *Ann N Y Acad Sci* 330:289, 1979.
7. Elliott P et al: The Small Area Health Statistics Unit: a national facility for investigating health around point sources of environmental pollution in the United Kingdom, *J Epidemiol Community Health* 46:345, 1982.
8. Fletcher DE: A mortality study of shipyard workers with pleural plaques, *Br J Ind Med* 29:142, 1972.
9. Hanninen H et al: Internal lead of aluminum and the central nervous system function of aluminum and the central nervous system function of aluminum welders, *Scand J Work Environ Health* 20:279, 1994.
10. Hughes JM, Weill H, Hammad YY: Mortality of workers employed in two asbestos cement manufacturing plants, *Br J Ind Med* 44:161, 1987.
11. Huuskonen MS et al: Finnish Institute of Occupational Health asbestos program 1987-1992, *Am J Ind Med* 28:123, 1995.
12. Jarvisalo J et al: Urinary and blood manganese in occupationally nonexposed populations and in manual metal arc welders of mild steel, *Int Arch Occup Environ Health* 63:495, 1992.
13. Klaas VE: A diagnostic approach to asbestosis, utilizing clinical criteria, high resolution computed tomography, and gallium scanning, *Am J Ind Med* 23:801, 1993.
14. Nosal RM, Wilhelm WJ: Lead toxicity in the shipbreaking industry: the Ontario experience, *Can J Public Health* 81:259, 1990.
15. Oksa P et al: High-resolution computed tomography in the early detection of asbestosis, *Int Arch Occup Environ Health* 65:229, 1994.
16. Puntoni R et al: Mortality among shipyard workers in Genoa, Italy, *Ann N Y Acad Sci* 330:353, 1979.
17. Roggli VL: Malignant mesothelioma and duration of asbestos exposure: correlation with tissue mineral fibre content, *Ann Occup Hyg* 39:363, 1995.
18. Sanden A, Jarvholm B: A study of possible predictors of mesothelioma in shipyard workers exposed to asbestos, *J Occup Med* 33:770, 1991.
19. Sanden A, Jarvholm B, Larsson S: The importance of lung function, non-malignant diseases associated with asbestos, and symptoms as predictors of ischemic heart disease in shipyard workers exposed to asbestos, *Br J Ind Med* 50:785, 1993.
20. Selikoff IJ, Lilis R, Levin G: Asbestotic radiological abnormalities among United States merchant marine seamen, *Br J Ind Med* 47:292, 1990.
21. Selikoff IJ, Nicholson WJ, Lilis R: Radiological evidence of asbestos disease among ship repair workers, *Am J Ind Med* 1:9, 1980.
22. Sheers G, Coles RM: Mesothelioma risks in a naval dockyard, *Arch Environ Health* 35:276, 1980.
23. US Department of Interior: *Minerals yearbook for 1990,* vol 1, Washington, DC, 1991, US Government Printing Office.
24. US Department of Labor, Bureau of Labor Statistics: *Industry wage survey: shipbuilding and repairing, October 1986* (Bulletin 2295), Washington, DC, 1988, US Government Printing Office.
25. Zavalic M, Bogadi-Sarc A: Lung functions and chest radiographs in shipyard workers exposed to asbestos, *Arch Hig Rada Toksikol* 44:1, 1993.
26. Zedd HC et al: Lead exposures during shipboard chipping and grinding paint-removal operations, *Am Ind Hyg Assoc J* 54:392, 1993.

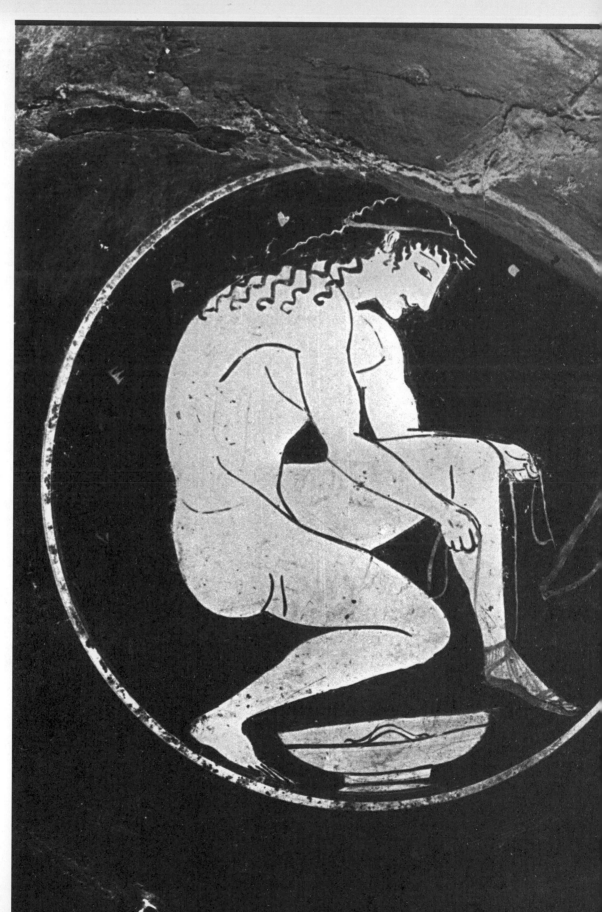

Greek vase painting. Youth lacing his sandals. Light figure on dark ground. Undated. (Courtesy Corbis-Bettmann)

35

Shoemakers

Robert S. Hoffman

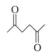

2,5-hexanedione   *benzene oxide*

- Hexacarbon neuropathy is a motor and sensory axonopathy caused by exposure to hexacarbons in glues and solvents

- Benzene is a potent hematologic toxin and is a proven leukemogen

- Carcinogens in tanned leather may account for the increased incidence of nasal adenocarcinoma

OCCUPATIONAL DESCRIPTION

The shoemaking industry may be one of the oldest professions. Despite debate over what type of footwear was first worn and when, it is widely accepted that most early cultures used some form of foot protection. Spanish archeological remains from a prehistoric culture document the use of grass sandals, and the ancient Egyptians wore sandals made from either palm leaves or papyrus.[28] Since ancient times, shoes have been made from many different materials, including naturally derived leather, wood, and cloth and synthetic fibers such as rubber and plastics.

Although many processes are now completely automated, hand craftsmanship remains an industry standard for the highest-quality products. A complete discussion of all the potential occupational exposures that might result from any step in the manufacture of the varied forms of footwear is clearly beyond the scope of this chapter. Thus, this section focuses on the most common exposures in the classic manufacture of leather shoes.

Risk assessment begins with an understanding of the manufacturing process and the different jobs involved in that process. Shoes are comprised of uppers and bottoms. The uppers are typically made of leather that has to be cut and molded into the proper shape. The bottoms include the heel and welt, the sole, and the insole. These items may be made of rubber, leather, wood, foam, or synthetic materials that must be cut and sized and then assembled by either nails, screws, stitches, or glue. Typical assembly uses a combination of these processes. The final product must then be dyed, polished, or waxed.

A comprehensive listing of job titles recognized by the International Labor Organization as involved with the manufacture of shoes is reviewed elsewhere.[36] For the purposes of this chapter, these job descriptions can be divided into a few major categories. Workers generally

Table 35-1 Potential toxic exposures for shoemakers

Toxic exposure	Source	Route of exposure	Chronic toxic effect(s)	Permissible exposure limit (TLV-TWA)
Benzene	Glues	Inhalation, some potential for dermal	Multiple myeloma, aplastic anemia, leukemia	1 ppm
n-Hexane	Glues	Inhalation	Peripheral neuropathy	50 ppm
Cyclohexane	Glues	Inhalation or dermal	Skin irritation	300 ppm
Isohexanes (2-methylpentane or 3-methylpentate)	Glues	Inhalation or dermal	Skin irritation	500 ppm
Methyl ethyl ketone	Glues	Inhalation	Exacerbation of effects of n-hexane	200 ppm
Toluene	Glues and dyes	Inhalation	Organic brain dysfunction; rare effects on bone marrow (possibly from benzene contamination)	50 ppm
Acetone	Glues	Inhalation	Heartburn, bronchitis, gastritis, eye irritation	750 ppm
Vinyl chloride	Plasticizer	Inhalation or dermal	Acroosteolysis, scleroderma, contact dermatitis	5 ppm
Leather dusts	Cutting and buffing	Inhalation	Nasopharyngeal adenocarcinoma	No specific standard (see general dust standards)

perform jobs whose principal functions are the cutting, glueing, sewing, dyeing, buffing, or polishing of various parts of the shoe. In addition to those workers who manufacture shoes, similar risks are incurred by individuals who repair shoes by using the same chemical or mechanical processes. The greatest risk for occupational toxicity occurs in the glueing process as workers are exposed to solvents. These chemicals have a strong association with the generation of significant medical illness. The other risk to be discussed is exposure to leather dust in the cutting areas.

POTENTIAL TOXIC EXPOSURES

In the late 1930s, an association between exposure to benzene and hematologic toxicity was noted.[22] Subsequently, multiple studies demonstrated that whenever benzene was used as a solvent in the shoe industry or elsewhere, exposure was sufficient to cause aplastic anemia, multiple myeloma, and acute leukemias.[6,17,39] Because of this clear association between exposure and disease, use of benzene as a common solvent was outlawed in 1963.[36] Although it is no longer commonly used, occupational risks from benzene persist, both from its presence in small amounts as a nondeclared constituent of other solvents[19] and as a result of the potentially long (more than 20 years) latency period between exposure and disease.[33]

Other solvents such as aromatic, aliphatic, and halogenated petroleum distillates replaced benzene as the principal solvents in glues on other products. While the use of these agents is not associated with significant hematologic toxicity, they are by no means nontoxic. As early as 1957, polyneuropathies were seen in shoe workers.[34] These disorders were originally attributed to small quantities of

triorthocresylphosphate (TOCP) found in glues.[1] By the 1970s, however, excellent epidemiologic studies in Italy excluded TOCP and suggested that n-hexane was the etiologic agents in shoemakers' polyneuropathy.[1,34] In the United States, a similar syndrome was described in shoe workers exposed to methylethylketone and toluene.[13] This disorder is now known as hexacarbon polyneuropathy and has been described in association with exposure to various straight-chained six-carbon molecules.

Other potential exposures of consequence in the shoemaking industry include the solvents (2-methylpentane, 3-methylpentane, acetone, and toluene), plasticizers (vinyl chloride), and leather dusts (Table 35-1).

CLINICAL TOXICOLOGY
Benzene

Benzene is a simple aromatic hydrocarbon with the chemical formula C_6H_6. It was widely used in dyes and glues because of its excellent properties as an organic solvent. At the present time, acute exposure to benzene is uncommon and results only from occupational accidents. After acute exposure, patients complain of dizziness, light-headedness, or vertigo, as benzene has immediate effects on the central nervous system. Other central nervous system findings may include headache, euphoria, altered consciousness, or seizures.[15] Arrhythmias that may be seen result largely from sensitization of the heart to endogenous catecholamines,[26] exacerbated by the hypoxia that may result from displacement of ambient oxygen.

Chronic exposure to benzene is a greater concern in that significant toxicity can occur at levels that are far below odor threshold. Occupational exposure results largely from inha-

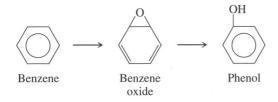

Fig. 35-1 Benzene metabolism.

lation, although ingestion produces similar toxicity in other settings. Dermal exposure has the potential to produce toxicity as well but has been poorly evaluated.[33] Signs and symptoms may occur rapidly, but latencies as long as 29 years have been described between last known exposure and overt toxicity.

Once absorbed, benzene is metabolized to phenol by aryl hydrocarbon hydroxylases in the liver and bone marrow. Benzene oxide is formed as an intermediate in this process (Fig. 35-1). This metabolite is an unstable electrophile that has the potential to bind to nucleic acids and block cell proliferation.[37] Benzene's direct effect on the DNA of shoe workers was recently demonstrated.[18] Sister chromatid exchange studies were performed in peripheral blood from 11 female shoe workers and compared with control subjects. Occupational exposure to benzene was confirmed by measuring preshift and postshift phenol concentrations in the urine. The authors reported a significant increase in dicentric chromosomes in the exposed workers. In addition, a higher number of sister chromatid exchanges were noted in the benzene-exposed workers, and this number tended to correlate with magnitude of exposure. The net result of this effect on DNA is destruction of the marrow. In a study of 217 Turkish shoe workers, nearly 25% were found to have some hematologic abnormality that was consistent with benzene toxicity.[5]

Initially after exposure, hypocellularity is noted in the marrow of experimental animals and correlates clinically with the aplastic crisis seen in humans. Patients present with pallor, fatigue, petechiae, bruising, bleeding, and infection. Depressions in the erythrocyte line alone or (more typically) multiple cell lines can be seen both peripherally and on bone marrow biopsy. Normal red blood cell indices are usually described, although macrocytosis has been reported.

Assessment begins with a history and physical examination. Emphasis should focus on other potential sources of bone marrow dysfunction and on findings of anemia or pancytopenia. Exposure to benzene can be confirmed (if the patient is still working) by the presence of phenol in the urine. Normal individuals excrete less than 10 mg/L of phenol. Although false-positive results may occur in individuals using phenol-containing medicines (such as Chloraseptic),[8] in their absence, levels above 200 mg/L are highly suggestive of recent benzene exposure. Determination of urinary phenol may be useful even if the patient and employer are unaware of benzene exposure because benzene may be present as a contaminant of other solvents used in the industry. This fact is supported by the demonstration of significant benzene exposures in 33 female shoe workers with no declared exposure to benzene.[19] Urinary determinations of phenylmercapturic acid and t,t-muconic acid have also been suggested as determinants of benzene exposure.

Adjunctive tests such as a urine analysis, stool guaiacs, a reticulocyte count, haptoglobin, and LDH can be useful to exclude hemolysis or peripheral losses as a mechanism for profound anemia. Urine analysis might also be helpful in cases of suspected multiple myeloma, so long as a complete protein evaluation (electrophoresis) can be performed. A bone marrow biopsy is indicated in most patients in whom a clear etiology for the hematologic abnormality is lacking. A predominance of acute myelogenous leukemia is noted in benzene-exposed individuals.[39] Other hematologic neoplasms, such as chronic myelogenous leukemia, acute granulocytic leukemia, acute monocytic leukemia, and multiple myeloma, have all also been associated with benzene exposure.[33] The incidence of leukemia in Turkish shoe workers in one study was at least 13/100,000, a relative risk of greater than 2 when compared with the population at large.[6]

Unfortunately, once discovered, there is very little therapy to offer beyond what is considered to be standard care for these disorders. Patients who are diagnosed while still at work should be removed from further exposure. Any discussion of the suggested therapies for leukemias, aplastic anemia, and multiple myeloma is clearly beyond the scope of this chapter. Five-year survival rates on the order of 30% have been reported for aplastic anemia. In general, thrombocytopenia and lymphoid marrow are felt to suggest a poorer prognosis. Patients with leukemia tend to have similar outcomes. Referral to a hematologist should be considered at the first indication of any benzene-related hematologic abnormality.

Toluene

Toluene, or methyl benzene, was one of the early benzene substitutes used in industry. Very few data are available with regard to specific adverse effects of toluene in the footwear industry (see Chapter 25 for a more detailed discussion).

Hexacarbon Neuropathy

Straight-chained hydrocarbon molecules such as n-hexane (C_6H_{14}), n-pentane, and n-heptane supplanted benzene as common solvents in the shoe industry. Significant neurologic toxicity has been described only with n-hexane. While ingestion and dermal exposure may produce symptoms in other settings, inhalation is the most typical route of toxicity in the workplace.[4] As with benzene, acute severe occupational exposure to n-hexane is uncommon, resulting only from accidental spills or breakdown of exhaust system. Patients may complain of light-headedness, headache, or confusion. Severe central nervous system depression may occur with high

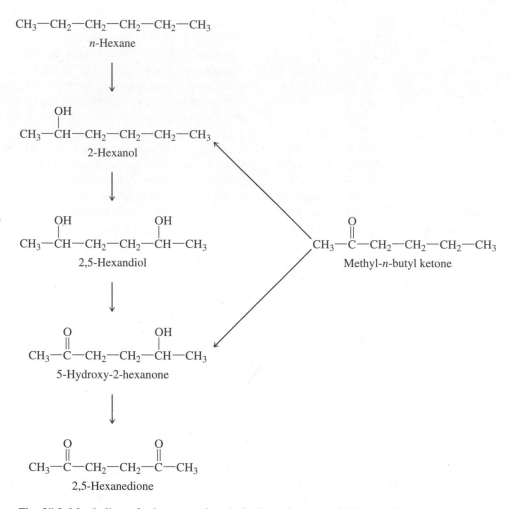

Fig. 35-2 Metabolism of n-hexane and methyl-n-butyl ketone to 2,5-hexanedione.

concentrations or prolonged exposures. Some euphoric effects that have been described may be responsible for the abuse potential of agents containing n-hexane.

Much like benzene, chronic toxicity results from n-hexane metabolites rather than from the parent compound. Once absorbed, n-hexane is metabolized by the mixed function oxidase system of the liver to form the secondary alcohols 2-hexanol and 2,5-hexanediol. Sequential oxidation of the 2,5-hexanediol alcohol groups to ketones forms 5-hydroxy-2-hexanone and the 2,5-hexandione. It has been proposed that the last metabolite, 2,5-hexanedione, is responsible for the neurotoxicity, but administration of each of the metabolites to animals produces similar symptoms as long as subsequent metabolism occurs. In addition, methyl-n-butyl ketone (formerly used as a solvent in other industries) produces similar symptoms presumably because of its metabolism to 2,5-hexanedione (Fig. 35-2). Shoe workers' polyneuropathy has also been associated with exposure to methyl-ethyl-ketone (a five-carbon molecule),[13] but probably results both from the compound's ability to increase mixed function oxidase activity,[7] and its common contamination with small amounts of methyl-n-butyl ketone.

The clinical features of shoemakers' polyneuropathy have been known for almost 40 years. Although the disorder was initially reported to be more prevalent in women, subsequent studies have demonstrated that this was related to job title and not gender. In a series of 122 shoe workers with polyneuropathy, a seasonal variation was noted in the onset of cases, with most new cases manifesting during the winter and spring.[1] This finding helped implicate both volatile hydrocarbons and poor ventilation as causes of the disorder. Although the disorder typically occurs following several years of exposure, cases have been reported after as little as a few months at the workplace.[1,34] The incidence of polyneuropathy is striking in some series. Ninety-eight cases of neuropathy were found by screening 654 employees of Italian shoe factories.[29]

The clinical course of this polyneuropathy is summarized as follows:[34] The syndrome begins with a prodrome of nausea, anorexia, and weight loss, followed by progressive paresthesias of the lower extremities, with the most severe symptoms noted distally. Approximately 1 month later, flaccid symmetric paralysis of all four extremities is seen, with loss of reflexes and muscular atrophy. A hypochromic anemia has also been noted at this stage and resolves within 2 or 3 months. Neurologic improvement occurs gradually, with several months of removal from exposure. By 1 year, most patients have complete clinical recovery. Residual clinical deficits and electromyographic abnormalities may persist indefinitely.[1,34]

Light and electron microscopy of biopsy specimens taken from the sural or peroneal nerves of affected workers shows characteristic changes.[34] Axonal swelling is prominent in both myelinated and nonmyelinated fibers and is attributed to accumulation of neurofilaments. The myelin sheaths over swollen axons are somewhat thinned but otherwise appear normal. Nerve degeneration occurs distal to the swelling. Although myelin degeneration is uncommon, it has been reported.

Once again, the diagnosis begins with a history of exposure and clinical findings suggestive of a mixed sensory and motor peripheral neuropathy. Other etiologies for peripheral neuropathy, such as repetitive motion injury, diabetes mellitus, alcoholism, and vitamin deficiencies, need to be excluded. The clinical laboratory is more useful for defining these other conditions, as abnormalities (other than the anemia mentioned) are not expected with hexacarbon neuropathy. Electromyography should always show slowed motor and sensory conduction velocities in affected individuals.[34] In fact, impaired conduction has been demonstrated even in clinically asymptomatic shoe workers exposed to solvents.[9] In one study, the incidence of polyneuropathy was related to the amount of glue used per worker per day and the degree of ventilation. In addition, age and total duration of exposure had a negative impact on conduction velocity. Besides corroborating the previously described effects of n-hexane on motor and sensory nerve conduction,[24] abnormalities of somatosensory evoked potentials have been demonstrated in 15 women from a shoe factory.[25] This finding suggests that n-hexane may have central nervous system (CNS) neurotoxic effects as well. Clinical findings of CNS dysfunction, such as spasticity or increased deep tendon reflexes, have been noted in some n-hexane-exposed workers as well.[29]

After a general medical history, physical examination, and laboratory evaluation, workers who present with signs and symptoms suggestive of a peripheral neuropathy should be referred for electromyographic studies. These studies help to confirm and document impairment and may exclude other etiologies for the patient's symptoms. Exposure to n-hexane should be definitively confirmed. While air monitoring of the workplace may be sufficient to define exposure risk, biologic monitoring is always preferable in that it confirms exposure. Numerous studies have demonstrated an excellent correlation between the urinary elimination of n-hexane metabolites and the degree of occupational exposure.[4,10,16,24,30] Unfortunately, screening for 2,5-hexanedione alone is somewhat nonspecific, as levels can be elevated after methyl-n-butyl-ketone exposure as well. Thus, urinary screening requires evaluation of multiple metabolites. Most experts suggest that optimal testing is accomplished by comparing urinary levels of n-hexane metabolites taken immediately before the start of work with those taken at the end of the day. An alternative method of monitoring involves evaluation of exhaled n-hexane. Several studies have demonstrated that the quantity of exhaled n-hexane correlates quite well both with ambient n-hexane levels and measurements of urinary metabolites.[31,32] Again, as with urine testing, since n-hexane and its metabolites are cleared fairly rapidly after exposure, testing has minimal utility for patients who have been out of the workplace for any significant period of time. Under these circumstances, workplace air levels would be more revealing.

The obvious problem with measuring either urinary or respiratory n-hexane elimination is that, although it documents exposure, it does not indicate impairment. Governa and colleagues evaluated 163 workers of 8 small shoe factories to determine whether peripheral polymorphonuclear (PMN) leukocyte activity could be used as a more sensitive marker of physiologic impairment than other tests.[14] They hypothesized that PMNs might have impaired chemotaxis since hexacarbon-induced peripheral neuropathy involved dysfunction of the cytoskeletal apparatus, and this mechanism is important for chemotaxis. Their results demonstrated a strong negative correlation between PMN chemotactic ability and urinary elimination of 2,5-hexanedione. Unfortunately, neither of these tests correlated with nerve conduction studies in the asymptomatic workers. Thus, either urinary or respiratory measurements of 2,5-hexanedione elimination or PMN chemotactic studies are adequate to define exposure. Nerve conduction studies appear to be the best way to identify early disease, even in asymptomatic individuals.

Treatment begins with removal from exposure. No specific therapy has been shown to be effective, and supportive care is all that is required. Referral is indicated more for diagnosis than for therapy. Since this is an axonopathy, recovery takes months to years and is often incomplete. Repeated physical examinations and nerve conduction studies can be used to document progress.

Effects of Mixed Hydrocarbon Exposure

A significant percentage of the shoe industry's workforce is women of childbearing age. They are often assigned to gluing and other tasks that predispose to hydrocarbon exposure. Several recent studies have evaluated the risks that this exposure poses to fertility. In Finnish women, spontaneous abortion rates were evaluated with regard to occupational exposures to solvents as a risk factor.[20] Exposed women had a relative risk of spontaneous abortion greater than 2. Although the numbers were too small to validly subdivide, toluene-exposed shoe workers appeared to have a risk of spontaneous abortion more than nine times that of controls. In a follow-up study, the same authors demonstrated that female shoe workers had a significantly increased time to pregnancy, indicating impaired fertility.[35]

The implications for care here are clear-cut. If a worker in the footwear industry suffers from either repeated spontaneous abortions or fertility problems, an evaluation for solvent exposure is indicated. This evaluation may be as simple as a good occupational history and site visit to the employee's job. Alternatively, exposure monitoring may be indicated. Either personal air space sampling devices or urinary monitoring usually suffices. In these circumstances, most of the hydrocarbons of interest (toluene, n-hexane, methyl-ethyl-ketone, etc.) have well-described protocols for air space or urinary biologic monitoring. Other causes of infertility should be evaluated, and referral to a gynecologist or endocrinologist would be appropriate.

Certain hydrocarbons, such as toluene, are known to have effects on the renal system. Several researchers have attempted to determine whether occupational exposure to these agents in the footwear industry is associated with renal dysfunction. One study measured proteinuria, albuminuria, urinary β-glucuronidase, and serum creatinine in 182 workers exposed to solvents in shoe factories and compared them with a group of former workers and a control group.[23] Although total protein excretion and β-glucuronidase were elevated in the exposed workers, none had albuminuria. The authors suggested the presence of a mild reversible tubular lesion. A similar study compared renal function in 59 solvent-exposed women shoe workers with controls.[40] The only abnormality found was an elevated urinary beta-N-acetylglucosaminidase in hydrocarbon-exposed workers. The authors concluded that long-term moderate exposure to solvents in this setting is not associated with a significant risk of renal impairment.

Similarly, the pulmonary effects of hydrocarbon exposures are better defined in other industrial settings (see Chapters 10 and 25). Pulmonary function was studied, however, in a cohort of 134 shoe factory workers with varying job titles.[27] Some degree of pulmonary toxicity (restrictive lung disease) was seen in leather workers (exposed to methylethylketone, dusts, and solvents), rubber workers (exposed to rubber dust, sulfur, carbon black, silicates, zinc oxide, and plasticizers), and plastics workers (exposed to vinyl chloride) compared with the tailors. The greatest impairment of lung function was observed in the plastic workers.

The office evaluation for pulmonary complaints should begin with a basic occupational history and physical examination. Special emphasis should be placed on the use of personal protective devices and ventilation-exhaust systems if dusts are involved. Other common causes of respiratory illness (such as smoking) should be sought. A chest radiograph and peak expiratory flow rate may be indicative of the problem. If further (formal pulmonary function) testing is required, referral to a pulmonologist may be indicated. Treatment involves protection from continued exposure and the use of bronchodilators and inhaled steroids as may be indicated.

Dust Exposure

Leather dust results primarily from cutting, grinding, and polishing processes. The high-speed grinders that are used to shape and smooth bottoms liberate substantial amounts of dust. In addition to the pulmonary toxicity associated with most dust exposures (see Chapter 32), leather dust has unique toxicity. Although the specific carcinogen in leather dust is unknown, it is thought to result from the tanning process. Leather is tanned either by chrome salts or by welting, which uses vegetable extracts. It is this latter process that is believed to produce (or activate) the carcinogen in leather dust.[3] When records from Florence covering the years 1963 to 1977 were retrospectively reviewed to identify cases of primary cancer of the nasal cavity and paranasal sinuses, a total of 66 cases were identified, 7 of which occurred in shoemakers.[11] The tumors in shoemakers occurred after many years of employment, with an average latency of 37 years, and were all of an adenocarcinoma cell type. A similar study was performed for the years between 1963 and 1967 in Wales and England.[2] The authors identified 266 cases of nasal cancer in leather workers, which corresponded to a relative risk of greater than 4 when compared with the general population. If shoemakers were considered individually among all leather workers, their relative risk was greater than 7 when compared with the general population. Once again, as previously described, a very high incidence of adenocarcinomas was noted in this population. The same authors did a broader survey covering the years from 1950 to 1979.[3] Although they noted that the number of exposed workers had declined with time, the incidence of nasal carcinoma was not declining. Relative risks as high as 7.8 were described for some job descriptions. The high-risk occupations included those that involved greater dust exposure and used vegetable-tanned leather.

Patients present with typical findings of nasal carcinoma and should be evaluated and managed accordingly. Long-term care and follow-up should be guided by specialists from otolaryngology and oncology.

Tumors of Unclear Pathogenesis

Clinicians who care for workers in the footwear industry should be aware of associations with other neoplasms. These associations are more poorly defined than nasal carcinoma in that neither specific job titles nor potential carcinogens have been adequately identified. When all cancers of the lower urinary tract that occurred during an 18-month period in Massachusetts were reviewed, 79 of the 668 cases identified occurred in leather workers, giving a relative risk of 2.[12] Although many cancers were noted in association with finishers (a high dust area), the association was not as clear as that for nasal carcinoma. In one review, the strong association between occupational bladder cancer and exposure to aromatic amines such as 2-naphthylamine and benzidine is noted.[38] Although the author also notes shoe and leather work as an occupational risk for bladder cancer, there is no firm relationship between these known etiologic agents and the footwear industry. Finally, a higher than expected incidence of non-Hodgkin's lymphoma has been found in men in the shoemaking or shoe repair industry.[21] Relative risks were 1.8 and 1.7 for shoe repairers and shoemakers, respectively.

CONCLUSION

Shoemakers and shoe repairers have well-defined occupational exposures that result in a number of clearly identifiable syndromes. Most cases of significant toxicity occurred years ago and abroad. With the current industrial hygiene standards in the United States, toxicity should be significantly limited. Unfortunately, because some of the syndromes have long latencies between exposure and disease, cases of consequential toxicity will still be identified currently and in the years to come.

REFERENCES

1. Abbritti G et al: Shoe-makers' polyneuropathy in Italy: the aetiological problem, *Br J Ind Med* 33:92, 1976.
2. Acheson ED, Cowdell RH, Rang EH: Nasal cancer in England and Wales: an occupational survey, *Br J Ind Med* 38:218, 1981.
3. Acheson ED, Pippard EC, Winter PD: Nasal cancer in the Northamptonshire boot and shoe industry: is it declining? *Br J Cancer* 46:940, 1982.
4. Ahonen I, Schimberg RW: 2,5-Hexanedione excretion after occupational exposure to n-hexane, *Br J Ind Med* 45:133, 1988.
5. Aksoy M et al: Haematological effects of chronic benzene poisoning in 217 workers, *Br J Ind Med* 28:296, 1971.
6. Aksoy M, Erdem S, Dincol K: Leukemia in shoe-workers exposed chronically to benzene, *Blood* 44:837, 1974.
7. Altenkirch H, Stoltenburg G, Wagner HM: Experimental studies on hexacarbon neuropathies induced by methyl-ethyl-ketone, *J Neurol* 219:159, 1978.
8. Baselt RC: Benzene. In *Disposition of toxic drugs and chemicals in man,* ed 2, Davis, Calif, 1982, Biomedical Publications.
9. Buiatti E et al: Relationship between clinical and electromyographic findings and exposure to solvents, in shoe and leather workers, *Br J Ind Med* 35:168, 1978.
10. Cardona A et al: Biological monitoring of occupational exposure to n-hexane by measurement of urinary 2,5-hexanedione, *Int Arch Occup Environ Health* 65:71, 1993.
11. Cecchi F et al: Adenocarcinoma of the nose and paranasal sinuses in shoemakers and woodworkers in the province of Florence, Italy (1963-1977), *Br J Ind Med* 37:222, 1980.
12. Cole P, Hoover R, Friedell GH: Occupation and cancer of the lower urinary tract, *Cancer* 29:1250, 1972.
13. Dyro FM: Methyl ethyl ketone polyneuropathy in shoe factory workers, *Clin Toxicol* 13:371, 1978.
14. Governa M et al: Human polymorphonuclear leukocyte chemotaxis as a tool in detecting biological early effects in workers occupationally exposed to low levels of n-hexane, *Hum Exp Toxicol* 13:663, 1994.
15. Harrington TF: Industrial benzol poisoning in Massachusetts, *Boston Med Surg J* 177:203, 1917.
16. Imbriani M et al: n-Hexane urine elimination and weighted exposure concentration, *Int Arch Occup Environ Health* 55:33, 1984.
17. Infante PF et al: Leukaemia in benzene workers, *Lancet* 2:766, 1977.
18. Karacic V et al: Possible genotoxicity in low level benzene exposure, *Am J Ind Med* 27:379, 1995.
19. Karacic V, Skender L, Prpic-Majic D: Occupational exposure to benzene in the shoe industry, *Am J Ind Med* 12:531, 1987.
20. Lindbohm ML et al: Spontaneous abortions among women exposed to organic solvents, *Am J Ind Med* 17:449, 1990.
21. Linet MS et al: Non-Hodgkin's lymphoma and occupation in Sweden: a registry based analysis, *Br J Ind Med* 50:79, 1993.
22. Mallory TB, Gall EA, Brickley WJ: Chronic exposure to benzene (benzol). III. The pathologic results, *J Ind Hyg Toxicol* 21:355, 1939.
23. Mutti A et al: Organic solvents and chronic glomerulonephritis: a cross-sectional study with negative findings for aliphatic and alicyclic C5-C7 hydrocarbons, *J Appl Toxicol* 1:224, 1981.
24. Mutti A et al: n-Hexane-induced changes in nerve conduction velocities and somatosensory evoked potentials, *Int Arch Occup Environ Health* 51:45, 1982.
25. Mutti A et al: Neurophysiological changes in workers exposed to organic solvents in a shoe factory, *Scand J Work Environ Health* 8(suppl 1):136, 1982.
26. Nahum L, Hoff H: Mechanism of sudden death in experimental acute benzol poisoning, *J Pharmacol Exp Ther* 50:336, 1934.
27. Oleru UG, Onyekwere C: Exposures to polyvinyl chloride, methyl ketone and other chemicals: the pulmonary and non-pulmonary effect, *Int Arch Occup Environ Health* 63:503, 1992.
28. Parmeggiani L: Footwear industry. In *Encyclopedia of occupational health and safety,* ed 3, Geneva, 1983, International Labor Organization.
29. Passero S et al: Toxic polyneuropathy of shoe workers in Italy. A clinical, neurophysiological and follow-up study, *Ital J Neurol Sci* 4:463, 1983.
30. Perbellini L, Brugnone F, Faggionato G: Urinary excretion of the metabolites of n-hexane and its isomers during occupational exposure, *Br J Ind Med* 38:20, 1981.
31. Periago JF et al: Biological monitoring of occupational exposure to n-hexane by exhaled air analysis and urinalysis, *Int Arch Occup Environ Health* 65:275, 1993.
32. Periago JF et al: Correlation between concentrations of n-hexane and toluene in exhaled and environmental air in an occupationally exposed population, *J Appl Toxicol* 14:63, 1994.
33. Rinsky RA et al: Benzene and leukemia: an epidemiologic risk assessment, *N Engl J Med* 316:1044, 1987.
34. Rizzuto N, Terzian H, Galiazzo-Rizzuto S: Toxic polyneuropathies in Italy due to leather cement poisoning in shoe industries. A light- and electron-microscopic study, *J Neurol Sci* 31:343, 1977.
35. Sallmen M et al: Reduced fertility among women exposed to organic solvents, *Am J Ind Med* 27:699, 1995.
36. Scarpelli A et al: Exposure to solvents in the shoe and leather goods industries, *Int J Epidemiol* 22(suppl 2):S46, 1993.
37. Snyder R et al: Bone marrow depressant and leukemogenic actions of benzene, *Life Sci* 21:1709, 1977.
38. Tola S: Occupational cancer of the urinary bladder, *J Toxicol Environ Health* 6:1253, 1980.
39. Vigliani EC, Saita G: Benzene and leukemia, *N Engl J Med* 271:872, 1964.
40. Vyskocil A et al: Urinary excretion of proteins and enzymes in workers exposed to hydrocarbons in a shoe factory, *Int Arch Occup Environ Health* 63:359, 1991.

Smelters and Metal Reclaimers

Francis J. DeRoos

Pb

- Lead toxicity affects hematopoetic and neurologic organs most prominently

- Standards for workplace monitoring and exposure limits are well defined

OCCUPATIONAL DESCRIPTION

Smelting is defined as the refining and production of metals. Smelting can utilize either the raw mine ore (termed *primary* smelting), or recycling of sources rich in the desired metal such as cans, batteries, old appliances, and automobiles (termed *secondary* or *reclamation* smelting). In smelting, the valuable metal's elements are separated from the worthless material by pyrometallurgical or hydrometallurgical processes.

Pyrometallurgical processes, as the name implies, utilize high temperatures to separate the less valuable materials from the molten collection of desired metal known as the *matte*. This same technique has been used for hundreds of years in the initial preparation of metals in foundries and is used almost exclusively in secondary smelting. Pyrometallurgical techniques are also used to prepare ore for further refining with hydrometallurgic processing. An example of this preparation process is sulfatizing roasting used to extract copper and nickel. In this process, the main contaminant, iron sulfide, is converted to iron oxide to allow for easy conversion of the valuable material into its metallic form for extraction.[40]

Hydrometallurgical processes take advantage of chemical properties such as solubility, electrical charges, reactivity with oxygen, and melting points to separate the desired metal from the worthless material. By modifying the surrounding environment with pressure, heat, electricity, or the addition of chemicals such as oxygen or solvents, the prized metals can be more easily extracted. Examples include electrolysis

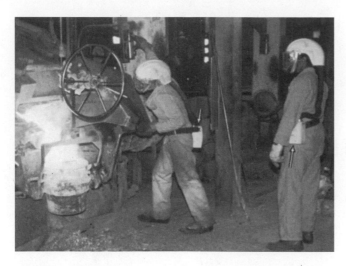

Fig. 36-1 Filling a ladle with molten brass. Tests of air in the breathing zone of each worker revealed no detectable lead with use of the filtered air supplied through the battery-powered devices *(arrows).* (From Zenz C, Dickerson OB, Horvath EP: *Occupational medicine,* ed 3, St Louis, 1994, Mosby.)

in copper refining and gas reduction of the leaching solution in nickel production.

Founding, in contrast, consists of pouring molten metal into a mold, cooling it, and producing a consistently shaped product. A typical foundry has several specific divisions: metal melting and pouring, molding, coremaking, and cleaning and finishing. The first step is actually a smelter, using pyrometallurgical techniques, incorporated into the founding process. The process begins by placing charges or layers of coke (a solid residue of impure carbon obtained from coal after removal of volatile material by destructive distillation), limestone, and a metal source of either scrap metal or blocks of crude iron, called *pig iron,* into a furnace. In iron founding, this is typically a tall, vertical furnace known as a *cupola.* Periodically, new charges of coke and metal are fed into the furnace until it is full and the desired temperature has been reached. Next the slag, consisting of nonmetallic impurities, that has collected on the surface of the molten metal is skimmed off. The furnace is then tapped, and the molten metal is removed and transferred either into a holding furnace or directly into ladles for immediate mold pouring.

Molds are cavities created in easily shaped material such as sand, into which molten metal is poured to produce a casting (Fig. 36-1). The internal cavities within the final casting are known as *cores.* They must be strong enough to withstand the pouring process but not too strong to be removed during cleaning. Silica sand is the most commonly used compound in these processes, although other sands, such as chromite, olivine, and zircon, can be used. This sand is mixed with binders such as clay, oils, sodium silicate, and many chemicals, including phenol-formaldehyde, furfuryl alcohol, polyurethane, and diisocyanate, which increase the

strength of the mold or core.[30] This mixture of sand and binders is then poured into the desired pattern and hardened with various techniques. With the "hot-box" method, curing is initiated with heat or acid. In "cold-box" systems, gases such as carbon dioxide, amines (trimethylamine, dimethyl-ethylamine), and sulfur dioxide are used as catalysts to harden the resins. In "no-bake" techniques, the curing catalyst is added to the sand initially, and time alone allows polymerization of the resin and sets the mold.[30] To ease the removal of the hardened mold, the pattern is often dusted or sprayed with a powder. Traditionally, this parting powder has been silica dust but, due to the high risk of silicosis, other agents such as talc or other liquid compounds are now being used.

Cleaning and finishing remove the sand, chemical residues, and excess metal from the casting. The initial step, termed the *knock-out stage,* involves dropping the cooled castings onto a vibrating screen. This initial jarring impact and the subsequent shaking dislodge most of the molding and core sand, which fall into a hopper below for reclamation and reuse. Next, the large pieces of unwanted metal such as the sprue, which is the vertical pouring channel into the mold, are removed with direct hammer blows. The casting is then subjected to abrasive cleaning, either in a tumbling mill or with high-pressure blasting with sand or steel shot. Final cleaning of burrs, embedded sand, and other blemishes is performed with pneumatic chisels and grinders.[30]

MAJOR JOBS IN SMELTING

The smelting process includes many different jobs. The first step is the organization of the raw materials, which typically occurs outdoors and involves hauling, stacking, and sorting various ores and materials. Next, the starting materials are reduced to more manageable sizes, typically with abrasive cutting or compression. The furnace is then loaded, tended, and tapped, as previously described. Because of the constant exposure to high temperatures, all the machinery and equipment require significant maintenance and cleaning.

WORKERS INVOLVED: EPIDEMIOLOGY

There are approximately 8248 "scrap and waste material establishments" registered by the U.S. Bureau of the Census. They employ an estimated 93,158 workers. In addition, more than 320,000 workers are potentially exposed as employees in U.S. foundries.[30] However, the actual number of sites where reclamation and smelting occur, in addition to the number of exposed workers, is unknown because the reclamation industry is small and difficult to regulate. In other countries, small, home-based reclamation smelters pose a significant exposure risk not only to the employees themselves but also to the surrounding community.[29]

Potential Toxic Exposures

The numerous potential intoxicants present in the working environment of smelters include metal dusts and fumes,

Table 36-1 Potential toxic exposures for smelters and metal reclaimers

Toxic exposure	Source	Route of exposure	Toxic effect(s)
Lead dust, fumes	Abrasive cutting, smelting, mold pouring	Respiratory	Anemia, peripheral neuropathy, encephalopathy, renal insufficiency, renal carcinoma (?), hypertension (?), teratogenic (?)
Arsenic trioxide	Copper smelting	Respiratory	Peripheral neuropathies, lung carcinoma
Metal oxides	Abrasive, thermal, cutting, smelting	Respiratory	Metal fume fever (fever, fatigue, myalgias)
Sulfur dioxide	Smelting	Topical, respiratory	Ocular and pulmonary irritation, chronic bronchitis
Carbon monoxide	Smelting	Respiratory	Hypoxia, acute neurologic impairment, delayed neurologic sequelae
Silica dust	Cast, mold production	Respiratory	Silicosis
Polycyclic aromatic hydrocarbons	Mold pouring	Respiratory	Carcinogenic

gases, and various chemicals either used initially or produced as by-products during the process (Table 36-1). The predominant exposures in this industry depend on many variables, such as what processes are being used, the type of metal being refined, the quality of the equipment and automation in the work environment, ventilation, and if any foundry work is being done at the smelting site. Many serious toxic exposures take place during routine maintenance of equipment and during system malfunctions.

Lead dust and fumes. Because inhalation is the most important route by which most metals are systemically absorbed, the greatest risk in the metallurgic industry is metal dust and fumes. The best example of an industry at high risk for this type of exposure is the lead reclamation industry.[20,28] This is because of both the economics of the lead reclamation industry and the nature of the lead reclamation process itself.

Lead is an integral part of the manufacturing of many products, including electric storage batteries, brass and bronze, radiators, solders, cables, outdoor paints, pottery glazes, and ammunition (Fig. 36-2). It is estimated that worldwide approximately 8.9 million metric tons of lead are produced annually. In 1985, the United States consumed more than 1.1 million metric tons of lead.[45] More than 60% of that was used in the manufacture of electric storage batteries, and, not surprisingly, these batteries have become the reclamation smelting industry's greatest source of raw material. As the demand for lead increases, so does the need for secondary smelting. In fact, in 1985, 55% of total U.S. production of lead was a result of lead recycling efforts.[45] The emphasis on secondary lead smelting can only increase as industrial lead consumption rises while domestic U.S. mining resources shrink and extraction becomes more costly. In addition, public concern about the environmental impact of mining and the "environmentally friendly" image of any form of recycling will continue to encourage lead reclamation smelting.

The distinct differences between primary and secondary lead production are important in understanding the signifi-

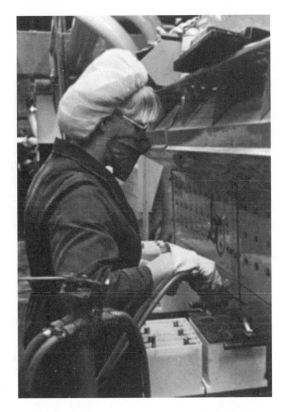

Fig. 36-2 The assembly of electric storage batteries exposes the worker to lead oxide dust. The risk can be reduced substantially by effective local exhaust ventilation. (From Zenz C, Dickerson OB, Horvath EP: *Occupational medicine,* ed 3, St Louis, 1994, Mosby.)

cant health risks involved in lead reclamation. Primary smelting sites, where pig lead is produced from raw ore, tend to be very large but few in number. This economy of scale allows for factories to be designed as highly mechanized and computerized and with excellent environmental control. This level of technology provides significant benefits by minimizing employee exposure to potential toxins. In addition, these smelters are highly visible and therefore can easily be evaluated for adherence to industry safety guidelines.

Secondary smelters, in contrast, tend to be small, "back-yard" or cottage industry operations and are numerous. They often work with refurbished or used equipment and have difficulty improving the working conditions. In the smallest operations, employees may be poorly trained about potential risks or the importance of personal and worksite hygiene. In 1984, an analysis of the size characteristics of U.S. foundries revealed that only 82 foundries employed more than 500 workers while at least 2633 such sites employed fewer than 50 workers (Fig. 36-3).

A second factor contributing to the high risk of metal dust and fumes exposure is the nature of the lead reclamation process itself. Lead dusts are aerosolized during moving and stacking the materials to be refined (typically, used electric storage batteries), abrasive cutting of large recycled metal sources, furnace charging, and cleaning of the final castings. Because of the high temperatures utilized, lead fumes are produced that can be emitted from the furnace, particularly during slagging or tapping.

Other dust and fume exposures. In addition to the potentially toxic dust and fumes generated from the primary metal being extracted, the other metals and compounds that "contaminate" or are often associated with the primary metal or production can also generate significant exposure and toxicity. Copper smelting, for example, produces arsenic trioxide, a known neurotoxin. Workers with a high risk of exposure to arsenic trioxide tended to have elevated levels of arsenic in hair, nail, and urine specimens. Impaired nerve conduction can also be demonstrated in this setting.[16] In iron founding, manganese is used to reduce the oxygen and sulfur content in the molten steel. Manganese dust and fumes are minor eye and upper airway irritants acutely; however, chronic intoxication can produce a parkinsonian-like syndrome.[13]

Metal fume fever. A common result of exposure to metal fumes is metal fume fever. This acute but self-limited condition is caused by inhalation of fumes of metal oxides, which are produced under high temperatures such as during abrasive or thermal cutting or during smelting. It is most frequently caused by zinc oxide, although other metals including cadmium, copper, and magnesium have also been associated with a clinical picture consistent with metal fume fever. Metal fume fever is characterized by sore throat, chills, fever, myalgias, and fatigue. The first symptoms usually occur between 4 and 12 hours after the exposure, can last several hours, and then dissipate spontaneously with only limited residual muscular stiffness or aches.[22] Fortunately, this debilitating syndrome has not been associated with any chronic disease states (see Chapter 37).

Toxic gases. Smelting can also produce significantly large quantities of toxic gases sulfur dioxide and carbon monoxide. Sulfur dioxide is formed when charges containing large amounts of sulfur are smelted. Sulfur dioxide is a significant ocular and respiratory irritant, and acute exposure

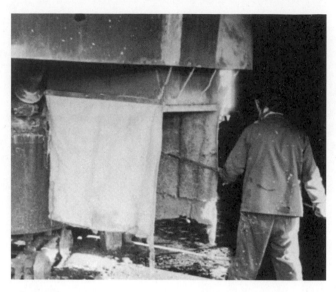

Fig. 36-3 Secondary lead smelting often is performed under primitive conditions in small smelters. The emptying of the furnace gives rise to highly dangerous concentrations of lead fumes in the air. (From Zenz C, Dickerson OB, Horvath EP: *Occupational medicine,* ed 3, St Louis, 1994, Mosby.)

can cause severe bronchospasm or even frank asphyxiation. Long-term exposure to sulfur dioxide may lead to chronic bronchitis.

Carbon monoxide (CO) is an odorless, colorless gas that can produce severe intoxication, in many cases insidiously. It is produced by incomplete combustion of any carbon-containing compound, particularly in the preheating of the initial furnace charge in these industries.[47] Acutely, CO avidly binds to hemoglobin, which greatly impairs oxygen-carrying capacity. In addition, CO exerts a significant oxidative stress against vascular endothelial cells. This precipitates a cascade of events that ultimately results in increased leukocyte adherence, lipid membrane peroxidation, and impaired cerebral function.[44] Symptoms of acute exposure can present rapidly and include headache, nausea, dizziness, lethargy, angina, confusion, coma, and death. Delayed neuropsychiatric sequelae occur in some patients who sustain significant acute exposures. These sequelae can be almost any neurologic abnormality, including chronic headaches, inability to concentrate, emotional instability, dementia, movement disorders, and peripheral neuropathies.[19] Carbon monoxide poisoning should be suspected in any smelting or foundry worker who presents with vague and nonspecific complaints, particularly neurologic ones. The smelting environment should have adequate ventilation and self-contained respiratory apparatus available, and workers should be educated about the symptoms and dangers of CO poisoning (see Chapter 15).

Silica dust. One of the more common exposures in foundry workers is silica dust. This dust is produced when sand is reclaimed upon cleaning of the castings. The free crystalline silica is first inhaled and deposited in the lung to initiate a reactive fibrotic response that, over time, results in a pneumoconiosis known as *silicosis*. The severity of this silica-related fibrosis is generally proportional to the duration and level of exposure to fine respirable silica crystals.[15] Some evidence suggests that silicosis may predispose workers to bronchogenic lung cancer.[35]

Other chemicals. The smelting and foundry environment is filled with many different chemical compounds and their decomposition products. This complex chemical milieu makes it extremely difficult to identify specific agents that have significant human toxicity. Several of these chemicals are significant irritants to either the mucous membranes or skin. The prime offenders are amines, ammonia, formaldehyde, furfurayl alcohol, and hexamethyleneteramine. Other agents considered carcinogenic include formaldehyde (nasopharyngeal cancer) and polycyclic aromatic hydrocarbons (PAHs) (see Chapters 23, 31, and 49).

The PAHs are formed when molten metal is poured into molds and there is incomplete pyrolysis of the organic binders. Some PAHs, particularly benzo*[a]*pyrene, have been demonstrated to be carcinogenic in animal studies and are considered human carcinogens.[1] Epidemiologic studies, however, have had difficulty demonstrating a strong link between cancer and PAH exposure.[2]

CLINICAL TOXICOLOGY OF LEAD
Pharmacodynamics

Lead enters the body via the gastrointestinal and respiratory tracts. Gastrointestinal absorption of lead is typically 10% to 15% of the total quantity ingested, although it can be dramatically greater in pregnant women, children, patients with iron deficiency, and those experiencing fasting states. Lead is well absorbed from the lung, and this route of exposure predominates in occupational settings. The actual quantity of lead absorbed depends on particle size, respiratory volume and rate, and intrinsic mucociliary and alveolar clearance mechanisms. Approximately 35% to 40% of total inhaled lead actually enters the blood.[33]

Once within the blood, lead avidly binds to erythrocytes. Over the next 4 to 6 weeks, it is distributed to those tissues that receive relatively high blood flow, including the kidney, liver, and brain. Redistribution of this lead is determined by the afinity of each specific tissue for lead. Bone has, by far, the greatest affinity for lead, and more than 90% of the total body burden of lead can be found here in the form of lead phosphate.[36] These deposits of lead within bony tissue exist in two compartments, one deeply incorporated within the compact bone matrix and immobile, and the other bound to the surface of the newly forming hydroxyapatite bone, typically trabecular bone, and capable of being mobilized. This second compartment persists for months or possibly years after an exposure.

Biophysically, lead resembles calcium, which may explain its high affinity for bone.

The body has no active process to eliminate lead, so it relies predominantly upon passive elimination via routine epithelial cell shedding and glandular secretions. Such sites of elimination thus include the biliary tract, the gastrointestinal tract, and glomerular filtration within the kidney.[7]

Pathobiology

General toxicity. Lead, like most heavy metals, is an extremely complex toxin. The biochemical effects of lead tend to fall into three major categories. The major toxicity of lead is related to its binding to various electron donors, particularly sulfhydryl groups. This sulfhydryl binding causes altered protein structure and enzymatic function. The second group of effects results from lead's biochemical and biophysical similarity to calcium. This similarity allows lead access into critical cellular pathways, particularly within the mitochondria and in second messenger systems. The result is that lead tends to competitively antagonize calcium's action. Finally, lead appears to affect nucleic acids by a yet undefined mechanism. This interplay with nucleic acids raises the strong concern that lead exposure could cause various chromosomal abnormalities.

Hematologic toxicity. Anemia is one of the most prominent and most extensively studied hallmarks of lead toxicity. Lead poisoning produces anemia by two mechanisms. By inhibiting heme synthesis and accelerating erythrocyte destruction, lead intoxication can produce significant anemia. The enzyme most susceptible to inhibition by lead is δ-aminolevulinic dehydratase, which converts δ-aminolevulinic acid into porphobilinogen. This inhibition correlates directly with the blood lead concentrations (BPb), and approximately 50% of this enzyme's activity is inhibited in the face of a BPb of 15 μg/dl.[23] Ferrochelatase, which forms heme by catalyzing the transfer of iron from ferritin into protoporphyrin, is also inhibited by lead. Inhibition of this enzyme results in the accumulation of free erythrocyte protoporphyrin or zinc protoporphyrin (FEP) and urinary elimination of coproporphyrin (Fig. 36-4).

While inhibition of heme synthesis is more pronounced as a result of chronic exposures, the increased erythrocyte destruction produced by lead is more pronounced in acute poisoning. The lead-induced hemolysis is caused by increased membrane fragility that is due to the inhibition of Na/K ATPase and pyrimidine 5′-nucleotidase. This inhibition of pyrimidine 5′-nucleotidase also impairs elimination of degrading RNA, which can be manifested as basophilic stippling.[49]

Neurologic toxicity. Although lead-induced anemia has been the most extensively studied manifestation of lead poisoning, the effects of lead on the nervous system are of the most clinical concern. Lead encephalopathy may present as irritability, behavioral changes, depression, ataxia, con-

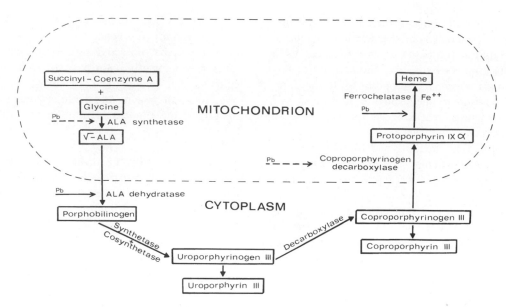

Fig. 36-4 Schematic outline of heme synthesis. The steps where the lead-induced inhibition is strong and well established are indicated by solid arrows. Dotted arrows indicate steps where inhibition is less marked. (From Hemberg S: Lead. In Zenz C, editor: *Occupational medicine,* ed 3, St Louis, 1994, Mosby.)

fusion, delirium, or seizures. These manifestations may develop slowly over weeks to months or may present acutely and dramatically over days after a severe exposure.[48]

While acute lead encephalopathy is the most dramatic and obviously devastating manifestation of lead toxicity, it is fortunately rarely seen today. A much greater concern is the serious long-term neurologic sequelae from subclinical exposures, first described more than 50 years ago in a case series of 20 children who suffered acute lead intoxication and were discharged from the hospital as "cured." On follow-up, all but one of these children had significant neuropsychiatric difficulties including poor reading, attention deficits, expulsion from school, sensorimotor deficits, and seizures.[9] Landmark work by Needleman and colleagues first established an association between mildly elevated BPb (above 25 μg/dl) and decreased intelligence testing in asymptomatic children.[31] Subsequent studies have confirmed this association with BPbs as low as 10 μg/dl.[5] Follow-up on this cohort demonstrated persistence of this association manifested as difficulties with reading and learning, as well as increased incidence of failure to complete secondary school.[32]

Accumulating evidence tends to indicate that lead may also affect cognitive functioning of adults. These abnormalities have been recently demonstrated with specific neuropsychiatric testing. This testing was able to identify the most severe deficits as a decrease in sensory motor reaction times and poor short-term memory.[43] Other studies have found fatigue, altered mood, and short-term memory loss in lead-exposed workers and correlated the severity of these abnormalities with increasing BPb.[46]

The neurotoxicity of lead involves disruption of neurotransmitter release by altering intracellular calcium second messenger systems. Impairment of synaptic communication appears to be associated with the behavioral changes seen in adults and may result in imprecise dendrite formation—and, ultimately, cognitive deficits—in children. This altered intracellular communication may also affect the microvasculature, increase blood-brain barrier permeability, and ultimately produce cerebral edema.[21]

In addition to its effects on the central nervous system, lead can also poison the motor neurons within the peripheral nervous system. The subsequent palsy was historically a common consequence of occupational lead poisoning but fortunately has become a rare entity. The clinical characteristics may include myalgias, muscular tenderness, easy fatigability, fine tremor, and an asymmetric extensor muscle palsy. Classically, a wrist or foot drop was seen to affect the worker's dominant side. Pathologic changes associated with lead palsies include segmental demyelination and axonal degeneration. Recent studies have observed subclinical impairment in motor nerve conduction associated with BPbs as low as 40 μg/dl.[41]

Renal toxicity. The renal toxicity of lead is characterized by two stages. The first stage is characterized by acute reversible changes within the proximal tubule cells. At BPbs as low as 25 μg/dl, their biosynthetic function is altered, resulting in impaired hydroxylation, and hence activation, of vitamin D. In addition, enhanced uric acid reabsorption results in hyperuremic acid gout. At higher blood lead levels, dense intranuclear inclusions made up of sulfhydryl-rich protein-lead complexes form, and mitochondrial swelling is seen. The second stage involves chronic, progressive destruction of these cells that results in nonspecific interstitial fibrosis and tubular atrophy.[6]

Several epidemiologic studies have demonstrated an association with chronic lead exposure and an increased risk of chronic renal disease.[27] Unfortunately, these studies have also demonstrated a strong association with a significant confounder—namely, hypertension—and low-level lead exposure.[37] The hypertensive effects of lead are due, in part, to renal effects (possibly by altering the renin-angiotensin system) and to a direct effect upon the vascular smooth muscle (possibly by altering calcium utilization).[8]

Reproductive toxicity. There is growing evidence that high-dose lead exposure is detrimental to reproductive function in both males and females. Decreased sperm count and abnormal sperm morphology have been associated with BPbs above 50 μg/dl.[3] Some studies suggest that this effect may be reversible.[17] In females, lead easily crosses the placenta, and high-dose exposures have been associated with an increased number of miscarriages.[39] In addition, abnormal fetal cognitive development has been linked to placental cord BPbs as low as 15 μg/dl.[5] Further well-designed epidemiologic studies are needed to confirm and clarify the significance of these associations.

Carcinogenesis. There is some animal evidence that renal malignancies may be produced as a result of high-dose lead exposures. While one recent human cohort study found an excess of renal cancer deaths in a cohort of smelter workers, many others have not demonstrated this link.[42] Further investigations are required before a definitive conclusion can be reached.

Diagnosis

The early symptoms of lead toxicity are typically nonspecific, although they do involve the neurologic and gastrointestinal systems. These symptoms may include difficulty with concentration or sleep, fatigue, irritability, headache, vague abdominal discomfort, nausea, anorexia, or constipation. In acute exposures, bone pain, severe recurrent abdominal pain (known as *lead colic*), and acute encephalopathy can be seen. Because these symptoms are so nonspecific, incorrect diagnosis is common. The disorders often confused with lead toxicity include sickle cell pain crisis, acute abdomen requiring exploratory laparotomy, and infectious encephalitis. Chronic exposures tend to present insidiously with the nonspecific neurologic and gastroenterologic disturbances previously mentioned or with such vague complaints as arthralgias, fatigue, weight loss, depression, decreased libido, impotence, or peripheral motor and sensory nerve dysfunction.[4]

Physical examination may, on occasion, reveal signs of acute encephalopathy and cerebral edema such as papilledema, deep coma, and posturing. Pallor may be noted in severely anemic patients. A bluish discoloration along the gums, known as a Burton's lead line, is rarely noted. This lead line is formed by precipitation of lead sulfide produced by lead binding to the sulfhydryl groups found in dental plaque. It represents merely lead exposure and poor dental hygiene, but not necessarily poisoning. The neurologic assessment is critical and may reveal mild tremors, peripheral nerve deficits, and impaired cerebellar function. Most patients with significant lead exposures, however, do not present initially with severe neurologic symptoms, and only extensive neuropsychiatric testing can document actual impairment.

The diagnosis of lead intoxication differs greatly in children and adults. In children, a definitive diagnosis is established in any patient with a BPb higher than 10 μg/dl and necessitates intervention.[11] This definition was established because of the overwhelming evidence of the impaired cognitive development and vitamin D activation caused by even low-level lead exposures. Regarding adults, there is no absolute BPb above which they are considered lead poisoned. The clinical presentation, in conjunction with evidence of end-organ functional impairment, is essential to establish the diagnosis of adult lead poisoning.

As previously mentioned, the enzymes involved in heme synthesis—namely, δ-aminolevulinic acid dehydratase and ferrochelatase—are inhibited by lead. This association has encouraged δ-aminolevulinic acid dehydratase activity assays, urine β-aminolevulinic acid levels, and serum erythrocyte protoporphyrin levels to be used as biologic markers of lead exposure. Unfortunately, all of these assays have significant limitations. Delta-aminolevulinic acid dehydratase activity is so sensitive to lead exposure that a relatively low BPb of 30 μg/dl causes near complete inhibition, thus making it impossible to distinguish between higher levels of exposure. In the urine, δ-aminolevulinic acid levels are not significantly elevated until the BPb is above 40 μg/dl, making this an insensitive screening tool.[23]

The FEP is extremely inexpensive and easy to perform, and it becomes abnormal at BPbs as low as 17 μg/dl. Unfortunately, since the Centers for Disease Control lowered the BPb at which children are considered lead intoxicated from 25 μg/dl to 10 μg/dl, the FEP is no longer sensitive enough as a screening tool. In addition, other disease states, including iron deficiency anemia and thalessemias, can elevate the FEP. However, FEP is still useful in occupational and chronic exposure settings because it represents the average lead exposure of the past 3 months and is considered to be adequately sensitive for adult screening.

The single best diagnostic test for acute lead exposures is the BPb, which has become the standard screening tool for all lead exposures because of the vast body of literature that established associations between elevated BPbs and impaired cognitive development and renal dysfunction.

Currently, x-ray fluorescence (XRF) is being evaluated as a noninvasive and rapid method to assess total body lead burden.[18] This technology is based on the concept that the

Table 36-2 Adult blood lead determinations and subsequent interventions based on the U.S. OSHA lead standard[34]

Blood lead level*	Intervention
>60 μg/dl† or if the average of the last three blood samples or all blood samples over the past 6 months (whichever is longer) is ≥50 μg/dl† (unless the last blood sample was ≤40 μg/dl)	Immediate medical removal of employee, BPb determination every 1 month
>40 μg/dl but <BPb requiring removal	BPb determination in 2 months
<40 μg/dl	BPb determination in 6 months, BPb at which an employee who has been medically removed may return to work*

*FEP level is recommended whenever a BPb is performed.
†Required confirmation BPb within 2 weeks.

majority of lead is deposited within the bone and that this store may be a reasonable and readily available marker for chronic lead exposure.

The chelation challenge test is another method to assess the total body burden of lead. It involves measuring the excretion of lead in the urine after an intramuscular dose of calcium disodium ethylenediaminetetraacetic acid calcium disodium EDTA. Recently, this practice has been more closely scrutinized and fallen somewhat out of favor.[12,23] In addition, several studies suggest that this mobilized lead can be redistributed into the brain and nervous tissue and may lead to greater neurotoxicity.[14]

The Lead Standard

In 1978, the United States lead standard was introduced into law by OSHA in order to reduce workplace exposures, prevent severe lead poisoning by early detection with BPb screening, and to assure appropriate medical care to those patients with elevated BPb. The standard requires employers to maintain certain workplace standards of environmental control and employee training, to perform routine employee and environmental lead monitoring, and to pay for all medical monitoring and therapy and continue the salary of any employee who is removed from the workplace for lead exposure reasons.[34]

A medical surveillance program must be established for any high-risk occupation in which the employees may be exposed to lead in the air above 30 μg/m³ for more than 30 days per year. These employees must be offered BPb and FEP tests at specific times (Table 36-2). Prophylactic chelation therapy to lower BPb and FEP prior to routine screening is considered unethical and illegal. The

employee must be removed from the workplace if there is a BPb of at least 60 μg/dl, if the average of the last three BPbs or all BPbs over the previous 6 months (whichever is over a longer time period) is at least 50 μg/dl, or if the employee has a medical condition, such as renal disease, which may be adversely affected by lead exposure.[38] Once removed, the employee must undergo monthly lead screening tests, and only after two consecutive BPbs are no higher than 40 mg/dl may he or she return to previous work duties.

Treatment

Once a worker has been identified as lead intoxicated, the primary therapy is cessation of the exposure, including both decreasing the potential environmental lead exposure by improving ventilation and modifying the patient's personal hygiene habits and optimizing personal respirator use (see Table 36-2).[34]

The decision to initiate chelation therapy in adults depends on many factors: the severity of clinical symptoms, degree of end-organ dysfunction, the actual blood lead level, and whether the exposure is acute or chronic. In general, however, chelation therapy is probably indicated in most patients with BPb higher than 80 μg/dl. Chelation therapy involves binding a potentially toxic substance, such as lead, with another substance to form a relatively nontoxic compound that can be safely eliminated from the body. Chelating drugs reduce the total body burden of lead primarily from tissues such as the erythrocytes, muscle, liver, kidney, and trabecular bone. Unfortunately, in patients with long-term exposures, the majority of the body stores remain tightly bound within the compact bone and the brain. Throughout this discussion, remember that while chelators effectively remove lead from the body, it is unclear exactly to what extent chelation therapy actually benefits the lead-poisoned patient, particularly with regard to neurotoxicity.[26]

Specific chelation therapy for lead sometimes begins with the use of 2,3 dimercapto-1-propanol (British antilewisite or BAL), 2 to 3 mg/kg intramuscularly every 4 hours. The BAL is suspended in peanut oil, removes both the intracellular and extracellular lead, and is eliminated via the bile.[25] One of the most important adverse effects of BAL is an allergic reaction to the peanut oil base. Consequently, patients with known allergies to peanuts should never receive this drug. Other important adverse reactions include hemolysis in the face of glucose-6-phosphate dehydrogenase deficiency, hypertension, vomiting, and hyperesthesias, particularly of the face and scalp.

This initial dose of BAL is followed 4 hours later with initiation of a continuous intravenous infusion of 50 mg/kg of calcium disodium EDTA. If it is infused prior to BAL administration, it loses efficacy and may cause harm by redistributing lead into the central nervous system.[14] Renal function and fluid status must always be closely monitored because calcium disodium EDTA is a known nephrotoxin. In addition, trace essential minerals including zinc, copper, and iron wind up being chelated along with the lead. This necessitates limiting the duration of the first course of therapy to 5 days.[10] During therapy, 24-hour urine collections should be used to assess the effectiveness of therapy. During the week after chelation therapy, the BPb tends to rebound as the lead redistributes, and repeat BPb analysis should be obtained to assess the need for further chelation therapy.

In 1991, a new oral chelating agent known as 2,3 dimercaptosuccinic acid (DMSA) (Succimer, Chemet) was approved for use in children demonstrating BPb higher than 45 µg/dl. Based on extensive animal data and limited but growing human clinical experience, its efficacy at lowering the total body lead burden appears equal or superior to BAL and calcium disodium EDTA, with fewer adverse effects.[24] As our understanding of DMSA evolves, it may be utilized in adults and ultimately replace current chelation practices.

Consultation, Referral, Follow-Up Care

All workers at risk for lead exposure should be enrolled in a medical surveillance program. These programs should follow the guidelines established by OSHA's lead standard. (see Table 36-2).[34] All patients with elevated BPbs or signs and symptoms possibly related to lead exposure should be carefully evaluated by a physician familiar with lead toxicity and its treatment. Decisions concerning more frequent surveillance, follow-up, or therapy should be based upon the OSHA lead standard and prudent clinical judgment.

REFERENCES

1. Agency for Toxic Substances and Disease Registry: *Toxicological profile for polycyclic aromatic hydrocarbons,* Washington, DC, 1990, US Department of Health and Human Services.
2. Andjelkovich DA et al: Mortality of iron foundry workers. II. Analysis by work area, *J Occup Med* 34:391, 1992.
3. Assennato G et al: Sperm count suppression without endocrine dysfunction in lead-exposed men, *Arch Environ Health* 41:387, 1986.
4. Balestra DJP: Adult chronic lead intoxication, *Arch Intern Med* 151:1718, 1991.
5. Bellinger D et al: Longitudinal analysis of prenatal and postnatal lead exposure and early cognitive development, *N Engl J Med* 316:1037, 1987.
6. Bernard BP, Becker DE: Environmental lead exposure and the kidney, *J Toxicol Clin Toxicol* 26:1, 1988.
7. Booker DV et al: Uptake of radioactive lead following inhalation and injection, *Br J Radiol* 42:457, 1967.
8. Boscolo P, Carmignani M: Neurohumoral blood pressure regulation in lead exposure, *Environ Health Perspect* 78:101, 1988.
9. Byers RK, Lord EE: Late effects of lead poisoning on mental development, *Am J Dis Child* 66:471, 1943.
10. Cantilena LR, Klaassen CD: The effect of chelation agents on the

excretion of endogenous metals, *Toxicol Appl Pharmacol* 63:344, 1982.
11. Centers for Disease Control: *Preventing lead poisoning in young children,* Atlanta, 1991, Department of Health and Human Services.
12. Chisolm JJ: Mobilization of lead by calcium disodium edetate: a reappraisal, *Am J Dis Child* 141:1256, 1987.
13. Cook DG, Fahn S, Brait KA: Chronic manganese intoxication, *Arch Neurol* 30:59, 1974.
14. Cory-Slechta DA, Weiss B, Cox C: Mobilization and redistribution of lead over the course of CaEDTA chelation therapy, *J Pharmacol Exp Ther* 243:804, 1987.
15. Davis GS: Pathogenesis of silicosis: current concepts and hypothesis, *Lung* 164:139, 1986.
16. Feldman RG et al: Peripheral neuropathy in arsenic smelter workers, *Neurology* 29:939, 1979.
17. Fisher-Fischbein J et al: Correlation between biochemical indicators of lead exposure and semen quality in a lead-poisoned firearms instructor, *JAMA* 257:803, 1987.
18. Gerhardsson L et al: In vivo measurements of lead in bone in long-term exposed lead smelter workers, *Arch Environ Health* 48:147, 1993.
19. Ginsberg MD: Carbon monoxide intoxication: clinical features, neuropathology, and mechanisms of injury, *Clin Toxicol* 23:281, 1985.
20. Gittleman JL et al: Lead poisoning among battery reclamation workers in Alabama, *J Occup Med* 36:526, 1994.
21. Goldstein GW: Neurologic concepts of lead poisoning in children, *Pediatr Ann* 21:384, 1992.
22. Gordon T, Fine JM: Metal fume fever, *Occup Med* 8:505, 1993.
23. Graziano JH: Validity of lead exposure markers in diagnosis and surveillance, *Clin Chem* 40:1387, 1994.
24. Graziano JH et al: Controlled study of meso-2,3-dimercaptosuccinic acid for the management of childhood lead intoxication, *J Pediatr* 120:133, 1992.
25. Howland MA: Dimercaprol (BAL). In Goldfrank LJ et al, editors: *Goldfrank's toxicologic emergencies,* ed 5, East Norwalk, Conn, 1994, Appleton and Lange.
26. Kosnett MJ: Unanswered questions in metal chelation, *J Toxicol Clin Toxicol* 30:529, 1992.
27. Kristensen TS: Cardiovascular diseases in the work environment. A critical review of the epidemiologic literature on chemical factors, *Scand J Work Environ Health* 15:245, 1989.
28. Lilis R et al: Prevalence of lead disease among secondary lead smelter workers and biological indicators of lead exposure, *Environ Res* 14:255, 1977.
29. Matte TD et al: Lead exposure from conventional and cottage lead smelting in Jamaica, *Arch Environ Contam Toxicol* 21:65, 1991.
30. National Institute for Occupational Safety and Health: *Recommendations for control of occupational safety and health hazards—Foundries,* Washington, DC, 1985, US Government Printing Office.
31. Needleman HL et al: Deficits in psychologic and classroom performance of children with elevated dentine lead levels, *N Engl J Med* 300:689, 1979.
32. Needleman HL et al: The long-term effects of exposure to low doses of lead in childhood. An eleven year follow-up report, *N Engl J Med* 322:83, 1990.
33. Nokzaki K: Method for studies on inhaled particles in human respiratory system and retention of lead fume, *Ind Health* 4:118, 1966.
34. Occupational safety and health standard: occupational exposure to lead (29 CR 1910.1025), *Fed Reg* 42:52952, 1978.
35. Paivon JC et al: Silica and lung cancer: a controversial issue, *Eur Respir J* 4:730, 1991.
36. Philip AT, Gerson B: Lead poisoning, part I: incidence, etiology, and toxicokinetics, *Clin Lab Med* 14:423, 1994.
37. Pocock SJ et al: Blood lead concentration, blood pressure, and renal function, *BMJ* 289:872, 1984.

38. Rempel D: The lead-exposed worker, *JAMA* 262:532, 1989.

39. Rom WN: Effects of lead on the female and reproduction: a review, *Mt Sinai J Med* 43:542, 1976.

40. Roto P: Smelting and refining. In Parmeggiani L, editor: *Encyclopedia of occupational health and safety,* vol 2, 1992 International Labor Organization, Geneva, Switzerland.

41. Seppalainen AM et al: Early neurotoxic effects of occupational lead exposure: a prospective study, *Neurotoxicology* 4(2):181, 1983.

42. Steenland K, Selevan S, Landrigan P: The mortality of lead smelter workers: an update, *Am J Public Health* 82:1641, 1992.

43. Stollery BY et al: Short term prospective study of cognitive functioning in lead workers, *Br J Ind Med* 48:739-749, 1991.

44. Thom SR: Leukocytes in carbon monoxide-mediated brain oxidative injury, *Toxicol Appl Pharmacol* 123:234, 1993.

45. US Department of the Interior: *Minerals yearbook for 1990,* vol 1, Washington, DC, 1991, US Government Printing Office.

46. Valciukas JA et al: Central nervous system dysfunction due to lead exposure, *Science* 201:465, 1978.

47. Virtamo M, Tossavainen A: Carbon monoxide in foundry air, *Scand J Work Environ Health* 2:37, 1976.

48. Whitefield CL, Ch'ien LT, Whitehead JD: Lead encephalopathy in adults, *Am J Med* 52:289, 1972.

49. Wintrobe MM: The anemia of lead poisoning. In Wintrobe MM, editor: *Clinical hematology,* ed 8, Philadelphia, 1981, Lea & Febiger.

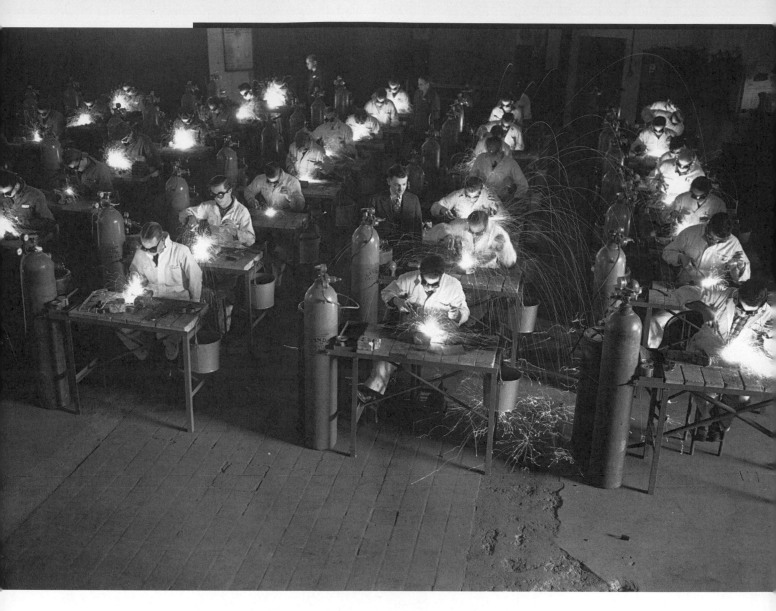

An impressive view of one of the "class rooms" at the
Academy of Aeronautics, Laguardia Airport, showing
some of the students of aviation mechanics at work in a
mass welding session. The school is training civilians
and military personnel. It was announced by the war
department in Washington that 300 enlisted men would
take the course here. March 7, 1941.
(Courtesy UPI/Corbis-Bettmann)

37

Welders

Amy J. Behrman

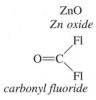

ZnO
Zn oxide

O=C
Fl
Fl
carbonyl fluoride

- Primary route of exposure is inhalational

- Inhalation of metal fumes produces several unusual clinical syndromes in welders with different acute and chronic effects

- Inhalation of non-metallic dusts and gases in the welding worksite can produce additional clinical syndromes and diseases

- Toxic exposures to welders are frequently mixed, and it can be difficult to determine which welding fume components are responsible for a clinical presentation

OCCUPATIONAL DEFINITIONS AND DESCRIPTIONS
Background

Welding is defined as the process of joining metal surfaces by heating them. The process can involve multiple simple or complex technologies. Welding is essential and ubiquitous in industrialized societies; it has been a widely used technique for most of this century. Globally, an enormous population of workers face multiple potential toxic exposures while welding. It is conservatively estimated that 800,000 workers worldwide[42] and 200,000 in the United States[40] work full-time in welding and joining. A much larger number of workers do welding on an intermittent or part-time basis.[40,49] Understanding the health risks and toxic exposures to which welders are subject requires a basic understanding of welding techniques. A representative group of these are briefly described here.[42,49]

Welding Techniques

Gas welding and cutting. Gas welding uses a burning fuel to melt and fuse the base metals. (The base metals are the surfaces being welded.) When a high-velocity oxygen source is added, the technique can be used to cut metals instead.

Arc welding. Arc welding employs an electric arc as the heat source to melt and fuse the base metals and any "filler," which is usually derived from a consumable electrode (welding rod). The temperature of the arc can average 4000° F. There are many variations of arc welding.

Shielded metal arc welding (SMAW; manual metal arc welding, MMA) utilizes a short consumable electrode coated with gas-generating material. The shielding gas protects the weld from oxidative weakening. In addition, molten fluxes derived from the rod carry potentially weakening impurities away from the weld.

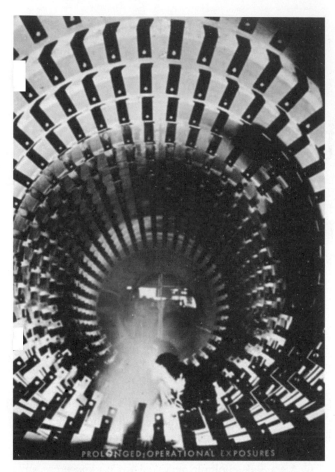

Fig. 37-1 An example of prolonged occupational exposure. (From Zenz C, Dickerson OB, Horvath EP: *Occupational medicine,* ed 3, St Louis, 1994, Mosby.)

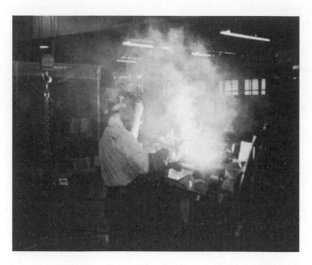

Fig. 37-2 Production welding before exhaust system was installed. Note dense fumes, which are mainly iron oxide. (From Zenz C, Dickerson OB, Horvath EP: *Occupational medicine,* ed 3, St Louis, 1994, Mosby.)

Potential Toxic Exposures

Welders are exposed to a wide range of metals and nonmetals with varying and sometimes additive toxic effects. In addition, welders are commonly exposed to physical hazards including heat, electrical current, noise, vibration, light (visible, infrared, ultraviolet), and ergonomic stresses. Most toxic exposures are inhalational. The degree of exposure to any specific compound depends on the composition of the base metals, electrodes, and fluxes as well as individual conditions of ventilation, positioning, and use of personal protective equipment[18,42] (Fig. 37-1).

Welding produces a "plume" of gases, fine particulates, and metal fumes (Fig. 37-2). Metal fumes are small (less than 1 micron) particles of metal or metal oxides produced when vaporized metal condenses in the air above the weld. Particles in this size range deposit in the terminal bronchioles and alveoli and clear slowly.[42] Particles may combine in the air to form larger aggregates, which deposit more proximally and are less biologically active. Table 37-1 summarizes potential toxic exposures in welding and joining.

Welders who present with occupational toxic syndromes have often been exposed to more than one of the substances listed in Table 37-1. Exposure histories are often incomplete, making the exact contribution of a given toxin to a clinical presentation unclear. In addition, variations in welding technique, use of personal protective equipment, local ventilation, and exposure to common nonoccupational toxins (such as cigarettes) greatly affect individual exposure levels and symptoms.* The following section describes some of the diseases associated with toxic exposures in welding and joining and discusses the probable contributions of specific compounds to each syndrome.

Gas metal arc welding (GMAW) is a semiautomatic process utilizing a continuously fed steel wire electrode and a "shield" of inert gas (metal inert gas welding, MIG) or active gas (usually carbon dioxide–inert gas mixtures, MAG) to protect the weld from oxygen.

Gas tungsten arc welding (GTAW; tungsten inert gas welding, TIG) utilizes a nonconsumable tungsten electrode, a continuously fed filler wire, and an inert shielding gas. Plasma-arc welding is similar to TIG but utilizes a plasma induced by the constriction of heated gas to shield the weld. Submerged arc welding fuses the base metals with the heat of an arc that is completely shielded beneath, or submerged in, a blanket of flux.

Joining methods. Soldering and brazing take place at a temperature below the melting point of the base metal. The join is achieved with a filler metal that has a lower melting point. Brazing uses an alloy or hard solder (which may contain copper, zinc, silver, or cadmium) that melts above 450° C. Soldering utilizes a filler material (typically a lead, zinc, or silver alloy) that melts below 450° C. Fluxes are added to protect the soldered material. Flux cores may be corrosive (acid) or noncorrosive (typically, the highly allergenic pine resin, colophony).

*References 6, 10, 13, 31, 35, 41, 45.

Table 37-1 Potential toxic inhalational exposures for welders, braziers, and solderers

Toxin	Source	Acute effects	Chronic effects
Iron oxide	Steel welding	Metal fume fever (MFF)	Siderosis
Zinc oxide	Galvanized steel	MFF	Bronchitis, dermatitis
Cadmium	Solder, welding rods	Pneumonitis, adult respiratory distress syndrome (ARDS), renal failure	Renal dysfunction, liver dysfunction, carcinogenesis
Chromate	Stainless steel welding	Bronchitis, mucosal irritation	Carcinogenesis
Manganese	Welding rods	MFF	CNS toxicity
Nickel	Nickel alloy welding	MFF	Carcinogenesis
Lead	Brazing, soldering, welding*	Gastroenteritis, CNS toxicity, renal failure	Neuropathy, CNS toxicity, renal failure, hypertension, anemia
Aluminum	Welding	MFF	CNS toxicity
Beryllium	Beryllium alloy welding	ARDS	Pneumonitis, berylliosis, carcinogenesis
Ozone	Arc welding	Bronchitis, pneumonitis, ARDS	
Nitrogen oxides	Welding	Bronchitis, ARDS	Chronic bronchitis (?)
Carbon monoxide	Welding*	CNS toxicity, cardiovascular	CNS toxicity
Asbestos	Worksite (shipyard)	Asbestosis	Lung cancer, mesothelioma (pleural and peritoneal)
Silica	Worksite	Acute silicosis	Accelerated and chronic silicosis, pulmonary fibrosis
Phosgene	Chlorinated hydrocarbons	ARDS, pneumonitis	
Fluoropolymers	Polymers, esp. Teflon	Polymer fume fever, pneumonitis	Interstitial fibrosis
Colophony	Solder flux	Bronchospasm	Asthma
Aminoethyl ethanolamine	Solder flux	Bronchospasm	Asthma

*Overt toxicity is rarely described in welders.

CLINICAL TOXICOLOGY IN WELDERS AND JOINERS
Metal Fume Fever

Metal fume fever (MFF) is the best characterized, the most frequently described, and a unique toxic syndrome in welders. It has been recognized as an occupational disease of metal workers since the early nineteenth century.[40] It is known among welders by a variety of vivid names that attest to its prevalence and presentation: metal malaria, brass founder's ague, brass chills, zinc chills, welder's ague, zinc fever, foundry fever, galvanized shakes, Monday morning fever, spelter shakes, and "the smothers."

The MFF is an acute, self-limited, systemic syndrome that occurs 4 to 12 hours after exposure to metal fumes.* Patients classically present with high fever, chills, sweats, malaise, myalgias, arthralgias, nonproductive cough, and a sweet or metallic taste in the mouth. They may complain of dyspnea, chest discomfort, nausea, vomiting, abdominal pain, or headache. Laboratory studies show a leukocytosis with a predominance of polymorphonuclear cells (PMNs) and moderately elevated lactic dehydrogenase (LDH). Chest x-rays and lung exam are usually normal.

Symptoms resolve spontaneously in 24 to 48 hours, and treatment is generally supportive and noninterventional. Many welders believe milk can prevent or ameliorate symptoms.[18] Although MFF is clearly an unpleasant and temporarily disabling experience, no long-term sequelae have been documented. It is probably reported to physicians 1500 to 2000 times yearly in this country.[18] Since the disease is understood by most welders to be self-limited, it seems likely that it is under-reported.

Most often, MFF is associated with exposure to zinc oxide fumes, but identical presentations have been reported after exposure to fumes of chromate, manganese, nickel, aluminum, copper, silver, tin, and magnesium.[42] The differential diagnosis includes viral syndromes, pneumonia, sepsis, hypersensitivity or chemical pneumonitis, and polymer fume fever.

The pathophysiology of MFF is unclear. It is known that MFF can occur after a first exposure to metal fumes or after repeated exposures.[37] Tachyphylaxis is well documented, and there is a reported tendency for attacks to be worst at the beginning of the work week[37,40,50] (hence "Monday morning fever").

One theory holds that MFF involves a delayed hypersensitivity response wherein inhaled metal fumes cause inflammation of the respiratory tract, modify lung proteins, and induce an antibody response to the altered proteins.[31,32,36,37,40] Alternatively, metal oxides have been hypothesized to form complexes with lung proteins capable of directly eliciting an antibody response. For example, one welder developed immediate and delayed angioedema and urticaria after zinc oxide exposure in the setting of typical MFF symptoms.[14]

*References 3, 4, 13, 18, 37, 40, 42.

However, immune mechanisms for MFF have not been well documented in additional clinical or experimental studies. Other researchers have focused on the similarity of MFF symptoms to those caused by exogenous and endogenous pyrogens. Animal studies in the 1920s demonstrated that a MFF-like syndrome could be produced with inhaled zinc oxide[18] and that the process involved the induction of endogenous pyrogen(s). Serum from rabbits exposed to zinc fumes was later shown to reproduce fever when injected into unexposed recipient animals.

Experimental zinc oxide fume exposure produced MFF symptoms without changes in pulmonary function in human volunteers. Bronchoalveolar lavage (BAL) fluid from similarly exposed rats and guinea pigs developed inflammatory changes with significant increases in total cells, LDH, and protein.[17] This inflammatory response of MFF might be mediated by cytokines, specifically those known to be involved in other pyrogenic responses: tumor necrosis factor (TNF) and interleukins 1, 6, and 8 (IL-1, IL-6, IL-8).[3] In one study,[3] a dose-dependent increase in BAL PMNs occurred in human volunteers exposed to welding fumes without demonstrable changes in pulmonary function or BAL cytokine levels. Subsequent studies with more sensitive cytokine assays[4] were able to detect significant increases in TNF, IL-6, IL-8, and PMNs in human BAL fluid after a similar exposure to welding fumes. Again, there were no changes in pulmonary function or airway reactivity associated with BAL changes.

In 1995, the same investigators assayed BAL in human subjects after exposure to purified, quantified zinc oxide fume.[13] They were able to demonstrate exposure-dependent increases in two proinflammatory cytokines (TNF and IL-8) and PMNs in subjects as opposed to controls. The weight of evidence now therefore supports a cytokine-mediated mechanism for MFF, although details remain to be elucidated.

Tachyphylaxis to metal fumes may also involve cytokine mechanisms, such as those mediating tolerance to endotoxin-induced fever. It has also been proposed that metal fume tolerance might involve the induction of metallothioneins.[18,23] Metallothioneins can be induced by metals including zinc, and their induction is associated with increased metal excretion.[27] They appear to play an important role in the homeostasis of essential metals and could be protective in overexposures.

Polymer Fume Fever

Polymer fume fever (PFF) is a febrile illness that occurs after industrial or household exposure to thermal decomposition products of fluoropolymers, most notably polytetrafluoroethylene (PFTE, Teflon). It has also been described in welders working on or near PFTE-coated materials.[43]

Like MFF, PFF is a delayed-onset, flulike, self-limited syndrome. As in MFF, patients may have fever, headache, myalgias, cough, dyspnea, chest discomfort, and leukocytosis. They do not report the metallic taste of MFF but more often complain of mucosal irritation of the eyes, mouth, and throat. The chest x-ray is either normal or shows diffuse infiltrates. Spirometry shows variable abnormalities.[43] Diagnosis is based on exposure history and clinical presentation. Urine fluoride levels are useful to estimate chronic exposure but not to elucidate acute illness. It may progress to chemical pneumonitis or to frank adult respiratory distress syndrome (ARDS). Tachyphylaxis does not occur. Treatment is supportive; inhaled steroids are useful for treating bronchospasm.

Fluoropolymer pyrolysis products are complex mixtures of smaller fluorinated compounds, including carbonyl fluoride (COF_2). Hydrolysis of carbonyl fluoride in the lung produces hydrofluoric acid (HF), an intense irritant that undoubtedly contributes to the pneumonitis. It seems likely that classic, reversible PFF may be due to the small particulates also present in polymer pyrolysis fumes. It has been induced in animals and humans under experimental conditions, but the specific pyrogen has not been identified.

Welding chloropolymer paints may produce a similar clinical syndrome. Fever, dyspnea, mucosal irritation, and airway reactivity developed in two welders working on steel painted with chloropolymers. Both had persistent airway dysfunction months after their acute illnesses.[46] The paints also contained zinc, but it was present in low concentration. The authors argued that chlorinated pyrolysis products, rather than metal fumes, were responsible for the symptoms observed. Analysis of the welding fume from the painted steel demonstrated hydrochloric acid (HCl) but not phosgene ($COCl_2$, an intense irritant). Zinc was not measured.

Chemical Pneumonitis

Acute chemical pneumonitis has been reported after occupational exposure to welding-associated compounds including phosgene, fluoropolymers, beryllium, nitrogen oxides, and, most commonly, ozone and cadmium fumes.[16,42] Although the syndrome is much less common than MFF, the clinical consequences are markedly worse.[16,30,39] Acute chemical pneumonitis presents with fever, headache, dyspnea, cough, myalgias, and nausea. It occurs a few hours after the exposure to irritant gases or particles in the plume. Severe cases may progress to ARDS. Restrictive pulmonary disease develops with diffuse bilateral infiltrates, hypoxia, and granulocytosis.

The differential diagnosis includes MFF, hypersensitivity pneumonitis, sepsis, and pneumonia. Treatment is supportive and frequently requires ventilation. Survivors may have normal lung function or residual deficits.[48] It is critically important to distinguish early chemical pneumonitis, with its potential for rapid deterioration and death, from the benign MFF it resembles. Blood cadmium levels may be markedly elevated in welders' chemical pneumonitis[16] but are unlikely to be available during the initial workup. Patients with apparent MFF and a history consistent with likely exposure to high concentrations of ozone (GMAW on aluminum base) or cadmium (cadmium-silver alloy in rods or solder) should be held for observation. Cadmium toxicity may also cause renal tubular injury and liver damage.

Hypersensitivity Pneumonitis

Hypersensitivity pneumonitis probably occurs less often than chemical pneumonitis in welders, although the true incidence of both is unknown. True hypersensitivity pneumonitis occurs only after repeated exposure to an offending agent and classically presents with a history of increasingly severe episodes. It may be difficult in the acute situation to differentiate from MFF and chemical pneumonitis. The presentation is similar, with delayed onset, dyspnea, cough, hypoxemia, leukocytosis, and diffuse infiltrates. Workers with this condition typically become symptomatic at levels of exposure where most co-workers are unaffected.

Given the variety of potential toxins and the variability of compounds to which welders are exposed, it may be difficult to determine which compound or metal is responsible for an individual's reaction. A careful history of the materials in use and a knowledge of plume components in different welding processes should enable the clinician to identify at least the most likely reactive substances.

Siderosis

Arc welders' siderosis (or pneumoconiosis) has been recognized since 1936,[11] when Doig and McLaughlin documented the presence of small, radiodense nodules in the lungs of asymptomatic steel welders. Welders with these abnormalities did not appear to have excess mortality,[42] but, on the rare occasions that autopsies were performed, lung histology was notable for the presence of iron deposits without accompanying fibrosis. It appears that the micronodules seen on x-ray films are produced by the accumulation of iron particles without any significant contribution by scarring. Although isolated cases of fibrosis with siderosis have been reported, these represent mixed-dust pneumoconioses.[42] Many welders have had extensive exposure to more reactive dusts, such as silica and coal.

Pulmonary function tests in individuals with radiographic evidence of siderosis are normal.[29] The course of siderosis is also notable for the fact that radiographic abnormalities may improve after exposure ceases, presumably due to macrophage clearance activity.

Pulmonary Function Testing

A number of studies[6,49] have suggested that welders may have a higher prevalence of pulmonary symptoms than nonwelders. A large number of studies have examined pulmonary function in welders from many countries. Comparison of these studies is difficult as they differ markedly in methodology (cross-sectional, longitudinal, cross-shift), analysis of variables (smoking, atopy, exposure to different welding plume components, exposure to other worksite toxins, ventilation, use of personal protective equipment), and follow-up. Welders with significant respiratory symptoms probably leave this physically demanding field and confound studies

that do not control for outmigration. When pulmonary function deficits are detected in these studies, it is extremely difficult to associate the deficits with specific toxins.

The relatively frequent complaints of pulmonary symptoms in welders do not correlate with easily demonstrable acute changes in lung function. Acute and recurrent pulmonary function changes have been demonstrated in several studies. Welding seems to cause mild increases in airway obstruction, as well as mild restrictive and mixed ventilatory defects on the job.[12,41] However, many studies have failed to find any acute or transient changes in pulmonary function.[1,33] In fact, one study has shown small but significant improvements in airway flow rates during welding.[42]

Asthma has been well described in association with compounds like colophony and aminoethyl ethanolamine, found in solder flux. (Hobbyists as well as professional joiners are at risk.) Individual case reports of asthma produced and reproduced by welding fume exposure exist, but larger studies have tended not to show an increased risk of asthma among welders[42,49] (as opposed to joiners). The SWORD (Surveillance of Work-related and Occupational Respiratory Disease project) reporting system collects cases identified by pulmonary and occupational physicians in Britain. An analysis of this data found a significant increase in risk of asthma in the occupational group that included welders.[34] However, this set also included solderers, and it is not clear how large a contribution welding fumes made to the findings.

Welders are at increased risk for developing mild but statistically significant chronic obstructive pulmonary disease (COPD), even when studies controlled for both asbestos exposure and cigarette smoking as independent risk factors.* Again, the relative contributions of dusts and welding plume components to the development of bronchitis cannot yet be determined. Most studies indicate that welding and smoking together pose a greater risk than either alone. (For a complete review of the epidemiology of chronic pulmonary function abnormalities in welders, see reference 42.) Most of these studies are cross-sectional and may underestimate disease prevalence because of the selective loss of symptomatic workers. Other studies failed to reproduce this effect.[42] It seems likely that chronic airway obstruction does occur more often in welders than in controls, but the degree of impairment is generally mild.

Pneumonia

A recent British study[7] showed strikingly more mortality from lobar pneumonia in welders than in the general population. This effect was consistent in four successive cohorts from 1959 to 1990. The increased death rate was restricted to working-age men. The fact that the excess risk disappeared after age of retirement suggested that reversible effects from metal fumes (or other welding-associated toxins such as ozone and nitrogen oxides) may increase suscepti-

*References 6, 9, 20, 21, 28, 47.

Table 37-2 Recent studies of lung cancer in welders

Population	Findings	Confounding variables
Pooled data on welders from nine European countries[44]	Increased risk for lung cancer deaths in welders, which increased with the duration of exposure for SS and MS workers	Study did not control for cigarette smoking or asbestos exposure; unrecognized asbestos exposure
German welders[2]	Increased lung cancer deaths	Unrecognized asbestos exposure
Norwegian MS welder's excess lung cancer deaths, not fully accounted for by exposure to asbestos or cigarettes[10]		
Meta-analysis of five studies of SS welders[45]	An increased risk for lung cancer death	All five considered the effects of smoking and asbestos in their analyses
French welders (part of the IARC cohort)[35]	Lung cancer deaths were significantly increased in MS welders as compared with controls or SS welders	Used only "shipyard" histories to control for asbestos exposure
Welders in Illinois[26a]	Significant associations between welding and lung and stomach cancer	Unrecognized asbestos exposure
Case-control study of welders in Germany[26]	No excess risk of lung cancer in welders that was not accounted for by their careful controls for asbestos and smoking	

bility to major lung infection or worsen the severity of disease. Further epidemiologic and experimental studies are needed to verify these observations and explain the pathophysiology of the effect, which could involve mild COPD, direct mucosal injury, or modification of local immune responses in welders.

Lung Cancer

The association between employment as a welder and death from lung cancer was first noted in 1954[5] and has been confirmed many times. This association is all the more striking since welders tend to have a lower overall mortality than the general population, a finding that probably reflects selection bias for this heavy manual work ("healthy worker effect"; see Chapter 22).

Welders have nonuniform exposure to compounds in the worksite (asbestos, possibly silica) and welding plume (nickel, hexavalent chromium, cadmium) that are known to be carcinogenic in other occupational settings. The MMA welding of stainless steel (SS) is known to generate high levels of hexavalent chromium. The MMA SS welders have a higher incidence of chromatid breaks in peripheral lymphocytes than controls,[24] and MMA welders of mild steel (MS) had a higher incidence of DNA-protein cross-links.[8] In addition, antibodies to oxidized DNA bases were elevated in MS welders versus controls,[15] although this did not reach statistical significance. By contrast, peripheral blood cytogenetic damage was decreased versus controls in SS welders using TIG, MIG, and MAG techniques in a Norwegian study.[25]

The International Agency for Research on Cancer (IARC) has categorized welding fumes as "possibly carcinogenic to humans."[22] Doubt as to the carcinogenicity of welding fumes persists because of two major confounding risk

factors: cigarette smoking and asbestos exposure. Several studies have indicated that cigarette smoking is more prevalent in welders than in the general population.[10,31,45] Asbestos is a pulmonary carcinogen with an effect potentiated by direct exposure to cigarette pyrolysis products. Asbestos is a recognized hazard for shipyard workers such as welders; some researchers therefore differentiate between shipyard and nonshipyard welders in an attempt to control for the effects of asbestos. However, welders referred for lung biopsy or BAL show a high degree of asbestos body retention with no difference between high-exposure shipyard welders and those without known histories of shipyard work or known asbestos exposure.[38] This suggests that unrecognized asbestos exposure in welders may be substantial. Many additional studies of lung cancer epidemiology in welders have been published since the IARC review of 1990.[22] A sample of these are reviewed in Table 37-2.

In conclusion, the current data are still contradictory. Some studies strongly suggest a role for welding plume components in carcinogenesis. Others show that the confounding effects of tobacco use and sometimes unrecognized asbestos exposure are considerable and may account for some, or even all, excess lung cancer deaths in welders. In addition, there is some variable evidence for differential risk in welders who use different techniques (MMA, GMAW) or work on different materials (MS, SS). Further longitudinal evaluations of welding populations with controls for techniques, welding materials, occupational exposure to asbestos and other carcinogens, and tobacco exposure are needed to identify and control specific carcinogens.

Aluminum Neurotoxicity

Neurotoxicity from chronic aluminum exposure is recognized in human populations (dialysis patients) and animal models. A study of Finnish aluminum workers[19] showed them to have increased serum and urine aluminum levels. There was an indication on neuropsychologic testing that short-term memory function and attention might be adversely affected in individuals with higher internal aluminum loads. These findings were inconclusive but argue for further study.

REFERENCES

1. Alcesson B, Skerfving S: Exposure in welding of high nickel alloy, *Int Arch Occup Environ Health* 4:489, 1985.
2. Becker N, Chang-Claude J, Frentzel-Beyme R: Risk of cancer for arc welders in the Federal Republic of Germany: results of a second follow-up (1983-8), *Br J Ind Med* 48:675, 1991.
3. Blanc PD et al: An experimental human model of metal fume fever, *Ann Intern Med* 114:930, 1991.
4. Blanc PD et al: Cytokines in metal fume fever, *Am Rev Respir Dis* 147:134, 1993.
5. Breslow L et al: Occupations and cigarette smoking as factors in lung cancer, *Am J Public Health* 44:171, 1954.
6. Chinn DJ et al: Respiratory health of young shipyard welders and other tradesmen studied cross sectionally and longitudinally, *Occup Environ Med* 55:33, 1995.
7. Coggon D et al: Lobar pneumonia: an occupational disease in welders, *Lancet* 344:41, 1994.
8. Costa M, Zhitkovich A, Toniolo P: DNA-protein cross-links in welders: molecular implications, *Cancer Res* 3:460, 1992.
9. Cotes JE et al: Respiratory symptoms and impairment in shipyard welders and caulker burners, *Br J Ind Med* 46:292, 1989.
10. Danielsen TE et al: Incidence of cancer among welders of mild steel and other shipyard workers, *Br J Ind Med* 50:1097, 1993.
11. Doig AT, McLaughlin AG: X-ray appearances of the lungs of electric welders, *Lancet* 1:771, 1936.
12. Donoghue AM et al: Transient changes in the pulmonary function of welders: a cross sectional study of Monday peak expiratory flow, *Occup Environ Med* 51:553, 1994.
13. Duschner WG: Pulmonary responses to purified zinc oxide fume, *J Investig Med* 43:371, 1995.
14. Farrell FJ: Angioedema and urticaria in acute and late phase reactants to zinc fume exposure with associated metal fume fever-like symptoms, *Am J Ind Med* 12:331, 1987.
15. Frenkel K et al: Occupational exposures to Cd, Ni, and Cr modulate titers of antioxidized DNA base autoantibodies, *Environ Health Perspect* 102(suppl 3):221, 1994.
16. Fuortes L et al: Acute respiratory fatality associated with exposure to sheet metal and cadmium fumes, *Clin Tox* 29:279, 1991.
17. Gordon T et al: Pulmonary effects of inhaled zinc oxide in human subjects, guinea pigs, rats, and rabbits, *Am Ind Hyg Assoc J* 53:503, 1992.
18. Gordon T, Fine JM: Metal fume fever, *Occup Med* 8:505, 1993.
19. Hanninen H et al: Internal load of aluminum and the central nervous system function of aluminum welders, *Arch Environ Health* 20:279, 1994.
20. Hunnicutt TN et al: Spirometric measurements in welders, *Arch Environ Health* 8:661, 1954.
21. Hunting KL, Welch LS: Occupational exposure to dust and lung disease among sheet metal workers, *Br J Ind Med* 50:432, 1993.
22. IARC Working Group on the Evaluation of Carcinogenic Risks to Humans: *Chromium, nickel, and welding: IARC monographs on the evaluation of carcinogenic risk to humans,* Lyons, France, 1990, IARC, World Health Organization.
23. Jahroudi N et al: Cell-type specific and differential regulation of the human metallothionein genes, *J Biol Chem* 265:6506, 1990.
24. Jelmert O, Hansteen I, Langard S: Chromosome damage in lymphocytes of stainless steel welders related to past and current exposure to manual metal arc welding fumes, *Mutat Res* 320:223, 1994.
25. Jelmert O, Hansteen I, Langard S: Cytogenetic studies of stainless steel welders using the tungsten inert gas and metal inert gas methods for welding, *Mutat Res* 342:77, 1995.
26. Jockel K, Ahrens W, Bolm-Audorff U: Lung cancer risk and welding: preliminary results from an ongoing case-control study, *Am J Ind Med* 25:805, 1994.
26a. Keller, Howe HL: Cancer in Illinois construction workers: A study, *Am J Ind Med* 24:223-230, 1993.
27. Kido T et al: Dose-response relationship between urinary cadmium and metallothionein in a Japanese population environmentally exposed to cadmium, *Toxicology* 65:325, 1991.
28. Kilburn K, Warshaw R: Pulmonary functional impairment from years of arc welding, *Am J Ind Med* 87:62, 1989.
29. Kleinfeld M et al: Welder's siderosis: a clinical roentgenographic and physiological study, *Arch Environ Health* 19:70, 1969.
30. Lucas PA et al: Fatal cadmium fume inhalation, *Lancet* 2:205, 1980.
31. McCord CP: Metal fume fever as an immunologic disease, *Int Ind Med Surg* 27:101, 1960.
32. McMillan G: Metal fume fever, *Occup Health* 38:148, 1986.
33. McMillan GH, Heath J: The health of welders in naval dockyards: acute changes in respiratory function during standardized welding, *Ann Occup Hyg* 22:19, 1979.
34. Meredith S: Reported incidence of occupational asthma in the United Kingdom, 1989-90, *Environ Community Health* 47:459, 1993.
35. Moulin JJ et al: A mortality study among mild steel and stainless steel welders, *Br J Ind Med* 50:234, 1993.
36. Mueller EJ, Seger DL: Metal fume fever: a review, *J Emerg Med* 2:271, 1985.
37. Offermann PV, Finley CJ: Metal fume fever, *Ann Emerg Med* 21:872, 1992.
38. Pairon J et al: Retention of asbestos bodies in the lungs of welders, *Am J Ind Med* 25:793, 1994.
39. Patwardhan JR, Finch ES: Fatal cadmium fume pneumonitis, *Med J Aust* 29:962, 1976.
40. Perry GF: Occupational medicine forum, *J Occup Med* 36:1061, 1994.
41. Sastogi SK et al: Spirometric abnormalities among welders, *Environ Res* 56:15, 1991.
42. Sferlazza SJ, Beckett WS: The respiratory health of welders, *Am Rev Respir Dis* 143:1134, 1991.
43. Shusterman DJ: Polymer fume fever and other fluorocarbon pyrolysis-related syndromes, *Occup Med* 8:519, 1993.
44. Simonato L et al: A historical prospective study of European stainless steel, mild steel, and shipyard welders, *Br J Ind Med* 48:145, 1991.
45. Sjogren B et al: Exposure to stainless steel welding fumes and lung cancer: a meta-analysis, *Occup Environ Med* 51:335, 1994.
46. Sjogren B et al: Fever and respiratory symptoms after welding on painted steel, *Scand J Work Environ Health* 17:441, 1991.
47. Sjogren B, Ulfvaren B: Respiratory symptoms and pulmonary function among welders working with aluminum stainless steel and railroad tracks, *Scand J Work Environ Health* 11:27, 1985.
48. Townsend RH: A case of acute cadmium pneumonitis: lung function tests during a four year follow-up, *Br J Ind Med* 25:68, 1968.
49. Wang ZP et al: Asthma, lung function, and bronchial responsiveness in welders, *Am J Ind Med* 26:741, 1994.
50. Zenz C, Dickerson OB, Horvath EP: *Occupational medicine,* ed 3, St Louis, 1994, Mosby.

38

Cl F
| |
H—C—C—O—CH₃
| |
Cl F

methoxyflurane

- Waste anesthetic gases continues to be a significant source of toxicity and a reproductive hazard

Zookeepers and Veterinarians

Susan E. Farrell

OCCUPATIONAL DESCRIPTION

Illness and adverse health effects associated with veterinary medicine and animal handling were reported as early as 1947: in the United Kingdom, during the 1930s and 1940s, four of eight veterinary researchers developed an illness like multiple sclerosis after working with lambs afflicted with "swayback disease," a neurologic disease of the central nervous system. In a more recent review and discussion of these cases,[4] the Cambridge veterinarians' work on this animal disease transmission, histopathology, and chemistry was described, and common exposure to laboratory fumes, dust, chemicals, or the infectious agent itself was postulated as causative in the associated human illness. This report helps to underscore the fact that professions that involve the care, handling, or study of animals bring the worker in contact with a multitude of potentially harmful occupational exposures.

Today's veterinarian or animal handler encounters a variety of occupational hazards, each of which presents its own risk of toxicity, but which, in combination, may have synergistic adverse effects. In many veterinary clinics and hospitals, the routine use of inhalational anesthesia for surgical procedures may expose personnel to waste anesthetic gas, the scavenging of which is commonly suboptimal. In addition, the use of ionizing radiation for both diagnostic and therapeutic uses may place personnel at risk for the toxicities related to excess radiation exposure. Obviously, a myriad of infectious diseases are associated with mammals, reptiles, and birds, many of which are pathogenic in humans and cause illness that may be very uncommon in other occupational groups. The numerous chemical therapeutic

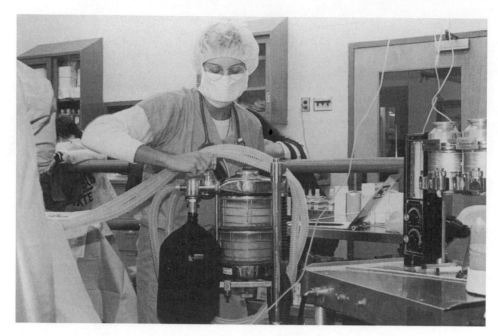

Fig. 38-1 The veterinary anesthetist is repeatedly exposed to trace concentrations of anesthetics. (From Steele LJ, Wilkins JR: Occupational exposures and risks of spontaneous abortion among female veterinarians, *Int J Occup Environ Health* 2:26, 1996.)

options used in animal health care may present a potential source of allergens or irritants to susceptible humans, and the risk of trauma associated with animal behavior and care is an exposure unique to veterinary medicine and related fields.

POTENTIAL TOXIC EXPOSURES
Anesthetic Gases

Veterinary care workers may be exposed to the anesthetic gases through leakage of the waste gas from the anesthetic system[21] (Fig. 38-1). In general, liquid anesthetic is vaporized, mixed with oxygen and nitrous oxide to the desired concentration, and inhaled by the patient. A Y-connector at the patient's endotracheal tube or mask allows collection of exhaled gases, containing carbon dioxide and unabsorbed anesthetic. In a semiclosed rebreathing system, these exhaled gases are collected, carbon dioxide is absorbed by a soda lime–containing canister, and the remainder of the waste gas is recycled, with the addition of oxygen and any necessary amounts of anesthetic. A pop-off valve is generally present on the carbon dioxide canister, where excess pressure in the system may be relieved by allowing the escape of waste gases. In a nonrebreathing system, waste gases are immediately expelled into the room after the animal exhales. In most cases, a reservoir bag is attached to the system to prevent a buildup of gas and resultant pressure. The presence of a scavenging system to collect waste anesthetic gases from the area of the pop-off valve helps to eliminate gas from the room atmosphere.

Leakage of waste anesthetic gas may occur at various points in the anesthetic system, including poorly fitting endotracheal tubes and face masks and leaky tubing or reservoir bags. Improper practices, such as use of excessive anesthetic gas flow, emptying of reservoir bags into the room air environment, poor ventilation, and lack of scavenging of gas released at pop-off valves, increase waste gas in the room environment. Several studies have been performed to analyze quantitatively the waste anesthetic gas concentrations in veterinary operating and recovery rooms, with attention to the concentrations in the breathing areas of veterinary personnel and to areas of excess leakage from the anesthetic system itself.

A 1980 survey of Colorado veterinary hospitals and clinics found that inhalational anesthetics were used by more than 80% of practices, mostly during small animal surgeries.[21,29] Of small animal surgery, 92% was performed under methoxyflurane anesthesia. Anesthetic gas concentrations that were measured in various areas of the procedure room showed that the average concentration of methoxyflurane during small animal surgeries was less than 2 ppm. In four unscavenged, semiclosed rebreathing systems, the average concentration of halothane (Fig. 38-2) ranged from 4 to 4.8 ppm. In one large animal surgery, the average concentration of halothane ranged from 10.4 ppm in the area of the veterinary operator to 20.9 ppm in the area of the anesthetist. Reported average concentrations of nitrous oxide ranged from 18.6 to 35 ppm. The average time of exposure was 5 to 10 hours per week. Factors that increased the concentration of waste anesthetic gas in the ambient air of

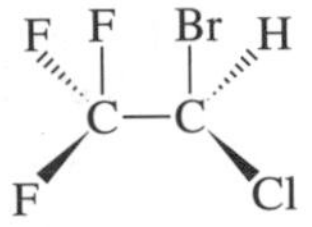

Fig. 38-2 Halothane structure.

workers were increased animal size, high anesthetic gas flow rate, and use of nonrebreathing systems, which directly vented waste gas into the room. The most leakage occurred at the pop-off valves and around endotracheal tubes. Poorly maintained machines were also more liable to leak gases. Scavenging equipment to collect waste anesthetic gas was present in only 3 of 28 operating systems but, when present, greatly reduced the room concentrations.

Similar studies have been performed in different regions of the United States[11,26,27] and in the United Kingdom.[6] These surveys took place in small and large veterinary hospitals, teaching hospitals, and research facilities. As expected, specialist surgeons were likely to have greater exposures,[11] as they spent a greater percentage of their time operating. In addition, surgeries scheduled in rapid succession in the same room led to a buildup of gases.[12] Waste gas concentrations were measured in ranges from 1.1 to 18 ppm[27] and 1.45 to 2 ppm[26] for halothane and from 0.52 to 0.55 ppm for methoxyflurane. In one study,[6] 77% of measured halothane concentrations were less than the recommended 2 ppm 8-hour time-weighted average (TWA). Of measured nitrous oxide concentrations, 86% were less than 100 ppm 8-hour TWA, but only 5% were less than the recommended 25 ppm. In almost every survey, exposures exceeded National Institute of Occupational Safety and Health (NIOSH) standards during some period of anesthesia.

All of these studies noted that the concentrations of waste anesthetic gas were increased when mask induction or maintenance was used to deliver anesthesia or when induction chambers were used, from which the animal was removed for surgery, saturated with anesthetic gas. Frequent disconnections of the endotracheal tube or other connections of the system leaked gas. Dumping reservoir bags into the room atmosphere was a significant contributor to this type of leakage. High flow rates increased pressure in the system and thus leakage at any loose or ill-fitting connections, especially the pop-off valves. For example, flow rates of 3 to 12 L/minute were associated with halothane concentrations of 8.9 ppm[26] in worker breathing zones. Other sources of increased waste included (1) extubation of animals immediately after anesthesia without diluting the animal's inspired gas with oxygen to limit exhaled waste gas and (2) careless spills during the filling of anesthetic vaporizers. Charcoal filters installed to absorb waste gas had minimal impact, as they were not changed and renewed frequently enough and do not absorb nitrous oxide.

Methods of minimizing exposure to waste anesthetic gases incorporate both mechanical and human factors. Anesthesia machines should be maintained well and undergo frequent routine evaluation for leak sources. The use of adequate room ventilation with rapid air exchange, especially in combination with scavenging systems that collect and evacuate anesthetic gases from personnel areas, dramatically reduces gas concentrations. In one of the previously mentioned studies,[27] installation of scavenging systems in two facilities reduced average halothane concentrations from 20 ppm to 1.1 ppm and from 4.7 ppm to 1.7 ppm, respectively, in the two facilities.

Proper procedural practices during animal anesthesia can have an additive benefit in decreasing waste anesthetic gas concentrations. These practices include minimizing chamber and mask use to induce anesthesia, using the minimal required gas flow rates, minimizing disconnections of the system during anesthesia, dumping reservoir bags only into scavenging systems, and diluting animal expired gas with oxygen. Finally, routine monitoring of the work environment for excess waste anesthetic gas may be performed using infrared analyzers or dosimeters that may be sent to appropriate laboratories for off-site analysis.

Ionizing Radiation

Because of the potential dangers associated with this occupational exposure, the National Council on Radiation Protection and Measurements outlined its regulations for the use of x-ray machines in veterinary settings.[20] These recommendations are intended to limit exposure, based on the maximum permissible dose. Reduction of radiation may be accomplished by increasing the distance of the worker from the source, decreasing the duration of exposure, and proper protection for exposed personnel through the use of barriers.

Under these guidelines, the restraint of an animal during radiography should be accomplished with the use of chemical or physical restraints and as rarely as necessary by human holding. Pregnant females and females under the age of 18 are not recommended to hold animals during radiography. When portable x-ray equipment is used, the operator should be able to stand at least 6 feet from the source. Decreasing the duration of exposure can be accomplished through several means. The radiation dosage is controlled by the kilovolt and milliamperage of the radiation energy, as well as the time over which the subject is exposed. Collimators should be used to "cone down" the useful beam of radiation to the size of the film cassette, which should also be as small as necessary. X-ray equipment should be contained in a protective tube housing, with a filter to absorb preferentially the lower energy portions of the x-ray. Thus, the greater the filtration, the greater the average energy of the beam, and the smaller the dose per a given x-ray. Whenever possible, radiography should be preferred over fluoroscopy to limit excessive exposure. Protective barriers should be available to all personnel who come in contact with ionizing radiation in the workplace. Lead aprons, neck bibs, and gloves with a thickness of at least 0.25 mm of lead should be used whenever necessary. Animals undergoing radiation therapy, which requires a greater amount of radiation, should be treated in lead-lined chambers. Occupied areas should be protected from scatter radiation with the use of lead-lined walls and doors, and the useful beam should be directed toward unoccupied areas of the clinic or hospital whenever possible. Personnel monitoring with film badges to assess cumulative exposure should be done. All of the previously mentioned methods are recommended to minimize the occupational exposure to ionizing radiation in the veterinary setting.

Chemical Exposure and Allergy

Veterinarians and animal handlers employ—and are exposed to—multiple chemicals and medications that are used to treat animals and animal environments. Flea control products applied to animals or sprayed in animal housing may cause significant medical illness if improperly used. These products are regulated as pesticides by the Federal Insecticide, Fungicide, and Rodenticide Act and are registered by the United States Environmental Protection Agency.[1] Organophosphate insecticides may represent the greatest potential chemical occupational hazard.[13] Acute excessive exposure to organophosphates can cause severe cholinergic crisis secondary to their binding and inactivation of cholinesterase. Symptoms may range from blurred vision, headache, and weakness to severe bronchospasm, pulmonary edema, abdominal cramping, diarrhea, and paralysis. Conversely, chronic low-level exposure is associated with subtle neurologic abnormalities.

In one report,[5] veterinary workers reported neuropathic pain, muscle weakness, and numbness associated with unprotected exposure to fenthion, a pesticide. In a telephone survey from California,[1] veterinary workers were questioned regarding flea control product use and adverse health effects. Products used included organophosphates, carbamates, pyrethrins, pyrethroids, d-limonene, linalool, and pennyroyal. The most frequently reported symptoms were ocular burning and excessive tearing, skin rash, flushed skin, and excess fatigue. These symptoms were generally associated with spraying and sponging of flea products. Protective rubber gloves and aprons were used by only 29% and 21% of workers, respectively. Diarrhea, muscle twitching, and mental status changes occurred more frequently when workers did not practice self-decontamination by washing hands or showering.

Several other chemical agents are used in veterinary practice.[15] Formaldehyde, which is used as a tissue sterilant and preservative for pathology specimens, may cause ocular irritation, dermatitis, and respiratory sensitization similar to asthma. Ethylene oxide is used as a sterilant for surgical instruments. It has been implicated as a mutagen and

potential carcinogen and, after inhalational exposure, associated with gastric cancer and leukemia. Finally, aerosols of clipper lubricant, grooming oils, and coat conditioners contain hydrocarbons that may cause skin and respiratory irritation. Resin-fiberglass cast materials may shed fiberglass particles when sawed, and such particles have been associated with the development of mesothelioma.

Therapeutic medications used in animal care may cause harmful side effects after excess human exposure. Antineoplastic drugs absorbed via inhalation or dermal absorption may act as mutagens, carcinogens, or teratogens.[15] Other veterinary drug mishaps that have been reported include accidental injection of xylazine, an animal sedative, causing 8 hours of coma, bradycardia, and mild hypotension,[23] and ingestion of equine phenylbutazone, a nonsteroidal antiinflammatory drug, causing coma and respiratory and renal failure.[16]

Many of the antibiotics used in veterinary practice have been implicated as causes of contact dermatitis.[5,22] The most common offending agents included penethamate, penicillins, and streptomycin.

Occupational respiratory disease in veterinarians is more likely related to allergens such as animal dander and to urinary and blood proteins, which may cause immune-mediated asthma or hypersensitivity pneumonitis.[8,10]

CLINICAL TOXICOLOGY
Reproductive Hazards

As more women enter the field of veterinary medicine, the occupational exposures associated with this field have an important bearing on the pregnant practitioner.[15] Exposure to waste anesthetic gas has been proposed to increase the incidence of spontaneous abortion and of multiple congenital abnormalities, including strawberry hemangiomata, cardiac defects, hypospadias, pyloric stenosis, inguinal hernias, and congenital hip dislocations.[7] Exposure to ionizing radiation has been reported to cause spontaneous abortion and congenital malformations involving the optic and central nervous systems. As previously mentioned, there is no level below which zero risk can be determined, but a maximum permissible dose of approximately 500 mrem over the period of gestation has been suggested.[7,18]

One study has investigated the adverse reproductive outcomes associated with these exposures.[9] In a survey of female veterinarians' pregnancies, the authors found no higher crude rates for adverse pregnancy outcomes in female veterinarians than in the general public. Odds ratios for adverse pregnancy outcomes were not found to be significant for exposure to waste anesthetic gas, alone, or to ionizing radiation, alone. However, the combination of the two exposures appeared to slightly increase the risk for adverse pregnancy outcomes. Shortfalls of this survey were noted to be the estimations of waste gas and radiation exposure, which were not actually quantified.

Infectious agents encountered in animal care that are most dangerous to the unborn child include toxoplasmosis and listeriosis. Primary maternal *Toxoplasma* infection acquired during the second trimester may subsequently infect the fetus via the placenta and result in fetal parasitemia. Spontaneous abortion, premature birth, and encephalitis may occur if the fetus is born alive. Sequelae in the infant include seizures, neuropsychiatric retardation, hydrocephalus, microcephaly, and deafness. Approximately one third of women who acquire toxoplasmosis during pregnancy do not infect the fetus.[7] Similarly, listeriosis infection may induce fetal death, listerial sepsis, meningitis, or hydrocephalus.

Carbon monoxide exposure during pregnancy can cause profound fetal hypoxia, leading to fetal death, or neurologic sequelae in live newborns. One situation in which carbon monoxide exposure may be excessive is in farrowing houses, where sows are housed in winter and artificial heat is employed without adequate ventilation.[7]

Finally, maternal exposure to any of the previously mentioned chemicals or medications may cause injury to the fetus. Of particular risk is exposure to prostaglandins, particularly PGF_2:[7] These agents are used to synchronize the estrus cycles in cattle for the purpose of various reproductive manipulations. Dermal absorption can lead to smooth muscle contractions that cause premature labor and spontaneous abortion.

Controversy exists regarding the potential hazards to pregnant women in veterinary medicine. Animal care workers are exposed to multiple occupational hazards, many simultaneously, and the contribution of each individual exposure to overall risk is not well known. There has been no dose-response relationship elucidated for most of these exposures, but, in combination, their potential for adverse effects may be additive or synergistic.

Studies to evaluate overall adverse reproductive effects provide conflicting results. One survey of veterinarians compared with lawyers noted no significant difference in overall rate of spontaneous abortion.[24] However, female veterinarians who performed more than five x-rays per week had a slightly greater incidence of spontaneous abortion, and children of veterinarians had a slightly increased rate of birth defects. Another study of childhood malignancies matched with parental employment[17] noted a slightly increased risk for all cancers in children of medical workers, including veterinarians. Risk factors for this outcome were hypothesized to be drug, anesthetic, and infectious exposures.

Knowledge and understanding of occupational exposures and their risk of adverse health effects should prompt appropriate protective wear and practices. Female veterinarians were questioned regarding their exposure to occupational hazards.[28] Although 83% reported exposure to waste anesthetic gases, 27% of those did not use scavenging systems to minimize their exposure. Although 82% reported radiation exposure, 41% did not wear film badges to quantitate exposure. Weekly pesticide use in their practice was reported by 52%. Women were noted to have made greater attempts to minimize their exposures during pregnancy, especially over the last three decades, as more information regarding adverse effects has become available.

Mortality in Veterinarians

Over the last two decades, studies have been done to examine mortality rates in veterinarians and to determine if they experience increased risks for various causes of death. Causes of veterinarian deaths from 1966 to 1977 and from 1947 to 1977 were studied and compared with expected death rates in the general population by using proportionate mortality ratios.[2,3] The authors found that the proportionate mortality ratios for white male veterinarians during these years were significantly greater for Hodgkin's and non-Hodgkin's lymphoma, leukemia, brain cancer, melanoma, and motor vehicle accidents. The increase in melanoma and motor vehicle accidents was noted in large animal practitioners and hypothesized to be secondary to excess sun exposure and a large proportion of time spent traveling to deliver on-site care. The increase in leukemia and lymphoma deaths was hypothesized to be secondary to unsafe exposure to ionizing radiation, animal viruses, or chemicals. This finding has been noted in other mortality studies in agricultural workers who have significant animal contact.[19] In a more recent study of 450 male and female veterinarian deaths in California,[14] standardized proportionate mortality ratios for white males were increased for malignant melanoma, colon cancer, and suicide. Standardized proportionate mortality ratios for females were increased for suicide.

CONCLUSION

Veterinarians, zookeepers, and laboratory animal handlers are exposed to several occupational hazards that have the potential to cause important adverse health effects and disease. At present, these effects have been reported with varying incidence but have not been well quantified in relation to given exposures. Education regarding preventable exposure, along with proper training practices, use of protective barriers, and regular health screening, may limit occupational illness in these workers.

REFERENCES

1. Ames RG et al: Health symptoms and occupational exposure to flea control products among California pet handlers, *Am Ind Hyg Assoc J* 50:466, 1989.
2. Blair A, Hayes HM Jr: Cancer and other causes of death among U.S. veterinarians, 1966-1977, *Int J Cancer* 25:181, 1980.
3. Blair A, Hayes HM Jr: Mortality patterns among US veterinarians, 1947-1977: an expanded study, *Int J Epidemiol* 11:391, 1982.

4. Dean G, Mcdougall EI, Elian M: Multiple sclerosis in research workers studying swayback in lambs: an updated report, *J Neurol Neurosurg Psychiatry* 48:859, 1985.

5. Falk ES, Hektoen H, Thune PO: Skin and respiratory tract symptoms in veterinary surgeons, *Contact Dermatitis* 12:274; 1985.

6. Gardner RJ, Hampton F, Causton FS: Inhalation anaesthetics: exposure and control during veterinary surgery, *Ann Occup Hyg* 35:377, 1991.

7. Gold CTK, Beran GW: Occupational hazards to pregnant veterinarians, *Iowa State Veterinarian* 45:55, 1983.

8. Grammar LC, Patterson R: Occupational immunologic lung disease, *Ann Allergy* 58:151, 1987.

9. Johnson JA, Buchan RM, Reif JS: Effect of waste anesthetic gas and vapor exposure on reproductive outcome in veterinary personnel, *Am Ind Hyg Assoc J* 48:62, 1987.

10. Lutsky I et al: Occupational respiratory disease in veterinarians, *Ann Allergy* 55, 2:153, 1985.

11. Manley SV et al: Occupational exposure to waste anesthetic gases in veterinary practice, *California Veterinarian* 9:14, 1982.

12. Manning NF: Coping with a buildup of waste anesthetic gases, *J Am Vet Med Assoc* 195:288, 1989.

13. Metcalf RL et al: Neurologic findings among workers exposed to fenthion in a veterinary hospital—Georgia, *MMWR Morb Mortal Weekly Report* 34:402, 1985.

14. Miller JM, Beaumont JJ: Suicide, cancer, and other causes of death among California veterinarians, 1960-1992, *Am J Ind Med* 27:37, 1995.

15. Moore RM Jr, Davis YM, Kaczmarek RG: An overview of occupational hazards among veterinarians, with particular reference to pregnant women, *Am Ind Hyg Assoc J* 54:113, 1993.

16. Newton TA, Rose SR: Poisoning with equine phenylbutazone in a racetrack worker, *Ann Emerg Med* 20:204, 1991.

17. Olsen JH et al: Parental employment at time of conception and risk of cancer in offspring, *Eur J Cancer* 27:958, 1991.

18. Pavlov H, Heneghan MA: Human radiation risk factors in veterinary medicine, *Sem Vet Med Surg (Small Anim)* 1:185, 1986.

19. Pearce N, Reif JS: Epidemiologic studies of cancer in agricultural workers, *Am J Ind Med* 18:133, 1990.

20. *Radiation protection in veterinary medicine,* Report No 36, Bethesda, 1970, National Council on Radiation Protection and Measurements.

21. Ruby DL, Buchan RM, Gunther BJ: Waste anesthetic gas and vapor exposures in veterinary hospitals and clinics, *Am Ind Hyg Assoc J* 41:229, 1980.

22. Rudzki E: Contact sensitivity to systemically administered drugs, *Dermatol Clin* 8:177, 1990.

23. Samanta A, Roffe C, Woods KL: Accidental self administration of xylazine in a veterinary nurse, *Postgrad Med J* 66:244, 1990.

24. Schenker MB et al: Adverse reproductive outcomes among female veterinarians, *Am J Epidemiol* 132:96, 1990.

25. Schuchman SM, Frye FL, Barrett RP: Toxicities and hazards for clinicians in small animal practice, *Vet Clin North Am* 5:727,1975.

26. Short CE, Harvey RC: Anesthetic waste gases in veterinary medicine: analysis of the problem and suggested guidelines for reducing personnel exposures, *Cornell Vet* 73:363, 1983.

27. Ward GS, Byland RR: Concentration of halothane in veterinary operating and treatment rooms, *J Am Vet Med Assoc* 180:174, 1982.

28. Wiggins P: Prevalence of hazardous exposures in veterinary practice, *Am J Ind Med* 16:55, 1989.

29. Wingfield WE et al: Waste anesthetic gas exposures to veterinarians and animal technicians, *J Am Vet Med Assoc* 178:399, 1981.

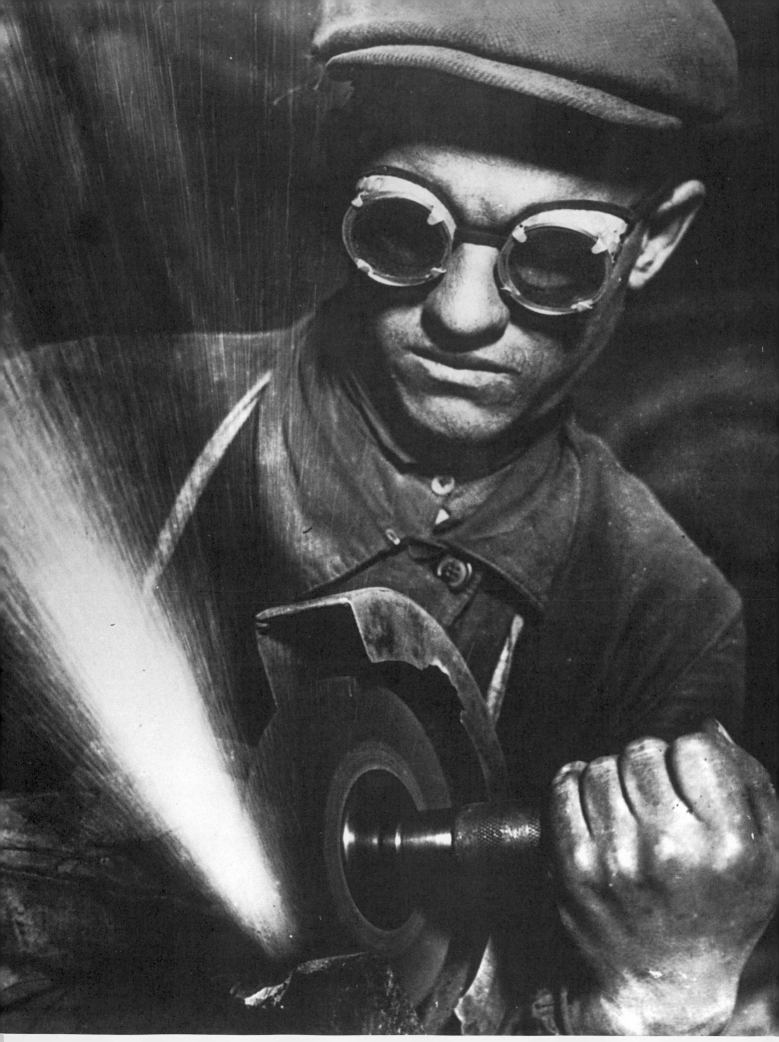

Section Two

Industrial Toxicology

Section Editor

Michael I. Greenberg

Worker grinding stone. Undated.
(Courtesy Corbis-Bettmann)

CH₃ structure label:

O₂N   NO₂

NO₂

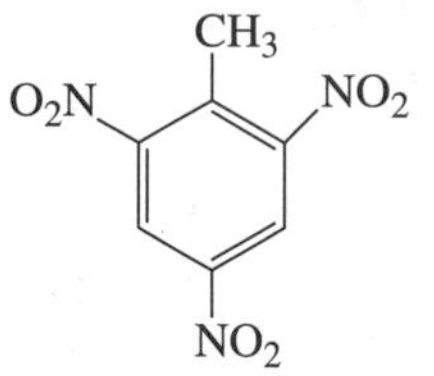

2,4,6-trinitrotoluene
(TNT)

- Acute exposure to nitrates can cause hypotension, coronary insufficiency, and methemoglobinemia

- Withdrawal vasospasm may occur in nitrate-tolerant workers who are away from work for 24 to 48 hours

- Preemployment screening, clinical monitoring, and elimination of dermal exposure are important actions to reduce occupational nitrate toxicity

Dynamite and Explosives

Surajit Suntornthan

Natalie M. Cullen

Dynamite is a widely used explosive agent. It currently consists of about 60% ammonium nitrate and sodium nitrate, 20% to 25% ethylene glycol dinitrate (EGDN), up to 5% nitroglycerin (NTG), 10% dinitrotoluene (DNT), 3% nitrocellulose, and a few percent of sawdust, chalk, and rhodomin. Ever since dynamite has been produced, the most significant toxic agent to dynamite workers has been nitrate esters or nitrate compounds.

Dynamite consists of NTG, a nitration of glycerin, which was originally synthesized in 1847 by an Italian chemist. He found that NTG detonated easily with shock, trauma, and impact. In 1867, Alfred Nobel incorporated NTG and diatomaceous earth, in an absorption process, to form dynamite. This process reduced the explosion hazard of pure NTG yet still had the characteristics of the explosive to detonate. However, this material was still hazardous to handle. Therefore, since the nineteenth century, mixtures composed of oxidizers and absorbent materials have been added to dynamite to decrease the potential danger and hazard.

Nitroglycerin, which freezes at 13° C, has unreliable explosive characteristics when it becomes frozen. The EGDN, which is produced by nitration of ethylene glycol, has been added to NTG to lower the freezing point. This additive has made dynamite much more stable. Increasing proportions of EGDN have been added to all dynamite produced since the 1920s. Ammonium nitrate, an oxidizer, has been used in formulations of dynamite since 1933. Trinitrotoluene (TNT), discovered in 1902, was also used as a component of dynamite because of its excellent explosive

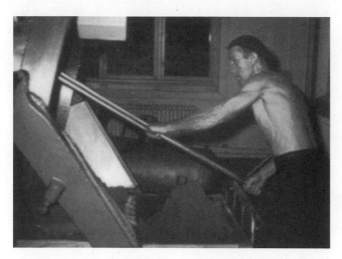

Fig. 39-1 A dynamite kneader from the 1950s. No protective equipment was used in that era. (From Zenz C, Dickerson OB, Horvath EP: *Occupational medicine,* ed 3, St Louis, 1994, Mosby.)

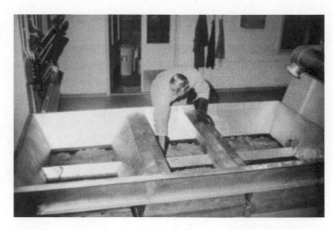

Fig. 39-2 A dynamite worker inspecting the kneaded mass. (From Zenz C, Dickerson OB, Horvath EP: *Occupational medicine,* ed 3, St Louis, 1994, Mosby.)

capacity. In the 1960s it was replaced by dinitrotoluene (DNT) to reduce explosion hazards.[28]

In the manufacturing processes of dynamite, blasting oil is produced by the mixture of NTG, EGDN, and DNT with sulfuric and nitric acids. The oil then is mixed with oxidizing salts (which mostly are ammonium nitrate and sodium nitrate), nitrocellulose, fillers (such as sawdust and chalk), and rhodomin.

In 1882, shortly after Nobel had begun producing dynamite, the first report on its occupational hazard was published.[29] During that time, the workers were usually exposed to the various compounds of dynamite directly and without protection. Many processes of dynamite production, such as kneading, rolling, and packing dynamite sticks, were done bare-handed and shirtless, especially in summertime when the factories were oppressively hot (Figs. 39-1 and 39-2). The toxic risk was increased, not only because the workers would vasodilate and absorb more of the chemicals transdermally, but also because they would have minimal protection from explosion.

In modern manufacturing, each part of the production process is performed in widely separated buildings to reduce the explosion hazards. Several manufacturing processes are automated, enclosed, and remote controlled. These measures have limited human injury. Limited quantities of explosive materials and restricted numbers of workers are allowed in any area of these factories. The greatest exposures to the substances may occur among mixers, cartridge fillers, and cleanup or maintenance workers, who appear to be at the highest risk for toxic exposure in the dynamite manufacturing industry.

Dynamites, which contain the alkyl nitrates, are only about 10% of the blasting agents used in the United States. In 1976, approximately 250 million pounds of dynamite contained 5% to 50% nitroglycerin, ethylene glycol dinitrate,

or both. About 8000 workers are exposed to these materials in the United States.[30]

The first occupational hazard report from dynamite in the United States was published shortly after the first report of a dynamite accident in 1890.[6] Some miners and tunnel workers developed severe headaches, difficulty breathing, weak pulse, pallor, drowsiness, weakness, diaphoresis, nausea, vomiting, dizziness, and/or asphyxiation after handling and inhaling dynamite and the by-products of dynamite explosions. The symptoms also developed in the workers' families, who laundered and ironed their clothes and bedclothes.[25] An increased pulse rate and alcohol intolerance were also described, as was the onset of tolerance among the workers and their families.

In addition, nearly 5% of the dynamite workers developed angina. Two of these workers died suddenly, although one death occurred 6 months after the last exposure to nitroglycerin.[24] In a study at a dynamite plant in Pennsylvania, the incidence of sudden death in workers aged 32 to 50 was about 15 times greater than the expected rate for this age group over a 4-year period.[23] More recently, a study reported 9 deaths from cardiovascular and cerebrovascular disease, compared with the national average of 4.5 expected, during 1965 to 1967 among male workers with at least 1 year exposure to dynamite and 20 years of induction-latency time.[20] Other studies have supported the increased incidence of cardiovascular and cerebrovascular mortalities among workers who have been exposed to alkyl nitrates, including nitroglycerin, ethylene glycol dinitrate, and 1,2-propylene glycol dinitrate (PGDN).[4,10,15,16,18]

CLINICAL TOXICOLOGY

Most of the substances involved in the dynamite and explosive industry are nitrate compounds. Nitroglycerin and the entire group of related compounds cause smooth muscle relaxation. Clinically, the vascular bed is most noticeably affected, although bronchial, biliary, gastrointestinal (GI), and uterine smooth muscles are also relaxed. Other common findings associated with nitrate exposure include headache, dizziness, fatigue, shortness of breath, nausea, vomiting, hypotension, palpitation, tachycardia, and angina pectoris. Some workers may be susceptible to arrhythmia and sudden death secondary to nitrate exposure.[31] There are two clinically significant vascular syndromes of occupational nitrate toxicity: acute vasodilatation and withdrawal vasospasm.

Acute Vasodilatation Effects

Exposure in the explosive industries to nitrate esters, NTG, EGDN, and propylene glycol dinitrate, which act directly on the smooth muscle of the arterial bed, can cause immediate arterial vasodilatation of variable onset and duration. Symptoms can occur related to vasodilatation, such as throbbing headache, skin flushing, light-headedness, orthostatic hypotension with reflex tachycardia, nausea, vomiting, abdominal cramps, and alcohol intolerance, as well as mental confusion, delirium, bradypnea, paralysis, and convulsions.

In addition, nitrates can be converted to nitrites in vivo. These nitrites can cause methemoglobinemia formation that is clinically demonstrated as cyanosis. Circulatory failure and death may occur.[2] Typically, the onset of action occurs in approximately 1 minute, with the maximum vascular effect in 5 minutes, disappearing in about 30 minutes, although this schedule may be quite variable.

Headaches in workers who make or use dynamite usually have a throbbing character and frequently begin in the forehead and move to the occipital region. The headaches may continue for 1 to 2 hours, or even for 3 to 4 days.[6,8,25,27,37] A sensation of facial heat and actual flushing may occur initially. Patients presenting with the headache may be restless and unable to sleep and show signs of depression. Dizziness, impaired vision, nausea, and vomiting, as well as occasional diarrhea, sweating, and abdominal pain, may accompany the headaches. Headaches may be precipitated or worsened by drinking alcohol, which can also cause hallucinations or mania.[27,34]

Systemic hypotension, especially a drop in systolic pressure, can result from sufficiently high acute NTG exposure. The patient may show signs of confusion and syncope. Hypotension may aggravate or incite cardiac ischemia or cerebrovascular disease and may even cause seizures secondary to cerebral ischemia. The generalized peripheral vasodilatation, combined with reflex tachycardia, causes rapid runoff, decreased ventricular relaxation, and a longer period of coronary blood flow, which may reduce coronary artery perfusion pressure and precipitate angina in heavily exposed individuals with preexisting coronary conditions. However, there is no study that firmly supports NTG independently causing "acute" or "acute on chronic" coronary artery disease. Tolerance seems to develop after a variable period of time. In addition, after a period away from

work, typically on Monday or after vacations, the paradoxic occurrence of cardiac arrest after reexposure to nitrates has been reported.[24] However, fatalities from hypotension are rare. After a week of exposure, workers become tolerant. This tolerance is short-lived; when they returned to work after 2 or more days away from work, the symptoms may recur. Many workers usually have acute blood pressure changes on Monday morning or after a few days away from the factory, although they may not complain of headache.[30,36] Once the tolerance occurs, workers have been known to avoid the Monday headache by placing a piece of dynamite under their headbands, sucking occasionally on a piece of dynamite, or inhaling the fumes from their workclothes over the weekend.[27]

Withdrawal Vasospasm

Workers regularly exposed to nitrates develop tolerance and may suffer angina or myocardial infarction owing to rebound coronary vasoconstriction upon sudden withdrawal of the drug. The vascular system of the habituated workers may develop a dependence on nitrates. Withdrawal from the exposure can be accompanied by vasospasm. Some workers who have become accustomed to nitroglycerine and, in particular, to ethylene glycol dinitrate due to exposure while manufacturing explosives have suffered from angina pectoris during withdrawal from exposure (on weekends or on vacations). Withdrawal affects both men and women and occurs principally in young workers. The angina typically lasts several minutes but can recur for several hours; it has been noted to last as long as 3 or 4 days in severe cases. The chest pain may be associated with palpitations and difficulty with breathing (ranging from mild shortness of breath to frank respiratory failure). These symptoms disappear when the patient returns to work, inhales fumes from workclothes, or administers sublingual nitroglyccrin.[1,22,24,26]

The most serious effect of withdrawal of NTG for a few days in chronic exposure is acute myocardial infarction and sudden death. This effect can occur even in those in whom coronary artery disease could not be proven by either arteriography or autopsy.[1,20,33,36] Often, acute withdrawal symptoms are seen in the young as well as in those with known disease. Death has been reported in workers as young as 32[30] despite the relative absence of cigarette smoking. Some nonspecific symptoms of malaise and weakness as well as the chest pain may be noted prior to sudden death, but most victims have no preceding symptoms.[3,26] Coronary vasospasm has been the postulated mechanism for these postwithdrawal symptoms.[12,21]

Other Chronic Effects

Other symptoms of chronic poisoning may include severe headache, hallucinations, and skin rashes.[2]

Increased incidence of chronic cardiovascular and cerebrovascular diseases has been associated with longtime dynamite work, usually greater than one year of exposure and 20 years of latency since first exposure.[16,17] In these studies, death rates from coronary artery disease increased about twofold, and the risk continued long after exposure ended. In addition, a threefold increased risk for sudden cardiac death in younger men with current or recent exposure was observed. The pathogenic mechanism remains unclear. The elevation of diastolic blood pressure and the promotion of atherosclerosis by the nitrate esters have been postulated and supported by animal evidence,[15] but many investigations have shown no differences in blood pressure between dynamite workers and controls. Differences have been noted only between the Monday parameters, which may be low, and those later in the week, which may increase because of compensatory mechanisms.[11,30]

Toxicity of TNT and DNT

The acute toxic effects of trinitrotoluene and dinitrotoluene exposure are similar to those of other nitrates. These agents, which can be absorbed in harmful amounts by the oral, inhalation, or dermal routes, can induce methemoglobinemia (which results in cyanosis) and hypotension accompanied by headache, irritability, dizziness, weakness, nausea, vomiting, dyspnea, drowsiness, unconsciousness, and possible death.

Prolonged exposure can cause hemolytic anemia secondary to methemoglobinemia. Skin exposure to trinitrotoluene can produce dermatitis and eczema. Trinitrotoluene can also form an irritant vapor. Other reported effects are decreased visual acuity, increased risk for cataract formation, increased mortality risk from ischemic heart disease, peripheral sensory neuropathy, and joint pain. It can also produce hepatitis and has been associated with aplastic anemia.

Toxicity of Other Agents

Ammonium nitrate and sodium nitrate, both oxidizing agents, can produce toxicity consisting of methemoglobinemia, hemolysis, dermal injury, and pulmonary injury.

Tetryl and amatol are frequently responsible for causing dermatitis. The face, collar line, wrists, and hands are chiefly affected. Especially with tetryl, exposed skin characteristically develops a yellow hue.

Picric acid (trinitrophenol), used in manufacturing rocket fuel, explosives, and fireworks, can produce skin irritation and sensitization. Inhalation of picric acid can produce weakness, headache, coma, nausea, vomiting, diarrhea, and myalgia. Hemolysis can occur, as well as renal damage and liver damage. Exposure to picric acid causes tissues (particularly skin and eyes) to turn yellow. It can also cause dermatitis and skin sensitization. Corneal injury is possible after exposure to acid dust.

Cyclonite (cyclotrimethylenetrinitramine) dust, known as hexogen HMX-RDX and RDX, can produce ocular and skin irritation, as well as irritation of the respiratory tract. Exposed workers may complain of headaches, irritability, seizures, and coma.

Toxicokinetics

Nitroglycerin and other organic nitrate compounds are well absorbed through mucous membrane, intact skin, and lung.[5,9,35] The vapor pressure of ethylene glycol dinitrate is higher than that of nitroglycerin. Therefore, workers who manufacture or use these vaporized mixtures are at greater toxic risk with ethylene glycol dinitrate than with nitroglycerin. The skin and pulmonary systems are important routes of exposure that can cause serious health hazards for dynamite manufacturing workers. Absorption of nitrate esters through these routes causes significant toxicity.[19] Nitric esters are readily reduced in the body to nitrites, which distribute rapidly to tissues from the bloodstream. The half-life time for EGDN in erythrocytes in vitro has been suggested to range from 20 to 40 minutes.[13]

DIAGNOSIS
Examination

The diagnosis of toxicity from nitroglycerin and related nitrate compounds is suggested by hypotension with reflex tachycardia and headache. In the setting of withdrawal vasoconstriction, a symptom of angina should be elicited. The patient's occupational history (type and duration of exposure) and clinical presentation are important guides for the diagnosis. Evidence of vasodilatation, including orthostatic hypotension and reflex tachycardia, should be measured. Yellow skin staining is useful for confirming the exposure.

Recommended Lab Tests and Procedures

Serum or plasma levels of nitrates are not commercially available and are not clinically useful. The Kodak Ektachem analyzer may report an increased total serum CO_2 (HCO_3). An elevation of 0.6 mEq/L in serum HCO_3 for each mmol of nitrate is observed in the presence of serum nitrates.

Twelve-lead electrocardiograms (ECG) should be performed in the patient with acute vascular effects. Although ECGs taken during episodes of pain are frequently normal, changes in ST and T waves have been noted. Potential abnormalities include changes in ST and T waves, first-degree heart block, intraventricular conduction delay, bundle branch block, atrial fibrillation, or old myocardial infarction. Some of these changes have persisted even after the worker's removal from the exposure.[16,22,24,26]

Although exercise ECGs have demonstrated ischemic changes only occasionally,[22,24] treadmill ECGs have been included in the screening program since 1970. The risk of death from coronary artery disease seems to eventually decline and return to normal.

Catheterization and angiography, in addition to showing structurally normal coronary arteries (with or without coronary artery spasm), have demonstrated elevations of end-diastolic pressure, decreased left ventricular ejection fraction, ventricular dilatation, and cardiomyopathy. Therefore, this study should be considered an important aspect of evaluating patients with symptomatic exposure.[22,24,32,33]

Because these agents also oxidize hemoglobin, the methemoglobin level should be measured. Cubital vein samples do not seem to be suitable for biologic monitoring of the total exposure. There appears to be a false elevation secondary to skin exposure to nitrates, which convert to nitrites and cause increased methemoglobinemia in vitro.

MANAGEMENT AND TREATMENT

The treatment approach to the patient is dictated by the clinical presentation. In the case of acute toxicity, removing the patient from the exposure and administering supplement oxygen, if available, are first. Monitoring for the development of systemic signs or symptoms is imperative, as is referral to a medical facility if symptoms occur. If respiratory distress occurs, such as cough or difficulty in breathing, evaluation for respiratory tract irritation, bronchitis, or pneumonitis is important. Administer symptomatic treatment, including 100% humidified supplemental oxygen with assisted ventilation as necessary.

Treat hypotension with supine Trendelenburg positioning. Fluid resuscitation with 10 to 20 ml/kg of isotonic intravenous crystalloid fluids should be administered to patients with evidence of marked vasodilatation, postural hypotension, or shock. If the patient is unresponsive to these measures, dopamine should be administered at 2 to 5 μg/kg/minute and to start and increased at a rate of 5 to 10 μg/minute as needed. Norepinephrine can be started at 0.1 to 0.2 μg/kg/minute and titrated as needed to the desired response.

If seizures occur, administer diazepam (Valium), 5 to 10 mg initially, which may be repeated every 15 minutes as needed up to 30 mg intravenously. If seizures are uncontrollable or recur, administer 15 to 18 mg/kg phenytoin initially, by very slow venous push, or dilute to 50 mg/ml, not to exceed 0.5 mg/kg/minute or 50 mg/minute, and then 100 mg orally or intravenously every 6 to 8 hours. Intravenous phenytoin must be administered slowly because it is diluted with propylene glycol, which causes cardiac toxicity when given rapidly.

Decontamination includes removal of contaminated clothing and shoes. Carefully wash the exposed skin with copious soap and water. Irrigation of exposed eyes with copious amount of tepid water or saline should be done for at least 15 minutes or until symptoms resolve. If irritation, pain, swelling, lacrimation, or photophobia persists, the patient should be seen in a health care facility.[7] A physician may need to examine the area if irritation or pain persists after washing.

If the patient is cyanotic and symptomatic, or if the methemoglobin level is higher than 30% in an asymptomatic patient, administration 1 to 2 mg/kg of 1% methylene blue is indicated via slow intravenous route. Additional doses may be required.

In the appropriate exposure-withdrawal setting (8 to 72 hours since the last exposure), evidence of ischemia by history or ECGs implies significant vasoconstriction, which should be managed conventionally. Nitroglycerin should be administered acutely via the dermal, sublingual, or intravenous route to treat the severe withdrawal symptoms of the nitrate-habituated worker; subsequent withdrawal can then be managed in a supervised medical setting. General management of the chronic vascular effects is the same as care for coronary artery disease related to any other cause.

PREVENTION

In the early times of dynamite production, workers accustomed to nitrate exposure learned to use a piece of dynamite inserted into their hat bands for preventing the symptoms of withdrawal through the weekend. Because this method may cause the chronic effects, reduction of exposure to nitrate is the best preventive measure available. Protection of workers from inhalation of vapors or skin contact is required. If the exposures can be kept at a level below the threshold of the vasoactive effect, which varies for each agent, the workers may not need to use nitrates or other vasodilators to prevent the withdrawal symptoms.

For many of those agents, including EGDN, dermal exposure can be the major source of systemic absorption; therefore, sole control of the air concentration is inadequate to control the exposure. Because rubber is not an ideal material for protective gloves in EGDN exposure, the National Institute of Safety and Health has recommended cotton or cotton-lined gloves for prevention of nitrate ester absorption: "If plastic or rubber gloves are used, cotton liners must be worn underneath them." However, occasionally some workers have remarked that they got less symptomatic (mainly headache) if they did not use the rubber gloves at all. Therefore, rubber gloves with inner cotton liners changed and disposed of as frequently as once or twice an hour have been recommended to diminish the skin resorption.[18]

No screening test is effective in reducing morbidity or mortality or predicting susceptibility in individuals. It is still recommended that, before beginning work in the explosives manufacturing industry, each potential nitrate-exposed worker should be screened with physical examination including both resting and exercise ECGs. Individuals with known or suspected coronary artery disease, cardiomyopathy, or life-threatening arrhythmias should not be assigned to work where significant exposure to nitroglycerin may occur.[14] However, there have been reports of sudden death in young and previously healthy workers who have passed the screening tests. In addition, the false-positive rate for these tests is likely to be unacceptable in a working population.

The workers should have knowledge about the toxicity of these agents. In addition, they should be regularly asked about the presence of the symptoms related to vasodilatation such as headache and light-headedness. If symptoms are present, action should be taken to identify and reduce the exposure.

Biologic monitoring may have a place for some of these agents. Such methods are particularly attractive because of the large role of dermal absorption in determining the internal dose. Unfortunately, the urine and serum levels of nitrates and their associated metabolites have not been adequately studied to validate these measurements as biologic measures. It has also been reported, but not confirmed, that measurement of serum EGDN from the arm vein may represent the local concentration resulting from skin absorption and, hence, overestimate the systemic levels.

Before exposure levels were controlled, nitrate-habituated explosives workers had significant concern surrounding nitrate-withdrawal deaths. This led to precautions that reduced exposure to nitrates in munitions production. Continued vigilance is required to keep exposures low as new agents and processes are introduced.

REFERENCES

1. Ben-David A: Cardiac arrest in an explosives factory worker due to withdrawal from nitroglycerin exposure, *Am J Ind Med* 15:719, 1989.
2. Budavari S, editor: *The Merck Index,* ed 11, Rahway, NJ, 1989, Merck.
3. Carmichael P, Lieben J: Sudden death in explosives workers, *Arch Environ Health* 7:424, 1963.
4. Craig R et al: Sixteen-year follow-up of workers in an explosives factory, *J Soc Occup Med* 35:107, 1985.
5. Craun GF, Greathouse DG, Gunderson DH: Methemoglobin levels in young children consuming high nitrate well water in the United States, *Int J Epidemiol* 10:309, 1981.
6. Darlington T: The effect of the products of high explosive, dynamite and nitroglycerin in the human system, *Med Rec* 38:661, 1980.
7. Department of Transportation: *1993 Emergency response guidebook. A guidebook for first responders during the initial phase of a hazardous materials incident,* Washington, DC, 1993, US Department of Transportation.
8. Einert C: Exposure to mixtures of nitroglycerin and ethylene glycol dinitrate, *Am Ind Hyg Assoc J* 24:435, 1963.
9. Fibuch EE, Cecil WT, Reed WA: Methemoglobinemia associated with organic nitrate therapy, *Anesth Analg* 58:521, 1979.
10. Forman SA, Helmkamp JC, Bone CM: Cardiac morbidity and mortality associated with exposure to 1,2 propylene glycol dinitrate, *J Occup Med* 29:445, 1987.
11. Forsman S et al: Medical examination of workers engaged in the manufacture of nitroglycerin and ethylene glycol dinitrate in the Swedish explosives industry. In *Proceedings of the XII Int Congr Occup Health, Helsinki* 3:254, 1957.
12. Foulger JH: The industrial nitroglycerin-nitroglycol question, *J Occup Med* 20:789, 1978.
13. Gotell P: Environmental and clinical aspects of nitroglycol and nitroglycerin exposure, *Occup Health Saf* 45:50, 1976.
14. Hathaway GJ et al: *Chemical hazards of the workplace,* ed 3, New York, 1991, Van Nostrand Reinhold.
15. Hogstedt C, Anderson K: A cohort study on mortality among dynamite workers, *J Occup Med* 21:553, 1979.
16. Hogstedt C, Axelson O: Nitroglycerine-nitroglycol exposure and the mortality in cardiocerebrovascular diseases among dynamite workers, *J Occup Med* 19:675, 1977.
17. Hogstedt C, Davidsson B: A cohort study on mortality among dynamite workers, *J Occup Med* 21:553, 1979.
18. Hogstedt C, Davidsson B: Nitroglycol and nitroglycerin in a dynamite industry 1958-78, *Am Ind Hyg Assoc J* 41:373, 1980.
19. Hogstedt C, Stahl R: Skin absorption and protective gloves in dynamite work, *Am Ind Hyg Assoc J* 41:367, 1980.
20. HSDB: *Hazardous substances data bank,* Bethesda, Md, 1993, National Library of Medicine; CD-ROM Version, Denver, 1993, Micromedex.
21. Keogh JP: Nitroglycerin induced heart disease, *J Occup Med* 21:153, 1979.
22. Klock JC: Nonocclusive coronary disease after chronic exposure to nitrate: evidence for physiologic nitrate dependence, *Am Heart J* 89:510, 1975.
23. Kristensen TS: Cardiovascular diseases and the work environment. A critical review of the epidemiologic literature on chemical factors, *Scand J Work Environ Health* 15:245, 1989.
24. Lange RL et al: Nonatheromatous ischemic heart disease following withdrawal from chronic industrial nitroglycerin exposure, *Circulation* 46:666, 1972.
25. Laws GC: The effects of nitroglycerin upon those who manufacture it, *JAMA* 31:793, 1898.
26. Lund RP, Haggendal J, Johnsson G: Withdrawal symptoms in workers exposed to nitroglycerin, *Br J Ind Med* 25:136, 1968.
27. Maccherini I, Camarri E: Nitroglycerin poisoning, *Med Lav* 50:193, 1959.
28. Myer E: Chemistry of hazardous materials. In *Oxidation-reduction phenomena,* Englewood Cliffs, NJ, 1977, Prentice Hall.
29. Nevitt B (1882): from Munch JC, Friedland B, Shepard M: Glyceryl trinitrate. II: chronic toxicity, *Ind Med Surg* 34:940, 1965.
30. NIOSH 78-167: *Criteria for a recommended standard: nitroglycerin and ethylene glycol dinitrate,* Washington, DC, 1978, US Government Printing Office.
31. Proctor N, Hughes J, Fischman M: *Chemical hazards of the work place,* ed 2, Philadelphia, 1988, JB Lippincott.
32. Przybojewski JZ: Myocardial infarction complicating dilated (congestive) cardiomyopathy in an industrial nitroglycerin worker. A case report, *S Afr Med J* 69:381, 1986.
33. Przybojewski JZ, Heyns MH: Acute myocardial infarction due to coronary vasospasm secondary to industrial nitroglycerin withdrawal, *S Afr Med J* 64:101, 1983.
34. Schwartz AM: The cause, relief, and prevention of headaches arising from contact with dynamite, *N Engl J Med* 235:541, 545, 1946.
35. Sundell L, Gotell P, Alexlson O: Effect of nitroglycerin and nitroglycol exposures. In Zenz C, editor: *Occupational medicine: principles and practical applications,* Chicago, 1975, Year Book.
36. Symanski H: Schwere Gesundheitsschädigungen durch berufliche Nitroglykoleinwirkung, *Arch Hyg Bakterol* 136:139, 1952.
37. Trainor DC, Jones RC: Headaches in explosive magazine workers, *Arch Environ Health* 12:231, 1966.

40

Fertilizer

José Eric Díaz Alcalá

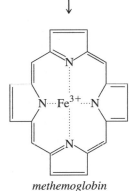

hemoglobin

↓

methemoglobin

- Nitrogen fertilizers can cause acute methemo-globinemia, although this is rare

- Anhydrous ammonia is a highly caustic substance that can cause immediate respiratory and dermatologic toxicity during occupational exposure

The fertilizer industry produces chemicals that are put in soil to improve the quality or quantity of plant growth. There are three basic types of fertilizers: organic, slow release, and soluble inorganic synthetic. In general, a fertilizer is usually a combination of nitrogen, phosphate, potassium, and other mineral nutrient materials. A fertilizer that contains all three primary elements (N-P-K) is called a *complete* or *complex fertilizer*.[24] At times, the product is classified by three numbers in a row (e.g., 3-5-92), representing the percentages of nitrogen (N), phosphorus (P), and potassium (K) by weight, respectively (see boxes on p. 328).

Organic fertilizers are obtained from plants and animals or from human waste (e.g., sewage sludge). The first manufactured fertilizer was derived from organic wastes and naturally occurring minerals including nitrogen from guano, Chilean nitrate, bonemeal, hooves, and horns; phosphorus from bone products and coprolites; and small amounts of potassium salts.[15] The inorganic fertilizers are basically divided into insoluble and water-soluble synthetic fertilizers. Slow-release fertilizers labeled as water-insoluble nitrogen (WIN) have a very high percentage of nitrogen that is released slowly. The rate of release for WIN fertilizers can be partially controlled by its granular size and membrane coating. In contrast, the nitrogen in soluble synthetic fertilizers is readily available. Furthermore, other main raw materials used in the production of inorganic fertilizers are ammonia, rock or mineral phosphates, potassium salts, and magnesium sulfate.[15] Some fertilizers may also contain poisons used to destroy pests of any sort (e.g., herbicides, insecticides, fungicides, rodenticides) and other additives for fortification (e.g., iron, copper, or zinc).

In general, liquid and granular forms of fertilizers are most commonly used to spread on the soil. Granular products are preferred in most circumstances because they

---

Sources of Nitrogen

- Bone meal
- Ammonium nitrate
- Ammonium sulfate
- Diammonium phosphate
- Fishmeal

- Monoammonium phosphate
- Processed sewage
- Seaweed
- Sulfur-coated urea
- Urea

Sources of Phosphorus

- Bonemeal
- Diammonium phosphate
- Monoammonium phosphate

- Processed sewage
- Superphosphate

Sources of Potassium

- Muriate of potash

- Sulfate of potash

Trace Elements

- Boron
- Calcium
- Copper
- Cobalt
- Iron
- Magnesium

- Manganese
- Nickel
- Sulfur
- Zinc
- Molybdenum

---

are easy to store and to apply. Other forms include sludge from animal waste and aerosolized anhydrous ammonia. More recently, as supplies of farmyard manure have fallen, the reuse of municipal sewage sludge and effluent (waste water) for agricultural purposes are becoming more prevalent. It has emerged as a means of waste disposal as well as a water resource for irrigation. Reusing the sewage reduces the cost of partially effective methods of waste treatment and serves as a simple alternative to conventional disposal methods. It can improve the chemical and physical properties of the soil, and it is a good source of plant nutrients. Sewage effluent usually contains more nitrogen, phosphorus, and potassium and lower salt concentrations than irrigation water from wells or surface reservoirs. (High salt concentrations are detrimental to plant growth.[11]) Not all sources of sewage have identical composition and vary with the geochemical characteristics of the area. Cleaning, processing, storing, and utilizing sewage sludge can be dangerous. Toxic gases may be formed, and toxic dusts may be present that could ultimately result in significant acute and chronic

toxicity.[19] Another potential problem associated with sewage application is the accumulation of heavy metals (e.g., Cd, Zn, Ni, and Pb[1,11]), pathogens (bacteria, viruses),[11] and refractory synthetic organic compounds (industrial contaminants)[11] that could enter the human food chain and pose a potential public health hazard. Those individuals processing the sewage could suffer a direct acute effect secondary to the direct exposure to heavy metals, pathogens, and refractory synthetic organic compounds.

Anhydrous ammonia and aqua ammonia are frequently used as inexpensive fertilizer. Anhydrous ammonia fertilizer is the third largest volume chemical produced in the United States, where 30% of this volume is used as a fertilizer.[21] It is also the most concentrated nitrogen source available from a fertilizer. Anhydrous ammonia compounds are usually a common cause of medical attention visits secondary to its toxicity. No known national databases record injuries or deaths due to exposure; therefore, no statistics are available. Anhydrous ammonia compound is stored and supplied to farmers in liquid form in pressurized tanks ranging in size from 5000 to 90,000 gallons at the retail distributors and 250 to 2000 gallons at the customer site. This liquefied gas is sprayed directly onto the fields. Exposure can occur during storage, transfer, and application or during connection of a tank to spraying equipment. A recent hazard and operability study of anhydrous ammonia application found that additional safety features, accurate operator procedures, and legitimate preventive equipment maintenance need to be developed and implemented to reduce the risks.[21]

CLINICAL TOXICOLOGY
Acute Exposure

In general, liquid and granular fertilizers have a low degree of toxicity. If ingested, they can cause mild gastrointestinal irritation. Methemoglobinemia may develop because of the presence of nitrates in some of them.

Anhydrous ammonia, a source of nitrogen, is extremely water soluble and forms a strong alkaline solution. In the liquid form, it is extremely caustic and causes serious burns to the skin and mucous membranes. Potential life-threatening situations can result, depending on the route, concentration, and period of exposure. Ultimately, liquefaction necrosis of tissues results from penetration and damages deep tissues. The most severe health risk is due to inhalation, compromising the respiratory system in the short and long term. Acute toxicity resulting from processing and using sewage waste is due to asphyxiation, cellular hypoxia, and acute pulmonary toxicity. The mechanism depends on the major toxic gas or dust involved.

Other fertilizers contain several additive combinations (e.g., herbicides, insecticides, heavy metals) that by themselves could be toxic. If sufficient quantities of these ingredients are involved, specific toxicity may develop. In some circumstances, it is also postulated that synergistic action of various compounds or the production of some toxic complexes—salts (e.g., copper, cobalt, and nickel) with ammonium compounds—may be the explanation of toxicity, for example, the combination of some heavy metal. After ingestion of a liquid preparation known as Kasvu, containing inorganic compounds such as heavy metal salts, ammonium compounds, and nitrates, a patient subacutely developed renal, hepatic, and respiratory failure with fatal results. Neither hemolysis nor methemoglobinemia developed, despite a high content of nitrates. Toxicologic experiments in animals showed similar results when the same preparation was used.[22]

Of the many pesticides available, organophosphate and carbamate are the insecticides that are commonly encountered in the United States. Routes of entry that could cause significant toxicity include inhalation, ingestion, and percutaneous absorption. Both toxins are lipid soluble, and the molecular targets consist of cholinesterase inhibition, particularly acetylcholinesterase (AChE), an enzyme that controls the transmission of nerve impulse at synapses. Acute classical cholinergic signs and symptoms that may develop after inactivation of AChE because of the accumulation of acetylcholine at the neuroreceptor site include headache, dizziness, weakness, nausea, vomiting, salivation, abdominal cramping, diarrhea, sweating, miosis, muscle fasciculation, tremor, seizure, and coma. Organophosphate pesticides cause muscarinic, nicotinic, and central nervous system (CNS) effects, whereas carbamate pesticides cause predominantly muscarinic effects.

Eye. In general, eye contact with any fertilizer may produce irritation. Eye injuries constitute the most serious hazard in regard to permanent disability when dealing with ammonia fertilizers. Alkaline fertilizers can produce severe eye injury, and its severity (disability) is in accordance to the amount, concentration, and duration of the exposure. A high pH has a definite pathologic biochemical action on living tissues: saponification of fats and structural alteration of proteins. The determining factor between the alkaline solutions concerning speed and extent of penetration into the eye is the water solubility of the chemical. In ammonia solutions exposure, animal studies and case reports in humans have detected ammonia or an increased pH in the aqueous humour within 5 to 30 seconds after contact.[12]

The pathologic picture of an ammonia eye injury begins upon contact, starting with epithelium slough and destruction and then corneal stroma edema. Clinically, the patient's injured eye may exhibit conjunctival hyperemia, lacrimation, and photophobia. The patient may exhibit a dull-looking cornea and may complain of severe eye pain. In severe cases, damage continues deeper to produce further inflammatory swelling, hemorrhaging, thrombosis, and, later on, neovascularization of the contacted areas. At this stage of severity, it is possible that the corneal nerves have been destroyed, producing anesthesia. Within hours or days of the injury, increased intraocular pressure (e.g., secondary glaucoma), cataractous changes in the lens, and atrophy of the whole globe or complete fusion of the affected areas into a mass of vascular granulation tissue have been noted.[12] Corneal opacity may develop slowly within a few weeks after the accident secondary to inflammatory cell infiltration with fibrous tissue scarring. When the cornea and adjacent areas are severely damaged, thrombosis of near vessels makes a poor bed for a corneal transplant.

Respiratory tract. Along with the skin, the upper and lower respiratory tract is a very common route of chemical exposure. Inhalation of dust of fertilizer mixtures can cause mild irritation of oral or nasal mucous membranes. The degree of irritation relates to the warning properties and water solubility of the chemical involved. Highly water-soluble chemicals (e.g., ammonia) most likely manifest with early strong warning signs (e.g., odor detection) and symptoms (e.g., lacrimation, hyperemic mucosa, cough, and headache) at low concentrations, and they are not usually associated with delayed onset of respiratory tract toxicity.

Alkaline fertilizers can cause adult respiratory distress syndrome (ARDS), bronchiolitis obliterans, and chronic bronchiectasis if inhaled in their gaseous form. Pulmonary fibrosis may also result after primary insult is survived. Pulmonary syndromes after contact with anhydrous ammonia differ according to exposure times and concentrations. High concentration (~2500 to 6500 ppm or greater) for short periods of time can result in an immediate feeling of suffocation and inability to speak due to laryngeal edema associated with stridor. These patients are likely to have serious burns to the upper airway that may progress to upper airway obstruction. Exposure to continuous lower concentrations (~100 to 2500 ppm) of ammonia vapor results in burns of the entire tracheobronchial tree. At lower concentrations, the upper respiratory irritation effects can be tolerated somewhat longer, leading to an increased cumulative dose in the lower respiratory tract. Once the vapor gets up to the small airways, it causes alkali burns on the mucosal surfaces, which lead to acute pulmonary edema. Gradual deterioration of pulmonary function can continue for months after the initial injury despite supportive treatment. Generally, severe lung exposures with these toxic chemicals may have an acute lung toxicity manifestation that could turn for the worse with time or have a long latency period before overt disease appears.[19]

Occupational asthma caused by sensitization to many of the additive substances to fertilizers has been reported. In the agricultural products merchant arena, a natural fertilizer containing castor bean was associated with seasonal asthma and rhinitis while the fertilizer was in storage. Six months later, the patient reported chronic bronchitis without asthma.[16]

The processing of sewage waste or liquid manure can cause pulmonary toxicity, cellular hypoxia, and asphyxiation. Toxic gases are commonly produced from the decadence of the organic waste by anaerobic degradation by facultative microbes. Hundreds of gases may be formed; fixed gases of methane, ammonia, carbon dioxide, carbon monoxide, and hydrogen sulfide are the most important.[19] High levels of hydrogen sulfide (H_2S), carbon dioxide (CO_2), and ammonia can occur, particularly during agitation of the manure material. A highly toxic colorless gas that is heavier than air, H_2S may give a characteristic rotten egg odor warning at low levels. However, at higher levels the olfactory system may be fatigued and paralyzed, and danger may go undetected. It causes cellular asphyxia or hypoxia by inhibition of the cytochrome oxidase system and is also a mucous membrane irritant. The acute clinical effects progress from nonspecific upper airway irritation signs and symptoms (e.g., sore throat, cough, and burning of eyes, nose, and throat) to systemic effects that consist of headaches, nausea and vomiting, dizziness, confusion, seizure, and coma. Death results from the toxic effect of sulfides on brain stem respiratory centers, asphyxia, and cardiac failure. Methane, CO_2, and nitrogen inert gases displace oxygen in ambient air to cause hypoxia. Carbon dioxide levels may result in asphyxiation but do not seem to cause any acute pulmonary toxicity.[19]

Sewage waste may contain toxic dusts that could affect the pulmonary system. Toxic dusts from animal dander, fecal material, and animal feeds may be present in respirable sizes. Also included in these dusts are pollens and mold spores. Asthma, bronchitis, bronchiolitis, airway obstruction, and organic dust toxic syndrome have all been reported by animal confinement workers.[19]

Gastrointestinal. Ingestion of fertilizer usually causes no symptoms other than nausea, vomiting, abdominal cramps, and diarrhea. Voluminous diarrhea has been described in superphosphate fertilizer poisoning.[6] Ingestion of 20 g (1 tablespoon) of a typical fertilizer mixture per kilogram is expected to produce gastrointestinal irritation.[24]

Neurologic. Particular neurologic effects have not been associated with fertilizer exposure. Ruminants that were accidentally intoxicated with urea fertilizer by ingestion and later died presented acutely with nonspecific signs and symptoms including muscular tremors, labile response to external stimuli, very aggressive behavior when examined, and sleepiness when left undisturbed. Urea toxicosis was illustrated by biochemical data and by extensive environmental search.[3] Urea is the innocuous end point of nitrogen metabolism in mammals; it is mainly formed in the liver and, later on, renally excreted. Hepatic encephalopathy may happen because of an impaired liver metabolism of the nitrogen excess. In ruminants, urea can be converted by bacteria to ammonia and carbon dioxide in the gastrointestinal tract. Ammonia, in contrast to urea, is the toxic substance that is rapidly absorbed and eventually detoxified

in the liver. Urea poisoning can occur only if the rate of ammonia production exceeds detoxification.

Clinical signs of superphosphate toxicosis, such as progressive CNS depression, apparent blindness, ataxic gait, marked teeth grinding, and severe diarrhea, ending in coma and death, were observed in ewes that accidentally ingested the preparation.[6]

Some organophosphate pesticides (e.g., trichlorphon and merphos), despite appropriate and aggressive treatment, can also cause delayed and chronic central and peripheral neurotoxicity that is not due to AChE inhibition. Symmetric distal and spinal cord tract axonal degeneration (demyelination) is caused by inhibition of a neuronal esterase, which appears to have a role in lipid metabolism. The clinical neuropathic findings are primary distal and sensorimotor in nature and usually starts about 1 to 2 weeks after appropriate treatment. Moreover, an intermediate syndrome has also been described, which appears 24 to 96 hours after an acute cholinergic crisis. It is a paralytic condition with a major effect on proximal limb and respiratory muscles without sensory impairment that may be associated with insufficient pralidoxime therapy.[9]

Hematologic. Hematopoietic alterations associated with nitrogenous product exposure are life-threatening if not detected and treated in time. Drug-induced methemoglobinemia and hemolysis are frequent conditions encountered in excessive nitrate exposure. The ingested, inhaled, and dermal doses of toxin required to induce methemoglobinemia are highly variable. An important environmental source for methemoglobinemia is groundwater contamination of well water with nitrogen-based fertilizers, which can cause infant death known as *well water methemoglobinemia* or *blue baby syndrome.*[23] Another source of the nitrate-nitrite compounds is decomposition of wastes containing organic nitrogen to ammonia (NH_3), which is then oxidized to nitrite (NO_2-) and nitrate (NO_3-). Methemoglobinemia may develop by conversion (reduction) of nitrate to highly reactive nitrite, in part by fecal microorganisms in the intestine when it was ingested. In addition, higher gut pH enhances the conversion of ingested nitrate to nitrite by allowing the growth of sufficient numbers of nitrate-reducing bacteria. Nitrate-nitrite toxicosis[2] could develop after they are absorbed in the bloodstream. Both nitrogen derivatives are oxidants, but nitrites are tenfold more toxic, converting hemoglobin (Hb) to methemoglobin (MHb). The effects of nitrite are the same whether nitrite-containing compounds are ingested or inhaled or nitrite is produced in vivo from nitrate.[14]

The MHb is an oxidized form of Hb. Methemoglobin inducers act by oxidizing ferrous (Fe^{2+}) to ferric (Fe^{3+}) iron Hb. Methemoglobin is not capable of oxygen transport and induces a functional anemia. Methemoglobinemia leads to a hemolytic anemia that is characterized by Heinz body formation, which is visible on special peripheral blood stains with the dark illumination method. Hemolysis occurs most frequently in patients with low tolerance for oxidative stress (e.g., glucose-6-phosphate dehydrogenase [G6PD] deficiency). In uncompromised adults, a small amount of methemoglobinemia is generally not a problem because they have adequate and mature enzymatic reduction mechanisms to maintain constant equilibrium (e.g., MHb reductase and glutathione reductase).

Nonspecific signs and symptoms (e.g., anxiety, headache, dizziness, and nausea, progressing to dyspnea, confusion, seizures, and coma) are caused by the impaired blood oxygen transport system and cellular hypoxia. Severe and life-threatening signs and symptoms most likely correspond to a higher measured MHb in most individuals.

Dermatologic. The most commonly observed dermal response to chemical exposure is contact dermatitis. The inflammation induced by exposure of the skin to an offending chemical may arise as an irritant (nonimmunologic) or an allergic dermatitis. Practically, any substance may have a direct irritant effect on the skin. For the most part, irritant dermatitis is secondary to exposure to corrosives (acids and alkalis), solvents, soap, and detergents. Allergic dermatitis is an expression of cell-mediated delayed hypersensitivity to the chemical involved; it is more likely if associated with metals (e.g., nickel, chromium, cobalt, and organomercurials). Furthermore, chemical burns could take place upon exposure to corrosives, phosphorus, and many other substances.

Allergic contact dermatitis and irritant skin reaction can develop to various materials produced in or used for agriculture. That is why it is extremely important to be familiar with the process methods, raw materials, and contaminants of fertilizers. Reported instances include irritant dermatitis due to pesticides, which are additives to many commercial fertilizers. Only a few are known to cause allergic contact dermatitis (e.g., parathion, malathion, and dichlorvos).[9] Skin irritation may develop specifically in repeated and prolonged exposure. Allergic contact dermatitis from fertilizers is not as well documented as irritant skin reaction. Allergic contact dermatitis, not in an irritable state, has been reported from use of calcium ammonium nitrate,[17] and cobalt- and nickel-containing fertilizers.[18]

Musculoskeletal. Skeletal fluorosis has been described in workers in superphosphate fertilizer production.[24] The fluoride and phosphate are thought to play a role in superphosphate poisoning. Fluoride toxicity results from direct cytotoxic and metabolic effects impairing oxidative phosphorylation, glycolysis, blood coagulation, and neurotransmission. In general, superphosphate fertilizer contains 30% calcium pyrophosphate, 10% calcium orthophosphate, 45% calcium sulfate, 5% water, 1% to 3% sodium fluoride, and up to 10% other components.[6] Symptoms of more serious intoxication include skeletal muscle weakness, tetany contractions, respiratory muscle weakness, and cardiac arrhythmias that could be associated with hypoglycemia, hypocalcemia, hyperkalemia, hypomagnesemia, and acute proximal renal tubular necrosis with hypercalciuria.

Chronic Exposures

Carcinogenicity. The genotoxicity of commonly used fertilizers is relatively less known. Some studies are trying to investigate at the chromosomal level for types of break distribution, randomness, or nonrandomness. Many of the carcinogens have been shown to cause breaks mostly at specific sites in a nonrandom fashion. Chromosomal breaks in bone marrow cells of fertilizer-fed mice were found in a nonrandom distribution when associated with urea and superphosphate and randomly distributed when associated with muriate of potash.[4]

The long-term effects of nitrates are of great concern and controversy. Carcinogenic *N*-nitroso compounds may be formed endogenously in humans by complex mechanisms. The major pathway of nitrogen excretion in humans is as urea, which is synthesized in the liver and renally cleared. Theoretically, then, prolonged diurnal exposure to airborne nitrate during fertilizer production could thus generate more endogenous nitrosation than nitrates from food. Workers exposed to nitrate fertilizers showed doubled concentrations of nitrate in their saliva as compared with people who were not occupationally exposed. It is still not known whether this process results in human cancer.[10]

A link between nitrate exposure and gastric and esophageal carcinoma and a possible association between occupational exposure to phosphate fertilizers and lung cancer have been suggested but not borne out by studies providing clear evidence of such relationships.[14,19,24] Non-Hodgkin's lymphoma has also been associated with elevated levels of nitrate in farming communities.[19] Recent studies among workers employed during the 1940s to 1980s for more than 1 year in a manufacturing site of nitrate fertilizer have shown no excessive risk of total cancer, stomach cancer, or lung cancer. No association was found between cumulated exposure to nitrate and gastric cancer, and there was no association between duration of employment or time since first employment and incidence of gastric cancer.[7,8,10,25] Despite the increase in nitrogen fertilizer used in industrialized countries, gastric cancer mortality has fallen on average by 30% since the early 1950s. Furthermore, in developing countries, the rates are mostly falling in a similar fashion.[5]

N-nitroso compounds may also be a causative factor in bladder cancer. Patients with clinical signs of bladder cancer tend to have high levels of urinary *N*-nitroso compounds. In theory, infection of the bladder with bacteria capable of both reducing nitrate and catalyzing nitrosation combine with the

---

Laboratory Studies to Consider

- Examination of blood color
- Calculated versus measured arterial saturation gap
- Methemoglobin level
- Hemoglobin and hematocrit level
- Peripheral smear (Heinz bodies)
- Serum free hemoglobin and haptoglobin level
- Urinalysis dipstick for occult blood and nitrite
- Sulfhemoglobin blood level
- Hemoglobin electrophoresis test
- Serum electrolytes and glucose levels
- Renal function test
- Liver function test
- Plasma and red blood cell cholinesterase activity

---

local irritation and ulceration of the epithelium to enhance the malignant potential of nitrates. In the Nile Delta, where annual fertilizer application is excessive, elevated urinary nitrate and *N*-nitroso compound concentrations are formed in relatively healthy young men infected with reducing bacteria and suffering from schistosomiasis.[5] In addition, a significant increase in prostate cancer incidence exists among nitrate fertilizer workers but not among other fertilizer workers.[10]

DIAGNOSIS

As with many acute toxins, rapid, assertive treatment is imperative and bedside tests may be helpful. If methemoglobinemia is suspected, an initial bedside qualitative determination can be made by placing a drop of blood on a filter paper with a control drop of blood nearby pending quantitative results: MHb is much darker in color than Hb, and it imparts a dark, brownish, or slate gray coloration to blood and tissues. If approximately 10% to 15% of MHb is suspected, then the affected blood has a chocolate brown color appearance in comparison with the control blood. A tube of MHb-containing blood does not turn red when shaken in air or when oxygen is bubbled through it, whereas blood that is dark because of a high content of normal deoxyhemoglobin turns red. For quantitative corroboration of MHb and oxygen saturation, arterial whole blood should be drawn for cooximeter blood gas analysis. If the diagnosis of methemoglobinemia is correct when the patient is treated with methylene blue, a major clinical improvement should be observed relatively fast. If that is not the case, the physician should explore the possibilities of other etiologies in a timely fashion (see box above). The differential diagnosis includes other causes of cellular hypoxia such as carbon monoxide, cyanide, severe sulfhemoglobinemia, and hydrogen sulfide. Measurements of biologic nitrate or nitrite levels in blood, urine, or saliva are not clinically useful. However, urinary and salivary nitrate-nitrite concentrations can be important indicators of exposure requiring remedial action.[14]

MEDICAL MANAGEMENT

The physician must carefully consider the possibility of toxicity secondary to fertilizer additives. In the case of carbamate and organophosphate pesticide poisoning, early and aggressive treatment consists of decontamination concurrently with resuscitative and antidotal measures. Treatment with atropine to block cholinergic effects at the muscarinic sites is considered a crucial primary antidote in both types of pesticides. In addition, early pralidoxime (2-PAM) administration is the antidote of choice to control nicotinic and CNS manifestations. It reactivates cholinesterase before an irreversible complex is achieved with the enzyme (AChE-phosphate). Successful recovery does not depend exclusively on de novo synthesis of the AChE, which takes an extended time to generate. The ChE-carbamate complex is spontaneously reversible and does not require 2-PAM therapy.

Inhalation Exposure

Immediately move patient from the toxic site to a fresh air environment. Carefully observe patients for development of any local and systemic signs or symptoms (e.g., cough, dyspnea, or hypoxemia) and administer symptomatic treatment as indicated. Administer 100% humidified supplemental oxygen with or without assisted ventilation if required. If severe pulmonary damage is suspected, early and aggressive supportive medical management is needed, which may include mechanical ventilation, oxygen, β-2 agonist, steroids, and antibiotics. Serial chest radiograph, arterial blood gases, and pulse oximetry may provide the only clue of impending pulmonary failure.

Dermal Exposure

Immediately remove contaminated clothing, and wash exposed skin with soap and copious water. Care providers must wear appropriate protective gear at all times to minimize exposure. There is rarely a need for chemical neutralization; heat generated by the neutralization reaction can potentially worsen injury.

Exposed eyes should be promptly irrigated with copious amounts of room temperature tap water or saline for at least 15 to 20 minutes or 1 liter per eye. Repeat as needed until the tear pH normalizes and signs and symptoms resolve. Local anesthetic eyedrops facilitate the irrigation process. Do not instill any neutralizing solution into the eye. Ideally, flushing of the eyes should start within seconds of exposure and continue until the patient reaches medical attention. Complete elimination of the chemical may be impractical, but a rapid, copious irrigation is essential in minimizing damage by limiting the duration of exposure. Close ophthalmology follow-up is warranted in all cases and especially if irritation, pain, swelling,

lacrimation, photophobia, and worsening of visual acuity persist after irrigation.

Oral or Parenteral Exposure

Emesis and gastric lavage are contraindicated in alkaline fertilizer ingestion and may increase gastrointestinal mucosal injury. In other fertilizer ingestions, if a massive and life-threatening exposure is suspected, immediate gastric lavage is indicated once airway protection is undertaken. Otherwise, administration of activated charcoal without emesis is a sufficient decontamination strategy.

Methemoglobinemia and Sulfhemoglobin

Therapy is directed toward reduction of MHb to Hb to provide sufficient oxygen transport for survival, since MHb is unable to carry either oxygen or carbon dioxide. In general, treat patients who are cyanotic, symptomatic, or if MHb concentration is greater than 30%. Under normal circumstances, a mildly elevated MHb level (15% to 20%) resolves spontaneously. The normal value of MHb is 0.5% to 2.5% of total Hb. Administer 100% oxygen to all cyanotic patients while preparing for methylene blue therapy to fully saturate all remaining normal hemoglobin. Methylene blue is a thiazine dye that reverses drug-induced methemoglobinemia. The therapeutic dosage is 1 to 2 mg/kg/dose (0.1 to 0.2 ml/kg/dose of 1% solution) intravenously over 5 to 10 minutes; it may be repeated in 30 to 60 minutes. It has a rapid onset of action, and maximal effect should be expected within 30 minutes. In excessive doses (more than 7 mg/kg), methylene blue is an oxidizing agent that could worsen the clinical condition. In addition, methylene blue therapy, to be successful, requires the presence of adequate amounts of G6PD and nicotinamide-adenine dinucleotide phosphate (NADPH) met Hgb reductase. Methylene blue should not be administered to a patient with known G6PD deficiency, as severe hemolytic anemia may develop. If the diagnosis is correct, a major improvement should be noticed shortly after administration. For severe, life-threatening MHb, especially for complicated or poor responders, treatment options include exchange transfusion and hyperbaric oxygen therapy (HBO). Ultimately, successful medical management is reached only when the nitrate source is identified and eliminated totally from the patient's environment.

In theory, ascorbic acid could be an adjunct therapy against methemoglobinemia. Ascorbic acid reduces MHb to Hb by a NADPH-dependent pathway[13] but is of very limited value in life-threatening situations because of its slow action.[2] A balanced diet with vitamins C, A, and E (nitrite scavengers) is helpful since it appears to protect against the development of methemoglobinemia and may inhibit the formation of carcinogenic *N*-nitrosamines.[10,25]

In cases of H_2S intoxication, there is controversy about the efficacy of antidotal treatment with nitrites. Potential benefit with nitrite therapy relies on the production of MHb, which has a greater affinity for sulfide than does the cytochrome oxidase. In theory, sulfmethemoglobin (SMHb) formation is far less toxic than H_2S, and cellular aerobic metabolism should be expected to resume. SMHb may undergo autooxidation-reduction to ferrohemoglobin and various toxic sulfur oxides. The induction of MHb alone does not fully explain nitrite effectiveness in H_2S poisoning. Additional hypotheses for the efficacy of nitrite include vasodilatation, direct stimulation of cytochrome oxidase, and MHb-independent inhibition of the binding of sulfide to cytochrome oxidase.[20] In severe cases, a reasonable modality to consider is HBO, which has improved clinical status in some cases.

H_2S can react with Hb to form sulfhemoglobin (SHb), in which sulfur incorporates into the porphyrin ring. In SHb, no therapy has proven to be of benefit. Methylene blue administration has no proven therapeutic effect. In general, SHb is usually not a fatal disorder,[14] and aggressive supportive management is sufficient. Formation of SHb reduces the oxygen-carrying capacity of the Hb, but there is a decreased affinity for oxygen in the remaining unaltered Hb, thereby facilitating unloading oxygen to the tissues. In severe, life-threatening SHb situations, HBO therapy is a rational medical management alternative to be considered.

CONCLUSION

Physicians must be aware of the need for immediate and proper emergency treatment methods for fertilizer toxic exposure, but preventive measurements by far are the most important factor in minimizing or eliminating injuries. Use of materials such as fertilizers is not without serious hazards. Their composition should be known before direct contact or use. Vigorous law enforcement can reduce injuries, in conjunction with more rigid standards for safety in the use of these chemicals by the fertilizer industry. Development and distribution of an accurate and complete material safety data sheet (MSDS) can identify health and safety information about these hazardous chemicals.

It is also important for manufacturers to educate their employees and their customers in proper operating procedures for storage, transfer, and use of these fertilizers through frequent, up-to-date safety seminars. Handling and transfer equipment should be engineered for fail-safe operation to minimize further human error and negligence injuries. At all times, proper personal protective equipment (e.g., full-face shield and chemical-type eye protection) must be worn and universal precautions followed. Finally, adequate first aid equipment (e.g., copious emergency water) must be available at the site of injury prior to transferring the patient to a medical facility for further evaluation and management.

REFERENCES

1. Berrow ML, Webber J: Trace elements in sewage sludges, *J Sci Fd Agric* 23:93, 1972.
2. Burrows GE: Nitrate intoxication, *Am Vet Med Assoc* 177:82, 1980.

3. Caldow GL, Wain EB: Urea poisoning in suckler cows, *Vet Rec* 128:489, 1991.

4. Chaurasia OP: Randomness of chromosome breaks in bone marrow cells of fertilizer-fed mice, *Mus musculus, Cytobios* 67:7, 1991.

5. Conway GR, Pretty JN: Fertilizer risks in the developing countries, *Nature* 334:207, 1988.

6. East NE: Accidental superphosphate fertilizer poisoning in pregnant ewes, *J Am Vet Med Assoc* 203:1176, 1993.

7. Fandrem SI et al: Incidence of cancer among workers in a Norwegian nitrate fertiliser plant, *Br J Ind Med* 50:647, 1993.

8. Fraser P: Nitrates: epidemiological evidence, *IARC Sci Publ* 65:183, 1985.

9. Fuortes LJ et al: *Cholinesterase-Inhibiting Pesticide Toxicity,* Washington, DC, 1993, US Department of Health and Human Services.

10. Hagmar L et al: Cancer morbidity in nitrate fertilizer workers, *Int Arch Occup Environ Health* 63:63, 1991.

11. Hamilton DL, Brockman RP, Knipfel JE: The agricultural use of municipal sewage, *Can J Physiol Pharmacol* 62:1049, 1984.

12. Helmers S, Top FH, Knapp LW: Ammonia and eye injuries in agriculture, *Sight-Saving Review* 41:9, 1971.

13. Henretig FM: Cyanosis unresponsive to oxygen administration in three children, *Pediatr Emerg Care* 1:205, 1985.

14. Kross BC, Ayebo A, Hall A: *Nitrate/nitrite toxicity,* Washington, DC, 1991, US Department of Health and Human Services.

15. Mattingly GEG: Inorganic fertilisers, *Education in Chemistry* 16:41, 1979.

16. Merget R et al: Seasonal occupational asthma in an agricultural products merchant—a case report, *Allergy* 49:897, 1994.

17. Pasricha JS, Gupta R: Contact dermatitis due to calcium ammonium nitrate, *Contact Dermatitis* 9:149, 1983.

18. Pecegueiro M: Contact dermatitis due to nickel in fertilizers, *Contact Dermatitis* 22:114, 1990.

19. Shaver CS, Tong T: Chemical hazards to agricultural workers, *Occup Med* 6:391, 1991.

20. Snyder JW et al: Occupational fatality and persistent neurological sequelae after mass exposure to hydrogen sulfide, *Am J Emerg Med* 13:199, 1995.

21. Spencer AB, Gressel MG: A Hazard and operability study of anhydrous ammonia application in agriculture, *Am Ind Hyg Assoc J* 54:671, 1993.

22. Takki S, Heinonen J, Taskinen E: Poisoning caused by a mixture of plant-nutrient substrates, *Arch Toxicol* 28:270, 1972.

23. Tarcher AB: *Principles and practice of environmental medicine,* New York, 1992, Plenum.

24. Temple AR et al: Fertilizers, *Tomes Medical Management—Micromedex* 86:1, 1995.

25. Zandjani F et al: Incidence of cancer among nitrate fertilizer workers, *Int Arch Occup Environ Health* 66:189, 1994.

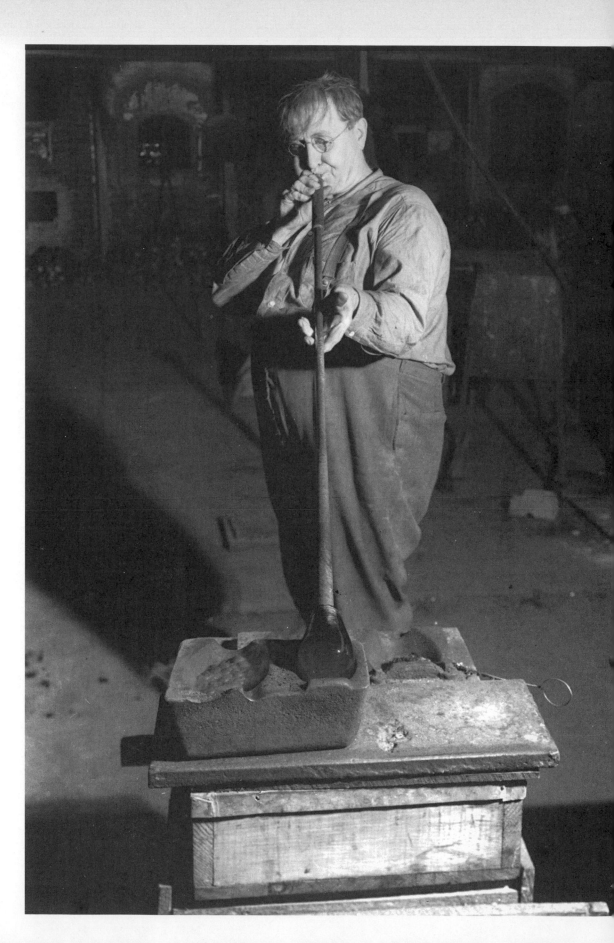

Glass blower. The bottle begins to take shape. First preliminary blowing. Undated. (Courtesy Corbis-Bettman)

Glass Manufacture

Natalie M. Cullen
Christine M. Stork

As
arsenic

HF
hydrofluoric acid

- Lead is a significant toxin for professional glassmakers, hobbyists, and family members of each of these groups

- Other metals including arsenic, manganese, and nickel are potential toxins for those working in glass production

- Heat related illness can be a problem for glassmakers working in areas with poor environmental control of ambient temperature

OCCUPATIONAL DESCRIPTION

Glass is defined (by Morey in 1938) as "an inorganic substance in a condition which is continuous with, and analogous to, the liquid state but which, as the result of having been cooled from a fused condition, has attained so high a degree of viscosity as to be, for all practical purposes rigid."[22] The American Society for Testing Material (de-Jong, 1989) defines *glass as* "an inorganic product of fusion that has cooled to a rigid state without crystallizing."[22]

Glass is found naturally in the form of obsidian, pumice (foam glass), and tektites (glass pieces, probably from meteorites). Smelting, historically noted as early as 3500 to 2000 BC, has consisted of melting tektite and then allowing it to cool. Melting of these and other raw materials forms the basis for modern-day glassmaking.

The major component of glass is silica. Many chemical mixtures technically form glass, but the major four types are soda-lime-silica, lead-potash-silica, borosilicate, and others. Soda-lime-silica is the most abundant and most versatile. It is used for flat glass, low-cost containers and glassware, and light bulbs. The lead-potash-silica is used in the production of heavy crystal, optical glass, and much hand-blown art glass. It is easy to cut and polish and is highly refractive. Its lead content makes it valuable in the electronics industry, as its inherent properties provide effective electrical resistance and radiation protection. The low thermal expansion makes bromosilicate useful for laboratory glassware as well as in domestic ovens.

Silica is the sand formed by crushed rock quartz and is the major ingredient of glass manufacturing. Often this sand is not pure silica; it may be mixed with sodium (soda ash or salt cake), potassium (carbonate or nitrate), limestone/dolomite, boric acid, or borate. Cullet is broken or crushed glass (waste glass) that is almost always added during smelting. Other chemicals seen in glass manufacturing include contaminants (ferric oxide being the most frequent, followed by titanium dioxide, zirconium dioxide, and chromium oxides), decolorizers (selenium, oxides of manganese, cobalt, and nickel), colorizers (transitional metal oxides: cobalt, nickel, chromium, iron, manganese, copper, vanadium, and cadmium), and aids for different purposes (fluorides to reduce viscosity and aid in melting, zirconium dioxide to raise the softening point, cerium oxide to stabilize against ultraviolet (UV) discoloration).

The process of glassmaking consists of three basic steps: melting, fining, and homogenizing. Melting occurs in tanks at temperatures in the range of 1200-1650° C. The processes of decarbonation, desulfurization, and dehydration also occur at this stage. Cullet (waste glass) is added to the cold batch to reduce the heat needed to melt raw materials and reduce dust during batching. Fining, the process of removing bubbles, can be accomplished either chemically (with sodium sulfate or arsenic and antimony trioxide) or by varying the temperature (increased temperature causes decreased viscosity and bubble expulsion, whereas decreased temperature causes gas absorption). Homogenization, which is the blending process, occurs as the mixture is adequately stirred. These steps can be either fully automated or completely manual; generally speaking, the more specialized the glass, the less automated the procedure. Based on the widely disparate processes involved in this industry, it is easy to see that the exposure of workers to heat and chemicals can be extremely variable.

Essentially five major types of glass are produced today: flat glass, containers and pressed ware, art glass, special glass (including optical, ophthalmic, electronic), and fiberglass. These are formed by blowing, pressing, drawing, or casting the molten glass. Glassblowing as a process is usually reserved for art objects or objects with complicated shapes. Shapes can be obtained by either handforming or by partially automated techniques. The blowing itself is either via mechanical means or by mouth. Pressing techniques are used to produce relatively flat objects. Press molds are usually made of cast iron, bronze, steel, or superalloys. Molds often require lubrication with any of the following lubricants: mineral oil, graphite, or other organic materials—tallow, oleic acid. Any of these substances may present significant health risks. Drawing is used for sheet glass. Grinding and polishing procedures are necessary in many techniques because imperfections are inevitable. Floating occurs when molten glass is poured into a molten bath of tin. In this process, the molten glass is drawn vertically to create flat glass similar to sheets or plates. Unlike plate or sheet glass, float glass has a fired finish that is free of distortion because the glass conforms to the perfect surface of the tin. Sulfur dioxide may be used at this point to further decrease the risk of marking. This produces mirror-quality glass in large quantities.

Annealing is the process of uniformly heating the glass product to reduce internal stress. This process is necessary for all forms of glass. Secondary processes for glass production include cutting, polishing, grinding, heat/chemical processing, and coating. Grinding removes the outer surface. Both natural (quartz, sandstone, diamond, garnet, and corundum) and synthetic (silicon carbide, aluminum oxide, and boric oxide) abrasives are used along with water or other solutions. Liquids are necessary to carry the abrasive and also as a cooling vehicle. Polishing is done either mechanically or chemically. Mechanical polishing is accomplished with fine powder abrasives such as rouge or ferric oxide and cerium oxide. Chemical or acid polishing uses sulfuric acid, hydrofluoric acid, or flame polishing. Enamels or metals may be applied either decoratively or as a means of transmission or reflection of light for electrical semiconductors, resistors in electrical circuits, defrosting agents, or aircraft glazing.

POTENTIAL TOXIC EXPOSURES

All of the chemicals and materials thus far discussed represent a source of potential health hazards for workers in the glass manufacturing industry. However, the greatest risk for acute health problems, is thermal exposure (heat-related illness and burns) during the melting process and chemical burns. Prior to the 1960s, there was also the risk of asbestos exposure. Until that time, asbestos insulated the vats used in melting; however, this is no longer the case. Silica, the most abundant chemical used in glassmaking, is of minimal risk because of its relatively inert properties. Silicosis, which is a lung disease that many industrial workers acquire if exposed to silica particles, seems to be a minimal health risk to the glassworkers because silica dust and particles are in limited quantities. Although glass is mostly silica, in the glass manufacturing industry, silica is found either in its molten state or as a solid. Silica particles small enough to enter the small airways to cause silicosis are rarely found in large enough quantities to be a significant risk in this population. Lead may increase the risk of cancer when combined with other chemicals used in this industry. Minimal health risks can occur during the melting process because of the following contaminants: ferric oxide, titanium oxide, zirconium dioxide, and chromium oxides. Decolorizers such as manganese and nickel, as well as colorizers (nickel, manganese, copper), appear to present a significant cancer risk to workers. In addition, the chemicals used in the fining process, arsenic and antimony, are also carcinogens. Selenium, used as a decolorizer, may actually have a preventive role in the development of cancer in this population.[22] Another health concern, specifically in glassblowers, is the development of respiratory abnormalities secondary to chronically elevated airway pressures. This same phenomenon occurs in vocalists and musicians who play wind instruments.[33]

Perhaps one of the most significant exposures that individuals involved in glass manufacture face involves hydrofluoric acid. The clinical toxicology of this and related compounds is discussed below.

CLINICAL TOXICOLOGY

Historically, a vast array of chemicals were used in the glass manufacturing industry. Consequently, toxic exposures can be diverse and significant. This chapter discusses how the major components needed to make glass today are potential health risks in this industry.

Acute health risks in the glass manufacturing industry are rare. The physical conditions of the factories, specifically high ambient temperatures, may cause problems such as heat-related illness and thermal burns. Burns may also occur chemically secondary to the use of hydrofluoric and sulfuric acids used in polishing and etching. Other acute health injuries or acute toxic exposures in this industry are extremely rare and should be considered on a case-by-case basis.

The majority of health problems in the glass manufacturing industry appear to be related to chronic low-level toxic exposures to chemicals that result in an increased risk of stomach cancer, colon cancer, and cardiovascular disease. There also appears to be an increased prevalence of lung cancer.[22] Toxic manifestations can also occur from exposure to polycyclic aromatic hydrocarbons, which are generated by oil furnaces and in mineral oils used to lubricate molds. As mentioned earlier, glassblowers specifically suffer an increased risk of chronic cough, wheeze, bronchitis, chronic obstructive pulmonary disease, and change in airway pressures.

Chemical exposures in the glass manufacturing population are generally extremely complex events. The complexity is due to low-level, multisubstance exposures over prolonged periods. This is partly due to what appears to be a very low job turnover rate in the industry. The risk of toxicity also appears to be greater in this industry than in many others because of the general dependence on manual skills as opposed to automation. The combination and interaction of multiple chemicals may enhance the development of the carcinogenic process. This is noted by the increased frequency of specific cancers that occur with certain combinations of chemicals.[32] For example, stomach cancer is strongly associated with exposure to arsenic, copper, nickel, manganese, and, to some extent, lead and chromium. A decrease in stomach cancer is associated with exposure to antimony, cadmium, selenium, and zinc. The combined exposure to manganese and chromium has demonstrated a dose-related increase in frequency in stomach cancer that appears to be minimal with the combination of nickel and copper. Likewise, any combination of chemicals with arsenic seems to increase the risk of stomach cancer. Colon cancer is an increased risk to those exposed to antimony and, to some extent, lead, especially in combination.[22] No metals, with perhaps the exception of arsenic, have been noted to increase the risk of lung cancer. There has

been some speculation that low-level lead, as well as arsenic, may increase the risk of lung cancer and that nickel may actually be protective, but these hypotheses have yet to be substantiated. Cardiovascular illness is uniformly influenced by the chemicals used in this industry, although there may be evidence that the risk is somewhat increased with the exposure to nickel and copper.[22] Therefore, exposure to certain metals and their combinations is again a complex matter. Further basic science and epidemiologic studies are needed to delineate the risk of each chemical individually and in combination in order to fully elucidate carcinogenic potential.

HYDROGEN FLUORIDE
Workplace Exposures

Work place concentrations of HF correlate linearly to serum fluoride in a study of asymptomatic HF workers who were tested pre and post 8 hour shifts.[17] Industrial accidents have also been reported with HF. Approximately 3000 persons were evacuated from a Texas community after a HF spill.[31] Of those presenting to the emergency department, the most common complaint was eye irritation, followed by throat burning and headache.

Pathophysiology

Unlike many dangerous acids, HF is a weak acid. The toxicity associated with HF exposure is caused by the formation of fluoride ions after primary dissociation and, to a lesser degree, hydrogen ions. Once in contact with human tissue, HF slowly dissociates and penetrates tissue via a nonionic diffusion gradient with a permeability constant similar to water. Fluoride ions then form a stable bond by combining with calcium or magnesium in tissue and bone. HF burns are also unique in that they readily produce systemic toxicity. In fact, a topical burn as small as 2.5% body surface area (BSA) burn has been reported to cause death. A 14-month-old who sustained an 11% BSA burn with an 8% solution of HF developed systemic toxicity and full thickness burns.[6] The systemic toxic effects of HF occur when fluoride complexes to cause hypocalcemia and hypomagnesemia and enables potassium influx through calcium dependent channels.[9]

Approximately 1-2 grams of calcium gluconate dissolved in 30 g of a water soluble jelly should be applied liberally and kept in contact with the exposed tissue. Because the appearance of the burn may not correlate with tissue damage, pain relief is the endpoint of therapy.

If topical calcium fails to provide pain relief, intradermal injections of calcium gluconate may be attempted. This may not be possible in certain areas, such as under the finger tips. Intraarterial calcium may be employed in patients where either intradermal calcium fails to provide pain relief or in which intradermal therapy is not possible.[28] The dose is 10 mL of a 10% solution of calcium gluconate dissolved in 40 mL of normal saline and infused intraarterially over 4 hours. This mode of therapy is often successful, but the risks of intraarterial infusion and damage of tissue due to calcium need consideration.[10,27] Some authors have also described an intravenous regional calcium gluconate infusion using Bier's method (Bier block).[14] However, this mode of calcium administration carries with it significant risks of an acute intravenous load of calcium.

If systemic signs of toxicity manifests (hypocalcemia or hypomagnesemia), intravenous replacement therapy should be given. A study evaluating the effect of intravenous magnesium in rabbits and rats for the treatment of hydrofluoric acid burns found wound improvement with magnesium treatment, however, further study is required to substantiate their results.[8,30]

The less common routes of HF exposure are ocular, pulmonary, and enteral exposures. These exposures must be treated aggressively because they may result in a large degree of morbidity and mortality. The use of calcium and/or magnesium salts in the eye remains controversial because of the potential ocular damage that may result from CaF.

Treatment

The administration of a cation able to complex the fluoride ion neutralizes HF. Temporizing therapy in the field may make use of readily available solutions such as Epsom salt (magnesium sulfate) or benzalkonium chloride applied to the affected area. Once medical attention is available, patients suspected of hydrofluoric acid exposure should first be given a trial of calcium gluconate. Calcium gluconate is the calcium salt of choice because it is less irritating to the tissues than calcium chloride.

In an experiment with rats given a 20% hydrofluoric acid burn, simple irrigation with water and application of 2.5% calcium gluconate gel was effective.[16] In a retrospective review of 237 cases of dilute (6-11%) hydrofluoric acid dermal exposure, 219 experienced symptoms, 3 of which developed into fingertip necrosis. Early application of calcium gluconate gel hastens the resolution of pain.[26] Several studies have been performed in an attempt to identify the most efficacious method of calcium administration. In a pig model, topical therapy is efficacious for superficial burns and subcutaneous injection is necessary for deeper burns of the dermis or sub-dermis. The use of depilatories that degrade skin integrity and enhance the ability of hydrofluoric acid to penetrate the skin limit the usefulness of this model.[11] For late therapy, calcium gluconate may be beneficial even one week after initial application, whereas treatments with benzalkonium chloride, A and D ointment, aloe gel, and magnesium gel are not.[5] Finally, topical magnesium was less effective than calcium for the treatment of dermal HF burns in one rabbit model study.[6]

Heat exposure and thermal burns are cause for major health concerns in the glass manufacturing industry. The body produces heat as a by-product of energy production. This increase in body temperature is closely regulated by the brain but may be altered in certain circumstances, such as exposure to increased ambient temperatures. The mecha-

nisms used to help keep the body temperature stable include conduction (2% of the body heat loss), convection (minimal body heat loss), radiation (up to 65% body heat loss in cool ambient temperatures but may actually be a means of heat gain with high ambient temperatures), and evaporation (0.58 kcal/ml of water evaporated—major mechanism of heat loss as ambient temperatures rise). Elevated ambient temperatures predispose workers to heat illnesses such as heat cramps, syncope, exhaustion, and stroke. Other predisposing factors for these heat illnesses are dehydration, manual labor, and lack of acclimatization to the environment, as well as underlying diseases (e.g., cardiac disorders, gastroenteritis, skin diseases that do not permit adequate sweating) and medication and drug use (e.g., anticholinergics, neuroleptics, β-adrenergics). Another potential problem in heat-related illness is occlusive, vapor-impermeable clothing or dressings that inhibit evaporation and conductive cooling.

Heat cramps actually represent a mild form of heat illness. These cramps, unlike those that afflict athletes, usually occur after strenuous work during a period of rest. The frequency is greatest during the first few days of work in a hot environment. These muscle cramps may be confused with hyperventilation syndrome. Carpopedal spasm, as occurs in hyperventilation, is associated with muscle cramping, as well as paresthesias and circumoral tingling. The paresthesias and circumoral tingling are the most notable differentiating factors between these two disease processes. The causes appear to be secondary to mild dehydration and insufficient salt intake. The best treatment is prevention: gradually increased heat exposure and maintaining adequate fluid and salt balance. Heat edema is inconsequential clinically but may also be seen during the first few days of exposure to heat. Deep vein thrombosis, thrombophlebitis, lymphedema, and congestive heart disease must be ruled out; once malignant causes have been ruled out, the swelling can be considered self-limiting. Heat syncope may occur secondary to a hot environment. This self-limiting condition is secondary to significant venous blood pooling in the periphery that leads to a decreased venous return to the heart. Often, on becoming syncopal, the patient assumes a horizontal position, which tends to increase blood flow to the thorax and heart and also cardiac output. Consequently, symptoms tend to resolve, and the worker may not seek medical attention. In this setting, the greatest concern is the safety of the patient and those around the area if syncope occurs. The laboratory diagnosis of these illnesses involves identifying low serum and urine sodium and chloride in association with the symptoms previously mentioned. The specific treatment involves removal from the heat source as well as adequate fluid replacement. Fluid should be replaced orally with a 0.1% to 1.2% salt solution (either 2 to 4 10-g salt tablets or ¼ to ½ tsp of salt in one quart of water). If symptoms are severe, 0.9% to 3% saline solution may be given intravenously. Salt tablets should not be ingested without first being dissolved in water because they may cause stomach erosion.

Heat exhaustion and heat stroke are significantly more serious displays of heat illness that can occur in the glass manufacturing industry due to high ambient temperatures in the plant. Heat exhaustion is thought to be caused by a combination of water or salt depletion and heat stress. Heat stress occurs during the body's exposure to excessive heat in the nonadapted state. Symptoms that characterize this illness include malaise, fatigue, headache (often frontal), vertigo, impaired judgment with other mental functions intact, and moderately elevated temperature (below 40° C [104° F]). Typically, the condition is resolved with the administration of fluids, either orally or intravenously (depending on the degree of dehydration and electrolyte abnormalities), and removal of the patient to a cool environment. Heat stroke is the most serious clinical situation in the spectrum of diseases known as heat illness. Heat stroke consists of all the symptoms of heat exhaustion, but in addition has central nervous system (CNS) involvement. It can include altered mental status, coma, and seizures, as well as multisystem tissue damage and end-organ dysfunction. The body's core temperature usually is recorded at levels greater than 41° C or 105° F. The severity of this disease is a product of time and temperature. The hallmark of heat stroke is CNS involvement, often with accompanying brain edema. All major organs show signs of ischemia because of a functional hypovolemia secondary to cutaneous vasodilatation. Anhydrosis may occur in 50% or more of these patients. Excessive cardiovascular demands are manifested by tachycardia as high as 170 to 200 beats per minute. Rhabdomyolysis and renal failure can occur and must be managed aggressively. Hepatic damage is so consistently found with heat stroke victims that its absence should cast serious doubt about the diagnosis. Coagulopathy is often seen in severe cases. Heat stroke occurs as the thermoregulatory responses fail. The differential diagnosis includes drug-induced heat illness, meningitis and encephalitis, thyroid storm, and serious infections. Malignant hyperthermia or neuroleptic malignant syndrome must also be considered in the appropriate setting. The mainstay of treatment, as for all the heat illnesses, is cooling and supportive care. Heat stroke is truly a medical emergency, and the patient requires close monitoring in an intensive care setting. The best treatment is prevention. Total body water deficits must be calculated and half replaced in the first 8 hours and the second half replaced in the following 16 hours. Icewater immersion has been shown to be the most effective method of cooling because it uses the principle of thermal conductivity. This technique utilizes the following principle: When objects are in contact (human body and water), heat flows from the hotter to the cooler object. This basic physics principle is often expressed as "the flow of heat." Evaporation using cool mist and air currents (fans) is another method that appears to be less effective. Ice packs, cooling blankets, and gastrointestinal (gastric or rectal)

lavage seem to have no significant benefit in cooling core temperature.[24] More heroic and extraordinary methods include cardiovascular bypass and peritoneal dialysis. These measures are generally reserved for those who are resistant to standard therapy. Antipyretics are contraindicated and should be avoided. Salicylates uncouple oxidative phosphorylation, which increases metabolic rate, CO_2 production, glucose utilization, and heat production. This may actually worsen hyperthermia. They may also cause or worsen a preexisting coagulopathy.

Thermal burns are another significant health concern in the glass manufacturing industry. High-temperature vats are used to melt silica and cullet to produce molten glass. During such processes, workers can sustain thermal burns. Burns are usually classified by degree (% body surface area, BSA) and depth (partial or full thickness). Partial-thickness burns are further subclassified into first and second degree; full-thickness burns are subclassified as third or fourth degree. *First-degree burns* are defined as heat injury to the epidermis causing minimal injury (i.e., redness of the skin). *Second-degree* is defined as a thermal injury to the epidermis as well as the dermis. The depth can be superficial or deep. Usually, there is some injury to the hair follicles, sweat glands, and stratum germinativum (the layer in the skin where new epithelial cells are formed), but these adenexal structures remain intact. Third-degree burns damage structures below the epidermis, dermis, and adenexal structures. If the burn is deep enough to cause injury to the muscle, fascia, or bone it is classified as a fourth-degree burn. Generally, full-thickness and deep partial-thickness burns require eventual referral to a plastic surgeon for skin grafting. The determination of %BSA of the burn is critical in the evaluation of a burn patient because it has important significance for the overall treatment and prognosis. Body surface area can be calculated in several ways. The most widely used is either the "rule of 9" or the "rule of palms." The former assigns values in multiples of 9 to 11 different body regions and an additional 1% to the perineum. The latter assumes that the surface area of one's palm is equal to approximately 1% of the total body surface and estimates the burn size according to how many "palms" have been injured. These two methods help to estimate the BSA injured by the thermal exposure in an attempt to establish adequate fluid replacement, which is imperative, especially in extensive burns.

Treatment of thermal burns is dictated by the degree and extent of the burn. Several basic considerations should always be addressed: First, and probably most important in all but minor burns, is fluid resuscitation. The Parkland formula (4 ml/kg/%BSA burn) is the most common method of calculating fluid deficit. Crystalloid solution, usually normal saline or Ringer's lactate, is the fluid of choice. Half of the total fluid requirement is given in the first 8 hours and the rest over the next 16 hours. Care should be taken to prevent excessive cooling in extensive burns, but cooling may be helpful in first-degree and superficial second-degree burns. Ice should be avoided in all cases because of possible increased injury to already injured tissue. The wound should be dressed with silver sulfadiazine (barring any relevant allergies), which increases comfort by decreasing air currents around the wound. It also decreases the likelihood of infection. An often overlooked consideration is tetanus status. The patient whose last immunization was more than 10 years ago should receive prophylaxis. Certainly all but very mild burns should be referred to a primary care physician, emergency department, or the closest burn center, depending on severity. Outpatient care can be arranged if the wound is partial thickness and less than 15% BSA or full thickness less than 2% BSA. Close follow-up is necessary to avoid infection or treat it, should it occur. Hospitalization should also be considered for those patients who have burns on the face (possibility of airway compromise), hands, feet, or perineum or who have significant underlying medical problems.[11]

Another health concern, especially for art glassworkers, is ultraviolet (UV) keratitis. The most effective prevention is protective glasses. The treatment is similar to any corneal abrasion. Referral to an ophthalmologist is imperative.

Glassblowers are subject to a specific health risk, namely, altered respiratory function, secondary to the high airway pressures they sustain. Continually altering airway pressures is necessary for blowing glass. The size of the glass blown seems to have a great deal of influence on the mouth pressure; more pressure is needed to blow a large ball of glass than a small amount.[33] These respiratory effects seem to be specific for this population. They have excessive chronic respiratory symptoms (such as chronic bronchitis, chronic sinusitis, and nasal bleeding) and acute symptoms (such as dry throat, dry nose, and eye irritation) that appear to be secondary to the direct irritation from inhalation of heat and chemicals. Thermal injury appears to affect the central airways. Inhalation of dusts (e.g., silica, lead), gases, hydrocarbons, and heat also seems to cause airway irritation. In contrast, these individuals have improved lung performance, probably due to excessive inspiratory maneuvers used just prior to blowing the glass into shape. It is universally felt that the physiology of these changes is due to increased recruitment and inflation of otherwise atelectatic areas of the lung. Most data demonstrated that glassblowers have increased vital capacity (VC), residual volume (RV), total lung capacity (TLC), and expiratory flow rates. Smoking is more the rule than the exception in this population, and its effects have an undefined influence on these parameters. Those who have worked longer than 10 years seem to show significant "across shift" changes (acute changes during the course of a workshift), including increased RV with normal DLCO, which implies that these changes are not consistent with emphysema. These changes seem to be physiologic, not pathologic, because they do not seem to progress to illness. Because this point remains unclear, further investigation seems warranted.[33]

CONCLUSION

As with any industry, the glass manufacturing industry includes many toxic hazards. Most of the acute health risks, such as heat illness, UV keratitis, and chemical burns, can be avoided with proper material handling and prevention. The risks of cancer appear to be related to long-term exposures that are inherently more difficult to control. Meticulous care should be taken to follow all guidelines to prevent illness in this industry.

REFERENCES

1. Bender JR: Science, public policy, and stewardship, *Regul Toxicol Pharmacol* 20:s2, 1994.
2. Bentur Y, Tannenbaum S, Jaffe Y, et al: The role of calcium gluconate in the treatment of hydrofluoric acid eye burn, *Ann Emerg Med* 22:1488-1490, 1993.
3. Beryllium, cadmium, mercury, and exposures in the glass manufacturing industry: working groups views and expert opinions, Lyons, 9-16 February, 1993, *IARC Monogr Eval Cardiog Risks Hum* 58:1, 1993.
4. Bordelon BM, Saffle JR, Morris SE: Systemic fluoride toxicity in a child with hydrofluoric acid burns: case report, *J Trauma* 34:437-439, 1993.
5. Bracken WM, Cuppage F, McLaury RL, et al: Comparative effectiveness of topical treatments for hydrofluoric acid burns, *J Occup Med* 27:733-739, 1989.
6. Burkhart KK, Brent J, Kirk MA, et al: Comparison of topical magnesium and calcium treatment for dermal hydrofluoric acid burns, *Ann Emerg Med* 24:9-13, 1994.
7. Cappell MS, Simon T: Fulminant acute colitis following a self-administered hydrofluoric acid enema, *Am J Gastroenterology* 88:122-126, 1993.
8. Cox RD, Osgood KA: Evaluation of intravenous magnesium sulfate for the treatment of hydrofluoric acid burns, *J Toxicol Clin Toxicol* 32:123-136, 1994.
9. Cummings CC, McIvor ME: Fluoride-induced hyperkalemia. The role of Ca^{++} dependent K$^+$ channels, *Am J Emerg Med* 6:1-3, 1988.
10. Dowbak G, Rohrich RJ: A biochemical and histologic rationale for the treatment of hydrofluoric acid burns with calcium gluconate, *J Burn Care Rehabil* 15:323-327, 1994.
11. Dunn BJ, MacKinnon MA, Knowlden NF, et al: Hydrofluoric acid dermal burns, *J Occup Med* 34:902-909, 1992.
12. Exposures in the Glass Manufacturing Industry, *IARC Monogr Eval Carcinog Risks Hum* 58:347, 1993.
13. Goldfrank L et al, editors: *Goldfrank's toxicologic emergencies,* ed 5, Norwalk, CT, 1994, Appleton & Lange.
14. Henry JA, Hla KK: Intravenous regional calcium gluconate perfusion for hydrofluoric acid burns, *J Toxicol Clin Toxicol* 30:203-207, 1992.
15. Kampstrup O: Carcinogenicity assessment of synthetic vitreous fibers: international regulatory perspective, *Regul Toxicol Pharmacol* 20:s182, 1994.
16. Kono K, Yoshida Y, Watanabe M, et al: An experimental study on the treatment of hydrofluoric acid burns, *Arch Environ Contam Toxicol* 22:414-418, 1992.
17. Kono K, Yoshida Y, Watanabe M, et al: Serum fluoride as an indicator of occupational hydrofluoric acid exposure, *Occup Environ Health* 65:s95-s98, 1993.
18. Kronenberg RS et al: Asbestos-related disease in employees of a steel mill and a glass bottle manufacturing plant, *Toxicol Ind Health* 7:73, 1991.
19. Lee DC, Wiley JF, Snyder JW: *Treatment of inhalational exposure to hydrofluoric acid with nebulized calcium gluconate, J Occ Med* 35(5):470, 1993.

20. Lockey JE, Wiese NK: Health effects of synthetic vitreous fibers, *Clin Chest Med* 13:329, 1992.

21. McCulley JP, Whiting DW, Petitt MG, et al: Hydrofluoric acid burns of the eye, *J Occup Med* 25:447-450, 1983.

22. Meeting of the IARC working group on beryllium, cadmium, mercury, and exposures in the glass manufacturing industry, *Scand J Work, Environ Health* 19:360, 1993.

23. Proceedings of symposium on synthetic vitreous fibers: scientific and public policy issues, Arlington, Virginia, 2-3 March, 1994, *Regul Toxicol Pharmacol* 20:s1, 1994.

24. Rosen P, Barkin RM, editors: *Emergency medicine: concepts and clinical theory,* ed 3, St Louis, 1992, Mosby.

25. Rubinfeld RS, Silbert DI, Arentsen JJ, et al: Ocular hydrofluoric acid burns, *Am J Ophth* 114:420-423, 1992.

26. Saadi MS, Hall AH, Hall PK, et al: Hydrofluoric acid dermal exposure, *Vet Hum Toxicol* 31:243-245, 1989.

27. Siegel DC, Heard JM: Intra-arterial calcium infusion for hydrofluoric acid burns, *Aviat Space Environ Med* 63:206-211, 1992.

28. Vance MV, Curry SC, Kunkel DB, et al: Digital hydrofluoric acid burns: treatment with intraarterial calcium infusion, *Ann Emerg Med* 15:890-896, 1986.

29. Webster RW: *Legal medicine and toxicology,* Philadelphia, Saunders 1930; 389.

30. Williams JM, Hammad A, Cottington EC, et al: Intravenous magnesium in the treatment of hydrofluoric acid burns in rats, *Ann Emerg Med* 23:464-469, 1994.

31. Wing JS, Sanderson LM, Brender JD, et al: Acute health effects in a community after a release of hydrofluoric acid, *Arch Environ Health* 46:155-160, 1991.

32. Wingren G, Axelson O: Epidemiologic studies of occupational cancer as related to complex mixtures of trace elements in art glass industry, *Scand J Work, Environ Health* 19(suppl 1):95, 1993.

33. Zuskin E et al: Respiratory function in workers in employment in the glassblowing industry, *Am J Ind Med* 23:835, 1993.

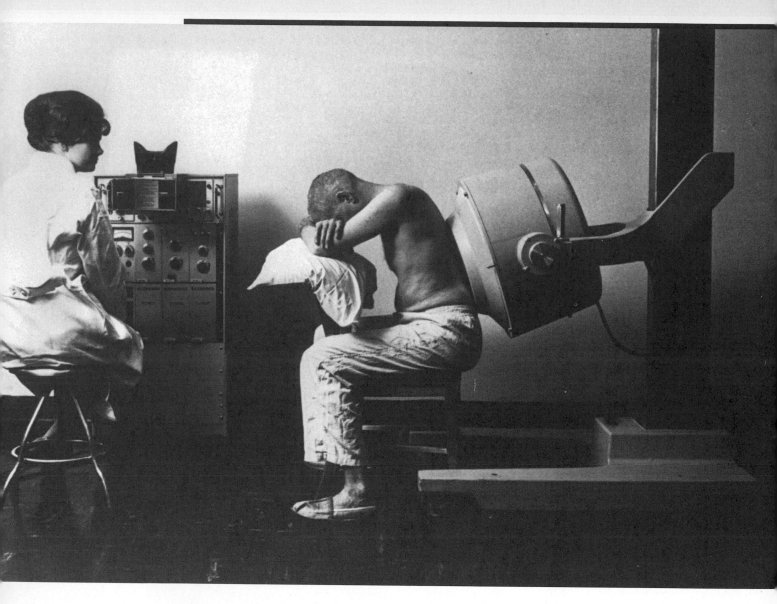

Gamma photographs being made of kidney function.
Undated. (Courtesy Corbis-Bettmann)

$$O=C-C-C-C=O$$
glutaraldehyde

- Hospitals represent a setting in which workers from many occupations share toxic exposures from a limited number of sources

- Occupational toxicity in the health care industry often results from the chemicals required to control the spread of infection (cleaning agents, sterilants)

Health Care

Leon Leleu

Peter T. Jezukaitis

Michael I. Greenberg

OCCUPATIONAL DESCRIPTION

This chapter discusses people who work in hospitals, health care laboratories, clinics, and nursing homes, including medical assistants, technicians, housekeeping personnel, administrative personnel, central supply personnel, security personnel, food service personnel, groundskeepers, mechanics, biomedical engineering personnel, and visitors to the hospital, but not physicians, nurses, or pharmacists. Of course, these people could potentially be exposed to virtually any toxin that exists or could exist in the hospital environment, certain specific health hazards exist for each of these groups in particular. In general, the hazards that exist for these individuals can be broken into the following broad categories: infectious hazards, chemical hazards, physical hazards, and allergic sensitization hazards (see box on p. 346). The health hazards regarding infectious agents within the hospital environment are significant. A complete and thorough discussion of the pathophysiology, diagnosis, treatment, and prevention of these diseases is well beyond the scope of this book, but Table 42-1 chronicles the most commonly encountered hospital and laboratory-acquired respiratory (only) pathogens.

POTENTIAL TOXIC EXPOSURES

Even absent the obvious infectious hazards in the hospital and health care environment, significant toxic health hazards exist for the workers. Exposure depends on the specific tasks performed by the worker, but some hazards can affect all workers in that environment. The health care worksite is unusual in that significant numbers of nonemployees are present daily as visitors to the facility. Consequently, a variable, though significant, portion of the public at large could be exposed to any toxin in these work environments. While factories and other worksites in the private sector usually strive to restrict public access to the worksite, hospitals, clinics, and nursing care facilities are generally accessible to the public, in some cases, 24 hours per day. In these instances, the potential for exposure to toxins is expanded manyfold because the public has so much generally free access to the physical plant. In addition, hospitals and long-term care facilities usually function 24 hours each day for 365 days each year. This continual operation not only expands the numbers of individuals who could potentially become affected by worksite-related toxins, but also significantly expands the contact time to the public in general for these toxins.

CLINICAL TOXICOLOGY
Housekeeping and Cleaning Functions

The chemical toxic hazards in these environments can be broken down into the categories listed in Table 42-1.

Housekeeping and cleaning are crucial functions in these health care environments. Routine cleaning is carried out, usually on a 24-hour-per-day basis by a staff of housekeeping personnel. In addition, some cleaning functions are performed by other personnel who are assigned to patient care duties such as nurses, medical assistants, technicians, and aides. The most important of the toxic health hazards that might affect these individuals with regard to cleaning tasks and cleaning materials are reviewed in Chapter 9. These personnel may be exposed to a wide range of potentially toxic substances. The most commonly involved materials are listed in the box at left on p. 347.

Allergic Sensitization

Allergic sensitization is one of the most important mechanisms that cause toxicity and disability in health care workers. The clinical spectrum of allergic sensitization includes rhinitis, nonspecific bronchial hyperreactivity (NSBH), and asthma. Mechanistic discussions of allergic sensitization have divided potential antigens into substances of high molecular weight—usually greater than 20,000—and low molecular weight—usually less than 5000—daltons. The high-molecular-weight antigens are typically animal and plant proteins, whereas the low-molecular-weight group generally involves chemicals and drugs. Both classes of antigens play roles as potential sensitizers in hospital and health care workers.

The box at right on p. 347 lists substances found in the health care setting that are often associated with allergic sensitization. Although the list includes chemically diverse agents, the majority of allergic sensitization in these work settings is due to laboratory animal allergy and pharmaceutic exposure.

Dusts of pharmacologic origin. Allergic reactions from exposure to pharmacologic dusts has been recognized as a significant health hazard in hospital pharmacy and laboratory settings.[16] Reports of ipecac-induced asthma in pharmacists appeared in the literature as early as 1920, but pharmacists are not the only health care workers who might be exposed to these pharmacologic dusts.[1] Pharmacy assistants, nurses, and others, too, could be exposed, depending on the particular health care setting.[2]

Health Care Employment Hazards

INFECTIOUS	CHEMICAL HAZARDS
Measles, mumps, rubella	Acids/alkalis
Varicella	Ethylene oxide
HIV disease	Glutaraldehyde
Viral illnesses	Hazardous drugs
Tuberculosis	Mercury
Legionnaires' disease	Methyl methacrylate
	Organic solvents
ALLERGIC SENSITIZATION	Nitrous oxide
Allergy due to pharmaceutic dusts	**PHYSICAL HAZARDS**
	Ionizing radiation
Latex allergy	Asbestos

Table 42-1 Hospital and laboratory-acquired respiratory (only) pathogens

Common name	Causative organism	Mode of spread	Reservoir
Q fever	*Coxiella burnetii*	Airborne	Chick embryos
Psittacosis	*Chlamydia psittacia*	Airborne	Bird excreta
Histoplasmosis	*Histoplasma capsulatum*	Airborne	Bird excreta
Tuberculosis	*Mycobacterium tuberculosis*	Airborne	Infected specimens
Blastomycosis	*Blastomyces dermatitidis*	Airborne	Not known
Coccidioidomycosis	*Coccidioides immitis*	Airborne	Infected specimen; contaminated glassware
Glanders	*Pseudomonas mallei*	Skin inoculation	Culture material
Anthrax	*Bacillus anthracis*	Airborne	Vaccine prep
Hemorrhagic fever with renal syndrome	*Francisella tularensis*	Fomites	Fomites
Tularemia	Hantaan virus	Airborne	Culture material

Modified from Harber P, Schenker MB, Balmes JR: *Occupational and environmental respiratory disease,* St Louis, 1996, Mosby.

The most common toxic effect of these materials is contact irritant dermatitis, although allergic skin manifestations may also occur. Solvents that contact the skin are capable of causing defatting of the subcutaneous fat on repeated exposures. Consequently, there is a high incidence of irritant hand dermatitis reported for hospital cleaning workers. If these materials are used in confined spaces, used in the wrong concentrations, combined inappropriately, or used with the wrong equipment, the possibility for adverse toxic exposures is enhanced.

Often, cleaning personnel in these types of health care settings receive little formal training regarding the materials they are using, and mistakes can lead to potentially very serious exposures that could affect not only the cleaning personnel themselves but also other employees and visitors alike. A case in point is chlorine-containing compounds, which commonly cause upper and lower respiratory tract symptoms. Their effects may be enhanced in people who have a preexisting respiratory problem or who are otherwise sensitized. A condition of occupational asthma may result from these exposures.

Perhaps the quintessential adverse reaction for cleaning personnel who use chlorine compounds occurs when chlorine-containing bleaches are mixed with ammonium solutions.[9] The ensuing chemical reaction liberates chloramine gas, which is extraordinarily noxious. Exposure to chloramine gas in a poorly ventilated closed space can lead to coma and death via asphyxiation.

The more serious sorts of exposures to cleaners tend to be instigated by cleaning procedures that stem from surface contamination by infectious agents, blood, or body fluids. The emotional drive to "sterilize" what is often a wide surface area after contamination with a potentially infectious agent often leads to "overcleaning" of the affected area. As a result, excessive amounts of chlorine, alcohol, and ammonium-containing materials, as well as surface disinfectants, often are used. This setting expands the possibility of significant skin and respiratory exposures to cleaners and to others in the immediate area.

In the health care setting, surface overcleaning is tempting to inadequately informed staff and is pervasive. Such overzealousness occurs routinely and is a potential source for toxic exposures to cleaning personnel and others in health care settings.

Another familiar setting for "overcleaning" occurs when a patient on a bed or stretcher is found to be infested with body lice, head lice, or scabies. In this setting, personnel are often driven by an emotional fear of being infested, even though they may have had absolutely no direct contact with the individual patient or patients in question. The most common locale for this scenario is the emergency department or the outpatient clinic. Often, after the ritualized process of overcleaning, personnel self-treat with topical antiparasitic medications in hopes of "prophylactically" preventing themselves from being infested by the ectoparasites. An additional emotional aspect drives this behavior in that personnel are acutely aware of not wishing to carry these parasites home to their spouses, children, and pets. Such use of these agents is not clinically indicated. Moreover, staff needs to be taught that these ectoparasites do not "jump" from person to person and generally are not transmitted via fomites. Rather, direct skin-to-skin contact or sharing of clothing or personal hygiene equipment (e.g., combs, brushes) is the most common means for transmission. This is not to say, however, that health care personnel could not be infested with any ectoparasite in the course of the performance of their normal duties. Inappropriate or aggressive overuse of the lindane (organochlorine) containing parasiticides can cause local skin reactions. In addition, about 10% of these topical preparations is absorbed, but significantly enhanced skin absorption can occur if these medications are not used properly. For instance, if used on large areas of abraded skin or if applied after washing with hot (rather than warm) water, systemic absorption can be enhanced. Lipid solvents

---

Potentially Toxic Substances

Chlorine-containing bleaches
Non–chlorine-containing bleaches
Solvents
Phenols
Caustics
Quaternary ammonium compounds

Some causes of allergic sensitization in hospital and laboratory workers

ANIMAL PROTEINS

Dander, excreta, secretions, serum

ENZYMES

Bacillus subtilis, papain, pepsin, pancreatic extracts

PHARMACEUTICALS

Antibiotics (penicillin, tetracycline, sulfuramides)

OTHER PHARMACEUTICALS

Psyllium, salbutamol, methyldopa, cimetidine, enflurane, piperazine, chloramine, isoniazid

STERILIZING AGENTS

Chloramine, sulfone chloramide, hexachlorophene, formaldehyde, glutaraldehyde

ORGANIC CHEMICALS

Acrylates, amines, colophony, latex

Modified from Harber P, Schenker MB, Balmes JR: *Occupational and environmental respiratory disease,* St Louis, 1996, Mosby.

also increase skin absorption of these toxins. Central nervous system toxicity can occur in this setting and may, in extreme cases, lead to mental confusion, seizures, and coma.

Cleaning personnel may become exposed to toxins in other ways as well. The most important involves the aerosolization of toxins that occurs when certain spills are vacuumed. The classic exposure of this nature is the heavy metal mercury, which is present in many different settings throughout the health care venue. The most common location for this metal, of course, is in sphygmomanometers and thermometers, although it is present in other pieces of biomedical equipment as well. When a mercury spill occurs, the first impulse is to vacuum it up, as the particles of mercury distribute over a wide area when they strike a hard surface. The most problematic setting is a mercury spill onto a carpeted surface, in which case personnel are tempted to use a vacuum-cleaning device to try to clean up the spill. Unfortunately, this method of cleaning very efficiently volatilizes the spilled mercury into the breathable air. With extensive spills, both cleaning personnel and others are exposed to potentially harmful inhaled mercury. Written policies should be in place to address mercury spills and the professional and safe correction of the problem.

Phenol, also known as *carbolic acid,* is a common disinfectant typically used to clean glassware and medical instruments. Contact with phenol can cause severe skin burns and permanent hypopigmentation. If high concentrations are inhaled, effects can range from simple irritation to severe systemic toxicity, including seizures, coma, and death. Urinary phenol levels can be monitored in exposed workers to determine overexposure.

Groundskeepers

In the health care venue, groundskeeping personnel may come in contact with any of the toxins that are routine for such workers. For a complete discussion of these toxic hazards, see Chapter 17.

Maintenance Personnel

In these venues, routine maintenance and repair functions include carpentry, metal work, welding, soldering, electrical repairs, tile work, carpet work, painting, and paint removal. These tasks do not generally present toxic hazards significantly different from those faced by workers performing the same tasks in other locations.

Central Supply Personnel

Those individuals employed in the supply areas of health care establishments may have exposure on an accidental basis to many different toxins. Each exposure must be dealt with on an individual basis, and speculating which toxins present the most serious or potentially severe exposure would be futile. In many settings, supply personnel are involved with sterilization of medical supplies and equipment. In that case, certain toxins of special concern bear consideration.

While sterilization of surgical equipment and other items is an important function, most items are sterilized via the use of pressurized steam. However, certain materials and pieces of equipment could be damaged by steam under pressure and are sterilized by either the glutaraldehyde or ethylene oxide. Glutaraldehyde, a substance chemically similar to formaldehyde, is discussed in Chapter 23.

Ethylene oxide is the more important process chemical in sterilization and toxic exposures.[8] Modern ethylene oxide sterilizers in hospitals are usually in isolated locations and have alarms to detect excessive ethylene oxide in the atmosphere. Older systems have been found to allow leakage of large volumes of ethylene oxide into the breathable air.[3,4] For discussion of adverse health effects from ethylene oxide exposure, see Chapter 8.

Administrative Staff

The administrative staff of health care institutions tend to be rather heterogeneous. It is not unusual to find physicians and nurses fulfilling administrative and provider roles concomitantly. Consequently, these "administrators" may be exposed to the very same toxins as other physicians and nurses and also those toxins that might affect more traditional administrative personnel. For exposures to be expected for administrative personnel, see Chapters 24, 51, and 52. The potential for these personnel to be exposed to significant toxic insults in the course of their work is usually minimal. One toxin of note for these individuals involves white board markers, which were initially available with hydrocarbon solvents as pigment vehicles. In the closed-in setting in which many white boards are used (typically a small conference room with poor ventilation), the solvents represent a potential skin sensitizer and minimal respiratory irritant. Recently, the hydrocarbon content of these products has been reduced or eliminated completely, thus ameliorating the problem to a large extent.

Operating Room Staff

Operating room staff are exposed to anesthetic gases, blood-borne pathogens, cytotoxic drugs, antibiotics, solvents, cleansers, and detergents, hazards that are completely discussed in other chapters. Another important toxin for these personnel is methyl methacrylate, an ester of methacrylic acid.

Methyl methacrylate monomers and polymers are used widely and found specifically in bone cements, spray adhesives, bandage solvents, artificial eyes, dentures, and contact lenses. The acute exposure to methyl methacrylate can result in ocular and mucous membrane irritation at concentrations as low as 125 ppm.[14] At higher concentrations, various systemic symptoms, including headache, limb heaviness, light-headedness, and lethargy, have been reported. Pulmonary edema can occur, and cardiac arrest has also been reported after exposure to methyl methacrylate. In one report, a nurse developed hypertension, difficult breathing, and a red skin eruption following repeated exposures to surgical glue that contained nearly 100% of the methyl methacrylate monomer.

Chronic methyl methacrylate exposure usually results in contact sensitization and "toxic dermatitis." This dermatitis is specifically characterized by the appearance of paresthesia and actual tenderness that persists after the rash is gone. The complaint of chronic cough has been noted in exposed workers. In addition, chronic exposure to methyl methacrylate has resulted in the development of occupational asthma. For a complete discussion, see Chapter 16.

Technicians

Technicians are utilized in many different areas of health care facilities. Their exposures to toxic hazards depend specifically upon the type of work they perform. However, several specific exposures for specific technicians are noteworthy.

X-ray technicians have a controllable exposure to ionizing radiation. A subset of this group is also exposed to ultrasound. While the hazards of x-ray exposure are well described, those associated with ultrasound are not. See Chapters 59 and 60 for discussion of these exposures.

X-ray technicians can also be exposed to those noted above. These typically include x-ray film developers and fixers. X-ray developers contain glutaraldehyde, a chemical discussed elsewhere in this text. Skin irritation and respiratory function impairment have been noted with other fixer and developer components, including alkaline glutaraldehyde, formaldehyde, acetic acid, hydrochloric acid, ammonium thiosulfate, and sulfur dioxide.[18] Because developers are typically used in confined, poorly ventilated areas, the possibility of respiratory effects is not surprising.[7] Other symptoms referable to exposure to these substances include severe headache, sore throat, hoarseness, nasal discharge, ocular soreness, fatigue, sinusitis, nausea, joint pain, paresthesia, and shortness of breath (see Chapter 27).

The best treatment for these exposures is obviously prevention. However, properly ventilated work areas and appropriate use of personal protective equipment are also essential. For the most part, symptomatic treatment suffices for the majority of these toxic effects. Occasionally, more extensive care is required.

Redevelopment and Decommissioning

Hospitals, especially large ones, present an ever-changing work environment in that, in the United States and the world over, governmental initiatives and funding resources have not allowed the building of new hospitals. As a result, rather than replacement, old and outmoded hospital areas are refurbished and remodeled. Toxic exposures can occur during construction and refurbishment, and occupants may be exposed to contaminants from such construction activities. Not only are hazardous substances introduced into the hospital environment by such construction but also areas of the hospital that have contained toxic materials in the past may be disturbed, and the toxic materials are thereby disseminated. The prime example is construction in old hospital buildings that may contain asbestos. The release of old and friable asbestos fibers into the air systems in a hospital or other health care facility can have profound and widespread effects on the workforce. If proper risk assessment and risk communication protocols are not followed, mass hysteria and other group reactions could occur. See Chapter 55 for a more complete discussion of this prodigious toxic exposure. Additional problematic toxic exposures during hospital construction might include cytotoxic drugs stored in construction areas and mercury hazards in repair shops that are being refurbished.

PATHOGENESIS AND PRESENTATION

The clinical presentation of drug allergies in health care workers includes allergic rhinitis, contact dermatitis, upper respiratory irritation, conjunctivitis, and asthma. Allergy caused by pharmacologic dusts is usually due to skin contact or inhalation, in contrast with an oral or injected exposure, as is usual in patients. The route for sensitization is a major determinant in antigen distribution. The route of exposure ultimately determines the target organ(s) affected. The immunogenicity and molecular weight of the allergen are other very important determinants of the immunologic response.

Prevention of symptomatology is best achieved through appropriate workplace hygiene via the proper use of vertical laminar flow hoods. Other efforts to contain drug dust generation must take place as well. Worker education regarding employment choices and safe work practices for sensitized workers are essential for prevention. A simple history of atopy is generally not sufficient as a screening tool to determine allergic potential in workers.

LABORATORY ANIMAL ALLERGY

Laboratory animals are routinely present in university hospitals and larger community hospitals where research programs are undertaken.[5] Technicians, physicians, veterinarians, cleaning personnel, and other workers may well come into significant contact with these animals during the course of their work duties.

Laboratory animal allergy (LAA) was first identified in the mid-1970s and has received increasing attention as an occupational hazard.[13] It is defined as a type I-IgE mediated hypersensitivity reaction due to skin or respiratory exposure to animal allergens. The published prevalence of the condition in exposed animal workers ranges up to 30%.[15]

Allergens from animal body fluids (urine and saliva) and dander appear to influence the onset of symptoms. Risk factors for LAA development have been difficult to define, but a history of atopy alone may not be associated with an increased risk of developing LAA.

Some investigators have noted that LAA may first present as rhinitis rather than as symptomatic asthma. The majority of symptoms reported by affected workers are rhinitis, upper airway irritation, and skin rashes. Note that asthma symptoms is glaringly absent from the list.

Environmental surveillance for the presence of airborne allergens may be helpful in a program of hazard control. One group performed a prevalence survey of LAA, correlated this to airborne rat urinary allergen concentration by job task, and found a significant association.

One study of more than 500 animal handlers determined that approximately 25% of workers reported LAA symptoms and 30% of those had to stop work because of the severity of their symptoms. The current approach of using gowns and gloves when the offending agent is likely an airborne allergen seems of little use. These authors suggest keeping the allergen close to the cage by using dustless bedding, reducing use of bedding, or using local exhaust ventilation (hoods) when cleaning cages. The use of respiratory protection for workers might also be considered, especially for those with rhinitis who have not yet developed full-blown occupational asthma.

REFERENCES

1. American Society of Hospital Pharmacists: ASHP technical assistance bulletin on handling cytotoxic and hazardous drugs, *Am J Hosp Pharm* 47:1033, 1990.
2. Boulet L: Increases in airway responsiveness following acute exposure to respiratory irritants, *Chest* 94:476, 1988.
3. Bousquet J, Michel F: Allergy to formaldehyde and ethylene-oxide, *Clin Rev Allergy* 9:357, 1991.
4. Bryant HE, Visser ND, Yoshida K: Ethylene oxide sterilizer use and short-term symptoms amongst workers, *Occup Med* 39:101, 1989.
5. Cockcroft A et al: Allergy in laboratory animal workers, *Lancet* 2:827, 1981.
6. Corrado OJ, Osman J, Davies RJ: Asthma and rhinitis after exposure to glutaraldehyde in endoscopy units, *Hum Toxicol* 5:325, 1986.
7. Cullinan P et al: Occupational asthma in radiographers, *Lancet* 340:1477, 1992.
8. Glaser ZR: Ethylene oxide: toxicology review and field study results of hospital use, *J Environ Pathol Toxicol* 2:173, 1979.
9. Hattis RP et al: Chlorine gas toxicity from mixture of bleach with other cleaning products—California, *JAMA* 266:2529, 1991.
10. Hendrick DJ, Lane DJ: Occupational formalin asthma, *Br J Ind Med* 34:11, 1977.
11. Katzman M et al: High incidence of bronchospasm with regular administration of aerosolized pentamidine, *Chest* 101:79, 1992.
12. Kern DG: Outbreak of the reactive airways dysfunction syndrome after a spill of glacial acetic acid, *Am Rev Respir Dis* 144:1058, 1991.
13. Kibby T, Powell G, Cromer J: Allergy to laboratory animals: a prospective and cross-sectional study, *J Occup Med* 31:842, 1989.
14. Lozewicz S et al: Occupational asthma due to methyl methacrylate and cyanoacrylates, *Thorax* 40:836, 1985.
15. McCoy G: Psittacosis among the personnel of the hygienic laboratory, *J Infect Dis* 55:156, 1934.
16. McDiarmid MA, Gurley HT, Arrington D: Pharmaceuticals as hospital hazards: managing the risks, *J Occup Med* 33:155, 1991.
17. McDiarmid MA et al: Efficacy of engineering controls in reducing occupational exposure to aerosolized pentamidine, *Chest* 102:1764, 1992.
18. Nethercott JR, Holness DL, Page E: Occupational contact dermatitis due to glutaraldehyde in health care workers, *Contact Dermatitis* 18:193, 1988.

Match Production

P_4S_3
phosphorus sesquisulfide

$KClO_3$
potassium chlorate

- The treatment for dermal exposure to yellow (white) phosphorus is 2% copper sulfate

- Potassium chlorate exposure can cause methemoglobinemia

- Red phosphorus is essentially non-toxic

Timothy Erickson

OCCUPATIONAL DESCRIPTION

The use of matches in our society is widespread. From igniting fires and barbecue grills to smoking tobacco products, the public demand for matches is enormous, resulting in a major international industry. Match manufacturing developed during the nineteenth century to provide the public with an inexpensive and accessible way to create a flame.[39]

The use of phosphorus in matchmaking represents one of the most important and intriguing historical perspectives in occupational medicine. In the early years, matchmakers were poorly paid and lived in extreme poverty. The majority of the workforce was women and children.[46] In the development of the modern match, different contents and manufacturing techniques were attempted but ultimately prohibited due to the health risks to both matchworkers and users.[39] The present-day industry involves the production of individual "strike anywhere" matches and safety matches, which supply a frictional striking surface on the matchbook or box. Today, most match manufacturing plants are fully automated, and the construction of boxes and folders and the printing of labels are done within the same factory.

POTENTIAL TOXIC EXPOSURES

Historically, the match industry's use of yellow (white) phosphorus as the major chemical component in matchheads resulted in chronic exposure in workers and significant occupational toxicity. This led to legislation enacted in the early twentieth century to outlaw the use of yellow phosphorus in the match industry.[1,10,15] Hunter referred to the early years of match production as "the greatest tragedy

Match Contents

I. Matchheads
  A. Safety matches
    1. Potassium chlorate
    2. Antimony trisulfate
    3. Sulfur
    4. Glue
    5. Powdered glass
  B. Strike-anywhere matches
    1. Phosphorus sesquisulfide
    2. Manganese trisulfide
  C. Potassium bichromate (France)
II. Striking surface
  A. Red phosphorus
  B. Sand
  C. Glue
III. Matchstick/splint
  A. Wood
    1. Pine
    2. Poplar
    3. Aspen
  B. Cardboard
  C. Paraffin
  D. Ammonium phosphorus/boric acid
IV. Matchboxes
  A. Wood veneer
  B. Cardboard

in the whole story of occupational disease."[46] The industry has now turned to less toxic alternatives such as potassium chlorate, red phosphorus, and phosphorus sesquisulfide in present-day production.

Although variations exist depending on the specific brand, most safety matchheads contain potassium chlorate (200 mg per 20 matches). Other additives include antimony trisulfide, sulfur, glue, and powdered glass. The heads for strike-anywhere matches contain phosphorus sesquisulfide and trace amounts of manganese trisulfide.[21,39] In France and other European nations, certain matchheads are comprised of potassium bichromate[44] (see box above). The striking surface of the matchbook or box consists primarily of red phosphorus, sand, and glue. The matchstick or splint is commonly constructed of wood (pine, poplar, or aspen) or cardboard with paraffin. The wood splints are impregnated in a bath of ammonium phosphate or boric acid (to temper afterglow) and coated with paraffin wax (to assist burning). Most match boxes are constructed of thin wood veneer or cardboard.[39,45]

Many of the by-products of match production, such as sawdust and fumes from match pastes, can cause nonspecific irritative disorders affecting primarily the upper respiratory tract. As a result, production materials should be kept in closed containers and the plant equipped with an adequate ventilation system.

Additionally, the manual handling of combustible pastes can result in contact dermatitis. Thus, employees working with these products should have hand protection. Skin and particularly facial eczema has been reported in workers who make strike-anywhere matches and their users. This eczematous condition has been attributed to the matches' phosphorus sesquisulfide and bichromates.[7,19,51]

Finally, there is a significant risk of fire and explosion in the mixing of matchhead pastes during production, as well as in the handling of individual matches. This risk appears to be the greatest when matches are manually handled and boxes are hand filled.[39] In this setting, the worker is not only susceptible to potentially serious burns of the hand but to significant smoke inhalation injury and carbon monoxide poisoning. Phosphorus is also capable of spontaneous ignition when exposed to air as it oxidizes.[21,24]

CLINICAL TOXICOLOGY
Yellow (White) Phosphorus

Pathobiology. The material known as yellow phosphorus is actually a translucent substance that in some lights gives a white appearance. When aged or in combination with oils, it may appear slightly yellowish. The terms *yellow phosphorus* and *white phosphorus* are commonly used interchangeably to refer to the same substance. Yellow phosphorus was discovered in 1674 by the German chemist Hennig Brandt, who extracted the metal when attempting to make gold from human urine. Although the experiment was deemed a failure, he did make a livelihood for himself by demonstrating the glowing properties of phosphorus. In addition, Brandt sold it to the public as a therapeutic agent.[46] Although no longer used to manufacture matches,[43] occupational exposures to yellow phosphorus can still be found in the production of rodenticides, bronze alloys, semiconductors, munitions, pyrotechnics (fireworks), and fertilizer.[15,40,43,46,62] When readily available as the phosphorus paste in match production, it was often used as a suicidal and homicidal poison.[5,6]

Although some believe there are three distinct types of toxicity due to phosphorus rather than a continuum of stages,[14] acute ingestion of yellow phosphorus has classically been described as three continuous stages.[21] After significant exposure, the worker suffers severe gastrointestinal (GI) symptoms associated with the development of garlicky breath odor, vomiting, diarrhea, and abdominal pain. On occasion, the vomitus and stools following ingestion has been described as luminescent with an "explosion of smoke from the mouth."[18,21] Some have labeled the phenomenon as the "smoking stool syndrome."[49] With severe toxicity, neurologic symptoms such as lethargy, stupor, and coma with cardiovascular collapse can accompany the GI phase (stage 1). This first stage is followed by a quiescent period (stage 2) within 2 or 3 days. The last stage (stage 3) usually consists of central nervous system (CNS) depression, encephalopathy, hepatorenal failure, and death.[12,14,21] Fatalities may result days after exposure but have been reported to be delayed for up to several weeks. As little as 1 mg/kg of yellow phosphorus can be fatal after oral ingestion. According to American Conference of Governmental Industrial Hygienists (ACGIH) guidelines, the threshold limit value (TLV)–time-weighted average (TWA) for this substance is 0.1 mg/m^3 or 0.02 ppm 8 hour.

Chronic industrial exposure (average 5 years; range 1 to 18 years[46,62]) can result in degenerative bony changes and subsequent osteomyelitis. This process most often targets the mandible and predisposes the worker to "phossy jaw" or "Lucifer's jaw" (named after the Lucifer match designed in 1829). The first recorded case of this disorder, more properly described as *mandibular phosphorous necrosis,* was reported by Lorinser of Vienna in 1844. In 1885, phossy jaw was seen among workers in a Japanese Lucifer match factory that utilized yellow phosphorus.[36] The first symptom of classic phossy jaw is odontalgia.[23] Changes in the periosteum of the mandible occur and may also be noted in the long bones. This can lead to abnormal fragility and pathologic fractures. At the height of the period when phossy jaw was common, mortality rates were as high as 20%, and death was usually attributed to septicemia.[46]

Yellow phosphorus toxicity in the match industry results primarily from the volatilization of the phosphorus in the course of production and processing and it's subsequent inhalation.[24] This route of exposure is far more common than oral ingestion of phosphorus. Airborne exposure can result in severe upper respiratory tract and eye irritation. Dermal exposure can result in second- and third-degree burns on contact and has resulted in systemic toxicity.[29]

Phosphorus is readily absorbed from the GI tract and is highly fat soluble. In addition, it is easily absorbed via burned, abraded, or otherwise denuded skin. Most commonly, the renal and hepatic systems are adversely affected by phosphorus toxicity. However, significant changes in calcium and phosphorus levels in the blood can also occur. These changes can be marked and may lead to death due to acute reversal of calcium-phosphorus ratios in the blood and subsequent arrhythmias and cardiovascular collapse.

Biochemistry. Yellow phosphorus is a protoplasmic poison that acts by uncoupling oxidative phosphorylation. The toxic effects of this form of phosphorus tends to target the GI tract, liver, kidney, and bone.[15,21] Early sudden death due to cardiovascular collapse may be associated with a postulated direct cardiotoxic effect.[12] In addition, hypocalcemia can follow phosphorus exposure. This, too, is postulated as a possible contributing factor in early sudden death.[12]

Diagnosis. Any worker who might have a significant occupational exposure to yellow phosphorus should have preplacement baseline tests as well as periodic reevaluations of electrolytes with serum phosphorus and calcium levels, renal and liver function tests, complete blood count, coagulation profile, and electrocardiogram.[47] The potential for inhalation exposure probably warrants a preplacement chest radiograph and arterial blood gas.[45] Any worker who has had chronic exposure and subsequently develops jaw or tooth pain should have a mandibular series of radiographs.

Management. Early GI decontamination is essential after phosphorus ingestion, and gastric lavage is preferred over ipecac in acute oral ingestions because of the corrosive effects of phosphorus.[45] Hypotension should be corrected with fluid replacement or blood products if bleeding is evident. Vasopressors may be used for refractory hypotension. Parenteral calcium replacement may be required. Hepatic or renal failure should be treated with supportive measures and hemodialysis when indicated.

Workers with acute inhalation exposure to phosphorus should be promptly removed from the source of exposure. They should also receive supplemental humidified oxygen therapy as soon as possible.

Exposed eyes should be irrigated with copious tepid water immediately at the worksite. If ocular pain persists, irrigation should be continued and the worker transported to an appropriate medical facility for a complete eye examination.

Phosphorus burns to the skin tend to be deep and extremely painful.[62] In fact, these properties have been exploited in the use of phosphorus as a chemical warfare agent.[2] After a skin burn, a firm eschar is typically produced, surrounded by an area of vesiculation. If loose particles of yellow phosphorus are adherent, they should be brushed from the skin. Covering burned skin with wet dressings or immersing burned extremities in water may give symptomatic relief. Because yellow phosphorus ignites at 34°C, some suggest covering the particles embedded in the skin with mineral oil.[15] Irrigation with 2% copper sulfate may be useful and is recommended prior to the removal of the phosphorus.[47] The rationale for its use is based on a chemical reaction that binds and sequesters the phosphorus and thereby prevents further burning due to oxidation. The granules of Cu_3P_2 are black and decompose easily.[63] Embedded particles should be delicately removed with metal forceps.[28] Surgical debridement is often required after significant dermal burns from phosphorus.

Consultation and Referral. With the high mortality rate that may result from severe yellow phosphorus toxicity (47% in patients with significant CNS and GI toxicity),[15,32] any symptomatic exposed worker should be observed in a monitored, intensive care setting. Significant dermal burns may require plastic surgery consultation.

RED PHOSPHORUS

Since modern matches no longer contain yellow phosphorus, chronic phosphorus poisoning is today seldom encountered.[17,21] Red phosphorus was introduced as a substitute for its yellow counterpart and is regarded as sufficient insurance against systemic phosphorus intoxication and bony necrosis in match factories. Red phosphorus is a nonvolatile, nonabsorbable, insoluble substance that is considered to be essentially nontoxic after oral ingestions. It also generates less vapor and is slower burning than yellow phosphorus.[6,21,24] In 1891, at a large London match factory, Barker was the first to use nontoxic red phosphorus by turning out over 6 million boxes per year. However, it was not until 1906 at the Berne Convention that yellow/white phosphorus was made illegal throughout Europe. In the United States, 25 years later a prohibitive tax was finally placed on yellow phosphorus to outlaw its import and export.[46]

POTASSIUM CHLORATE
Pathobiology

Chlorates are used in the manufacture of dyes, explosives, printed fabrics, weed killers, antiseptics, and matches. With modern-day matches, the principal toxic hazard relates to their content of chlorate rather than phosphorus.[21] However, it is estimated that fewer than 20 wooden matches (330 mg) or 2 books of paper matches (220 mg) do not contain enough potassium chlorate to be harmful to a child.[45,58] Acute doses of as little as 7.5 to 35 g of potassium chlorate have been reported to be fatal in adults; however, people who have ingested as much as 150 g have survived.[9] Chlorates are odorless compounds. Their usual toxicity develops after exposure via ingestion or inhalation. Acute ingestion may result in nausea, vomiting, and abdominal pain.[25,31] In addition, liver toxicity with jaundice and hepatomegaly has been reported.[52] With significant inhalational exposure, dyspnea and cyanosis resistant to oxygen therapy may be noted, with the development of methemoglobinemia.[25,31,52] Additionally, chlorates are directly nephrotoxic, and acute renal failure has been described.[31,52] Seizures have been reported in fatal cases.[56]

Biochemistry

Chlorate compounds can cause a significant local irritant effect, usually targeting the respiratory and gastric mucosa. These chemicals are very potent oxidizing agents, and exposure to them can result in hemolysis in conjunction with methemoglobin formation.

Diagnosis

In a match worker who is presenting with dyspnea and cyanosis resistant to oxygen therapy, methemoglobinemia and exposure to chlorates should be strongly considered. In addition to routine laboratory data, an arterial blood gas and methemoglobin level should be immediately obtained. Chlorate levels can be measured but are not readily available or clinically practical in the acute setting. Urine is considered the best determinant, but blood levels can also be assessed.[41]

Management and Treatment

Gastric decontamination measures are indicated for recent ingestion in patients who have not already vomited.[45] Activated charcoal should be administered in standard doses.

If inhalation exposure occurs, the worker should be immediately removed from the site of exposure to fresh air. Oxygen therapy is administered if the worker remains symptomatic. Although ocular exposures to powdered or 5% aqueous solutions of potassium chlorate are well tolerated, exposed eyes should be irrigated with copious amounts of tepid water.[22] With chlorates, skin absorption is minimal, but contaminated skin should, nevertheless, be washed thoroughly with soap and water. If the worker is exhibiting symptomatic methemoglobinemia or if the methemoglobin level exceeds approximately 30%, the administration of intravenous 1% methylene blue is recommended at 1 to 2 g/kg. In some cases, the methemoglobinemia may be refractory to methylene blue therapy.[52] In this setting, methylene blue is theorized to catalyze chlorate to chlorite, which may increase the methemoglobinemic action of the chlorate.[50] In addition, chlorate inactivates G6PD, thus decreasing NADPH and rendering methylene blue ineffective. As a result, exchange transfusion in conjunction with dialysis may be considered in severely intoxicated patients. Some sources recommend sodium thiosulfate administration to inactivate the chlorate ion to a less toxic chloride compound (dose: 2 to 5 g in 200 ml 5% sodium bicarbonate).[25] However, an in vitro study demonstrated that sodium thiosulfate did not prevent chlorate-induced methemoglobinemia.[53]

Consultation and Referral

Any worker who remains symptomatic after chlorate exposure should be removed from the site of exposure and taken to a health care facility for evaluation, oxygenation, decontamination, and supportive care. If the worker has significant methemoglobinemia, requiring antidote therapy with methylene blue, monitoring in an intensive care setting is recommended.

POTASSIUM BICHROMATE
Pathobiology

Oral ingestion of this hexavalent chromium compound can produce GI corrosion and hemorrhage,[26,33,34,60] acute multisystem shock, bleeding, hepatorenal failure,[27,34,48] and death.[26] In France, certain match heads may contain potassium bichromate. A 3-year-old ingested 40 matchheads (approximately 5 g of potassium bichromate) and developed renal failure a few days after the ingestion.[44] Inhalation of these compounds has also been implicated in causing nasal mucosa ulceration and perforation (chrome holes).[11,13] In addition, asthma, anaphylactoid reactions, metal fume fever,[54] and pulmonary edema have been described.[33] In the chronic setting, an increased incidence of lung cancer has been associated with chronic exposure to hexavalent chromium.[38] However, an increased mortality risk from cancer was not observed in a recent group of chromate workers who had been employed under modern, well-sanitized conditions.[42] Chromate dermatitis and eczema have also been observed in people who make or even use matches containing potassium bichromate.[19]

Biochemistry

The hexavalent chromium salts are very strong oxidizing agents that can penetrate the skin and mucosal membranes. On contact with skin, a reduction reaction from hexavalent to trivalent chromium occurs. This trivalent compound can react with skin proteins to form antigenic compounds. Corrosive burns can result from these chemical reactions, which cause denaturation of tissue protein.[35]

Diagnosis

The presence of chromium and chromium complexes in biologic specimens can be determined with chromatographic and colorimetric techniques.[55] Patch testing has been used to determine chromium sensitivity in the occupational setting. After a significant inhalational exposure, a chest radiograph is recommended.

Management and Treatment

To dilute and remove the potentially corrosive chromates, acute ingestions may be managed with the insertion of a small-bore oral gastric tube if the patient is alert and cooperative. This decision should be based on the time since exposure and the amount and concentration of chromate ingested. To date, the benefit of activated charcoal has not been evaluated in chromate poisoning. Induction of vomiting with syrup of ipecac is contraindicated because of the caustic nature of the compound.[45] Some sources advocate a controversial treatment, an orally administered ascorbic acid solution.[33,57] The proposed mechanism is that ascorbic acid reacts with hexavalent chromium salt to form the less toxic trivalent form.[30]

After an acute inhalational exposure, the worker should be removed from the exposure site. If in respiratory distress, oxygen therapy should be initiated. Severe corneal injury may result from ocular contact with solid or concentrated solutions of hexavalent salts.[22] Therefore, exposed eyes should be immediately irrigated with copious amounts of tepid water for at least 15 minutes. For skin exposure, the area should be washed with water or 10% ascorbic acid. Chronic chrome ulcers typically heal in several weeks with no specific treatment.

Workers with significant toxicity may require fluid resuscitation, blood products, and pressor agents. The efficacy of dialysis in chromate poisoning–induced renal failure is questionable.[4,26] Chelation with various agents may be attempted but has not been shown to be efficacious in most cases. In one study, dimercaprol (BAL) did not change renal clearance of hexavalent chromium in dogs.[16] Calcium ethylenediaminetetraacetic acid (EDTA) does not adequately chelate hexavalent chromium.

Consultation and Referral

Endoscopic consultation should be obtained emergently in workers with a definite ingestion, stridor, dysphagia, or drooling. Extreme caution should be used when performing endoscopy in this setting. The endoscopist should be especially careful not to pass beyond the first circumferential burn.[61] If burns are found, the worker should be followed 10 to 20 days later with a barium swallow or esophagogram. If the patient is in renal failure, a nephrologist should be consulted. Any severely toxic patient should be monitored in an intensive care setting.

ANTIMONY TRISULFIDE
Pathobiology

Antimony is a common additive to safety matches that is also used in manufacturing smoke bombs, military ammunition, illuminating shells, explosives, and pyrotechnics. Its most common use is in metallurgy to harden metals such as lead, zinc, and copper and to increase corrosion resistance.[37] It was originally added to matches to provide a less toxic alternative to yellow phosphorus.[6] Acute oral exposures are unusual because there are few oral preparations. Most exposures are chronic and related specifically to occupational exposures. Potential poisoning is greatest in antimony mining and the preparation of metallic antimony alloys. Symptoms of metallic antimony toxicity include skin rashes (antimony spots),[59] inflammation of the cornea, mucosal membrane irritation, and metal fume fever.[17] As in arsenic poisoning, abdominal cramps, nausea, vomiting, and watery diarrhea may occur. More severe toxicity may include cardiovascular disturbances and seizures.[37] At the worksite, conditions in which nascent hydrogen can react with antimony to form stibine (SbH_3) should be avoided. Stibine is an extremely toxic substance that can cause GI symptoms, headache, hemolysis, hematuria, and death.[45] Other forms of antimony in descending order of toxicity are metallic antimony, trisulfide, pentasulfide, trioxide, pentoxide.[18]

Biochemistry

Although chemically related to bismuth, antimony's principal toxicologic properties more resemble those of arsenic. Some initial studies indicate that antimony may act by interfering with cellular metabolism by combining with sulfhydryl groups after respiratory exposure.[45]

Diagnosis

Serum concentrations of antimony in normal subjects approximate 3 µg/L. A normal urinary level is approximately 0.8 µg/L. Urine assay may be used to assess clinical symptoms. Levels of 1 mg/L indicate a potentially harmful antimony exposure.[20]

Management and Treatment

Treatment for antimony exposure is primarily symptomatic. General gastric decontamination principles should be followed. Eye or skin exposures should be irrigated with copious tepid water. Inhalation-exposed workers with metal fume fever should be removed from the worksite into fresh air, and oxygen therapy should be given to symptomatic workers. There are no specific antidotes, although BAL and D-penicillamine[3] have been used as chelating agents with some success.[2] Dimercaptosuccinic acid (DMSA) may be the most effective chelator available, although there is no literature demonstrating its efficacy in antimony poisoning.[45]

Consultation and Referral

Any symptomatic worker should be removed from the source of exposure. If elevated antimony levels are detected, chelation therapy may prove beneficial.

FIRE OR EXPLOSION

A significant explosion and fire hazard exists in the match production industry. In 1993, a warehouse in Shenzhen, China, that stored a number of hazardous materials, including an enormous supply of matches, caught fire. A series of explosions resulted. More than 4000 firefighters, police, and soldiers were needed to extinguish the blaze, which destroyed 8 of 10 warehouses over an area of 20,000 square meters. Stemming from this disaster, 80 deaths were reported.[8] This incident points out the need for precautions in this industry. For instance, workers should be clothed in fire-resistant attire, and the factory should have state-of-the-art fire alarm and sprinkler systems.[39] In case of a fire or explosion, specific plans should exist for the workforce to be evacuated from the plant. Exposed victims should receive supplemental oxygen therapy for smoke inhalation, as well as monitoring of carbon monoxide when indicated. In the case of elevated carbon monoxide levels and/or neurologic symptoms at the scene, hyperbaric oxygenation is recommended.

REFERENCES

1. Andrews JB: Phorphorous poisoning in the match industry in the United States, *Bull U S Bureau Labor Stats* 20:31, 1910.
2. Bailly R et al: Experimental and human studies on antimony metabolism: their relevance for the biological monitoring of workers exposed to inorganic antimony, *Res Commun Chem Pathol Pharmacol* 32:355, 1981.
3. Basinger MA, Jones MM: Structural requirements for chelate antidotal efficacy in acute antimony intoxication, *Res Commun Chem Pathol Pharmacol* 32:355, 1981.
4. Behari JR, Tandon SK: Chelation in metal intoxication. Removal of chromium from organs of potassium chromate administered to rats, *Clin Toxicol* 16:33, 1980.
5. Campana M: Phosphorus poisoning (suicide)—fatal gastrointestinal hemorrhage, *J Chim Med* 4:610, 1958.
6. Chevallier A: Amorphous phosphorus used as a substitute for common phosphorus and methods to be applied in practice for the prevention of intoxication, *Ann d'Hygiene Publ Med Legale*, p 124, 1955.
7. Chiarenza A, Gallone C: Match dermatitis, *Contact Dermatitis* 7:346, 1981.
8. Chinese crackers, *Hazard Cargo Bull* 14:96, 1993.
9. Cochrane WJ, Smith RP: A fatal case of accidental poisoning by chlorate of potassium: review of the literature, *Can Med Assoc J* 42:23, 1940.
10. Dearden WF: The causation of phosphorus necrosis, *BMJ* 2:408, 1901.
11. Deng JF, Fleeger AK, Sinks T: An outbreak of chromium ulcer in a manufacturing plant, *Vet Hum Toxicol* 32:142, 1990.
12. Diaz-Rivera RS et al: Acute phosphorus poisoning in man: a study of 56 cases, *Medicine(Baltimore)* 29:269, 1950.
13. Dingle AF: Nasal disease in chrome workers, *Clin Otolaryngol* 17:287, 1992.
14. Diseases caused by phosphorus and its toxic compounds. In *Early detection of occupational diseases* Geneva, 1986, World Health Organization.
15. Ellenhorn MJ, Barceloux DG (editors): *Medical toxicology diagnosis and treatment of human poisoning,* New York, 1988, Elsevier.
16. Ellis EN et al: Effects of hemodialysis and dimercaprol in acute dichromate poisoning, *J Toxicol Clin Toxicol* 19:249, 1982.
17. Finkel AJ, editor: In *Hamilton and Hardy's industrial toxicology,* ed 4, Boston, 1983, John Wright PSG.
18. Fletcher G, Galambos J: Phosphorus poisoning in humans, *Arch Intern Med* 112:846, 1962.
19. Fregret S: Book matches as a source of chromate, *Arch Dermatol* 88:114, 1963.
20. Friberg L, editor: *Handbook on the toxicology of metals,* Amsterdam, 1979, Elsevier/North-Holland Biomedical Press.
21. Gosselin RE, Smith RP, Hodge HC (editors): *Clinical toxicology of commercial products,* ed 5, Baltimore, 1984, Williams & Wilkins.
22. Grant WM, editor: *Toxicology of the eye,* Springfield, Ill, 1986, Charles C Thomas.
23. Hamilton A: Phosphorus. In *Industrial poisons in the United States,* New York, 1929, Macmillan.
24. Heimann H: Phosphorus and compounds. In *Encyclopedia of occupational health and safety,* vol 2, 1983.
25. Helliwell M, Nunn J: Mortality in sodium chlorate poisoning, *BMJ* 1:1119, 1979.
26. Iserson KV et al: Failure of dialysis therapy in potassium dichromate poisoning, *J Emerg Med* 1:143, 1983.
27. Kaufman DB, DiNicola W, McIntosh R: Acute potassium dichromate poisoning, *Am J Dis Child* 119:374, 1970.
28. Kaufman T, Ullmann Y, Har-Shai Y: Phosphorus burns: a practical approach to local treatment, *J Burn Care Rehabil* 9:174, 1988.
29. Konjoyan TR: White phosphorus burns: case report and literature review, *Mil Med* 148:881, 1983.
30. Korallus U, Hazdorf C, Lewalter J: Experimental bases for ascorbic acid therapy of poisoning by hexavalent chromium compounds, *Int Arch Occup Environ Health* 53:247, 1984.
31. Lee DB et al: Haematological complications of chlorate poisoning, *BMJ* 2:31, 1970.
32. McCarron MM, Gaddis GP, Trotter AT: Acute yellow phosphorus poisoning from pesticide pastes, *Clin Toxicol* 18:693, 1981.
33. Meert KL et al: Acute ammonium dichromate poisoning, *Ann Emerg Med* 24:748, 1994.
34. Michie CA et al: Poisoning with a traditional remedy containing potassium dichromate, *Hum Exp Toxicol* 10:129, 1991.
35. Milner JE: Ascorbic acid in the prevention of chromium dermatitis, *J Occup Med* 22:51, 1980.
36. Miura T: Occupational health history of yellow phosphorus intoxication in Japan, *J Sci Labour* 61:221, 1985.
37. Musur M: Antimony toxicology in industry, *Ochrona Pracy* 19:10, 1964.
38. Norseth T: The carcinogenicity of chromium and its salts, *Br J Ind Med* 43:649, 1986.
39. Nyunt KM: Match industry. In *Encyclopedia of occupational health and safety,* vol 2, 1983.
40. O'Donoghue JL: Carbon monoxide, nitrogenous compounds and phosphorous. In Raton B (editor): *Neurotoxicity of industrial and commercial chemicals,* vol 1, Boca Raton, Fla, 1985, CRC Press.
41. Oliver JS, Smith H, Watson AA: Sodium chlorate poisoning, *J Forensic Sci Soc* 12:445, 1972.
42. Pastides H et al: A retrospective-cohort study of occupational exposure to hexavalent chromium, *Am J Ind Med* 25:663, 1994.
43. Phosphorous necrosis under control, *Br Dent J* 76:343, 1944.

44. Picaud JC et al: Acute renal failure in a child after chewing match heads, *Nephron* 57:225, 1991.
45. *Poisindex(R) substance identification,* 1996, Micromedex.
46. Raffle PB, McCallum RI, Murray R (editors): *Hunter's diseases of occupations,* London, 1987, Edward Arnold Publishers.
47. Rom WN, editor: *Environmental and occupational medicine,* ed 2, Boston, 1992, Little, Brown.
48. Sharma BK, Singhal PC, Chugh KS: Intravascular hemolysis and acute renal failure following potassium dichromate poisoning, *Postgrad Med J* 54:414, 1978.
49. Simon FA, Pickering LK: Acute yellow phosphorus poisoning: "smoking stool syndrome," *JAMA* 235:1343, 1976.
50. Singlemann E, Steffen C: Increased erythrocyte rigidity in chlorate poisoning, *J Clin Pathol* 36:719, 1983.
51. Steele MC, Ive FA: Recurrent facial eczema in females due to "strike anywhere" matches, *Br J Dermatol* 106:477, 1882.
52. Steffen C, Sitz R: Severe chlorate poisoning: report of a case, *Arch Toxicol* 48:281, 1978.
53. Steffen C, Wetzel E: Pathophysiologic aspects of chlorate poisoning, *Hum Toxicol* 4:541, 1985.
54. Stoke J: Metal fume fever in ferro-chrome workers, *Cent Afr J Med* 23:25, 1977.
55. Suzuki Y: Anion-exchange high-performance liquid chromatography of chromium (VI) and chromium (III) complexes in biological materials, *J Chromatogr* 415:317, 1987.
56. Timperman J, Maes R: Suicidal poisoning by sodium chlorate: a report of three cases, *J Forens Med* 13:123, 1966.
57. Walpole IR et al: Acute chromium poisoning in a 2 year old child, *Aust Paediatr J* 21:65, 1985.
58. Wasserman GS, Green VA, Wise GW: Nondrug ingestions in pediatrics, *Clin Toxicol* 7:401, 1974.
59. White GP, Mathias CT, Davis JS: Dermatitis in workers exposed to antimony in a melting process, *J Occup Med* 35:392, 1993.
60. Wood R et al: Acute dichromate poisoning after traditional use of puratives: a report of seven cases, *S Afr Med J* 77:640, 1990.
61. Zargar SA et al: The role of fiberoptic endoscopy in the management of corrosive ingestion and modified endoscopic classification of burns, *Gastrointest Endosc* 37:165, 1991.
62. Zenz C, editor: *Occupational medicine principles and practical applications,* Chicago, 1988, Year Book Medical.
63. Zong-Yue S et al: Treatment of yellow phosphorus skin burns with silver nitrate and copper sulfate, *Scand J Environ Health* 11:33, 1985.

44

Natural Gas

Harold E. Hoffman
Tee Lamont Guidotti

H₂S
hydrogen sulfide

- "Sour gas" is natural gas containing sulfur or carbon dioxide in high levels, making the gas "acid" or "sour"

- The H₂S-induced acute central toxicity leading to reversible unconsciousness is called "knockdown"

- "Gas eye", or keratoconjunctivitis, is a superficial inflammation of the cornea and conjunctiva that is often recurrent in workers in sour gas plants

- Sulfhemoglobinemia is a rare but extremely serious consequence of H₂S exposure

OCCUPATIONAL DESCRIPTION

The natural gas industry produces, processes, and transports natural gas to consumers. Because it is very economical, natural gas is the main heating fuel in Canada and many other countries. This gaseous form of petroleum is formed underground in reservoirs of gas or from gas dissolved in crude oil. Processing removes water, sulfur compounds, and liquid hydrocarbons. Large quantities of fluids (gases and liquids) are transported in pipelines under high pressure. Leaks, deliberate release, and work procedures such as maintenance and sampling release measurable amounts of natural gas into the workplace.

Homes, buildings, and industries require natural gas for fuel and as a raw material. The burning of natural gas may expose people to its contaminants and products of combustion. Injuries, accidents, and deaths occur regularly from exposure to natural gas in western Canada.[10]

The composition of natural gas varies between fields and wells, but the composition even varies with the well depth at a location.[34] For example, natural gas in Alberta contains 0% to 90% hydrogen sulfide.[9,12] As it comes from the well, natural gas contains oil, condensate, and gases.[25] It is primarily a mixture of light hydrocarbon gases with typical carbon numbers C1 to C4. Methane, ethane, propane, butane, carbon dioxide, and nitrogen comprise 99.5% of the natural gas by volume.[40] Other hydrocarbons include isobutane, normal butane, isopentane, normal pentane, hexane, heptane, and octane. Oxygen, hydrogen sulfide, sulfur, mercaptans, carbon dioxide (CO_2), carbon disulfide (CS_2), carbonyl sulfide (COS), helium, selenium, arsenic, mercury amines, water vapor, halogens, helium, radon, and polychlorinated biphenyls (PCBs) are often present.[12,30,46,57] Natural gas sold for fuel (sales gas)

Table 44-1 Sales gas specifications

Item	TCPL	A&S	US	BC	CWNG
H_2S (mg/m³)	23	6	6	23	23
CO_2 (Mol%)	2	2	1	—	—

From Petroleum Industry Training Service: *Basic natural gas chemistry.*

Table 44-2 Based mostly on the hydrogen sulfide content, natural gas is classified as follows by producers

	Dry natural gas	Low H_2S	High H_2S
Methane	10-90%	60-85%	60-85%
Ethane	1-17%	10-30%	10-30%
Propane	<8%	3-7%	3-7%
Butanes plus	<6%	1-5%	1-5%
Carbon dioxide	<3%	1-5%	1-5%
Hydrogen sulfide	0	<0.4%	7-40%

From Esso Occupational Health Division: *Material safety data sheet 4429 on raw gas (low H_2S),* Calgary, 1995, Imperial Oil Limited.

should not contain material hazardous to health, damaging to the pipeline, or limiting to marketability.[40] Sour natural gas contains carbon dioxide and/or hydrogen sulfide in amounts beyond the specifications of sales gas (Tables 44-1 and 44-2).

POTENTIAL TOXIC HAZARDS
Odorization

For fuel gas, government regulations often require the industry to inject 5 to 7 ppm of odorants, which allow for safer use by facilitating odor detection. However, odorants are not required for gas sold as process raw materials. Several contaminants in natural gas diminish the odor and reduce the ability of exposed people to detect the gas. Natural mercaptans oxidize synthetic mercaptans and thereby reduce their effectiveness. Oxides of nitrogen tend to consume the odorant.[33] Propane and butane mask the odorants.

Combustion Hazards of Natural Gas

When released, natural gas readily mixes with air to create a combustible atmosphere, and ignition of natural gas is a well-recognized explosive hazard. Oxidizing agents, including chlorine, bromine, pentafluoride, oxygen difluoride, and nitrogen trifluoride, burn or explode when mixed with natural gas.[2] Natural gas ignites spontaneously when mixed with chlorine dioxide.[2]

Natural gas workers and consumers may be exposed to the combustion hazards of natural gas from open flames or as the result of inadequately vented appliances. Incomplete combustion during home heating with natural gas may be a hazard due to the production of carbon monoxide (see Chapter 15).

The use of gas for cooking has been associated with a higher prevalence of respiratory disease in schoolchildren.[22] This has been attributed to the nitrogen dioxide produced by the burning of natural gas.[22] During poultry processing, for example, flames impinge on the carcasses to remove pinfeathers. This process has the potential to deposit chemicals on the meat.[43] Nitrogenated polycyclic aromatic compounds (PACs) form in the extremely oxygen-poor central region of the natural gas flame. Direct-acting mutagenic activity has been detected with these compounds.[5] Formaldehyde and soot are also possible by-products of combustion.[39]

Chemical Hazards Associated with "Sweet" Gas

Radon may be present at levels as high as 119 pCi/L in natural gas in pipeline distribution systems. The average radon concentration in natural gas at the point of consumer use is 20 pCi/L.[7] The National Health and Welfare Canada guideline for domestic radon levels is 22 pCi/l in air. Ambient air usually dilutes radon in natural gas to well below this level. Radon concentrates in the propane component of natural gas and in the natural gas liquids that are typically extracted in many gas plants. Processed gas and sales gas typically have much lower levels of radon. As radon decays rapidly during storage or transit, radon content decreases with distance from the production point.[7] The decay products of radon, such as bismuth-210, polonium-210, and lead-210, occur in sludge or scale in the equipment.[7] Workers who repair equipment are exposed to pipe scrapings that have radiation levels as high as 50 Bq/g (Becquerels/gram).[46] This is a potentially significant health concern.

Formaldehyde scavenges (removes) hydrogen sulfide. Traces of formaldehyde can reach the gas stream, go to meter stations, and contribute to a risk of exposure to this chemical.[46]

The oxides of nitrogen (NOx) are introduced into gas pipelines, typically, accidentally from sour gas processing facilities. Sodium nitrite produces oxides of nitrogen when used to scavenge hydrogen sulfide. Nitric oxide (NO) is a colorless, odorless gas that reacts in the presence of oxygen to produce nitrogen dioxide (NO_2). Nitrogen dioxide has a brown color and a noxious odor.

Ammonia, carbon monoxide, and acid fumes are usually minor components of natural gas. Sodium nitrite added to natural gas results in the formation of ammonia.[46] Decomposition of some hydrogen sulfide scavengers forms carbon monoxide.[46] Wells are treated with acid chemicals that can introduce acid fumes into the transmission facilities.[46]

Benzene, arsenic, and mercury occur in gas supplies.[40] Benzene, a known human carcinogen, is commonly found in very low levels in natural gas but may be found in concentrations up to 30 ppm, which is more than the Occupational Safety and Health Administration (OSHA) standard of 1 ppm.[40]

Table 44-3 Contaminants in natural gas

Contaminant	Source
Hydrogen sulfide	Naturally occurring (sour gas)
Mercaptan sulfur	Naturally occurring or odorant
Total sulfur	Naturally occurring or odorant
NO/NO_2	Hydrogen sulfide treatment
Formaldehyde	Hydrogen sulfide treatment
Arsenic	Naturally occurring
Benzene	Naturally occurring or suspect supplies
Radon	Naturally occurring
Mercury	Naturally occurring
Vinyl chloride	Landfill gas
Chlorinated HCs	Landfill gas
PCBs	Contaminated compressor lubricants

From Sosteck TI: Trace contaminants in natural gas, *Environmental Professional* 15:412, 1993.

Table 44-4 Hazards to workers introduced by natural gas production, processing, and transportation

Exposure	Source
Hydrogen sulfide	Raw gas
Mercaptans	Raw gas and extracted sulfur
Carbonyl sulfide	Raw gas and extracted sulfur
Hydrocarbons (C1 to C5)	Raw and product gas
Solvents	Maintenance and installation of equipment
Amines (principally monoetha-nolamine and diethanolamine)	Desulfuration
Elemental sulfur	Sulfur recovery
Methanol	Wax solvent, antifreeze
Demulsifiers (detergents)	Separation
Ethylene glycol	Dehydration
Corrosion agents	Pipeline and tank protection
Bactericidals	Production water, wastewater treatment
Defoamers	Separation
Asbestos	Plant insulation
Noise	

From Cottle MKW, Guidotti TL: Process chemicals in the oil and gas industry: potential occupational hazards, *Toxicol Ind Health* 6:41, 1989.

Polychlorinated biphenyls (PCBs) can be introduced by lubricants. Vinyl chloride and other chlorinated hydrocarbons (e.g., trichloroethylene, perchloroethylene) can come from landfill gas supplies.[40]

Diluents and contaminants adversely affect the quality of natural gas. Carbon dioxide, nitrogen, and helium are noncombustible gases that reduce the heating value. Potential contaminants can include water, free liquids (such as liquefied paraffins, crude oils, corrosion inhibitors), toxic gases (such as hydrogen sulfide), pipeline trash (pipe scale, sand, and dirt), and sludge[26] (Tables 44-3 and 44-4).

Table 44-5 Effects of exposure to hydrocarbon gases (C1-C4)*

Concentration of hydrocarbon gas	Effects
1000 ppm in air	No known effects from 12 hours exposure
2000 (C4)-5000 ppm (C1)†	Maximum exposure level before signs of intoxication may appear
20,000 (C4)-50,000 ppm (C1)	Intoxication, loss of coordination, reduced ability to reason and perform mental tasks
140,000 ppm	Asphyxia (oxygen reduced to 18%)
250,000 ppm	Asphyxia (oxygen reduced to 5.8%)
>250,000 ppm	Irreversible brain damage from lack of oxygen

From Evans HL: Occupational hygiene at an Alberta (Canada) natural gas processing plant, *Ann Occup Hyg* 33:145, 1989.
*C1 is methane. C4 is *n*-butane in practice but could be other unsaturated hydrocarbons with 4 carbon atoms such as *i*-butane, butene, and butyne.
†This means that 2000 ppm of butane or 5000 ppm of methane will have an equal effect. Ethane and propane are intermediate in potency.

CLINICAL TOXICOLOGY

Studies of natural gas distribution workers have not demonstrated mortality rates (standard mortality rates) higher than comparable populations.[21] Natural gas presents the physical hazards of fire and explosivity, common to all flammable gases.[40] The C1, C2, and C3 aliphatic hydrocarbons act as simple asphyxiants.[14] In high concentrations, they displace oxygen and cause hypoxia. Natural gas is irritating to the eyes and respiratory tract. Central nervous system effects include anesthesia, headaches, and dizziness (Table 44-5). Cold injury to the eyes and skin can result from exposure to rapidly expanding gas.

The hydrocarbon gases are fast acting, mild narcotic agents at levels below that causing oxygen deficiency. The one exception is methane, which causes narcosis only at concentrations that result in oxygen deficiency. At concentrations where the ambient oxygen is above 18%, narcotic effects are present for butane and propane, marginal for ethane, and absent for methane.[10] These gases also have poor warning properties, as the odor threshold is higher than the concentration causing physiologic effects[10] (Tables 44-6 and 44-7).

Sulfur oxides are strong irritants to the conjunctiva, the nasal mucosa, and the lungs. Exposure to 1 ppm for as little as 5 hours can cause bronchospasm in sensitive people.[19] Repeated or prolonged inhalation can lead to chronic bronchitis. Inclusion in an aerosol particle as sulfate or

Table 44-6 Narcosis thresholds for several hydrocarbons

Hydrocarbon	Predicted onset of narcosis (ppm)
Methane	300,000 ppm
Ethane	130,000
Propane	47,000
Butane	17,000

From Drummond I: Light hydrocarbon gases: a narcotic, asphyxiant, or flammable hazard? *Appl Occup Environ Hyg* 82:120, 1993.

Table 44-7 Toxic properties of pure methane (mixtures of hydrocarbons have additive narcotic effects)

Concentration of methane	Toxic properties
Less than 50,000 ppm	Not toxic
140,000 ppm (18% oxygen air limit)	Onset of hypoxia
300,000 ppm	Onset of narcosis

From Drummond I: Light hydrocarbon gases: a narcotic, asphyxiant, or flammable hazard? *Appl Occup Environ Hyg* 82:120, 1993.

Table 44-8 Effects of the oxides of nitrogen

Concentration	Health effect
Nitric oxide (NO)	
2 ppm	Threshold limit value set to prevent irritation and erosion of teeth
60-150 ppm	Immediate irritation of nose and throat, burning in the chest
100-150 ppm	Pneumonitis and pulmonary edema after 30-60 minutes exposure
200-700 ppm	Fatal after short exposure
Nitrogen dioxide (NO$_2$)	
25 ppm	Respiratory irritation and chest pain
50 ppm	Irritation to eyes and nose, pulmonary edema after 1 hour
80 ppm	Chest tightness after 3-5 minutes
100 ppm	Pulmonary edema and death after 1 hour

From Tiemstra E, Cirka L: *Trace constituents: experience of Nova Corporation of Alberta,* Gas Quality Measurement Conference, Institute of Gas Technology, 1990.

conversion to sulfuric acid in raindrops intensifies the response to sulfur dioxide.[19]

Acids are highly corrosive and irritating and give rise to local effects on the skin, eye, and other mucous epithelia when there is direct exposure to sufficient concentrations.[61] Sulfuric acid is 4 times more irritating than elemental sulfur in causing bronchospasm.[19] Sulfuric acid irritates mucosa at 0.125 to 0.50 ppm,[19] with repeated exposure leading to chronic bronchitis. Occupational exposure to strong inorganic-acid mists containing sulfuric acid is carcinogenic to humans (Group 1).[55]

Carbonyl sulfide (COS) is a respiratory irritant and also acts as a narcotic in high concentrations. Upon exposure to organic vapors, COS may produce hydrogen sulfide, sulfur dioxide, mercaptans, and other sulfur-containing compounds.[19]

Mercaptans occur in trace levels in raw sour gas and are reintroduced as odorizers before the natural gas enters the home. Mercaptans have a very offensive odor often associated with nausea and headache. High concentrations of mercaptans themselves can produce unconsciousness.[35]

Other trace components should be considered as possible causes for adverse health effects in this industry. The oxides of nitrogen include nitric oxide (NO) and nitrogen dioxide (NO$_2$), which are respiratory irritants (Table 44-8). Carbon dioxide is an asphyxiant in sufficient concentration. Radon levels tend not to be high enough to be a health hazard, unless deposited in equipment. Arsenic is present in traces in some natural gas. Mercury in Alberta natural gas occurs at levels less than 1.5 ppbw (parts per billion by weight),[28] which is not hazardous.

Selenium may be present in trace amounts that are of low toxicity. Organoselenium compounds, formed when sele-

nium combines with organic residues, produce greater toxicity because of the increased vapor pressure of the organoselenium compound.[19]

Formaldehyde is a very strong irritant of the respiratory tract and eyes and a potential carcinogen. Polychlorinated biphenyls (PCBs) affect the liver, cardiovascular system, nervous system, and skin and are considered possible carcinogens.

Hydrogen Sulfide and Sour Gas

Hydrogen sulfide (H$_2$S) is a common and potent toxic agent that is the primary chemical hazard in the gas production industry.

Occupational exposure to hydrogen sulfide is primarily a problem in the sour gas segment of the natural gas industry, which is limited to relatively few natural gas fields worldwide. Sour gas is natural gas containing sulfur or carbon dioxide in high levels that make the gas "acid" or "sour." In the formation of natural gas, prolonged degradation of underground organic material is reduced to hydrogen sulfide. It is most often a hazard in well drilling and servicing, pumping, and gas refining close to the source in the "oil patch," especially Texas, Oklahoma, and the Gulf Coast of the United States, Alberta, the North Sea, and the Middle East. Hydrogen sulfide is a variable constituent of sour gas that ranges from low concentrations to 85% and more. The problem is uniquely severe in the Canadian province of Alberta because of the heavy concentration of high-sulfur-content oil and gas fields in the province.[3]

The H$_2$S in sour gas is usually accompanied by concentrations of methyl mercaptans—CH$_3$SH, (CH$_3$)$_2$S, and (CH$_3$)$_2$S$_2$—and carbonyl sulfide (COS), which are usually regarded to be of low toxicity.[22,52] During gas processing, some of these compounds are converted to H_2S. Mercaptans are also added to natural gas as a safety measure to ensure detection of leaks.

Toxicology of Hydrogen Sulfide

Hydrogen sulfide is inhaled and enters the circulation directly across the alveolar-capillary barrier, where it dissociates, in part, into the sulfide ion, HS. Some remains as free H_2S in the bloodstream, and this fraction appears to interact with metalloproteins, disulfide-containing proteins, and thio-S-methyl-transferase, to form methyl sulfides. The sulfide ion binds to heme compounds and is itself metabolized by oxidation to sulfate.

Hydrogen sulfide interacts with a number of enzymes and other macromolecules, including hemoglobin and myoglobin. Because most macromolecules are held together by disulfide bonds, they are prone to disruption by aqueous sulfide. The critical target enzyme of H_2S is cytochrome oxidase, a family of related enzymes constituting the electron transport system in oxidative phosphorylation, the principal energy-generating system of cells. Oxygen is the final substrate of this system and is necessary to its function. The effect of H_2S in disrupting cytochrome oxidase activity is the same as oxygen deprivation or asphyxiation, except that it may act more quickly.[4,32]

The exposure-response curve for lethality is extremely steep for hydrogen sulfide. As an inhaled toxic substance, H_2S gives little margin of safety.[27] The primary determinant of toxicity is the concentration rather than the duration of exposure. Thus, H_2S does not follow Haber's law; that is, the product of the concentration and the duration of exposure needed to achieve a given effect is not constant. Higher concentrations are much more toxic, even with proportionally shorter exposure levels.

Acute Effects of Hydrogen Sulfide

The principal effects of H_2S and the approximate thresholds for these responses are summarized in Table 44-9. Acute central neurotoxicity, pulmonary edema, and the mucosal effects are well documented in association with H_2S. Odor followed by olfactory paralysis and keratoconjunctivitis are the characteristic effects of H_2S at lower concentrations.*

The H_2S-induced acute central toxicity leading to reversible unconsciousness is called a *knockdown*. Whether repeated or prolonged knockdowns are associated with chronic neurologic sequelae is highly controversial, but the evidence is strongly suggestive. Knockdowns can be acutely fatal as a consequence of respiratory paralysis and cellular anoxia. Respiratory paralysis may occur if exposure is prolonged, presumably as a direct consequence of sulfide toxicity inhibiting brainstem respiratory nuclei. Very high concentrations (500 to 1000 ppm) may be associated with a knockdown. A knockdown may be fatal if exposure is

*References 3, 4, 6, 13, 15, 23, 24, 29, 32, 37, 39, 45, 51, 52, 56.

Table 44-9 Health effects of hydrogen sulfide at various exposure levels

Concentration (ppm)	Effects
0.01-0.3	Odor threshold (highly variable)
1-5	Moderate offensive odor; may be associated with nausea, tearing of the eyes, headaches, or loss of sleep with prolonged exposure; healthy young male subjects experience no decline in maximal physical work capacity
10	8-Hour ocupational exposure limit in Alberta
15	15-Minute occupational exposure limit in Alberta
20	Ceiling occupational exposure limit evacuation level in Alberta; odor very strong
20-50	Keratoconjunctivitis (eye irritation) and lung irritation; possible eye damage after several days of exposure; may cause digestive upset and loss of appetite
100	Eye and lung irritation; olfactory paralysis, odor disappears
150-200	Sense of smell paralyzed; severe eye and lung irritation
250-500	Pulmonary edema may occur, especially if prolonged
500	Serious damage to eyes within 30 minutes; severe lung irritation; unconsciousness and death within 4 to 8 hours; amnesia for period of exposure; "knockdown"
1000	Breathing may stop within one or two breaths; immediate collapse

Data from Guidotti TL: Occupational exposure to hydrogen sulfide in the sour gas industry: some unresolved issues, *Int Occup Environ Health* 66:133, 1994; and US National Research Council, Committee on Medical & Biological Effects of Environmental Pollutants: Subcommitee on Hydrogen Sulfide: *Hydrogen sulfide*, Baltimore, 1979, University Park Press.

prolonged. If exposure is transient, as usually happens in the oil patch, recovery may be equally rapid and apparently complete.[3,4,6,13,15]

Pulmonary edema is also a well-recognized acute effect of H_2S toxicity, especially when exposure is prolonged. The prognosis for recovery is generally good if the patient can be supported through the acute episode.[3,4,6,13,15]

Acute inhalation of H_2S may be fatal, depending on the concentration and duration of exposure and the duration of anoxia.†

Hydrogen sulfide paralyzes the olfactory nerve and prevents perception of the otherwise strong smell. After a strong odor of rotten eggs, the odor disappears because of physiologic olfactory nerve fatigue. This removes a vital warning to, for example, oilfield workers caught in a cloud or entering a geographic land depression in which the gas has collected.[28,31,34,47,49]

†References 3, 6, 24, 39, 48, 52.

"Gas eye," or keratoconjunctivitis, is a superficial inflammation of the cornea and conjunctiva that is often recurrent in workers in sour gas plants who are exposed for prolonged periods to relatively low concentrations. A peculiar feature of this effect is that it can be associated with reversible chromatic distortion and visual changes. This effect is sometimes accompanied by blepharospasm, tearing, and photophobia.[15,22,44,49]

Another property of H_2S is its irritant effect on mucous membranes. The respiratory tract is particularly vulnerable because of its unprotected contact with the gas in air. Hydrogen sulfide has the ability to penetrate deeply into the respiratory tract because its solubility in water is relatively low, which renders it capable of causing alveolar injury leading to acute pulmonary edema.[15,49]

Although sulfhemoglobin may form after H_2S exposure, the development of clinically significant sulfhemoglobinemia is distinctly uncommon.[4]

Chronic Effects of Hydrogen Sulfide

Chronic central nervous system effects may be cumulative after several knockdowns. Whether these chronic effects represent the sequelae of minor brain damage resulting from anoxia or trauma is controversial. Investigators have found evidence for cognitive function abnormalities, labile affect and personality changes, and anosmia, with a suggestion of increasing severity associated with length of time unconscious.* Experimental studies in mice also suggest a cumulative effect in reducing brain cytochrome oxidase activity.[15]

Other possible effects of H_2S include respiratory, cardiac, ocular, and immunologic defense disorders, but the evidence that H_2S exposure leads to clinical disorders of these organ systems remains inconclusive.[3,15]

Long-term, low-level exposure to H_2S is a particular concern in communities located near sour gas facilities.[9,40] To date, these concerns have not been effectively addressed.

Treatment of Hydrogen Sulfide Exposure

Many antidotes to H_2S intoxication have been proposed, but few are in regular use or appear to be more than laboratory phenomena inadequate for human application. Thiosulfate is not indicated in H_2S intoxication, where it is a metabolite of sulfide and not a substrate for enzymatic oxidation of the toxic moiety, as in the case of cyanide intoxication.[45]

Hydrogen sulfide resembles cyanide in that both bind reversibly to cytochromes, although there appear to be differences at a biochemical level. For this reason, treatment with nitrites has been advocated as a therapeutic approach to H_2S toxicity, on the theory that the methemoglobin so generated would displace the sulfide as it does cyanide and thus regenerate the active cytochrome

oxidase. However, investigators studying the kinetics of nitrite as an antidote have concluded that it can be effective only within the first few minutes following exposure and may actually slow sulfide removal thereafter. A further practical problem with this approach is that it may add to the anoxic burden that already may exist from the cytochrome poisoning, respiratory paralysis due to central toxicity, and ventilation-perfusion mismatch associated with pulmonary edema. It may also induce hypotension and further complicate the anoxia with hypoperfusion. Administration of nitrites is usually begun with inhalation of amyl nitrite (for 30 seconds of every minute), followed by sodium nitrite intravenously, in the same dosages as for cyanide poisoning.[31,39,45]

Treatment with oxygen and supportive care alone has been recommended in order to avoid further complicating the toxic effects with iatrogenic anoxia and nitrite toxicity. However, confirmation that oxygen therapy alone works is limited to anecdotal reports, and experimental studies with H_2S-exposed mice did not show increased survival with oxygen alone. Unlike cyanide intoxication, there is no evidence that H_2S intoxication confers a risk on the rescuer during mouth-to-mouth resuscitation.[31,38]

Hyperbaric oxygen therapy is an attractive and logical option for treating H_2S intoxication, and anecdotal evidence suggests that it may be effective. Given the low morbidity of hyperbaric oxygen treatment in skilled hands, it is a prudent intervention if facilities are available.[36,54]

Combined treatment with hyperbaric oxygen and nitrite appears to be emerging as the treatment of choice.

Occupational Hazard Management for Hydrogen Sulfide

The OSHA permissible exposure level and the National Institute of Occupational Safety and Health–recommended exposure level for H_2S are both 10 ppm, 8-hour time-weighted average; OSHA also has a short-term standard of 15 ppm.

Studies on normal volunteers during exercise suggest that 5 ppm H_2S is easily tolerated and results in no detectable physiologic change. In the absence of well-conducted studies of community residents or low-level exposure of workers, this is the best evidence available that current occupational exposure standards are probably adequate (see Table 44-9).

Environmental Issues Associated with the Natural Gas Industry

In buildings, natural gas combustion products emanate from poorly vented appliances. Buildings sealed for energy efficiency prevent the dispersion of natural gas leaks.

In the environment, chronic low-level exposures to sour gas plant emissions may irritate the respiratory system enough to cause symptoms in children but not in adults.[13] In both children and adults, no reduction in respiratory function

*References 15, 18, 25, 38, 48, 50-53.

occurred.[13] Flare stacks release hydrogen sulfide (up to 375 ppm), carbonyl sulfide, carbon disulfide, and sulfur dioxide (from 275 to 3000 ppm).[47]

In general, however, natural gas is usually considered a preferred fossil fuel because it burns cleanly at the site of combustion (once the sulfur is extracted). All fossil fuels generate carbon dioxide, of course, but the energy produced per unit of carbon dioxide generated is less for natural gas than for other fuels.

CONCLUSION

Natural gas is an efficient fuel with hazards mostly associated with safe handling in the sweet gas industry and hydrogen sulfide in the sour gas industry. To date, there is no indication for an excess mortality in the industry as a whole or for a peculiar occupational disease of gas workers except for knockdowns associated with hydrogen sulfide in the "upstream" sour gas industry.

REFERENCES

1. Alberta Environment: *Sour-gas processing-plant applications: a guide to content,* Guide G-26, Calgary, 1981, Energy Resources Conservation Board.
2. American Gas Association: Material safety data sheet (sample) on natural gas.
3. Arnold IMF et al: Health implications of occupational exposures to hydrogen sulfide, *J Occup Med* 27:373, 1981.
4. Beauchamp RO Jr et al: A critical review of the literature on hydrogen sulphide toxicity, *Crit Rev Toxicol* 13:25, 1984.
5. Braun AG et al: Generation of biologically active substances in a natural gas flame, *Environ Health Perspect* 72:297, 1987.
6. Burnett WW et al: Hydrogen sulfide poisoning: review of 5 years' experience, *Can Med Assoc J* 117:1277, 1977.
7. Cahill RA, Coleman DD: Overview of the significance of radon in natural gas: an update. In Proceedings of the 1985 Joint Annual Meeting: *Impact of air toxics on the quality of life,* 1985, Air Pollution Control Association.
8. Cottle MKW, Guidotti TL: Process chemicals in the oil and gas industry: potential occupational hazards, *Toxicol Ind Health* 6:41, 1989.
9. Dales RE et al: Respiratory health of a population living downwind from natural gas refineries, *Am Rev Respir Dis* 139:595, 1989.
10. Drummond I: Light hydrocarbon gases: a narcotic, asphyxiant, or flammable hazard? *Appl Occup Environ Hyg* 8:120, 1993.
11. Esso Occupational Health Division: *Material safety data sheet 4429 on raw gas (low H₂S),* Calgary, 1995, Imperial Oil Limited.
12. Evans HL: Occupational hygiene at an Alberta (Canada) natural gas processing plant, *Ann Occup Hyg* 33:145, 1989.
13. Glass DC: A review of the health effects of hydrogen sulphide exposure, *Ann Occup Hyg* 34:323, 1990.
14. Gorman DF: Problems and pitfalls in the use of hyperbaric oxygen for the treatment of poisoned patients, *Med Toxicol Adverse Drug Exp* 4:393, 1989.
15. Guidotti TL: Occupational exposure to hydrogen sulfide in the sour gas industry: some unresolved issues, *Int Occup Environ Health* 66:153, 1994.
16. Jäppinen P et al: Exposure to hydrogen sulphide and respiratory function, *Br J Ind Med* 47:824, 1990.
17. Kangas J, Jappinen P, Savolainen H: Exposure to hydrogen sulfide, mercaptans, and sulfur dioxide in pulp industry, *Am Ind Hyg Assoc J* 45:787, 1984.
18. Kilburn K: Case report: profound neurobehavioural deficits in an oil field worker overcome by hydrogen sulfide, *Am J Med Sci* 306:301, 1993.
19. Klemm RF: *Environmental effects of the operation of sulfur extraction gas plants,* Calgary, 1972, Environment Conservation Authority, Alberta Government.
20. Langenkamp RD: *The illustrated petroleum reference dictionary,* ed 3, Tulsa, 1985, Penwell Books.
21. Liveright T, Stanbury M: An historical prospective study of mortality within a cohort of gas distribution workers, *Am J Ind Med* 4:651-657, 1983.
22. Malia RJ et al: Association between gas cooking and respiratory disease in children, *BMJ* 2:149, 1977.
23. Milby TH: Hydrogen sulfide intoxication: review of the literature and report of unusual accident resulting in two cases of nonfatal poisoning, *J Occup Med* 4:431, 1962.
24. Osbern LN, Crapo RO: Dung lung: a report of toxic exposure to liquid manure, *Ann Intern Med* 95:312, 1981.
25. Parra O et al: Inhalation of hydrogen sulphide: a case of sub-acute manifestations and long term sequelae, *Br J Ind Med* 48:286, 1991.
26. Petroleum Industry Training Service: Basic natural gas chemistry.
27. Prior M et al: Concentration-time interactions in hydrogen sulfide toxicity in rats, *Can J Vet Res* 52:375, 1988.
28. Province of Alberta, Energy Resources Conservation Board: Information Letter IL OG-72-06.
29. Public Health Service: *Criteria for a recommended standard occupational exposure to hydrogen sulfide,* DHEW(NIOSH) Publication No. 77-158, Atlanta, 1977, US Department of Health, Education, and Welfare, Centers for Disease Control.
30. Raisanen W: Practical field measurement of mercury in natural gas. In Proceedings of the 1985 joint annual meeting: *Impact of air toxics on the quality of life,* 1985, Air Pollution Control Association.
31. Ravizza AG et al: The treatment of hydrogen sulfide intoxication: oxygen versus nitrites, *Vet Hum Toxicol* 24:241, 1982.
32. Reiffenstein RJ, Hulbert WC, Roth SH: Toxicology of hydrogen sulfide, *Annu Rev Pharmacol Toxicol* 32:109, 1992.
33. Runge P: *Economics of gas quality,* 1990, Institute of Gas Technology Conference on Gas Quality Measurement.
34. Runion HE: Occupational exposures to potentially hazardous agents in the petroleum industry, *Occup Med* 3:431, 1988.
35. Sax NI: *Dangerous properties of industrial materials,* ed 6, New York, 1986, Van Nostrand Reinhold.
36. Smilkstein MJ et al: Hyperbaric oxygen therapy for severe hydrogen sulfide poisoning, *J Emerg Med* 3:27, 1985.
37. Smith RP, Gosselin RE: Hydrogen sulfide poisoning, *J Occup Med* 21:93, 1979.
38. Smith RP, Kruszyna R, Kruszyna H: Management of acute sulfide poisoning: effects of thiosulfate, oxygen, and nitrite, *Arch Environ Health* 31:166, 1976.
39. Snyder JW et al: Occupational fatality and persistent neurological sequelae after mass exposure to hydrogen sulfide, *Am J Emerg Med* 13:199, 1995.
40. Sosteck TI: Trace contaminants in natural gas, *Environmental Professional* 15:412, 1993.
41. Spitzer WO et al: Chronic exposure to sour gas emissions: meeting a community concern with epidemiologic evidence, *Can Med Assoc J* 141:685, 1989.
42. Stanbury M, Liveright T: Retirement disability among workers in natural gas distribution company, *Am J Ind Med* 4:641, 1983.
43. Steinmetz GF: *Harmonizing global standards for natural gas quality and appliance performance, appendix 1: AGA statement of gas quality issues,* Baltimore, 1990, Baltimore Gas and Electric Company, Institute of Gas Technology Conference on Gas Quality Measurement.
44. Stine RJ, Slosberg B, Beacham BE: Hydrogen sulfide intoxication: case report and discussion of treatment, *Ann Intern Med* 85:756, 19

45. Tansy MF et al: Acute and subchronic toxicity studies of rats exposed to vapors of methyl mercaptan and other reduced-sulphur compounds, *J Toxicol Environ Health* 8:71, 1981.

46. Tiemstra E, Cirka L: *Trace constituents: experience of Nova Corporation of Alberta,* Gas Quality Measurement Conference, Institute of Gas Technology, 1990.

47. Tollefson EL, Strosher MT: An investigation of flare stack emissions from a sour gas plant. In Proceedings of the 1985 joint annual meeting: *Impact of air toxics on the quality of life,* 1985, Air Pollution Control Association.

48. Turner RM, Fairhurst S: *Toxicology of substances in relation to major hazards: hydrogen sulphide,* London, 1990, HMSO.

49. Tvedt B et al: Delayed neuropsychiatric sequelae after acute hydrogen sulfide poisoning: affection of motor function, memory, vision, and hearing, *Acta Neurol Scand* 84:348, 1991.

50. U S National Research Council, Committee on Medical & Biological Effects of Environmental Pollutants: Subcommittee on Hydrogen Sulfide: *Hydrogen sulfide,* Baltimore, 1979, University Park Press.

51. Vannatta JB: Hydrogen sulfide poisoning: report of four cases and brief review of the literature, *J Okla State Med Assoc* 75:29, 1982.

52. Wang DX: [A review of 152 cases of acute poisoning of hydrogen sulfide; in Chinese], *Chin J Prev Med* 23:330, 1989.

53. Wasch HH et al: Prolongation of the P-300 latency associated with hydrogen sulfide exposure, *Arch Neurol* 46:902, 1989.

54. Whitcraft DD III, Bailey TD, Hart GB: Hydrogen sulfide poisoning treated with hyperbaric oxygen, *J Emerg Med* 3:23, 1985.

55. World Health Organization, International Agency for Research on Cancer: Occupational exposures to mists and vapours from strong inorganic acids and other industrial chemicals, *IARC Monogr Eval Carcinog Risks Hum* 54, 1992.

56. World Health Organization, International Programme on Chemical Safety: *Environmental health criteria 19: hydrogen sulphide,* Geneva, 1983, World Health Organization.

57. Zingaro RA et al: Measurement of arsenic in natural gas. In Proceedings of the 1985 Joint Annual Meeting: *Impact of air toxics on the quality of life,* 1985, Air Pollution Control Association.

SUGGESTED READINGS

Beck JF et al: Nitrite as antidote for acute hydrogen sulfide intoxication? *Am Ind Hyg Assoc J* 42:805, 1981.

Bhambhani Y et al: Comparative physiological responses of exercising men and women to 5 ppm hydrogen sulfide exposure, *Am Ind Hyg Assoc J* 55:1030, 1994.

Bhambhani Y, Sing M: Physiological effects of hydrogen sulfide inhalation during exercise in healthy men, *J Appl Physiol* 71:1872, 1991.

Brown WE: Experiments with anesthetic gases, propylene, methane, dimethyl ether, *J Pharmacol Exp Ther* 23:485, 1924.

Hoidal CR et al: Hydrogen sulfide poisoning from toxic inhalations of roofing asphalt, *Ann Emerg Med* 15:826, 1986.

Richardson DB: Respiratory effects of chronic hydrogen sulfide exposure, *Am J Ind Med* 28:99, 1995.

45

Pharmaceutical

David Lee

methotrexate

- Because all pharmaceuticals are, by definition, biologically active, exposed workers are potential candidates to experience toxicity

- Asthma and dermatitis are frequent manifestations of occupational toxicity in the pharmaceutical industry

OCCUPATIONAL DESCRIPTION

The pharmaceutical industry has been described as a special subset of the chemical industry.[14] A distinctive characteristic of the pharmaceutical industry is that it focuses on natural and synthetic agents that are almost all biologically active. Workers in this field are often exposed to multiple biologically active agents or various by-products during their development, production, and distribution. Occupationally related exposures has been reported as early as 1751, when Ramazzini reported deleterious health effects in workers involved in the production of opiate-containing medicinals.[5] In the modern medical literature, work-related poisoning has been reported as early as 1945, when Watrous and McCaughey described cases of arsenic toxicity at Abbott Laboratories.[35]

The pharmaceutical industry is varied and global. Different manufacturers may utilize diverse methods to produce similar drugs. Therefore, workers at a U.S. plant may be exposed to different additives and intermediate compounds than workers in a plant in Asia, although they may be producing the same drug. Many companies manufacture their specific pharmaceuticals through a batch process. In this method, workers have varying exposures to chemicals, and it would be unusual for one group of workers to have a chronic exposure to a single chemical.[34]

The pharmaceutical industry also encompasses a wide range of job descriptions, which may have varying risks to occupational exposures. These include workers in the research laboratories who are often exposed to various chemicals and animals, workers in the manufacturing process who are often exposed to the drug itself, and workers in packaging and distribution, for example, pharmacists, who suffer a different pattern of work-related injuries.

Although various disease processes have been attributed to work-related exposures or environments, the few studies that have examined this issue have not shown a definitive association between the pharmaceutical industry and increased mortality. Harrington and Goldblatt reviewed death records of workers in the pharmaceutical industry in England and noted no clear association between the type of work performed and excess mortality risk. They did note a trend for an increased incidence of colon cancer, but the authors felt that this increased risk was caused from nonoccupational sources. They also noted a trend for increased risk of suicide deaths, which they thought was consistent with other studies of "professional" populations and not specific for the pharmaceutical industry.[14]

Thomas and Decoufle also noted an increased risk of death by suicide and cancers in their study of a large, U.S.-based, pharmaceutical company. Using a proportionate mortality analysis that compared these workers with the general population, they noted increased numbers of various cancers. Cancer rates of malignancies of the large intestine, liver, kidney, and brain were elevated in men, and the cancer rate of breast malignancies were elevated in women. However, when epidemiologically compared to the general population, the authors also believed that these increased incidences were due to nonoccupational causes. Data on respiratory cancers, melanomas, and leukemias were inconclusive. Again, these authors noted a marked elevated risk for suicide by overdose. Like Harrington and Goldblatt, Thomas and Decoufle believed that this increased risk was due to worker familiarity and availability of drugs.[35]

The incidence of miscarriages as a reflection of worker health is another area that investigators have examined. Several authors have noted higher rates of spontaneous abortions in pharmaceutical laboratory workers.[13,33] Elevated rates of spontaneous abortions also appear in hospital and university laboratory workers.[32] Using questionnaires, Hansson and associates noted no difference in pregnancy outcomes in a Swedish pharmaceutical plant between plant workers and controls. The authors did note higher rates of perinatal death and major malformations in workers involved in chemical laboratory work.[13]

Taskinen and colleagues performed a register-based study on Finnish pharmaceutical workers. The authors found an increased incidence of spontaneous abortions in general, but it was not statistically significant. Increased odds ratios were noted in certain subgroups: workers exposed to methylene chloride, estrogens, or four or more organic solvents, and workers who had to perform continuous heavy lifting.[33]

POTENTIAL TOXINS

The three main afflicted organ systems in workers in the pharmaceutical fields are the musculoskeletal, dermal, and respiratory systems. Although different organ systems may be involved depending on the drug being manufactured, work-related injuries to these three systems far exceed injuries to other physiologic systems. Certain job requirements increase the risk of certain injuries. Rotgoltz and associates reported that more than two thirds of pharmaceutical factory workers complained of low back pain. Not surprisingly, this problem was much more prevalent in workers involved with packaging and distributing than in office workers or workers involved in manufacturing.[28] Slovak and Hill reported that 30% of pharmaceutical personnel exposed to research laboratory animals had types of laboratory animal allergies causing rhinitis or asthma.[31] Lahti and colleagues noted that janitorial and maintenance personnel may have higher risks of contact dermatitis because they are physically exposed to toxins when working on contaminated machinery or spillage.[17]

CLINICAL TOXICOLOGY
Dermal

As with other industries, the risk of occupational skin disease is associated with the amount of exposure. Incidence rates for skin disorders that require medical attention range from 0.1% to 6%.[30] Personnel involved in management tend to have lowest risk, followed by workers involved in manufacturing, and then by workers involved in research and maintenance, who have the highest risk. The most common body part affected is the dorsum of the hand and forearm, followed by skin diseases of the face and neck, probably because of the fine, powdery nature of manufactured drugs that allows airborne particulate distribution.[10]

The most commonly reported type of occupational skin disorder is allergic contact dermatitis. Sheretz reported that the incidence of this disease ranged from 0.1% to 1%. A host of drugs can cause it[30] (see box on p. 369). The classic presentation includes pruritic papules with weeping, crusted vesicles, and bullae with sharp margins. There may be linear streaks and angular corners suggestive of physical contact. Chronic changes include lichenification with scaling and fissuring. This is typically a cell-mediated, type IV, delayed immunologic response to a specific allergen. There are usually two phases in this disease. The first is sensitization, in which a worker becomes exposed and then allergic to a specific chemical. The second phase is elicitation, in which the worker is continuously exposed to the allergen, which causes a further immunologic response. The allergen is usually a small molecule of less than 500 daltons since it must penetrate the outer layers of the skin.[20] Certain workers are usually sensitized to specific allergens. Rydroft and colleagues noted that confirming specific allergen sensitivity may be difficult, especially with patch testing.[29]

Although not as commonly reported, irritant contact dermatitis is probably more prevalent, causing up to 80% of all dermatoses.[20] This disorder results from nonimmunologically mediated physical or chemical insult to the skin. Irritant contact dermatitis may be difficult to distinguish from allergic contact dermatitis. However, the

---

Specific Chemicals in the Pharmaceutical Industry Reported to Cause Contact Allergy

2-Aminothiazole	Ethyl
Albendazole[22]	Hydrazine
Alprenolol[10]	Hydroxylamine sulfate
2-Aminothiophenol[36]	2-Methyl-3-nitro-4-methoxymethyl-5-cyano-6-chloropyridine
Azathioprine[2]	α-Naphthyl acetonitrile[33]
Bumetamide[23]	Nicergoline[15]
2-Chloromethyl imidazoline hydrochloride	p-Nitrobromacetophenone
α-Chloromethyl naphthalene	Opium alkaloids[4]
6-Chloromethylpteridine hydrochloride[20]	Oxolamine[5]
Chlorophenoxamine	Oxprenolol[30]
Chloroquine[19]	Propranolol[30]
2,6-Dichloropyrimidine	Ranitidine base[16,32]
Dicyclohexyl-carbodiimide	Thiamine[21]
Diethyl-β-chloroethylamine[7]	p-Toluol chloride phenylhydrazone
	3,4,6-Trichloropyridazine[8]

---

rapid onset of symptoms usually leads to identification of the offending agent. Thus, strong irritants are usually well known. Weaker irritants often require recurrent or prolonged exposure to produce symptoms. Fisher reported frictional irritant contact dermatitis in pharmacists caused by repetitive irritation from opening and closing child-proof bottles. Sometimes certain environments are required to produce symptoms. For example, hot and wet environments can cause increased incidences of dermatitis since this situation allows greater skin penetration of chemicals. Chronic exposures can lead to hardening, an adaptive response by which the skin stops mounting an inflammatory response and the layers of the dermis become thickened, especially the stratum corneum. Confirmatory tests for irritant contact dermatitis are not commercially available, and the diagnosis is made on clinical grounds. When known irritating substances are used, protective procedures, including a closed or airtight production line and appropriate personal protective gear, should be employed.[20]

A third frequent skin disorder is contact urticaria. It consists of a wheal-and-flare phenomenon that can be classified into two types. The first is an immunologic reaction, which consists of type I, IgE-mediated hypersensitivity reaction.[20] The classic example is contact urticaria caused by the latex in rubber gloves used in research laboratories. The second is nonimmunologic, which is caused by a host of biologic mediators, not all of which are well understood. This does not require sensitization. A model is opiate pharmaceutical workers who develop opiate hypersensitivity.[5]

The treatment for all three disorders is similar. The main treatment is avoidance. Workers should be properly educated about skin care and avoidance of offending agents. Protective gear such as gloves and face masks are often the first line of treatment. Barrier creams are controversial. Soaps and cleansers should be as mild as possible. First-line medicinal treatment of the disorders include topical or systemic antihistamines and topical or systemic steroids.

Pulmonary

The most common occupational respiratory disorder in the pharmaceutical industry is occupational asthma. Many pharmaceutical compounds have been reported to cause occupational asthma or airway hyperreactivity (see box on p. 370).

Weissmann and Baur reported a classic study of occupational asthma.[38] They described 14 cases of asthma caused by occupational exposure of porcine pancreatic dust during the manufacturing of insulin. Workers complained of cough, wheezing, and other symptoms of airway obstruction. All of the workers were more symptomatic when exposed to the dust; they had more symptoms during the workweek and fewer symptoms during weekends. Pulmonary function tests showed obstructive and restrictive patterns. These findings prompted new protective measures at the manufacturing facility.[38]

Probably the best-studied occupationally induced asthma in the pharmaceutical industry is the allergic pulmonary symptoms associated with laboratory animal workers. Although this group is not solely confined to the pharmaceutical industry, the prevalence for laboratory animal allergy ranges from 11% to 30%.[6,37] Lutsky reports that the most common offending animal appears to be the rat, followed in decreasing order by mice, rabbits, guinea pigs, and hamsters.[4,37] Slovak and Hill reported that symptoms, which consisted of allergic contact dermatitis and allergic rhinitis, usually began within a few months of employment. Workers with positive skin prick tests were at risk to develop full-blown asthma. Therefore, some authors have recommended that preemployment screening for atopy be used for prospective workers who would handle animals. This

---

Pharmaceuticals Reported to Cause Occupational Asthma

Antibiotics	Cimetidine
Ampicillin	Hydralazine
Cephalosporins	Methyldopa
Penicillin	Opiate compounds
Penicillamine	Pancreatic extracts
Piperazine	Psyllium
Spiramycin	Salbutamol
Tetracycline	

---

screening would include questionnaires concerning allergy history and family history of allergies, and a skin prick test for environmental allergens and total IgE levels would be performed.[6]

Another well-studied cause of occupational asthma is psyllium. Psyllium is a hydrophilic mucilloid that expands exponentially when exposed to water. Psyllium dust has been reported to be 10 to 20 microns in diameter, and inhaled psyllium dust can cause airway obstruction and an immunologic response. McConnochie and colleagues reported that almost 50% of workers exposed to psyllium dust developed symptoms of chest tightness, wheezing, rhinitis, dermatitis, or conjunctival irritation. Workers who were atopic and had a positive radioallergosorbent test (RAST) and positive skin test to psyllium went on to develop severe respiratory symptoms.[4] Bardy and associates reported a 3.6% prevalence of occupational asthma in a pharmaceutical plant that prepared psyllium laxatives.[21] Marks and colleagues also reported a 3.2% incidence of psyllium-related occupational asthma, with a 7% incidence of allergy by skin prick testing.[19]

Antibiotics are frequently reported as a cause of occupational asthma in the pharmaceutical industry. Penicillin and penicillin-like compounds are the most commonly reported, although multiple other antibiotics have been associated with occupational asthma (see box above).[6-9,16,18,22,23]

Salbutamol, a long-acting, inhaled β-agonist, is an interesting cause of occupational asthma. High doses of salbutamol and intermediate products during the production of salbutamol have both been incriminated in causing asthma.[1,12] In the cases where intermediate products caused the asthma, salbutamol was used to treat the symptoms.

Pharmaceutical personnel who are at high risk to develop occupational asthma should be considered for preemployment evaluations and regular reevaluations at 6- to 12-month intervals. Evaluations should include careful histories and physicals, with specific attention to the development of allergic or irritant respiratory symptoms. Pulmonary function testing, chest x-rays, skin prick tests, RAST, and other immunologic tests should be considered in workers with significant symptoms.

Endocrine

There are various occupational health hazards in the production of synthetic hormones. Exposure to synthetic hormone as the cause of hyperestrogenism was reported as early as the 1971 in Poland.[4] It has also been reported on the U.S. mainland and in Puerto Rico.[15,34] Symptoms of synthetic hormone exposure included gynecomastia, impotence, and decreased libido in males and increased frequency of intermenstrual bleeding in females. Poller and associates noted increases in clotting times in workers exposed to estrogen-progesterone combinations.[27] Taskinen and colleagues also noted an increased odds ratio for spontaneous abortion in workers exposed to synthetic estrogens.[33]

Adrenocortical suppression has been associated with occupational exposure to synthetic glucocorticoids. Newton and associates reported 12 workers he had considered to have adrenocortical suppression secondary to chronic dermal absorption of exogenous glucocorticoids. He and other authors recommended strict guidelines for workers in the manufacture of these agents, including self-contained breathing apparatus, full decontamination at the end of each shift, measurement of ambient air levels of glucocorticoids, and consideration of routine tetracosactrin or cortisol testing.[25,26]

Other

Certain agents have been associated with various target organ damage. Albert and colleagues reported a case of hypoglycemia induced by inhalation of sulfonylureas.[2] Clonidine has been associated with hypotension and bradycardia in a plant supervisor not wearing the standard protective gear required for the factory workers (personal communication). Chloroquine has been associated with keratopathy due to topical dust exposure.[11] Tomei and associates studied 40 Italian workers who manufactured various hepatotoxic agents, including erythromycin, iodochloro-oxyquinoline, disinfectants, and preserving agents (prevan and parabenzoate). The authors noted elevated liver indices in those workers exposed to these agents.[36]

REFERENCES

1. Agius RM et al: Occupational asthma in salbutamol process workers, *Occup Environ Med* 51:397, 1994.
2. Albert F et al: Hypoglycemia by inhalation, *Lancet* 342:47, 1993.
3. Bardy JD et al: Occupational asthma and IgE in a pharmaceutical company processing psyllium, *Am Rev Respir Dis* 135:1033, 1987.
4. Beeson MF et al: Prevalence and diagnosis of laboratory animal allergy, *Clin Allergy* 13:433, 1983.
5. Biagini RE et al: Evaluation of cutaneous responses and lung function from exposure to opiate compounds among ethical narcotics-manufacturing workers, *J Allergy Clin Immunol* 89:108, 1982.
6. Brooks S: Occupational and environmental asthma. In Rom WN, editor: *Environmental and occupational medicine,* ed 2, Boston, 1992, Little, Brown.
7. Coutts II et al: Asthma in workers manufacturing cephalosporin, *BMJ* 283:950, 1981.

8. Davies RJ, Hendrick DJ, Pepys J: Asthma due to inhaled chemical agents: ampicillin, benzyl penicillin, 6 amino penicillinic acid and related substances, *Clin Allergy* 4:227, 1974.

9. De Hoyos A, Holness DL, Tarlo SM: Hypersensitivity pneumonitis and airways hyperreactivity induced by occupational exposure to penicillin, *Chest* 103:303, 1993.

10. Dooms-Goossens A, Deleu H: Airborne contact dermatitis: an update, *Contact Dermatitis* 25:211, 1991.

11. Eriksen LS: Chloroquine keratopathy in chloroquine workers after topical dust exponation. A case report, *Acta Opthalmol* 57:823, 1979.

12. Fawcett IW, Pepys J, Erooga MA: Asthma due to "glycyl compound" powder—an intermediate in production of salbutamol, *Clin Allergy* 6:405, 1976.

13. Hansson E et al: Pregnancy outcome for women working in laboratories in some of the pharmaceutical industries in Sweden, *Scan J Work Environ Health* 6:131, 1980.

14. Harrington JM, Goldblatt P: Census based mortality study of pharmaceutical industry workers, *Br J Ind Med* 43:206, 1986.

15. Harrington JM et al: The occupational hazards of formulating oral contraceptives—a survey of plant employees, *Arch Environ Health* 33:12, 1978.

16. Lagier F et al: Occupational asthma in a pharmaceutical worker exposed to penicillamine, *Thorax* 44:157, 1989.

17. Lahti A, Puurunen J, Hannuksela M: Occupational contact allergy to 2,4-diamino-6-chloromethylpteridine hydrochloride: an intermediate product in methotrexate synthesis, *Contact Dermatitis* 22:294, 1990.

18. Malo JL, Cartier A: Occupational asthma in workers of a pharmaceutical company processing spiramycin, *Thorax* 43:371, 1988.

19. Marks GB, Salome CM, Woolcock AJ: Asthma and allergy associated with occupational exposure to ispaghula and senna products in a pharmaceutical work force, *Am Rev Respir Dis* 144:1065, 1991.

20. Martini MC, Marks JG. Contact dermatitis and contact urticaria. In Sams WM, Lynch PJ, editors: *Principles and practice of dermatology,* New York, 1990, Churchill Livingstone.

21. McConnochie K, Edwards J, Fitfield R: Ispaghula sensitization in workers manufacturing a bulk laxative, *Clin Exp Allergy* 20:199, 1990.

22. McCullagh SF: Allergenicity of piperazine: a study in environmental aetiology, *Br J Ind Med* 25: 319,1968.

23. Menon MP, Das AK: Tetracycline asthma—a case report, *Clin Allergy* 7:284, 1977.

24. Moller NE, Nielsen B, von Wurden K: Changes in penicillin contamination and allergy in factory workers, *Contact Dermatitis* 22:106, 1990.

25. Newton RW et al: Adrenocortical suppression in workers manufacturing synthetic glucocorticoids, *BMJ* 1:73, 1978.

26. Newton RW et al: Adrenocortical suppression in workers employed in manufacturing synthetic glucocorticosteroids: solutions to a problem, *Br J Ind Med* 39:179, 1982.

27. Poller L et al: Effects of manufacturing oral contraceptives on blood clotting, *BMJ* 1:1761, 1979.

28. Rotgoltz J et al: Prevalence of low back pain in employees of a pharmaceutical company, *Isr J Med Sci* 28:615, 1992.

29. Rycroft RG et al: Dermatitis and patch testing problems from 2-amino-thiophenal, *Contact Dermatitis* 23:270, 1990.

30. Sherertz EF: Occupational skin disease in the pharmaceutical industry, *Dermatol Clin* 12:533, 1994.

31. Slovak AJ, Hill RN: Laboratory animal allergy: a clinical survey of an exposed population, *Br J Ind Med* 38:38, 1981.

32. Strandberg M et al: Spontaneous abortions among women in a hospital laboratory, *Lancet* 1:384, 1978.

33. Taskinen T, Lindbohm M-L, Hemminki K: Spontaneous abortions among women working in the pharmaceutical industry, *Br J Ind Med* 43:199, 1986.

34. Teichman RF, Fallon LF, Brandt-Rauf PW: Health effects on workers in the pharmaceutical industry: a review, *J Soc Occup Med* 38:55, 1988.

35. Thomas TL, Decoufle P: Mortality among workers employed in the pharmaceutical industry: a preliminary investigation, *J Occup Med* 21:619, 1979.

36. Tomei F et al: Liver damage in pharmaceutical industry workers, *Arch Environ Health* 50:293, 1995.

37. Venables KM et al: Laboratory animal allergy in a pharmaceutical company, *Br J Ind Med* 45:660, 1988.

38. Weissmann KJ, Baur X: Occupational lung disease following long-term inhalation of pancreatic extracts, *Eur J Resp Dis* 66:13, 1985.

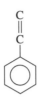

vinyl chloride

styrene

- Styrene causes neurologic, respiratory, and dermatologic toxicity and should be considered genotoxic

- Toluene diisocyanate is a potent sensitizing agent that can cause bronchospasm as well as dermatitis

46

Plastics

Scott D. Phillips

The plastics industry employs several hundred thousand workers involved in the production of more than 50 different commercial forms. The unique properties of plastics allow them to be molded into sheets, strands, pipes, fabrics, and many other forms. Plastics are of two types: thermoset (TS) and thermoplastic (TP). The thermoset plastics are rigid and lose form when heated. Thermoplastics can be heated without losing their characteristics.[26] Plastics, when heated sufficiently, pyrolize, which may lead to the formation of several new and potentially toxic compounds. This occurs in fires that involve plastic materials such as polyvinyl chloride (PVC).

More than three quarters of plastics are thermoplastics. Common TPs include PVC, polyethylene (PE), polypropylene (PP), and polystyrene (PS). Other familiar types include nylon (polyamide), Plexiglas (polymethylmethacrylate), and Teflon (fluorocarbon polymers). Plastics that are TSs include urea-formaldehyde, polyurethane, and epoxy resin.

ADDITIVES

Different chemicals are added to the plastic material during processing to create the many types and forms of plastics. These chemicals can provide wanted stability, durability, wearing strength, color, form, and other desirable features. These additives can be divided into groups based on their function in the material.

Plasticizers have a low order of toxicity. Examples include adipates, phthalates, sebacates, or stearates. Di(2-ethylhexyl)phthalate is used in the production of PVC and in the rubber industry. It is reportedly an animal carcinogen, causing hepatocellular tumors.[22] The PVC industry has substituted it for trimellitic anhydride (TMA), which may cause irritation[40] or immunologically mediated respiratory tract symptoms.

373

Other plasticizers include alkylsulfonic esters, chloroparaffins, polymeric plasticizers, and epoxidized soy bean oil, which is used mostly in the PVC industry.

Certain organic peroxides are used as hardeners in the plastic industry. Benzoylperoxide and dicumylperoxide are common hardeners for polyester plastics and polyethylene. They are reactive irritants and cytotoxic. Benzoylperoxide is a tumor promoter in mouse skin.[36]

These additives provide stabilization of the plastic against temperature or light. Among stabilizers, hydroquinone, organotin, benzophenones, lead stearates or inorganic lead, and cadmium compounds are used.[37]

Like fillers for many products, these agents are added to reduce production costs, alter hardness, or make the plastic opaque. Other physical characteristics include electrical properties, ultraviolet light resistance, processing characteristics, and reduced elasticity. Because of their higher specific gravity, they increase the density of the finished product. Fillers in plastic lower tensile strength, elongation, and tear strength.

Flame retardants include brominated or chlorinated organics and tri-chloroalkylphosphate esters. Toxicologically, the most important are the brominated flame retardants, the most common of which in the plastic industry has been tris(2,3-dibromopropyl)-phosphate (Tris-BP). Polybrominated biphenyl ethers have been substituted for the formerly common PBBs. Common chloro-organic flame retardants are chlorinated paraffins.

Pigments used in the plastic industry are both inorganic and organic. Heavy metals, such as chromium, cadmium, and lead compounds, have been used in both paints and plastics. Benzidine and benzidine-related organic compounds are still in use in some parts of the world. Many are carcinogens and should be respected for their toxicity.

Plastic foam is created by using foaming or blowing agents. Substances that give off gases at high temperature include azobisisobutyronitrile, azbisformamide, or oxybisbenzenesulfonyl hydrazides.[15] Trichloromonofluoromethane (FC 11) or difluoromonochloromethane (FC 22) have been used in the blowing of PU foam.

Polymerization may require a substance to initiate the process. Common chemicals that are used for this feature include benzoyl peroxide and didecanoyl peroxide.

Toluene Diisocyanate

Toluene diisocyanate (TDI) is used as a precursor in the production of polyurethane, polyamide, and simple polymers of isocyanates. It is manufactured by reacting toluene diamine with carbonyl chloride (phosgene). An important feature of isocyanates is that they contain the N=C=O group. All these compounds are collectively referred to as *polyurethanes*. Most TDI is used commercially for the production of polyurethane foams in the automobile and furniture industries. It is also used in floor varnishes, sealants, and elastomers. It is a highly volatile compound with poor olfactory warning properties. In the presence of reactive hydrogen, TDI forms toluene diamine. This may react further to form a urea. Foams of polyurethane are created by mixing polyhydroxy compounds with TDI. This can polymerize to form a spongelike mass.

Toluene diisocyanate may cause irritative symptoms of the eyes, upper respiratory tract, and skin. If severe, pulmonary irritation can lead to bronchitis and pulmonary edema. Exposure to TDI produces asthma symptoms in sensitized individuals.[1,39] In nonsensitized persons, TDI may cause an asthmalike reaction.[5] There is a dose-dependent response in nonsensitized individuals.[33,38] Symptoms include chest tightness, chills, cough, fever, headache, wheezing, and shortness of breath. The onset of these symptoms can be delayed up to 8 hours[1] and usually resolve within 24 to 48 hours.

Symptoms in sensitized individuals resemble other forms of bronchospasm. Once sensitization has occurred, persons exhibit symptoms at doses as low as 0.001 ppm. Once workers develop these symptoms, they usually cannot return to the workplace. Rates of sensitization in workers range from 4% to 15%.[1,9] Some exhibit the sensitized allergic reaction following the first exposure; others may become sensitized to TDI only after years of exposure. Neither atopy nor smoking increases risk of TDI sensitivity.[1] The mechanism of asthma induced by TDI is thought to be immunologic: IgE-mediated processes have been suggested, and IgE-specific TSH-displacing antibodies have been isolated in some sensitized workers.[23]

Respiratory irritation and asthmalike symptoms have been suggested to be dose related. These symptoms were reported in plants where TDI concentrations were below 0.1 ppm, but not in plants where levels were below 0.07 ppm.[17] Others have found both acute and chronic respiratory effects at levels as low as 0.003 ppm.[13,31] Although TDI may cause chronic respiratory impairment in both sensitized and nonsensitized persons, sensitization may lead to long-term pulmonary impairment even after removal from exposure.

A similar chronic finding is seen in workers who are not sensitized. In these, TDI causes the development of obstructive lung disease at low exposure levels.

TDS is reported to be mutagenic in bacterial test systems[34] due to the TDI amine analog 2,4-toluenediamine (TDA), formed during hydrolysis of isocyanates. Both TDI and TDA are considered carcinogenic in certain laboratory animals.[34] No epidemiologic studies of TDI workers have been published that examine the increased cancer risk in exposed workers. Recommendations for worker protection are provided in the National Institute of Occupational Safety and Health (NIOSH) criteria document on diisocyanates.[32] Other isocyanates do not have the toxicologic importance of TDA.

Isocyanates can react with a wide variety of compounds to produce rigid or flexible forms, surface coatings, adhesives, rubbers, and fibers.

Typical Agents Used in the Curing Process of Epoxy Resins

AMINES

Amidopolyamines
Diaminophenyl sulfone
Diethylene triamine
p-Phenylenediamine
Triethylamine

ACID ANHYDRIDES

Hexylhydrophthalic anhydride
Pyromellitic dianhydride

Table 46-1 The major types of styrene and the amounts of each form that are used

Type	Percent
Polystyrene	62
Acrylonitrile-butadiene-styrene and styrene-acrylonitrile	22
Styrene-butadiene latex	7
Styrene-butadiene rubber	7
Others	2

Modified from the National Institute of Occupational Safety and Health: *Criteria for a recommended standard: occupational exposure to styrene*, DHHS (NIOSH) Publication 83-119, Cincinnati, 1983, National Institute for Occupational Safety and Health.

Polymer Plastics

Polymer plastics are used for manufacturing films, sheets (PE), fibers, and molded goods (PP). The manufacture of PE and PP uses additives like antioxidants, slip-additives, antistatics, and silica.[35]

Polyvinyl chloride (PVC) is one of the most important of the modern plastics. Polyvinyl chloride resin is formed from vinyl chloride (VC), generally VC monomer.

Polymethyl methacrylate (PMMA, Plexiglas) belongs to the acrylic class of plastics,[20] as do the polyacrylamides. It is used for glazing, instrument panels, and protective goggles, as bone cement, and in dentistry and orthopedics. The polymerization begins with methacrylate (MA) in water. Hydroquinone is added as an inhibitor to impede spontaneous polymerizing. Methacrylate is irritating to eyes, skin, and mucous membranes and can cause sensitization.

Epoxy Compounds

Epoxies are TS plastic resins. They are usually formed by reacting a compound with an epoxy group with an alcohol. For example, epichlorohydrin can be reacted with bisphenol A.[24] Epoxies need to be cured after this reaction to give the desired TS structure. Commonly used curing agents are listed in the box above. Large amounts of curing agents are usually needed in this process, typically approaching the amount of resin.

The health effects are well described and typically involve sensitization. Epoxy bonds are very reactive and can alkylate DNA. Because of the structure-activity relationship concern, these agents are carcinogen suspects.

THE RUBBER INDUSTRY

The rubber industry encompasses both natural and synthetic polymers (elastomers). Common synthetic elastomers include acrylate-butadiene rubber (ABR), acrylonitrile-butadiene styrene (ABS), styrene-butadiene rubber (SBR), butadiene rubber (BR), chloroprene rubber (CR), butadiene-acrylonitrile rubber (BAR), and ethylene-propylenediene terpolymer (EPDM).

Several hundred additives may be used in the production of various rubbers. A single elastomer may contain up to 20 additives. The chemicals are categorized based on their function: curing agents, accelerators, antioxidants, activators, retarders, blowing agents, peptizing agents, antitacking agents, plasticizers, mold release agents, flame retardants, fillers or reinforcers, and organic. During the production process, they are added in the weighing and mixing stages of the process. During the curing stage, volatile compounds may evaporate. Potentially harmful new agents may be generated during the manufacturing process.

The vulcanization process allows cross-reaction between the curing agents and the polymer chains. Surveys[4,10,11] have identified approximately 500 well-defined chemicals in the rubber industry, and 25 more chemicals have been identified as by-products generated during several steps in the process.

Vapors that are generated during the curing of rubber tires may cause certain forms of pulmonary disease. Sampling during the tire vulcanization process detects styrene, toluene, ethyl benzene, and oligomers of butadiene. *N*-nitroso compounds, some of which are potent animal carcinogens, have been identified as air contaminants during certain processes.

Dermatologic effects from rubber chemicals are well known.[12] Paraphenylenediamine derivatives, mercaptobenzothiazole, and thiuram compounds are all sensitizing agents that cause dermatitis. Certain rubber chemicals have been proposed by the International Contact Dermatitis Research Group to be amenable to patch testing.[22]

Styrene

Styrene, or vinyl benzene, is used extensively in the plastics industry both as a solvent and as a monomer for plastics and synthetic rubber elastomers. Styrene is produced by formation of a double bond from ethyl benzene, creating vinyl benzene. Styrene has many uses (Table 46-1). About one third of styrene is consumed in polystyrene production. The next largest use is production of plastic polymers such as styrene-acrylonitrile (SAN) and acrylonitrile-butadiene-styrene (ABS). A small amount is used in styrene-butadiene

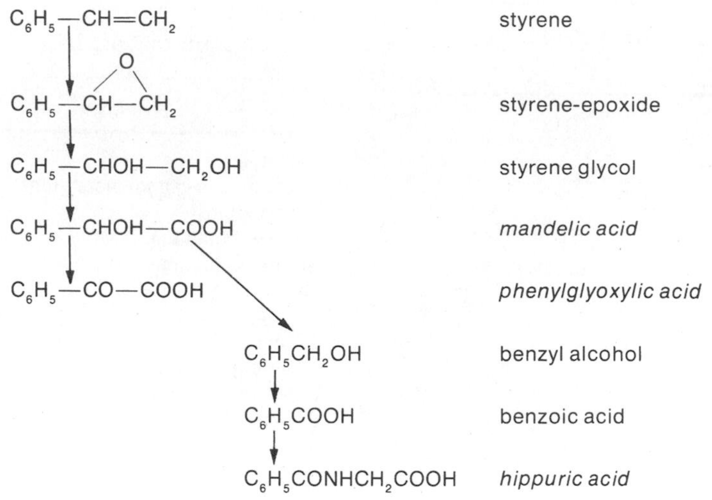

$C_6H_5-CH=CH_2$ — styrene

$C_6H_5-CH-CH_2$ (with epoxide O) — styrene-epoxide

$C_6H_5-CHOH-CH_2OH$ — styrene glycol

$C_6H_5-CHOH-COOH$ — *mandelic acid*

$C_6H_5-CO-COOH$ — *phenylglyoxylic acid*

$C_6H_5CH_2OH$ — benzyl alcohol

C_6H_5COOH — benzoic acid

$C_6H_5CONHCH_2COOH$ — *hippuric acid*

Fig. 46-1 Metabolism of styrene. (From Zenz C, Dickerson OB, Horvath EP: *Occupational medicine,* ed 3, St Louis, 1994, Mosby.)

rubber (SBR) and in polyester resins. Large amounts of styrene are consumed during the production of polyester plastics with fiberglass reinforcement in the manufacture of boats, swimming pools, and containers of various sizes. This production often is done in small manufacturing industries. The styrene content of the resin is approximately 40% (by weight). During production, as much as 15% of styrene may evaporate into the workroom air.

Styrene is absorbed well via the skin or by inhalation. It is further metabolized in the liver (Fig. 46-1). The epoxide form, like other epoxides, can bind to proteins and form adducts such as with DNA.[7,18] If the epoxide form continues to be metabolized, mandelic acid, phenyl glyoxylic acid, and hippuric acid can be measured in the urine. Prolonged skin exposure can cause dermatitis because of its fat-dissolving properties, typical of all organic solvents. Other symptoms and signs include upper respiratory tract irritation, mild shortness of breath, drowsiness, and impaired balance.[8] Slower reaction times have also been suggested. This finding is not unexpected, as it is an organic solvent, many of which result in central nervous system (CNS) depression.

Lymphocytes with increased sister chromatid exchanges and single strand breaks have been reported.[2,25] Chromosomal abnormalities have also been described in Europe.[2,16,19,27,28] Because of these findings, styrene (styrene epoxide) should be considered genotoxic.[7]

Adequate personal protective equipment should be worn when workers exceed the permissible exposure limit time-weighted average. Appropriate ventilation and exhaust systems should be constructed in the work area as effective engineering controls.

Butadiene

Butadiene is a colorless liquid and an irritating, flammable gas at higher temperatures. It is a coproduct in the manu-facture of ethylene. It is also produced by dehydrogenation of *n*-butane or *n*-butene.[3,14,29,30] Butadiene, when combined with styrene (styrene-butadiene rubber, SBR), and polybutadiene rubber (BR) still account for the two largest uses in the United States. The major use of butadiene is in the tire industry. Acrylonitrile-butadiene-styrene (ABS) resins are used to make high-impact-resistant pipes and parts for automobiles and appliances. In the United States, an estimated 65,000 workers are employed in this industry.

Human experiences and animal data attest to the absorption of 1,3-butadiene vapors by inhalation. Distribution is ubiquitous but by no means uniform. Volatile metabolites (3,4-epoxybutadiene monoxide, 3-butene-1,2 diol, and 3,4-epoxybutadiene 1-2 diol) are exhaled and identified by spectroscopy and radioactive label.

Butadiene has produced narcosis in larger exposures. Rats exposed to butadiene by inhalation were found to have benign and malignant tumors at various sites including testicular, thyroid, mammary, and uterine adenomas. Reasonable evidence supports this agent as a possible human carcinogen.

Chloroprene

Chloroprene, when polymerized, forms neoprene rubber. Chloroprene (2-chloro-1,3 butadiene) has produced alopecia, CNS depression, and possible liver injury after heavy exposure.[21]

CONCLUSION

This enormous industry uses many important and toxic chemicals. Workers in this industry face many health hazards and require proper medical surveillance and workplace controls. Specific engineering controls that are needed include adequate ventilation and exhaust systems with regular air monitoring and properly fitted personal protective equipment.

REFERENCES

1. Adams WG: Long-term effects on the health of men engaged in the manufacture of toluene diisocyanate, *Br J Ind Med* 32:72, 1975.
2. Andersson HC et al: Chromosomal aberrations and sister chromatid exchanges in lymphocytes of men occupationally exposed to styrene in a plastic-boat factory, *Mutat Res* 73:387, 1980.
3. Arce GT et al: In vitro and in vivo genotoxicity of 1,3-butadiene and metabolites, *Environ Health Perspect* 86:75, 1990.
4. Blum S et al: Stomach cancer among rubber workers: an epidemiologic investigation. In *Dust and diseases,* Park Forest South, 1990, Chicago, Pathotax.
5. Brugsch HG, Elkins HB: Toluene diisocyanate (TDI) toxicity, *N Engl J Med* 265:353, 1963.
6. Butcher BT et al: Inhalation challenge and pharmacologic studies of toluene diisocyanate (TDI)-sensitive workers, *J Allergy Clin Immunol* 64:146, 1979.
7. Byfalt Nordqvist M et al: Covalent binding of styrene and styrene-7,8-oxide to plasma proteins, hemoglobin and DNA in the mouse, *Chem Biol Interact* 55:63, 1985.
8. Carpenter CP et al: Studies on the inhalation of 1,3-butadiene with a comparison of its narcotic effect with benzol, toluol and styrene, and a note on the elimination of styrene in the human, *J Ind Hyg* 26:69, 1944.
9. Carroll KB et al: Asthma due to non-occupational exposure to toluene diisocyanate, *Clin Allergy* 6:99, 1976.
10. Case RAM, Hosker ME: Tumour of the urinary bladder as an occupational disease in the rubber industry in England and Wales, *Br J Prev Soc Med* 8:39, 1954.
11. Cronin E: *Contact dermatitis,* Edinburgh, 1980, Churchill Livingstone.
12. Delzell E, Monson RR: Mortality among rubber workers. III. Cause-specific mortality, 1940-1978, *J Occup Med* 23:677, 1981.
13. Diem JE et al: Five-year longitudinal study of workers employed in a new toluene diisocyanate manufacturing plant, *Am Rev Respir Dis* 126:420, 1982.
14. Fajan M et al: Occupational exposure of workers to 1,3-butadiene, *Environ Health Perspect* 86:11, 1990.
15. Fishbein L: Additives in synthetic polymers: an overview. In Jarvisalo J, Pfaffli P, Vainio H, editors: *Industrial hazards of plastics and synthetic elastomers,* New York, 1984, Alan Liss.
16. Fleig I, Thiess A: Mutagenicity study of workers employed in the styrene and polystyrene processing and manufacturing industry, *Scand J Work Environ Health* 4(suppl 2):254, 1978.
17. Hama GM: Symptoms in workers exposed to isocyanates. Suggested exposure concentrations, *AMA Arch Ind Health* 16:232, 1957.
18. Hemminki K: Covalent binding of styrene to amino acids, human serum proteins and hemoglobin. In Sorsa M, Norppa H, editors: *Monitoring of occupational genotoxicants,* New York, 1986, Alan Liss.
19. Hogstedt B et al: Increased frequency of chromosome aberrations in workers exposed to styrene, *Scand J Work Environ Health* 5:333, 1979.
20. Holmberg B: The toxicology of monomers in the polyvinyl plastic series. In Jarvisalo J, Pfaffli P, Vainio H, editors: *Industrial hazards of plastics and synthetic elastomers,* New York, 1984, Alan Liss.
21. International Agency for Research on Cancer: *IARC Monogr Eval Carcinog Risk Hum*; (Suppl 7), 1987.
22. International Agency for Research on Cancer: *IARC Monogr Eval Carcinog Risk Hum* 18, 1982.
23. Karol MH, Alarie Y: Antigens which detect IgE antibodies in workers sensitive to toluene diisocyanate, *Clin Allergy* 10:101, 1980.
24. Lyle W et al: Dimethyfromamide and alcohol intolerance, *Br J Ind Med* 36:63, 1979.
25. Maki-Paakkanen J et al: Single strand breaks, chromosome aberrations, sister chromatid exchanges, and micronuclei in blood lymphocytes of workers exposed to styrene during the production of reinforced plastics, *Environ Mol Mutagen* 7:27, 1991.
26. Martinmaa JM: Synthetic polymers: main classes of plastics and their current uses. In Jarvisalo J, Pfaffli P, Vainio H, editors: *Industrial hazards of plastics and synthetic elastomers,* New York, 1984, Alan Liss.
27. Meretoja T et al: Occupational styrene exposure and chromosomal aberrations, *Mutat Res* 56:193, 1977.
28. Meretoja T et al: Chromosome aberrations in lymphocytes of workers exposed to styrene, *Scand J Work Environ Health* 4(suppl 2):259, 1978.
29. Morrow NL: The industrial production and use of 1,3-butadiene, *Environ Health Perspect* 86:7, 1990.
30. Mullins JA: Industrial emissions of 1,3-butadiene, *Environ Health Perspect* 86:9, 1990.
31. Musk AW et al: Absence of respiratory effects in subjects exposed to low concentrations of TDI and MDI, *J Occup Med* 14:756, 1982.
32. National Institute for Occupational Safety and Health: *Criteria for a recommended standard for occupational exposures to diisocyanates,* Pub 78-215, Cincinnati, 1978, National Institute for Occupational Safety and Health.
33. National Institute for Occupational Safety and Health: *Criteria for a recommended standard: occupational exposure to styrene,* DHHS (NIOSH) Pub 83-119, Cincinnati, 1983, National Institute for Occupational Safety and Health.
34. National Institute for Occupational Safety and Health: *Toluene diisocyanate (TDI) and toluenediamine (TDA): evidence of carcinogenicity,* NIOSH Intelligence Bulletin 53, DHHS (NIOSH) Pub 90-101, Cincinnati, 1989, US U S Department of Health and Human Services.
35. Slovak AJM: Occupational hazards of polyethylene and polypropylene processing. In Jarvisalo J, Pfaffli P, Vainio H, editors: *Industrial hazards of plastic and synthetic elastomers,* New York, 1984, Alan Liss.
36. Staga TJ et al: Skin tumor–promoting activity of benzoyl peroxide, a widely used free radical-generating compound, *Science* 213:1023, 1981.
37. Stenius U et al: The role of GSH depletion and toxicity in hydroquinone-induced development of enzyme altered foci, *Carcinogenesis* 10:593, 1989.
38. Walworth HT, Virchow WE: Industrial hygiene experiences with toluene diisocyanate, *Am Ind Hyg Assoc J* 20:205, 1959.
39. Woolrich PF: Toxicology, industrial hygiene, and medical control of TDI, MDI, and PMPPI, *Am Ind Hyg Assoc J* 43:89, 1982.
40. Zeiss CR et al: A model of immunologic lung injury induced by trimellitic anhydride inhalation: antibody response, *J Allergy Clin Immunol* 79:59, 1987.

47

Railroad

Michael I. Greenberg

M-*cresol*

I-OH *pyrene*

- Phosphorus and sulfur-containing fumigants used in railcars pose a significant toxic hazard to rail workers

- Acute phosphine (fumigant) poisoning can cause CNS depression as well as pulmonary edema, myocarditis, and vascular collapse

- Diesel exhaust fumes pose a significant threat to rail workers and have resulted in the development of reactive airway dysfunction (RADS).

OCCUPATIONAL DESCRIPTION

The first railroads date back to the mid-1500s, when crude railcars were used in European mines. These early railroads consisted of wagons that men or animals pushed on wooden tracks. Later, iron tracks came into use and, with the advent of steam power, rail wagons were hauled by ropes connected to stationary engines. In 1804, the first successful railroad steam locomotive was used in England, and the Stockton and Darlington Railway became the first common carrier to use steam locomotives in 1825.

In the United States, the first railroads began their operation in 1830 (Baltimore and Ohio Railroad and the South Carolina Railroad). By 1855, railways linked the Midwest with the Atlantic seaboard, and in 1869 the first transcontinental route was completed to the Pacific coast.

During the last half of the nineteenth century, railroads became the predominant means for overland transportation. Technological advances came to the railroad industry exceedingly quickly, with more powerful locomotives resulting in greater speeds. Larger freight and passenger cars resulted in a marked expansion in transportation and trade and the invention of air brakes, automatic signaling, and the automatic coupler resulted in increased safety. Steam-powered underground railways (subways) were first built in 1863 in London, England, and electric power was introduced to rail transportation in the mid-1880s in the United States, Canada, and Europe. By 1900, electric power had replaced horsecars and cable cars as the chief form of urban transportation. Electrified, elevated, or subway lines were built in several European cities, as well as in Boston, Chicago, and New York City. Electrification spread early in the twentieth century to intercity railroad lines, and the diesel-electric locomotive eventually became dominant in the United States. By the 1950s, however, the automobile, bus, and airplane had replaced the railroad train as the principal passenger carriers in the United States.

Railroads offer essentially two types of passenger service: commuter service and intercity service. Commuter service is provided between cities and their suburbs. Intercity trains usually run between two large cities, known as *end points*. These end points are typically at least 100 miles apart. In some countries, intercity trains traverse an entire continent on a route that may pass through several countries.

While commuter trains usually have coaches designed to carry as many people as possible, freight cars tend to be much more specialized. Freight cars can be classified into three basic types: the boxcar, the open-top car, and the flatcar. Today, railroads use many variations of these basic types, along with many special cars designed to carry specific types of freight.

Boxcars carry merchandise or other freight that must be protected from the weather. Some boxcars use cushioned gear to protect fragile materials from damage. Cars with open tops primarily carry minerals, such as coal or iron ore. Many have hopper doors that allow the cargo to be unloaded through the bottom of the car. Others are designed to be unloaded by turning the entire car upside down using a car-dumper machine. Flatcars are essentially open cars with no side panels and are designed to transport a variety of freight, such as steel beams, lumber, heavy machinery, and construction equipment.

To better serve shippers and to compete with highway trucking, railroads utilize various special types of cars. In the United States, the movement of highway trailers or marine containers on intermodal flatcars has become the fastest-growing segment of the railroad business. Efficient double-stack trains carrying containers stacked one on top of the other became widely used during the 1980s. Other specialized cars include auto-rack cars, which carry up to 21 finished automobiles or small trucks; tank cars for hauling petroleum, liquid chemicals, and gases; covered hopper cars to carry grain or chemicals; and refrigerated boxcars, known as reefers, used to carry produce that can spoil.

The railroad industry has a long and impressive history. From the days of the steam engine until the modern diesel era, railroad workers have played a critical role in the economic development of all nations. Today, in the United States, more than 500,000 individuals are employed in some aspect of the railroad industry. With thousands of miles of track and thousands of cars of rolling stock currently operative in the United States, this industry stands as a crucial part of the modern economy.

POTENTIAL TOXIC HAZARDS

In the modern era, there are numerous potential toxic threats to individuals employed in the railroad industry. These potential hazards include both acute toxic threats and chronic hazards. These toxic threats can be best considered by examining the industry from the point of view of the locations of these potential toxins. Railroad personnel can be assumed to consist essentially of those individuals working in repair and maintenance roles, those working in railyards, in the transfer of goods and materials between trucks and railcars and between railcars, and finally those who actually operate the rolling stock. While some of the hazards may overlap these somewhat artificial classifications, others are specific to these categories.

During the steam engine era, railroad workers were often exposed to asbestos in the course of their jobs, especially those workers employed in the machine shops. Workers who ripped out old insulation from steam boilers and replaced it with new insulation probably suffered the greatest exposure. These particular asbestos exposures were largely eliminated when diesel engines replaced steam locomotives. When the tissue asbestos content in workers whose only known exposure to asbestos was in the railroad yards during the steam era was analyzed, the median uncoated fiber content was found to be similar to that of shipyard workers who were not employed as insulators. However, the median asbestos body count in these rail workers was indeed considerably less than that of the shipyard workers. This finding is probably related to the fact that chrysotile asbestos was the predominant asbestos form used in the railroad yards. Histologically confirmed asbestosis was noted in only 10% of these workers.

Workers in both the repair shops and the railyards can have significant exposure to diesel fumes, diesel fuels, lead, carbon monoxide, and oxides of nitrogen. Those workers who transfer chemicals between cars and from truck to railcar may suffer accidental exposure to any one of a host of chemicals and potentially toxic materials that are frequently transported by rail (Fig. 47-1). Those workers who actually operate and ride on the trains are also at risk for these same exposures. One additional special exposure that these workers may be at risk for is the toxic substances used as fumigants, rodenticides, and pesticides inside the rail cars.

CLINICAL TOXICOLOGY
Fumigants

Fumigants of all types (including pesticides) are commonly employed in the rail industry to protect foodstuffs from insect and pest damage during storage and transport. Carbon tetrachloride and carbon disulfide mixtures were the primary fumigants used during rail transport prior to the mid 1980s, but these products have been banned by the U.S. Environmental Protection Agency (EPA). These original fumigants subsequently were replaced by fumigation processes utilizing phosphorus- and sulfur-containing compounds.

Aluminum phosphide, a highly efficacious insecticide, is being used to an increasing extent by the grain industry. When placed into a loaded boxcar, aluminum phosphide pellets react with water in the grain to produce phosphine, an extremely toxic gas. This chemical reaction takes place rapidly, usually in 5 minutes or less. Consequently, the U.S. Department of Transportation (DOT) has required that, after a loaded car is fumigated, it must not be allowed in service for at least 48 hours.[16-20] Once the phosphine gas has completely dissipated, the product in the railcar is considered to be nontoxic. Entry into a fumigated railcar prior to the completion of this period of decontamination can be fatal.

Phosphine is rapidly absorbed through the respiratory tract. Symptoms of phosphine toxicity, which can have their onset almost immediately after an acute exposure, include fatigue, headache, nausea, vomiting, abdominal pain, cough, and shortness of breath. Acute phosphine poisoning can result in the development of central nervous system depression, acute pulmonary edema, myocarditis, vascular collapse, and hypotension. Aluminum phosphide and phosphine cannot be detected in blood or urine by any assay. Treatment following an acute exposure is essentially symptomatic and supportive. The effects of long-term exposure are thought to include genotoxicity.[11]

The EPA and DOT have both promulgated published guidelines on the placement of appropriate warning signs on transport vehicles or freight containers and railcars that have been fumigated or otherwise treated with toxic chemical substances. These guidelines are highly variable with regard to the wording, graphic symbols, languages used, and the size and placement of such signage. At this point, commercial carriers are required to conform to only one or the other (not both) agency's set of regulations and guidelines.

Surveillance for poisoning that occurs in freight railcars is complicated by lack of uniform reporting guidelines.[1] In addition, it is often quite difficult to attribute any given adverse health effect specifically to such an exposure. Although a number of states (currently 25 states) require reporting of illnesses caused by pesticide chemicals, follow-up of such case reports is not consistent. Many such cases are detected through the Sentinel Event Notification System for Occupational Risk (SENSOR) program of the Centers for Disease Control's National Institute for Occupational Safety and Health (NIOSH).

As an example of one state's current practice, Texas mandates reporting of occupationally related pesticide exposures, including those who apply fumigants, agricultural workers, and grain inspectors. California mandates that physicians report all illnesses caused by pesticides to local health officers. Nonetheless, deaths resulting from illegal or inappropriate entry into fumigated rail transport cars have not been widely reported, perhaps, in part, because state-based surveillance systems to identify such incidents are not uniform in the United States currently.

Since railcar fumigation is such a widespread practice, preventive measures need to be uniform.[5,6] From the point of prevention, appropriately placed, highly visible warning signs printed in English and other languages that incorporate symbols may prevent unnecessary deaths following railcar fumigation.[10,15] In addition, prevention includes adequate locking for all points of entry on railcars.

Diesel Exhaust Fumes (DEF)

Acute effects. Accurately assessing the potential risks for exposure to diesel exhaust fumes (DEF) is problematic.

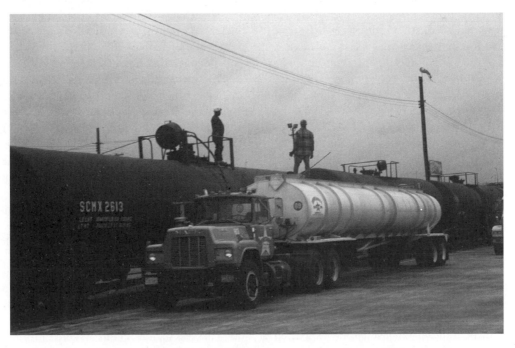

Fig. 47-1 Transfer of hydrofluric acid from railcar to truck at intermodal transport site.

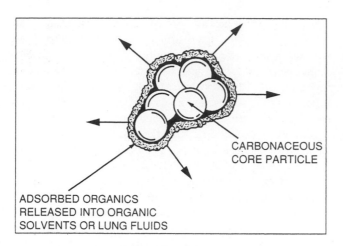

CARBONACEOUS
CORE PARTICLE

ADSORBED ORGANICS
RELEASED INTO ORGANIC
SOLVENTS OR LUNG FLUIDS

Fig. 47-2 Schematic representation of a diesel exhaust particle. (From Harber P, Schenker MB, Balmes JR: *Occupational and environmental respiratory disease,* St Louis, 1996, Mosby.)

However, as with most toxic exposures, the potential risks can be either acute or chronic effects.

The nature of any acute exposure to DEF is dependent on the concentration of the fumes and the amount of fresh air ventilation available to dilute the fumes. When such an exposure occurs in a closed space with inadequate ventilation, if the worker is not properly protected with appropriate respiratory protection, death could occur from carbon monoxide exposure in relatively short order (see Chapter 15). In addition, a relatively acute exposure to high levels of DEF could result in a clinically significant reactive airways dysfunction syndrome (RADS) as described later in this chapter. Acute exposure to high concentrations of DEF can be life-threatening and must be avoided at all costs. There is no substitute for appropriate, properly fitted personal protective equipment and adequately ventilated work areas. Work area monitoring to detect elevations of carbon monoxide levels may be appropriate, depending upon the specific work site. Although the acute effects of DEF exposure can be life-threatening, it is the chronic effects of DEF that are of widespread concern.

Chronic effects. The material known as *diesel exhaust* is a heterogeneous mixture of carbonaceous particles and gases (Fig. 47-2). These particles are made up of a carbonaceous center, similar to carbon black, with various hydrocarbon molecules adsorbed to its surface. It is important to note that the relatively small size (less than 0.05 μm in diameter) of these particles makes them easily respirable and readily presented to the most distal alveolar sites in the tracheobronchial tree.

The potential adverse health effects of diesel exhaust particles have been the focus of many research investigations over the past two decades. This spate of research stemmed originally from a specific EPA directive that indicated that organic solvent extracts of diesel exhaust particles appeared

to be mutagenic for bacteria. Since the publication of that directive, several in vitro studies have demonstrated that extracts of diesel exhaust particles are potentially mutagenic in mammalian cells as well as in lower forms. In addition, such extracts have also been shown to exert a clastogenic effect on animal chromosomes. The chromosomal studies have specifically sought to classify the chemicals present in extracts of diesel exhaust that might account for mutagenicity. Studies such as these have made it possible to compare the potency of diesel exhaust extracts with extracts of cigarette smoke, roofing tar, and coke oven emissions. Since diesel exhaust extracts appear to be mutagenic in vitro and this in vitro activity is comparable with that from extracts of known human carcinogens, it becomes most important, then, to ascertain how such in vitro activity might translate into clinically significant health risks for workers who may be exposed on the job.

A number of animal inhalation studies have attempted to determine the carcinogenic potential of diesel exhaust. In these studies, laboratory animals were exposed to rather high concentrations of diesel exhaust fumes. With exposure to diesel exhaust at high concentrations for at least 7 hours per day, for at least 5 days per week, for at least 24 months, an increase in the incidence of pulmonary neoplasia was noted. In other studies, rats were exposed to DEF after its particulate matter had been specifically removed via filtration. Only those animals exposed to the exhaust mixtures that contained the particulates demonstrated an increased incidence of lung tumors. As a result of these studies, it is generally assumed that the presence of particles per se in DEF appears to be a necessary condition to produce lung tumors in rats. However, in murine models, studies did not demonstrate the same carcinogenic response. Inhalation of diesel exhaust fumes produced consistent significantly increased rates of appearance of lung tumors in rats only!

Several epidemiologic studies involving diesel exhaust fume exposure in humans have been conducted. Only two studies have demonstrated a statistically supportable association between lung cancer and inhalation of diesel exhaust. Both these studies reported on workers who were enrolled with the U.S. Railroad Retirement Board. The duration of exposure in these studies was reflective of the rapid dieselization of railroads in the U.S. after the Second World War, which resulted in a 95% use of diesel engines across the board by 1959.

One particular case control study demonstrated a statistically significant increase in the relative odds for lung cancer in workers under age 64 who had had 20 years or more of diesel exhaust exposure at death.[13,14] Another cohort study evaluating the same associations reported a statistically significant (although rather small) elevation in the relative risk for lung cancer (1.45) in exposed individuals. However, these studies suffer from significant design weaknesses, such as failure to correct for the fact that many of the study participants were smokers. In addition, there may not have been an entirely accurate and complete assessment of the exhaust exposure history. Nonetheless, such studies currently represent the best evidence that diesel exhaust may be carcinogenic in humans.

The International Agency for Research on Cancer (IARC) has classified diesel exhaust as being carcinogenic in animals and noted that it is probably carcinogenic to humans. However, it is problematic to accurately estimate the specific risk for humans based on available data. Various estimates for the risk for lung cancer in this setting range from approximately 100 to 3800 cases per year per $\mu g/m^3$ of diesel exhaust exposure. Estimates of diesel exhaust fume exposure for the U.S. population have been as high as 30 $\mu g/m^3$, the hypothesis for a Manhattan street lined with skyscrapers if only 1 of every 5 vehicles present was powered by diesel engines. Workers using diesel-powered equipment can have much greater potential exposures, depending upon the setting in question. In the coal mining industry, for example, there is great concern about the concentration of exhaust in dieselized coal mines, where the total respirable dust standard is 2000 $\mu g/m^3$, a substantial part of which could be diesel exhaust.

Risk assessment for DEF-exposed humans based primarily on animal data is difficult at best.[3] Such exercises are seriously complicated by the use of extrapolation from one species to another. While reproducible studies in animals might serve to clarify some of the issues, still, estimating risks for potentially carcinogenic air pollutants, such as DEF, is complex and somewhat unreliable (see Chapter 51).

Reactive Airway Dysfunction

Consequent to exposure to diesel exhaust fumes, several railroad workers have reportedly been diagnosed as suffering from what has come to be known as *reactive airway dysfunction* (RADS). A discussion of this clinical syndrome is appropriate when considering the potential toxic hazards that railroad workers might be at risk for developing.

The variant of occupational asthma now known as RADS was originally described in the late 1960s. In 1968, reports of workers developed a new-onset asthma syndrome following exposure to various airborne materials.[8] These inciting agents included hydrogen sulfide, diethylene diamine, fumes from overheated plastics, and smoke and fumes from the combustion of a variety of other materials. The pathophysiologic mechanism responsible for this syndrome was identified as related to inflammatory bronchospasm. Original accounts of RADS described rapid onset of airflow obstruction, within hours after exposure to a bronchitis or bronchopneumonia that itself seemed to have been induced chemically. Symptoms seemed to reach a clinical zenith within the first week and to lessen over the ensuing months. Many patients suffering this syndrome

continued to manifest bronchial hyperresponsiveness for long periods. This prolongation of symptoms depends primarily on the corrosive properties of the original material responsible for inducing the process.

The first investigators to use the terminology *reactive airway dysfunction syndrome* were Brooks and Lockey,[2] who in 1981 described it as a form of "nonallergic work-related asthma" caused by a high-level irritant exposure. These investigators described a syndrome that included mucous membrane and ocular inflammation that was noted to be dependent primarily on the concentration and solubility of the agent in question. Workers were described who had been exposed to high concentrations of respiratory irritants and developed the type of persistent symptoms described previously. The persistent bronchial hyperreactivity was linked to the extensive chemically induced inflammatory response. Unfortunately, some of these individuals had evidence of significant confounding variables related to previous cigarette smoking or atopic disease.

There is controversy as to whether RADS is a variant of traditional occupational asthma. Several pathologic studies have suggested that RADS involves a distinct and different pathophysiologic basis. From the limited available data, the inflammatory characteristics of chronic RADS appear much less intense than in immunologically induced occupational asthma. What is unclear is the precise mechanism by which the asthmatic symptoms persist. Several theories have been proposed to explain this pathogenesis. One proposal is that, after the extensive inflammation that follows acute exposure, receptor reactivity "thresholds" are significantly lowered. This is thought to cause a state of continual bronchial hyperreactivity. Another hypothesis is that direct damage to the cell of the bronchial mucosa may lead to increased permeability that results in chronic airway hyperresponsiveness. Alternative hypotheses have proposed that the entire process may be due to neurologically mediated inflammation.

The clinical presentation of RADS is very different from allergic work-related asthma. In RADS, the exposure is usually noted to be acute and extreme in nature, typically a single, intense exposure episode with no observed latency period. The episode usually lasts only several minutes. The individuals affected often attribute the inciting exposure episode to a specific accident, incident, or circumstance that involves poor ventilation in conjunction with very high concentrations of a given toxin. Patients diagnosed with RADS are more likely to be male with no evidence of preexisting respiratory symptoms. The specific diagnostic criteria for RADS also stipulate no prior history of atopy.

The nature of the onset of symptoms is a critical factor in the correct diagnosis of RADS. The development of symptoms should be immediate or, at the very most, within a few hours of exposure. The symptoms must be severe enough for the exposed individual to seek immediate medical attention. When the onset of symptoms does not

---

Diagnostic Criteria for Reactive Airway Dysfunction Syndrome (RADS)

1. Total absence of preexisting respiratory disease in a nonatopic person
2. Documented exposure to excessive concentrations of corrosive or irritating gas, vapor, fumes, or dust
3. Abrupt onset of symptoms within minutes or hours (always within a 24-hour period), requiring urgent medical care
4. Persistence of asthmalike symptoms such as chest tightness, cough, or dyspnea
5. Normal or reversible airflow pattern on spirometry; reversibility is generally less than that seen in immunologically induced occupational asthma
6. Presence of moderate to severe bronchial hyperreactivity on methacholine challenge (<8 mg/ml)
7. Histopathology showing minimal lymphocytic inflammation without eosinophilia

---

From Occupational asthma and related disorders. In Rich RR, editor: *Clinical immunology,* St Louis, 1995, Mosby.

precipitate the need for immediate medical assistance, the incident is unlikely to represent irritant-induced asthma or RADS (see box above).

Creosote

Creosote oil is a wood preservative derived from coal tar that may be encountered in railyards as well as along the course of rail track. It is often used as a preservative for railroad ties and may be applied by rail workers in order to prolong protection for rail ties. Occupational exposure may take place by inhalation of creosote vapors or via skin contact. It is a recognized health hazard that causes toxic effects primarily to the skin and eyes. Creosote is noted to be a compound that is probably carcinogenic to humans.[4]

More than 100 different compounds have been analyzed in creosote oils; however, it is unclear which specific chemicals cause the adverse health effects. Analysis of polycyclic aromatic hydrocarbons (PAHs) in creosote impregnation plants has shown that naphthalene and its alkyl derivatives were the main volatiles found in the air, with concentrations 1000 times higher than the particulate PAHs. Pyrene was a major constituent of these PAHs of both stationary and airborne creosote.

Chemical exposures are an especially serious health concern whenever they involve PAHs because this class of compounds is widely considered to have strong human carcinogenic potential. Workers in industrial operations with high airborne concentrations of PAHs demonstrate excess rates of lung cancer, and workers exposed specifically to creosote have an excess of lip and skin cancer. Urinary levels of 1-hydroxypyrene (1-HP) are used to monitor exposure. This is true for both the parent compound pyrene as well as

a biomarker for total exposure to PAHs. The assay for 1-HP measures the absorption of pyrene or PAHs by all possible routes of entry. Dermal absorption is being increasingly recognized in studies on occupational exposure to PAHs. In creosote workers, the skin is probably the most important route of exposure to PAHs.[3,7,11,12]

Although exposure to creosote is typically associated with working outdoors, the urinary concentrations of 1-HP in creosote workers are very high in comparison with workers exposed to PAHs from other work environments, for example, at a coke plant, at an aluminum plant, and in asphalt road surfacing. Although it has yet to be studied, urinary 1-HP levels in railyard workers would be expected to be lower than those of creosote production workers.

Another complicating factor is that in humans the excretion process of 1-HP is biphasic, showing two relatively long half-lives: a shorter one (1 to 2 days) for the readily available (for metabolism and then excretion) body pyrene and a longer one (16 days) for the more slowly available components. Both elimination components imply pyrene accumulation, and consistent with this the average net increase in urinary 1-HP over a workday was less than the change within a working week or within the samples taken before shifts (Friday minus Monday values). The Monday morning concentrations of 1-HP were very high in all the men studied, a finding characteristic for creosote workers. The concentrations were so high that they exceeded not only the upper limits reported for normal 1-HP excretion of unexposed nonsmokers and smokers but also the biologic exposure limits proposed for coke oven workers.

It is not clear to what extent differences between people may cause variation in the urinary excretion rates of 1-HP. Alcohol consumption, medication, and age are known to have little effect on the elimination kinetics of 1-HP in humans. Also, the daily amounts of 1-HP excretion that may come from the diets seem relatively unimportant in creosote workers. Although smoking is known to increase the 1-HP concentrations in urine, it seems to be a negligible source of pyrene exposure in creosote workers.

Lead

All of the potential lead exposures suffered by railroad and railyard workers have not been completely defined to date. However, several specific sources for lead do exist in this industry and pose a significant hazard to workers. The pathophysiology of lead poisoning, the industrial monitoring of workers for exposure to lead, and the specific treatments for lead intoxication are beyond the scope of this chapter. However, it is extremely important that the potential sources for lead intoxication and exposure in any given industry be identified.

Many of the paint products used in railyards and rail shops contain lead. While domestic paints have essentially been cleared of all lead as of the late 1970s, many industrial outdoor paints still contain significant amounts of lead. In addition, most bridges and iron superstructures that traverse railyards or bridges that carry rail lines are painted, with high-lead-content paint. When these structures are disassembled, scraped, or prepared for repainting, significant amounts of lead can be found in the air spaces surrounding these sites. In addition, the ground and soil surrounding these sites are often heavily contaminated with lead. For railworkers who are physically present at or near such sites, the possibility for contact with significant lead exposures is obvious. Moreover, the painting and surface preparation of leaded areas may be performed by railroad employees themselves.

Another significant source of lead exposure for rail employees is in the machine shop, where locomotives and other rolling stock and equipment are repaired and refurbished. When grinding and sanding procedures are performed without proper personal protective equipment, significant lead exposures can result. When workers eat or smoke in leaded areas, they may continually self-intoxicate with lead particles that they ingest or inhale. Furthermore, workers can carry significant lead home to their families and thereby contaminate their home environments and potentially poison spouses, children, and pets.

Indeed, a worrisome lead hazard does exist in the rail industry. The problems related to appropriate biologic monitoring of workers and proper utilization of personal protective equipment, however, is not specific to this industry alone (see Chapters 4, 36, and 51).

Machine Shop Toxins

As noted previously, many important equipment repair and refurbishment functions arc carried out in railyard repair shops. The potential toxic hazards for the workers in these shops are legion: exposures to cutting and lubricant oils, degreasers, metal cleaners, detergents, solvents, welding fumes, metal cutting vapors, and others (see Chapters 21, 37, and 50).

REFERENCES

1. Alavanja MC et al: Proportionate mortality study of workers in the grain industry, *J Natl Cancer Inst* 78:247, 1987.
2. Brooks SM, Lockey J: Reactive airways dysfunction syndrome (RADS): a newly defined occupational disease [Abstract] *Am Rev Respir Dis* 123 (suppl):A133, 1981.
3. Cheng YS et al: Characterization of diesel exhaust in a chronic inhalation study, *Am Ind Hyg Assoc J* 45:547, 1984.
4. Cosma GN et al: Expression of the CYP1A1 gene in peripheral lymphocytes as a marker of exposure to creosote in railroad workers, *Cancer Epidemiol Biomarkers Prev* 1:137, 1992.
5. Elovaara E et al: Significance of dermal and respiratory uptake in creosote workers, *Occup Environ Med* 52:196, 1995.
6. Feldstein A, Heumann M, Barnen M: Fumigant intoxication during transport of grain by railroad, *J Occup Med* 33:64, 1991.
7. Floderus B, Tornqvist S, Stenlund C: Incidence of selected cancers in Swedish railway workers, 1961-79, *Cancer Causes Control* 5:189, 1994.
8. Gandevia B: Occupational asthma (Part 1), *Med J Aust* 2:332-333, 1970.
9. Garry VF et al: Human genotoxicity: pesticide applicators and phosphine, *Science* 246:251, 1989.
10. Jayaraman KS: Death pills from pesticide, *Nature* 353:377, 1991.
11. Karlehagen S, Andersen A, Ohlson CG: Cancer incidence among creosote-exposed workers, *Scand J Work Environ Health* 18:26, 1992.
12. Landrigan PJ: Health risks of creosotes, *JAMA* 269:1309, 1993.
13. Mancuso TF: Mesothelioma among machinists in railroad and other industries, *Am J Ind Med* 4:501, 1983.
14. Mancuso TF: Relative risk of mesothelioma among railroad machinists exposed to chrysotile, *Am J Ind Med* 13:639, 1988.
15. Morgan DP: Recognition and management of pesticide poisonings, ed 4, pub EPA-540/9-88/001, Washington, DC, 1989, US Environmental Protection Agency.
16. U S Environmental Protection Agency: *Guidance for the reregistration of pesticide products containing aluminum or magnesium phosphide as the active ingredient,* Report 540/RS-87-109, Washington, DC, 1986, U S Environmental Protection Agency.
17. U S General Accounting Office: *Pesticides on farms—limited capability exists to monitor occupational illnesses and injuries:* report to the chairman, Committee on Agriculture, Nutrition, and Forestry, U S Senate, Report GAO/PEMD-94-6, Washington, DC, 1993, U S General Accounting Office.
18. Wilson R et al: Acute phosphine poisoning aboard a grain freighter, *JAMA* 244:148, 1980.
19. Worthing CR, editor: The pesticide manual: a world compendium, ed 7, Suffolk, England, 1983, Lavenham Press.
20. Zaebest DD et al: Phosphine exposure in grain elevators during fumigation with aluminum phosphide, *Appl Ind Hyg* 3:146, 1988.

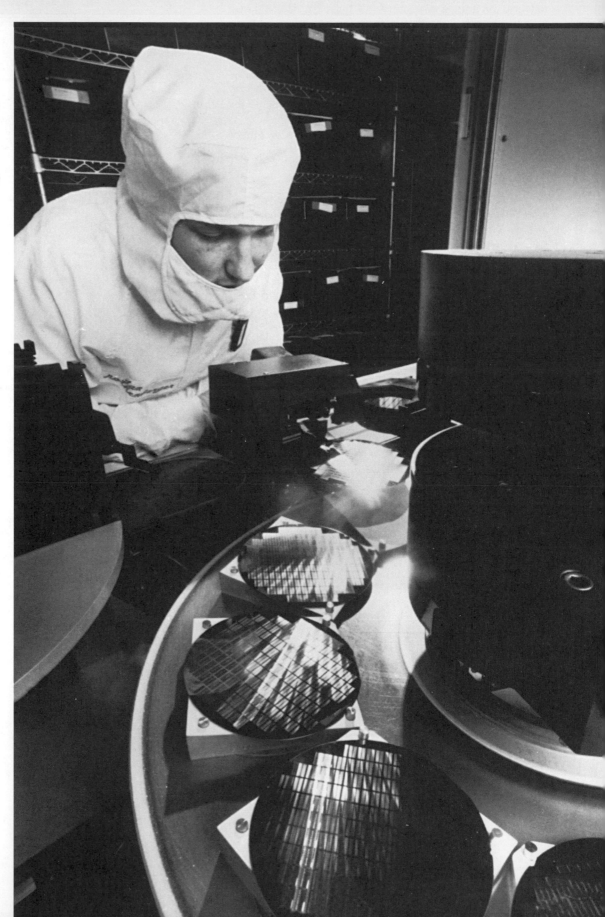

Essex Junction, Vermont. IBM manufacturing employee, Dan Rothenberger, checks the motion of a robotic arm as it positions silicon wafers for processing in an "ion implantation" machine. Each wafer will eventually be cut into about 170 individual computer memory chips.
(Courtesy Corbis-Bettmann)

48

Semiconductor

Lisandro Irizarry
Howard Blumstein

AsH$_3$
arsine gas

- Semiconductor manufacturers are required to develop strategies for the safe handling of gases used in the production process

- Arsine gas is rapidly absorbed via the inhalation route, but initial clinical signs of toxicity may be delayed for up to 24 hours

- Many genotoxic and fetotoxic chemicals are used in this industry, including solvents, heavy metals, and toxic gases

OCCUPATIONAL DESCRIPTION

Semiconductors are a pervasive but generally unseen aspect of everyday life. These dime-sized electronic circuits, etched on silicon, are critical to the operation of virtually all electronics and have developed into an essential element of our nation's economic and military security. In 1993, the United States regained from Japan its lead in the worldwide semiconductor market and maintained that lead in 1994 at 43.4%. In that year, merchant sales of semiconductors were in excess of $43 billion in the United States.[16]

The number of people directly involved in semiconductor manufacture is surprisingly small. The U.S. Department of Labor reported that 214,000 Americans worked domestically in 1993 for semiconductor companies, with probably no more than 30% of them involved in direct product handling.[16] The rest of these individuals are employed in a variety of engineering, support, sales, and administrative functions.

The technologic and economic benefits associated with the semiconductor industry have been accompanied by growing scientific and public concern for its workers. Semiconductor manufacturing is unique in its relatively large number and wide variety of toxic hazards. In addition, there is a relatively high toxicity involved with those compounds routinely handled by employees. The spectrum of potentially harmful substances tends to change rapidly with the development of new manufacturing processes within the industry, and there is frequently insufficient time to characterize potential health effects of these substances before they are brought into widespread industrial use.[9]

DEVICE MANUFACTURING

Semiconductor manufacturing can be divided into two groups of processes, each with its own unique toxic potential: (1) substrate manufacture and (2) device fabrication and interconnection.

Substrate Manufacture

Silicon is the basic substrate used to make more than 95% of wafers. Silicon is heated and exposed to high-purity hydrogen chloride gas to produce trichlorosilane. Trichlorosilane, in turn, reacts with hydrogen at high temperatures to produce "electronic grade" silicon, which has less than 1 parts per billion impurities.

Almost all crystal growth is done by what is known as the Czochralski method. A starter seed crystal of silicon is placed on the end of a rod, which is then dipped into molten silicon. The rod is rotated and slowly withdrawn, which allows silicon crystals to attach with resulting growth of the crystal. Depending on the electrical properties desired in the finished product, molten silicon may be "doped," or selectively contaminated with various different substances. Boron powder is used if an electron "deficient" melt is desired; the use of phosphorus or arsenic results in a surplus of electrons. Crystal growth occurs in an atmosphere with high concentrations of argon to prevent oxidation of the silicon crystal and the introduction of impurities from ambient air. Energy to heat the melt is supplied by radiofrequency.

Silicon wafers are produced by diamond saw slicing of the ingots, followed by rounding by automatic grinders. After these machining operations are complete, the wafer surface is chemically etched in a mixture of nitric, acetic, and hydrofluoric acids. These processes are followed by an additional etch with chromic acid and hydrofluoric acids. Standard precautions include eye and skin protection and ventilation hoods. The last step in wafer preparation is removing the silica colloid in a mixture of sulfuric acid or ammonium hydroxide solution. After they are polished and packaged, the wafers are ready to be fabricated into circuits.

While the vast majority of wafers are made of silicon, some special applications require the use of gallium arsenide. These special applications generally include optoelectronics, military hardware, and very-high-speed semiconductors. The main advantage of gallium arsenide over silicon is that electrons move 5 to 6 times faster in gallium arsenide. Unfortunately, gallium arsenide is much more hazardous than silicon to use and requires much more stringent control.

Device Fabrication

Device fabrication includes the vast majority of all chemical hazards encountered in the semiconductor industry. The fabrication of microscopic devices onto the surface of wafers is carried out in "clean rooms" and is accomplished by creating areas of altered electricity within the high-purity silicon substrate. Altering conductivity in selected areas of the silicon is essential in the process of creating microelectronic devices.

Electronic device manufacture requires a high level of contaminant control and is therefore carried out in clean rooms, which are designed to minimize deposition of contaminant particles onto the product and are not necessarily intended to serve a protective function for workers. Clean rooms are defined and designated according to the number of 0.5-micron-diameter particles present per cubic foot of air. Normal ambient air typically exceeds 500,000 particles per cubic foot of air. The original controlled environments created in the semiconductor industry were relatively airtight rooms in which air was continuously filtered and recirculated to remove particles. Airflow in these rooms was often turbulent. This turbulence allowed solvent vapors to accumulate to significant concentrations that put the worker at risk of exposure. In these circumstances, many air changes were often required before all particles were effectively removed from the room.

The evolution of clean room design has progressed from the original "mixed air" type to the introduction of clean work stations within the clean rooms and further to the modern vertical laminar flow clean rooms. Clean work stations use high-efficiency particulate air (HEPA) filters and vertical laminar flow, which together effectively remove all particles larger than 0.05 microns. This technique protects the product under the hood from any particles but can expose the worker to vapors generated beneath the hood. Optimally, each work station should have a separate, externally vented exhaust system. The state of the art in clean room ventilation is vertical laminar flow ventilation, in which air is pumped through HEPA filters in the ceiling and captured through the floor, thereby eliminating the need for individual work station ventilation hoods. The entire volume of air within a workspace can be recycled in approximately 6 seconds. Because of the lack of individually vented hoods, gases released in this environment are quickly distributed throughout the entire room and pose a significant risk to all workers.

The first step in device fabrication, oxidation, involves the formation of silicon dioxide over the surface of the silicon wafer. The next step, photolithography, establishes the pattern of the circuit on the wafer. Circuit patterns are "written" onto the silicon dioxide by applying a protective layer, the "photoresist," to the surface of the wafer. Subsequently, it is exposed through a mask of the unprotected areas with ultraviolet or some other form of radiation. Next, the unprotected silicon dioxide is etched away with either hydrofluoric acid (wet etching) or ionized gases (dry etching). At this point, there exist specific areas where the silicon dioxide layer has been removed to reveal bare silicon. This silicon can then be contaminated or "doped" with various types of elemental particles with a resultant change in the electrical conductivity of the silicon wafer, as discussed previously. This doping is accomplished by either ion implantation or diffusion. Another layer of silicon is now applied to the wafer to cover or "bury" the area of silicon that was altered or doped. These processes are repeated several times until the final circuit patterns are established. The last step is to wire together the devices to create electronic circuits. This is done by depositing patterns of metal by the same photolithographic techniques used to create the devices.[5]

POTENTIAL HAZARD EXPOSURE

Semiconductor manufacturing requires very low levels of external contamination of materials and devices. This level of environmental control tends to reduce operator exposure to toxins. Previous studies have shown that local process controls necessary to produce high-quality devices have actually enhanced worker safety in general.[19,20] Production protocols are designed to control toxic exposures associated with routine operations to well below recommended limits. However, because of poorly designed or implemented controls, equipment failure, lack of maintenance, poor work practices, or improper training, preventable exposures from the large number of hazardous toxic materials and processes used in this industry can and do occur.[20] Although these control methods, when properly implemented, protect equipment operators and production workers, maintenance employees commonly circumvent controls in the course of their duties. These workers are the ones who are at the greatest risk for injuries and illnesses.

The goal of chemical control systems is to minimize the risk of accidental or routine employee exposure. It can be accomplished in various ways. Choosing the least hazardous chemicals and production processes is the best control because the hazard is kept entirely away from the workers. Such control is often difficult to implement because many chemicals, such as the various dopants, are chosen for their individual specific properties and are difficult to substitute. Simple containment by enclosing or isolating a hazardous process is common practice in the industry and is a function of the degree of automation. The primary problem with containment controls is that over time the enclosure may lose its effectiveness, either through predictable aging or by human tampering or misuse. Systematic inspection and maintenance procedures are necessary if effective control is to be assured. Ventilation is most appropriate when these methods are not practical. Local exhaust systems for chemical storage cabinets and some process equipment are important for protecting the workplace from release of gases, but the presence of ventilation equipment does not necessarily ensure safety because its effectiveness is based on design, employee work practices, and adequate maintenance. Failure of contaminant control systems is common in industry and must be considered when evaluating employee complaints.

Hazards by Production Process

Although the semiconductor manufacturing industry has often been considered a "clean" industry, extreme hazards are associated with the chemicals used as well as with the processes employed in manufacturing. Process optimization requires stringent control of the clean room environment. Ambient temperature is maintained at about 74° F (23.3° C). Humidity is kept as close as possible to 35% to protect wafers from condensation and accumulation of water droplets. Air is constantly kept moving at about 100 linear feet per minute. These three factors in combination can give rise to multiple health problems, including dermatoses, upper respiratory problems, asthma, and ocular irritation.

Clean room garments provide protection to wafers from external contamination. These garments are worn over or in place of street clothes to prevent shedding of contaminant particles from workers. Chronic exposure to some of the garment materials or to the detergents used in their cleaning has resulted in chronic dermatitis in some susceptible individuals.

Air filtration within the clean room removes ions and therefore increases the accumulation of static electricity on surfaces. Accumulation of low doses of static electricity can cause significant damage to the surface of exposed wafers. Ionization systems used in clean rooms to prevent the accumulation of static electricity generate ozone. Although the quantity of ozone generated is usually of little significance, failure of ventilatory systems can result in ozone accumulation within the clean room.

The most hazardous processes in semiconductor production are photolithographic operations, etching processes, and ion implantation. These processes involve many risk factors, including toxic gases, solvents and photoreactive polymers, metals, acids and alkalis, and radiation. Table 48-1 lists the most common hazards in the production process.

Gases. Every semiconductor manufacturer must develop a strategy for the safe handling of gases. The first step in safe gas handling is to identify every gas used and the potential of each to cause injury or illness. This step may be the most important in the entire sequence of controls. The extensive use of highly toxic dopant gases such as arsine, phosphine, and diborane with threshold limit values in the low ppm ranges is accompanied by the possibility of an accidental release into the workplace and into the community. Arsine is a colorless, odorless, nonirritating gas that is 2.5 times denser than air. It has poor olfactory warning properties and evolves from arsenic compounds upon addition of an acid. Acute arsine toxicity has been associated with a mortality in the range of 25%. Exposures from 25 to 50 ppm arsine for 0.5 hours and to 10 ppm for longer periods are lethal.[1] Arsine is rapidly absorbed via the lungs after inhalation. Clinical signs and symptoms appear 2 to 24 hours after exposure and may include headache, malaise, dyspnea, abdominal pain with nausea and vomiting, hepatomegaly, hemolysis with hemoglobinuric renal failure, and death. The mechanism for sudden death after arsenic exposure is probably respiratory arrest caused by central nervous system (CNS) depression. Cessation of exposure, fluid hydration, and general support are the mainstays of treatment. Hemodialysis and even ex-

Table 48-1 Hazards by production process

Production area	Particulates	Metals	Solvents	Acids	Caustics	Flammable gases	Systemic and respiratory toxins
Polycrystalline silicon	X		X	X		X	
Single crystal ingot	X	X		X			X
Wafer preparation	X		X	X	X		
Oxidation						X	
Photolithography			X	X	X		X
Etching				X			X
Junction formation		X				X	X
Metalization	X						

Table 48-2 Common reactive gases in semiconductor manufacturing

Gas	TLV-TWA (mg/m^3)*	Health hazards
HCl	7.5†	Corrosive, pulmonary edema
HF	2.6†	Corrosive, pulmonary edema
H$_3$PO$_4$	1.0	Corrosive, pulmonary edema
NH$_3$	25 ppm‡	Corrosive, nasal/oral/laryngeal burns, pulmonary edema
O$_3$	0.2†	Pulmonary edema; subacute exposure causes chronic bronchitis, asthma exacerbation
NO$_2$	5.6	Corrosive, pulmonary edema

Data from Wald PH, Jones JR: Semiconductor manufacturing: an introduction to processes and hazards, *Am J Ind Med* 11:203, 1987; and ACGIH: 1987.

*Threshold limit values–time-weighted average for worker exposed 8 hours/day, 5 days/week.

†Denotes ceiling limit, maximum exposure at any time.

‡TLV in parts per million.

change transfusion may be considered in the most severe cases.

Phosphine and diborane are also extremely toxic in low doses. These gases are primarily local pulmonary irritants that can cause coughing, cyanosis, and noncardiac pulmonary edema. Table 48-2 lists common reactive gases in the industry.

Solvents. Solvents are used in many different operations, including cleaning, degreasing, photo mask operations, etching, and stripping. Most solvents have only limited toxic effects. Low dose exposure, by either ingestion or inhalation, may be associated with fatigue, concentration difficulties, and headaches. Long-term low dose exposures may be accompanied by CNS depression, neuropathy, hematopoietic and reproductive effects, and liver and kidney damage.[1]

Glycol ethers are vehicles for photoactive polymers and are the most toxic of all solvents used in semiconductor manufacture. They have been reported to produce teratogenic and reproductive effects in animals.[2,4,17] The exact mechanism(s) by which glycol ethers may cause reproductive toxicity is not known. Studies have suggested that interference with DNA or RNA synthesis may be involved.[4,12,17] The current hypothesis is that they interfere with the availability of one-carbon units for incorporation into purine and pyrimidine bases. Glycol ethers are metabolized to biologically active ethylene glycol ethers and their acetates by hepatic alcohol dehydrogenase. The clinical presentation of acute exposure can be expected to be similar to that seen with ethylene glycol exposure. High dose glycol ether exposure can result in persistent nausea and vomiting, with CNS agitation, followed by the gradual onset of lethargy and then coma, which often appears within 4 to 8 hours of severe exposure. Diffuse neurologic abnormalities may be noted, including nystagmus, ataxia, myoclonic movements, absent reflexes, and seizures. Tachycardia, accompanied by arrhythmias, is often seen, as well as a prolonged QT on electrocardiogram due to systemic hypocalcemia. Specific treatment consists of preventing the metabolism of glycol ether and ethylene glycol by inhibiting alcohol dehydrogenase and extracorporeal removal.[2] The action of alcohol dehydrogenase in the liver is the first rate-limiting step in the breakdown of these compounds to toxic metabolites. Ethanol is the preferential substrate for alcohol dehydrogenase and, if administered in sufficient concentration, allows the unchanged primary alcohols to be renally eliminated. An optimal blood ethanol level should be attained quickly by administering an intravenous loading dose, and this level should be maintained until the blood level of ethylene glycol reaches zero. This is best accomplished with an intravenous loading dose of 0.8 g/kg of ethanol, followed by maintenance doses of 130 mg/kg per hour. Although the intravenous route is preferred, ethanol may also be administered orally. All of the toxic metabolites are effectively removed by hemodialysis. Hemodialysis should be performed on any patient who is symptomatic, has a significant metabolic acidosis, has a blood level of ethylene glycol greater than 25 mg/dl, or has renal compromise. The solvents commonly used in production are listed in Table 48-3.

Table 48-3 Common solvents utilized in semiconductor manufacturing

Solvent	Threshold limit value (ppm)	Toxicity (mg/kg)
Ethylene glycol ethers		
2-Methoxy ethanol	5	2460
2-Ethoxy ethanol	5	3000-5500
2-Ethoxy ethylacetate	5	3900
Carbon tetrachloride	10	1770
Freon		>20 not toxic
Tetrachloroethylene	25	4000 ppm
Trichloroethylene	50	538
Methylene chloride	50	2136
Chloroform	50	908
Methyl isobutyl ketone	50	
Ethylene glycol	50	4700
Isopropanol	400	5045
Toluene	100	5000
Xylene	100	4300
N-Butylacetate	150	13,100
1,1,1-Trichloroethane	350	750
1,1-Dichloroethane	200	725
Methyl alcohol	200	13,000
Acetone	750	9750
Ethanol	1000	21,000

Table 48-4 Common dopants in semiconductor manufacturing

Gas	TLV-TWA (mg/m^3)*	Health hazards
Arsine	0.16	Acute hemolysis, hemoglobinuria, renal failure
Diborane	0.11	Pulmonary edema, CNS effects, metal fumelike fever
Borotriflorane†	2.8	Dissociates to corrosive acids
Phosphine	0.42	Pulmonary edema, headache diarrhea, nausea, vomiting, possible CNS and myocardial depression
Indium	0.1	
Thallium	0.1	
Geranium (tetrachloride)	0.63	
Antimony	0.5	
Selenium compounds	0.2 (as selenium)	
Selenium hexafluoride	0.16	
Arsenic‡	0.01	

Data from ACGIH 1987 and Wald PH, Jones JR: Semiconductor manufacturing: an introduction to processes and hazards, *Am J Ind Med* 11:203, 1987.

*Threshold limit values–time-weighted average for worker exposed 8 hours/day, 5 days/week.

†Denotes ceiling limit, maximum exposure at any time.

‡Known human carcinogen.

Metals. Metallic impurities, also called *dopants,* are added to the silicon wafers as discussed previously. Crystal ingot production incorporates materials such as arsenic, antimony, nickle, chromium, cadmium, lead, tellurium, mercury, zinc, germanium, gallium, and indium. These metals may be used in their elemental form, as halogenated compounds, or in other forms. In contrast with metals such as arsenic, lead, cadmium, and mercury, relatively little is known about the mechanisms of toxicity of these other agents, either alone or more commonly as binary or trinary compounds. Table 48-4 lists the commonly used dopants.

One compound that has developed increased importance in the production of integrated circuits is gallium arsenide. Its benefit involves its ability to allow electrons to move 5 to 6 times faster than silicon does. In addition, gallium arsenide has a significantly lower power of heat dissipation. Up to 1984, it was generally thought that gallium arsenide was biologically inert and that health hazards encountered during its production were primarily associated with the use of arsenic as a raw material.[1] A number of experiments have shown that gallium arsenide dissociates in the lung or gut to gallium and arsenic, with the latter acting metabolically as an inorganic arsenic species.[5,21-23] The metabolism and potential for toxicity of arsenic are further complicated by the in vivo transformation of inorganic forms by methylation to monomethyl and dimethyl arsenic. This is presumed to be a detoxification process, but the roles, if any, that these metabolites play in clinical toxicity remains poorly defined.

Exposures to arsenic in the semiconductor industry are unlikely to result in acute symptoms. More concern has been raised regarding the chronic effects of arsenic exposure. Early features of chronic exposure involve the gastrointestinal tract and the skin. In humans, chronic exposure to organic arsenic induces a series of characteristic changes in skin epithelium ranging from hyperpigmentation and hyperkeratosis to squamous cell carcinoma. Chronic exposure to inorganic arsenic compounds may lead to neurotoxicity of both the peripheral and central nervous systems. Neurotoxicity begins with sensory changes in stocking-glove distribution, paresthesias, and muscle tenderness followed by weakness, progressing from proximal to distal muscle groups. Arsenic-related peripheral neuropathy may be progressive and involve both sensory and motor neurons; these effects appear dose related. Liver injury may manifest itself initially with jaundice, which may progress to cirrhosis and ascites. Occupational exposure to airborne inorganic arsenic particles is associated with lung cancer, usually of the epidermoid bronchogenic carcinoma type. Studies of arsenic carcinogenesis in animals have shown a positive correlation that is greater in those exposed to arsenic plus other carcinogenic agents.[14] These data indicate that trivalent arsenic produces marked alterations in gene expression patterns in several cell types and therefore may create a situation that may permit other carcinogenic substances to act more effectively.[3]

Acids and alkalis. Acids and alkalis are used in semiconductor production mainly in wet-etching processes and in the neutralization of wastes from etching baths. All of these substances are capable of causing irritation of the skin and eyes and damage to the lungs, stomach, and mucous membranes after inhalation or ingestion.

The most dangerous and widely used acid in this industry is hydrofluoric acid (HF). The concentration, route of exposure, contact time, and premorbid state of affected tissues are correlated with the onset and the severity of injury. It is the effect of the highly electronegative fluoride ion binding to enzymes and the structural components of cell membranes that is thought to cause damage to tissues, as opposed to the effects of the hydrogen ion. Because of this property, hydrofluoric acid is able to produce severe ocular and dermal injury as well as life-threatening systemic toxicity with minimal external tissue damage. As the chemical does not cause immediate pain, there may be no warning signal to the individual that the chemical is on the skin; therefore, prolonged exposure can take place. Fatalities have been reported resulting from dermal exposure to as little as 2.5% of body surface area.[18] In addition, significant exposure can take place after the inhalation of hydrofluoric acid vapor.

Initially, after dermal exposure to HF, the skin may appear normal or mildly erythematous, but as ischemia progresses, the skin becomes blanched, with frank necrosis following in those with untreated exposure. Concentrated solutions of HF produce immediate symptoms, whereas those exposed to less concentrated solutions may not begin to experience symptoms for 12 hours or more after exposure. Appropriate initial management includes copious washing of the affected area with water in order to limit the severity of exposure. Therapy for minor to moderate HF burn injuries includes either the application of a calcium gluconate gel or local tissue infiltration with calcium gluconate. The use of magnesium sulfate has also been advocated. The calcium gluconate gel can be made by adding 3.5 g calcium gluconate powder to 5 oz of a water-soluble surgical jelly. Treatment for severe burns is intradermal injection of 10% calcium gluconate directly into the affected tissues. These injections should be administered with a 25- or 30-gauge needle and in amounts no greater than 0.5 ml/cm^2 of involved tissue. The end point of the infiltration procedure is pain relief, which often is almost immediate. If the pain recurs, the procedure may be repeated. If pain is refractory to intradermal instillation of calcium gluconate, then intraarterial infusion of calcium gluconate remains a viable alternative. The technique for intraarterial administration involves placement of a standard intraarterial catheter proximal to the injury.

After arterial placement has been confirmed, 10 ml of a 10% solution of calcium gluconate is mixed with 50 ml of D5W and infused slowly with a pump over approximately 4 hours.

While ingestion of hydrofluoric acid is unlikely within the semiconductor industry, pulmonary exposure remains a serious concern. Inhaled hydrofluoric acid is extremely irritating. It can produce transient coughing and choking, followed by an asymptomatic period that may last from a few hours to 1 or 2 days. After the asymptomatic period, there may be coughing, dyspnea, cyanosis, and possibly pulmonary edema. Exposure may result in chronic pulmonary symptoms such as hoarseness and coughing that can take months or even years to resolve. Inhalation of high concentrations of hydrofluoric acid can result in the rapid development of atelectasis, hemorrhage, and death. Treatment entails removal of the worker from the site of exposure, administration of humidified air or oxygen, and transportation to the nearest health care facility. Monitoring the patient for the development of laryngeal edema, pneumonitis, pulmonary edema, hemorrhage, and other signs of systemic toxicity may be necessary for up to 48 hours. Lee and colleagues treated 12 workers at the site of exposure with nebulized calcium gluconate, and none of the patients experienced any ill effects from this therapy.[10]

Reproductive Hazards

Adverse reproductive outcomes are a significant public health problem. Awareness has been increasing of the potential for occupational and environmental exposures to hazardous substances that may adversely affect the reproductive outcome in both males and females. First, numerous teratology studies in animals implicate a variety of chemical substances commonly used in the electronics industry as embryo-fetal toxins or teratogens. Second, epidemiologic studies of workers in other industries suggest associations between increased rates of spontaneous abortions or birth defects and exposure to substances commonly used in the electronics industry. Third, recent studies of pregnancy outcome in women drinking water contaminated with substances used in the electronics industry have suggested a potential association between these chemicals and the occurrence of spontaneous abortion and birth defects.[15]

The microelectronics industry, which employs large numbers of women, is often described as a "clean industry." Paradoxically, many potential genotoxic and fetotoxic chemicals are used in semiconductor manufacturing. Analysis of reproductive outcomes among Finnish women showed that the frequency of spontaneous abortion was increased in electronics plants.[6] A subsequent case control study demonstrated a significant increase in the rate of spontaneous abortion among women with exposure to occupational organic solvents.[7] Other studies have supported these findings.[8,11] Rudolph and Swan reviewed the potential reproductive hazards presented by the materials and physical factors common in this industry. The authors concluded that both male and female employees in this industry are exposed to factors known to cause reproductive disorders in numerous animal teratology studies and in epidemiologic studies of workers in other industries.[15] Pastides and associates described the risk of adverse reproductive outcomes and the prevalence of general illness symptoms in workers in semiconductor facilities. Increased spontaneous abortion rates were observed for women working in the diffusion and photolithographic processes.[13]

CONCLUSION

The evolution of the semiconductor first began in 1948 with the development of the transistor, which replaced the inefficient vacuum tube. The rapid growth and advancing technology of the industry since that time have made it difficult to adequately study and characterize the toxicology of the various substances used in semiconductor manufacturing. Certainly, knowing specifically what an affected employee was working with and at what levels can be critical to the diagnosis, treatment, and prevention of future problems. However, toxicologic information is almost always focused exclusively on single-substance exposures. This information is less useful in an industry where exposure to multiple substances is common. The semiconductor industry must evaluate the nature and extent of materials commonly used in the manufacture of semiconductors and related devices and consider health and safety in selecting materials and fabrication methods. Consequently, health professionals should become familiar with the manufacturing process and possible hazards from exposure.

REFERENCES

1. Bauer S et al: Health hazards in the semiconductor industry. A review, *Pol J Occup Med Environ Health* 5:299, 1992.
2. Browning RG, Curry SC: Clinical toxicology of ethylene glycol monoalkyl ethers, *Hum Exp Toxicol* 13:325, 1994.
3. Fowler BA et al: Cancer risks for humans from exposure to the semiconductor metals, *Scand J Work Environ Health* 19:101, 1993.
4. Hardin BD: Reproductive toxicology of glycol ethers, *Toxicology* 27:91, 1983.
5. Harrison RJ: Gallium arsenide: state of the art reviews, *Occup Med* 1:49, 1986.
6. Hemminki K et al: Spontaneous abortions among women employed in the metal industry in Finland, *Int Arch Occup Environ Health* 47:53, 1980.
7. Hemminki K, Franssila E, Vaino H: Spontaneous abortions among female chemical workers in Finland, *Int Arch Occup Environ Health* 45:123, 1980.
8. Huel G, Mergler D, Bowler R: Evidence for adverse reproductive outcomes among women microelectronic assembly workers, *Br J Ind Med* 47:400, 1990.
9. LaDou J: Health issues in the microelectronics industry: state of the art reviews, *Occup Med* 1:1, 1986.
10. Lee DC, Wiley JF, Snyder JW: Treatment of inhalation exposure to hydrofluoric acid with nebulized calcium gluconate, *J Occup Med* 35:470, 1993 (letter).
11. Lipscombe JA et al: Pregnancy outcomes in women potentially exposed to occupational solvents and women working in the electronics industry, *J Occup Med* 33:597, 1991.
12. Mebus CA, Welsch F: The possible role of one carbon moieties in 2-methoxyethanol and 2-methoxyacetic acid-induced developmental toxicity, *Toxicol Appl Pharmacol* 99:98, 1989.
13. Pastides H et al: Spontaneous abortion and general illness symptoms among semiconductor manufacturers, *J Occup Med* 30:543, 1988.
14. Pershagen G, Bjorklund NE, Nordberg G: Carcinomas of the respiratory tract in hamsters given arsenic trioxide and/or benzo(a)pyrene by the pulmonary route, *Environ Res* 34:227, 1984.
15. Rudolph L, Swan S: Reproductive hazards in the microelectronics industry, *Occup Med* 1:135, 1986.
16. Semiconductor Industry Association: Status report and industry directory 1996-1997, San Jose, Calif, 1996, Semiconductor Industry Association.
17. Snyder R, Andrews LS: Toxic effects of solvents and vapors. In Klassen CD, editor: *Casarett and Doull's toxicology, the basic science of poisons*, ed 5, New York, 1996, McGraw-Hill.
18. Tepperman PB: Fatality due to acute systemic fluoride poisoning following a hydrofluoric acid skin burn, *J Occup Med* 22:691, 1980.
19. Wade R, Williams M: *Semiconductor industry study*, Sacramento, 1981, California Department of Industrial Relations, Division of Occupational Safety and Health, Taskforce on the Electronics Industry.
20. Wald PH, Jones JR: Semiconductor manufacturing: an introduction to processes and hazards, *Am J Ind Med* 11:203, 1987.
21. Webb DR, Spies IG, Carter DE: In-vitro solubility and in-vitro toxicity of gallium arsenide, *Toxicol Appl Pharmacol* 76:96, 1984.
22. Webb DR, Wilson SE, Carter DE: Pulmonary clearance and toxicity of respirable gallium arsenide particulates intratracheally instilled into rats, *Am Ind Hyg Assoc J* 48:660, 1987.
23. Yamauchi H, Takahashi K, Tamamura Y: Metabolism and excretion of orally and intraperitoneally administered gallium arsenide in the hamster, *Toxicology* 49:237, 1986.

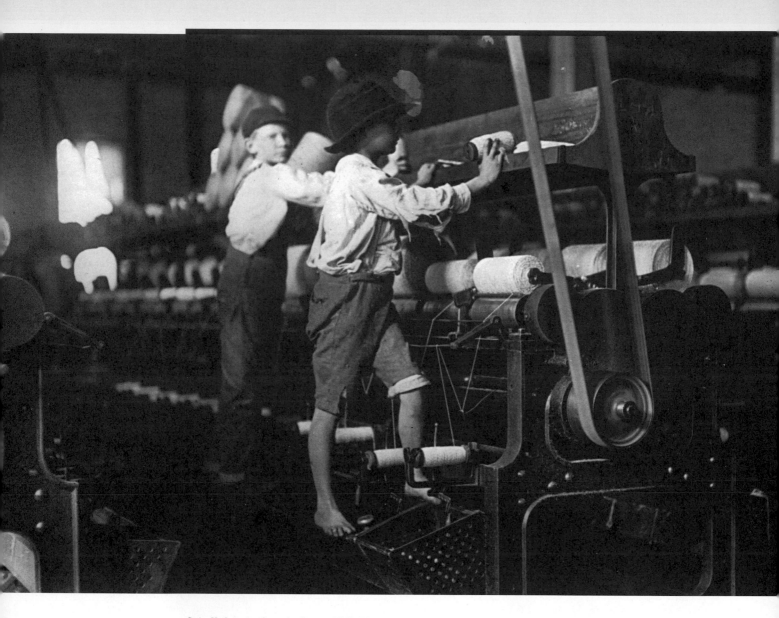

Spindle boys in Georgia Cotton Mill. Photo by Lewis Hines. Undated.

(Courtesy Corbis-Bettmann)

49

Textile Manufacture

Michael I. Greenberg

aniline

benzidene

- Formaldehyde exposure can occur with the use of dimethylol dihydroxy ethylene urea as a crease-resistant treatment in textiles

- Byssinosis is a respiratory syndrome resulting from inhalation of cotton, hemp, or flax dusts

- Workers exposed to direct brown 95, direct black 38, and direct blue 6 excrete high levels of benzidene

- Exposure to carbon disulfide (CS_2) causes the development of accelerated atherogenesis

OCCUPATIONAL DESCRIPTION

The textile production industry is one of the oldest and most technologically complex of all industries. The manufacture of textiles probably has its origin roughly around the year 8000 BC, when organic materials (grasses) were the first substances used to make a form of yarn. Certainly, cloth, carpets, and tapestries, thousands of years old, have been discovered in many parts of the world. Relics of such ancient fabrics have been found in many countries and are on display in museums, universities, and private collections around the world.

Near the close of the eighteenth century, the Industrial Revolution brought the development of machines and the beginnings of mass production of textiles. Now, the industry has grown to the point where production of textiles is one of the most important industries in the world, as well as in many parts of the United States. In the late 1980s, nearly 750,000 Americans were estimated to be engaged in textile manufacturing, without taking into account the estimated large numbers of people who might participate in this industry in a clandestine, "off the books," or otherwise illegitimate manner. Nevertheless, over the past two decades, much of the basic textile industry has shifted to developing countries, where the numbers of workers cannot be ascertained.

The production of textiles includes all of the following processes: spinning, weaving, knitting, dyeing, and finishing of various natural and synthetic fibers. The technology used in these processes varies from the simplest and even primitive looms found in cottage (home) industries to processes involving sophisticated, automated, and computerized machines in modern factories.

Raw cotton bales are received and opened, and then the cotton may be blended with other fibers. The cotton then goes to the picking machines, which moves the fibers to the "cards." During these first stages, fibers may be transported by the use of air currents in a process known as *blowing*. Fibers of cotton are then carded. From the card, the fiber strands go to the drawing frame and then are moved onto a device called a *roving frame*. The product of this process, called *roving,* then goes to the spinning frame, where so-called warp yarn and filling yarn are made. The next processes, which precede weaving, are meant specifically to prepare the yarn for the weaving process. Warp yarn on the spinning frame is transferred from a bobbin to a large spool. A large number of these packages are placed on a warping machine to make a beam of yarn. For the process known as *beaming,* two specific types of winding machines are used, a spooler and a warper. Several beams are run together on the last machine before weaving, called a *slasher.* During this process, a hot solution of starch is applied to the warp yarn to reduce breakage and damage in the weaving. Yarn, especially wool, may undergo a dyeing process prior to being woven on a loom. The term *finishing* refers specifically to any of the final processes, including dyeing, finishing, and inspecting the fabric.

POTENTIAL TOXIC EXPOSURES

Textile workers can be exposed to dusts (both natural and synthetic) generated from the textile products in various stages during the textile manufacturing process. While the spinning, weaving, and knitting operations involve only limited use of chemicals, other processes depend on chemicals. The most important chemicals used in spinning, knitting, and weaving are "sizing agents" like starch and the various polymers used as lubricants to prevent tangling of the yarn.

Specifically, cotton textile workers can be exposed to mineral lubricants used in the spindles during an operation known as *mule spinning,* which involves twisting yarn to thicken it. Because of the adverse exposure potential, the mule spinning process was discontinued in Europe in the 1960s, and many countries have enacted legislation prohibiting oils for mule spinning. In addition, other countries have limited the practice to the use of less harmful animal or vegetable oils only. Nonetheless, mule spinning may still be practiced in other parts of the world, and thus textile workers may have a continuing exposure to inhalation and skin contact with mineral lubricants as a result of mule spinning.

Another potential hazardous exposure for textile workers involves exposure to dyestuffs, products whose purpose is to add color to materials. The term *dyestuffs* applies to both dyes and pigments. At present, most textile dyes are synthetic products.

The first synthetic dye, mauve, was discovered in 1865. The synthetic dyestuff industry developed rapidly soon after this discovery with the introduction of another very important dye, magenta. Subsequently, development of the water-soluble azo dyes represented a landmark in the synthetic dye industry. The most important dye structures include triphenylmethane compounds, indigoid and azo structures, azines, thiazines, anthraquinone derivatives and phthalocyanines. A crucial technological advance occurred in the 1950s with the discovery of "reactive" dyes, which react directly with the fiber itself. Reactive dyes produce textiles with specific color fastness that had not been possible with the earlier water-soluble dyes.

Approximately 38,000 different colorants and dyes exist in the textile industry. These dyes involve more than 9000 different chemical structures. World production of dyestuffs was estimated to be 600,000 to 700,000 tonnes (active substance) in 1978, of which 50% to 60% were used for textiles. In 1986, more than 107,000 tonnes of textile dyes were produced in the United States.

One of the most commercially important dyes is the benzidine-based dye group. Due to health concerns discussed later in this chapter, production of benzidine-based dyes decreased drastically in the United States during the 1970s, but they may still be widely used elsewhere in the world.

Another important source for potential toxicity to textile workers involves the finishing processes. These finishing treatments are intended to enhance the properties of textiles and include crease-resistant, flame-retardant, water-repellent, antisoiling, and antimicrobial treatments.

Crease-resistance treatments are the most widely used process for textiles such as cotton and viscose because these fibers are the most likely of all to wrinkle significantly. Formaldehyde-based resins have been extensively used since the early 1950s, to produce "permanent press" fabrics. The first such resin was urea-formaldehyde resin, which first came on the market in 1933. Melamine-formaldehyde resins are used for crease resistance treatments in the textile industry today.

A new class of crease-resistant finishing agent for textiles was introduced in the United States in the late 1940s. These chemicals were the cyclic ethylene ureas including dimethylol ethylene urea, which reacts directly with cellulose fibers. Application of finishing agents increased gradually as the popularity of permanent press garments grew during the 1950s. In 1959, dimethylol dihydroxy ethylene urea was formulated, and it is currently the most widely used crease-resistant finishing agent. This chemical is made from urea, formaldehyde, and glyoxal and during production releases significantly less formaldehyde than the earlier urea and melamine resins. In the 1980s, the release of formaldehyde from dimethylol dihydroxy ethylene urea was further reduced by alkylation. Other low-formaldehyde processes continue to be developed.

The addition of flame retardants in the production of textiles dates back to antiquity, when seawater, clay, and

Table 49-1 Chemicals used in textile-manufacturing processes

Process	Associated chemical(s)
Water repellents	Fluorocarbons, silicones, zirconium emulsions
Antistatic agents	Polyethylene glycols, epoxy resins
Antisoiling agents	Aluminum, silicon and titanium oxides, starch, fluorocarbons, polymers
Antimicrobial agents	Quaternary ammonium compounds, tributyltin oxide
Antimildew agents	Pentachlorophenyl laurate, copper and zirconium compounds
Softeners	Tensides, polyethylene glycol, polysilicates

vinegar in combination were utilized to form primitive flame retardants. Over the last 30 years, considerable research has sought to develop effective fire-retardant textiles for use in work clothes, upholstery, space and aeronautical research, and military textiles. Currently, the most widely used flame retardants are inorganic salts and reactive phosphorus and nitrogen compounds. Despite the fact that they tend to dissolve during normal laundering processes, inorganic salts are attractive agents because they are easier to apply during manufacturing. In addition, these compounds tend to be less toxic than the organic reactive flame retardants.

Organic Solvents

Aliphatic hydrocarbons are often used to clean parts and equipment in textile mills and plants. Stoddard's solvent, mineral spirits, and kerosene are examples of such chemicals commonly used for this purpose. Specifically, 1,1,1-trichloroethane, a chlorinated hydrocarbon, is used to clean metal parts. In addition, it is often used for "spot-cleaning" of cloth. Exposure to any of these solvents may cause defatting and resultant skin irritation leading to pruritic dermatitis. In addition, these materials can be very potent central nervous system depressants. The chlorinated solvents also have potential hepatic and renal toxicity. Studies involving textile workers exposed specifically to 1,1,1-trichloroethane have not detected any problems. Solvents of essentially historical importance include carbon disulfide, a known neurotoxicant widely used in the past in the production of the synthetic fiber viscose rayon, and methyl *n*-butyl ketone, a substance known to cause sensorimotor neuropathies in exposed workers.

Other Processes

Other processes of importance used in the textile industry today include application of water repellents, antistatic agents, antisoiling agents, antimicrobial agents, antimildew agents, and softening agents (Table 49-1).

CLINICAL TOXICOLOGY
Dusts and Byssinosis

Byssinosis is a respiratory syndrome that occurs as the result of inhaling dust that is produced when cotton, flax, or hemp is handled. Byssinosis probably represents one of the most significant health problems in the entire textile industry today.

The precise pathogenesis of byssinosis is unclear, but it does involve the development of clinically significant bronchoconstriction.[1,3,9] This bronchoconstriction is thought to be related to endogenous histamine contained within the cotton bract itself. In addition, it is assumed that a direct release of histamine from pulmonary mast cells contributes to the development of the clinical signs and symptoms.

Byssinosis was first reported in England but was not generally recognized in the United States until the late 1960s. This is when it became recognized as a major occupationally related health problem. Byssinosis has evolved to become a significant regulatory and political issue, particularly where textiles are manufactured or processed.

When cotton is first picked, a large quantity of torn and chopped-up leaves and stems are mixed in with the cotton fibers. Automated picking of cotton tends to produce a great deal of this sort of contamination and certainly significantly more than occurs with hand-picked cotton. It has been theorized that the bract leaf located just below the cotton boll itself may contain vasoactive chemicals. It is these chemicals that are specifically capable of inducing bronchospasm. Other theories hold that bacteria growing in the cotton dust itself can produce endotoxins during storage and that this endotoxin is responsible for producing the bronchospastic response associated with byssinosis. There does seem to be an association between the prevalence of byssinosis and measured levels of endotoxin in cotton dust and in workplace air.[10,11]

Clinically, byssinosis is first manifested by complaints described as chest "tightness," which is sometimes associated with a continual cough, shortness of breath, and occasionally wheezing. These symptoms typically occur on the first day of the workweek. Early in the development of the disease, symptoms have their onset only occasionally. Often the earliest symptoms occur during excessively humid weather. This early form of byssinosis is classified sometimes as grade ½ byssinosis. Over time, a distinct progression of symptoms is noted to occur. Following the initial stage (grade ½), the next stage is grade I. This stage usually involves complaints of chest tightness on most work days or at least on all first work days of the week (typically Monday). During the ensuing several years, symptomatology may progress to grade II byssinosis, characterized by symptoms on days other than Monday. In this stage, symptoms still are generally worse at the start of the week, with many workers noting some degree of improvement toward the end of the week. This progression of symptoms is extremely important to the clinician, as a tendency for symptoms to improve as the week progresses differentiates byssinosis from nonspecific airway reactivity. In nonspecific settings, symptoms do not improve and may actually worsen as the workweek progresses.

If ongoing exposure to the dust responsible for the problem is completely eliminated or at least significantly decreased, the symptoms of grade II byssinosis can be reversed. However, if the relevant exposure continues, symptoms can and do progress to become grade III byssinosis. The hallmark of this stage is a clinical picture of chronic bronchitis. Grade III byssinosis usually continues to worsen to the point of clinical irreversibility. At this point, the patient has developed significant chronic airway obstruction.

An Occupational Safety and Health Administration (OSHA) standard specifically addresses dust exposure for workers. Since this OSHA dust standard requires the measurement of both forced expiratory volume (FEV_1) and forced vital capacity (FVC) in cotton dust–exposed workers, it is crucial for the clinician to understand the clinical correlations at play. On the first day of the work week, the bronchospasm (which is typically reversible at that stage) seen with byssinosis can be demonstrated by the use of spirometry performed prior to the start of the worker's shift. Spirometric parameters can then be measured again 5 to 6 hours later to determine if there has been any diminution in FEV. Despite the fact that most clinicians agree that the measurement of FEV_1 provides poor sensitivity, FEV_1 measurements are often used to demonstrate bronchial hyperreactivity to cotton dust. A 10% decline in FEV is generally considered to be sufficient evidence that a worker is significantly reactive to cotton dust. It is important to note that OSHA considers FEV_1 declines of as little as 5% to be clinically significant. In these cases, OSHA requires that such individuals be placed into a program of increased surveillance.[30]

Although byssinosis still represents a significant health problem in the cotton textile industry, it has been replaced in importance by chronic obstructive pulmonary disease (COPD) in cotton textile workers. Textile workers often smoke cigarettes, and some studies have shown that the adverse health effects of smoking and inhalation of cotton containing dust are additive. Perhaps one of the most pressing clinical questions in the industry today is whether smoking, cotton dust, or a combination is the cause of chronic obstructive pulmonary disease in cotton textile workers. The answer to this question is not easy because of its health and compensation implications. Recently, one study suggested that smokers may be susceptible to adverse effects following lower levels of cotton dust exposure than are nonsmokers.[31]

Perhaps the most important question for the clinician is what advice is most appropriate to give to cotton textile workers who have developed COPD. When COPD has been diagnosed in these workers, it is more than reasonable to strongly counsel them to stop smoking immediately. An organized smoking cessation program would be optimal. These workers have often been involved in the textile industry for many years. While simply changing jobs may represent the best possible solution and provide for elimination of exposure, such a change often may not be a viable option. It may be possible to transfer afflicted individuals to areas in the textile plant or mill that do not involve exposure to cotton dust. When total elimination of exposure to cotton dust is not achievable, use of one of the several different types of respirators currently in use in the textile industry should be considered.

Textile-related Occupational Asthma

On occasion, a textile worker with a recognized (or unrecognized) history of atopy reacts to cotton dust exposure on the job with acute or subacute asthma symptoms. This is thought to be due to pollens as well as other contaminants, which may be found in microscopic or macroscopic quantities in cotton dust. A complete allergy workup may or may not identify these antigens. The use of spirometry before and immediately following the work shift may be useful in determining the presence of a significant drop in FEV_1 during the time of exposure. The only obvious solution to this problem is total removal from exposure. Many, if not most, of these individuals leave the textile industry because of the severity of their symptoms and the clear-cut association with exposures at work. In addition, some of the commonly encountered dyes are of low molecular weight and can induce asthma in exposed workers (see the next section).

Other pulmonary conditions noted in workers in the cotton textile industry include "mill fever" and "weaver's cough." Both of these disorders may be due to inhalation of microorganisms found as contaminants of air conditioning systems in mills and processing plants.

Dyestuffs

The chemicals that are the most widely used in the textile industry are the dyes that impart color to yarn or cloth (Table 49-2). Several adverse health effects and potential

Table 49-2 Important classes of textile dyes and related compounds

Class of dye	Major use
Acid dyes	Wool, polyamides
Basic (cationic) dyes	Cotton
Direct dyes	Cotton, viscose
Disperse dyes	Synthetics
Reactive dyes	Cotton, wool
Mordant dyes	Wool
Sulfur dyes	Cotton
Vat dyes	Cotton, wool
Optical brighteners	All fibers
Dye carriers	Polyester, wool

adverse effects have been defined for this group of substances.

Two primary production processes are used today to dye fabrics and textiles. *Continuous* processes are used for large cotton materials and for carpets, as well as for fabrics that contain 100% synthetic fibers. *Noncontinuous* processes are generally used for all other materials.

In the dyeing process, the dye molecules penetrate the pores of the swollen fibers and are retained there by chemical or physical forces. Cotton is generally dyed after the yarn has been woven or knitted into fabric; wool yarn is usually dyed before these processes are undertaken.

The dyes developed for use with cotton can be divided into three main groups: (1) water-soluble dyes, (2) dyes soluble by alkaline reduction, and (3) dyes formed on the fiber. Water-soluble textile dyes are *direct* dyes that have an affinity for cellulose fibers. *Reactive* dyes react chemically with cellulose fibers. All water-soluble dyes in the textile industry are electrolytes. Dyes soluble by alkaline reduction include the "vat" and sulfur dyes. Dyes formed on the fiber include azo and oxidation dyes obtained from the oxidation of various amines.

Polyester fabric is usually dyed with "disperse" dyes. These compounds contain different chemicals called *chromophores* and use carrier compounds. The purpose of these carrier compounds is to improve the ability of the polyester material to accept the dyes. Some of these carrier compounds include biphenyl, chlorinated benzene, naphthalene, naphthalene derivatives and phthalimides.

Wool and polyamides are normally dyed with acid dyes, metal complex dyes, or chromium dyes.

Reactive dyes are known to cause a form of occupational asthma. The typical history is that an employee who mixes or applies these dyes develops wheezing or symptoms of asthma relatively quickly following exposure. At first, the symptoms appear to be mild. However, the symptoms get progressively worse. Fatal anaphylactic reactions can occur in workers who had previous wheezing upon exposure. Consequently, any initial reaction upon exposure must be treated cautiously, with careful clinical follow-up a must. The following low-molecular-weight dyes have been reported to be associated with the development of asthma or asthma symptoms in exposed workers: anthraquinone, paraphenyl diamine (used in the fur industry), hexafix brilliant yellow, drimaren brilliant blue, and cibachrome brilliant scarlet.

Today, many of the commonly used textile dyes are supplied as pastes rather than as powders. As a result, this form tends to diminish the potential for aerosolized exposure and subsequent sensitization.

The azo-type, benzidine, and benzidine derivative dyes have been widely used in the textile industry, and their potential toxicity and carcinogenic properties are of great concern.[14] The metabolism of these dyes has been studied extensively.[15-18] Significant detoxification and metabolic activation take place in vivo, with both oxidative and reductive pathways involved in these processes. The majority of these dyes undergo reduction catalyzed by enzymes of the intestinal microorganisms or hepatic enzymes, including microsomal and soluble enzymes. Many of the azo dye substances in common use today have highly charged substituents such as sulfonates. These tend to resist enzymatic attack and are generally poorly absorbed from the intestinal tract. In addition, they provide poor access to the liver, which is the major site of the mixed-function oxidase system. The lipophilic dyes, which are often carcinogenic, readily access oxidative enzymes and are activated by mixed-function oxidase systems. Biochemical reduction of the carcinogenic dyes usually leads to diminution or complete loss of carcinogenic activity. In contrast, most of the highly charged water-soluble dyes become mutagenic only after reduction. Even then, most of the fully reduced amines require oxidative metabolic activation. An outstanding example is the potent human bladder carcinogen benzidine, which derives from the reduction of several azo dyes. Many problems regarding mutagenic and carcinogenic activation remain to be solved. At the present time, it is apparent that both oxidative and reductive pathways yield toxic products.

Benzidine and benzidine derivatives. There are many specific dyes of concern in this category but of special note are direct brown 95, direct black 38, and direct blue 6. The latter two dyes have also been used in hair color dyes (see Chapter 19). Workers exposed to these dyes excrete high levels of benzidine into their urine as these compounds are actively metabolized to benzidine itself. Consequently, there exists a cancer risk for these workers. One of the most famous studies to address the issue of benzidine and related compounds' carcinogenic ability looked at Japanese kimono painters and dyers who habitually "pointed" their brushes by passing the brushes through their pursed lips, resulting in dye exposure and presumed ingestion. This population had more bladder cancer than what might be expected in an unexposed population. Consequently, these compounds should be handled with great caution in the workplace. They should be regarded as carcinogenic, and the numbers of workers exposed to them should be strictly limited within any given work site (see Chapter 56).

The dyestuffs used in the textile industry present other medical concerns. Recent reports indicate a statistically significant excess mortality attributable to pernicious anemia within the textile industry. Those individuals whose deaths were attributed to pernicious anemia within the industry were more than twice as likely to have worked in textile mills than anyone else.

Flame Retardants

Organic flame retardants, such as tetrakis (hydroxymethyl) phosphonium chloride and *N*-methylol dimethylphosphonyl propionamide, react with cellulosic fibers to form chemical

Industries in Which Formaldehyde Exposure Can Occur

Agricultural workers	Fur processors
Anatomists	Furniture makers
Beauticians	Glue and adhesive makers
Biologists	Hide preservers
Bookbinders	Histology technicians
Botanists	(including necropsy
Chemical production	and autopsy technicians)
workers	Hobbyists
Cosmetic formulators	Ink makers
Crease-resistant textile	Lacquerers and lacquer
finishers	makers
Disinfectant makers	Medical personnel
Disinfectors	(including pathologists)
Dress goods shop	Mirror manufacturers
personnel	Paper makers
Electrical insulation	Particle board makers
makers	Photographic film makers
Embalmers	Plastics workers
Embalming fluid makers	Plywood makers
Fireproofers	Rubber makers
Formaldehyde production	Taxidermists
workers	Textile mordanters and
Formaldehyde resin	printers
makers	Textile waterproofers
Foundry employees	Varnish workers
Fumigators	Wood preservers

From United States National Institute for Occupational Safety and Health.

bonds that are stable and maintain themselves through many launderings. The first compound of this type was introduced in the early 1950s and has given rise to a number of variants. One of the most widely used and most durable flame retardants, Pyrovatex CP, was patented in 1965.

In the 1970s, tris (2,3-dibromopropyl) phosphate was commonly used as a flame retardant for textiles, specifically for children's pajamas in the United States. Eventually, this chemical was discovered to have both carcinogenic and mutagenic properties. As a result, production of it was discontinued by the end of the 1970s.

Crease Resisters

Formaldehyde. Formaldehyde is a colorless gas with a very pungent and characteristic odor. It is readily soluble in water, ethyl alcohol, and diethyl ether. As a commercial product, it is most commonly formulated as a 30% to 50% solution in water to produce formalin. Formaldehyde is produced in great quantities in many countries. In 1992, approximately 12 million tonnes were produced worldwide. This chemical finds use in many different industries (see box above), including leather production, rubber and cement production, and foundry work. One of its most prolific uses is in the textile industry.[2]

Formaldehyde is generally used in the textile industry to attain a permanent press finish. Consequently, textile workers may become exposed to formaldehyde during the finishing of cloth. Less commonly, exposures can result during the sewing of cloth. Because of the exposure potential while large quantities of fabric are manufactured and treated with formaldehyde, time is alloted in the production process to allow for "off-gassing" to release formaldehyde from the material.[4] Alternatively, sometimes, the formaldehyde is physically washed from the fabric. In either case, the procedures involved with removal of formaldehyde from the fabric can pose a special threat of exposure to workers.

Formaldehyde is a well-known cause of ocular and airway irritation. In addition, it can cause certain skin reactions, including contact dermatitis via either allergic or irritant mechanisms. Patch testing with a 1% to 2% aqueous solution of formaldehyde can help to differentiate these two common forms of contact dermatitis. Occasionally, contact with formaldehyde results in urticaria, which is thought to occur by both allergic and nonallergic mechanisms, depending upon the clinical setting. The allergic type of dermatitis usually results in lesions in noncontact areas, and the nonallergic contact urticaria generally is limited to the area of skin that actually came into contact with the formaldehyde. Because the concentration of residual formaldehyde on the fabric surface is carefully controlled (generally limited to less than 300 ppm), contact dermatitis from just wearing finished fabrics is unusual.[5]

Upper respiratory and eye irritation can be expected when air concentrations of formaldehyde exceed 1 ppm.[6] Currently, the OSHA permissible exposure limit (PEL) is 0.75 ppm, and the majority of textile manufacturers maintain operating formaldehyde levels below 0.5 ppm. Workers who are exposed to formaldehyde are required by OSHA to complete a questionnaire designed to assess whether symptoms are present that may be due to formaldehyde exposure when levels exceed 0.5 ppm.[7] Certain individuals can develop specific respiratory sensitization to formaldehyde that result in rhinitis or an asthmalike picture. The symptoms of the former condition may be quite similar to allergic rhinitis. However, after relatively high exposures, a pure asthma picture may emerge, including the development of IgE and IgG antibodies. In most cases of formaldehyde-related asthma, the specific causal mechanisms are not clearly or completely understood. There are no simple diagnostic laboratory tests to help the clinician in the diagnosis of formaldehyde-induced asthma. Skin tests that use dilute formaldehyde solutions have not been standardized, and inhalation challenge tests with formaldehyde can be dangerous unless they are conducted under very carefully controlled conditions.[8] The best diagnostic option for the occupational clinician is a physical examination in conjunction with spirometry both prior to and immediately following the work shift. In this way, both clinical and spirometric differences can be compared before and after exposure.

Following studies that demonstrated the ability of formaldehyde to produce nasal cancer in small laboratory animals, formaldehyde has been identified as an animal carcinogen. It is unclear, however, if the carcinogenic effects are due primarily to specific cytotoxic effects or if genotoxic mechanisms are at play. Of course, it is possible that both types of effects may come together to produce neoplasia. Although epidemiologic studies have not shown a consistent association between the development of cancer in humans and formaldehyde exposure, the suspicion of an association remains strong based on animal data (see Chapters 23 and 56).

Synthetic Fibers

Polyester, acrylic, nylon, rayon, and polypropylene have long been considered essentially biologically inert. In fact, during early studies of byssinosis, workers exposed to synthetic fibers were used as controls for studies of cotton-exposed workers. Preshift and postshift spirometry showed no changes due to acute exposure to synthetic workers. Furthermore, the mean FEV of synthetic fibers workers was normal, yet that of cotton workers was lower. However, a recent longitudinal study showed a surprising and unexplained result: Workers in synthetic fiber mills had greater annual decline in FEV than workers in cotton mills. This result cannot be explained by our knowledge of synthetic fibers. Additional research will be necessary both to validate the results and to explain them if validated.

Viscose rayon. The chemical carbon disulfide (CS_2) is prominent in the production process of the synthetic fiber viscose rayon.[12] Specifically, CS_2 is used in the conversion process of cellulose to rayon fiber and cellophane. In addition, CS_2 has also been used in the vulcanization of rubber, the extraction of fats, and the manufacture of sulfur matches.[13,16]

During the early years of rubber manufacturing as well as the early days of rayon production, extremely high levels of CS_2 resulted in severe CNS disorders including acute mania and narcosis. Since the inception of stricter regulatory controls, however, ambient levels of CS_2 have diminished, and, at present, acute exposures are rare.[21] However, these changes have allowed the emergence of chronic exposure to low levels of CS_2 and the consequent clinical effects.

The most common clinical effect of chronic CS_2 exposure is a distal sensorimotor neuropathy. It attacks the long axons in the CNS and the peripheral nervous system preferentially. A clinically apparent encephalopathy discernible via neuropsychiatric testing and associated with cerebral atrophy has also been observed following chronic exposure to low CS_2 levels in textile workers.[22-26]

Exposure to CS_2 has been clearly shown to accelerate the rate of atherogenesis and is associated with increased levels of low-density lipoproteins and hypertension. Consequently, it is unclear if the encephalopathic effects of CS_2 are due to the effect of accelerated atherogenesis or to the direct CNS toxicity of this chemical. Chronic low-level exposure to CS_2 has also been reported to be associated with testicular atrophy, impotence, and a variety of poorly understood visual disorders.

The metabolism of CS_2 is noteworthy in that it may be excreted or exhaled unchanged or actually undergo complex metabolic alteration.[27] This metabolic alteration predominantly results in the production of dithiocarbamate and trithiocarbonate compounds.[28,29] This is significant in that the isolation of 2-thiothiazolidine-4-carboxylic acid (TTCA) in the urine of workers exposed to CS_2 has led to the use of it as a means to assay exposure to CS_2 in the workplace since TTCA remains in the urine for several days after exposure.

Organic Solvents

Methyl *n*-butyl ketone toxicity. A fabric printing plant in Ohio was the setting where human exposures revealed the neurotoxicity of methyl *n*-butyl ketone. Sensorimotor neuropathies developed in workers exposed to the solvent during the months that followed the substitution of methyl *n*-butyl ketone for methyl isobutyl ketone in a solvent mixture. The neurotoxicity of methyl *n*-butyl ketone, as well as its potentiation by methylethylketone (MEK), were confirmed in experimental animals. We now appreciate that methyl *n*-butyl ketone and *n*-hexane are metabolized to the same toxic metabolite, 2,5-hexanedione.

SUGGESTED READINGS

1. Claude J et al: Life-style and occupational risk factors in cancer of the lower urinary tract, *Am J Epidemiol* 124:578, 1986.
2. Malker HSR et al: Occupational risks for bladder cancer among men in Sweden, *Cancer Res* 47:6763, 1987.
3. Schoenberg JB et al: Case-control study of bladder cancer in New Jersey. I. Occupational exposures in white males, *J Nat Cancer Inst* 72:973, 1984.
4. Siemiatycki J et al: Associations between several sites of cancer and nine organic dusts: results from an hypothesis-generating case-control study in Montreal, 1979-1983, *Am J Epidemiol* 123:235, 1986.

REFERENCES

1. Beckett WS et al: Women's respiratory health in the cotton textile industry: an analysis of respiratory symptoms in 973 non-smoking female workers, *Occup Environ Med* 51:14, 1994.
2. Cassitto MG et al: Carbon disulfide and the central nervous system: a 15-year neurobehavioral surveillance of an exposed population, *Environ Res* 63:252, 1993.
3. Christiani DC et al: Pulmonary function among cotton textile workers. A study of variability in symptoms reporting, across-shift drop in FEV1, and longitudinal change, *Chest* 105:1713, 1994.
4. Chu CC et al: Polyneuropathy induced by carbon disulphide in viscose rayon workers, *Occup Environ Med* 52:404, 1995.
5. Dement JM, Brown DP: Lung cancer mortality among asbestos textile workers: a review and update, *Ann Occup Hyg* 38:525, 1994.
6. Drexler H et al: Carbon disulphide. I. External and internal exposure to carbon disulphide of workers in the viscose industry, *Int Arch Occup Environ Health* 65:359, 1994.
7. Drexler H, Goen T, Angerer J: Carbon disulphide. II. Investigations on the uptake of CS2, *Int Arch Occup Environ Health* 67:5, 1995.

8. Egeland GM et al: Effects of exposure to carbon disulphide on low density lipoprotein cholesterol concentration and diastolic blood pressure, *Br J Ind Med* 49:287, 1992.

9. Fishwick D, et al: Respiratory symptoms and dust exposure in Lancashire cotton and man-made fiber mill operatives, *Am J Respir Crit Care Med* 150:441, 1994.

10. Gibbs GW: The assessment of exposure in terms of fibres, *Ann Occup Hyg* 38:477, 1994.

11. Glindmeyer HW et al: Exposure-related declines in the lung function of cotton textile workers. Relationship to current workplace standards, *Am Rev Respir Dis* 144:675, 1991.

12. Gold EB, Sever LE: Childhood cancers associated with parental occupational exposures, *Occup Med* 9:495, 1994.

13. Graham DG et al: Pathogenetic studies of hexane and carbon disulfide neurotoxicity, *Crit Rev Toxicol* 25:91, 1995.

14. Howard K: Dyestuffs and bladder cancer, *N Z Med J* 106:391, 1993 (letter).

15. Kremer AM et al: Airway hyper-responsiveness and the prevalence of work-related symptoms in workers exposed to irritants, *Am J Ind Med* 26:655, 1994.

16. Krstev S, Perunicic B, Farkic B: The effects of long-term occupational exposure to carbon disulphide on serum lipids, *Eur J Drug Metab Pharmacokinet* 17:237, 1992.

17. Levine WG: Metabolism of azo dyes: implication for detoxification and activation, *Drug Metab Rev* 23:253, 1991.

18. Morgan DL et al: Summary of the National Toxicology Program benzidine dye initiative, *Environ Health Perspect* 102(Suppl 2):63, 1994.

19. Moya C, Anto JM, Taylor AJ: Outbreak of organising pneumonia in textile printing sprayers (Collaborative Group for the Study of Toxicity in Textile Aerographic Factories), *Lancet* 344:498, 1994.

20. Nilsson R et al: Asthma, rhinitis, and dermatitis in workers exposed to reactive dyes, *Br J Ind Med* 50:65, 1993.

21. Phillips M: Detection of carbon disulfide in breath and air: a possible new risk factor for coronary artery disease, *Int Arch Occup Environ Health* 64:119, 1992.

22. Riihimaki V et al: Assessment of exposure to carbon disulfide in viscose production workers from urinary 2-thiothiazolidine-4-carboxylic acid determinations, *Am J Ind Med* 22:85, 1992.

23. Roman E et al: Pernicious anaemia in the textile industry, *Br J Ind Med* 48:348, 1991.

24. Sailstad DM et al: Evaluation of an azo and two anthraquinone dyes for allergic potential, *Fundam Appl Toxicol* 23:569, 1994.

25. Sanz P, Prat A: Toxicity in textile air-brushing in Spain, *Lancet* 342:240, 1993 (letter).

26. Swaen GM, Braun C, Slangen JJ: Mortality of Dutch workers exposed to carbon disulfide, *Int Arch Occup Environ Health* 66:103, 1994.

27. Vanhoorne M, De Bacquer D, De Backer G: Epidemiological study of the cardiovascular effects of carbon disulphide, *Int J Epidemiol* 21:745, 1992.

28. Vanhoorne M, de Rouck A, de Bacquer D: Epidemiological study of eye irritation by hydrogen sulphide and/or carbon disulphide exposure in viscose rayon workers, *Ann Occup Hyg* 39:307, 1995.

29. Vanhoorne M, Vermeulen A, De Bacquer D: Epidemiological study of endocrinological effects of carbon disulfide, *Arch Environ Health* 48:370, 1993.

30. White NW, Cheadle H, Dyer RB: Workmens' compensation and byssinosis in South Africa: a review of 32 cases, *Am J Ind Med* 21:295, 1992.

31. Zuskin E et al: A ten-year follow-up study of cotton textile workers, *Am Rev Respir Dis* 143:301, 1991.

50

OH

n-nitrosodiethanolamine

- Exposure to machining fluids occurs via two main routes: 1) inhalation and 2) dermal contact

- Prevention for irritant contact dermatitis includes engineering controls and product substitution, as well as barrier glove use and after-work application of emollient creams

- There appears to be an association between bladder cancer and employment in the tool and dye industry

Tool and Die and Machinists

Dennis B. Phillips

OCCUPATIONAL DESCRIPTION

The tool and die industry consists of a broad variety of jobs and related job tasks. There were 359,000 machinists and tool programmers in 1992 according to the Bureau of Labor Statistics. As the name suggests, there are two major operational categories. The operations may be performed separately, or in conjunction with one another. For example, if plans call for the production of a large number of a particular hand tool, a die (or set of dies) may be created specifically to allow casting and production of that particular tool. Simply stated, a die is a mold that is used to create a cast. A tool usually implies a hand-type of tool, with a wide range of complexity.[12] For both dies and tools, there are three major jobs of concern. One job is creation of a new tool or part "from scratch." Another major job is a modification procedure to an existing die or tool. Repair of damaged existing tools or dies is the third major job (see the first box on p. 404).

Knowledge of the general processes and process flows within operations enables an individual to understand the range of tasks, skills needed to perform those tasks, potential hazards, and potential toxic exposures within the tool and die trade. The second box on p. 404 reviews the major jobs associated with the generation of new tools or dies. Figure 50-1 and the third box on p. 404 represent overall process flows for the generation of new metal dies and new tools. Also presented is the general process for hot-forging (Fig. 50-2) and the types of metal machining operations for the forming and working of metal (see the box on p. 405).[9,45]

General Operations for Die Workers and Toolmakers

A. Die operations
  • Generation of new dies
  • Modification of existing dies
  • Repair of damaged existing dies
B. Tool operations
  • Generation of new tools
  • Modification of existing tools
  • Repair of damaged existing tools
  • Engraving of tools

General Process Flow for Creation of a New Metal Die

A. Metal production fabrication (forming and working)
  • Foundry operations
  • Forging
  • Metal machining
  • Welding
  • Heat treating
  • Nondestructive testing
B. Metal preparation
  • Abrasive blasting
  • Metal degreasing
  • Acid and/or alkali cleaning of metals
  • Grinding, polishing, and buffing
C. Metal finishing
  • Electroplating
  • Metal thermal spraying
  • Painting
D. Assembly

General Product Generation Jobs Performed By Tool and Die Workers for Metals, Plastics, and Rubber Products

  • Fabrication
  • Preparation
  • Finishing
  • Assembly

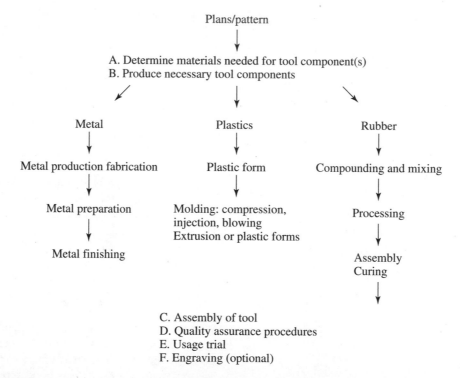

Fig. 50-1 Summary flow chart for general operations for production of a new hand tool.

Training programs (apprenticeships or technical schools) impart skills necessary to perform all the general operations within the tool and die industry. The "generalist" tool and die worker (a "journeyman" once program completion and certification are achieved) may continue using all these skills for a company or may "specialize" in one (or more) of the operations. Companies produce different products and have different requirements for the tool and die employee. Both special operations and general tool and die operations can be performed within a particular company. Tool and die

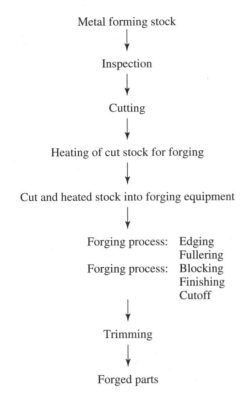

Metal forming stock

↓

Inspection

↓

Cutting

↓

Heating of cut stock for forging

↓

Cut and heated stock into forging equipment

↓

Forging process: Edging
Fullering

Forging process: Blocking
Finishing
Cutoff

↓

Trimming

↓

Forged parts

Fig. 50-2 General process flow associated with hot-forging operations.

Metal Machining Operations

Cutting
- Blanking
- Piercing or punching
- Edge improvement

Sawing
- Reciprocating units
- Circular units
- Continuous units

Abrasive grinding
- Rough grinding
- Precision grinding

Drilling and boring
- Counterboring
- Spot facing
- Countersinking
- Reaming

Milling
- Seven different types

Lathing, Planing, Shaping, Slotting
- Turning machines—lathes
- Planers
- Shapers and slotters
- Broaching

Honing

Lapping

Mass Finishing

Super Finishing

department functions may differ, even among companies producing similar products.

The tradeworker within the tool and die industry may be called upon to work with both natural and man-made materials and substances. Production, repair, and modification of tools and dies (in various subassembly parts) consisting of metals, plastics, and rubber are ubiquitous for these workers.

POTENTIAL TOXIC EXPOSURES

Workers within the tool and die industry have the potential to be exposed to numerous hazards and toxins from the various operations and jobs performed. Characterizing exposures (agents, intensity, duration, and frequency) is difficult for a variety of reasons, and generalizations concerning toxicology of the industry as a whole are therefore arduous.

In order to appreciate the vast amount of potential toxic exposures, this section is divided into metal and nonmetal work. The various operations and jobs are presented with their potential toxic exposures (see the box on pp. 406-408).[9,26,45,47] Some potential toxic exposures overlap operations or jobs, and brief reviews of some of them are given in the following sections. The threshold limit values (TLV)–time-weighted average (TWA) levels given are for the United States.

Common Potential Toxic Exposures: Metals

Chromium is a hard metal. It is naturally occurring and a required trace metal for humans. The absorption of chromium is dependent on the valence and solubility of the particular chromium species. The valence also is an important determinant for toxicity (including carcinogenesis). The principal route of water-soluble chromium Cr(IV) elimination is in the urine. Workers with chronic exposures may maintain elevated urine concentrations for many years. Chromates may cause allergies (and manifestations of such), ulcers of the skin and nasal septa, and perforation of the nasal septa. There have been reported human nasal and lung cancers. The TLV-TWA for water-soluble Cr(IV) compounds is 0.05 mg/m^3.[2,21,46]

Nickel is a hard, silver-colored metal. It is insoluble in water. Nickel alloys have been noted to cause pulmonary effects (asthma, fibrosis, and pulmonary edema) in welders using the alloy. Nickel and its inorganic compounds are not absorbed through unbroken skin to cause any systemic toxicity but are known to cause contact dermatitis in sensitized individuals (general population nickel sensitization prevalence is 2.5% to 5%). Nickel exposure has not been clearly associated with human respiratory cancer in any of the industries using nickel. The TLV-TWA is 1 mg/m^3 for the metal and insoluble compounds and 0.1 mg/m^3 for the soluble compounds as nickel.[2,46]

Common Potential Toxic Exposures: Chemicals

Acids and bases belong to substances known as corrosives or caustics. Acids and bases are either organic (contain carbon atoms) or inorganic. Their classification may be according to their charge or according to the number of dissociated H$^+$ or OH$^-$ ions per molecule of the parent compound. Acids and bases may exist in their pure form, as salts, or as anhydrides. Acids and bases are highly

Common Potential Toxic Exposures: Operations and Jobs

I. Metal operations
   A. Metal production fabrication (forming and working)
      Products of combustion
      - Carbon monoxide
      - Aldehydes
      - Nitrogen oxides
      - Sulfa oxides
      - Larger hydrogen molecules (including polynuclear aromatics)
      Nuisance dusts
      Metal fumes and dusts
      Die lubricants
      - Various chemical composition categories to consider
      Oil decomposition products
      - Oil mist
      - Carbonaceous particulates
      - Vapors
      Acids and alkalis
      - Inorganic and acid liquids: sulfuric, hydrochloric, nitric, hydrofluoric, nitric-hydrofluoric, phosphoric, sulfuric nitric
      - Airborne gases, mists, vapors for acid baths: nitrogen oxide, nitric, sulfuric, hydrogen fluoride, nitrogen oxide, sodium cyanide, hydrochloric, hydrogen chlorate
      - Alkaline cleansers: borax, potassium hydroxide, ortho silicate, sodium carbonate, sodium hydroxide, sodium meta
      Machining fluids
      - Mineral oils: >80% mineral oil, <20% additives
      - Emulsified oils: 3%-10% mineral oil, emulsifiers, additives
      - Synthetic machining fluids: chemically active ingredients in aqueous solutions
      Additives
      - Methylchloroisothiazolinane/methylisothiazolinane (Kathon) (biocide)
      - Alkanolamine borates (corrosion inhibitors)
      Contaminants
      - n-Nitrosodiethanolamine (a chemical product of nitrite)
      Radiation
      - Nonionizing (infrared and ultraviolet)
      - Ionizing
   B. Metal preparation
      Abrasive blasting
      - Silica
      Acid cleaning of metals
      Alkaline cleaning of metals (see acid and alkaline above)
      Metal degreasing
      - Cold degreasing: petroleum hydrocarbon (prior to 1960)
      - Chlorofluorocarbon halogenated solvents (from 1950s to now)
      - Hydrochlorofluorocarbon (beginning late 1980s)
      - Vapor-phase degreasing:
         Chlorofluorocarbon
         Hydrocarbonfluorocarbon
      Grinding, polishing, and buffing
      - Dusts: workpiece or abrasive
   C. Metal finishing
      Electroplating
      - Air contaminants from bath:
         Acid: chromium, copper, nickel, tin
         Alkaline-cyanide salt based: cadmium, copper, brass, bronze, silver, zinc
      - Air contaminants from mist, gases, vapors:
         cyanide salt
         cadmium salt
      - Air contaminants from fumes: lead
      - Ingestion of particulates
      - Dermal exposure:
         Cyanide   1° Irritants
         Solvents   Sensitizers
      Metal thermal spraying
      - Metal fumes
      - Gases
      - Nonionizing radiation
      Painting
      - Solvents: liquids and vapors
      - Paint pigments

II. Nonmetal operations
   A. Foundry molding and coremaking
      Silica sands*
      Olivine sand†
      Zircon sand†
      Chromite sand†
      Acetaldehyde
      Acrolein
      Ammonia
      Aniline
      Benzene
      Carbon monoxide
      Carbon dioxide
      Formaldehyde
      Hydrogen cyanide
      Hydrogen sulfide
      Meta-xylene
      Napthalene
      Phenols
      Bentonite suspension
      Graphite
      Metal stearates
      Mica
      Mineral oil
      Molybdenum disulfide
      Oleic acid
      Polyethylene
      Polyvinyl alcohol
      Silica flow

*Commonly used in U.S. operations.
†European community substituting for silica sands.

Common Potential Toxic Exposures: Operations and Jobs—cont'd

Silicones
Soya lecithin
Stearic acid
Sulfur dioxide
Talc
Toluene

B. Plastic manufacturing and products

1. Common plastic polymers

Polymer	Thermal degradation products of polymer
Fluoro polymers	Carbonyl fluoride
	Hydrogen fluoride
	Perfluoroisobutylene
Phenolic	Ammonia
	Cyanide
	Formaldehyde
	Nitrogen dioxide
Polyethylene	Carbon monoxide
Polystyrene	Styrene
	Benzene
Polyurethane	Aldehydes
	Ammonia
	Cyanide
	Isocyanates
	Nitrogen dioxide
Polyvinyl chloride	Dioxins
	Furans
	Hydrochloric acid
	Phosgene
	Vinyl chloride

2. Additives (14 general classes, approximately 2500 chemicals)
   - Antioxidants
   - Antistatic agents
   - Blowing agents
   - Colorants
   - Curing agents
   - Fillers and reinforcements
   - Flame retardants
   - Heat stabilizers
   - Initiators
   - Lubricants and flow control agents
   - Optical brighteners
   - Plasticizers
   - Solvents
   - Ultraviolet light absorbers

C. Rubber manufacturing

1. Dusts
   - Raw materials handling:
     Natural or synthetic rubber (16 major types)
     Additives
     Antioxidants
     Retarders
     Antidegradents
     Processing oils
     Reinforcing agents
     Fillers

2. Potential process toxic exposures
   - Raw materials handling: dusts
   - Milling:
     Vapors
     Hot rubber aerosols
     Additives and compounding agent dusts
     Talc or soapstone dusts
   - Extruding and calendaring:
     Volatilization of rubber and additive/compounding agent
     Volatile organic compounds
     Solvents (heptane, hexane, isopropenol, methanol, naphtha, and toluene)
     (See milling)
   - Component assembly:
     Solvents (heptane, hexanes, isopropenol, methanol, naphtha, and toluene)
     Uncured tire components
   - Vulcanizing:
     Solvent-based lubricants (hexane, neotene, isopropenol, naphtha, toluene)
     Curing fumes
   - Finishing:
     Rubber dust
     Solvent vapors

3. Potential compounding toxic exposures
   - Vulcanizing agents:
     Aromatic nitrogen compounds
     Benzole peroxide
     Dicumyl peroxide
     Diisocyanates
     Dioximes
     Dinitrio compounds
     Dithiocarbomates
     Dithio phosphates
     Merpholine
     Phenols
     Sulfur
     Tetraethylthiuran disulfide
     Tetramethylthiuran sulfide
   - Accelerators (major groups):
     Carbamates
     Mercapto group
     Naphthyl group
     PPD group
     Thiurams
     Miscellaneous
   - Activators:
     Zinc oxide is the most common
     Others are lead oxide, magnesium oxide, sodium carbamate
     Solubilizing agents—stearic acid, lauric acid

Continued.

Common Potential Toxic Exposures: Operations and Jobs—cont'd

- Retarders:
    - Organic acids
    - Anhydrides
    - Phthalimides
- Antidegradants and antioxidants:
    - Amines
    - Phenols
    - Thioesters
- Processing aids:
    - Aromatic processing oils with PAH
    - Mercaptan derivatives
    - Thiophenols
    - Mercaptobezothazole
- Reinforcing agents:
    - Carbon black
    - Amorphous silica
- Miscellaneous agents:
    - Ammonium phosphate
    - Antimony oxide
    - Brominated aromatics
    - Chlorinated paraffins
    - Clay fillers
    - Fluorinated hydrocarbons
    - Magnesium hydroxide
    - Mica
    - Organic solvents
        - Acetones
        - 1,1,1-Trichloroethene
        - Methyl ethyl ketone
        - Methylene chloride
        - Trichloroethyl
    - Polyethylene glycols
    - Silicon
    - Talc

---

reactive compounds. Industrial exposures are usually accidental and most commonly involve skin and eye contact, followed by inhalation and then ingestion. Local dermal effects by acids produce coagulation necrosis with eschar formation. The local dermal effect of bases is due to liquefaction necrosis. Systemic effects are limited to those absorbable agents (anions of arsenic, cyanide, fluoride, heavy metals, plus ammonia and hydrazine) and are agent-specific. Threshold limit values are available for specific substances.[21,46]

Organic solvents are volatile compounds that can be divided into aromatic and aliphatic classes. Solvent hazards and toxic effects are related to the vapor pressure and intrinsic solvent chemical properties. A vapor-hazard ratio is used to help determine the potential of human exposure. The main target organs for toxicity are the skin, central and peripheral nervous systems, liver, and kidneys. Dermal and mucous membrane irritant effects are also common. Chronic exposure has been associated with central nervous system (CNS) effects. The TLVs are available for the specific solvent.[2,46]

Formaldehyde may be a gas, powder, or liquid. Exposure may occur by ingestion, inhalation, or absorption. It is a normal metabolite of the body. Formaldehyde is normally converted and excreted as carbon dioxide in the air (via pulmonary excretion) and formic acid in the urine. Acute dermal effects range from mildly irritant to corrosive (dependent upon solution concentration), or sensitization may occur. Acute upper and lower respiratory irritant effects may occur. If sensitization has taken place, allergen rechallenge may result in dermal, upper respiratory, or lower respiratory effects. There has been no preponderance of evidence that formaldehyde causes cancer in humans. The TWA is 1 ppm.[6,33,35]

Cyanide may be a gas, liquid, or inorganic salt solid. The major occupational exposures occur from inhalation and dermal contact. There is rapid mucous membrane and inhalation absorption. Cyanide impairs oxidative phosphorylation and thereby causes energy deprivation. There are still issues, however, concerning whether cyanide toxicity is mainly caused by cellular inhibition of cytochrome oxidase and the resultant intracellular hypoxia or because of other biochemical processes. Humans detoxify cyanide by converting cyanide to thiocyanate. A two-stage antidote strategy involves the enhancement of cyanide to thiocyanate conversion by use of exogenous sodium thiosulfate and then induction of methemoglobinemia.[22,46,49] Treatment, though, depends on the availability of the antidotes available among different countries due to statutory and regulatory differences.[3]

Common Potential Toxic Exposures: Gases

Carbon monoxide is a tasteless, colorless, odorless gas whose optimal exposure setting occurs wherever fuel is burned and there is insufficient ventilation. There is a normal physiologic amount of carboxyhemoglobin present in individuals. The carboxyhemoglobin level in tobacco smokers is higher than that in nonsmokers. Carbon monoxide is rapidly absorbed by the lungs and attaches to hemoglobin. Carbon monoxide has a 250 times greater affinity for hemoglobin than oxygen. Carbon monoxide decreases the number of available hemoglobin binding sites and shifts the oxyhemoglobin dissociation curve to the left. It inhibits cytochrome oxidase. Carboxyhemoglobin levels provide evidence of exposure but do not correlate with severity of intoxication. The acute and the chronic effects can mimic virtually any neurologic or psychiatric illness. Heart tissues (and thus effects) are also very susceptible to carbon monoxide exposure. Treatment involves the removal from the external carbon monoxide source, high-dose supplemental oxygenation, and possibly hyperbaric oxygen.[46,48]

Common Potential Toxic Exposures: Physical

Infrared radiation (IR) is emitted by all matter. Three arbitrary subareas (near, middle, and far) can be used to divide the spectrum. Wavelengths below 1400 nm can affect the lens of the eye and cause cataract formation. However, sufficient duration, intensity, and frequency of the correct IR is required for cataract formation.[46,51]

Ultraviolet (UV) radiation has limited penetration into human tissue. The UV radiation in welding operations emits photons with sufficient energy to produce ozone and oxides of nitrogen from the dissociation of oxygen and nitrogen molecules. Ozone is irritating to the respiratory system. At wavelengths shorter than 0.3 μm, UV overexposure can cause photokeratitis. The UV dermal effects may range from no changes to erythema, increased pigmentation, darkening of pigment, and changes in cellular growth.[46,51]

CLINICAL TOXICOLOGY

The broad range of potential toxins for tool and die industry workers was shown in the previous section. Although many of these toxins are worthy of in-depth clinical toxicology discussion, only three are discussed in detail here.

1. Tool and die workers commonly encounter machining fluids, and a clinical toxicology review of machining fluids is given in this section.
2. Contrary to common assumptions, tool and die trade workers may be responsible for the generation of molds (and cores) from nonmetals, and they sometimes make and repair silica-sand-based molds (and cores). Silica and silicosis are therefore discussed here.
3. Many industries (and workers) are concerned about carcinogenesis in the workplace and the industry. In this regard, a review of cancer in the tool and die industry is presented.

Machining Fluids

Machining fluids are specifically designed fluids applied at the interface between a cutting tool and the stock metal piece. Machining fluids have six basic functions: (1) cooling the interface, (2) lubricating the interface, (3) flushing away metal chips from the interface, (4) extending tool life, (5) improving the surface finish, and (6) improving the dimensional stability of the part during machining.[9,40]

There are three major forms of machining fluids: mineral oil, emulsified oil, and synthetics. Each major form has groups of additives blended with the major form.[40]

Mineral oil forms have a mineral oil paraffinic or naphtheric base of 60% to 100% composition. For mineral oils less than 100% mineral oil composition, other additives, such as polar additives (animal and vegetable oils, fats, waxes along with esters, fatty oils and acids, poly or complex alcohols), extreme pressure lubricants (sulfur-free sulfurized fat, chlorine, sulfur chlorinated mineral oil or fatty oil, phosphorus), and germicides,[36] are blended.

Emulsified oil forms contain a 50% to 90% mineral oil base with water dilution. Additives include emulsifiers (petroleum sulfurates, amine soaps, rosin soaps, naphthnic acids), polar additives (sperm oil, lard oil, esters), extreme pressure lubricants, corrosion inhibitors (polar organics), germicides, and dyes.[36]

The synthetic oil forms have various water bases ranging from 50% to 80% of the concentrate. A true synthetic contains no oil, whereas semisynthetics may contain mineral oil amounts from 5% to 25% of the concentrate. The additives include corrosion inhibitors (inorganics such as borates, nitrites, nitrates, and phosphates or organics such as amines and nitrites), surfactants, lubricants (esters), dyes, and germicides.[36] Studies have specifically identified alkanolamine borates (corrosion inhibitors), methylchloroisothiazolinone/methylisothiazolinone (a biocide), and n-nitrosodiethanolamine (a byproduct of nitrite additives) as specific products that cause dermal toxicity. The former two are common causes for contact dermatitis.[7,48] The latter is a potent animal carcinogen.[24]

The mineral oil–based machining fluids have been used for many decades, with peak use in the 1960s. Since the 1960s, emulsified and synthetic machining fluid use has risen greatly.[9,40]

Exposure to machining fluids occurs via two main routes: inhalation and dermal contact or absorption (Figs. 50-3 and 50-4). Data concerning the concentration of machining fluid aerosols show a reduction in air concentration of machining fluid aerosols over the past decades from various U.S. and Swedish studies.[9]

Some of these same studies evaluated air concentrates of polycyclic aromatic hydrocarbons (PAHs) in bulk oil and oil mist, plus the oil mist itself for changes, sensitizing potential, irritancy, and skin carcinogenicity over a 5-year period. These studies were negative for PAH buildup (bulk and oil mist fraction) and the oil properties (sensitivity potential, irritancy, skin carcinogenicity).[9]

Another study phase noted aerosol size for machining fluids was greater with spraying and splashing of machine fluids than fine aerosols generated by shear forces and high temperatures at the cutting point.[9]

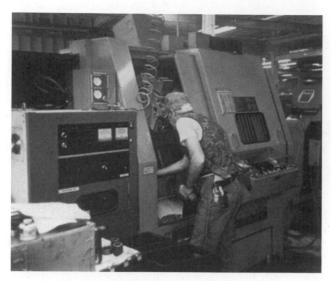

Fig. 50-3 A semiautomatic lathe with complete enclosure to protect the worker from cutting and cooling fluids. (From Zenz C, Dickerson OB, Horvath EP: *Occupational medicine,* ed 3, St Louis, 1994, Mosby.)

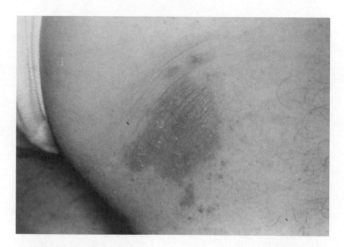

Fig. 50-4 Irritant contact dermatitis on the thigh of a machinist. The lesion developed from inadvertently placing a rag still moist with solvent in the pocket of work trousers. (From Zenz C, Dickerson OB, Horvath EP: *Occupational medicine,* ed 3, St Louis, 1994, Mosby.)

Dermal effects of machining fluids are dermatitis (primarily irritant) and folliculitis.[13]

Irritant contact dermatitis (ICD) is a nonallergic reaction of the skin caused by dermal exposure to an irritating substance or substances. If a substance has a sufficient degree of concentration and dermal contact duration, then any substance may act as an irritant. Although ICD accounts for approximately 80% of occupational contact dermatitis, ICD is also the most frequent nonoccupational contact reaction.[8,13]

There are two basic types of irritants. The first type is classified as "mild" (marginal) and is characterized by requiring repeated or prolonged dermal contact to produce inflammation. The category includes most solvents, soaps, and detergents. The second type is the "strong" irritant, characterized by its ability to injure the skin immediately upon dermal contact. Strong irritants are acids or alkalis.[4] Symptoms of ICD include "stiff"-feeling (inelastic) skin, discomfort related to dryness, pruritus secondary to inflammation, and pain if fissures, blisters, or ulcers are present.[4] For the mild irritants, ICD signs reveal erythema, microvesiculation, and oozing acutely but dryness, thickening, and fissuring with chronic exposure. For the strong irritant, ICD signs include blisters, erosions, and ulcers.[4]

Detailed inquiry concerning contactants in all environments (name of the substance, work, hobbies, and so on) must be conducted, along with a job site and workstation analysis.

Preventive measures for ICD include primary industrial hygiene controls of engineering out the exposure, or substitution of another product may be undertaken. Personal protective equipment (tertiary control) includes barrier glove (with dermal glove liner) use and consideration of after-work-application of emollient creams. After-work emollient cream reduces the prevalence of cutting fluid dermatitis, although small studies do not demonstrate a statistically significant difference. Barrier creams do not appear to be effective.[18,19]

Allergic contact dermatitis (ACD) is a manifestation of delayed hypersensitivity (type IV). It results from the exposure of sensitized individuals to contact allergens.[4,13] The mechanism includes the binding of a chemical group(s) to an epidermal protein to form a complete antigen. This complete antigen then reacts with sensitized T-lymphocytes. A release of mediators from the T-lymphocytes attracts inflammatory cells that are involved in the eczematous response.[13]

The incubation period after initial sensitization to an antigen ranges between 5 and 21 days. The reactive time after reexposure to that same specific antigen is 12 to 48 hours.

Additional factors contribute to the development of ACD: genetic predisposition, local antigen, concentration, exposure duration, cutaneous permeability, and immune tolerance. Also in consideration are the presence of other dermal diseases, heat, cold, occlusion, pressure, and friction.[4,13] Machining fluids may have common sensitizing allergens present such as formaldehyde, formaldehyde-containing release agents, rosins, and leachates of chromium, nickel, and cobalt.[8,9,13,40,41]

The primary ACD symptom is pruritus. The signs for mild ACD are similar to those for ICD but usually include grouped or linear vesicles or blisters. More severe ACD may reveal edema, involvement of other body areas secondary to hand transfers, and less severe ACD signs involving scalp, palms, and soles. Allergic contact dermatitis also is noted to have a gradual eruption appearance over a period of several days. In general, any dermal eruption with an unusual appearance should suggest ICD or ACD.[4,20]

During the assessment, the same inquiry and investigations given for ICD must occur for ACD. Patch testing for contact allergens in ACD is essential for specific identification of causative agents.[4]

Preventive measures for ACD include a thorough dermal wash as soon as possible after antigen exposure.[4]

Treatment for contact dermatitis (CD) can be divided into acute and chronic active dermatitis regimens. For an acute, mild to moderate, exudative or vesicular CD, therapy includes cold compresses 4 to 6 times a day with aluminum acetate or aluminum chloride. Soothing shake lotions can be applied, along with oral antihistamines. After the vesicles have subsided, topical corticosteroid cream, lotion, or aerosol can be applied.[4]

For an acute irritant reaction, forceful and prolonged water irrigation is indicated. Postirrigation treatment is performed as per burn protocols.[4]

Acute, severe edema and bullae call for topical corticosteroid treatment, plus tepid tub baths with cornstarch or colloidal oatmeal bath 2 or 3 times per day and early and aggressive system corticosteroids over 2 to 3 weeks (unless a secondary dermal skin reaction is present, or another contraindication to systemic steroid use exists).[4]

For chronic CD, a 5-minute soak to the affected area with immediate hydrophobic emollient (e.g., petrolatum) application is suggested. A dermatologist should be consulted for use of iodochlorhydroxyquin preparations, ultraviolet phototherapy, or photochemotherapy.[4]

Folliculitis secondary to mineral oil dermal exposures has been reported. Most types of folliculitis not involving the face are superficial and do not represent a serious problem. The face is a common site for deep folliculitis. Treatment of a superficial folliculitis is aggressive topical hygiene and use of topical local antibiotics. Treatment of facial folliculitis is dependent upon location, duration, and recurrence.[4,8,9,36]

Respiratory effects of machining fluids can be divided into three major categories: cancers, upper tract noncancerous disorders, and lower tract noncancerous disorders.[8]

Respiratory tract cancer has been evaluated in workers with exposures to machining fluids with inconsistent and inconclusive results. Upper respiratory tract disorders have not been conclusively demonstrated. Lower tract fibrosis and pneumonia are not consistently demonstrated. A risk of occupationally related asthmas and bronchitis has been suggested, but studies conducted on this topic have not been conclusive.[8,9]

SILICA
Pathobiology

Silica (SiO_2) is the most abundant mineral on earth. It exists in crystalline and amorphous forms. Of the crystalline forms, quartz is the most common and stable. Other crystalline silica forms are tridymite and cristobalite.[1] Amorphous silica is noncrystalline. It occurs as diatomite or vitreous silica.[5]

The crystalline silica materials produce the chronic pulmonary condition termed *silicosis,* a type of pneumoco-

niosis. The term *pneumoconiosis* refers to lung diseases resulting from the inhalation of dust (usually inorganic in nature). The tridymite and cristobalite forms appear to have greater fibrogenic potency than the quartz form.[31]

The gross pathology of silicosis notes that the silicotic lung is firm and blacker than normal. The lung surface is nodular and coarse, with fibrotic areas of the visceral pleura. Cutting the lung reveals palpable intrapulmonary nodules, especially in the upper lobes. Nodule diameter size depends on the type of silicosis (2 to 6 mm for simple silicosis, 10 to 20 mm for conglomerate or progressive massive).[5]

The type of microscopic pathology found depends on the stage and type of silicosis. Prenodule, silicotic nodule, and progressive massive fibrotic lesions are the major divisions noted. The nodule has a central zone hyalinized with concentrically arranged collagen fibers, with the peripheral zones whirled or less organized. Birefringent crystals (silicates) may be noted centrally more than peripherally. Nodule coalescence forms the progressive massive fibrotic basis. These centers may then cavitate.[44]

There is a histologic pattern difference between acute and chronic silicosis. Acute silicosis rarely has nodules but may have silicoproteinosis (alveolar filling with proteinaceous material)[5] (see Chapter 32).

Biochemistry and Pathogenesis

Inhalation of crystalline silica particles with favorable alveolar space deposition characteristics (particle diameter between 0.5 μm and 3 μm) produces an interaction between the silica particle and the alveolar macrophage. A recurrent cycle of macrophage phagocytosis of the silica particle, cell death, release of intracellular enzymes, and reuptake of the silica particle by another macrophage perpetuates the inflammatory process. There is gradual accumulation of cells and production of collagen. Hyalinization then occurs.[32]

The fibrogenic effect of the silica may be due to the elaboration of several inflammatory mediators by alveolar macrophages.[31] However, since pulmonary fibrosis is not a large feature of acute silicosis, acute silicosis pathogenesis may differ from that of classic or chronic silicosis (acute silicosis has been noted to have the alveoli filled with an amorphous lipoproteinaceous exudate).[5]

Diagnosis and Classification

The diagnosis of silicosis usually depends on historical and roentgenographic evidence. A history of significant exposure to free silica is required.[32]

Silicosis may be classified into one of three major groups: classic silicosis, accelerated silicosis, and acute silicosis. A basic understanding of each type is necessary; however, there are similarities in the clinical diagnosis in all of them. There are three requisites of a clinical silicosis diagnosis[5]: The first requisite is physician exposure assessment that has shown adequate exposure data to cause silicosis. The second requisite is the presence of chest radiographic abnormalities consistent with silicosis. The third is the absence of illnesses that mimic silicosis.[32]

If one or more requisites are missing or inadequate or the case is atypical, other diagnostic tests and procedures may be used for investigation (open lung biopsy, bronchoalveolar lavage, and scanning electron microscopy with analytic techniques).[5]

Classic silicosis is the most frequent presentation. The exposure duration is usually 20 or more years, with exposure intensity classified as low to moderate. The chest radiograph allows classification of extent of classic silicosis.[5] Severe classic silicosis without progressive massive fibrosis may cause respiratory impairment (with accompanying dyspnea on exertion), but most cases are without pulmonary symptoms as impairment.[32] Progressive massive fibrosis (PMF) can cause respiratory impairment (and pulmonary symptoms). It causes restriction in the lung volumes, decreased pulmonary compliance, and decreased gas transfer. As the pathology progresses, the symptoms worsen (dyspnea on exertion to dyspnea at rest). The risk of spontaneous thorax also increases as PMF progresses, or pulmonale may develop. The risk of infection with mycobacterial agents is a concern with silicosis.[4]

Accelerated silicosis gives a greater exposure intensity history, with a shorter exposure duration than classic silicosis (5 to 10 years). Accelerated silicosis notes the progression of the disease, and other findings or syndromes are also present (positive serum antinuclear antibodies, scleroderma, systemic lupus erythematosus, and rheumatoid arthritis).[4]

Acute silicosis is the most devastating form of the disease. The exposure profile is one of excessive free crystalline silica concentrations for less than a few years. The clinical course includes dyspnea, pulmonale development, and pulmonary achexia. Lung studies (function tests and diffusing capacity) also follow a progressively worsening course. This type is frequently fatal.[4]

The chest radiograph does not correlate well with the exposure duration. The International Labor Office International Classification of Radiographs of the Pneumocosis is used to classify each chest radiograph by a specially trained chest radiograph reader (B-reader). High-resolution computed tomography scans of the chest can be helpful for classification and diagnosis in any of the silicosis types.[4,44]

Classic silicosis chest radiographic appearance includes rounded opacities of 1 to 10 mm diameter in the upper lung zones. With advanced silicosis stages, the middle and lower lung areas may become involved also. Roentgenographic progression of simple disease, or from simple to complicated, can usually be expected within 5 years.[32]

Chest radiographs of PMF note greater than 10 mm diameter upper lung zone coalesced lesions that cause subpleural air space enlargements due to retraction, loss of upper lung volumes, hilar elevation, and large emphasematous changes.[5,15,32]

Calcification of pulmonary nodules is rare. Lymph nodes may calcify and produce an eggshell appearance. Enlargement of lymph nodes is common and may occur before pulmonary nodulation.[32]

Silicosis must be differentiated from disorders producing similar roentgenographic appearances, including sarcoidosis, cancer, diffuse carcinomatosis, infectious granulomas, mycobacterium infections, and other pneumonocoses.[32,44]

Despite the complex pathophysiology of silicosis, in simple silicosis the clinical tests of ventilatory function are often normal. Series of symptomatic silicosis include restrictive, obstructive, and mixed ventilatory impairment. Complicated silicotic cases show reduced diffusing capacities and exercise-induced hypoxia. Lung compliance is usually reduced. Terminal silicotic cases have severe restrictive impairments. Severe hypoxema dominates the last phase of the disease. The diffusing capacity tests note declination of diffusion as the pulmonary involvement increases.[32]

Management and Treatment

Surveillance for associated complications is required. Because of the association between silicosis and pulmonary tuberculosis, yearly tubercular tests (intermediate purified derivative tests) are important. Evaluation for mycobacterial infection (purified protein derivative, chest radiograph, acid-fast smears, cultures) should occur with worsening respiratory symptoms and worsening chest radiograph. Treatment based on diagnosis and current accepted protocols should occur.[5,15,32] Atypical mycobacterial infections may also occur, and treatment of such per currently accepted protocols should be undertaken.[15,32]

Immune-mediated complications (previously mentioned) should be investigated when signs or symptoms of such occur. Rheumatologic consultation is advised for diagnosis and treatment.

A number of silica nephropathies have also been reported in known silicotic individuals. Renal specialists should be consulted for diagnostic confirmation and treatment and surveillance protocols.[5]

Some studies have suggested an increase in pulmonary neoplasms in silicotics; however, causality has not been established from the studies to date.[5,44]

There is no effective therapy for silicosis. Current treatment is palliative toward the symptoms of the associated organ-system conditions.[5,15,32,44] Consultation with the appropriate specialist (e.g., cardiology, pulmonary) is advised.

Silicosis prevention (primary preferred) is the best approach to dealing with silicosis. The current TLV-TWA is 0.1 mg/m^3 respirable dust.[2]

TOOL AND DIE INDUSTRY CANCER REVIEW

A discussion of potential toxic exposures would not be complete without information regarding cancer. Tool and die workers have been investigated regarding cancer, and a brief review of the results is presented in this section.

The American Cancer Society has recently (January 1995) revised their cancer facts and figures for the United States. This document presented individual state cancer facts and specific cancer type data. The American Cancer Society listed occupational sources as risk factors (or possible risk factors) for the following cancers: lung, lymphoma, skin, and bladder.[11] The three most common target organs of known occupational carcinogens are, first, skin, then lung, and, third, bladder.[23]

In the 1960s, a survey of cancer in relation to occupation was performed by the National Institute of Occupational Safety and Health (NIOSH) to identify possible relationships between occupations and cancer. The study contained job titles, and the tool and die industry was represented by the job titles *toolmakers, diemakers,* and *setters.* In this survey, these jobs had some noted relationships with multiple myeloma and cancer of the testis.[14]

Since that NIOSH report, other studies have been performed to obtain information concerning cancer and the tool and die industry. The previously reported increase in multiple myeloma and testicular cancer relative risks have not been borne out, but associations between multiple myeloma and benzene[38] and between testicular abnormalities and dibromochloropropane were noted.[50]

The tool and die industry has been noted to have an association with risk of bladder cancer, but the potential etiologic agent is unknown.[42]

Other studies have not specifically used the job classifications of diemakers, toolworkers, or toolmakers. Through broader classification terms (such as "metal workers" or "metal fabrication"), the tool and die worker may be included in such studies; however, job operations, tasks, and exposures may differ. The "metal worker" job literature notes an inconsistency for the occurrence of colon and colorectal cancers. The "metal fabricating" job classification literature gave little evidence to suggest the potential contribution for the development of gallbladder cancer.[34]

Another approach to evaluate cancer potential for the tool and die industry workers is to evaluate the substances the workers are potentially exposed to in the workplace and to note any association between the substance and types of cancer. A tool and die worker may be exposed to the documented respiratory carcinogens beryllium, chromium, and nickel. However, the processes associated with the development of reported respiratory cancers and the associated exposure intensity, duration, and frequency for these metals are not the reported processes or metal exposures seen within the tool and die industry.[16]

Of particular concern is the potent experimental carcinogen, n-nitrosodiethanolamine.[27] This nitrosamine was a common contaminant of metal working lubricants up until the late 1970s at levels as high as 2% by weight. This led to a flurry of research to identify the extent of human exposure.[27] Patterns of carcinogeneity in machinists have not been identified. Although n-nitrodiethalamine concentrations have been reduced dramatically, they have not been eliminated, and surveillance should be continued.[24]

Long-term exposure to cutting oils may lead to skin cancers, particularly scrotal cancers.[30] The cutting oils containing more polycyclic aromatic hydrocarbons (PAHs) (poorly refined oils) show a form of dose-response relationship regarding PAHs and carcinogenicity.[39] There are conflicting studies for other cancers (bronchus, larynx, stomach, nonscrotal skin, and lip) with cutting oils exposure.[37,43]

Solvents are found in the tool and die industry (metal degreasing operations, painting operations, plastic and rubber operations). The halogenated hydrocarbons common in these operations have been shown to be carcinogenic in animal systems. However, human carcinogenicity studies are not convincing. There are some spot reported increased specific cancers in select worker groups, but no definite conclusions can be drawn.[17,43]

Carcinogenesis related to chronic inorganic acids and bases revealed some association between lung cancer and chromium compounds.[25] However, these workers were involved in producing chromium pigments, a process not noted to be performed by tool and die workers.

In summary, there appears at this time to be an association with risk of bladder cancer for workers within the tool and die industry. The etiologic agent of such a risk is currently not known. There is potential for the development of other cancer types. However, other cancer types currently are not supported by the literature as cancer specific for the industry as a whole.

REFERENCES

1. Amdur MO, Doull, J editors: *Casarett and Doull's toxicology,* ed 3, New York, 1986, Macmillan.
2. American Conference of Governmental Industrial Hygienists: *Documentation of the threshold limit values and biological exposure indices,* ed 6, Cincinnati, 1991, ACGIH.
3. *Antidotes for poisoning by cyanide,* New York, 1993, Cambridge University Press.
4. Arndt KA: *Manual of dermatologic therapeutics,* ed 3, Boston, 1983, Little, Brown.
5. Balaan ME, Banks DE: Silicosis. In Rom WM, editor: *Environmental and occupational medicine,* ed 2, Boston, 1992, Little, Brown.
6. Bordana EJ, Montanaro A: The formaldehyde fiasco: a review of the scientific data, *Immunol Allergy Prac* 9:11, 1987.
7. Bruze et al: Occupational allergic contact dermatitis from alkanolamine boratesin metal working fluids, *Cont Derm* 32:24-27, 1995.
8. Burge PS: *Proceedings of a conference on the health effects of cutting oils and their control,* University of Birmingham, England, April 1989.
9. Burgess WA: *Recognition of health hazards in industry, a review of materials and processes,* ed 2, New York, 1995, John Wiley.
10. Burns PB, Swanson GM: Stomach cancer risk among black and white men and women: the role of occupation and cigarette smoking, *J Occup Environ Med* 37:10, 1995.
11. *Cancer facts & figures,* 1995, American Cancer Society.
12. Cralley LJ, Cralley LV, editors: *Industrial hygiene aspects of plant operations,* vol 2, *Unit operators and product fabrication,* New York, 1984, Macmillan.

13. Davidson CL: Occupational contact dermatitis of the upper extremity, *Occup Med* 9:59, 1994.

14. Deoufie P: *A retrospective survey of cancer in relation to occupation,* Cincinatti, National Institute of Occupational Safety and Health, Department of Health, Education, and Welfare, 1991.

15. Duffell GM: Pulmonotoxicity: toxic effects in the lung. In Williams PL, Bivser JL, editors: *Industrial toxicology,* New York, 1985, Van Nostrand Reinhold.

16. Frank AL: Occupational cancers of the respiratory tract, *Occup Med* 2:71, 1987.

17. Gerr F, Letz R: Solvents. In Rom WN, editor: *Environmental and occupational medicine,* ed 2, Boston, 1992, Little, Brown.

18. Goh CL, Gan SL: Efficacies of a barrier cream and an after work emollient cream against cutting fluid dermatitis in metal workers: a prospective study, *Cont Derm* 31:176-180, 1994.

19. Goh CL, Gan SL: The incidence of cutting fluid dermatitis in a metal fabrication factory: a prospective study, *Cont Derm* 31:111-115, 1994.

20. Goldner R: Work-related irritant contact dermatitis, *Occup Med* 9:37, 1994.

21. Goyer RA: Toxic effect of metals. In Klaassen CD, Amdur MO, Doull J, editors: *Casarett and Doull's toxicology,* ed 3, New York, 1986, Macmillan.

22. Hall AH, Rumack B: Clinical toxicology of cyanide, *Am J Emerg Med* 15:1067, 1986.

23. Hueper WC: *Occupational and environmental cancers of the urinary system,* New Haven, Conn, 1969, Yale University Press.

24. Keefer LK: Persistance of n-nitrosodiethanolamine contamination in American metal-working lubricants, *Fd Chem Toxic* 28(7):531-534, 1990.

25. Langard S, Virgander T: Occurrence of lung cancer in workers producing chromium pigments, *Br J Ind Med* 40:71, 1983.

26. Lewis R, Sullivan JB: *Toxic hazards of plastic manufacturing.* In Sullivan JS, Krieger GR, editors: *Hazards materials toxicology,* Baltimore, 1992, Williams & Wilkins.

27. Liginsky W, Reuber MD, Martinez WB: Potent carcinogenicity of nitrosodiethanolamine in rats, *Nature Land* 288:589-590, 1980.

28. Loeppky RN, Hansen TJ, Keefer LK: Reducing nitrosamine contamination in cutting fluids, *Fd Chem Toxic* 21:607-613, 1987.

29. Madden SO, Thiboutout DM, Marks JG: Occupationally induced allergic contact dermatitis to methylchloroisothiazolinone/methylisothiazolinone among machinists, *J Am Acad Dermatol* 30:272-274, 1994.

30. Maikener CR: Health effects of oil mists: a brief review, *Toxicol Ind Health* 5:429, 1989.

31. Menzel DS, Amdur MO: Toxic responses of the respiratory system. In Klaassen CD, Amdur MO, Doull J, editors: *Casarett and Doull's toxicology,* ed 3, New York, 1986, Macmillan.

32. Morton Z, Jones RN, Weill H: Silicosis, *Am Rev Respir Dis* 113:643, 1976.

33. National Research Council: *Formaldehyde and other aldehydes,* Washington, DC, 1981, National Academy Press.

34. Neugut AI, Wylie P: Occupational cancers of the gastrointestinal tract, *Occup Med* 2:137, 1987.
35. Niemela R, Vainio H: Formaldehyde exposure in work and the general environment: occurrence and possibilities for prevention, *Scand J Work Environ Health* 7:95, 1981.
36. O'Brien DO, Frede JC: *Guidelines for the control of exposure to metal working fluids,* NIOSH Pub 78-165, Cincinnati, 1978, Department of Health, Education, and Welfare.
37. Park R, Krebs J, Mier F: Mortality at an automotive stamping and assembly complex, *Am J Ind Med* 26:449, 1994.
38. Rinsky RA, et al: Benzene and leukemia: an epidemiologic risk assessment, *N Engl J Med* 316:1044, 1987.
39. Roy TA et al: Correlation of mutagenic and dermal carcinogen activities of mineral oils with polycyclic aromatic compound contents, *Fundam Appl Toxicol* 10:466, 1988.
40. Ruane PJ: *Proceedings of a conference on the health effects of cutting oils and their control,* University of Birmingham, England, April 1989.
41. Rycroft RJG: *Proceedings of a conference on the health effects of cutting oils and their control,* University of Birmingham, England, April 1989.
42. Schulte PA et al: Occupational cancers of the urinary tract, *Occup Med* 2:85, 1987.
43. Schwarz-Miller J, Rom WN, Brandt-Rauf PW: Polycyclic aromatic hydrocarbons. In Rom WM, editor: *Environmental and occupational medicine,* ed 2, Boston, 1992, Little, Brown.
44. Silicosis and Silicate Disease Committee: Diseases associated with exposure to silica and nonfibrous silicate minerals, *Arch Pathol Lab Med* 112:673, 1988.
45. Soule RD: Metal machining. In Cralley LJ, Cralley LV, editors: *Industrial hygiene aspects of plant operations,* vol 2, *Unit operations and product fabrication,* New York, 1984, Macmillan.
46. Sullivan JS, Krieger GR, editors: *Hazards material toxicology,* Baltimore, 1992, Williams & Wilkins.
47. Sullivan JB, VanErt M, Lewis R: Chemical hazards in the tire and rubber manufacturing industry. In Sullivan JS, Krieger GR, editors: *Hazards materials toxicology,* Baltimore, 1992, Williams & Wilkins.
48. Thom S, Keim L: Carbon monoxide poisoning: a review of epidemiology, pathophysiology, clinical findings and treatment options including hyperbaric oxygen therapy, *Clin Toxicol* 12:281, 1985.
49. Vogel SN, Sultar TR, Ten Eyck RP: Cyanide poisoning, *Clin Toxicol* 18:367, 1981.
50. Whorton MS: Health effects of dibromochloropropane. In Rom WN, editor: *Environmental and occupational medicine,* ed 2, Boston, 1992, Little, Brown.
51. Wilkening GM: Nonionizing radiation. In Clayton GD, Clayton FE, editors: *Patty's industrial hygiene and toxicology,* ed 4, New York, 1991, John Wiley.

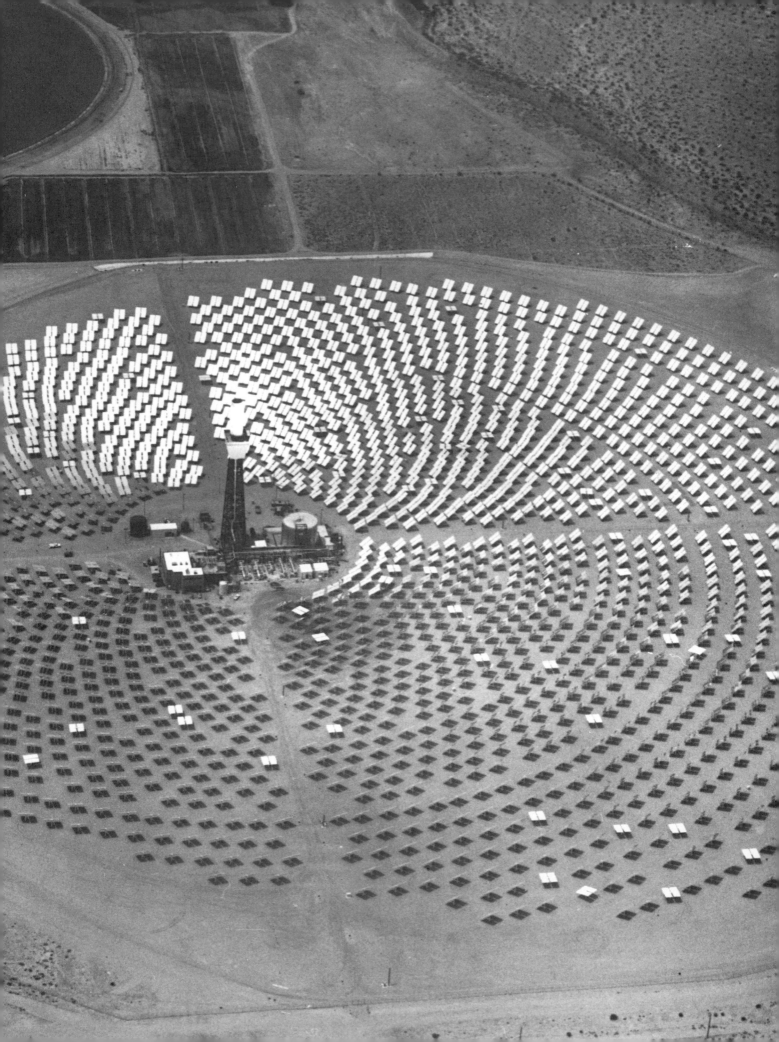

Environmental Toxicology

Section Editor

Scott D. Phillips

*Solar One, the world's largest solar power pilot plant at
10,000 kilowatts, nears completion in the Mojave Desert.
The facility consists of a 300-foot "power tower"
surrounded by about 1800 heliostats or giant movable
mirrors that reflect the sun on the tower to produce steam.
The project is located on 75 acres. August 27, 1982.*

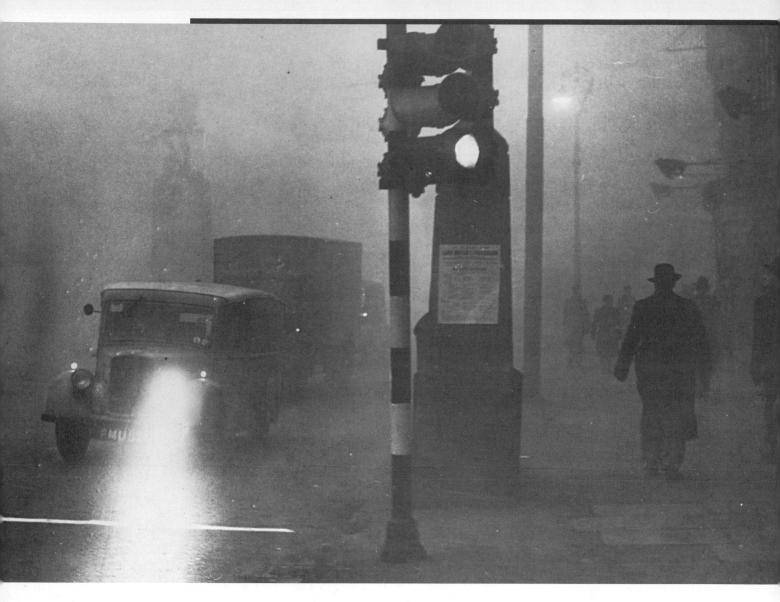

Traffic moves slowly with lights aglow as smog descends
over the British capital during daytime hours.
Policeman helps children find their way across the street
on their way to school. Government agencies probe
methods of reducing smog problem. December 6, 1953.
(Courtesy UPI/Corbis-Bettmann)

51

O=O—O •
ozone

air pollution

- Ozone, sulfur dioxide, oxides of nitrogen and particulates may aggravate reactive airways disease

- Combustion of fossil fuels is largely responsible for oxide generation

Outdoor Air Pollution and Issues of Quality

Scott D. Phillips

Jeffrey Brent

Since air pollution is a complex mixture of toxic chemicals and particles, rarely can exposure to only one type of pollutant occur. Each of us is affected by this exposure regardless of occupation. However, occupations resulting in greater time in heavily traveled areas have the greatest exposures. Large segments of the population are exposed to the criteria pollutants. Thus, traffic police, tunnel workers, and urban construction workers receive greater doses of outdoor air pollution than those working in indoor environments. As this is a ubiquitous exposure, primary care providers are likely to be asked questions regarding the health effects of air pollution. This chapter reviews the adverse effects of outdoor air pollution on human health.

ENVIRONMENTAL DESCRIPTION

In areas where thermal inversions and air currents occur in conjunction with heavy local traffic, such as Denver, Phoenix, and Salt Lake City, concentrations of air pollutants may reach levels that could, potentially, cause adverse health conditions. Thermal inversions are temperature changes that, when associated with certain air patterns, result in air—and air pollution—being trapped over an area. Typically, these areas have significant production of pollutants. There have been many instances of excess deaths throughout the world because of thermal inversions that trapped toxic pollutants.

419

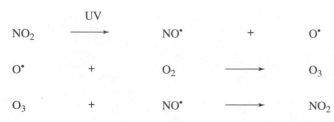

Fig. 51-1 Generation cycle of ozone photochemically by the action of ultraviolet radiation on nitrogen dioxide.

As a result of these episodes and appropriate concern about the adverse effects of air pollution, clean air legislation has been enacted.

As we will see in this chapter, there are several types of air pollutants, each involving mixtures of chemicals and particulates. For example, *smog* now refers to a type of photochemical pollution. Originally coined to refer to a mixture of fog and smoke, such as that characterizing London in the preregulatory era, the term *smog* has evolved. In a more common and more contemporary sense, *smog* refers to the results of sunlight acting on atmospheric gases (oxides of nitrogen, hydrocarbons, sulfur dioxide, and carbon monoxide) typically derived from automobile exhaust. This type of air pollution is more prevalent in areas of greater industrialization or traffic, particularly those prone to air inversions. Ozone (O_3) is a major product of photochemical smog, generated by the reaction shown in Figure 51-1. The generation of O_3 is self-propagating.

Separating the components of air pollution is not a valid method in examining overall health effects. Though each may have specific effects on the respiratory tract, they act in concert. For example, gases attach to particulates that, if of respirable size, may be delivered deep into the lung.

The extent of delivery of toxicants into the respiratory tract is a function of size and solubility. Large particulates are filtered out in the upper airway; smaller ones penetrate deeper. It is generally thought that water-soluble substances are removed from the airstream in the upper airway, thereby causing more proximal effects. Conversely, lipid-soluble chemicals tend to travel more distally. Thus, sulfur dioxide that has high water solubility causes upper airway irritation. Less soluble gases such as ozone and nitrogen dioxide penetrate to deeper levels of the airways. This "rule" applies when the subject is resting. Exceptions include mouth breathing, which tends to deliver more volume than nasal breathing, and increased minute ventilation. Working under conditions of high exertion with increased minute ventilation overcomes the solubility issues and delivers a greater proportion of the dose of soluble material distally. This phenomenon has been best studied in firefighters.[46,49]

LEGISLATION

Given the concern about decreasing outdoor air quality in the 1950s, Congress passed the first federal clean air act in 1955,

Table 51-1 National ambient air quality standards

Pollutant	Primary standards to prevent adverse health effects	Type of average
Ozone	0.12 ppm (235 µg/m³)	Maximum daily 1-hr average*
PM_{10}	50 µg/m³	Annual arith mean†
	150 µg/m³	24 hr†
Sulfur dioxide	0.03 ppm (80 µg/m³)	Annual arith mean 24 hr‡
Nitrogen dioxide	0.053 ppm (100 µg/m³)	Annual arith mean
Carbon monoxide	9 ppm (10 mg/m³)	8 hr‡
	35 ppm (40 mg/m³)	1 hr‡

*The O_3 standard is attained when the expected number of days per calendar year with a maximum hourly average concentration >0.12 ppm is ≤1 (averaged over the previous 3 years).
†Particulate standards use PM_{10} (particles ≤10 µm in diameter) as the indicator pollutant. The annual standard is attained when the expected annual arithmetic mean concentration is ≤50 µg/m³; the 24-hr standard is attained when the expected number of days per calendar year >150 µg/m³ is ≤1.
‡Maximum quarterly average.

known as the Air Pollution Control Act. In 1965 the Motor Vehicle Air Pollution Control Act was passed, thereby establishing national standards for the control of motor vehicle emission. The Clean Air Act (CAA) was originally enacted in 1963 and has been amended several times. The U.S. Environmental Protection Agency (EPA) is the primary federal agency charged with the responsibility for enforcing the mandates of the act. However, there is also input from state and local authorities regarding the control of air pollution and thus a multifaceted regulatory framework. The most recent amendment to the CAA provides new goals for attaining required air standards. It is primarily the responsibility of the individual states to achieve the mandated emission reductions. Should the states not be able to meet these goals, the EPA will assume the task of meeting the mandated objectives.

One of the more important aspects of the CAA is the mandate to establish standards for airborne pollution, the national ambient air quality standards (NAAQS) (Table 51-1). The NAAQS were developed to define the allowable airborne concentration of substances called *criteria pollutants* (see box on p. 421) that may exist but would be anticipated to have no adverse health effects. In addition to the primary standards of criteria pollutants, there are secondary standards, which were enacted to provide a measure of protection to plants and animals within the environment. In the United States, areas are given one of three designations related to the standard: attainment, nonattainment, or unclassifiable within the standards. The CAA requires areas in the attainment of the standard to prevent significant deterioration (PSD). These mandates are known as the *PSD requirements*.

EPA Criteria Pollutants	
Carbon monoxide	Ozone
Lead	Particulates
Nitrogen dioxide	Sulfur dioxide

Obviously, the primary concern within the NAAQS are for areas of the country classified as in nonattainment of the standards.

In an area of nonattainment, standards are utilized for local municipalities to come into compliance with the CAA. For areas of nonattainment, further inquiry is undertaken to determine the degree of air pollution control that will be required. This is, in part, determined by the population statistics and the U.S. Census Bureau in that area. The severity of nonattainment is then determined, and remediation goals are varied, depending on the pollutant. For example, oxides of sulfur, nitrogen, and lead require control strategies in order to reach required standards. Carbon monoxide and particulate matter (PM) have two levels of classification. One of the more complicated criteria pollutants is ozone, which has a classification structure reflecting five levels of severity. The 1990 amendments to the CAA extend its scope to address issues of acid rain and atmospheric ozone depletion.

ENVIRONMENTAL TOXICOLOGY OF AMBIENT AIR POLLUTION

Recent research by Dockery and colleagues[3] has evaluated the effects of air pollution on mortality, while controlling for other individual risks. This Harvard Six Cities Study was a 14-year mortality follow-up of 8111 adults in six U.S. cities. The study controlled for individual risks including demographics, smoking, educational level, age, average body mass index, job exposure to dust or fumes, and environmental factors other than ambient air pollution. Total inhalable particulates, fine particles, sulfate particles, aerosol acidity, sulfur dioxide, nitrogen dioxide, and ozone effects on health were evaluated. The six cities were Watertown, Massachusetts; Harriman, Tennessee, including Kingston; St. Louis, Missouri; Steubenville, Ohio; Portage, Wisconsin, including Wyocena and Pardeeville; and Topeka, Kansas. Data on ambient air pollution concentration were obtained from monitors in these cities. The results of this study suggest that, of the factors considered, mortality rates were most strongly associated with cigarette smoking. However, after adjusting for smoking and other risk factors, a statistically significant, although weak, association between air pollution and mortality was documented. Adjusted mortality rate ratio for the most polluted of the cities compared to the least polluted was 1.26 (95% CI, 1.08 to 1.47). Air pollution was positively associated with death from lung cancer and cardiopulmonary disease, but not with death from aggregate other causes.

This increased mortality was most strongly associated with air pollution with fine particulates containing sulfates. Total particulates were not associated with mortality.

A major concern regarding ambient air pollution is the possibility of exacerbating preexisting asthma. Inducers of asthma are agents that increase airway inflammation or cause bronchospasm. Certain nonspecific spasmogens such as histamine and methacholine are capable of causing constriction of airway smooth muscle directly. Additional nonspecific spasmogens include exercise, hyperventilation, laughing (which results in cooling and drying of the airway mucosa), fog, metabisulfite, sulfur dioxide (SO_2), and bradykinin. Air pollutants may affect the airways of asthmatic subjects in a variety of ways. Pollutants may act as inciters or triggers when the airways are hyperresponsive, resulting in transient airway narrowing. They may act as an inducer to increase airway inflammation and therefore airway hyperresponsiveness, which may persist beyond the exposure time. Pollutants may also have a direct toxic effect on the airways and lead to asthmalike symptoms in normal individuals. They may affect the immune system and result in sensitization or increased allergic responses in the airway.

Respiratory symptoms related to air pollution are difficult to interpret because of socioeconomic factors, coexistent aeroallergens, cigarette smoking, industrial contributions, and the difficulty in diagnosing the asthma, for example, by questionnaire. In Switzerland, there was no relationship between levels of air pollutants and respiratory symptoms in children except for an association with total suspended particles. In the United States, no evidence suggests the prevalence of asthma is higher in Los Angeles than any other areas of the country, despite the extent of air pollution in that city. This is also noted in polluted versus nonpolluted areas of Sydney, Australia. An interesting comparison has been done following the reunification of Germany, comparing two populations of exposure to very different air pollutants. Eastern Germany, with industrialized towns such as Mipzig and Erfurt, has high concentrations of SO_2 in particulates, whereas the western cities such as Munich and Hamburg have low levels of SO_2 and particulates but higher levels of nitrogen oxides (NO_x). The prevalence of asthma and allergic diseases are reported to be higher in Munich than in Mipzig but the prevalence of bronchitis was higher in Mipzig.[52] Differences are reported, based on questionnaires, in the frequent asthma attacks of Hamburg residents compared to less frequent attacks of Erfurt residents. There was also higher prevalence of indoor allergens in Duesenberg, West Germany, than in Leuna, East Germany. This suggests indoor exposure to allergens may be more important in determining asthma than exposure to outdoor air pollution such as SO_2 or particulates.

OZONE

Ozone, the major active product of photochemical smog, has effects almost totally restricted to the respiratory system, where it is a potent oxidant and irritant. This effect of ozone is tempered by its vanishingly short atmospheric persistence.

Paradoxically, at a time when stratospheric ozone depletion is a major environmental concern, low-altitude ambient ozone levels are rising. Because ozone derives principally from photochemical smog, its formation is dependent on ambient levels of nitrogen oxides, volatile organic compounds, and sunlight. Because motor vehicles are the major source of nitrogen oxides, ozone levels tend to be high in regions of high use. Automobile ozone-generating photochemical reactions are promoted by sunlight and high temperatures. Thus ambient ozone levels tend to be highest in the summer.

Ozone has low water solubility; therefore, it tends to exert most of its pulmonary effects on the lower respiratory tract. Several studies have addressed the relationship of ozone concentration in the ambient atmosphere with hospital visits for asthma or other respiratory problems. These have had variable findings,[31] while others have not.[23] A study of emergency asthma visits by children at an inner city hospital in Atlanta between June and August of 1990 found that they were significantly higher on days when the 1-hour maximum ozone level exceeded 0.11 ppm. No relationship was found when the level of ozone was less than 0.11 ppm or with the mean 8 hours daily maximum of ozone. Asthmatics and patients with chronic obstructive pulmonary disease do not appear to be more sensitive to ozone than the general population, with progressive fall in airflow and increases in airway resistance in all populations as ozone levels rise.[24] Tachyphylaxis to these effects occurs with repeated exposures.[13]

The role of pulmonary inflammation in ozone-induced respiratory illness appears to be due to the ability of ozone to cause the release of inflammatory mediators from the epithelial cells lining the respiratory tract and macrophages.[18,39,48] In addition to its local effects, ozone has been shown to modulate the immune response[19] in a manner that depends on the time course and the dose. This includes impaired function of natural killer lymphocytes.[6] The effects of ozone on mucociliary clearance are imprecisely understood. Animal models tend to show decreased particle clearance induced by ozone. Humans appear to show the opposite response, with enhanced particle clearance with exposure to moderate levels of ozone.[16] Although ozone clearly has detrimental effects on pulmonary function, studies correlating its ambient concentrations with respiratory effects must be interpreted cautiously. As an end product of photochemical smog (see box), ozone's presence may be a measure of other chemical entities generated in these reactions.

The present NAAQS for ozone is 0.12 ppm (as a 1-hour maximum concentration), which is paradoxically higher than the American Council of Governmental Industrial Hygienists (ACGIH) 8-hour threshold limit value (TLV) time-weighted average (TWA) or the permissible exposure limit (PEL) (both 0.1 ppm). A large proportion of the United States has not attained these NAAQS. Atmospheric ozone levels tend to be highest in the late morning or afternoon. Despite the frequency of nonattainment of the standards, analysis of dose-response data indicates that the present NAAQS are too high. Ozone-induced respiratory symptoms occur at, or below, the current 0.12 ppm standard.[27,37,47,51] Animal[38] and human[11] studies suggest that chronic exposure to ozone may cause permanent decline in pulmonary function.

It has been recently suggested that ozone can cause a sustained elevation of intracytoplasmic calcium.[36] This effect is completely blocked by verapamil and is due both to release from intracellular storage and to influx from the extracellular fluid. Studies are underway to establish the nature of the secretagogue that may be causing the influx of calcium and the relationship between intracellular calcium accumulation and asthma.

SULFUR DIOXIDE

Sulfur dioxide not only has direct toxic effects but also contributes to acid rain and the formation of "sulfates." The latter are acidic particles that may result in adverse respiratory effects. These particles are known as *acid aerosols*. Sulfur dioxide is a natural contaminant of fossil fuels and hence is emitted through their combustion, usually from point sources such as power plants and industrial settings. These emissions increased until the introduction of the CAA in 1970 and declined thereafter. Anthropogenic activities are responsible for approximately half of the SO_2 produced. The remainder derives from the natural decay of organic matter.

Once in the atmosphere, SO_2 is oxidized to sulfuric acid (H_2SO_3) and sulfuric acids. This occurs when the gas is attached to particles or is dissolved, for example, in rain. Most sulfates are less than 1 μm in diameter, but SO_2 may dissolve in fog droplets, which are in the 10-μm-diameter range, resulting in "acid fog." Because of the droplet size and solubility, these would be expected to be deposited in the upper airway,[50] particularly the nasal passages. The dissociation of the sulfurous acid formed from the hydration of SO_2 yields bisulfite (HSO_3), which is a bronchoconstrictor.[14]

When levels of SO_2 are especially high, asthmatic subjects may have increased symptoms after exertion. Since SO_2 is an irritant gas, it may trigger bronchial constriction. There is also evidence to support the notion that sulfate particles may incite asthma when concentrations are high. However, it appears that asthma prevalence is not related to the level of sulfates. Rather, those with asthma may be more susceptible to the effects of air pollution with sulfates.

Sulfur dioxide causes chest tightness and immediate bronchial constriction, but the concentration required depends to some extent on the degree of underlying airway hyperresponsiveness. In normal subjects, concentrations greater than 5 ppm are usually required to provoke bronchial constriction. For asthmatics, bronchial constriction may develop at concentrations greater than 1 ppm. Furthermore, with moderate exercise, asthmatic patients may have bronchial constriction with concentrations of 0.25 ppm. This incremental effect of these low concentrations of SO_2 on exercise-induced asthma appears to be similar, irrespective of the severity of asthma.

The effect of SO_2 on preterm labor was recently evaluated in a prospective cohort in China. It was thought that total suspended particulates (TSPs) and SO_2 may contribute to an excess risk of preterm labor. However, these data must be regarded as preliminary.[54]

In a recent EPA study of an area with over a half million population in urban areas, it was estimated that the potential annual health benefits for eastern Canada, from the reduction of U.S. SO_2 emissions, would be $1 billion annually starting in 1997. Reductions in premature deaths would account for 88% (RR 1.15, 95% CI 1.09-1.22) of health care dollar savings, while reductions in chronic bronchitis would account for 9%.[50] However, methodologic consideration casts doubt on the precision of these numbers.

The sulfur in acid rain is derived from sulfur dioxide in air pollution. Though acid rain may have deleterious health effects in people, it may contribute to the growth of plants as an essential nutrient. Some plants such as wheat and oilseed rape, which require a large amount of sulfur for growth, improve in areas of acid rain. The effect on crops is more apparent in Europe than in the United States. High-sulfur acid rain is most common in areas burning high-sulfur fossil fuels, such as the eastern United States.

OXIDES OF NITROGEN

Nitrogen oxides, generally designated as NO_x, are comprised of nitric oxide (NO), nitrogen dioxide (NO_2), and nitrogen tetroxide (N_2O_4). Most ambient NO_x derives from the combustion of fossil fuels, particularly in motor vehicles. As noted earlier, nitrogen oxides are largely responsible for atmospheric ozone generation in photochemical smog (see Fig. 51-1).

Following inhalation, NO_x undergoes hydration reactions leading to the formation of nitric (HNO_3) and nitrous (HNO_2) acids. Nitrogen dioxide also provokes free radical production and local oxidative injury, mostly involving lipid peroxidation.[29] Atmospheric NO_x may be converted to nitrous and nitric acids, which contribute to acid aerosols and acid rain.

Nitrogen oxides have been evaluated in several studies for their effect on lung function in asthmatic subjects. Some studies have shown an increase in airway hyperreactivity,[4,28,30] while others have found no effect on pulmonary function.[7,17,22] Differences in these studies may represent different methodologic techniques as well as individual responses among asthmatic subjects to NO_x. More studies are needed to determine real effects of NO_x on asthmatic subjects.

Normal subjects exposed to high concentrations of NO_x have small and inconsistent pulmonary effects. Exposures to concentrations of less than 1 ppm have not had any significant effects. Long-term exposure of asthmatic patients, including some with severe asthma, to NO_x in concentrations of 0.3 and 0.6 ppm and to ambient air in Los Angeles with an NO_x content of 0.09 ppm had no effect on airway function. Even in the patients with the most severe asthma, there was no significant evidence that NO_x effects are potentiated by other pollutants such as ozone or particulates. However, NO_x concentrations of 0.4 ppm for 6 hours have caused increased interleukin 8 and tumor necrosis factor-α (TNF-α). Small increases in airway responsiveness have been reported at concentrations of 0.1 to 0.3 ppm. There do not appear to be any differences in the responsiveness of normal and asthmatic subjects. It has been reported in concentrations of 0.08 to 0.12 ppm for over 6 hours that there is an increased airway hyperresponsivity in normal subjects. This mechanism with increased neutrophils in bronchoalveolar lavage suggested ozone provokes an inflammatory response that is present up to 18 hours after exposure. Exposure of asthmatic subjects to 0.12 ppm of ozone for 1 hour caused a small increase in airway response to inhaled allergens, although there is no increase in exercise-induced bronchial constriction. Areas with high concentrations of ozone of 0.4 ppm for 4 hours have increased the eosinophilic inflammatory response to intranasal applied allergens in atopic subjects. Most studies suggest that ozone concentrations that may be present during the summer months may have a small effect on airway responsiveness that may be associated with increased airway inflammation.

ACID AEROSOLS

As noted previously, acid aerosols are suspended particles principally containing sulfur acids. To a lesser extent, nitrogen acids are present on them as well. The sulfur acids are primarily sulfurous acid and sulfuric acid from SO_2 and SO_3.

Inhalation of sulfuric acid fog at relevant concentrations has little or no effect on airway function in either normal or asthmatic individuals. However, pulmonary morbidity and mortality are increased at high concentrations. There have been three classic episodes of major air pollution associated with cold weather and still wind causing polluted air to become trapped or inverted. These occurred in the Meuse Valley in Belgium in 1930,[15] Donora, Pennsylvania in 1948,[8] and London in 1952.[26] There has also been a similar description in Yokahama, Japan, where increased asthma symptoms among U.S. military personnel and their families corresponded to periods of smog. However, these effects were not seen to the same extent in resident Japanese asthmatic patients. Minimal to no asthmatic symptoms were seen in the infamous London smog exposure of 1952.

Data from summer camp studies on the pulmonary effects of ambient conditions of children indicate decrements of expiratory flow parameters with increased amounts of local acid aerosols.[37] Similarly, the Harvard Six Cities studies demonstrate a correlation between atmospheric acidity and respiratory morbidity in children.[47]

LEAD

Although leaded gasoline is no longer available in the United States, there has been a contribution of airborne lead from the combustion of alkyl lead fuel additives in gasoline. The elimination of leaded gasoline resulted in a marked reduction in ambient levels of airborne lead.[51] However, leaded gasoline is still available for local agricultural uses in equipment and extensively used in countries outside the United States. Average blood lead levels have correlated closely with airborne lead levels.[27] If ambient lead levels continue to decline, lead may cease to be a major concern in air quality.

CARBON MONOXIDE

Carbon monoxide is a by-product of incomplete combustion of carbon-based fossil fuels. Quantitatively, it is the major air pollutant of industrialized society. However, most ambient CO derives from nonanthropogenic sources, particularly the decomposition of organic matter. Through 1983 to 1984, the U.S. EPA conducted an exposure survey on population-based samples of nonsmoking adults from Washington, DC, and Denver, Colorado.[1] In this study it was found that the activity contributing most to overall exposure of nonsmokers to carbon monoxide was motor vehicle travel. Travel time exposures averaged 5 ppm, and average subjects spent a mean of 2 hours per day in transit. Automobile exhaust continues to be the major source of carbon monoxide production; however, it is also generated from cigarette smoking, manufacturing, wildfires, power equipment, barbecuing, and space heating. In occupations requiring significant time in and about traffic (tunnel workers, police officers) or near combustion sources (concrete cutters and power equipment operators), chronic carbon monoxide may result a lowering of the angina threshold. The long-term neuropsychiatric sequelae, if any, of chronic carbon monoxide exposure are unknown. The rate of accumulation of carbon monoxide is dependent on the inspired concentration of carbon monoxide, the minute ventilation of the subject, and the diffusing capacity into the bloodstream. The last is generally very high and thus nonlimiting. However, this can be significantly reduced in patients with chronic obstructive pulmonary disease.

Carbon monoxide is one of the few inhaled pollutants that is not responsible for local effects in the lungs and appears to exert its effect only through systemic dissemination. Studies have demonstrated increased cardiovascular symptoms in patients with angina.[2] Although implicated as a possible cause of atherosclerosis in humans, it does not appear to be responsible for atherosclerosis in animal models. Probably largely as a result of clean air legislation and reduced reliance on fossil fuels, CO levels in the atmosphere are declining.

PARTICULATES

Particulate air pollution is a complex mixture of substances, including carbon particles (from fossil fuel combustion), dust, and acid aerosols. Particulate air pollution has been described as total suspended particulate matter (TSP) or particulate matter (PM). Size is a major determinant on the health effects of inhaled particulates and determines how deeply they will penetrate into the respiratory tract. Particles less than 10 μm in aerodynamic diameter (PM_{10}) may be inhaled into the alveoli, where there is slow mucociliary clearance. Larger PM tends to be filtered out in the upper respiratory tract.

The current 24-hour NAAQS for PM_{10} is 150 μg/m^3. The annual arithmetic mean standard is 50 μg/m^3. This has been reduced in the state of California to 50 μg/m^3. It is estimated by the EPA that 45% of the U.S. population reside in counties where the PM_{10} exceeds 50 μg/m^3.[9]

Schwartz[40] compared the patterns of death in the Harvard Six City Study to the London smog epidemic of 1952. They examined death certificates from Philadelphia on 5% of the days with the highest particulate level of air pollution and 5% of the days with the lowest particulate of air pollution during the years of 1973 through 1980. They found that there was also little difference in weather between the high and low pollution days, but TSP concentrations averaged 141 μg/m^3 on high pollution days versus 47 μg/m^3 on low pollution days. The relative risk of dying on high pollution days was 1.08 ($p < .001$). The relative increase was higher for chronic obstructive pulmonary disease (COPD) (1.25) and pneumonia (1.13). This paralleled the pattern seen in London in 1952, and the age pattern of relative risk of deaths was also similar. Thus, the effects of TSP are statistically significant but slight.

Particulates in air pollution are divided into two general categories, depending on particle size. Larger (nonrespirable) particles tend to be derived from erosion and abrasion nonpoint sources (e.g., agricultural tilling, dirt roads). Smaller (hence respirable) particles occur from both stationary and mobile point sources, such as fossil fuel combustion engines, and power plants). The smaller particles also tend to be acidic, which affects their toxicity.

The toxicity of particles is a function of their surface-to-mass ratio, which increases with diminishing size. Particles are described by their size in microns. The term PM_{10} is used to describe particles that are less than 10 μm in diameter. There are more recent data to suggest that the PM_{10} (NAAQS) standard may not be protective, and a smaller particulate size standard has been suggested by many authors.* Recently, another particulate measure has emerged that appears to be significant; it is referred to as the $PM_{2.5}$.

*References 3, 12, 20, 21, 25, 35, 40-45.

This designation refers to all particles with a diameter of equal to or greater than 2.5 µm.

A prospective cohort study found an association between particulates and mortality.[33] A study of children in the Utah Valley, an area of elevation of over 4500 feet with frequent thermal inversions, found that particle concentrations correlated with more frequent hospital admissions.[32] Emergency department visits and asthma medication use in Seattle[45] were found to be associated with increased levels of particulates, those below the PM_{10}. Though not as significant, smaller impairments in lung function have been seen in patients with obstructive lung disease after exposure to high levels of particulates.[34] A growing body of evidence supports lowering particulate standards to include $PM_{2.5}$.

Recently, it has been suggested that the increased prevalence of asthma may be related to an increase of latex particles in the atmosphere.[53] Latex antigens are extractable from rubber tires and are abundant in air samples. These shed particles are smaller from radial tires than from bias tires.[5] These particles may contribute to allergic responses directly or in conjunction with other particulates. Further studies are ongoing to evaluate this causal link. Environmental legislation and controls of particulate emissions have been responsible for decreasing the TSP in the atmosphere.

CONCLUSION

The health impact of ambient air pollution is significant in terms of its toxicants and number of individuals exposed. Millions of people are exposed to ambient air contamination throughout the world on a daily basis, with increased morbidity and perhaps mortality (Fig. 51-2). We have discussed the increase in cardiorespiratory mortality, asthma morbidity, increased respiratory infections, decreased lung function, and altered immune response. The notable air pollutants include both primary (CO_2, NO_x, Lead, SO_2, PM) and secondary (ozone) contaminants. While the combustion of fossil fuels is largely responsible for the production of CO and NO_x, SO_2 is generated from the burning of high-sulfur-content coal in power plants. There are many other air contaminants that may be emitted. They tend to be most concentrated about stationary sources of pollution but must be considered to evaluate a specific site.

Number of persons living in countries with air quality levels above the primary national ambient air quality standards in 1991

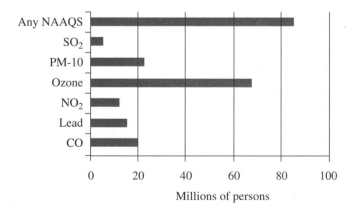

Fig. 51-2 Number of people living in counties with measured air quality above primary National Ambient Air Quality Standards. Figures based on 1991 air quality data. (Reproduced from Document No. 450-12-92-001 of the U.S. Environmental Protection Agency Office of Air Quality Planning and Standards.)

REFERENCES

1. Akland GG et al: Measuring human exposure to carbon monoxide in Washington, DC, and Denver, Colorado, during the winter of 1982-1983, *Environmental Science Technology* 19:911, 1985.
2. Allred EN et al: Short-term effects of carbon monoxide exposure on the exercise performance of subjects with coronary artery disease, *N Engl J Med* 321:1426, 1989.
3. Archer VE: Air pollution and fatal lung disease in three Utah counties, *Arch Environ Health* 45:325, 1990.
4. Bauer MA et al: Route of inhalation influences airway responses to 0.30 ppm nitrogen dioxide in asthmatic subjects, *Am Rev Respir Dis* 133:A171, 1985 (abstract).
5. Bogdan L, Albrechinski TM: *Characterization of tire wear particles,* EPA Publ No 82-153586, Washington, DC, 1981, US Dept of Commerce.
6. Burleson GR, Keyes LL, Stutzman JD: Immunosuppression of pulmonary natural killer activity by exposure to ozone, *Immunopharmacol Immunotoxicol* 11:715, 1989.
7. Bylin G et al: Effects of short-term exposure to ambient nitrogen dioxide concentrations on human bronchial reactivity and lung function, *Eur J Respir Dis* 66:205, 1985.
8. Ciocco A, Thompson DJ: A follow-up on Donora ten years after: methodology and findings, *Am J Public Health* 51:155, 1961.
9. *Current estimates from the National Health Interview Survey United States, 1991: data from the National Health Interview Survey,* series 10, No 184, 1992.
10. Dockery DW et al: An association between air pollution and mortality in six U.S. cities, *N Engl J Med* 329:1753, 1993.
11. Euler GL et al: Chronic obstructive pulmonary disease symptom effects of long-term cumulative exposure to ambient levels of total oxidants and nitrogen dioxide in California Seventh-Day Adventist residents, *Arch Environ Health* 43:279, 1988.
12. Fairley D: The relationship of daily mortality to suspended particulates in Santa Clara County, 1980-1986, *Environ Health Perspect* 89:159, 1990.
13. Farrell BP: Adaptation in human subjects to the effects of inhaled ozone after repeated exposure, *Am Rev Respir Dis* 119:725, 1979.
14. Fine JM, Gordon T, Shepard D: The roles of pH and ionic species in sulfur dioxide- and sulfite-induced bronchoconstriction, *Am Rev Respir Dis* 136:1122, 1987.
15. Firket J: The cause of the symptoms fund in the Meuse Valley during the fog of December, 1930, *Bull Acad R Med Belg* 11:683, 1931.
16. Foster WM, Costa DL, Langenback EG: Ozone exposure alters tracheobronchial mucociliary function in humans, *J Appl Physiol* 63:996, 1987.
17. Hazucha MJ et al: Effect of 0.1 ppm nitrogen dioxide on airways of normal and asthmatic subjects, *J Appl Physiol* 54:730, 1983.
18. Hunter JA et al: Predominant generation of 15-lipoxygenase metabolites of arachidonic acid by epithelial cells from human trachea, *Proc Natl Acad Sci USA* 82:4633, 1985.
19. Jakab GJ et al: The effects of ozone on immune function, *Environ Health Perspect* 103(Suppl 2):77, 1995.
20. Katsouyanni K et al: Air pollution and cause specific mortality in Athens, *Epidemiol Commun Health* 44:321, 1990.

21. Kinney PL, Ozkaynak H: Associations of daily mortality and air pollution in Los Angeles County, *Environ Res* 54:99, 1991.

22. Klinman MT et al: Effects of 0.2 ppm of nitrogen dioxide on pulmonary function and response to bronchoprovocation in asthmatics, *J Toxicol Environ Health* 12:815, 1983.

23. Koening JQ et al: The effects of ozone and nitrogen dioxide on pulmonary function in healthy and adolescent asthmatics, *Res Rep Health Eff Inst* 14:5, 1988.

24. Kreit JW et al: Ozone-induced changes in pulmonary function and bronchial responsiveness in asthmatics, *J Appl Physiol* 66:217, 1989.

25. Lipfert FW et al: *A statistical study of the macroepidemiology of air pollution and total mortality,* Upton, Long Island, NY, 1988, Brookhaven National Laboratories.

26. Logan WPD: Mortality in the London fog incident 1952, *Lancet* 336, 1953.

27. Mahaffey KR et al: National estimates of blood lead levels: United States, 1976-1980; association with selected demographic and socio-economic factors, *N Engl J Med* 307:573, 1982.

28. Moshenin V: Airway responses to nitrogen dioxide in asthmatic subjects, *J Toxicol Environ Health* 22:371, 1987.

29. Mustafa MG, Tierney DF: Biochemical and metabolic changes in the lung with oxygen, ozone, and nitrogen dioxide toxicity, *Am Rev Respir Dis* 118:1061, 1978.

30. Orehek J et al: Effect of short-term low-level nitrogen exposure on bronchial sensitivity of asthmatic patients, *J Clin Invest* 57:301, 1976.

31. Pope CA: Respiratory hospital admissions associated with PM_{10} pollution in Utah, Salt Lake, and Cache Valleys, *Arch Environ Health* 46:90, 1991.

32. Pope CA et al: Respiratory health and PM_{10} pollution, *Am Rev Respir Dis* 144:668, 1991.

33. Pope CA et al: Mortality risks of air pollution: a prospective cohort study, *Am Rev Respir Dis* 147:A13, 1993.

34. Pope CA, Kanner RE: Acute effects of PM_{10} pollution on pulmonary function of smokers with mild to moderate chronic obstructive pulmonary disease, *Am Rev Respir Dis* 147:1336, 1993.

35. Pope CA, Schwartz J, Ransom MR: Daily mortality and PM10 pollution in Utah Valley, *Arch Environ Health* 46:211, 1992.

36. Qu QS, Chen LC: Modulation of Ca^{2+} influx by a mediator released from human tracheal epithelial cells exposed to ozone in vitro, *Am J Physiol* 268:L558, 1995.

37. Raizenne ME et al: Acute lung function responses to ambient aerosol exposures in children, *Environ Health Perspect* 79:179, 1989.

38. Rieser KM et al: Long-term consequences of exposure to ozone. II. Structural alterations in lung collagen of monkeys, *Toxicol Appl Pharmacol* 89:314, 1987.

39. Salari H, Wong A: Generation of platelet activating factor (PAF) by a human lung epithelial cell line, *Eur J Pharmacol* 175:253, 1989.

40. Schwartz J: Particulate air pollution and daily mortality in Detroit, *Environ Res* 56:204, 1991.

41. Schwartz J: What are people dying of on high pollution days? *Environ Res* 64:26, 1994.

42. Schwartz J, Dockery DW: Increased mortality in Philadelphia associated with daily air pollution concentrations, *Am Rev Respir Dis* 145:600, 1992.

43. Schwartz J, Dockery DW: Particulate air pollution and daily mortality in Steubenville, Ohio, *Am J Epidemiol* 135:12, 1992.

44. Schwartz J, Marcus A: Mortality and air pollution in London: a time series analysis, *Am J Epidemiol* 131:185, 1990.

45. Schwartz J et al: Particulate air pollution and hospital emergency room visits for asthma in Seattle, *Am Rev Respir Dis* 147:826, 1993.

46. Sparrow D et al: The effect of occupational exposure on pulmonary function, *Am Rev Respir Dis* 125:319, 1982.

47. Speizer FE: Studies of acid aerosols in six cities and in a new multicity investigation: design issues, *Environ Health Perspect* 79:61, 1989.

48. Standiford TJ et al: Interleukin-8 gene expression by a pulmonary epithelial cell line. A model for cytokine networks in the lung, *J Clin Invest* 86:945, 1990.

49. Taskin DP et al: Respiratory status of Los Angeles fireman: one-month follow-up after inhalation of dense smoke, *Chest* 71:445, 1977.

50. US Environmental Protection Agency: *Environmental Protection Agency report on the health effects of acid rain,* Washington, DC, 1996, Environmental Protection Agency.

51. US Environmental Protection Agency: *Air quality criteria for lead,* vols 7, 11, Publ No EPA-600/8-83/028, Research Triangle Park, NC, 1986, US Environmental Protection Agency.

52. Wichmann HE et al: Health effects during a smog episode in West Germany in 1985, *Environ Health Perspect* 79:89, 1989.

53. Williams PB et al: Latex allergen in respirable particulate air pollution, *J Allergy Clin Immunol* 95:88, 1995.

54. Xu X, Ding H, Wang X: Acute effects of total suspended particles and sulfur dioxides on preterm delivery: a community-based cohort study, *Arch Environ Health* 50:407, 1995.

52

4-phenylcyclohexene

- The most important early data in an IAQ investigation are competently taken medical histories from affected individuals

- Most IAQ problems are related to improperly functioning HVAC systems

Indoor Air Quality

Franklin D. Aldrich

More than 200 years ago, Benjamin Franklin acknowledged the salutary effect of open windows upon sleep.[17] His opinion challenged a prevailing eighteenth-century notion that sleeping in fresh air was unhealthy, a view that would change during the next century. Among other benefits, fresh air in large volume was found to reduce the spread of airborne infections. Tuberculosis sanitaria operated on the principle that exposure to air and abundant sunlight hastened recovery from consumption. For the next 100 years, more or less, the quality of air indoors closely matched that of ambient air outdoors. Central heating gradually replaced fireplaces, stoves, and charcoal-heated bed warmers. Screened, openable windows and doors admitted fresh air, as needed; area fans circulated it and drew stale air out. Central air conditioning was rare until after the Second World War. In the early 1970s, design and construction of office and institutional buildings changed radically because of sharply rising energy costs. Building codes were rewritten to specify increased thermal insulation, double-glazed windows, and central heating, ventilating, and air conditioning (HVAC) systems. Older existing buildings were insulated and fitted with windows that did not open. Central HVAC was installed.

Private residences are not exempt from indoor air quality (IAQ) problems. Newer, state-of-the-art homes with close HVAC control of interior climate may have, in miniature, perturbations of IAQ like those in large, institutional buildings.

The character of work in industrialized nations has changed during the past generation. As jobs in manufacturing have decreased in number, white-collar jobs have increased. Manufacturing employees are being replaced by people doing "information processing" in its broadest sense. Members of the latter group occupy offices and deal with information in print and electronic formats, rather than with the production of goods. These demographic facts underlie much of today's concern with the effect of IAQ on health. Estimates of annual health care costs attributed to IAQ problems range up to $1 billion and for lost white-collar workplace productivity, $10 billion.[8,50] Thus, IAQ can have a major economic impact on builders, employers, makers of construction materials, building operators, and building occupants. When a building's interior environment does not meet the building occupants' needs, their comfort, morale, and health may be affected.

Ideal HVAC systems maintain reasonable temperature and humidity throughout a building, in all seasons, while controlling the introduction of fresh outside air and the exhausting of stale air. As building design philosophy changed in the early 1970s, materials technology advanced also. New buildings embodied new synthetic polymers, fibers, fabrics, and surface finishes. Many of these materials contribute volatile organic compounds (VOC) or particulates to indoor air. This fact is one basis for many IAQ problems.

Thermal comfort and humidity are important in the indoor environment. Temperatures between 18° and 22°C, with relative humidity from 30% to 60%, likely define an optimum comfort zone for light indoor work, although there are no definitive standards. Long-term excursions of relative humidity above 60% favor the proliferation of microflora and the colonization of HVAC cooling towers, drip pans, filters, and ducts. It has been common practice to line metal HVAC ducts with man-made fibrous mats for sound deadening. By trapping moisture and contaminants, these materials provide a growth medium for fungi and bacteria. This sets the stage for continuing release of biologic products that can cause allergic syndromes or infectious diseases in susceptible persons. Operation of a modern multistory building is a complex task requiring constant attention to HVAC system maintenance and to potential sources of contaminants. Unfortunately, the design, operation, and maintenance of HVAC systems may be less than ideal.

Air Pollutants and Sources

Volatile organic compounds. Virtually any organic compound can be found in indoor air (Table 52-1).[4,5] Substances with sufficiently high vapor pressure at room temperature may be present as vapor. Substances of low vapor pressure, if finely divided, may exist as particulate aerosols. Many reports have cataloged hundreds of indoor VOC entities in indoor environments, identified by sorbent trapping and analysis by gas chromatography/mass spectrometry (GC/MS).

The VOC composition of indoor air may be a unique "fingerprint" if little or no fresh air is introduced into the building. However, in a properly balanced HVAC system, fresh air is constantly being mixed with circulating air.

Table 52-1 Representative classes of organic substances in indoor air

Substance class	Typical sources
Alcohols	Adhesives, cleaning compounds, lacquers, paints
Aldehydes	Adhesives, fabrics, particleboard, plywood
Alkanes	Adhesives, cleaning agents, paints, waxes
Amines	Adhesives, floor coverings, humidifier water
Aromatics*	Adhesives, paints, photocopy processes
Esters	Adhesives, floor coverings, lacquers
Glycol ethers	Cleaning agents, epoxies, lacquers, paints, polishes
Haloalkanes	Cleaning agents, degreasers
Haloaromatics	Pesticides
Ketones	Lacquers, paints, particleboard, plywood
PAHs†	Fuel combustion
Phthalates	Polyvinyl plastics

From Levin HL: Building materials and indoor air quality, *Occup Med* 4:657, 1989.
*Includes benzene and substituted derivatives.
†Polynuclear aromatic hydrocarbons.

Therefore, the indoor VOC profile reflects, in some degree, outdoor VOC composition. This fact accounts for the occasional appearance indoors of ozone, nitrogen oxides, carbon monoxide, and sulfur dioxide, which are often associated with outdoor air. Figure 52-1 illustrates the similarity of, and the subtle differences between, the VOC compositions of outdoor and indoor air samples obtained simultaneously.

Xerography, blueprint, offset printing, photo processing, and operation of electronic devices can contribute significant quantities of VOC to white-collar environments.[10] Many technologies have typical VOC profiles; this fact can be helpful in IAQ investigations.

Health hazards presented by airborne VOC are those intrinsic in the individual substances. Benzene, for example, is a known human carcinogen, as is benzo[*a*]pyrene. Both substances may be found indoors, traceable to vehicle exhausts in outdoor air or to indoor fossil fuel combustion.[32] Neurobehavioral toxicity, manifested as memory impairment, motor incoordination, or personality change, is associated with solvent exposures.[33] However, the pharmacologic significance of very low-level solvent exposures remains unresolved.

Threshold limit values (TLVs) are established for many workplace chemicals.[1] Threshold limits represent "safe" maximum airborne concentrations of substances to which most persons can be exposed for 8 hours daily and 40 hours weekly, without adverse effect. The TLV values have regulatory status in many jurisdictions but apply only to specific substances or their mixtures in industrial settings. It is important to understand that in ambient indoor air, in nonmanufacturing settings, VOC usually exist at concentrations several orders of magnitude below TLV levels, yet,

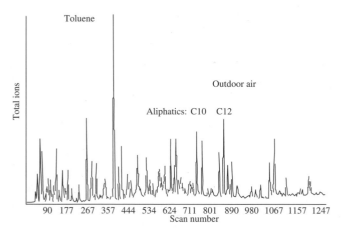

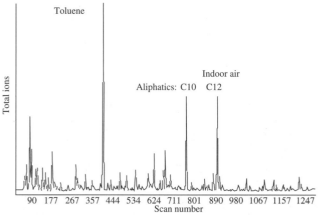

Fig. 52-1 Comparative ion chromatograms of volatile organic compounds in simultaneously collected outdoor and indoor air samples. Locale: southern Arizona, in summer.

under proper conditions, some VOC may be identifiable in breath and blood samples from persons who breathe the air. At this time of writing, there are no U.S. regulations governing indoor VOC in nonmanufacturing environments.

Volatile organics in indoor air may exist below odor threshold or may contribute to obvious odor problems.[34] Examples of the latter, originating outside the building, include vehicle exhaust gases, paint, or pesticide fumes entrained with outdoor air into an HVAC air intake plenum. An elegant example of VOC air pollution arising indoors is 4-phenyl cyclohexene contaminating new carpet backed with styrene-butadiene latex foam. This highly odorous chemical is thought to be generated by means of a Diels-Alder reaction between styrene and 1,3-butadiene.[48] At parts-per-billion levels it can cause a variety of symptoms, including headache, nausea, and eye and mucous membrane irritation in occupants of newly carpeted buildings.

Particulates. Particulates of respirable size, 10 μm mass median diameter (mmd) or smaller, may originate in many ways. Environmental tobacco smoke (ETS) is likely the most important indoor particulate. It contains extremely small particles, down to 0.3 μm mmd, and is a complex mixture of

mutagens, carcinogens, and toxic, irritant gases and vapors.[16] Its contribution to total suspended particulates is well documented.[28] Wood and coal fires emit particulates and combustion gases. House dust contains pollens, shedded skin cells, food crumbs, fibers, animal danders, aeroallergens, and a variety of environment-specific particles, such as those generated by hobby, construction, and remodeling activities. In farming areas, many pesticides are present in household dusts.[48]

Fibers. Asbestos fibers are of most concern because of their known fibrogenic and carcinogenic potential. The mineral was once applied routinely in new construction because of its excellent fireproofing qualities. Once applied, asbestos is stable and unlikely to become airborne unless physically disturbed. However, in recent years a campaign has been mounted to remove old asbestos lagging and pipe insulation from buildings and schools. Any physical removal activity generates asbestos fiber aerosols. Asbestos removal, therefore, is a hazardous operation. It is subject to strict safety procedures to protect workers and to minimize environmental release of fibers.

Glass fiber matting and textiles are widely used in commercial and home construction. Fibrous glass aerosols can cause skin and respiratory tract irritation. To date, however, epidemiologic studies have not revealed any chronic health effects caused by airborne fibrous glass.[26]

Bioaerosols. "Bioaerosol" implies airborne living organisms, or substances derived from them. Representative bioaerosol sources include algae, arthropods, bacteria, flowering plants, fungi, protozoa, and viruses. Each of these sources can contribute unique allergens, pathogens, or toxins to the environment.[42] Body parts and feces from the common house dust mite, *Dermatophagoides* spp., are potent allergens in sensitive persons. They are nearly ubiquitous in household dust when relative humidity is maintained above 50%.[37]

Illnesses Associated With Indoor Air Pollution

Building-related illnesses. In this category are diseases with definable causes that can be diagnosed by routine history, physical examination, and clinical laboratory procedures. They are called *building-related* because they may appear in the context of buildings in which affected individuals work or live.[35,36] The diseases, however, also may occur in individuals who have no occupational or residential association with any "building."

Hypersensitivity pneumonitis. Hypersensitivity pneumonitis, or extrinsic allergic alveolitis, is an immune-mediated response to external allergens. Inflammation of lung parenchyma, including alveoli and terminal airways, results from repeated inhalation of allergens by susceptible individuals. Many allergens have been described, including organic dusts, aerosolized proteins, molds, and animal danders.[7,9] Bagassosis, humidifier lung, and woodworker's lung are only three examples of "classical" hypersensitivity pneumonitis. The first is caused by moldy sugar cane residue (bagasse), the second is caused by fungi growing in HVAC humidification systems, and woodworker's lung is caused by dusts of oak, cedar, and mahogany.

Onset of hypersensitivity pneumonitis may be gradual or sudden. Acute onset involves cough, fever, chills, malaise, and shortness of breath within a few hours after exposure to antigen. The syndrome may resolve spontaneously within a few days, if reexposure to the antigen does not occur.

Subacute disease may appear insidiously over a few weeks, with gradually worsening cough and dyspnea. Continued antigen exposure may prolong the illness, and progression to severe dyspnea and cyanosis may mandate hospital care. Interstitial lung disease may follow continued, unresolving pneumonitis, with fibrosis as an end-stage result. A diagnosis of hypersensitivity pneumonitis is suggested by a history of antigen exposure, with subsequent appearance of symptoms consistent with the disease. Physical signs are nonspecific, as are chest roentgenograms early in the course of the illness. Pulmonary function tests may reveal restrictive changes, lung volume loss, and decreased compliance. Resting hypoxemia may be present. Obstructive changes indicate progressive disease. Routine hemograms are not diagnostic but may show elevated neutrophil and decreased lymphocyte counts. Eosinophilia is usually not present. Identification of serum precipitins against offending antigens is helpful because their presence may indicate significant exposure.[23]

Humidifier fever. This entity is related to hypersensitivity pneumonitis but is caused by endotoxins elaborated by gram-negative bacteria.[30] It has some of the constitutional symptoms of hypersensitivity pneumonitis but is without major pulmonary involvement. Fever, chills, and malaise are prominent. Fever begins within 8 hours of exposure. The syndrome lasts about 24 hours, is self-limited, and usually subsides without specific treatment.[25]

Asthma and rhinitis. Bronchospasm is the hallmark of asthma, manifested as expiratory wheezing and reduced airflow. Common indoor air pollutants, including ozone, nitrogen dioxide, sulfur dioxide, and tobacco smoke, are frequent causes of asthma reported in a recent survey.[22,31] Environmentally caused asthma may involve immune complexes formed between immunoglobulin E (IgE) and high-molecular-weight antigens or may arise from haptens such as isocyanates, amines, and metals.[12]

Rhinitis (atopic, nonseasonal, or perennial) results from antigen-antibody reactions in allergic individuals, but, as with asthma, simple irritants also may cause it. Symptoms include nasal discharge, sneezing, tearing, and itching nasal mucosa. Physical signs include boggy, pale mucous membranes, periorbital swelling, and watery discharge. Asthma and rhinitis may display immediate or delayed reaction patterns, depending upon the degree of antigen participation.[9,11,12]

Legionnaires' disease. This disease was named in 1977, following a 1976 outbreak of epidemic pneumonia among American Legion conventioneers at a Philadelphia hotel, in which 29 of 182 affected men died.[18] *Legionella pneumophila* eventually was implicated in this event. The organism is a gram-negative, aerobic, motile, pleomorphic, rod-shaped organism, ubiquitous in aqueous environments. Typically, it grows in cooling towers, standing water, heat exchangers, hot tubs, and humidifiers, as well as in lakes and ponds. Growth is enhanced by stagnation, infrequent decontamination, and temperatures of 36° to 70° C.

Legionnaires' disease is a fulminant pneumonia with abrupt onset of malaise, weakness, headache, and myalgia. Fever and rigors may appear within 24 hours, with body temperatures often exceeding 40° C. Cough is usually nonproductive or with thin sputum or scant hemoptysis. Accompanying diarrhea, nausea, vomiting, and abdominal pain are common. Central nervous system signs and symptoms, including lethargy, hallucinations, delirium, and obtundation, may indicate toxic encephalopathy.[5]

Pontiac fever. Pontiac fever is named for a 1968 epidemic in a Michigan office building, involving 144 persons. Fever, chills, headache, and myalgia are prominent features of this self-limited, influenza-like illness.[24] Pneumonia is not present, but mild gastroenteritis may be. *Legionella pneumophila* is associated with the disease, as can be confirmed by rising antibody titers to that organism in infected persons. Contaminated HVAC systems, cooling towers, and steam lines have been implicated.[19] It is not known why a single species of pathogen may cause two diseases so different in severity as Legionnaires' disease and Pontiac fever.

Behavioral syndromes. The illnesses in this category are less well defined than those classified as building related. However, many individuals who claim illness due to indoor air pollution do manifest sick-building syndrome, mass psychogenic illness, or multiple chemical sensitivity. None has rigid diagnostic criteria or characteristic physical or laboratory findings. The diagnoses are made by first excluding allergic, infectious, or toxic processes and then assessing the circumstances and emotional status of affected persons.

Sick-building syndrome. The constellation of symptoms now known as *tight building syndrome, sick-building syndrome,* or *SBS* was first encountered in the early 1970s as a feature of early indoor air pollution episodes. It is a group of nonspecific, recurring symptoms that prevail among office workers when they are in their work environment but usually abate when they are absent from it. Characteristically, the syndrome includes headache, dizziness, fatigue, eye-nose-throat irritation, nasal congestion, nosebleeds, chest tightness, dry skin, nausea, and difficulty concentrating. Not all these symptoms may occur simultaneously. Notably lacking in individuals with SBS are abnormal physical findings. Clinical laboratory tests usually reveal no abnormalities. The diagnosis of SBS is best made by a history of symptom exacerbation while in a problem building and symptom remission while away from the building. Typically, SBS affects *groups* of persons at the same time, rather than individuals, although this is not a rigid criterion for SBS diagnosis. Odor complaints may or may not be present. The cause(s) of SBS remains elusive, but there is an apparent association between "inadequate ventilation" and emergence of the syndrome. Inadequate ventilation means (1) inadequate removal of stale air, (2) inadequate distribution of air to occupied spaces, or (3) insufficient fresh air introduced into the building. However, a Canadian study of 1546 individuals in four office buildings revealed no relationship between reported sick-building symptoms and the volume of outdoor air supplied to the buildings.[29]

Other factors, including mold, ETS, or other pollutants, show minor associations with SBS.[79] To date, no specific, highly correlated cause for SBS has been identified. It is recorded that women predominate among SBS patients, but the role of gender bias in reporting health effects is unclear.[4,44] One authority advocates abandoning the term *sick-building syndrome* because of its inexact definition.[21]

Mass psychogenic illness. Similar to those of sick-building syndrome, the symptoms of mass psychogenic illness (MPI) typically spread quickly across a population of workers. In contrast to SBS, which may be localized to one or more areas of a building and spread slowly, MPI "recruits" victims rapidly. Odors are frequent stimuli for MPI events, particularly if an odor is perceived as unusual or is not easily identified. An outbreak may begin when one person who becomes ill attributes the cause to a workplace condition.[6,8] Incidence patterns may not be congruent with known HVAC air distribution pathways. A pattern of person-to-person communication may be revealed by careful questioning of affected individuals.[20]

Multiple chemical sensitivity. In 1987, this syndrome was named and described as "an acquired disorder characterized by recurrent symptoms, referable to multiple organ systems, occurring in response to demonstrable exposure to many chemically unrelated compounds at doses far below those established in the general population to cause harmful effects. No single widely accepted test of physiologic function can be shown to correlate with these symptoms.[15] Features of the MCS syndrome include headache, malaise, fatigue, dizziness, loss of ability to concentrate, nausea, mucosal irritation, and abdominal pain. First occurrence of the symptoms is usually associated with a single, specific exposure event, but subsequent recurrences may be triggered by reexposure to the same agent, or others, at levels much lower than those encountered originally.[13] The syndrome of MCS is similar to that of sick-building syndrome, but the key difference may be that SBS symptoms are present only when the affected individual is within a problem area or building, whereas the MCS patient may continue to be symptomatic in a variety of settings.

In its most extreme expression, MCS renders the patient a chemical cripple, unable to function in the workplace or elsewhere, because of reaction to "chemicals" in the environment.

Synonyms for MCS originate from alternative medicine, which is the province of clinical ecology. Examples include environmentally induced illness, chemical hypersensitivity syndrome, complex allergy, cerebral allergy, twentieth-century disease, total allergy syndrome, allergic toxemia, and ecologic illness.[49] Each of these terms begs definition and reflects the confusion that surrounds MCS and its characterization. Simply put, at this time, no proven diagnostic tests can identify MCS patients. Although these patients may indeed feel very ill under certain circumstances, there are no reliable clinical markers for the syndrome.

Despite the attention given to MCS in recent years by the medical, environmental, legal, and journalistic communities, no effective, specific therapy has emerged to help those who claim to be afflicted. Suggested therapies range from environmental isolation to acupuncture.[3] The prescription by alternative medicine practitioners of "safe" environments can have devastating social and economic consequences for MCS patients. The isolation and lifestyle changes such environments require typically specify that living quarters must be free from all synthetic polymers, fabrics, and surface finishes. Only "organic" food is to be consumed, and distilled water is used for drinking and bathing. Further prescription may specify a living location far removed from vehicular traffic, industrial operations, agricultural activities, and urban smog.

Rational treatment for MCS patients focuses upon the individual, rather than on the environment. Paramount is nonjudgmental acceptance of the reality of the patient's symptoms.[45,46] A thorough history and physical examination, supplemented by judicious use of laboratory tests, are necessary to rule out physical disease, environmentally caused or otherwise. Further evaluation is guided by the patient's reaction to his or her disease. Consultation with a psychiatrist or occupational or environmental medical specialist may yield valuable insight.

The MCS syndrome has been recognized as a potentially disabling condition in some jurisdictions, and by the U.S. Social Security Administration and Department of Housing and Urban Development. The latter agency contributed funds for the construction of an "Ecology House," intended to be a safe environment for MCS patients. After tenants occupied this building, some complained of no improvement or actual worsening of their symptoms.[42]

Investigating Indoor Air Quality Problem Situations

An ideal IAQ investigating team has at least one health professional who is an excellent interviewer and history taker. The "history of the present illness" is pivotal information in the investigation. It must be obtained skillfully by individuals who are not simply recording amanuenses and who can ask questions insightfully, interpret the information obtained, and use it to guide further study of the environment or of affected individuals.

Questions of ventilation, airborne particulates, and VOC can be addressed by an industrial hygienist, who should also be a team member. The hygienist plays a key role in communicating with building managers and facilities professionals who are responsible for operating and maintaining the HVAC system. Investigating industrial processes and operations, if part of the IAQ situation under study, is another responsibility of the industrial hygienist. When environmental sampling is to be done, the hygienist is the logical person to supervise or conduct that activity.

Available to the consulting team, but not necessarily a primary member of it, should be an experienced ventilation engineer to help assess problems that may be identified with the client's HVAC system.

Crisis management. Most IAQ problems that require consultants' services are crisis situations with two variables: technical problems and people problems. Both variables must be solved before the crisis can be resolved.[62] At the heart of these situations is the risk to health as perceived by those caught in the crisis. Because most crisis participants are in that role involuntarily, their reactions are likely to include anger or outrage.[38,39] Therefore, the IAQ consulting team must interpret the risk situation as well as investigate its cause. It is important for the client to appoint a crisis manager, who should be an effective communicator and ombudsperson within his or her organization, to work closely with the IAQ investigation team.

General rubrics [6,8]

1. Meet with management. This is an opportunity to assess management's understanding of its IAQ problem. Explain the complex relationships between the building itself, its HVAC system, pollutant sources, and people. Outline your approach to the investigation, and invite management's ideas, but do not be pressured into testing you deem unnecessary or excessive.

2. Limit the number of consultants. Too many experts, literally, can spoil the investigation.

3. Designate one chief consultant, experienced in IAQ issues, to coordinate the investigation and communicate with management, the media, and employees.

4. Hold meetings with groups of employees. Be open and candid about the investigation in order to dispel rumors by honest discussion. Invite employees to participate in your investigation by agreeing to be interviewed about their concerns.

5. The most important early data in any IAQ investigation are competently taken medical histories from affected individuals. The information gleaned can guide collection of environmental data or reduce the need for costly, time-consuming procedures, such as VOC or bioaerosol assays.

6. Do not rely on questionnaires for history taking. Observing employees' interview behavior may provide valuable clues to the nature of the crisis situation. Personal contact can be reassuring for those under stress. Some recommend questionnaires, but their use reduces rapport between investigators and respondents.[37,48] Interviewers may use checklists for recording information. However, a respondent's offhand remark has sometimes identified an IAQ problem's root cause.

7. If the number of affected persons is large, ask them to assemble in an area apart from the main workplace. Then, you have a sequestered forum for question-and-answer sessions and interviews.

8. If you feel that employees need medical evaluation beyond history taking, arrange for them to be seen in one clinic or by a single physician who is knowledgeable in environmental or occupational medicine. Doing this reduces the likelihood of speculative diagnosis or misattribution of cause. If the client has an in-house medical department, it is appropriate to enlist its collaboration.

9. If you are convinced that no significant health hazard exists, do not recommend closing a work area because closure increases anxiety among employees and complicates reopening the area later.

10. Avoid being pressured into reaching a premature conclusion about the cause of the IAQ problem. Your credibility diminishes if you have to change your mind later.

Finding the cause

1. Personal interviews and history taking from employees are vital parts of the investigation. Interview enough employees to be confident that your sample is representative. That may mean 10, 100, or more interviews, depending upon the size of the problem at hand.

2. A walk-through survey should include all areas of the problem building, including detailed inspection of the HVAC system and its level of maintenance. All team members should participate in the walk-through. Too often, the investigating team's inspection of a problem building or workplace is cursory or incomplete. That fact explains the failure of many IAQ investigations. Invite the building engineer or facilities manager to accompany you. Ask if the HVAC system is operated in accordance with ASHRAE Standard 62-1989, which specifies that a minimum of 20 cubic feet/minute of fresh air *per person* be supplied to occupied office areas.[2] Do not fail to study *all* parts of the HVAC system, including air intakes, as potential entrainment points for contaminated outside air.

Often, computer rooms or data processing centers are equipped with stand-alone air handlers that maintain local temperature and humidity only, without connection to the building's main HVAC system. In these areas, be certain that the air handlers' drip pans, sumps, and filters are clean and free from microbial overgrowth. These environments are intended primarily for electronic equipment. When, as sometimes happens, human workstations are introduced into them without readjustment of HVAC to allow for fresh air makeup, IAQ complaints emerge predictably.

3. Environmental sampling, at minimum, should include temperature, relative humidity, and ambient carbon dioxide levels in problem and nonproblem areas of the building. Colorimetric detector tubes are adequate for CO_2 grab samples. Carbon dioxide levels above about 1000 ppm suggest inadequate fresh air supply to the area. Detector tubes are also available for many key VOC pollutants and are useful for rough approximation of VOC levels. Be alert for pollutants originating from specialized operations, such as printer and blueprint rooms, machine shops, carpentry and paint shops, chemical laboratories, photo darkrooms, and kitchens and dining areas. Quantitative assays for VOC and bioaerosols are specialized undertakings and, in many cases, may be postponed or omitted, depending upon the complaint patterns revealed in employee interviews.

If clinical judgment suggests the collection of quantitative VOC or bioaerosol data, the sampling should be conducted simultaneously in the problem area, in a nonproblem area, and outdoors. Samples so obtained allow direct comparison of VOC species and levels, as well as microorganism colony counts. If, for example, the colony count in a problem area is fivefold that of a nonproblem area or outdoors, that is presumptive evidence of colonization of the problem area. If counts in problem and nonproblem areas are nearly equal and not markedly elevated above outdoor counts, it is likely that there is no indoor organism proliferation. Particulate collection is accomplished by gravimetric or optical methods, some of which are direct-reading. Bioaerosol sampling methods involve collection of spores or organisms on agar culture media by means of impingement or filtration techniques.

Portable ionization detectors and gas chromatographs are available for real-time VOC assays in the field. Beyond this, formal determination of airborne VOC requires field collection and storage of adsorbed samples, with later desorption and analysis by gas chromatography/mass spectrometry.

4. When you have formulated a working hypothesis about the problem, schedule a preliminary meeting with management and employee representatives. Present your findings succinctly. Help all parties understand their perceived problem in terms of general IAQ principles, and try to place the identified problem(s) in the perspective of familiar examples. If some data are uncertain or inconclusive, acknowledge this fact.

Address risks in general terms, recognizing that "involuntary" risks carry more emotional impact than "voluntary" ones, such as smoking and skydiving. "Zero" risk is improbable in any life situation; your task is to make this point without alarming your audience. Perceived threat to health caused by IAQ problems is usually an emotional issue that requires tactful handling by the investigators and management. Work closely with the client's crisis manager to formulate a credible response plan for dealing with employee concerns and with queries from outside sources, including news media.

5. Your final report to management should await the assembling and evaluation of all data. Assuming that your preliminary meeting successfully addressed all parties' major concerns, there is usually no need to rush your final report. A valuable point to make is that very few indoor air pollutants have any regulatory values in nonmanufacturing workplaces. Your final report should document all sampling and analytic methods used for environmental VOC, bioaerosol, or particulate measurements.

Concluding your report should be recommendations for dealing with the IAQ problems your investigation identified and for preventive measures and periodic monitoring to prevent recurrence.

REFERENCES

1. American Conference of Governmental Industrial Hygienists: *Documentation of the threshold limit values and biological exposure indices,* Cincinnati, 1991, ACGIH.
2. American Society of Heating, Refrigeration and Air Conditioning Engineers: *Standard 62-1989: Ventilation for acceptable indoor air quality,* Atlanta, 1989, ASHRAE.
3. Arnetz BB et al: A nonconventional approach to the treatment of "environmental illness," *J Occup Environ Med* 37:838, 1995.
4. Bachmann BO, Myers JE: Influences on sick building syndrome in three buildings, *Soc Sci Med* 40:245, 1995.
5. Bernstein MS, Locksley RM: Legionella infections. In Wilson JD et al, editors: *Harrison's principles of internal medicine,* ed 12, New York, 1991, McGraw-Hill.
6. Boxer PA: Indoor air quality: a psychosocial perspective, *J Occup Med* 32:425, 1990.
7. Brooks BO, Aldrich FD: Indoor air pollution: immunological interactions. In H Knöppel, P Wolkoff, editors: *Chemical, microbiological, health and comfort aspects of indoor air quality: state of the art in SBS,* Dordrecht, 1992, Kluwer.
8. Brooks BO, Davis WF: *Understanding indoor air quality,* Boca Raton, Fla, 1992, CRC Press.
9. Brooks BO et al: Immune responses to pollutant mixtures from indoor sources, *Ann N Y Acad Sci* 641:199, 1992.
10. Brooks BO et al: Chemical emissions from electronic products. In Bendz D, Allensby B, editors: *Proceedings of the IEEE symposium on electronics and the environment,* Washington, DC, 1993, Institute of Electrical and Electronics Engineers.
11. Brooks SM: Host susceptibility to indoor air pollution, *J Allergy Clin Immunol* 94:344, 1994.
12. Chan-Yeung M, Malo J-L: Occupational asthma, *N Engl J Med* 333:107, 1995.
13. Cohn JR: Multiple chemical sensitivity or multi-organ dysesthesia, *J Allergy Clin Immunol* 93:953, 1994.
14. Cooper KR, Alberti RR: Effect of kerosene heater emissions on indoor air quality and pulmonary function, *Am Rev Respir Dis* 129:629, 1984.
15. Cullen MR: The worker with multiple chemical sensitivities: an overview, *Occup Med* 2:655, 1987.
16. First M: Constituents of sidestream and mainstream tobacco smoke and markers to quantify exposure to them. In Gammage RB, Kaye SB, editors: *Indoor air and human health,* Chelsea, Mich, 1985, Lewis.
17. Franklin B: *The art of procuring pleasant dreams,* London, 1771.
18. Fraser DW et al: "Legionnaires' disease": description of an epidemic of pneumonia, *N Engl J Med* 197:1189, 1977.
19. Friedman S et al: Pontiac fever outbreak associated with a cooling tower, *Am J Public Health* 77:568, 1987.
20. Guidotti T, Alexander R, Fedoruk M: Epidemiologic features that may distinguish between building-associated illness outbreaks due to chemical exposure or psychogenic origin, *J Occup Med* 9:148, 1987.
21. Hodgson M: The sick-building syndrome, *Occup Med* 10:167, 1995.
22. Hoffman R, Wood EC, Kreiss K: Building-associated asthma in Denver office workers, *Am J Public Health* 83:89, 1993.
23. Hunninghake GW, Richardson HB: Hypersensitivity pneumonitis. In Wilson JD et al, editors: *Harrison's principles of internal medicine,* ed 12, New York, 1991, McGraw Hill.
24. Kaufman AF et al: Pontiac fever: isolation of the etiologic agent (*Legionella pneumophila*) and demonstration of its mode of transmission, *Am J Epidemiol* 114:337, 1981.

25. Kreiss K: The epidemiology of building-related complaints and illness, *Occup Med* 4:575, 1989.

26. Lee I et al: Man-made vitreous fibers and risk of respiratory system cancer: a review of the epidemiologic evidence, *J Occup Environ Med* 37:725, 1995.

27. Levin HL: Building materials and indoor air quality, *Occup Med* 4:657, 1989.

28. Lofroth GR et al: Characterization of environmental tobacco smoke, *Environ Sci Technol* 23:610, 1989.

29. Menzies R et al: The effect of varying levels of outdoor air supply on the symptoms of sick building syndrome, *N Engl J Med* 328:821, 1993.

30. Olenchock SA: Endotoxins. In Morey PR, Feely JC Sr, Otten JA, editors: *Biological contaminants in indoor environments, STP 1071,* Philadelphia, 1990, ASTM.

31. Ostrow BD et al: Indoor air pollution and asthma. Results from a panel study, *Am J Respir Crit Care Med* 149:1400, 1994.

32. Perry R, Gee IL: Vehicle emissions and effects on air quality: indoors and outdoors, *Indoor Environ* 3:224, 1994.

33. Ross HL: The behavioral effect of indoor air pollutants, *Occup Med* 10:147, 1995.

34. Ruth JH: Odor thresholds and irritation levels of several chemical substances: a review, *Am Ind Hyg Assoc J* 47:A-142, 1986.

35. Samet JR, Marbury MC, Spengler JD: Health effects and sources of indoor air pollution. Part I, *Am Rev Respir Dis* 136:1486, 1987.

36. Samet JR, Marbury MC, Spengler JD: Health effects and sources of indoor air pollution. Part II, *Am Rev Respir Dis* 137:221, 1988.

37. Samimi BS: The environmental evaluation: commercial and home, *Occup Med* 10:95, 1995.

38. Sandman P: Medicine and mass communication: an agenda for physicians, *Arch Intern Med* 85:378, 1976.

39. Sandman P: Emerging communication responsibilities of epidemiologists, *J Clin Epidemiol* 44(Suppl 1):41S, 1991.

40. Seltzer JM: Building-related illnesses, *J Allergy Clin Immunol* 94:351, 1994.

41. Seltzer JM: Creating healthy indoor environments. A road map for the future, *Occup Med* 10:229, 1995.

42. Seltzer JM: Biologic contaminants, *Occup Med* 10:1, 1995.

43. Simon GE et al: Immunologic, psychological, and neuropsychological factors in multiple chemical sensitivity. A controlled study, *Ann Intern Med* 119:97, 1993.

44. Soine L: Sick building syndrome and gender bias: imperiling women's health, *Soc Work Health Care* 20:51, 1995.

45. Sparks PJ et al: Multiple chemical sensitivity syndrome: a clinical perspective. I. Case definition, theories of pathogenesis, and research needs, *J Occup Environ Med* 36:718, 1994.

46. Sparks PJ et al: Multiple chemical sensitivity syndrome: a clinical perspective. II. Evaluation, diagnostic testing, treatment, and social considerations, *J Occup Environ Med* 36:731, 1994.

47. Starr HG et al: Contribution of household dust to human exposure to pesticides, *Pestic Monit J* 8:209, 1974.

48. Sullivan JB Jr, Van Ert M, Krieger GR: Indoor air quality and human health. In Sullivan JB Jr, Krieger GR, editors: *Hazardous materials toxicology: clinical principles of environmental health,* Baltimore, 1992, Williams & Wilkins.

49. Terr A: "Multiple chemical sensitivities": immunologic critique of clinical ecology theories and practice, *Occup Med* 2:683, 1987.

50. Woods JE: Cost avoidance and productivity in owning and operating buildings, *Occup Med* 4:753, 1989.

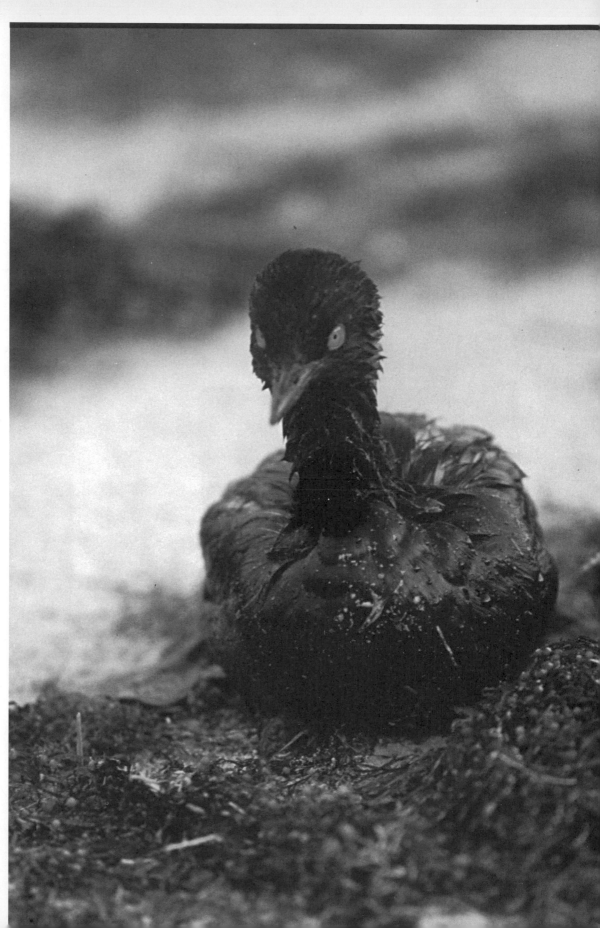

An oil-soaked cormorant sits on the beach near the Saudi Arabian-Kuwait border unable to walk or swim. Iraq continues to dump oil into the sea from Kuwait's al-Ahmadi terminal. The slick is now more than 30 miles long and heading south. January 27, 1991. (Courtesy Reuters/Corbis-Bettmann)

53

Br Br Cl
H—C—C—C—H
H H H

1, 2-dibromo-3-chloropropane

- Water is supplied from surface waters (lakes and streams), or groundwater

- Nonpoint sources of water pollution are more difficult to evaluate and control

Water Pollution

Hernan F. Gomez
Scott D. Phillips

Human life has always been, and always will be, dependent on the presence of clean, fresh water. Of the approximately 1.4 billion cubic kilometers of this planet's water supplies, fresh water comprises a relatively modest 3%.[21] Of this 3% about two thirds is in glaciers (and therefore unavailable), polar ice caps, and snowfields, particularly in Antarctica.[21,26,39] This represents enough water contained in frozen form to raise the Earth's sea level 170 feet if the ice and snow were to suddenly and completely melt.[36] Less than 1% of water is contained below the earth's surface as groundwater,[26] thus leaving only a tiny fraction (approximately 0.3%) of the earth's freshwater reservoirs readily available for human use as surface water resources.[21,26,39] A glossary of terms is found in the box on p. 438.

The basic source of all water on earth is precipitation in the form of rain, snow, and sleet.[26] About 70% of the precipitation that reaches land areas is evaporated or transpired (through vegetation) directly back into the atmosphere.[26] Ten percent soaks in and becomes groundwater, and the remainder runs off into lakes, streams, and rivers.[26] The earth's surface and groundwater ultimately flow into the world's oceans and seas.[26] Evaporation may then take place from large bodies of water with subsequent precipitation returning water back to the land. A fundamental concept of the field of hydrology is the hydrologic cycle, the circulation of water among the ocean, atmosphere, and land (Fig. 53-1).[26] Chemical movement occurs between phases or media: between air and water, soil and water, or soil and air. Chemicals move in a dynamic nature between phases, depending on many factors.

Water pollution is defined as any physical, biologic, or chemical change in water quality that adversely affects

Glossary of Water Terms

ABSORB: To take in. Many things absorb water.

ACID RAIN: The acidic rainfall that results when rain combines with sulfur oxides emissions from combustion of fossil fuels (coal).

ADSORPTION: The adhesion of a substance to the surface of a solid or liquid. Adsorption is often used to extract pollutants by causing them to be attached to such adsorbents as activated carbon or silica gel. Hydrophobic, or water-repulsing, adsorbents are used to extract oil from waterways in oil spills.

AERATION: The process of bubbling air through a solution, sometimes cleaning water of impurities by exposure to the air.

ALLUVIAL: 1. Pertaining to or composed of alluvium, or deposited by a stream or running water. 2. Said of a placer formed by the action of running water, as in a stream channel or alluvial fan; also, said of the valuable mineral, e.g., gold or diamond, associated with an alluvial placer.

ALLUVIUM: A general term for deposits made by streams on river beds, flood plains, and alluvial fans; esp. a deposit of silt or silty clay laid down during time of flood. The term applies to stream deposits of recent time. It does not include subaqueous sediments of seas and lakes.

AQUA: Prefix meaning water.

AQUEDUCT: A pipe or conduit made for bringing water from a source.

AQUIFER: A water-bearing stratum of permeable rock, sand, or gravel.

ARTESIAN AQUIFER: An aquifer where the water is under sufficient head (pressure) to cause it to rise above the zone of saturation if the opportunity were afforded for it to do so.

ARTESIAN WELL: A well tapping a confined or artesian aquifer in which the static water level stands above the top of the aquifer. The term is sometimes used to include all wells tapping confined water. Wells with water levels above the water table are said to have positive artesian head (pressure), and those with water level below the water table, negative artesian head.

BIOCHEMICAL OXYGEN DEMAND: The oxygen used in meeting the metabolic needs of aerobic microorganisms in water rich in organic matter.

BIODEGRADATION: The technology that uses microorganisms to degrade contaminants.

CFC/HCFC: Chlorofluorocarbon (CFC) and hydrogen chlorofluorocarbon (HCFC) are considered major contributors to the destruction of the earth's ozone layer.

CHLORINATED HYDROCARBONS: These include a class of persistent, broad-spectrum insecticides that linger in the environment and accumulate in the food chain. Among them are DDT, aldrin, dieldrin, heptachlor, chlordane, lindane, endrine, mirex, hexachloride, and toxaphene.

CONDUIT: A natural or artificial channel through which fluids may be conveyed.

CONTAMINATION (WATER): Damage to the quality of water sources by sewage, industrial waste, or other matter.

EFFLUENTS: Something that flows out, usually a polluting gas or liquid discharge.

EUTROPHICATION: The process of enrichment of water bodies by nutrients. Eutrophication of a lake normally contributes to its slow evolution into a bog or marsh and ultimately to dry land. Eutrophication may be accelerated by human activities that speed up the aging process.

FILTRATION: The mechanical process that removes particulate matter by separating water from solid material, usually by passing it through sand.

FLOCCULATION: The process of agglomeration of finely divided particles into larger particles. The larger particles in turn rapidly settle (sedimentation) during the water purification process.

---

living organisms or makes water unsuitable for desired uses (Table 53-1).[21] Even without human interference, there has always been a natural influx of pollutants into water. Naturally caused contamination, as in the case of poison springs, took place long before humans started to influence our planet's ecosystems.[21] Human activities have led to fresh water pollution since well before the twentieth century.[21] Since pollution is, to a large extent, a question of dilution of potential toxins, many substances can become pollutants that threaten an ecosystem if the concentration is too high.[21] This chapter explores many of the ways humans have polluted their drinking and recreational waters, as well as progress made in controlling pollution through federal legislation and water purification technologies.

WATER SOURCES

There are three primary sources of drinking water: groundwater, surface water, and the earth's atmosphere (protected runoff). For water supply purposes, water generally comes from surface waters (such as lakes and streams) or groundwater. Each source has its advantages and disadvantages. Until relatively recently, groundwater was considered to be almost a standard of water purity.[21] The use of groundwater is widespread, and it continues to be one of the cleaner forms of water for various reasons. Groundwater is essentially precipitation that does not evaporate or run off into a river. It "percolates" through soil and permeable rocks until it is held back by an impermeable layer of rock or clay.[21] This process, known as *infiltration,* along with the constant rising and falling of the water table and the length

Glossary of Water Terms—cont'd

FLOW: The rate of water discharged from a source given in volume with respect to time.

GROUNDWATER: The supply of fresh water found beneath the earth's surface (usually in aquifers), which is often used for supplying wells and springs.

HAZARDOUS WASTE: By-products of society that can pose a substantial or potential hazard to human health or the environment when improperly managed. Possesses at least one of four characteristics (ignitability, corrosivity, reactivity, or toxicity) or appears on special EPA lists.

HEAVY METALS: Metallic elements with high atomic weights, such as mercury, chromium, cadmium, arsenic, and lead. They can damage living organisms at low concentrations and tend to accumulate in the food chain.

HYDROCARBONS: Chemical compounds that consist entirely of carbon and hydrogen, such as petroleum, natural gas, and coal.

HYDROLOGIC CYCLE (WATER CYCLE): The cycle of water movement from the atmosphere to the earth and back to the atmosphere through various processes, including precipitation, infiltration, percolation, storage, evaporation, transpiration, and condensation.

INFILTRATION: The gradual downward flow of water from the surface into soil material.

LANDFILL: A disposal facility where waste is placed in or on land.

LEACHING: The process by which soluble materials in the soil, such as nutrients, pesticide chemicals, or contaminants, are washed into a lower layer of soil or are dissolved and carried away by water.

MAXIMUM CONTAMINANT LEVEL (MCL): Maximum permissible level of a contaminant in water that is delivered to any user of a public water system.

MAXIMUM CONTAMINANT LEVEL GOAL (MCLG): A nonenforceable concentration of a drinking water contaminant that is protective of adverse human health effects and allows an adequate margin of safety.

NONPOINT SOURCE POLLUTION: Forms of pollution caused by sediment, nutrients, and organic and toxic substances originating from land use activities that are carried to lakes and streams by surface runoff. Nonpoint source pollution occurs when the rate of materials entering these waterbodies exceeds natural levels.

ORGANIC WASTE: Natural materials, such as food and yard waste, that decompose naturally.

PERCOLATION: The movement of water through the subsurface soil layers, usually continuing downward to the groundwater or water table reservoirs.

PERCOLATION WATERS: Waters that pass through the ground beneath the earth's surface without a definite channel. It is presumed that groundwaters percolate.

POINT SOURCE: A stationary source of a large individual air or water pollution emission, generally of an industrial nature.

POINT SOURCE POLLUTION: This type of water pollution results from the discharges into receiving waters from easily identifiable "points." Common point sources of pollution are discharges from factories and municipal sewage treatment plants.

POTABLE WATER: Drinkable water.

RADON: A radioactive, colorless, odorless gas that occurs naturally in the earth. When trapped in buildings, concentrations build up, and it can cause health hazards such as lung cancer.

REFERENCE DOSE (RfD): An estimate of a daily exposure to the human population that is likely to be without appreciable risk of deleterious effects over a lifetime.

SUBSURFACE WATER: All water below the ground surface.

SURFACE WATER: Water on the earth's surface exposed to the atmosphere, e.g., rivers, lakes, streams, oceans, ponds, and reservoirs.

WATERSHED: The area of land that contributes surface runoff to a given point in a drainage system.

---

of time that infiltrated water stays and moves in the ground, ensures, under usual circumstances, a high degree of water purity.[21] Thus it is normally free of suspended solids, bacteria, and other disease-causing organisms that may afflict other sources of water.[26] It does not require extensive treatment except in those relatively few areas where it has become polluted. Suitable groundwater may be obtained via collection from springs that flow to the surface or through drilled wells extending into aquifers.[26] In some regions of the world, groundwater is available close to the surface in geologic formations that allow the water to be extracted easily and economically. Aquifers composed of sand, fractured rock, or porous limestone are easily pumped.[36] The quality of groundwater is determined by the aquifer from which it is derived. Since groundwater close to the surface may be more vulnerable to contamination, it is often necessary to drill a well through several aquifers before a suitable water quality is found.[36]

Surface water refers to water on the earth's surface such as rivers, lakes, streams, oceans, and reservoirs, which are exposed to the atmosphere. Some regions of the world are fortunate enough to be blessed with an abundant supply of surface water, and indeed most of the world's great cities are located next to large bodies of surface water. Lake Superior, for example, has provided an excellent source of clean water for years for cities such as Duluth, Minnesota, that are fortunate enough to be located nearby.[36] Surface supply sources usually require extensive purification before use, and industrial pollution has increased the costs of purification.[26] Surface waters tend to vary considerably in quality throughout North America. In the northeastern United States surface waters are generally soft (low in minerals) and low in

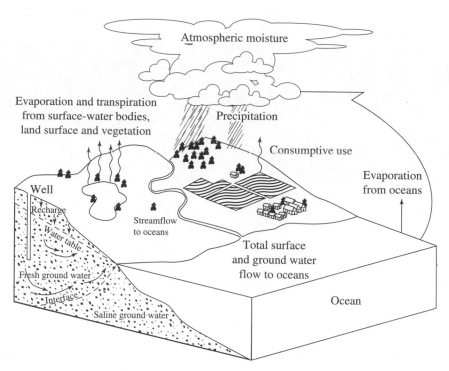

Fig. 53-1 The hydrologic cycle. (From Council on Environmental Quality: *Environmental trends,* Washington, DC, 1989, Executive Office of the President.)

Table 53-1 Personal and domestic uses of water

Domestic use	Examples	Waste characteristics
Personal use	Drinking, cooking, bathing, laundering	Waste food products, miscellaneous soiled materials
Waste carriage	Human excreta: fecal and urine	May harbor infectious organisms
Recreational uses	Swimming, boating, sailing	Discharges of oil and gasoline into lakes and rivers
Irrigation	Agriculture uses approx. 140 billion gallons each day	Highest water use in AZ, KA, CA, NB, and TX

From Moeller DW: Water and sewage. In Moeller DW, editor: *Environmental health,* Cambridge, Mass, 1992, Harvard University Press.

turbidity, whereas, surface waters in the midwest and western United States have a generally high turbidity.[36] Regional climatic differences may have an important influence on surface waters. The increased evaporation rates of the dry Southwest have resulted in a tendency toward increased salt concentrations.[36] Evaporation rates of as high as 10 feet per year are common in this part of the country. Overall there is a concern in many parts of the world about the local adequacy of surface water supplies, particularly in agricultural areas where demands for irrigation may be high.[26]

Another freshwater source is the atmosphere through protected watersheds (protected runoff). Protected runoff is another important source of water for some cities (such as New York City, Boston, and Lisbon). These communities have established protected watersheds that collect the precipitation that falls on them and use this source as part of their drinking water supply.[26] The water is generally disinfected by chlorination before use. Individual households may also take advantage of precipitation as a water source by collecting the rain falling on the roof of a house and storing it in a cistern for use as needed.[26] Although it is a relatively small water reservoir, it has the most rapid turnover rate.[21] Within the hydrologic cycle, the atmosphere provides the important mechanism of distributing freshwater and replenishing terrestrial reservoirs.[21] Much like groundwater, water collected from the atmosphere has largely been considered a naturally clean source of water. Such an assumption is flawed by the presence of chemicals in the atmosphere. Acid rain is the most common pollution phenomenon with regard to atmospheric water.[21] Acid rain is capable of dissolving minerals found in soil, which may then be carried into lakes and streams.[26] An unusual source of freshwater for a community is that of Boulder, Colorado. This city obtains much of its water from snowmelt from the Arapahoe Glacier in the Rocky Mountains. The water is filtered for the removal of potentially harmful endemic contaminants (e.g., *Giardia lamblia*) and chemically treated to add hardness. Water from snowmelt is naturally quite soft and can be corrosive to pipes. Population growth has resulted in the addition of water sources originating from the western slope of the Rocky Mountains.

WATER POLLUTANTS

"Pure water" is relatively rare in nature. When it evaporates, it soon becomes contaminated with aerosols and gaseous impurities that are present in the atmosphere.[21] Groundwater and surface water, by contrast, naturally contain dissolved minerals and organic matter. Nonetheless, the immense increase in human activities during and after the Industrial Revolution has had at least two major consequences with regard to the environment.[21] First, the release of pollutants has increased tremendously, particularly since the 1950s.[21] Second, people have begun to release man-made industrial pollutants of a completely different nature, many of which are characterized by high toxicity and slow degradability.[21] Many modern pollutants are extremely stable and thus may remain in the environment for centuries.[21] Since groundwater-bearing aquifers may take thousands of years to turn over their water content, it becomes extremely difficult, if not impossible, to purify an aquifer once it has become contaminated.[21]

For a closer analysis of freshwater pollutants, it is helpful to divide them up into five major categories: infectious agents, organic chemicals, inorganic chemicals, radioactive materials, and acid rain. Both organic and inorganic chemicals can be further subcategorized with regard to their relative persistence in the environment.[21] The primary biologic hazard of domestic wastewater is associated with endemic pathogenic microorganisms. Infectious agents consist of bacteria, viruses, and parasites. The main source of these pathogens is human waste, which enters the water cycle with insufficient treatment and thus contaminates the drinking water of a local community.[21] Raw domestic waste water contains millions of microorganisms in each milliliter of volume.[36] The introduction of disinfection in the developed nations shortly after 1900 has eliminated many infectious diseases that are transmitted through the ingestion of water.[26] Thus, the transmission of infectious disease through drinking water tends to be a more prevalent problem in Third World countries. Nonetheless, First World regions such as North America are by no means immune to this problem. The April 1993 outbreak of cryptosporidiosis in Milwaukee remains an unpleasant memory for most of the inhabitants since nearly 400,000 persons were afflicted by this outbreak.[35] Theories regarding the etiology of this outbreak include human error, the possibility of malfunctioning monitoring equipment in an aging Milwaukee plant, and contaminated water intake points.[35] This outbreak was particularly devastating for HIV-positive and other immunosuppressed residents. In general, although the effects of water contaminated with infectious diseases can have an alarming immediate effect, they do not bear the lasting and devastating effect on the ecosystem that pollutants found in the other categories can have.[23]

The category containing organic chemicals includes pesticides, fertilizers, plastics, detergents, solvents, oil, and gasoline. Toxic organic chemicals enter the water cycle through two methods: improper disposal of industrial and household wastes, or as the result of runoff of pesticides from agricultural or other areas where chemicals might be applied to land surface.[23] Contamination of drinking water with organic chemicals has been increasingly recognized as a public health concern with the discovery of 1,2-dibromo-3-chloropropane in drinking water in California's Central Valley and solvents in water in New Jersey in 1979.[8] The pesticide 1,2-dibromo-3-chloropropane was injected into the soil to kill nematodes since 1955. Overall, about 1.4 million kg were applied annually in California before its use was halted in 1977, when male workers were found to have an elevated incidence of sterility and reduced sperm counts.[8] Drinking water surveillance in California found that approximately 2500 wells were contaminated with this organic toxin. This toxin is representative of the particularly difficult problem of environmental persistence in view of its estimated half-life in soil of 141 years.[6]

The solvent group includes toxins such as trichloroethylene and perchloroethylene, which have been suggested by some to be associated with an increased incidence of leukemia and non-Burkitt's, non-Hodgkin's lymphoma.[9] These results must be interpreted with caution due to possible misclassification of exposure from individuals. Though the typical adult consumes approximately 2 L of water a day, exposure to volatile compounds in water can occur by routes other than direct ingestion, such as inhalation of contaminants transferred to the air from showers, baths, toilets, dishwashers, washing machines, and stoves.[5,30] Dermal absorption of contaminants may occur while a person is washing, bathing, and showering.[5,30] A New Jersey community had benzene levels in drinking water as high as 1.5 ppm, resulting in sufficient airborne contamination to produce a cancer risk estimate of 1 in 1000 excess cases.[4]

The pesticide group includes toxins and contaminants such as organochlorine pesticides (such as DDT), polychlorinated biphenyls, and dioxins. These substances are fat-soluble and therefore have in common a tendency to bioaccumulate in the food chain.[21] They are absorbed from contaminated water and are concentrated into the tissues of aquatic organisms. The toxin concentration then increases with every rise in the food chain until it reaches humans, the organism at the end of the food chain (Fig. 53-2).

The inorganic chemical category contains naturally occurring substances such as asbestos, arsenic, selenium, and radionuclides such as radium, radon, and uranium.[5] It also includes environmental contamination with the human production of acids, caustics, salts, and metals.[21] Heavy metals, for example, are found in sediment from the nearshore urban and industrialized centers of the Great Lakes. The heavy metal (including Cr, Cu, Pb, and Zn) concentrations in these areas are frequently at concentrations well above geologic background values.[20] Wetlands in mining districts in the western United States are frequently impacted by heavy metal–contaminated sediments.

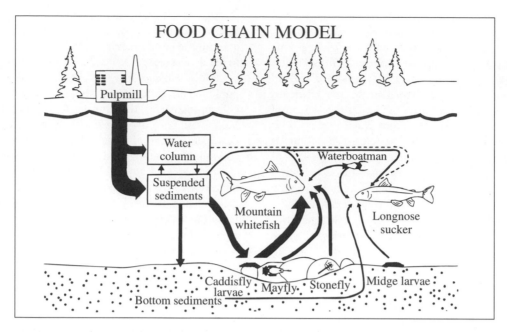

Fig. 53-2 Food-chain bioaccumulation model for 2,3,7,8-tetrachlorodibenzo-p-dioxin and 2,3,7,8-tetrachlorodibenzofuran in mountain whitefish and longnose suckers to show the importance of transport vectors, sediment ingestion, and food prey. (From Owens JW, Swanson SM, and Birkholz DA: Bioaccumulation of 2,3,7,8-Tetrachlorodibenzo-p-Dioxin, 2,3,7,8-Tetrachlorodibenzofuran and extractable organic chlorine at a bleached-kraft mill site in a northern Canadian river system, *Environ Toxicol Chem* 13:352, 1994.)

Asbestos is the commercial designation given collectively to a group of natural mineral fibers that contain hydrated magnesium silicates.[18] Commercial asbestos is obtained from asbestos-bearing rocks mined in open-pit or underground mines. The rock is then crushed, and asbestos fibers are separated and washed in a process known as *milling*.[18] Asbestos, which has many commercially useful properties such as strength, durability, and resistance to degradation by heat and chemicals, was first added to cement for use in pipes at the turn of the century in Europe.[5] Asbestos fibers added strength and durability to asbestos-cement pipes. Asbestos-cement proved to be popular for water distribution systems throughout Europe, and asbestos-cement pipe was first used in the United States in the 1930s. Since an estimated 65 million people may receive their drinking water via asbestos-cement pipe, concern regarding the theoretical possibility of asbestos-contaminated water has been raised.[5] Overall, asbestos-cement pipe has been shown to be quite durable: Asbestos-cement pipes do not rust and can tolerate high water pressures. It has been shown, however, that under certain water conditions (e.g., water with a low pH, low calcium level, and low level of dissolved solids) the calcium carbonate of the cement may be dissolved and asbestos fibers released.[29] Asbestos is found in very low concentrations as a normal contaminant in drinking water in many areas of the United States. Much of it comes from water that passes over natural formations of asbestos-containing rock, although some may come from asbestos-cement pipes.[18] Unlike the clearly documented cancer risk of long-term aerosol asbestos particle exposure, asbestos fibers in drinking water have not been shown pose significant health hazards.[17,28]

Arsenic is found in the environment in both organic and inorganic forms. Arsenic occurs in all geologic materials. For example, arsenic readily substitutes for silicon, ferric iron, and aluminum in crystal lattices of silicate minerals.[19] The major source of arsenic to the environment appears to be volcanos with total atmospheric emissions estimated at 31×10^9 g/year.[19] The primary use of arsenic in the United States has been in insecticides,[13] which subsequently may become a nonpoint source of water contamination via groundwater contamination or surface runoff. Although arsenate (As^{+5}) is the principal form of inorganic arsenic found in drinking water,[5] the arsenite (As^{+3}) form is the more acutely toxic form of arsenic and may also be found in groundwater.[19] Improvements in sample collection and analytic techniques have suggested that arsenite is more prevalent in groundwater than was previously believed.[19] The usual scenario for finding arsenate in groundwater is in alluvial types of water systems. Such wells do not yield enough water for a municipal supply; thus, persons affected tend to be those with family wells.[19] The bone marrow, skin, and peripheral nervous system may become involved after acute or chronic exposure. Basal cell cancer and squamous cell cancer have been reported after prolonged exposure. The Occupational Safety and Health Administration (OSHA) has linked arsenic to cancer of skin, lungs, lymph glands, and bone marrow.[31] It has also been associated with bladder, kidney, prostate, lung, and liver cancer.[7,13]

The use of halogens remains one of the most important public health breakthroughs in the purification of water. Chlorination of water has resulted in a rapid decline in the incidence of gastrointestinal disease; however, the use of chlorine products for disinfection relies on the release and killing power of free chlorine, which may then react with organic compounds present in the water to produce chlorinated hydrocarbons.[5] Thus, the chlorination of surface waters produces small amounts of chloroform and other potentially toxic by-products.[34] Although chlorination of water by treatment plants is generally regarded as safe, concern has been raised that the long-term ingestion of these agents by large numbers of people may have potential adverse health effects. Studies have provided mixed support for an association between chlorination and the risk of bladder and colon cancer.[5,27]

Radioactive materials form the fourth and final category.[20] Radioactive material can be the result of natural phenomena, as in the case of the naturally occurring radon gas, or it can be the result of nuclear waste products, such as uranium derivatives or other contaminated materials. Overall radioactivity as a source of water pollution is extremely rare.[21] Radon, a radioactive gas derived from decaying radium, is found in land formations throughout the United States. The decay series begins with uranium-238 and goes through four intermediates to form radium-226. Radium-226 subsequently decays to form radon-222 gas. The gas is colorless and odorless, and it emits harmful radioactive α-particles.[14] The EPA estimates that indoor radon exposure is responsible each year for 5000 to 20,000 deaths from lung cancer.[40] Although all histologic types have been noted, most radon-related lung cancers are bronchogenic.[16] There are several sources of radon: soil, water, building materials, and natural gas. Radon in the soil on which a structure is built is the most common reason for increased indoor radon levels.[2] In the home, exposure to radon may occur by the direct ingestion of drinking water or via inhalation after radon has volatilized from tap water or seeped into living spaces from soil and bedrock located directly beneath the house's foundation.[5] Although the EPA is required under the 1986 Safe Drinking Water Act to regulate radon and other radionuclides in drinking water, it does not have any legal authority to regulate the much higher risk of radon in indoor air.[5] Thus, the main risk from radon in homes remains unregulated; however, ingested radon represents a higher cancer risk than that of many other regulated organic contaminants in drinking water.[5]

The actual sources of water pollution are also categorized into point and nonpoint sources.[21] Point sources are stationary sources of water pollution and are generally of an industrial nature. An example is the discharge of pollutants from drainpipes of factories into bodies of water. Since point sources are easily identified and the contents of pollution discharges from point sources are fairly uniform, the regulation and monitoring of a point source discharge are relatively easy. An example of point source pollution is discharge from the McCormick & Baxter Creosoting Company site in Portland, Oregon. Sediments near the site are contaminated by several groups of potentially toxic chemicals, including polycyclic aromatic hydrocarbons, polychlorinated dibenzo-*p*-dioxins, polychlorinated dibenzofurans, and metals.[33] Another example of point source pollution may be found in the pulp and paper industry. Pulp mills function to extract from wood and process cellulose fibers, which is subsequently used for the manufacture of paper, cardboard, and fiberboard. The majority of pulp mills operating in the United States use the sulfate or "kraft" method.[25] The kraft method utilizes sodium sulfide and an enormous number of other chemicals, many of them chlorinated, to digest pulp and bleach paper. Sulfur released as H_2S is mainly responsible for the rather unpleasant odor associated with pulp mills. The kraft pulping process results in the production of a large amount of contaminated water, which is then discharged with little treatment into a body of water.[25] Hundreds of these chemicals have been identified and have been associated with various stages of bleaching within the kraft mill.[38] The compounds identified in bleached kraft pulp mill effluents include resin acids, organic acids and their chlorinated derivatives, small-chain volatile chlorinated organics, chlorinated phenols, and large polycyclic compounds, including polychlorinated dibenzo-*p*-dioxin and dibenzofurans.[25]

Nonpoint forms of pollution are caused by sediment, nutrients, and organic and toxic substances originating from land use activities, which are carried to lakes and streams by surface runoff. Nonpoint source pollution occurs when the rate of materials entering these waterbodies exceeds natural levels. Regulation of nonpoint source pollutants is much more difficult because there is no specific location of discharge and are often episodic in nature.[21] Examples of nonpoint sources include surface runoffs in chemically treated agricultural areas. An example is nitrate and nitrite water contamination. Groundwater contamination with nitrates and nitrites from nitrogenous fertilizer and organic wastes from livestock excrement is relatively common.[5,37] The primary public health concern of nitrate contamination from excessive nitrate levels in drinking water (usually well water) is the development of methemoglobinemia in infants.[5] Illness and death secondary to methemoglobinemia was first recognized in 1947.[10]

After ingestion of nitrate-contaminated water, nitrate is converted to nitrite in the gastrointestinal tract of the infant. The nitrite is then absorbed and reacts with the infant's hemoglobin to form methemoglobin and thus reduce the oxygen-carrying capacity of the blood. The manifestation of illness and degree of cyanosis are associated with the amount of hemoglobin available, as well as the percent oxidized to methemoglobin.[11,37] Young children are particularly vulnerable since fetal hemoglobin more readily forms methemoglobin than adult hemoglobin.[11] Well owners are therefore advised to use bottled water for infant drinking and formula preparation.[5]

Acid rain is another common example of a nonpoint source of water pollution. Acid rain is acidic rainfall that results when rain combines with sulfur oxides emissions from combustion of fossil fuels. Coal and oil combustion leads to the formation of sulfuric and nitric acid in the atmosphere. Once in the atmosphere, these substances may be distributed over long distances away from the original source. Smaller bodies of water such as lakes are particularly vulnerable since they generally have low biologic activity and may contain little alkaline material as a neutralizing agent.[21] If the pH in a body of water sinks low enough, aquatic life can be limited to a few resistant species of fungi and mosses.[21] Lime may be added to small streams to increase the pH.

In contrast to the reduction in plant life seen in lakes affected by acid rain, phosphor-based fertilizers and sewage may result in a process known as *eutrophication*.[21] Since phosphate is a limiting nutrient for freshwater flora, rising levels of phosphate result in an increase in plant growth.[21] Eutrophication is a man-made acceleration of a natural process. Eutrophication of a lake normally contributes to its slow evolution into a bog or marsh and ultimately to dry land. Eutrophication of freshwater lakes with phosphate accelerates this aging process. The high biologic productivity of a eutrophic body of water ultimately leads to a thick growth of water plants and algae, which may lead to increased decaying organic matter. The decaying matter stimulates increased oxygen consumption by aerobic bacteria and thus decreases the oxygen content of the affected lake. This drop in oxygen content finally leads to a sharp decrease in the fish population.[21]

WATER PURIFICATION

The preparation of water for human consumption is a major industry in industrialized countries. There are approximately 60,000 municipal water purification systems in the United States alone.[26] The combined output of these systems is 40 to 50 billion gallons per day, or 160 to 200 gallons daily per capita.[26] The main purpose of a water purification system is to collect water from an appropriate water source, purify it to drinking quality if necessary, and distribute it to consumers. Most groundwater sources do not require treatment; therefore, the processes described here pertain to the collection and purification of surface water supplies.[26] Various methods have been developed to remove the numerous forms of pollution from wastewater. These water treatment methods fall into three general categories: physical, biologic, and chemical.[36]

The physical treatment category includes screening, sedimentation, flocculation, filtration, reverse osmosis, distillation, and cooling. The screening, flocculation, and filtration processes are designed for the removal of particulate matter.[36] The size of the particulate matter to be removed dictates the method to be used. The smallest particles, for example, bacteria (which may be as small as 1 μm), are treated by various means so that they may clump together to form larger particles. This preparation allows easy removal through sedimentation or filtration.[36] In sedimentation, the water is placed in large storage (or settling) tanks for a predetermined period of time, which allows particulate matter and sludge to settle to the bottom. The settled material is then removed from the settling tank and sent for disposal.[26]

The steps of rapid sand filtration include raw water storage, chemical treatment and rapid mixing, flocculation and sedimentation, filtration, disinfection and fluoridation, and finally clear well storage[26] (Fig. 53-3). After clear well storage, the water is ready for distribution to municipal consumers. Raw water storage reduces turbidity and bacteria early in the water purification process. Storage also provides the community a water reserve, should the municipal water supply become temporarily contaminated with bacteria or toxins.[26] Chemical treatment of wastewaters, introduced several decades ago, was generally required in light of increasingly stringent standards for water decontamination. The chemical treatment of water involves the use of coagulating agents such as lime, aluminum, ferric salts, or synthetic polyelectrolytes. These chemicals serve to flocculate and settle organic colloids and phosphorus.[36] In the United States, the chemical called *alum* or $Al_2(SO_4)_3$; cd $14H_2O$ is most commonly used. Ferric chloride ($FeCl_3$) is also commonly used as a coagulant. Both substances are used in the rapid mixing portion of the water purification process to form a gelatinous mass called floc.[26] Once the coagulation process has been completed, the water is gently agitated to allow the floc to further agglomerate into larger particles, which are then allowed to settle to the bottom of the tank. The settled floc (or sludge) is then removed and sent to disposal[26] (see Fig. 53-3). To remove any remaining traces of floc, the treated water is passed through a filtration process consisting of several feet of sand. The final filtration process may consist of further flocculation and sedimentation before the purification process is finalized.[26] The final step, disinfection and fluoridation, is done prior to clear storage and distribution to municipal consumers. Chlorine may be added for disinfection and can be utilized to convert ammonia to nitrogen gas, which is subsequently lost from the water due to its insolubility.[36] Ozone can also be used as a disinfectant; however, ozone is expensive and, unlike chlorine, does not leave a protective residual in the water supply.[26]

Slow sand filtration is a simple, commonly used process whereby water is passed through a layer of sand 2 to 3 feet in depth. A biologic growth develops within the sand and acts to remove particulate matter from the wastewater. This

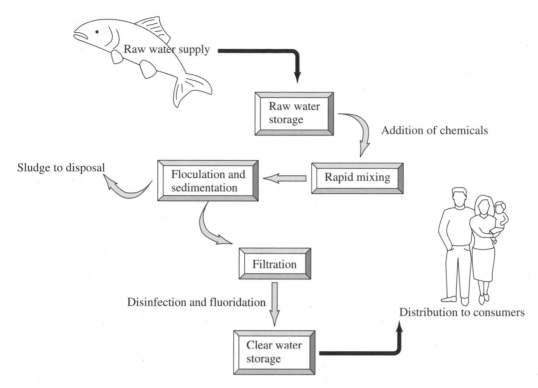

Fig. 53-3 Principal steps in the water purification process. (Reprinted by permission of the publisher. From Moeller DW: *Environmental health,* Cambridge, Mass, 1992, Harvard University Press, Copyright 1992 by the President and Fellows of Harvard College.)

relatively simple method removes most bacteria and other infectious organisms, including the cysts of *Giardia lamblia.*[26] A filter bed area of 2000 square feet may provide approximately 100,000 gallons of treated water per day.[26] Rapid sand filtration is a several-step process designed to provide high-quality drinking water in a relatively rapid fashion.

One of the more common tertiary water treatments is activated charcoal adsorption. Activated charcoal is effective in removing unwanted odors and tastes from purified water.[26] When water is brought into contact with the activated charcoal, particulate matter is adsorbed onto the charcoal and thus removed from the water. In some cases, the charcoal can be "regenerated" by burning off the organic material in incinerators.[36] Activated charcoal can be placed on the surface of sand filters, mixed with chemical coagulants, or placed in an adsorption bed separate from sand filters.[26] An activated charcoal bed may require a depth of 9 feet to be effective.[26]

WASTEWATER

In ancient times, the disposal of domestic waste was largely an individual problem. As the population grew and formed communities, it became clear that an organized collection system was required. Thus, by the beginning of the Roman Republic, the renowned Cloaca Maxima (main drain or great sewer) was built to give combined sewer service to the

Roman Forum and part of the city.[15] The Cloaca Maxima remains the oldest monument of Roman engineering. So sound was the stone construction, so ample the dimensions, that this sewer is still in use today.[15] In modern times, wastewater is generally directed to water treatment plants through gravitation flow in underground collection systems. Underground collection systems were an improvement over open drainage ditches, which were a common source of infectious disease.[36] The purification of municipal sewage is not discussed in this chapter, but thorough reviews of this subject are available elsewhere.[26,36]

Water usage and wastewater go hand in hand, with the first leading to the second.[36] Wastewater production has increased during the twentieth century, with urbanization and industrialization intensifying the problem.[36] People in the developed nations use water for a wide variety of purposes, many of which are indirect or almost unnoticed—and wasteful.[26] In 1985, approximately 400 billion gallons of water per day were withdrawn from American water sources such as aquifers and streams for use as public water supply, agriculture, and industry,[26] 75% of which (307 billion gallons) were eventually released into rivers and streams. Another 23% (92 billion gallons) was consumed and incorporated into manufactured products and agriculture.[26] Direct human use accounts for only about 3% of water used in this country.[26] The pollutants in domestic wastewater usage generally originate from food prepara-

Table 53-2 Selected examples of industrial waste characteristics and treatment

Industries	Origin of major wastes	Major characteristics	Treatment and disposal
Canned goods	Trimming, culling, juicing, and blanching of fruits and vegetables	High in suspended solids, colloidal and dissolved organic matter	Screening, lagooning, soil absorption, or spray irrigation
Dairy products	Dilutions of whole milk, separated milk, buttermilk, and whey	High in dissolved organic matter, mainly protein, fat, and lactose	Biologic treatment, aeration, trickling filtration, activated sludge
Brewed and distilled beverages	Steeping and pressing of grain, residue from distillation of alcohol, condensate from stillage evaporation	High in dissolved organic solids, containing nitrogen and fermented starches or their products	Recovery, concentration by centrifugation and evaporation, trickling filtration; use in feeds
Meat and poultry products	Stockyards, slaughtering of animals, rendering of bones and fats, residues in condensates, grease and wash water, picking of chickens	High in dissolved and suspended organic matter, blood, other proteins, and fats	Screening, settling and/or flotation, trickling filtration
Pharmaceutical products	Mycelium, spent filtrate, and wash waters	High in suspended and dissolved organic matter, including vitamins	Evaporation and drying, feeds
Yeast	Residue from yeast filtration	High in solids (mainly organic) and BOD	Anaerobic digestion, trickling filtration
Coffee	Pulping and fermenting of coffee bean	High BOD and suspended solids	Screening, settling, and trickling filtration
Fish	Reflects from centrifuge, pressed fish, evaporator, and other wash water wastes	Very high BOD, total organic solids, and odor	Evaporation of total waste, barge remainder to sea
Soft drinks	Bottle washing, floor and equipment cleaning, syrup storage tank drains	High pH, suspended solids and BOD	Screening, plus discharge to municipal sewer
Textiles	Cooking of fibers, desizing of fabric	Highly alkaline, colored, high BOD and temperature, high suspended solids	Neutralization, chemical, and biologic treatment, and trickling filtration
Leather goods	Unhairing, soaking, deliming and bating of hides	High total solids, hardness, salt, sulfides, chromium, pH precipitated lime, and BOD	Equilization, sedimentation, and biologic treatment
Acids	Dilute wash waters; many varied dilute acids	Low pH, low organic content	Upflow or straight neutralization, burning when some organic matter is present

From Nemerow NL: *Theories and practices of industrial waste treatment,* Reading, Mass, 1963, Addison-Wesley.
BOD, Biologic oxygen demand.

tion, household and body cleansing functions, and bodily excretions.[36] Water meeting drinking water quality standards is presently routinely used for irrigating lawns, washing automobiles, cleaning streets, fighting fires, and recreational purposes.[26] Table 53-1 summarizes nonindustrial domestic uses of water.

Industrial processes routinely result in water pollution when portions of the intended product or a by-product escape or are released intentionally in bodies of water.[36] An example may be found in the manufacture of paper. Much of the wood sugar and lignin (which may account for 50% of wood by weight) are dissolved in the manufacturing process and are carried off as wastewater.[36] The cellulose fibers are harvested and account for the remaining 50% of the original wood product.[36] Table 53-2 contains a brief summary of the origin and character of industrial wastewaters.

Domestic and industrial uses of water contribute organic and nonorganic chemicals into water discharge. These discharges are usually in a suspended state in the form of colloids or particles.[36] Assays have been developed to measure indirectly the amount of organic material contaminating the water supply. Measuring the amount of organic matter provides an indication of how effective a given treatment process may be in purifying the water supply. This is accomplished indirectly by using the biochemical oxygen demand (BOD) test. The BOD test is a measure of the oxygen used by microorganisms that oxidize organic matter biochemically.[26,36] If untreated or partially treated wastewater is discharged into a well-oxygenated body of water, aerobic organisms begin to oxidize the organic matter biochemically.[26] This process results in the depletion of oxygen from the water. At the same time, oxygen is replenished in the water by the turbulent water flow and by plant life such as green algae. If the oxygen is depleted faster than it is replenished, the dissolved oxygen may become too low to support aquatic life.[26] This assay is conventionally performed over a 5-day period. Originally, the procedure was developed in England to simulate the microbial purification process in rivers. Since in England most rivers flow to the ocean in approximately 5 days, this period of time was selected for the test. This rationale may not apply well to all bodies of water in North America; nonetheless, the BOD assay has been a useful tool in the United States as well.[36] The chemical oxygen demand (COD) test may be performed in approximately 2 hours. This rapid assay was designed to overcome the 5-day time limitation of the BOD assay.[36] The wastewater is boiled in the presence of sulfuric acid, which rapidly oxidizes organic contaminants present in the sample. The oxidation in the water sample is then quantified.[36]

WATER QUALITY LEGISLATION

Concern over waterborne disease and uncontrolled water pollution resulted in the first of a series of federal water quality legislation beginning in the late nineteenth century. Largely through the result of federal legislation, significant advances have been made in the reduction of suspended particles, waterborne disease, and control of BOD. Surface water quality and groundwater quality are currently regulated in the United States through a variety of federal and state programs. The earliest legislative act aimed at improving water quality was the Rivers and Harbors Act of 1899. This early legislation prohibited the discharge of refuse into navigable waterways.[5] This was followed by the 1924 Oil Pollution Control Act and the Federal Water Pollution Control Act (FWPCA) of 1948.[8] The FWPCA of 1948 is considered to be the first major clean water legislation passed in the United States.[23]

In the latter half of the twentieth century, even as improvements have been made in water quality, so have the number and variety of pollutants released into the environment. By the early 1970s, more than 12,000 chemical compounds were known to be in commercial use, and many more were added each year.[8] As more has become known about human health effects from contaminated water, Congress continued to pass legislation aimed at reducing the new categories of pollutants. Thus, the FWPCA of 1948 was followed over time by other amendments enacted by Congress. New legislation has included the Water Quality Act of 1965 and the FWPCA Amendments of 1972.[23] The 1972 amendments to the FWPCA represented a substantial change in water pollution legislation, and the FWPCA was thus renamed the Clean Water Act (CWA). With the passage of the 1972 amendments, the program underwent a change to technology-based standards.[8] This act was intended to eliminate the discharge of pollutants into navigable waters and to make the nation's waters swimmable and fishable.[22]

Central to the act is the prohibition against discharge of any pollutant into a navigable waterway without a permit. The act covers point sources, such as sewage treatment facilities and factories, and the handling of dredged material from adjacent waters.[5] The aim of the CWA was to accomplish these goals through industrial discharge regulations, nonpoint source controls, municipal sewer system improvements, and ambient water quality standards.[22] A major breakthrough of the CWA was the requirement that industries discharging pollutants to a publicly owned treatment works must provide pretreatment to minimize water degradation at the point of ultimate discharge.[5]

Reflecting increasing government involvement in clean water regulation, the financial investment of the federal government has been substantial. The government has invested $56 billion in municipal sewage treatment from 1972 to 1989, with total federal, state, and local expenditures of more than $128 billion.[1] Similarly, private sector spending has also increased. In 1973, industry spent about $1.8 billion on water pollution controls. By 1986, this figure had jumped to almost $5.9 billion.[1] A close examination of current legislation reveals that the CWA is concerned mainly with the quality of water sources, that is, with regulating industrial and municipal discharges into rivers, streams, and lakes so that the nation's water bodies can meet certain levels of "designated use."[24] The Safe Drinking Water Act (SDWA), passed in 1974 (and its amendments of 1986), applies primarily to the quality of the water delivered to homeowners through municipal water systems: it does not consider the water sources but, instead, emphasizes the end product coming out of the water tap.[1,5,24] The SDWA also protects valuable aquifers and groundwater from environmental contamination.[5] To ensure drinking water quality, the EPA or the states set legally enforceable standards for contaminants in drinking water, maximum contaminant levels (MCLs), which are divided into two categories: primary, for chemicals that have adverse health effects, and secondary, for those that have undesirable aesthetic effects in the taste, odor, or appearance of the water.[5] Since 1991, the EPA has markedly increased the number of standards issued with the number of MCLs currently at 86.[5] The EPA also issues nonenforceable concentration guidelines, maximum contaminant level goals (MCLGs), which are the concentrations of drinking water contaminants thought to be protective of adverse human health effects plus an adequate margin of safety. The reference dose (RfD) refers to an estimate of daily exposure to the human population that is likely to be without appreciable risk of deleterious effects over a lifetime. Table 53-3 summarizes the MCLs, MCLGs, and RfDs of selected chemicals. To establish standards, toxicologists consider the data on a toxin's acute and chronic effects, neurotoxicity, teratogenicity, mutagenicity, and carcinogenicity. With noncarcinogenic contaminants, scientists often recommend that

Table 53-3 Environmental Protection Agency drinking water standards for selected chemicals

Chemicals	MCLG mg/L	MCL mg/L	RfD mg/kg/day
Aldicarb	0.007	0.007	0.001
Antimony	0.006	0.006	0.0004
Arsenic	—	0.05	—
Benzene	0.0	0.005	—
Beryllium	0.004	0.004	0.005
Cadmium	0.005	0.005	0.0005
Carbon tetrachloride	0.005	0.005	—
Cyanide	0.2	0.2	0.022
Dichlorobenzene p-	0.075	0.075	0.1
1,2-Dichloroethane	0.005	0.005	—
1,1-Dichloroethane	0.007	0.007	—
Diquat	0.02	0.02	0.0022
Endothall	0.1	0.1	0.02
Glyphosate	0.7	0.7	0.1
Heptachlor	0.0	0.0004	0.0005
Lindane	0.0002	0.0002	0.0003
Mercury (inorganic)	0.001	0.002	0.0003
Nitrate	10	10	1.6
Nitrite	1	1	0.16
Radon	0.0	300 pCi/L	—
Selenium	0.05	0.05	0.005
Styrene	0.1	0.1	0.2
Tetrachloroethylene	0.005	0.005	—
Thallium	0.0005	0.002	0.00007
1,1,1-Trichloro-ethane	0.2	0.2	—
Trichloroethylene	0.005	0.005	—
Turbidity, NTU	1-5		
Uranium	0.0	20 µg/L	0.003
Vinyl chloride	0.002	0.002	—

From Office of Water: *Drinking water regulations and health advisories,* Washington, DC, 1993, Environmental Protection Agency.
MCL, Maximum contaminant level; *MCLG,* maximum contaminant level goal; *RfD,* reference dose; —, under review.

the standard be set at a level up to 10,000 times below the "no observed adverse effect level" (NOAEL) in order to allow for differences in toxic responses between animal species and humans.[5]

The CWA, in contrast, is designed to eliminate water pollution in the rivers and lakes from which half of the population obtains its drinking water.[1] With the passage of amendments to the WQA in 1987, the program has resorted to a risk-based approach that deals with such issues as nonpoint source pollution, stormwater discharges, the National Estuaries Program, environmental toxin control, and sewage sludge management.[8] Under the WQA, the EPA has been considering approaches that would assist with toxin control at municipal sewage treatment plants. This includes the evaluation of existing sewage treatment technologies, and the development of new techniques to remove potential environmental toxins.[8]

Changes continue to be made to water legislation and will likely continue for the foreseeable future. More recently (April 1995), the Transportation and Infrastructure Subcommittee on Water Resources and the Environment of the U.S. House of Representatives voted to make some dramatic revisions to the CWA (HR 961, Clean Water Act Reauthorization).[3] Among its key provisions, the bill would revoke a requirement that public and private entities obtain federal permits to discharge stormwater into waterways. It would also require the EPA to conduct risk and cost-benefit analyses on major regulations and require the government to pay landowners whose property values decline because of federal wetlands regulations.[3] The bill also proposes an increase in federal funding for pollution prevention programs. Under the previous CWA authorization, the federal government was authorized to provide $2 billion a year to states in revolving loan funds that finance pollution prevention and cleanup projects; HR 961 would boost that authorization to $3 billion.[3]

The political and economic climate has influenced and will likely continue to play an important role in water legislation in this country. There clearly has been some success in reducing some forms of serious water pollution, especially from the more traditional sources of pollution such as industrial discharges into lakes and rivers (point sources of pollution). Nonpoint sources of pollution have been more difficult to control, and, in fact, in some instances there is evidence that we are going backward in efforts to restore the health of our aquatic ecosystems.[1] Today, although there may be consensus on what the major issues are—drinking water quality, watershed management, wetlands, and funding—there is an ongoing debate on what should be done to balance and ensure economic and personal health to the citizens of this country.[24] It is ultimately the responsibility of concerned Americans (the final recipient of clean water) to let their legislators know the importance of a prudent and judicious regulatory process.

REFERENCES

1. Adler R: The Clean Water Act: has it worked? *EPA Journal* 10:10, 1994.
2. American Academy of Pediatrics (Committee on Environmental Hazards): Radon exposure: a hazard to children, *Pediatrics* 83:799, 1989.
3. Benenson B: House panel easily approves revision of Clean Water Act, *Congressional Quarterly Weekly Report* 53:935, 1995.
4. Bishop BL, Rosenman KD, Patel DB: *An exposure-risk assessment for benzene in shower air,* Trenton, 1984, New Jersey Department of Health.
5. Brown JP, Jackson RF: Water pollution. In Brooks, Gochfeld, Heizstein et al, editors: *Environmental medicine,* St Louis, 1995, Mosby.
6. Burlison NE, Lee LA, Roseblatt DH: Kinetics and products of hydrolysis of 1,2-dibromochloropropane, *Environ Sci Technol* 16:727, 1982.
7. Chen CL, Kuo TL, Wu MM: Arsenic and cancers, *Lancet* 1:414, 1988.
8. Clark RM, Ehreth DF, Convery JJ: Water legislation in the U.S.: an overview of the Safe Drinking Water Act, *Toxicol Ind Health* 7:43, 1991.

9. Cohn P et al: Drinking water contamination and the incidence of leukemia and non-Hodgkin's lymphoma, *Environ Health Perspect* 102:556, 1994.

10. Comly H: Cyanosis in infants caused by nitrates in well water, *JAMA* 129:112, 1945.

11. Committee on Nutrition: Infant methemoglobinemia, *Pediatrics* 46: 475, 1970.

12. Council on Environmental Quality: *Environmental trends,* Washington, DC, 1989, Executive Office of the President.

13. Dart RC: Arsenic. In Sullivan and Krieger, editors: *Hazardous materials toxicology,* Baltimore, 1992, Williams & Wilkins.

14. Demers R: Overview of radon, lead and asbestos exposure, *AFP* 1(suppl):51, 1991.

15. Fuhrman RE: History of water pollution control, *Journal of the Water Pollution Control Federation* 56:306, 1984.

16. Harley N et al: Contribution of radon and radon daughters to respiratory cancer, *Environ Health Perspect* 70:17, 1986.

17. Harrington JM et al: An investigation of the use of asbestos cement pipe for public water supply and the incidence of gastrointestinal cancer in Connecticut, 1935-1973, *Am J Epidemiol* 107:96, 1979.

18. Holland JP: Asbestos. In Sullivan and Krieger, editors: *Hazardous materials toxicology,* Baltimore, 1992, Williams & Wilkins.

19. Korte NE, Fernando Q: A review of arsenic (III) in groundwater, *Critical Reviews in Environmental Control* 21:1, 1991.

20. Krantzberg G: Spatial and temporal variability in metal bioavailability and toxicity of sediment from Hamilton Harbour, Lake Ontario, *Environmental Toxicology and Chemistry* 13:1685, 1994.

21. Krautz J: Poisoning the fount of life: fresh water pollution and its consequences, *Contemporary Review* 265:144, 1994.

22. Krieger GR: Hazardous wastes. In Krieger GR, editor: *Accident prevention manual for business & industry,* Itasca, Ill, 1995, National Safety Council.

23. Krieger GR: United States Legal and Legislative Framework. In Krieger GR, editor: *Accident prevention manual for business & industry,* Itasca, Ill, 1995, National Safety Council.

24. Lewis B: At odds on environmental policy: the water debates, *Water Environment & Technology* 7:10, 1995.

25. Marty MA, Shusterman DJ: Toxic hazards of the pulp and paper industry. In Sullivan and Krieger, editors: *Hazardous materials toxicology,* Baltimore, 1992, Williams & Wilkins.

26. Moeller DW: Water and sewage. In Moeller DW, editor: *Environmental health,* Cambridge, Mass, 1992, Harvard University Press.

27. Morris RD et al: Chlorination, chlorination by-products, and cancer: a meta-analysis, *Am J Public Health* 82:955, 1992.

28. National Research Council, Committee on Nonoccupational Health Risks of Asbestiform Fibers: *Asbestiform fibers: nonoccupational health risks,* Washington, DC, 1984, National Academy Press.

29. National Research Council, Safe Drinking Water Committee: *Drinking water and health,* vol 4, Washington, DC, 1982, National Academy Press.

30. National Toxicology Program: *Toxicology and carcinogenesis studies of tribromomethane in F344/N rats and B C F mice (gavage studies),* NTP TR 350, Washington, DC, 1989, US Department of Health and Human Services.

31. Occupational Safety and Health Administration: *Health hazards of inorganic arsenic,* Washington, DC, 1979, OSHA.

32. Office of Water: *Drinking water regulations and health advisories,* Washington, DC, 1993, Environmental Protection Agency.

33. Owens JW, Swanson SM, and Birkholz DA: Bioaccumulation of 2,3,7,8-Tetrachlorodibenzo-p-Dioxin, 2,3,7,8-Tetrachlorodibenzofuran and extractable organic chlorine at a bleached-Kraft mill site in a northern California river system, *Environ Toxicol Chem* 13:352, 1994.

34. Pastorok RA et al: Ecological risk assessment for river sediments contaminated by creosote, *Environmental Toxicology and Chemistry* 13:1929, 1994.

35. Rook JJ: Formation of haloforms during chlorination of natural waters, *J Soc Water Treat Exam* 23:234, 1974.

36. Smith V: Disaster in Milwaukee: complacency was the root cause, *EPA Journal* 20:16, 1994.

37. Speece RE: Water and wastewater. In Purdom PW, editor: *Environmental health,* ed 2, New York, 1980, Academic Press.

38. Sullivan JB Jr et al: Health-related hazards of agriculture. In: *Hazardous materials toxicology,* Baltimore, 1992, Williams & Wilkins.

39. Suntio LR, Shiu WY, Mackay D: A review of the nature and properties of chemicals present in pulp mill effluents, *Chemosphere* 18:1249, 1988.

40. UNESCO: *Scientific framework of world water balance,* Technical papers in hydrology No 7, Paris, 1971, UNESCO.

41. Upfal M: Radon toxicity. In Samet JM, editor: *Case studies in environmental medicine,* Washington, DC, 1990, US Department of Health and Human Services.

54

Noise Pollution

David Koh
Swee-Cheng Foo

sound wave

- Ambient noise is one of the most common occupational disorders

- Frequency spectrum and intensity of a noise are important in assessing its adverse health effects

Sound is energy transmitted through air in wave form from compressions and rarefactions of the air adjacent to a vibrating surface. As the vibrating surface moves into the air, the adjacent air is compressed, creating a pressure peak above the prevailing atmospheric pressure. The air molecules in this pressure peak in turn compress the air molecules next to them, making the pressure peak move away from the site where it was generated. When the surface moves backward, the adjacent air is rarefied, creating a pressure trough relative to the prevailing atmospheric pressure that propagates forward the same way the pressure peak does.

When sound waves impinge on the hearing organs, they are interpreted as sound. Noise is unwanted sound. For a stationary observer, the number of pressure peaks (or troughs) passed in 1 second is the sound frequency in Hertz and the root-mean-square pressure of a sound is the sound pressure (amplitude) in $\mu N/m^2$ (μPa).

If a noise is made up of only one frequency alone, it is called a *pure tone noise*. When it consists of a spectrum of different frequencies with various sound pressures, it is a broad-band noise. Pitch is the subjective perception of a tone that enables the observer to identify the tone.

The rate of energy imparted to the sound wave by the sound source is called *sound power* and is measured in watts (W). When the sound power radiates away from the source in the form of a sound wave, the energy transmitted through a unit area of the imaginary surface perpendicular to its path is the sound intensity. This is measured in watts per square meter (W/m^2).

Both the frequency spectrum and the intensity of a noise are important for assessing its adverse health effects.

MEASUREMENT OF SOUND
Sound Power Level

Sound power level (L_w) in decibels (dB) is defined as

$$L_w = 10 \log(W/W_o) \qquad (1)$$

where W is the power of interest and W_o is the reference power of 10^{-12}W.

Sound power propagates away from the sound source through the air, even though there is no net air movement resulting from the sound wave. The sound power is a property of the source and is independent of the environment and distance of a observer.

Sound Intensity Level

Sound intensity level (L_I) in dB is defined as

$$L_I = 10 \log(I/I_o) \qquad (2)$$

where I is the intensity of interest and I_o the reference intensity 10^{-12}W/m^2.

Sound intensity is related to the sound power and distance of the observer from the source. When sound can radiate equally in all directions from a stationary point source (relatively small in physical size), the spherical surface at a distance r from the source receives sound energy uniformly. Hence, the sound intensity varies according to the inverse square distance from the source.

$$I = W/4\pi r^2 = P^2/p_o C \qquad (3)$$

$$L_I = L_w - 10 \log(4\pi r^2) \qquad (4)$$

where $p_o C$ is acoustic characteristic impedance.

Equation 4 indicates that the sound intensity level falls by 6 dB for every doubling of the distance from the source. However, in practice, the fall may differ from 6 dB due to environmental factors such as room acoustics, air absorption, and other factors.

Sound uniformly emitted in all directions is just an ideal condition that is seldom met with in practice. Sound from a source can be stronger in one direction than others because of the nature of the source or environmental factors (such as reflecting surfaces) when the source is sited on the floor, close to a wall, or in a corner. In such situations, Equation 4 can be modified by introducing a directivity factor (Q).

$$I = QW/4\pi r^2 \qquad (5)$$

$$Q = (I_\theta/I_{av})\,|_{r=r1} = (P_\theta/P_{av})^2\,|_{r=r1} \qquad (6)$$

where
I_θ = sound intensity at direction of interest at r_1
I_{av} = average I over the spherical surface at r_1
P_θ = sound pressure at direction of interest at r_1
P_{av} = average P over the spherical surface at r_1

If the distribution of sound power from a source is concentrated into a narrow direction instead of uniformly radiated over a spherical surface, the sound pressure level is raised. The Q values for some of the situations in a room and

Table 54-1 Values of directivity factors and their contribution to overall L_1

Source	Q value	Contribution to L_1
In center of large room (free field)	1	0 dB
In center of one wall	2	3 dB
In junction of two room surfaces	4	6 dB
In junction of three room surfaces	8	9 dB

the contribution to sound pressure levels are given in Table 54-1.

The auditory effects of noise are associated with the intensity of the sound exposed. As such, sound intensity would be a more relevant parameter to monitor for hearing conservation programs in industry. In practice, however, sound pressure levels (to be defined in the next section) are monitored instead, as sound intensity is more difficult to measure. For airborne noises, the values of sound pressure levels and intensity levels are numerically the same in dB values. Hence, sound pressure level meters become the instruments of choice for noise evaluation.

Sound Pressure Level

Sound pressure levels (Lp) in dB (10% of a Bel) are measured in a logarithmic scale with reference to a sound pressure of 20 µPa, the sound barely audible to human ears. Hence, sound pressure level is proportional to the logarithm of the ratio of pressures squared and is proportional to the sound power of the sound source.

$$\text{Sound pressure levels: } L_p = 10 \log(P/P_o)^2 \text{ dB} \qquad (7)$$

$$\text{Sound pressure ratio square: } (P/P_o)^2 = 10^{(L_p/10)} \qquad (8)$$

where $P_o = 20$ µPa. From Equations 3, 5, and 7, it is easily shown that

$$L_p = L_w + 10 \log(Q/4\pi r^2) \qquad (9)$$

$$Q = 10^{(P\theta - Pav)/10} \qquad (10)$$

This is a useful equation for predicting the sound pressure level produced by a machine if it is installed in the factory when the sound power of the machine is known. Alternatively, it can also be used to predict the sound pressure level of a machine after relocation when its sound pressure level before relocation is known.

Since sound pressure levels (dB) are in the logarithmic scale, they cannot be added arithmetically. In adding, subtracting, or averaging sound pressure levels, the squared ratios of sound pressures in µPa are added, subtracted, or averaged instead. The formulas for these arithmetic computations are:

$$\text{Adding: } L_{pt} = 10 \log[\Sigma 10^{(Lpi/10)}] \qquad (11)$$

$$\text{Subtracting: } L_{p2} = 10 \log[10^{(Lpt/10)} - 10^{(Lp1/10)}] \qquad (12)$$

$$\text{Averaging: } L_{pav} = 10 \log[(1/n)\Sigma 10^{(Lpi/10)}] \qquad (13)$$

Table 54-2 Rule of thumb for adding decibels

Difference between noises	Value added to the higher noise
0-1	3
2-3	2
4-9	1
≥10	0

Table 54-3 Rule of thumb for subtracting decibels

Difference between noises	Value subtracted from the higher noise
≤1	≥10
1	7
2	4
3	3
4-5	2
6-9	1
≥10	0

Note: This method is unreliable when the difference is less than 3 dB.

where
L_{pi} = the ith sound pressure level
L_{pt} = the total sound pressure level
L_{pav} = the average sound pressure level

Arithmetic operations on sound pressure levels in the logarithmic scale usually require a scientific electronic calculator, which may not be readily available. In many situations, only approximate solutions are required. Rules of thumb for quick and easy estimation of the results in adding, subtracting, or averaging sound levels are useful in these situations. The approximate methods for adding and subtracting of two sound pressure levels are given in Tables 54-2 and 54-3.

Approximate methods for estimating average sound pressure level are:

1. When the range of sound pressure levels is less than 5 dB, the average sound pressure levels can be approximated arithmetically.

$$L_{pav} = (1/n)\Sigma L_{pi} \text{ dB} \tag{14}$$

where i = 1 to n.

2. When the range of sound pressure levels is between 5 dB and 10 dB, the average sound pressure levels can be approximated by adding 1 to the arithmetic average.

$$L_{pav} = (1/n)\Sigma L_{pi} + 1 \text{ dB} \tag{15}$$

where i = 1 to n.

Example 1: What will the sound pressure level be if: (a) two machines of 90 dB (independently) are switched on together? (b) if a third machine emitting 95 dB is also switched on?

Solution:
$$(P_1/P_o)^2 = 10^9 \quad \text{for machine 1}$$
$$(P_2/P_o)^2 = 10^9 \quad \text{for machine 2}$$
$$(P_3/P_o)^2 = 10^{9.5} \quad \text{for machine 3}$$

(a) Two machines of 90 dB switched on:
$$\begin{aligned} L_p &= 10 \log(10^9 + 10^9) \\ &= 10 \log(10^9) + 10 \log(2) \qquad = 93 \end{aligned}$$
(b) For all three machines switched on:
$$\begin{aligned} L_p &= 10 \log(10^9 + 10^9 + 10^{9.5}) \\ &= 10 \log(10^9) + 10 \log(5.16) \qquad = 97.1 \end{aligned}$$

Example 2: Reworking example 1 using rule of thumb:
1. Adding noises from two 90 dB machines (difference 0 dB): 90 + 3 = 93 dB

2. Adding noise from the third machine (95 dB) to result in (1) (difference 2 dB): 95 + 2 = 97 dB
3. Graphic representation of the adding procedure:

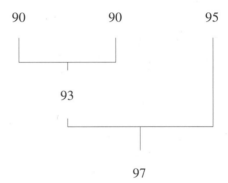

The result of 97 dB compares favorably with the exact method of 97.1 dB.

Sound Frequency

The number of pressure compressions or rarefactions observed by a stationary observer per second is the sound frequency (f) in Hz. The time taken by two successive pressure compressions or rarefactions is the period (T) in seconds. The distance between corresponding points on two successive pressure compressions or rarefactions is the wavelength (λ) in meters. The speed of the sound wave (c) depends on the characteristics of the carrying medium. It has a speed of 344 m/second in air at 20° C, 3048 m/second in concrete, and 5182 m/second in iron or steel.

The relationships between these parameters are:

$$\lambda = cT = c/f$$

where T = 1/f.

The sensitivity of the hearing organs is frequency dependent. The audible frequencies for human beings are between 20 Hz and 20 kHz. Hearing sensitivity in this audible range is not uniform, and the most sensitive frequency range coincides with the human speech range of 125 Hz to 8 kHz. Sound frequencies below 20 Hz (infrasound) and those above 20 kHz (ultrasound) are not audible to normal human beings.

NOISE RATING

The purpose of noise rating is to describe different noises in a form enabling them to be rated easily according to the risk associated with the effects of interest. The two commonly employed methods are noise frequency analysis and frequency weighting.

Frequency Analysis

Frequency analysis is commonly done on octave-band or ⅓ octave-band analyzers, where the bandwidth is a fixed percentage of the center frequency.

Octave band:

An octave band has a center frequency that is $(2)^{1/2}$ times of the lower cutoff frequency. The upper cutoff is twice that of the lower frequency.

$$f_o = (f_1 f_2)^{1/2} \qquad\qquad f_1 = (2)^{-1/2} f_o$$
$$f_2 = (2)^{1/2} f_o \qquad\qquad bw = f_2 - f_1$$
$$bw/f_o = 70.7\%$$

where
     f_1 = lower cutoff frequency
     f_2 = upper cutoff frequency
     f_o = center frequency b_w = band width

⅓ Octave band:

In the ⅓ octave, each octave is divided into three frequency geometrically equal frequency bands.

$$f_o = (f_1 f_2)^{1/2} \qquad\qquad f1 = (2)^{-1/6} f_o$$
$$f_2 = (2)^{1/6} f_o$$
$$bw = f_2 - f_1 \qquad\qquad bw/f_o = 23.2\%$$

where
     f_1 = lower cutoff frequency
     f_2 = upper cutoff frequency
     f_o = center frequency   bw = band width

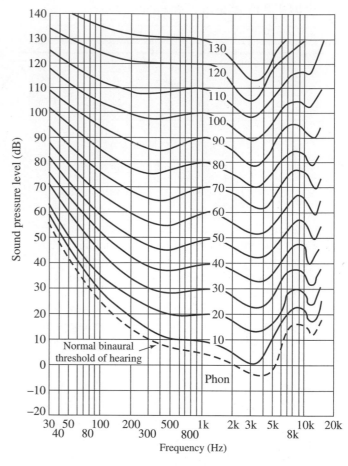

Fig. 54-1 Equal loudness contours for free-field binaural listening. (From Irwin JD, Graf ER: *Industrial noise and vibration control,* Englewood Cliffs, NJ, 1979, Prentice Hall.)

Loudness Levels

Since the sensitivity of human hearing organs to sound is frequency dependent, sound pressure levels of each frequency component in a given sound have to be measured to describe the sound fully. This makes it difficult to compare the loudness (or health risk potential) of two sounds (noises) with widely different frequency spectra. The loudness level of a sound is experimentally rated by a group of young subjects with normal hearing, comparing it with sound of 1000 Hz at different pressure levels. Sound loudness is measured in phons, which are numerically the same with the dB values of an equally loud 1000 Hz sound. Hence, a sound perceived to equal in loudness to a 10 dB, 1000 Hz sound has a loudness level of 10 phons. A set of standardized equal loudness contours are given in Figure 54-1.

Sound Levels and Frequency Weighting Curves

Sound levels (L) are noise indices adjusted for the frequency sensitivity of human ears. Weighting curves (networks) labeled A, B, and C are used. They are smoothed curves based on the equal loudness contours of 40, 70, and 100 phons, respectively. The two weighting curves most often used to evaluate noise hazard are A and C. Noise evaluation according to the A-weighting network appears to correlate well with the effects of noise (such as hearing loss and annoyance).

Most commercially available sound pressure level meters have the A and C networks built in and display the values of noise levels in dBA or dBC, according to the chosen weighting network. Noise level in dBA is used to evaluate the long-term risk to hearing organ damage or community response. Noise levels in dBC are used in peak level evaluation and in one of the methods for selection of hearing protectors.

As low-frequency noise is heavily discounted in the A-weighting network, the noise level difference between the dBA and dBC values is small for noise dominated by mainly high-frequency components. The difference between the dBA and dBC readings is large for noise dominated by low-frequency components (Fig. 54-2).

For describing a time-varying noise, L_{eq}, the time-weighted average sound level is used.

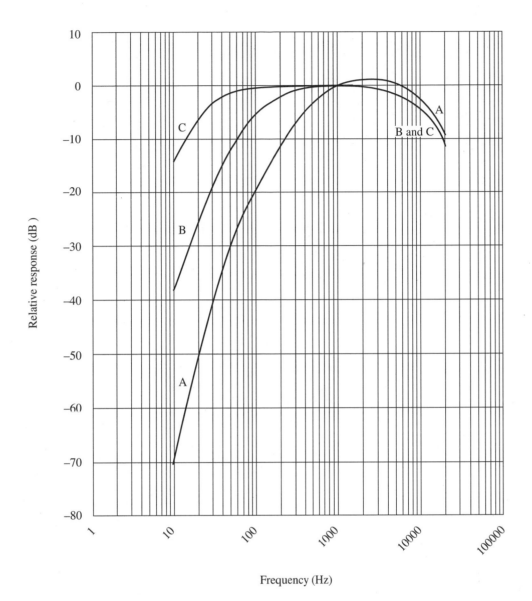

Fig. 54-2 Frequency response for the A, B, and C weighting networks.

$$L_{eq} = 10 \log \Sigma (P_i)(10^{L_i/10}) \text{ dBA}$$
where i = number of intervals, 1 to n
P_i = fraction of time spent in interval i
L_i = A-weighted level in time interval i

NOISE CRITERIA

Noise causes annoyance, interference with speech and telephone communication, community responses, hearing loss (temporary or permanent threshold shift), and other adverse health effects, which are discussed in detail later. Some of the most common criteria for the prevention of these effects are discussed here. A hearing conservation program is described later in the chapter.

The Preferred Noise Criteria

Preferred noise criteria (PNC) curves are a modified version of the noise criteria curves. They are formulated for rating the background noise in rooms for office work (Table 54-4). These curves are shown in Figure 54-3. Each curve specifies the maximum octave band sound pressure levels for a given PNC rating. The following steps are followed to rate a noise:

1. Use an octave band analyzer to obtain the octave sound pressure levels of the noise from 31.5 to 8000 Hz.
2. Plot the octave band sound pressure levels on the PNC chart and determine the point of highest penetration.

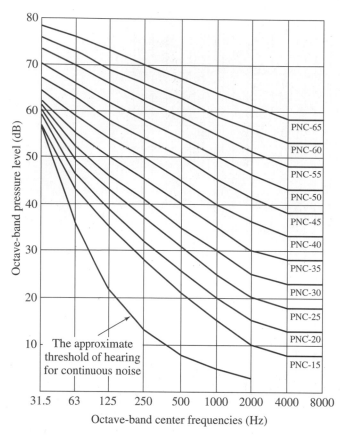

Fig. 54-3 Preferred noise-criteria curves. (From Beranek LL: *Noise and vibration control,* New York, 1971, McGraw Hill.)

Table 54-4 Recommended PNC criteria for indoor background noise

Environments	PNC curve
Sleeping quarters	25-40
Living quarters	30-40
Office or classroom	30-40
Recording studio	10-20
Retail store or restaurant	35-45
Laboratory	40-50
Computer room	45-55

The rating of the noise is given by the highest PNC curve penetrated by the octave band levels.

Speech Interference Criteria

Interference of speech communication by background noise can be evaluated by the preferred speech interference levels (PSIL) or noise levels in dBA. The simpler dBA noise levels method is discussed here. The voice levels required for effective speech communication depend on the background noise levels and the distance between the speaker and listener. The set of curves for rating the voice requirement in various background A-weighted noise is given in Figure

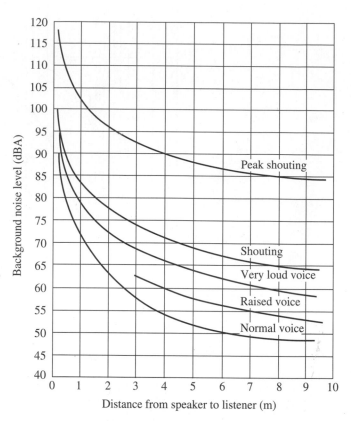

Fig. 54-4 Expected voice levels required for speech communication with various A-weighted background noise levels and separations between speaker and listener. (From Environmental Protection Agency: *Information of levels of environmental noise requisite to public health and welfare with an adequate margin of safety,* Report No 550/9-74-00, Washington, DC, 1974, Environmental Protection Agency.)

54-4. This chart can also be used to estimate the background levels by determining the ease of speech communication between two persons. For example, if two persons with normal hearing cannot establish effective speech communication within half a meter distance, the background noise is likely to exceed 85 dBA.

COMMUNITY RESPONSE

Studies of community response to neighborhood noise have reported from many countries (England, France, Germany, Sweden, Switzerland, and the United States). Annoyance data from these studies have been summarized by Schultz[48] (Fig. 54-5). The noise levels in community response are expressed in the day-night noise level (L_{dn}) in dBA, a 24-hour time weighted average noise level with a 10 dB nighttime penalty. The L_{dn} is designed to predict the long-term effects of environmental noise on the population and is computed by the following expression:

$$L_{dn} = 10 \log \{ \tfrac{1}{24} [(15)(10^{L_d/10}) + (9)(10^{(L_u + 10)/10})] \}$$

where L_d =   L in the 15 hours daytime period 0700 - 2200

        L_u =   L in the 9 hours nighttime period 2200 - 0700

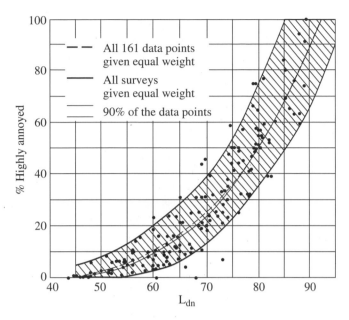

Fig. 54-5 Community annoyance to neighborhood noise: a summary of various survey data points. (From Schultz TJ: Social surveys on noise annoyance—further considerations. In Tobias JV, Jansen GJ, Ward WD, editors: *Proceedings of the Third International Congress on Noise as a Public Health Problem, Sept 25-29, 1978, Freiburg, Germany,* Rockville, Md, 1980, American Speech-Language-Hearing Association.)

The time-weighted average sound level over a 24-hour period, L_{eq}, has been used in Japan and many European countries for community noise. Schultz has shown that L_{dn} and L_{eq} are highly correlated ($L_{dn} = 1.03\ L_{eq} + 1.6$).[48]

OCCUPATIONAL EXPOSURE
Audible Noise

The American Conference of Governmental Industrial Hygienists (ACGIH) has set the threshold limit value (TLV) for noise exposure at 85 dBA for 8-hour days and 40-hour weeks to prevent noise-induced hearing loss. Noise exposure exceeding 140 dBC for unprotected persons is not permitted.

At this level, it is estimated that about 10% of the exposed workers suffer more than 25 dB hearing loss averaged over 0.5, 1, and 2 kHz. The TLV should protect the median of the population against a noise-induced hearing loss exceeding 2 dB after 40 years of occupational exposure for the average of 0.5, 1, 2, and 3 kHz.

The National Institute for Occupational Safety and Health has estimated that more than 9 million American workers are exposed to noise levels that are potentially hazardous to hearing.[36] Worldwide, many millions more are exposed to hazardous noise levels. The industries with excessive noise exposure range from the metalworking, engineering, woodworking, and textiles to mining, construction, repair work, and transport workers (e.g., airport staff).

A personal dosimeter or integrating sound level meter is preferred for occupational noise monitoring. All measure-

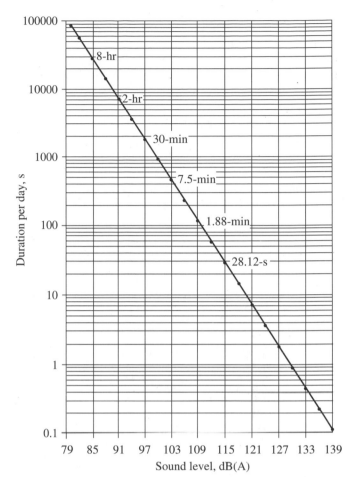

Fig. 54-6 ACGIH's threshold limit values for occupational noise exposure. (From ACGIH: *1994-1995 Threshold limit values for chemical substances and physical agents and biological exposure indices,* Cincinnati, 1994, American Conference of Governmental Industrial Hygienists.)

ment should be made on the A-weighting network with slow meter response. A meter with an additional built-in C-weighted peak level indicator is recommended. The dosimeter should be set at 3 dB exchange rate and an 8-hour criteria level of 85 dBA (100% dosage level). The noise exposure is excessive if the average sound level given by an integrating sound level meter exceeds the values in Figure 54-6 or the dosage by a dosimeter exceeds 100%.

Upper Sonic and Ultrasonic Acoustic Radiation

The ACGIH has recommended TLV values for preventing annoyance for noise from 10 to below 20 kHz and hearing loss for noise from 20 to 50 kHz (Table 54-5).

HEALTH EFFECTS OF NOISE
Effect on Hearing and the Vestibular System

Anatomy and physiology of the auditory system. An appreciation of the anatomy and physiology of the auditory pathway will assist in the understanding of the pathobiology of noise-induced hearing loss. The ear consists of the external ear, the middle ear, and the inner ear (Fig. 54-7).

The pinna is the visible portion of the external ear. It assists in collecting of sound waves and directing them to the external auditory meatus (EAM). The EAM is about 4 cm long and supported by cartilage at its outer third and by the bony skull in its inner two thirds. Sound waves traveling through the EAM impinge upon the tympanic membrane, which delineates the external and middle ear.

The middle ear is an air-filled chamber of about 1 to 2 cubic cm. It is connected to the oropharynx by the eustachian tube, which equalizes the air pressure of the middle ear to the external environment. Sound waves cause the tympanic membrane to vibrate. This vibration is transmitted via the

Table 54-5 Permissible airborne upper sonic and ultrasonic acoustic radiation exposure levels

⅓ octave center frequency (kHz)	⅓ octave-band level (dB)
10	80
12.5	80
16	80
20	105
25	110
31.5	115
40	115
50	115

ossicular chain of the malleus, incus, and stapes. The footplate of the stapes rests on the oval window on the inner wall of the middle ear. On this inner wall can also be found the round window, which is below the oval window. The round window is covered by a thin membrane, which distends outward as the oval window moves in, and vice versa.

The inner ear consists of the vestibulocochlear apparatus. The vestibular labyrinth is responsible for part of the equilibrium and balance functions. The three semicircular canals are at planes that are at right angles to each other.

The cochlea serves the function of hearing. It is snail-like in appearance, with two and a half turns. Within the cochlea is the organ of Corti, which has thousands of sensory hair cells. Sound pressure, which is transmitted via the ossicular chain and the oval window, causes movement of the fluid in the cochlea. This causes excitation of the hair cells along the basilar membrane of the organ of Corti, as well as production of electrochemical nerve impulses. The nerve impulses are transmitted along the eighth cranial nerve to the brain, which perceives the sound.

Pathobiology of acute effects of noise on hearing

Acute acoustic trauma. Sudden exposure to intense noise levels (usually impulse noises above 140 dB) or a blast injury can cause acute acoustic trauma. In severe cases, there may be a disruption of the conductive hearing pathway, with rupture of the tympanic membrane, disruption of the ossicular chain, or both. Direct damage to the cochlea or vestibular system can also occur.

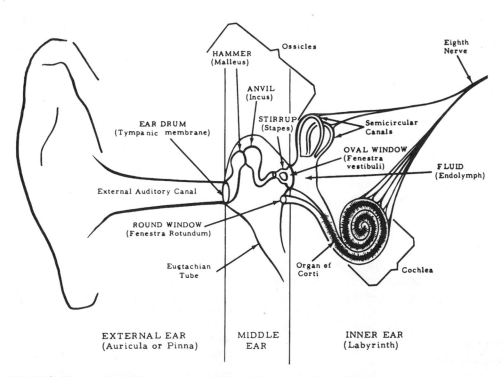

Fig. 54-7 The anatomy of the external, middle and inner ear. (From Niland J, Zenz C: Occupational hearing loss, noise and hearing conservation. In Zenz C, Dickerson OB, Horvath EP Jr, editors: *Occupational medicine,* ed 3, St Louis, 1994, Mosby.)

Common presenting symptoms include hearing loss, tinnitus, sound distortion, and pain. Occasionally, there may be sound sensitivity or hyperacusis. The acute hearing loss is often sensorineural but may be mixed if there is damage to the conductive hearing pathway. The frequencies affected may also be variable, depending on the type of injury.[5] Low-frequency loss is less common and appears to be limited to cases involving explosions.

Treatment of acute acoustic trauma. Unlike chronic noise-induced hearing loss, which is irreversible and for which no treatment exists, several methods of treatment have been utilized for cases of acute acoustic trauma that affects the cochlea. These include a stay in a silent environment,[13] the use of dextran,[5] and even hyperbaric oxygen.[42] The response to treatment has been variable.

Pathobiology of chronic effects of noise on the cochlea. The main effect of prolonged exposure to excessive levels of noise is on the cochlea, and the outcome is noise-induced hearing loss (NIHL). The biology of NIHL is not clearly understood.[2] Histologically, the pathologic finding in NIHL is a diffuse degeneration of the hair cells and nerves of the upper basal turn of the cochlea. The earliest changes are the loss of the stereocilia and deformity, swelling, and disintegration of the cell bodies. At a later stage, there is also some degeneration of the cochlear nerve fibers and changes in the central nervous system.

The site that is maximally affected is from the 9- to 13-mm region of the cochlea, which is the site most sensitive to 3 kHz to 6 kHz sounds. There are two common theories to explain the preferential action of sound at this site. The dual eddy theory or the jet theory is that strong mechanical destructive forces develop at this particular region of the cochlea during sound stimulation. The second theory is that this region is especially vulnerable to injury because of insufficient blood supply at the junction of the main cochlear artery and the cochlear ramus artery.[47]

It is further believed that the increased metabolic activity following sound stimulation depletes enzymes and glycogen stores, diminishes oxygen tension, decreases energy output, and causes reversible alterations in organelles of the sensory cells and nerve endings.[47] Functionally, this leads to the biochemical and metabolic exhaustion of the hair cells of the cochlea. This stage of injury manifests as auditory fatigue and temporary hearing threshold shift. A more intense stimulation over a prolonged period results in permanent hearing loss.

Clinical features of noise-induced hearing loss. Patients with NIHL typically present with a sensorineural hearing loss, due to damage to the hair cells of the cochlea. The hearing loss initially affects the higher frequencies and is usually bilateral and symmetric.

An exception to the symmetric picture is hearing loss due to exposure to firearms noise. In such cases, the hearing in the ear closer to the gun barrel (i.e., the left ear in right-handed persons) is usually affected more, as the other ear is farther away from the noise source and is also protected by the "head shadow."

Onset and effect on various frequencies. Noise-induced hearing loss has a gradual onset, and occurs after years of exposure to noise. The clinical picture is initially that of a high tone loss, affecting the 3 kHz, 4 kHz, or 6 KHz frequencies.[21] Frequencies below 3 kHz are almost never affected by occupational noise exposure without earlier effects on the higher frequencies.

Gradually, the lower speech frequencies are affected. The rate of deterioration of the hearing loss varies at different frequencies. At the 3, 4, and 6 kHz frequencies, hearing deteriorates rapidly in first 10 to 15 years and remains stable thereafter (Fig. 54-8). At the lower frequencies, such as 2 kHz, the most rapid change in hearing threshold occurs after 20 to 40 years of noise exposure.

Severity of hearing loss. A pure NIHL almost never produces a profound hearing loss. The low-frequency hearing threshold limits are usually about 40 dB, and the high-frequency limits are about 75 dB.[46]

Once the exposure to noise ceases, there is usually no further deterioration of hearing. A previous history of NIHL does not make the ear more susceptible to future noise exposure.

Tinnitus. Tinnitus may be an accompanying symptom among workers with NIHL. In a study of 647 noise-exposed workers confirmed as suffering from NIHL,[41] 23% complained of tinnitus. The tinnitus was bilateral in 42% of the cases. One third of affected workers complained that it affected daily activities such as telephone conversation and sleep. Cases of NIHL with tinnitus were found to have higher hearing thresholds than those without tinnitus.[41] However, other studies did not document any apparent relationship between tinnitus and severity of hearing loss.[54]

Vestibular dysfunction and noise exposure. Does noise cause a vestibular dysfunction? Several reports have studied the association between noise exposure and hearing loss, and vestibular and balance dysfunction.[26,27,49,56] The findings of 22 men with NIHL and 21 controls showed a symmetric, subclinical, and centrally compensated decrease in the vestibular end-organ response among the NIHL subjects.[49]

However, it is recognized that temporary vestibular symptoms may arise from exposure to high noise levels (the Tullio phenomenon). Some authorities feel that the symptoms do not persist after removal from noise exposure. A review by Hinchcliffe and associates[18] on noise exposure and possible vestibular malfunction concluded that such damage is possible, but the evidence is not strong enough to regard it as probable.

Risk factors and interactions. The most significant risk factor for NIHL is, of course, exposure to noise. The occupational health legislation of many countries specifies levels of 80 dB or even 85 dB as hazardous levels at which

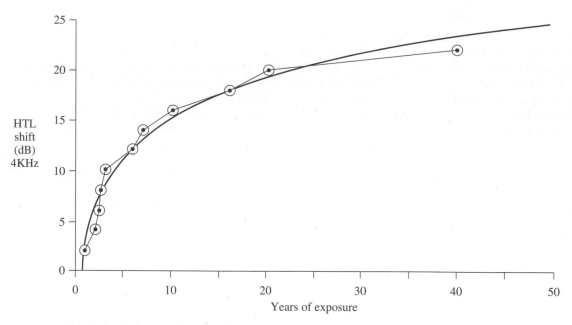

Fig. 54-8 Hearing loss as a function of years of exposure to noise (90 dBA) for the 5% most sensitive individuals. (From Australasian Faculty of Occupational Medicine and Australian Association of Audiologists in Private Practice: *Hearing surveillance in the workplace,* 1993.)

measures must be taken to protect workers' hearing. As to what is a "safe" level for hearing, a recent consensus conference on noise and hearing loss[35] agreed that a sound environment below 75 dB was not harmful.

Thus, at levels above 75 dB, damage to hearing can potentially occur. The degree of damage and the progression of the damage depend on several factors, including the sound level, the length of exposure, and individual susceptibility. Above a level of 140 dB, a single sound may produce permanent damage.

Solvent exposure. Some drugs and industrial solvents are recognized to be ototoxic. Recent studies have indicated that noise exposure combined with exposure to drugs or industrial solvents may produce more hearing loss that would be expected from a simple summation of individual effects.[37]

A study of the audiometric results of noise- and solvent-exposed workers[34] showed interaction between noise and toluene exposure. Compared to a nonexposed group of 50 workers, 50 noise-exposed workers had a relative risk (RR) of 4, 39 noise- and mixed solvent–exposed workers had an RR of 5, and 51 noise- and toluene-exposed workers had an RR of 11 for the risk of hearing loss.

The Copenhagen male study of 3284 male workers aged 53 to 74 years[25] reported that an exposure to solvents (of 5 years or more) among men not exposed to occupational noise was associated with an increased risk (RR 1.4, 95% CI 1.1-1.9) of self-assessed hearing problems. Occupational exposure to noise for 5 years or more had a greater effect than that of solvents RR 1.9 (95% CI 1.7-2.1). Among men

exposed to both solvents and noise, the effect of noise dominated, and no additional effect from solvents was noted.

Diabetes. It is believed that the vascular and metabolic changes caused by diabetes may increase the risk of cochlea damage from noise exposure. However, the results of studies have been conflicting.[20,23,54] Most occupational physicians do not believe that the evidence is strong enough to justify the exclusion of diabetic workers from noisy work.

Smoking. The role of smoking in increasing the risk of NIHL is another risk factor that has been studied.[8,11] While smokers were experimentally shown to experience a smaller temporary threshold shift than nonsmokers, the long-term effect of smoking on hearing loss was found to be in the other direction. Smokers have been reported to have a slightly higher risk for NIHL and a greater permanent hearing loss than nonsmokers in several studies.[8,11,54] This is believed to be due to cardiovascular changes resulting from smoking.

Other risk factors. Other studies have investigated various possible risk factors for NIHL, ranging from hyperlipoproteinemia, atherogenic diet, and eye color.[54]

Nonauditory Effects of Noise

Cardiovascular system. Is noise exposure associated with hypertension and other cardiovascular effects? A possible mechanism of action is the increased stress response to noise, as noise acts as a nonspecific stressor on humans. The resulting increase in adrenocortical hormones leads to an increased heart rate, high blood pressure, and eventually other cardiovascular diseases. The effects of noise on cardiovascular health have been studied among the general population exposed to environmental traffic and aircraft noise, as well as occupational groups exposed to higher levels of noise.

A review of the health effects of aircraft noise on the general population[45] concluded that there was sufficient evidence to show that noise from low-level flights was harmful to human health. The more important consequences were felt to be "stress-mediated physiologic effects, especially cardiovascular ones, and psychologic effects, particularly among children," rather than the effects on hearing acuity.

A large-scale study, the Speedwell study on the effects of traffic noise exposure and risk factors for ischemic heart disease among 2348 men aged 45 to 63 years, found significant associations between noise and potential ischemic heart disease risk factors, including increased total triglycerides, platelet count, and plasma viscosity. However, not all results supported the hypothesis that traffic noise increased the risk of ischemic heart disease, as noise exposure was significantly associated with decreased systolic and diastolic blood pressures.[7] Statistical analysis in the Caerphilly and Speedwell studies revealed a marginally increased risk of ischemic heart disease (RR 1.1) among men exposed to the highest noise levels (Leq, 6-22h = 66-70 dB[A]) compared to those exposed to the lowest noise (Leq, 6-22h = 51-55 dB[A]). However, the observed incidence of major ischemic heart disease over a 4-year period was lower (RR = 0.8) among men exposed to the highest noise.[8]

Among noise-exposed workers, a cross-sectional study of 2124 males with prolonged exposure to occupational noise showed no difference in systolic or diastolic blood pressure among workers exposed to 85 to 115 dB, those exposed to less than 85 dB noise levels, and office workers.[19] As expected, hearing loss prevalence in the group with the highest noise exposure was higher (16.5%) than in the group with lower noise exposure (7.5%) and the office workers (2.8%). The blood pressure of workers with hearing loss was similar to those with normal hearing.

Other studies have provided contrary results. A cross-sectional study of 1101 female textile mill workers in Beijing showed that noise exposure was a significant determinant of prevalence of hypertension.[57] Another study of 245 retirees with noise exposure of over 30 years[52] found that severe noise-induced hearing loss was an independent predictor of hypertension among older (aged 64 to 68 years) workers but not younger workers (56 to 63 years). Yet another cross-sectional study of 7901 subjects, 432 of whom were exposed to noise at work (more than 85 dBA) showed elevated blood pressure among exposed subjects.[31] The elevated blood pressure was no longer observed after adjustment for age, body mass index, and alcohol intake. However, taking the duration of exposure into account, the prevalence of hypertension increased for workers with prolonged exposure to noise (longer than 25 years), even after statistically

adjusting for the effects of age, body mass index, and alcohol. Noise exposure and hearing loss was associated with mean blood pressure and hypertension among 119 black workers but not among 150 white workers in an automobile assembly plant.[53]

Studies looking at the relationship between noise exposure and cardiovascular disorders face the difficulty that aging is simultaneously associated with increased degrees of hypertension and cardiovascular disease, noise exposure, NIHL, and presbyacusis. Many of the studies also lacked a nonexposed comparison group and had inadequate measures of noise exposure among the noise-exposed groups. As can be seen, the results of several studies on the subject, both population based and on occupationally noise-exposed groups, have been conflicting.

Subjective and behavioral effects of noise. Annoyance, irritation, a lowering of performance level, and sometimes even altered behavior to others may result from noise exposure. The extent and severity of these effects may be dependent on the sound levels, the frequencies generated, the exposure duration, the temporal variability, and the signal-to-noise ratio of the noise exposure.

In a review of subjective and psychophysiologic responses to noise and the effects of noise on performance among persons occupationally exposed to moderate intensity noise, it was concluded that, in many respects, research presented a rather inconsistent picture of these effects.[28] The reviewer felt that these nonauditory effects of noise may be serious enough to warrant as much attention in the occupational setting as in residential settings.

Noise and pregnancy. The critical period for damage to the cochlea of the fetus is the third trimester of pregnancy. Some amount of noise attenuation is provided by maternal tissues,[30] but this varies with the frequencies. A study of sound levels in the human uterus[43] indicated that low-frequency sounds (0.125 kHz) generated outside the mother were actually enhanced. A gradual increase in attenuation was noted with increasing frequencies, with a maximum attenuation of 10 dB at 4 kHz.

Therefore, the fetus is also exposed to environmental noise and may also be at risk for NIHL. A study of 131 children showed that those whose mothers were exposed to noise levels of 85 to 95 dBA for 8 hours were three times more likely to suffer high-frequency hearing loss than those whose mothers were exposed to lower noise levels.[30] A significant increase in the risk of hearing loss at 4 kHz was noted when the exposures involved a strong component of low-frequency noise.

Noise may also have other effects on the course and outcome of pregnancy. Experimental noise exposure (15 minutes of white noise at 90 dB) was found not to affect heart rate, arterial pressures, stress hormones, and uterine blood flow in normotensive and hypertensive pregnant women.[14]

With regard to adverse pregnancy outcomes, noise-exposed mothers were not found to be at increased risk for threatened abortion. However, the risk of pregnancy-induced hypertension was found to be increased among noise-exposed shift workers. The duration of pregnancy was also found to be shorter.[40] Noise, however, is unlikely to be an important environmental teratogen.[29]

Noise and accidents. There is evidence to suggest that noise can cause accidents. There are reports of accidents specifically caused by noise, such as the collapse of a motorway viaduct that killed three persons and injured several others (warning shouts were drowned out by the noise of concrete pumps and vibrators), a worker who lost his hand in a machine and did not receive any help because his screams were not heard above the loud noise, and a railway worker who did not hear an alarm while standing near a noisy machine and was fatally struck by a train.[55]

In addition, some cross-sectional studies have shown an association between noisy work areas and increased accident rates. Other studies have found reductions in accident rates with the introduction of a hearing conservation program. While these studies do not provide conclusive evidence, the findings offer suggestive evidence that noise can be a contributory factor in accidents.[55]

There are various possible ways by which noise can contribute to accidents. Noise can cause lack of attention among workers, and noise can mask auditory signals such as warning shouts, sirens, or machinery sounds that may indicate impending danger. Workers with NIHL can also have further difficulties in hearing warning signals and communication, especially when hearing protection is worn.

DIAGNOSIS OF NOISE-INDUCED HEARING LOSS
Patient History and Physical Examination

Details of the patient history to be elicited should include any complaints of hearing impairment or tinnitus and their duration. The history of both occupational and social noise exposure and any previous military history and exposure to gunfire noise should be documented. Noise exposures should be quantified in terms of general noise levels, the type and frequency of the noise, the exposure pattern during a typical work cycle, and the total duration of exposure. The job titles, type of work performed, type of industry in which the patient worked, and use of hearing protectors may offer some insight into the noise exposures. Social noise exposure may take the form of exposure to loud music, domestic machinery, transport vehicles, noisy hobbies, or hunting.

The patient's past medical history, including previous injuries, illnesses, history of medication and drug ingestion, and history of any otologic disease, should also be recorded. The presence of a positive family history of hearing impairment or otologic disease may be a significant factor. Details and results of previous otologic or audiometric examinations should also be asked for.

The physical examination should focus particular attention on a careful examination of the ear, nose, and throat, including otoscopic examination for abnormalities and removal of ear wax or other debris if needed. Examination of eye reflexes and observation for nystagmus may be necessary. The details of how to perform a physical examination of the ear, nose, and throat can be found in general ear, nose, and throat textbooks.

A case history. Figures 54-9 and 54-10 show two audiograms of a 43-year-old military pilot that are fairly typical of NIHL. The initial audiogram in 1983 (Fig. 54-9) already showed a pattern of bilateral high-frequency hearing loss due to aircraft noise exposure. The second audiogram in 1994 (Fig. 54-10) indicates a mild deterioration over a period of 10 years. The pilot still flies regularly with proper hearing protection.

Audiometry

Several types of audiometric assessment can be performed,[4] including:

1. Screening audiometry, in which pass-fail criteria for hearing thresholds are predetermined for given frequencies, such as 20 dB at 500 Hz to 4 kHz
2. Threshold audiometry, in which an averaging of responses is used to obtain a single threshold at a given frequency, with masking procedures if required
3. Diagnostic audiometry, in which thresholds are determined for air and bone conduction with application of masking procedures if there is an interaural difference of at least 40 dB in hearing threshold
4. Cortical evoked response audiometry, in which the ear is stimulated externally and the electrical activity of the brain is recorded to determine the hearing threshold
5. Brainstem response audiometry, in which acoustic nerve conduction is measured along the neural pathways to enable the site of the lesion to be determined

In addition, other tests for hearing, such as speech audiometry, are also available.

Protocol for Audiometric Assessment

A proposed protocol[4] for audiometric assessment is as follows:

1. There should be a quiet period of at least 16 hours before audiometric assessment to allow for recovery from any possible temporary threshold shift. If necessary, this may be achieved by the use of appropriate hearing protection while the patient performs work duties.
2. The ambient noise levels (in the audiometric test booth) for audiometric noise testing must not exceed prescribed limits at given frequencies.
3. The equipment (audiometer) must comply with prescribed standards in terms of facilities and regularity of calibration.
4. The threshold determination method must follow a specific standard technique, such as AS 1269 (Australian Standard AS 1269 (1989) Acoustics, Hearing Conservation Standards, Sydney).

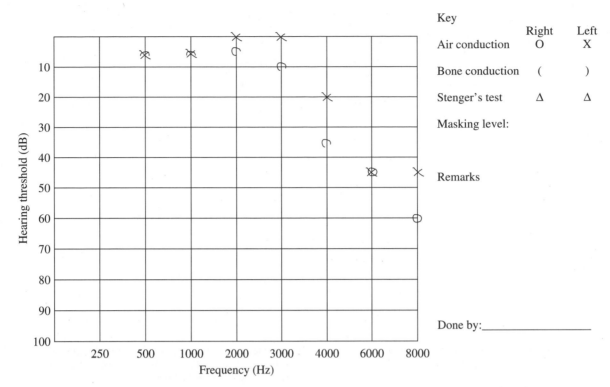

Fig. 54-9 Audiogram in 1983. (Courtesy Dr. R. Tan, Singapore.)

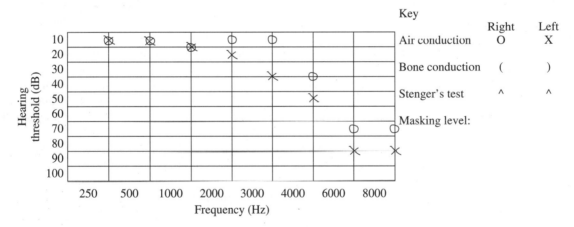

Fig. 54-10 Audiogram in 1994. (Courtesy of Dr. R. Tan, Singapore.)

5. Both ears should be inspected otoscopically to exclude any condition that would interfere with reliable testing. Persons performing these otoscopic examinations should be able to detect wax or debris, occlusion, significant infective conditions, or other coincidental pathology. It is also necessary to identify the presence of tinnitus. Referral for assessment of the nature and extent of tinnitus is needed when the audiometrist or other employee assesses the condition to be a significant handicap.

6. Preemployment or baseline audiometric assessment should include the frequencies 0.5 to 8 kHz in both ears. If hearing thresholds are equal to or greater than 25 dB at 3, 4, or 6 kHz in either ear, referral to audiologic or medical personnel is indicated. This is for evaluation of potential risk for further hearing impairment as well as for evaluation of fitness for carrying out work duties.

7. Monitoring audiometry for noise-exposed workers should include the frequencies 3 to 6 kHz in both ears, and testing should be done every 2 years. If no change occurs over two subsequent tests and noise exposure remains constant, further testing at 5-year intervals and at cessation of employment should be carried out.

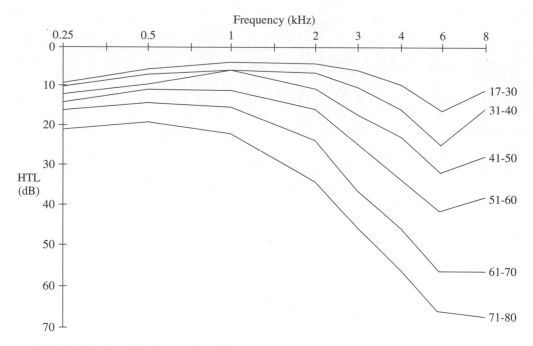

Fig. 54-11 Predicted hearing thresholds for men in nonmanual occupations. Each line represents the mean for the age band shown in the figure. (From Lutman ME, Spencer HS: Occupational noise and demographic factors in hearing, *Acta Otolaryngol Suppl (Stockh)* 476:74, 1991.)

8. Referral for audiologic opinion is indicated when either (a) hearing thresholds vary by 15 dB or more at 3, 4, and 6 kHz in either ear from the most recent previous test and no previous specialist opinion has been sought or (b) hearing thresholds at any point exceed 45 dB and no previous specialist opinion has been sought. Medical opinion should be sought by the audiologist if it is necessary to establish the likely cause of the hearing loss and the risk for further deterioration.

9. Reporting of the results should be done verbally at the time of testing and subsequently in writing.

Diagnostic Dilemmas

A thorough occupational history that documents prolonged exposure to hazardous levels of noise and a clinical examination and audiometric assessment that demonstrate a bilateral sensorineural hearing loss affecting the high frequencies can often confirm the diagnosis of NIHL. An assessment of the workplace and noise exposure measurements document noise exposure levels and offer further supportive evidence for the diagnosis.

However, the results of the history, examination, audiometric tests, and workplace assessment may sometimes not be conclusive. Often serial audiometric assessments may be required; occasionally, objective hearing tests may have to be performed.

Other causes of bilateral high-frequency sensorineural hearing loss have also to be considered in the differential diagnosis. This may range from presbyacusis to viral infections, ototoxic drugs, and other causes. At times, the clinical finding of a noise-exposed worker may be of a hearing impairment with a pattern different from that of a classical bilateral high-frequency sensorineural hearing loss. This may indicate that the hearing impairment may not be solely due to noise exposure.

Other causes of high-frequency sensorineural hearing loss. There are other causes of high-frequency sensorineural hearing loss that may mimic the audiometric findings of NIHL.

Presbyacusis. Hearing deteriorates with age. The effect of presbyacusis has to be taken into account in the assessment of the hearing thresholds of noise-exposed workers. In presbyacusis, the affected hearing thresholds are often at the high frequencies and the hearing loss is a sensorineural hearing loss. In fact, an international standard, ISO 7029, exists to describe the expected hearing thresholds as a function of age for otologically normal persons.

The hearing pattern in the different age groups in a typical population, as opposed to a stringently selected population of otologically normal persons, is characterized by an "excess aging" effect of between 10 to 15 years. In a study of a typical population that excluded persons with material conductive impairment,[32] the hearing thresholds of non–noise-exposed males in nonmanual occupational groups clearly showed an increase in hearing thresholds with age, the effect being more marked at the higher frequencies (Fig. 54-11).

Viral infections. Viral infections, especially upper respiratory tract viral infections, may be accompanied by hearing loss, tinnitus, and vestibular dysfunction. The hearing loss may be either temporary or permanent and may have a variety of patterns, including a 4 kHz dip. Rubella, mumps, measles, herpes, and other viral infections have also been known to cause such a hearing loss.

Ototoxic drugs. Well-recognized ototoxic drugs are streptomycin, the aminoglycoside antibiotics such as gentamicin and kanamycin, diuretics such as furosemide, and other drugs such as aspirin and quinine. The ototoxic effects are potentiated if excretion of the drugs is impaired, such as in renal failure. Under normal circumstances, high doses of ototoxic drugs, administered over prolonged periods, are required for ototoxic effects to be manifested. The hearing loss is often a high-frequency sensorineural hearing loss. Profound hearing loss may also be encountered.

Other conditions. Sensorineural hearing loss may occasionally result from a head injury. The hearing loss may vary from a 4 kHz dip following a mild concussion, to total deafness following a fracture of the cochlea.

Other conditions, such as a familial type of hearing loss, acoustic neuroma (which usually produces asymmetric hearing loss), or multiple sclerosis, could also present with hearing loss of different patterns, including a high tone sensorineural hearing loss.

Other patterns of hearing loss. Other patterns of hearing loss may indicate that factors other than noise may be responsible for the hearing impairment. For example, a conductive hearing loss is not caused by prolonged exposure to excessive noise, although it may be occupational in origin, such as barotrauma or other traumatic injury to the external or middle ear.

However, mixed conductive and sensorineural hearing loss suggests that the cause of the hearing impairment may not solely be due to noise exposure. A finding of profound sensorineural unilateral hearing loss with normal hearing in the other ear is also not likely to be compatible with a diagnosis of NIHL. Finally, variable and inconsistent audiometric findings may suggest functional or nonorganic hearing loss. Objective audiometric assessments may be required in such instances.

MANAGEMENT

At present, there is little that can be done to treat NIHL. The condition is irreversible and can be progressive if noise exposure is not curtailed. As such, the removal or protection of the worker from further exposure to hazardous noise levels should be part of the management of NIHL. Audiologic rehabilitation, including counseling and the provision of the appropriate hearing aids, can benefit persons suffering from NIHL.[17]

The use of hearing protection reduces both signal and noise equally but may alter the spectrum of noise reaching the ear and may also reduce ability to identify the direction of the noise source. This may interfere with the worker's ability to hear warning signals. One solution is to increase the signal-noise ratio of warning signals at work and perhaps to alter the frequency spectrum of warning signals. The use of visual signals to supplement auditory warning signals is another possibility.

Fitness for Work

There are generally very few occupations in which persons with hearing impairment have a severe enough hearing loss to be deemed unfit for employment.[50] However, some jobs, such as radio or sonar operators, have highly specific hearing requirements.

Compensation

Many countries have a workers' compensation scheme that allows persons suffering from NIHL to claim disability benefits. However, the laws in different countries prescribe different methods of evaluating the hearing loss and different criteria for impairment. Such laws are also reviewed and modified periodically. Even within a country such as the United States, there are different compensation schemes for NIHL in the different states.[33]

In general, compensation is payable for confirmed cases of NIHL with a documented history of noise exposure if hearing loss due to other causes has been excluded or adjusted for. The average hearing thresholds of both ears at the 0.5, 1, 2, and 3 kHz frequencies are usually considered in the final evaluation. In some countries or states, some adjustment may also be made for the effects of presbyacusis.

Repeated and careful testing of hearing ability may be necessary to establish the true hearing level. This is because some persons who claim for compensation for NIHL may be motivated to exaggerate their hearing loss in order to increase the claim amount. The cost per claim between 1979 and 1983 in Canada was estimated to be around $14,000.[3]

PREVENTION

As NIHL is irreversible, the approach to the problem of noise at the workplace is to control its levels and prevent the occurrence of NIHL. This can be achieved by a hearing conservation program. Several practical guides for the implementation of such a program are available.[36,38]

Hearing Conservation Program

The aim of a hearing conservation program (HCP) is to control the noise hazard in the work environment and to prevent NIHL. Noisy workplaces are required to have HCPs by federal and state occupational safety and health agencies, and companies failing to comply with the appropriate regulations are liable to citations and fines.[36] A successful HCP requires not only management commitment but also the enthusiastic support of all workers.

A senior manager should be responsible for the formulation of the hearing conservation policy and the overall supervision of the HCP. A written HCP policy should be

---

Essential Components of a Hearing Conservation Program

Noise exposure monitoring
Engineering and administrative controls
Hearing protection devices
Audiometric evaluation
Education and motivation
Record keeping
Program evaluation

From NIOSH: *A practical guide to effective hearing conservation programs in the workplace,* Publ No 90-120. Washington, DC, 1990, US Dept of Health and Human Services.

prepared to confirm the company's commitment to the program and to identify persons responsible for various components of the HCP. The essential components of a HCP are outlined in the box above.

Noise exposure monitoring. Noise exposure monitoring is needed to characterize and assess the hazard present. Its objectives are to determine whether hazards to hearing exist, to identify employees for inclusion in the HCP, to evaluate specific noise sources for noise control purposes, and to evaluate the noise control efforts.

A sound level meter is required for measuring steady-state noise, while a noise dose meter or an integrating or averaging sound level meter is needed to measure nonsteady noise (noise levels that fluctuate by more than 6 dBA). A true peak sound level meter is needed to measure impact noise.

Adequate samples should be taken, and the measurements taken should reasonably reflect typical production cycles. Results of noise levels should be properly recorded, and reported to the HCP implementer and employees in a clear and understandable manner.

A checklist of questions recommended by NIOSH to ensure that noise measurement is adequately performed includes the following:

Were the essential/critical noise studies performed?

Was the purpose of each noise study clearly stated? Have noise-exposed employees been notified of their exposures and apprised of auditory risks?

Are the results routinely transmitted to supervisors and other key individuals?

Are results entered into the health or medical records of noise-exposed employees?

Are results entered into shop folders?

If noise maps exist, are they used by the proper staff?

Are noise measurement results considered when procuring new equipment? Modifying the facility? Relocating employees?

Have there been changes in areas, equipment, or processes that have altered noise exposure? Have follow-up noise measurements been conducted?

Are appropriate steps taken to include (or exclude) employees in the HCP whose exposures have changed significantly?

Engineering and administrative controls. The noise hazard can be controlled at its source, along the pathway of its transmission, or at the site of the receiver. Engineering measures can be utilized to control noise emissions at the source. The pathway of sound transmission can be disrupted with enclosures or acoustic barriers or by the installation of sound-absorbing materials. The pathway can also be made longer by increasing the distance between the source and the receiver. Personal protective devices, regulation of exposure times, and work in an isolation booth are some measures to control the noise hazard at the level of the receiver.

Engineering controls should begin with employers specifying low noise levels for new equipment. Employees should learn to operate and maintain their machines to take full advantage of noise controls. Regular and proper maintenance to replace or adjust worn or loose machine parts or mufflers and lubrication of machine parts ensure that noise levels are kept at reasonable levels. For very noisy operations, substitution of machines or processes may have to be considered, such as hydraulic for mechanical presses, rotating shears for square shears, compression for impact welding, and pressing for rolling or forging.

Administrative controls, such as work scheduling to reduce work time in noisy processes and the provision of relatively quiet canteen and rest areas, can help in reducing noise exposures. Signs should be posted at noisy areas to inform workers of the noise hazard and to remind them that hearing protection should be worn. A checklist of questions to determine the adequacy of engineering and administrative controls[36] should include the following:

Have noise control needs been prioritized?

Has the cost-effectiveness of various options been addressed?

Are employees and supervisors apprised of plans for noise control measures? Consulted on various approaches?

Will in-house resources or outside consultants perform the work?

Have employees and supervisors been counseled on the operation and maintenance of noise control devices?

Are noise control projects monitored to ensure timely completion?

Has the full potential for administrative controls been evaluated? Are noisy processes conducted during shifts with fewer employees? Do employees have sound-treated lunch or break areas?

Hearing protection devices. Noise should ideally be controlled at its source or along its pathway of transmission. However, personal protective devices may be needed before noise levels are successfully reduced by engineering methods or when engineering methods are not feasible or practical.

Earplugs and ear muffs are the common types of hearing protection. The choice of hearing protection depends on several factors, such as the noise reduction rating of the hearing protector (at least 20 dBA for earplugs and 30 dBA for ear muffs), the noise exposure levels (earplugs if less than 100 dBA, ear muffs for levels up to 120 dBA, and both earplugs and ear muffs for levels at or above 120 dBA), and the comfort and fit of the protectors. It should be noted that, in most cases, the attenuations provided by hearing protectors at the workplace are less, and the standard deviations greater, than those quoted by the manufacturers from laboratory tests.[15]

Earplugs can be worn with spectacles and other headgear and can be either disposable or nondisposable. The disposable plugs are relatively comfortable to wear and fit all ear canal sizes. Nondisposable earplugs are available in different shapes and sizes, and the right size should be selected to fit the ear canal of the user. The correct method of using the earplug is to pull the pinna back and upward and then to insert the earplug in the ear canal.

Ear muffs tend to be more uncomfortable to wear, particularly in hot work environments, and are more expensive. However, ear muffs offer a greater noise reduction rating. They can also be easily worn and removed and are thus more convenient for situations where noise exposure is intermittent.

Hearing protection devices should be properly maintained and replaced when there is cracking or loss of shape and proper fit due to normal wear and tear. Workers should also wear the protection at all times in noisy areas. Using the protectors for part of the time offers only limited protection from the risk of developing NIHL. Regular inspections should be performed to ensure that workers use hearing protectors at noisy work areas. Those not wearing the hearing protection should be counseled and encouraged to use the protective devices.

The following checklist of questions should be considered to determine if the hearing protection device component of the HCP is successful.[36]

Have hearing protectors been made available to all employees whose daily average noise exposures are 85 dBA or above?

Are employees given a variety of protectors from which to choose?

Are employees fitted carefully with special attention to comfort?

Are employees thoroughly trained, not only initially, but at least once a year?

Are the protectors checked regularly for wear or defects and replaced immediately if necessary?

If employees use disposable hearing protectors, are replacements readily available?

Do employees understand the appropriate hygiene requirements?

Have any employees developed ear infections or irritation associated with the use of hearing protectors? Are there any employees who are unable to wear these devices because of medical conditions? Have these conditions been treated properly?

Have alternative types of hearing protectors been considered when problems with current devices are experienced?

Do employees who incur noise-induced hearing loss receive intensive counseling?

Are those who fit and supervise the wearing of hearing protectors competent to deal with the many problems that can occur?

Do workers complain that protectors interfere with their ability to do their jobs? Do they interfere with spoken instructions or warning signals? Are these complaints followed promptly with counseling, noise control, or other measures?

Are employees encouraged to take their hearing protectors home if they engage in noisy nonoccupational activities?

Are new types of protectors considered as they become available?

Is the effectiveness of the hearing protector program evaluated regularly?

Supervisor involvement

Have supervisors been provided with the knowledge required to supervise their subordinates' use and care of hearing protectors?

Do supervisors wear hearing protectors in appropriate areas?

Have supervisors been counseled when employees resist wearing protectors or fail to show up for hearing tests?

Are disciplinary actions enforced when employees repeatedly refuse to wear hearing protectors?

Audiometric evaluation. In many countries, noise-exposed workers are required to undergo periodic statutory medical examinations that include otologic and audiometric examinations. Audiometric evaluations are the means to determine if the HCP is successful and if NIHL is being prevented.

The audiograms have to be properly performed by trained audiometric technicians on calibrated audiometers and in audiometric booths with background noise sufficiently low to conform to acceptable standards. Pretesting instructions are important. Workers have to be instructed to avoid noise exposure for at least 16 hours before the test in order to minimize temporary threshold shift.

Audiometric testing includes air conduction testing and bone conduction testing if abnormal results occur at 4 kHz or below. A repeat audiogram may be necessary. Results should be compared to previous audiograms, if available. The worker should be informed of the results, counseled, and followed up when appropriate. The use of the following checklist is helpful to ensure that monitoring audiometry and record keeping are adequate.[36]

Has the audiometric technician been adequately trained, certified, and recertified as necessary?

Do on-the-job observations of the technicians indicate that they perform a thorough and valid audiometric test, instruct and consult the employee effectively, and keep appropriate records?

Are records complete? Are follow-up actions documented?

Are hearing threshold levels reasonably consistent from test to test? If not, are the reasons for the inconsistencies investigated promptly?

Are the annual test results compared to baseline to identify the presence of an OSHA standard threshold shift?

Is the annual incidence of standard threshold shift greater than a few percent? If so, are problem areas pinpointed and remedial steps taken?

Are audiometric trends (deteriorations) identified, both in individuals and in groups of employees?

Do records show that appropriate audiometer calibration procedures have been followed?

Is there documentation showing that the background sound levels in the audiometer room were low enough to permit valid testing?

Are the results of audiometric tests being communicated to supervisors and managers as well as to employees?

Has corrective action been taken if the rate of no-shows for audiometric test appointments is more than about 5%?

Are employees incurring standard threshold shift (STS) notified in writing within 21 days?

Referrals

Are referral procedures clearly specified?

Have letters of agreement between the company and consulting physicians or audiologists been executed?

Have mechanisms been established to ensure that employees needing evaluation or treatment actually receive the service, such as transportation, scheduling reminders?

Are records properly transmitted to the physician or audiologist and back to the company?

If medical treatment is recommended, does the employee understand the condition requiring treatment, the recommendation, and methods of obtaining such treatment?

Are employees being referred unnecessarily?

Education and motivation. A successful HCP requires the cooperative efforts of both management and employees. It is important to educate both on the hazards of noise, its control, and benefits of the HCP. Education and training should begin once the employee starts work and be a continuous process.

The HCP coordinator should be committed and motivated to ensure the success of the program. Workers and management should raise concerns and unresolved issues pertaining to the HCP to the coordinator, and all problems should be promptly addressed. An education and training checklist could have the following questions:[36]

Has training been conducted at least once a year?

Was the training provided by a qualified instructor?

Was the success of each training program evaluated?

Is the content revised periodically?

Are managers and supervisors directly involved?

Are posters, regulations, handouts, and employee newsletters used as supplements?

Are personal counseling sessions conducted for employees having problems with hearing protection devices or showing hearing threshold shifts?

Record keeping. Record keeping is an integral part of the HCP. If done properly, it is a valuable means to evaluate the effectiveness of the HCP. In many countries, proper record keeping is required by labor law. Various kinds of records need to be kept. Noise survey forms, medical histories, and audiogram results should be standardized, well maintained, and cross-referenced. Management needs to provide adequate resources for record processing, review, and storage. Confidentiality of medical records is another issue to be addressed.

Program evaluation. Every program for prevention needs to be continuously evaluated, and the HCP is no exception. Progress and activity reports should be prepared by the HCP coordinator. There are two basic approaches to program evaluation. The first approach is to assess the completeness and quality of the program's components, for example, by using a checklist of questions such as those given in this chapter. Second, the audiometric data should be evaluated. Management and employees must be willing to provide and accept feedback, acknowledge problems if they arise, and be motivated to jointly solve the problems.

Checklist for hearing conservation program administration

Have there been any changes in federal or state regulations? Have HCP policies been modified to reflect these changes?

Are copies of company policies and guidelines regarding the HCP available in the offices that support the various program elements? Are those who implement the program elements aware of these policies?

Are necessary materials and supplies being ordered with a minimum of delay?

Are procurement officers overriding the HCP implementer's requests for specific hearing protectors or other hearing conservation equipment? If so, have corrective steps been taken?

Is the performance of key personnel evaluated periodically?

If such performance is found to be less than acceptable, are steps taken to correct the situation?

Safety: Has the failure to hear warning shouts or alarms been tied to any accidents or injuries? If so, have any remedial steps been taken?

CONCLUSION

Noise is a pervasive and ubiquitous hazard in many workplaces. Millions of persons are at risk of developing NIHL, the main health effect of noise. Its other health effects, such as those on the cardiovascular and other organ systems and as a general nonspecific stressor, as well as the role of noise in the causation of accidents, are less well studied, but nonetheless believed to be a significant burden to the population.

Knowledge on how to prevent NIHL exists. Preventive measures are often not technically difficult and are, in many instances, practically achievable. Implementing these measures would probably also reduce the occurrence of the other adverse health effects of noise. What is lacking and needed is a widespread application of the knowledge of prevention into practice. If this is attained, irreversible and needless suffering of noise-exposed workers can be minimized or avoided altogether.

REFERENCES

1. ACGIH: 1994-1995 *Threshold limit values for chemical substances and physical agents and biological exposure indices,* Cincinnati, 1994, American Conference of Governmental Industrial Hygienists.
2. Alberti PW: Noise induced hearing loss, *BMJ* 304:522, 1992.
3. Alleyne BC et al: Costs of workers' compensation claims for hearing loss, *J Occup Med* 31:134, 1989.
4. Australasian Faculty of Occupational Medicine and Australian Association of Audiologists in Private Practice: *Hearing surveillance in the workplace,* April 1993.
5. Axelsson A, Hamernik RP: Acute acoustic trauma, *Acta Otolaryngol (Stockh)* 104:225, 1987.
6. Babisch W et al: Traffic noise and cardiovascular risk: the Speedwell study, first phase. Outdoor noise levels and risk factors, *Arch Environ Health* 48:401, 1993.
7. Babisch W et al: Traffic noise and cardiovascular risk: the Caerphilly and Speedwell studies, second phase. Risk estimation, prevalence, and incidence of ischaemic heart disease, *Arch Environ Health* 48:406, 1993.
8. Barone JA et al: Smoking as a risk factor for noise induced hearing loss, *J Occup Med* 29:741, 1987.
9. Barrs DM et al: Work related, noise induced hearing loss: evaluation including evoked potential audiometry, *Otolaryngol Head Neck Surg* 110:177, 1994.
10. Beranek LL: *Noise and vibration control,* New York, 1971, McGraw-Hill.
11. Dengerink HA, Lindgren FL, Axelsson A: The interaction of smoking and noise on temporary threshold shifts, *Acta Otolaryngol (Stockh)* 112:932, 1992.
12. Environmental Protection Agency: *Information of levels of environmental noise requisite to public health and welfare with an adequate margin of safety,* Report No 550/9-74-004, Washington, DC, 1974, Environmental Protection Agency.
13. Flottorp G: Treatment of noise induced hearing loss, *Scand Audiol Suppl* 34:123, 1991.
14. Hartikainen-Sorri AL et al: No effect of experimental noise exposure on human pregnancy, *Obstet Gynecol* 77:611, 1991.
15. Hempstock TI, Hill E: The attenuations of some hearing protectors as used in the workplace, *Ann Occup Hyg* 34:453, 1990.
16. Hetu R, Quoc HT, Duguay P: The likelihood of detecting a significant threshold shift among workers subjected to annual audiometric testing, *Ann Occup Hyg* 34:361, 1990.
17. Hinchcliffe R: Sound, infrasound and ultrasound. In Raffle PAB et al, editors: *Hunter's diseases of occupations,* ed 8, London, 1994, Edward Arnold.
18. Hinchcliffe R, Coles RRA, King PF: Occupational noise induced vestibular malfunction? *Br J Ind Med* 49:63, 1992.
19. Hirai A et al: Prolonged exposure to industrial noise causes hearing loss but not high blood pressure: a study of 2124 factory labourers in Japan, *J Hypertens* 9:1069, 1991.
20. Hodgson MJ et al: Diabetes, noise exposure, and hearing loss, *J Occup Med* 29:576, 1987.
21. Irwin J: Noise induced hearing loss and the 4 kHz dip, *Occup Med* 44:222, 1994.
22. Irwin JD, Graf ER: *Industrial noise and vibration control,* Englewood Cliffs, NJ, 1979, Prentice Hall.
23. Ishii EK et al: Is NIDDM a risk factor for noise-induced hearing loss in an occupationally noise exposed cohort? *Sci Total Environ* 127:155, 1992.
24. ISO 7029 Acoustics: *Threshold of hearing by air conduction as a function of age and sex for otologically normal persons,* Geneva, 1984, International Organization for Standardization.
25. Jacobsen P et al: Mixed solvent exposure and hearing impairment: an epidemiological study of 3284 men. The Copenhagen male study, *Occup Med* 43:180, 1993.
26. Juntunen J et al: Postural body sway and exposure to high-energy impulse noise, *Lancet* 2:261, 1987.
27. Kilburn KH, Warshaw RH, Hanscom B: Are hearing loss and balance dysfunction linked in construction iron workers? *Br J Ind Med* 49:138, 1992.
28. Kjellberg A: Subjective, behavioral and psychophysiological effects of noise, *Scand J Work Environ Health* 16(Suppl 1):29, 1990.
29. Kurppa K et al: Noise exposure during pregnancy and selected structural malformations in infants, *Scand J Work Environ Health* 15:111, 1989.
30. Lalande NM, Hetu R, Lambert J: Is occupational noise exposure during pregnancy a risk factor of damage to the auditory system of the fetus? *Am J Ind Med* 10:427, 1986.
31. Lang T, Fouriaud C, Jacquinet-Salord MC: Length of occupational noise exposure and blood pressure, *Int Arch Occup Environ Health* 63:369, 1992.
32. Lutman ME, Spencer HS: Occupational noise and demographic factors in hearing, *Acta Otolaryngol Suppl (Stockh)* 476:74, 1991.
33. Melnick W, Morgan W: Hearing compensation evaluation, *Otolaryngol Clin North Am* 24:391, 1991.
34. Morata TC et al: Effects of occupational exposure to organic solvents and noise on hearing, *Scand J Work Environ Health* 19:245, 1993.
35. National Institutes of Health: *Consensus development conference statement: noise and hearing loss,* Bethesda, Md, 1990, National Institutes of Health.
36. NIOSH: *A practical guide to effective hearing conservation programs in the workplace,* Washington, DC, 1990, US Dept of Health and Human Services (NIOSH) Pub No 90-120.
37. NIOSH: A proposed national strategy for the prevention of noise induced hearing loss. In: *Proposed national strategies for the prevention of leading work-related diseases and injuries,* Part 2, Washington DC, 1988, US Government.
38. Noise and Hearing Conservation Committee, American Occupational Medical Association: Guidelines for the conduct of an occupational hearing conservation program, *J Occup Med* 29:981, 1987.
39. Noise and hearing loss, *Lancet* 338:21, 1991.
40. Nurminen T, Kurppa K: Occupational noise exposure and course of pregnancy, *Scand J Work Environ Health* 15:117, 1989.
41. Phoon WH, Lee HS, Chia SE: Tinnitus in noise-exposed workers, *Occup Med* 43:35, 1993.
42. Pilgramm M: Clinical and animal experiment studies to optimize the therapy for acute acoustic trauma, *Scand Audiol Suppl* 34:103, 1991.
43. Richards DS et al: Sound levels in the human uterus, *Obstet Gynecol* 80:186, 1992.
44. Robinson DW: The audiogram in hearing loss due to noise: a probability test to uncover other causation, *Ann Occup Hyg* 29:477, 1985.

45. Rosenberg J: Jets over Labrador and Quebec: noise effects on human health, *Can Med Assoc J* 144:869, 1991.

46. Sataloff RT, Sataloff J: *Occupational hearing loss,* ed 2, New York, 1993, Marcel Dekker.

47. Schuknecht HF: *Pathology of the ear,* ed 2, Philadelphia, 1993, Lea & Febiger.

48. Schultz TJ: Social surveys on noise annoyance—further considerations. In Tobias JV, Jansen GJ, Ward WD, editors: *Proceedings of the Third International Congress on Noise as a Public Health Problem, Sept 25-29 1978, Freiburg, Germany.* Rockville, Md, 1980, American Speech-Language-Hearing Association.

49. Shupak A et al: Vestibular findings associated with chronic noise induced hearing impairment, *Acta Otolaryngol (Stockh)* 114:579, 1994.

50. Sinclair A, Coles RRA: Hearing and vestibular disorders. In Cox RAF, Edwards FC, McCallum RI, editors: *Fitness for work: the medical aspects,* ed 2, Oxford, 1995, Oxford University Press.

51. Smith AP: The combined effects of noise, nightwork and meals on mood, *Int Arch Occup Environ Health* 63:105, 1991.

52. Talbott EO et al: Noise-induced hearing loss: a possible marker for high blood pressure in older noise exposed populations, *J Occup Med* 32:690, 1990.

53. Tarter SK, Robins TG: Chronic noise exposure, high frequency hearing loss, and hypertension among automotive assembly workers, *J Occup Med* 32:685, 1990.

54. Touma JB: Controversies in noise induced hearing loss, *Ann Occup Hyg* 36:199, 1992.

55. Wilkins PA, Acton WI: Noise and accidents: a review, *Ann Occup Hyg* 25:249, 1982.

56. Ylikoski J et al: Subclinical vestibular pathology in patients with noise induced hearing loss from intense impulse noise, *Acta Otolaryngol (Stockh)* 105:558, 1988.

57. Zhao Y et al: A dose response relation for noise induced hypertension, *Br J Ind Med* 48:179, 1991.

55

$Mg_6Si_4O_{10}(OH)_8$

Chrysotile asbestos

- Asbestos remains a significant health concern, particularly in developing countries

- Asbestos exposure may cause asbestosis, mesothelioma, lung cancer, and several benign conditions

- Two major types of asbestos exist: Amphibole and crysotile. Most commercial asbestos in the United States is crysotile

- Crysotile asbestos is cleared from the body more readily than is amphibole. Amphibole tends to accumulate and is therefore more biologically dangerous

- Eighty-five percent of individuals who develop malignant mesothelioma have had a significant environmental or occupational exposure to asbestos

- A significant latent period, often 30 years or longer, characterizes the development of mesothelioma following asbestos exposure

Asbestos

John P. Holland

Dorsett D. Smith

PHYSICAL AND CHEMICAL PROPERTIES

Many different types of fibrous minerals occur naturally, but only those of commercial usefulness are referred to as *asbestos*. *Asbestos* is the collective name for a group of hydrated silicates that are found as mineral fibers in natural rock formations. The six distinct types of asbestos each have a different chemical structure and are divided into two major groups, serpentine and amphibole asbestos (Table 55-1).

The only type of asbestos in the serpentine group is chrysotile asbestos. Chrysotile asbestos comes from serpentine rock, which is the most common form of asbestos-forming rock in the world. This accounts for the fact that 95% of the asbestos used commercially is of the chrysotile variety. It is estimated that more than 40% of the land area of the United States is composed of minerals that may contain asbestos. In particular areas of this country, such as the Serpentine Hills of California, wind erosion releases significant amounts of airborne asbestos, but there has been no evidence of any health hazard in this area.

Chrysotile asbestos is a very flexible, long, snakelike fiber, a shape that makes it ideal for weaving into cloth. It is used in the formation of gaskets, as well as for making insulation blankets. The chrysotile fiber itself does not have low thermal conductivity, but because the fibers are easily separated, they trap air between them and thus have a high insulation value. The fibers are very heat resistant and therefore have been used extensively for the purpose of fire-proofing. In addition, chrysotile has fairly high tensile strength, which allows it to be woven into cloth and makes it a useful binding agent for ceramic materials. Chrysotile

471

Table 55-1 Taxonomy of naturally occurring mineral fibers

Group	Mineral	Formula
Commercially useful fibers or asbestos		
Serpentine	Chrysotile	$Mg_3Si_2O_5(OH)_4$
Amphibole	Amosite	$(Fe,Mg)_7Si_8O_{22}(OH)_2$
	Anthophyllite	$(Mg,Fe)_7Si_8O_{22}(OH)_2$
	Crocidolite	$Na_2Fe_3^{2+}Fe_2^{3+}Si_8O_{22}(OH)_2$
Contaminants	Actinolite	$Ca_2(Mg,Fe^{2+})_5Si_8O_{22}(OH)_2$
	Tremolite	$Ca_2(Mg,Fe)_5Si_8O_{22}(OH)_2$
Less commercially useful fibers or not asbestos		
Zeolite	Erionite	$NaK_2MgCa_{1.5}(Al_8Si_{28})O_{72} \cdot 28H_2O$
Others	Attapulgite	$(Al,Mg)_4(Si,Al)_8O_{20}(OH)_4 \cdot 2H_2O$
	Sepiolite	$(Mg,Fe)_8Si_{12}O_{30}(OH)_4 \cdot 4H_2O$
	Wollastonite	$CaSiO_3$

asbestos is not acid stable, but it is resistant to strong alkalis.

Amphibole asbestos represents a group of fibrous minerals forming needlelike fibers that have different crystalline structures and different physical properties than chrysotile. The amphibole asbestiform minerals tend to be more heat resistant than chrysotile and much more acid resistant, so they can be used in making acid-resistant filters. However, they are more vulnerable to strong alkalis. These crystalline silicates tend to form in amorphous riebeckite rock and are rich in iron. This makes them easily stainable with iron stains for lung section studies.

There are five types of amphibole asbestos: amosite, crocidolite, anthophyllite, actinolite, and tremolite. The only two that have been commercially important in the United States are amosite and crocidolite, which primarily came from mines in South Africa. In addition, tremolite has been a significant contaminant in most chrysotile asbestos mined in North America, as well as in commercial vermiculite and talc deposits in many parts of the world.

Asbestos fibers have a fixed diameter, which is dependent upon their crystalline structure, ranging from 0.01 to 3 μm. Amphiboles are straight, single, needlelike fibers that are found in natural mineral deposits stacked together with parallel orientations. In contrast, chrysotile fibers have a wavy shape, and in natural mineral deposits each chrysotile fiber is made up of concentric bundles of smaller fibrils. In natural mineral deposits, asbestos fibers have no fixed length and can be up to several centimeters long. The process of mining and milling (i.e., crushing) asbestos-bearing minerals, as well as natural weathering of minerals, tends to break the asbestos fibers into a variety of shorter lengths.[45]

HISTORICAL PERSPECTIVE
Production and Uses

Because of its unique physical properties, asbestos has had a wide variety of uses over the years. Asbestos fibers have been used in ceramics because of their strengthening properties. The earliest use of asbestos was probably in Finland, where indigenous anthophyllite asbestos was used to make clay pots as early as 2000 BC. At a later time, Charlemagne was said to use a tablecloth of asbestos that he threw into the fireplace to impress his guests. Marco Polo was said to have brought back asbestos products from the Orient, and Ben Franklin carried a purse made of asbestos that was often referred to as *salamander skin*. The term *asbestos* comes from the Greek and means "unquenchable."

With the advent of the industrial age and the invention of the steam engine, commercial applications rapidly developed for this easily available fiber. The mining of chrysotile began in Quebec in 1878, and production escalated very rapidly. By the late 1920s and early 1930s, it was required by law in the construction of certain types of ships with steam turbines and other high-temperature applications. It was also required for the fire protection of buildings as sprayed on steel beams. Asbestos was a natural product to be used for clutch and brake linings and other domestic products, such as ironing board covers, cooking mats, vinyl floor covering, ceiling tiles, wallboard, and wallboard joint compound.

All types of commercially used asbestos were used in the past as fireproofing sprayed on girders (such as in the construction of high-rise buildings), as pipe insulation, and in the form of insulating blankets over thermal structures. Because amphiboles are highly resistant to heat, amosite and crocidolite have been used preferentially for high-temperature applications such as for boiler insulation and steam lines in ships and power stations. In contrast, chrysotile asbestos has primarily been used in lower-temperature applications.

Because of its binding properties as a fiber and its resistance to chemical degradation, asbestos has been used extensively in cement pipes and cement sheeting. Its properties as a binder and as a fire retardant have also led to its use in a variety of building materials, including vinyl floor tiles, ceiling tiles, wallboard, siding, and roofing materials.

Because it can be woven into cloth, it has been used extensively in fire-retardant clothing, welding blankets, and theater curtains. It has also been used as a binder in paper. Because of their resistance to acids, amphibole fibers were used extensively for filters in chemical processes and in gas masks.[45] Industries and occupations that may be associated with significant asbestos exposures include construction, ship building, friction materials, insulation, fire proofing, and mining.

Chronology of the Recognition of Health Effects

With the increasing use of asbestos, early reports suggested there may be adverse health effects. At the turn of the century, the British inspector of factories noted that the fibers were small, needlelike, and irritating, and he suggested that it be banned.[2] The first documented case of asbestosis was reported by Murray in 1907.[38] This received very little mention until 1924, when Cooke described a better documented case that was unfortunately complicated by tuberculosis.[15] By the late 1920s, it became increasingly accepted that exposure to high concentrations of asbestos fibers caused interstitial lung disease, which was first called *asbestosis* by Cooke.[16] In 1929, the British government funded a study by Merewether and Price that found a high incidence of asbestosis in workers at British asbestos textile plants.[36] After this, asbestosis became accepted as a work-related condition in Great Britain, and studies were done in other countries to look for evidence of asbestosis. The most famous of these was the study of Dreessen in 1938, which evaluated South Carolina asbestos textile mills.[21] Dreessen was the first to suggest a threshold limit value of 5 million particles per cubic foot as a probable safe level of asbestos exposure.

Initial studies focused on workers involved in manufacturing asbestos products, and there was little evaluation of end users of asbestos products until the study by Fleischer and colleagues of American shipyard workers at the end of World War II.[24] This study found that shipyard insulators using asbestos products were often exposed to high levels of asbestos, but that average exposures were generally not above 5 million particles per cubic foot. Since very little asbestosis was found in this group, it was concluded by experts at the time that this type of work and these levels of exposures posed no significant health risks. The study has since been faulted because most of those studied had worked only a short time in the industry, not long enough for them to develop clinical asbestosis, which often has a latency period of 20 or more years. Unfortunately, this significant bias in the data tended to produce a false sense of security among health professionals in terms of risks from asbestos.

It is now recognized that the latency period for asbestos-related disease is related to both the duration and intensity of exposure as well as the fiber type and fiber size of the inhaled particles. In the asbestos textile mills studied by Merewether

and Price in 1929, some workers who had extremely heavy asbestos exposures developed significant asbestosis within 5 years of their first asbestos exposure. Similar exposures may have been common in the United States during this same time period. However, after the U.S. threshold limit value of 5 million particles per cubic foot was implemented in 1938, there was probably a significant drop in exposure levels, and the latency time from initial exposure until development of asbestosis was usually more than 20 years.

In the 1960s and 1970s, several large epidemiologic studies were published that had evaluated cohorts of workers with some of the largest historical asbestos exposures, such as shipyard insulators and asbestos textile mill workers. These studies clearly established the association between high asbestos exposures and the later development of asbestosis, lung cancer, and mesothelioma and led to more stringent regulation of asbestos exposures in the United States since the early 1970s. Some of these studies also provided quantitative data on asbestos exposure levels for the workers studied, which is the basis for most of the risk assessment models that have been used increasingly in recent years to guide government policies and regulations on asbestos. Since the 1980s, extensive scientific work has focused on trying to understand the cellular and biochemical mechanisms underlying asbestos-related diseases.

ROUTES OF EXPOSURE

Of the three routes of exposure (dermal, ingestion, and inhalation) to asbestos fibers, inhalation is responsible for most, if not all, of the serious health effects. It remains controversial whether ingestion of asbestos fibers results in adverse health effects, and dermal exposures result in only localized skin lesions.

Dermal and Ingestion Exposures

Historically, workers with a great deal of skin contact with asbestos, from handling this material with their bare hands, would sometimes develop nodular skin lesions termed *asbestos corns*. These benign lesions are a foreign body reaction from fibers embedded in the skin. No other type of dermal toxicity is associated with asbestos.[45]

Significant ingestion of asbestos fibers occurs as a part of inhalation exposures, since many inhaled asbestos fibers become trapped in respiratory mucus, which is then swallowed and passes through the gut. Breathing through the nose leads to the capture of some asbestos fibers in the mucus of the upper respiratory tract. These fibers are swallowed, along with asbestos fibers cleared from the lung by the mucocilliary elevation. Asbestos fibers are also sometimes ingested in food or drinking water (usually from water flowing over natural rock formations).

Ingested asbestos fibers appear to pass through the gut essentially unchanged and without significant systemic absorption. There is evidence that asbestos fibers can become embedded in the intestinal wall (such as in the cecum). Whether ingested asbestos fibers result in adverse health effects remains controversial.

Some studies have shown increased rates of colon cancer in cohorts of workers with high asbestos exposures. However, several other studies have not shown higher rates of colon cancer in cohorts or workers with documented asbestos-related pulmonary problems. A recent meta-analysis of epidemiologic studies investigating the relationship between asbestos exposure and colon cancer found no significant association between even very high levels of asbestos exposure and colon cancer. Studies of populations where the drinking water contains asbestos fibers have not shown increased rates of colon cancer.[28]

How Fibers Enter the Lung

Inhalation of asbestos fibers into the lungs is by far the most important route of exposure, accounting for most, if not all, adverse health effects associated with asbestos. While some inhaled asbestos fibers are captured in the mucus of the upper respiratory tract, a large percentage of fibers stay entrained in inhaled air and enter the lungs.

For a person who is breathing through the nose, almost all spherical particles over 10 μm in diameter are captured in the mucus of the upper respiratory tract and do not enter the lungs. However, fibers such as asbestos have aerodynamic properties that tend to keep many of them entrained in the airstream during inhalation so that a large proportion of longer fibers (some up to 20 μm in length) enter the lungs, as do many of the smaller fibers.

One reason such a large proportion of inhaled fibers enter the lung is the very small size of these fibers, with fiber diameters ranging from 0.01 to 3 μm. Because of the crystalline structure of the fibers, they break at various lengths. Electron microscope analysis shows the majority of fibers in most airborne asbestos samples are very short fibers under 5 μm in length, but fibers up to 100 μm long can be found in lung tissue samples.

Another reason a large proportion of asbestos fibers travel deep into the lung has to do with the concept of settling time and the aerodynamic properties of fibers. In the perfectly still air of an enclosed experimental chamber, fibers settle at a rate inversely proportional to the fiber diameter. In such a chamber, the mean settling time of asbestos fibers with a diameter of 0.1 μm is several hours. This very long settling time for asbestos fibers has two significant implications for exposed individuals: First, a person passing through a room where there are loose asbestos fibers settled on the floor probably provides enough air turbulence to entrain any settled asbestos dust into the air to create potential inhalation exposures. Second, once these fibers are airborne, it requires many hours of perfectly still air for them to settle. Therefore, in assessing the potential for occupational exposures, any loose asbestos fibers (such as in dust on the floor) can be assumed to present a potential inhalation exposure.

The Importance of Fiber Size

Traditionally, industrial hygiene monitoring for particulates has used cyclone devices to determine a respirable fraction (i.e., exposures to particles less than 10 μm in diameter that would bypass the filter of the nose). However, identification of such a respirable fraction is not meaningful in evaluating asbestos exposures because fibers stay airborne much longer than spherical particles of equal mass, as noted previously, so even long asbestos fibers may be inhaled into the lungs. Therefore, industrial hygiene monitoring of asbestos exposure is based on counting fibers captured on the filter of an air pump monitoring device.

The standard industrial hygiene monitoring technique for evaluating asbestos exposures is fiber counts with phase contrast light microscopy (which has a limit of resolution of 0.5 μm). The accepted procedure with this method is to count any particle captured on the filter as a fiber if it has a diameter over 0.5 μm, a length over 5 μm, and a length to width ratio over 3:1. Since the 1970s, two new techniques, scanning electron microscopy (SEM) and transmission electron microscopy (TEM) have allowed identification of much smaller asbestos fibers. Of these two techniques, TEM is preferred because it can see all asbestos fibers, whereas SEM misses fibers with diameters less than 0.1 μm. Identification of specific asbestos fiber types in a sample requires special methods; the current preferred method is electron probe analysis (EDXA).[11]

Studies of asbestos samples using TEM suggest that historical asbestos fiber counts with phase contrast microscopy, which could identify fibers with diameters less than 0.5 μm, vastly underestimated the total asbestos fiber counts. Recent research suggests that very short asbestos fibers (less than 5.0 μm in length) do not pose significant health risks in that they appear to be effectively phagocytized by macrophages and removed from the lung. In animal studies, these very short fibers are not fibrogenic or carcinogenic.[17] Research has shown that the asbestos fibers that are most toxic in producing asbestosis and other asbestos-related lung diseases are the very thin and long fibers (known as Stanton fibers), which are less than 0.25 μm in diameter and over 8 μm long.[50]

The TEM studies have shown that samples of asbestos taken from different asbestos products or manufacturing processes can contain quite different proportions of very short asbestos fibers (which are probably benign) and thin, longer asbestos fibers (which are the most toxic for producing asbestos-related disease). For example, manufacturing of asbestos cloth appears to break asbestos into thin, longer fibers, which may explain the increased rates of lung cancer and asbestosis seen in asbestos textile workers.[19]

Unfortunately, there is not a good correlation between the number or size of asbestos fibers seen on light microscopy and the number or proportion of Stanton fibers seen on TEM analysis. This lack of correlation creates a significant problem in estimating health risks based on light microscopy fiber counts because the most pathogenic fibers (i.e., the very thin, long Stanton fibers) are not visible with this technique. It also creates difficulty in interpreting the majority of epidemiologic studies of asbestos-exposed workers, which have generally measured asbestos exposures with light microscopy fiber counts or have estimated exposures based on job duties with no direct environmental measurements.

Clearance and Persistence of Fibers in the Lung

The lung has several clearance mechanisms for removing foreign materials, and all of these aid in removing asbestos fibers to some degree. Fibers can become trapped in the mucus that lines the conducting airways of the lung and are then removed as cilia on the bronchial epithelium sweep the mucus out of the lung until it is swallowed and passes through the gut.

Fibers that escape entrapment in the mucocilliary blanket become deposited in the respiratory bronchioles and alveolar spaces. Here, several other forms of clearance of asbestos fibers come into play. Smaller asbestos fibers under 5 μm in length can be phagocytized by macrophages, where they are chemically dissolved and removed from the lungs. Longer fibers, greater than 10 μm, are incompletely phagocytized and become covered with an iron protein coat. These coated fibers stain with iron stains, are called *ferruginous bodies,* and have a birefringent appearance. This reaction is not unique to asbestos but is seen with other fibrous materials such as aluminum silicate fibers. When the protein-coated fiber is an asbestos fiber, it is called an *asbestos body.*[10] Chrysotile fibers appear to be removed by macrophages more easily than amphiboles, which some researchers suggest is caused by chemical differences that allow chrysotile fibers to be more easily dissolved by macrophages. Some smaller fibers also penetrate the alveolar epithelial cells to the interstitial spaces, where they enter the lymphatic drainage and are removed to regional lymph nodes or moved out of the lung.

Those fibers that are not cleared from the lungs (by the mucocilliary elevator, phagocytosis, or lymphatic drainage) may stay deposited in the alveoli or may migrate to the interstitial tissue. Fibers can also migrate to the pleural surface and to the peritoneum, presumably by penetrating the diaphragm; they are believed to be the stimuli for mesothelioma. Amphibole fibers are considered more toxic than chrysotile in producing both asbestosis and mesothelioma, which may be partially related to the fact that chrysotile fibers are cleared from the lungs at a greater rate than amphiboles. Some also theorize that the needlelike shape of the amphibole fibers makes them more liable to migrate to the pleural surfaces, where they somehow stimulate formation of a mesothelioma.[52]

ASBESTOS-RELATED LUNG DISEASES

There are four main types of asbestos-related lung diseases: asbestosis, asbestos-related pleural disease, lung cancer,

and mesothelioma. Based on the mechanism of disease, these disorders can be further grouped into the two categories of fibrotic diseases and neoplastic diseases. The fibrotic diseases include asbestosis (a generalized interstitial fibrosis of the lung parenchyma) and several types of nonmalignant pleural reactions, including pleural effusions, diffuse pleural thickening, and pleural plaques. The neoplastic diseases are lung cancer (bronchogenic carcinoma) and mesothelioma (a malignant tumor of the pleura or peritoneum). The pathophysiology, clinical course, diagnosis, and treatment are described next for each of the four major types of asbestos-related lung disease.

Asbestosis

Epidemiology. Asbestosis, which is a diffuse interstitial fibrosis of the lung parenchyma, has been associated with exposures to high concentrations of asbestos fibers since the early decades of the twentieth century. Many epidemiologic studies of heavily exposed asbestos workers have documented a strong dose-response relationship between the extent of exposure and the prevalence and severity of asbestosis. These studies have typically found a latency period of 20 to 40 years between first asbestos exposure and the clinical manifestations of asbestosis (based on abnormal chest x-ray or pulmonary function test findings). However, there are case reports from earlier in the century of development of asbestosis in as few as 4 years after massive and persistent exposures.

It has been recognized since the early part of the twentieth century that workers heavily exposed to airborne asbestos fibers developed a generalized fibrosis of the lungs, referred to as *asbestosis.* The extent of historical exposures can only be estimated because industrial hygiene monitoring techniques for asbestos were developed only in the 1930s and were not extensively used until after World War II. Furthermore, the techniques for air sampling and counting asbestos fibers have evolved over the past several decades, so that it is often not possible to accurately compare exposure data from epidemiologic studies done during different time periods.

Most epidemiologic studies have focused on studying worker cohorts in jobs known to have very high and prolonged exposures (such as shipyard insulators). In these studies, the number of years worked in a high-exposure job is used as a proxy of asbestos exposure in lieu of industrial hygiene exposure data. Based on the data available, it is estimated that in the earlier part of this century exposures of up to 1000 fibers/ml were found in some industries, and exposures of 10 fibers/ml may have been common in high-exposure jobs until the 1970s. In 1972, the Occupational Safety and Health Administration (OSHA) began requiring respiratory protection when airborne asbestos levels were above its permissible exposure level (PEL). During the same time, the U.S. Environmental Protection Agency (EPA) began banning asbestos for certain applications, and the industrial use of asbestos in the United States has dropped steady since then.

Numerous epidemiologic studies of asbestos-exposed workers have shown a strong dose-response relationship between lifetime asbestos exposures (i.e., cumulative dose of fibers inhaled) and development of asbestosis. Amphibole fibers are more toxic (i.e., more potent) than chrysotile if the levels of airborne exposure are equivalent, and crocidolite is the most toxic of the amphiboles.

Analysis of asbestos fibers in lung tissue samples (done by chemically digesting the lung tissue and then counting the residual fibers) provides further evidence of a strong dose-response relationship and also supports the concept of a threshold effect for the development of asbestosis. Individuals with confirmed asbestosis have been shown to have asbestos fiber counts in lung tissue at least 100 times greater than persons living in urban areas with no occupational exposure.[14]

Asbestosis is seen more frequently in smokers than in nonsmokers with similar exposures. This may be related to decreased clearance of asbestos fibers from the lungs in smokers, since cigarette smoke causes a decrease in cilliary action in the respiratory epithelium.

Pathophysiology. There are no immediate effects from inhalation of asbestos fibers, even in high concentrations, because the pathophysiology requires many years of development before clinically detectable disease is present. The primary mechanism for the health hazards of the inhalation of asbestos fibers is related to the theory of "frustrated macrophage." The fibers are relatively chemically inert, and the short fibers are easily phagocytized and removed from the respiratory system. The longer fibers are too difficult to phagocytize and cause the release of lymphokines from the macrophage while it attempts to digest the longer fibers. Release of lymphokines from the macrophage is thought to be the source of the fibrotic reaction that ensues in the lung and can cause asbestosis.

Fibers that are more durable in the lung, such as crocidolite or amosite asbestos, tend to be more fibrogenic because of increased fiber persistence and perhaps because of their sharp, needlelike shape. Chrysotile fibers are more easily dissolved in the lung because they are not very acid stable. Most of the chrysotile fibers are removed so that higher concentrations of chrysotile exposure are required to produce an equivalent level of asbestosis. The cancer-causing potential of these fibers also seems to correlate with their fibrogenic potential.

Fibers that are long and thin appear to be most likely to cause not only asbestosis but mesothelioma as well. Stanton fibers are less than 0.25 μm in diameter and longer than 8 μm. These fibers tend to be particularly mesotheliogenic. They are not visible with the light microscope and therefore are not counted by standard light-phase microscopy techniques.

Persistence of asbestos fibers in the lung then stimulates an ongoing inflammatory response that leads to the diffuse peribronchiolar and perialveolar fibrosis that is the hallmark of asbestosis. The local inflammatory response that leads to asbestosis appears to occur when macrophages are unable to completely engulf and phagocytize large asbestos fibers (generally those over 5 μm in length). Chemical mediators released by the macrophages then stimulate an inflammatory response, including release of chemotactic factors to mobilize more macrophages to the area and release of fibronectin, which stimulates fibroblasts to lay down fibrous tissue in the area.

The intensity of this inflammatory response appears directly related to the number of asbestos fibers that persist in the alveolar and respiratory bronchiolar spaces, which depends both on how many fibers enter these spaces and the extent to which the fibers are cleared from the lungs. This may explain some of the differences in toxicity between asbestos fiber types in their ability to produce asbestosis.

Chrysotile, which is considered the least toxic in producing asbestosis, appears in animal models to be cleared from the lung to a greater degree than a similar inhaled dose of amphibole fibers of similar length. There is speculation that this difference may be partially caused by the chemical composition of chrysotile, which may allow it to be digested more easily by macrophages. In contrast, amphibole forms of asbestos (such as amosite and crocidolite) may exhibit greater toxicity for producing asbestosis primarily because they have a lower rate of clearance from the lung than chrysotile fibers.

In animal experiments, a local inflammatory response in the lungs is seen within several days after asbestos exposure. The inflammatory response continues as long as asbestos fibers persist in the lung and gets worse as the number of fibers increases. Studies of workers with histories of prolonged, high-level asbestos exposures but no x-ray evidence of asbestosis found 20% to 30% had evidence of an inflammatory response on analysis of bronchial alveolar lavage (BAL) fluid.[40] Unfortunately, the use of antiinflammatory drugs, such as corticosteroids, has so far not been shown to reduce the early inflammatory responses to asbestos exposure.

Recent research shows that the inflammatory response of asbestosis starts within weeks after the first exposure, and the process of fibrosis continues as long as it is stimulated by persistent asbestos fibers in the lung. The first symptoms of asbestosis are shortness of breath with exertion and decreased exercise tolerance. Autopsy studies show that, when symptoms first appear, there is already a significant degree of diffuse peribronchiolar fibrosis in the lung. Similarly, x-ray findings of interstitial fibrosis and spirometry evidence of restrictive lung disease frequently occur prior to the onset of symptoms.

Once the diagnosis of asbestosis is made, about 20% of patients have a progression of the disease to severe interstitial fibrosis; in the remaining patients, asbestosis

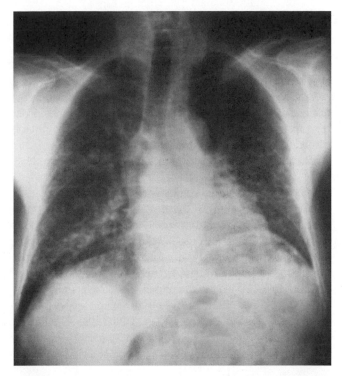

Fig. 55-1 Asbestosis x-ray. Chest radiograph of an asbestos worker showing more advanced abnormalities of the lung parenchyma. The coarse reticulation is diffuse and of higher density, and the cardiac silhouette is beginning to be ill-defined. (From Harber P, Schenker MB, Balmes JR: *Occupational and environmental respiratory disease,* St Louis, 1996, Mosby.)

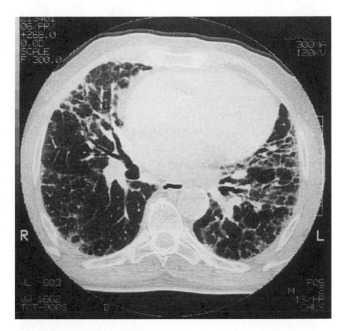

Fig. 55-2 Pleural CT scan of an asbestos worker with asbestosis and bilateral minimal pleural thickening. The honeycombing is prominent in the left lung field, and parenchymal changes of reticular nature are well appreciated. (From Harber P, Schenker MB, Balmes JR: *Occupational and environmental respiratory disease,* St Louis, 1996, Mosby.)

progresses slowly. Severe diffuse interstitial fibrosis leads to pulmonary hypertension and sometimes death from right-sided heart failure. Those who do not develop massive pulmonary fibrosis may develop shortness of breath with exertion and decreased exercise tolerance, but they tend to die of causes other than asbestosis. At the time of initial diagnosis of asbestosis, there is no accurate way to predict which patients will develop a rapid progression of their disease, except that it seems to occur more commonly in those with more severe disease at the time of diagnosis. Individuals with advanced asbestosis may have a higher incidence of pulmonary infections, but the reason for this is unclear.

Some scientists have claimed that detectable changes in midexpiratory flow rates at low lung volumes could be due to asbestos-related airway disease and that therefore such measurements might be of value in detecting early asbestosis. However, even though researchers have reported structural abnormalities of small airways in asbestos-exposed workers, clinical tests of small airways function have not been found clinically useful in detecting early asbestosis or any other abnormalities clearly related to asbestos exposure.

Diagnosis. The clinical presentation of asbestosis is no different than the clinical presentation for idiopathic diffuse pulmonary fibrosis. The patient's predominant complaint is shortness of breath. Cough does not occur early in the course

of the disease and is usually a very late complication of advanced interstitial asbestos-related fibrosis. Patients commonly have dry, crackly, late-inspiratory rales or "cellophane" rales at both bases. Lung function tests show a restrictive pattern with decreased diffusion and the chest x-ray demonstrates small, irregular opacities in the lower lobes (Fig. 55-1). If irregular opacities are also seen in the upper lobes, the diagnosis of asbestosis is much less likely. Computed tomography (CT) scanning has been used in an effort to find early disease and is a valuable adjunct to the diagnostic workup (Fig. 55-2). However, the only reliable finding on CT scan that is proof of asbestosis is honeycombing of the lung. Asbestos fibers or asbestos bodies on analysis of BAL fluid (Fig. 55-3) and the presence of pleural plaques on chest x-rays are considered markers of asbestos exposure, but these findings by themselves do not establish a diagnosis of asbestosis.[42]

The definitive diagnosis of asbestosis is made by histologic exam of lung tissue that shows characteristic diffuse peribronchiolar fibrosis and the presence of asbestos bodies or asbestos fibers. Such a tissue diagnosis can be obtained only by a thoracotomy and open lung biopsy; adequate tissue cannot be obtained by bronchoscopy.

There remains a lack of consensus on the specific clinical criteria for diagnosing asbestosis in its earliest stages. The

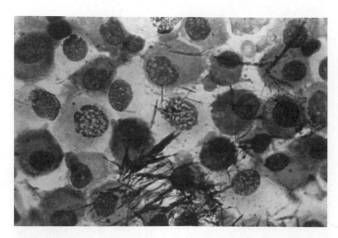

Fig. 55-3 Asbestos fibers in cytospin. Cytospin of a lung lavage in an asbestos worker showing several fibers, many of these longer than the average macrophage diameter (8 μm); Wright-Giemsa; magnification × 1000. (From Harber P, Schenker MB, Balmes JR: *Occupational and environmental respiratory disease,* St Louis, 1996, Mosby.)

American Thoracic Society (ATS) criteria for the diagnosis of asbestosis require a history of significant asbestos exposure, an appropriate interval between exposure and detection (usually over 20 years), and evidence on chest x-ray of interstitial fibrosis (i.e., small opacities of International Labor Organization [ILO] grade 1/1 or greater). Other findings that support the diagnosis of asbestosis include evidence of restrictive lung disease on spirometry (with a forced vital capacity [FVC] less than the lower limit of normal), an abnormally low diffusing capacity, and bilateral late or periinspiratory crackles at the posterior lung bases.[1]

A formal system grading the severity of asbestosis and other pneumoconioses on chest x-rays has been developed by the ILO, a component of the World Health Organization. This ILO classification includes a 12-point scale for rating the severity of interstitial fibrosis (ratings vary from –/0, which is clearly normal to 3/3, which is severe diffuse interstitial fibrosis) and a formal method for rating pleural lesions. This system has been useful both for epidemiologic research and for establishing the diagnosis of asbestosis (but it is not used for rating impairment). A standard system for grading interstitial fibrosis seen on high-resolution CT has not yet been developed.

The U.S. National Institute of Occupational Safety and Health (NIOSH) has a training program and certification exam for reading pneumoconiosis films by the ILO criteria. Physicians who pass this NIOSH exam are designated as B-readers. The OSHA asbestos standard specifies that chest x-rays done as part of required asbestos medical surveillance programs must be interpreted by a B-reader. The rationale for using B-readers is to increase objectivity and reduce intrarater variability in the interpretation of asbestosis-related x-ray changes. Several studies have shown there is still variability between B-readers who are interpreting the same sets of chest x-rays, but in most cases ratings of interstitial fibrosis by different B-readers are within 1 point of each other.

Impairment ratings for asbestosis are usually based on lung function test findings and sometimes on demonstration of decreased exercise capacity on electrocardiogram stress testing. The specific rules for rating impairment from asbestosis vary greatly for different state and federal compensation systems within the United States.

Treatment and prevention. There is no effective treatment for asbestosis, other than supportive measures such as treating any secondary lung infections. Therefore, the only effective intervention is to prevent asbestos fibers from entering the lung. Some clinicians recommend that persons with documented asbestosis be restricted from further work with asbestos, citing evidence from clinical and animal studies that continued exposure may lead to a worsening of the asbestosis. However, this remains controversial, since if proper work practices are followed, few if any asbestos fibers should be taken into the lungs. (See pp. 483-486 for a further discussion of public health and workplace prevention issues.)

Asbestos-Related Pleural Diseases

Epidemiology. Most large epidemiology studies of asbestos-exposed worker cohorts have reported increased prevalence of nonmalignant pleural changes, including benign pleural effusions, diffuse pleural thickening, pleural plaques, and a reaction of the visceral pleura known as *rounded atelectasis.*

These conditions appear to be more common in those with higher cumulative asbestos exposures and appear to have latency periods, since the first exposure is similar to that seen with asbestosis and asbestos-related malignancies. These pleural conditions are not precursors to asbestosis or asbestos-related malignancies. Therefore, asbestos-related pleural changes are frequently, but not always, found in persons with asbestosis and asbestos-related cancers, but these pleural changes are also often seen in asbestos-exposed persons with no other asbestos-related conditions. Therefore, many clinicians regard asbestos-related pleural changes as markers of prior asbestos exposure but not as an indicator of asbestosis or early cancer.

The degree of asbestos exposure needed to produce pleural changes is unclear. It appears to be more than the background level exposures seen in the general population but less than the very high cumulative exposures needed to produce asbestosis.

While asbestos-related pleural changes are often benign, persons with extensive amounts of pleural thickening or pleural plaque formation can develop clinically significant restrictive lung disease, which may cause functional impairment. This can result in significant reductions in lung function and may require surgical release of constricting fibrous tissues.[41]

Pathophysiology. Asbestos-related pleural disease can occur in many forms but is generally thought to be initiated when inhaled asbestos fibers small enough to penetrate alveoli deep in the lung are removed by the lymphatics to the visceral pleural surface. These fibers may then enter the pleural space, where they are absorbed by the lymphatics in the parietal pleura. Other fibers appear to become entrapped in the pleural membranes to cause pleural disease.

Some researchers speculate that the fibers sticking through the lung perhaps abrade the parietal pleural surface, particularly in areas of greatest respiratory excursion, such as the lower posterior lateral aspects of the chest and the diaphragm (which is where pleural plaques are commonly seen). Another theory is that the location of pleural plaques in this area is not related to respiratory movement but to a preferential pulmonary lymphatic flow to these areas.

Pleural plaques. Pleural plaques are areas of hyaline fibrosis that develop only on the parietal pleura, either over the chest walls or over the diaphragm. The pleural plaques are circumscribed flat plaques covered by a smooth, glistening membrane, so that they generally do not impede the motion of the lung in the chest and hence reduce lung function. The thickness and area covered by these plaques may vary considerably. Pleural plaques are generally considered a sign of exposure to asbestos but do not constitute a cause for alarm other than indicating that asbestos exposure may have occurred. However, in a small percentage of cases, extensive, thick plaques can result in significant restrictive lung disease and may affect a person's daily functioning.

Benign pleural effusions. In addition to parietal pleural reactions, there are visceral or visceroparietal reactions due to asbestos. One of the most common is benign asbestos pleural effusions, originally described in 1960. A study by Epler and associates[22] initially suggested that it was most common around 15 years after moderate levels of exposure to asbestos. However, more recent data suggest that benign pleural effusions can occur at any time after asbestos exposure, with some persons developing benign asbestos-related pleural effusions more than 50 years after moderate to heavy exposure. Asbestos-related pleural effusions tend to occur episodically, and their cause is unclear. Some data suggest a slightly increased risk of mesothelioma in these patients.

Diffuse pleural fibrosis. Benign asbestos effusions are thought to lead to diffuse pleural fibrosis, which is fairly common in patients who have had moderate exposure to asbestos. Most patients diagnosed with diffuse pleural fibrosis can recall no history of benign asbestos-related pleural effusions, which suggests that asbestos-related pleural effusions are often asymptomatic and go undetected. The diffuse pleural fibrosis occurs on the parietal pleura. It may be fairly localized or may encase the entire lung with a fibrous pleural peel that greatly impairs lung function.

The impact of the diffuse pleural fibrosis on lung function is difficult to estimate based on review of the chest x-ray and CT scan. In some individuals, small amounts of diffuse pleural disease may be associated with significant impairment; other persons with a moderate amount of diffuse pleural disease may have normal lung function. This process is independent of the development of asbestosis, although patients with asbestosis may develop dense areas of scarring of lung parenchyma that extend to the pleural surface and mimic diffuse pleural fibrosis. Recent studies suggest that diffuse pleural disease is the most common cause of impaired lung function in asbestos-exposed individuals.

Diffuse pleural disease can also produce mass lesions on chest x-ray by causing numerous invaginations of the lung parenchymal surface by fingers of pleural fibrosis. The retraction and concentric curling of segments of the lung near the pleural surface are known as *rounded atelectasis*. It appears on x-rays as a mass near the periphery of the lung. These conditions can advance to the point that they impair lung function, at which time the entrapped lung may be released surgically, the lung then uncoils, and usually lung function returns. Usually these focal masses are asymptomatic, are not associated with significant impairment of function, and can be treated conservatively if neoplasm has been excluded.[48]

In rare cases, inflammation associated with asbestos-related pleuritis and effusions may extend to the pericardium. These patients present with pericardial effusions and pericardial pain and commonly have associated pleural abnormalities. They may respond to corticosteroids, and the pericarditis is usually self-limited.

Diagnosis

Pleural plaques. Only about 10% to 15% of pleural plaques found at autopsy are visible on chest x-ray[49] because plaques must be tangential to the x-ray beam before they are visible. Later on, plaques may become calcified and are more frequently detected on x-ray, and most pleural plaques are visible on CT scan.[25] Since there are other causes of pleural plaques besides asbestos, only plaques that are bilateral, symmetric, and present in the subaxillary areas can generally be assumed to be related to asbestos exposure.

Asbestos-related pleural effusion. The presenting symptoms in persons with asbestos-related pleural effusions are often pleuritic chest pain and shortness of breath, although patients with smaller effusions are frequently asymptomatic. Asbestos-related pleural effusions may be unilateral or bilateral and may be associated with symptomatic pleuritis. The pleural effusions are usually confirmed by x-rays. If thoracentesis is done, the effusion fluid itself is exudative, usually with a normal glucose and without asbestos fibers. The fluid may be hemorrhagic or clear. On pathologic exam, the pleural surfaces are covered by a thin, fibrinous exudate.

Diffuse pleural fibrosis. Diffuse pleural fibrosis is usually evident on chest x-ray but is best seen on CT scan. Persons with severe pleural fibrosis that extends into the lung parenchyma often present with shortness of breath and may have restrictive changes on pulmonary function tests. On chest x-rays, these areas at the periphery of the lung often have a crow's-feet-like appearance or may produce dense focal masses that mimic a lung cancer. Usually, CT shows twisting and pulling of the bronchiolar-vascular bundle into the area of lung fibrosis that cause a "comet tail" sign, which is strongly suggestive of a benign focal pleural mass.[51]

Treatment. Benign pleural effusions usually resolve spontaneously, although larger effusions associated with breathing difficulties are often drained. There is no treatment for pleural plaques, and usually they do not affect function, in any case. Diffuse pleural effusion is also usually not treated, although a surgical release of these tissues is sometimes performed if pleural fibrosis entraps lung parenchyma (as in rounded atelectasis) and affects function.

Asbestos-Related Lung Cancer

Epidemiology. Several large epidemiologic studies since the 1960s have shown excess numbers of lung cancer (i.e., bronchogenic carcinoma) deaths in worker cohorts with many years of high-level asbestos exposure.[44] These bronchogenic carcinomas in asbestos-exposed cohorts cannot be distinguished from tumors associated with cigarette smoking on the basis of either their histologic type or their anatomic locations in the lung (the majority of tumors are in the large airways).[12]

For this reason, epidemiologic studies evaluating the association between asbestos exposures and lung cancer must be adequately controlled for the effects of cigarette smoking. Studies of occupationally exposed cohorts have typically done this by comparing lung cancer rates in the asbestos-exposed worker cohorts with lung cancer rates in non–asbestos-exposed comparison populations, while controlling for smoking by analyzing data separately for smokers and those who have never smoked.[43]

It is clear from several epidemiologic studies that, for worker cohorts with high historical asbestos exposures, those subgroups that have developed asbestosis also have higher than expected rates of lung cancer. This association between lung cancer and asbestosis holds true for both smokers and nonsmokers, although lung cancer rates are much higher in the smokers. In contrast, epidemiologic studies have not found increased rates of lung cancer in groups of workers without asbestosis, even when cumulative asbestos exposures have been high.

Rates of lung cancer in heavily exposed asbestos workers who are also cigarette smokers are much higher than would be expected from merely adding the estimated lung cancer risks for asbestos exposure alone and for cigarette smoking alone. This suggests some type of synergy between asbestos and smoking that leads to a relative risk for lung cancer nearly 50 times that of a nonsmoker with no asbestos

exposures (compared with a relative risk of about 5 for nonsmokers with heavy asbestos, and a relative risk of 10 for smokers with no asbestos history of exposure).[44]

Several studies have also shown that worker cohorts exposed to higher concentrations of amphibole fibers have higher lung cancer rates than those exposed to similar concentrations of chrysotile asbestos. Based on this, amphibole fibers—particularly crocidolite—are considered more toxic or pathogenic than chrysotile fibers for producing lung cancer. This pattern of increased toxicity of amphiboles also holds true for all the other asbestos-related lung diseases (asbestosis, pleural disease, and mesothelioma). Numerous animal and human studies suggest that the reason for this apparent higher toxicity is that the amphibole fibers have a longer persistence in the lung than chrysotile fibers (which are more easily chemically degraded and cleared from the lung).[18]

The latency period for asbestos-related lung cancer, defined as the time between the first asbestos exposure and clinical diagnosis of lung cancer, has been shown to be at least 20 years. Persons with relatively lower cumulative dose exposures tend to have longer latency periods of 30 to 40 years or even longer. This same relationship between cumulative dose and latency is seen with all the other asbestos-related lung diseases.

A classic study, which documented the increased rate of lung cancer and mesothelioma in asbestos-exposed workers, was done by Selikoff and Seidman who prospectively studied a cohort of asbestos insulation workers in the New York City area who had been continually employed in this trade from 1943 to 1963. The study began in 1963, and in the following years a very high proportion of the cohort died from lung cancer or mesothelioma.[46] This study was better designed than some earlier studies, since all subjects had at least 20 years of exposure prior to starting the study, which is the minimum latency period for most asbestos-related diseases. Also, this cohort was among the most-exposed occupational groups, with many having had expensive exposure to asbestos as insulators in shipyards during this time. This study, which documented greatly increased rates for lung cancer and mesothelioma in asbestos insulation workers, received a great deal of publicity and probably helped to pass legislation that authorized establishment of OSHA in 1972.

In recent years, there has been intense scientific debate on whether heavy asbestos exposure alone can cause lung cancer or whether the development of asbestosis is necessary before asbestos-related lung cancer can occur. A comprehensive review of data from all published animal studies shows that lung cancer does not develop in animals unless asbestosis is also present. This is consistent with several epidemiologic studies of asbestos-exposed workers that suggest asbestos-related lung cancers do not develop until there is clinical asbestosis. An autopsy study of South

African workers found that all the patients with asbestos-related lung cancer also had asbestosis.[47] A study from Mt. Sinai Hospital in New York City, which evaluated more than 100 patients with asbestos exposure and lung cancer, found all of these patients also had asbestosis.[32]

Studies by Doll in England in 1955,[20] Bohlig and colleagues in Germany in the 1960s[4], and Hughes and Weill,[29] who evaluated asbestos cement workers in the New Orleans, all found no increased incidence of lung cancer in asbestos-exposed workers, except in those subgroups with evidence of asbestosis on chest x-rays.

Pathophysiology. The precise mechanisms by which asbestos exposure leads to excess lung cancer rates is not clear, but several theories have been developed, based on both experimental and epidemiologic evidence. Current research suggests all types of cancer develop in a multistep process involving both tumor initiation and tumor promotion. Carcinogenesis is probably initiated by mutations of critical genes in the cell, with the number of mutations required to produce a cancer ranging between 5 and 20. The critical target genes thought to be important in the development of cancer are the protooncogenes and the tumor suppressor genes, which must either be lost or somehow inactivated to allow carcinogenesis to proceed. Once a cancer has been initiated, then other substances often act as tumor promoters and increase the rate of tumor growth.[29]

The current thinking is that asbestos acts as a promoter rather than an inducer of lung cancer and that asbestos-related lung cancers do not develop unless there has been an inflammatory response to asbestos sufficient to cause asbestosis. It has long been recognized that an intense inflammatory reaction in the lung can induce lung cancer; some speculate that asbestos-related lung cancer is a type of scar cancer secondary to asbestosis.

Recent research has shown that the asbestos-induced inflammatory response in the lung is mediated by lymphokines, which include a mixture of fibroblast growth factors, chemotactic factors, fibronectin, prostaglandins, platelet-derived growth factors, and active oxygen metabolites. Several researchers suggest these active oxygen species are causative agents for both asbestosis and asbestos-related malignancy. In laboratory experiments, cultures of alveolar macrophages exposed to asbestos release active oxygen metabolites, such as super oxide ion (O_{2-}) and hydrogen peroxide (H_2O_2); these same substances are found in the BAL fluid of patients with asbestosis. The release of lymphokines by macrophages also stimulates mitogenesis (i.e., cell division) in bronchial epithelial cells, and basic research on carcinogenicity suggests increased mitogenesis is associated with greater likelihood of mutagenic events and the initiation of cancer.[37]

There is some evidence from both animal studies and short-term bioassay techniques that asbestos is an incomplete carcinogen for lung cancer and may act primarily as a tumor promoter. Asbestos is not genotoxic by the Ames test, and rodent bone marrow assays for detection of chromosomal aberrations have been negative. Some researchers have suggested that asbestos fibers associated with fibrogenesis act as a tumor promoter and, as such, exert a synergistic effect on cancers induced by cigarette smoking. Tissue cultures exposed to both asbestos fibers and cigarette smoke have shown an increase in single strand breaks in DNA. This is consistent with both animal experiments and human epidemiologic studies that have shown higher rates of asbestosis and more asbestos-related chest x-ray abnormalities associated with smoking.[23] Animal and epidemiologic data also show that smoking increases fiber retention in the lung several fold.[13,53]

Taking all of this information into account presents fairly strong evidence that asbestos can act as a tumor promoter, although there is also some evidence that asbestos may have some direct mutagenic effects.

Diagnosis. Lung cancer patients are frequently asymptomatic when their cancer is first diagnosed, usually on the basis of an abnormal x-ray finding. Others with lung cancer present with symptoms such as a dry cough, hemoptysis, chest pain, or systemic symptoms related to cancer (such as weight loss, fever, or general malaise).

Since lung cancers often metastasize to the brain, the initial presentation is sometimes that of an intercranial mass with symptoms of mental confusion, headache, or even focal neurologic findings. Metastatic lung cancer is the most common type of brain tumor seen in smokers.

The preliminary diagnosis of lung cancer is usually from identification of a mass identified on chest x-ray. Further definition can often be provided by a CT scan of the chest. The diagnosis is usually confirmed with tissue biopsy, which is frequently obtained via bronchoscopy or needle biopsy through the chest wall. Although sputum cytology and cytologic analysis of BAL fluid can identify tumor cells, these techniques are not clinically useful as screening tests for lung cancer and are seldom needed to confirm the diagnosis.

Treatment and prevention. Despite the multiple treatments for lung cancer, these tumors tend to rapidly metastasize, so that a cure is frequently not possible. The focus of treatment is generally on increasing survival time and treating complications. Depending upon the tumor cell types, aggressive chemotherapy can lead to improved survivals in some patients of 1 to 2 years or more. At this time, there is no clear evidence that early diagnosis improves overall survival rates; therefore, screening programs for early detection of lung cancer have not been shown to be useful.

As with all other asbestos-related disease, the only effective preventive interventions are protecting individuals from asbestos exposures high enough to cause asbestos-related lung cancer and not smoking.

Asbestos-Related Mesothelioma

Epidemiology. Mesothelioma is the only malignancy besides bronchogenic carcinoma that has clearly been associated with asbestos exposure. Mesothelioma is the primary tumor of the mesothelial cells lining the pleura of the chest cavity or the peritoneal lining of the abdomen. Peritoneal mesotheliomas tend to occur in individuals with histories of heavier cumulative asbestos exposures, generally in those who had developed asbestosis. In contrast, pleural mesotheliomas can occur in patients with lower levels of asbestos exposure who do not have asbestosis.[7]

The minimal body burden of asbestos fibers at which mesothelioma develops cannot be accurately estimated, since about 10% to 20% of mesotheliomas are of uncertain etiology and are not associated with known occupational asbestos exposures. Other potential causes of mesothelioma include exposure to other naturally occurring mineral fibers (such as zeolite in Turkey), recurrent lung infections, radiation exposure, and possibly other occupational exposures.[39] The overall prevalence of mesothelioma is greater in heavily industrialized coastal areas of the United States, particularly around shipyards that used asbestos extensively in the past.[3]

Epidemiologic studies of asbestos-exposed worker cohorts have found no evidence that smokers are at any higher risk for developing mesotheliomas than are nonsmokers. Theoretically, rates of mesothelioma ought to be higher in smokers, who have decreased clearance of asbestos from the lungs, and some researchers suggest the inability to show such a relationship is due primarily to insufficient statistical power in existing studies.

Epidemiologic studies suggest that patients who worked in a shipyard during World War II for 3 months had an increased risk of mesothelioma. The latency period from inhalation of a threshold dose of asbestos to the development of a mesothelioma is usually greater than 20 years and can be as long as 60 years after the exposure.[33] Certain fiber types are much more likely to cause mesotheliomas; with crocidolite the most carcinogenic and amosite of intermediate toxicity.[26]

It has been a matter of debate as to whether exposure to chrysotile asbestos alone can produce mesotheliomas. In studies of asbestos miners and millers in Quebec who were exposed to chrysotile asbestos contaminated with tremolite, mesotheliomas were seen only in workers who had very high cumulative exposures, usually at doses sufficient to cause asbestosis. Animal studies by Wagner[52] found that asbestos from Zimbabwe (also known as Rhodesian asbestos), which is a pure form of chrysotile not contaminated with tremolite, does not produce mesotheliomas when injected in rats, whereas Canadian chrysotile contaminated with tremolite does cause mesotheliomas in rats. Based on this evidence, many researchers suggest that the tremolite contamination of chrysotile asbestos, rather than the chrysotile fiber itself, is the likely cause of the mesothelioma in the Quebec miners and millers and that mesotheliomas are primarily related to amphibole asbestos exposures.[9]

Pathophysiology. Both animal experiments and genotoxicity studies suggest that asbestos acts as an initiator in tissue cultures incubated with mesothelioma cells.[54] Experimental studies have shown a mesothelioma can be caused by injecting asbestos fibers into either the pleural or peritoneal spaces of animals. These studies have shown a threshold dose for the development of mesothelioma, since no mesotheliomas were seen in animals when the injected dose of asbestos was less then 100,000 fibers. Human epidemiologic studies also suggest there is a threshold dose for development of mesothelioma, which has been estimated to be approximately 5 fiber years (e.g., an expose of 1 fiber/cc for 5 years).[6] Cytogenetic analysis has revealed that there are nonrandom chromosomal alternations occurring in human mesotheliomas. It is generally thought that human chromosomes 1,3,5,6,7, are most likely the important ones involved in the initiation and promotion of carcinogenesis. The actual mechanism of asbestos-induced aneuploidy, which means either the gain or loss of an individual chromosome, is uncertain. It has been hypothesized that, as the macrophages undergo mitosis, the physical presence of fibers may interfere with the chromosomal segregation.[54] Indeed, analysis of asbestos-exposed cells in anaphase has revealed an increase in the number of cells with abnormalities. This would suggest that with mesothelioma cells asbestos may act as an initiator, whereas the data suggest that asbestos is primarily a promoter for lung cancer. It appears that the long, thin fibers are more active in producing cancer than the stubby, short fibers. Exactly why the long, thin fibers are more tumorigenic is unclear, but in part it is related to the greater biopersistence of these fibers in the human body. The shorter fibers are more likely to be removed by the normal phagocytosis by alveolar macrophages and, hence, have short retention times. A recent review by Lippmann[35] suggested that the rate of dissolution in lung fluids may affect the underlying fiber's carcinogenicity: glass wool is less than rock wool, which is less than chrysotile asbestos, which is less than amphibole asbestos. Lippman points out that the rates of dissolution are exactly in the reverse order of ability of these different fibers to produce cytotoxicity, lung fibrosis, and cancer.

Finally, a recent study has reported that DNA sequences similar to simian SV-40 virus have been found in most pleural mesotheliomas. The simian SV-40 virus is known to have been a contaminant of a polio vaccine, which was widely used in the 1950s. Most mesotheliomas that contain this DNA sequence have been associated with asbestos exposure, suggesting a possible synergistic effect of the simian SV-40 virus and asbestos in the development of mesothelioma.[8]

Diagnosis. The presenting symptoms of mesothelioma are usually pleuritic chest pain (seen in 70% to 80% of patients) and sometimes shortness of breath, but cough is not a prominent symptom. Chest x-rays and CT scans of the lung often show a pleural effusion and lobular pleural-based masses. Thoracentesis usually shows a bloody pleural effusion.

The definitive diagnosis of a mesothelioma is best obtained by a thorascopic or open lung biopsy. In most cases, it is possible to make a diagnosis with smaller needle biopsy specimens, but sometimes the tumor is so anaplastic that it is very difficult to differentiate from an epithelial lung cancer. Some patients with reactive pleuritis develop very atypical mesothelial cells, which makes a diagnosis by cytologic evaluation of the pleural fluid more speculative. Electron microscopy and special immunologic stains have proven to be quite helpful in distinguishing mesotheliomas from lung cancers.

Once the diagnosis of mesothelioma is established, the clinical course is short, averaging from 12 to 18 months from the time of diagnosis to death. There is no curative treatment available at this time. Surgery and chemotherapy for mesothelioma have not been shown to improve survival, although they may produce some temporary symptomatic relief. Radiation therapy and extremely aggressive surgery have not been successful.

PREVENTION AND PUBLIC HEALTH ISSUES
Public Health and Public Policy Issues

Since there is no effective treatment for asbestos-related diseases, the only effective intervention is primary prevention, that is, preventing the inhalation of asbestos fibers at levels likely to cause disease. Over the past two decades, there have been huge public health and public policy efforts in the United States and many other industrialized countries directed at reducing the use of asbestos in manufactured products and construction, proper maintenance or removal and disposal of asbestos materials now in place, and appropriate personal protection of workers and the general public from exposures to dangerous levels of asbestos.

The extent to which asbestos exposure poses a health threat to the general public in the outdoor air environment and as occupants of buildings containing asbestos has been a topic of intense controversy in recent years. Low levels of airborne asbestos are found in the outdoor (ambient) air in many parts of the United States, as well as inside a large percentage of U.S. public and private commercial buildings. It is also clear that these exposures to the general public are usually thousands of times lower than the historical exposures to worker cohorts who have had higher rates of asbestos-related diseases in epidemiologic studies.

The controversy revolves around both the levels of potential asbestos exposure to the general public (especially inside buildings) and the assumptions of the mathematical risk assessment models that have been used to estimate risks for asbestos-related disease from these types of low-level exposures. Over the past decade, there has been a great deal of concern in the United States about potential health risks from asbestos for children in schools and for occupants in other public or commercial buildings where asbestos has been found.[27]

Levels of Airborne Asbestos in the Outside Environment and Inside Buildings

Airborne asbestos enters in the outdoor environment both from natural sources and as a by-product of an industrial society. Asbestos can become airborne in the outdoor environment from erosion of outcroppings of asbestos-containing minerals, mainly from serpentine rock formations, which are common in many parts of the United States. Asbestos also enters the outdoor air environment as a result of industrial processes using asbestos, from wear or damage to asbestos-containing materials, and due to demolition of structures containing asbestos.

One survey estimated that asbestos-containing materials can be found in 20% to 40% of all U.S. public and private commercial buildings.[27] In the past, asbestos was often incorporated into vinyl floor tiles, acoustic ceiling panels, firewall board, exterior siding, and roofing materials. Asbestos was often sprayed on steel beams as fireproofing and was also sprayed on ceilings. Asbestos lagging and free-formed asbestos mud were frequently used as pipe and boiler insulation. Asbestos exposures to building occupants can occur when free asbestos fibers (also called *friable asbestos*) are released into the air from physical damage, mechanical wear, or thermal or chemical breakdown of asbestos-containing materials, or when these materials are intentionally removed.

Historical records on the production and use of asbestos indicate the majority of asbestos used in U.S. buildings was probably chrysotile; the amphibole asbestos materials (crocidolite and amosite) were used preferentially for some applications such as insulating high-pressure steam lines.

Surveys of U.S. buildings containing asbestos materials have frequently found a mixture of chrysotile and amphiboles. In addition, chrysotile from the mines of Quebec, which was the primary source of asbestos used in the United States has been shown to be contaminated with tremolite. Therefore, although more than 90% of asbestos in place in U.S. buildings is probably chrysotile, it is reasonable to assume for the purpose of public safety that most asbestos-containing materials in U.S. buildings contain some amphibole fibers. For this reason, risk assessments often assume an exposure to mixed fibers when estimating risks for low-level exposures to building occupants.

Surveys of public and commercial buildings have generally found very low levels of airborne asbestos in buildings where asbestos-containing materials were not damaged or deteriorated. In many cases, exposure levels in these buildings were similar to or lower than airborne asbestos

Table 55-2 Regulated and ambient levels of asbestos exposure

Title	Level
U.S. Public Health Service Standard, 1938	30 f/cc
ACGIH proposed standard, 1968	12 f/cc
ACGIH proposed standard, 1970	5 f/cc
OSHA proposed standard, 1972	2 f/cc
OSHA proposed standard, 1983	0.5 f/cc
OSHA proposed standard, 1986	0.2 f/cc
OSHA proposed standard, 1990	0.1 f/cc
Urban ambient air	0.0001 f/cc
Building with asbestos-containing material	0.0002 f/cc
Mining towns, Quebec	0.01 f/cc
San Benito County, California	0.3-5.3 f/cc
Epidemiologic studies of workers exposed to chrysotile asbestos without risk	1-5 f/cc

levels in the outside environment. However, higher levels were seen in buildings with certain types of asbestos materials, such as spray-on ceilings, and when the asbestos-containing materials were significantly damaged or deteriorated. Typical exposure levels found in U.S. schools and public buildings are shown in Table 55-2.[30]

There is no way to determine if suspect materials contain asbestos or what fiber types are present without laboratory microscopic analysis of the materials. Therefore, it is recommended that construction and maintenance personnel in buildings arrange for appropriate sampling and analysis of potential asbestos-containing materials before they are disturbed. Workers who are around asbestos-containing materials (such as for installation, repair, or removal of these materials) are covered by stringent OSHA regulations designed to minimize exposures to both workers and the environment.

Estimating the Health Risks of Low-level Asbestos Exposures

Adults in urban areas in industrialized countries probably all have a sizable body burden of asbestos fibers in their lungs from asbestos exposure in the outdoor environment. Autopsy studies of adults in urban areas of North America with no known occupational asbestos exposures and no evidence of asbestos-related disease, found fiber counts of about 1,000,000 fibers per gram of dry lung for both chrysotile and tremolite and about 10,000 fibers per gram of dry lung for both amosite and crocidolite asbestos.[10] Similar autopsy studies have found fiber counts about 10 times higher in adults living near the Thedford chrysotile asbestos mines in Quebec who had no occupational exposures to asbestos. Again, this group had no evidence of asbestos-related disease.

In contrast, individuals who have developed asbestosis have lung burdens of asbestos fibers at least 100 times those found in the nonoccupational exposed general public, and a number of studies also suggest that asbestos-related lung cancer only occurs at levels of exposure sufficient to cause asbestosis.

For all of these reasons, the primary controversy on the extent of health risks from very-low-level asbestos exposures revolves around the risk for developing mesothelioma, which has been shown to occur after asbestos exposures much lower than those needed to produce asbestosis.

It is recognized from both epidemiologic and animal studies that mesotheliomas can occur after much lower levels of asbestos exposure than those needed to cause asbestosis or lung cancer. Exposures to amphiboles, especially crocidolite, are generally considered to pose a greater potential for developing mesothelioma than chrysotile exposures of equivalent intensity. While mesotheliomas have been seen in miners who worked in the chrysotile mines of Quebec, these cannot be considered pure chrysotile exposures since the chrysotile asbestos taken from these mines is naturally contaminated with the amphibole tremolite.

There is disagreement among experts on whether a lower threshold dose of cumulative asbestos exposure exists for the development of asbestos-related mesotheliomas. Supporters of the threshold dose hypothesis point out that there has been no recorded increase in the incidence of mesothelioma in the non–asbestos-exposed U.S. general public (particularly women) over the past 30 years, in contrast to the dramatically increased incidence rates of mesothelioma seen in occupationally exposed U.S. and English workers during this time period.[31]

These experts contend that significant numbers of asbestos fibers are found in the lungs of members of the general public who are not occupationally exposed; therefore, excess mesothelioma cases should have been seen in the general public if the nonthreshold hypothesis were true, and extremely low-level asbestos exposures could cause mesothelioma. Supporters of the threshold model also cite a study in which no mesotheliomas were seen in residents of towns near the Thedford chrysotile mines in Quebec who were not occupationally exposed, even though these individuals had lung fiber counts for both chrysotile and tremolite that were 10 to 100 times the levels in adults who were not occupationally exposed in a large Canadian city.[33]

Several mathematical risk assessments have been developed to estimate health risks from very-low-level asbestos exposures. These have generally used epidemiologic data with high occupational exposures as the only known data points and estimated health risks at the very low levels found in buildings by using a linear extrapolation of this data. Such an approach has been criticized as a "one hit hypothesis" by those who suggest that a lower threshold exists for all the asbestos-related diseases.

Hughes and Weill developed a risk assessment for lung cancer and mesothelioma from asbestos exposure by using such a linear extrapolation, nonthreshold model.[30] They used data from seven large cohorts with occupational asbestos

Table 55-3 Risk assessment of exposure in buildings with asbestos-containing material

Risk	Common risks per million persons exposed
Cigarette smoking	1200
Bicycling (10-14 years old)	15
Playing high school football	10
Eating 4 tbsp peanut butter/day	8
Aircraft accidents	6
Whooping cough vaccination	1-6
Living 2 months with a smoker	1
Asbestos in schools (0.001 f/cc)	0.02-0.37
Asbestos in schools (0.001 f/cc) chrysotile	0.006-0.11

exposures, which they stated were the only studies of lung cancer and mesothelioma in asbestos-exposed persons that also provided some type of quantitative estimates of asbestos exposures. Their risk estimates for developing asbestos-related lung cancer and mesothelioma at different exposure levels are well known.[35] Despite extensive debate in the scientific literature concerning the risks of low-level asbestos exposure, however, the risk assessments used by U.S. government agencies (EPA and OSHA) in establishing regulations for asbestos are based on the nonthreshold linear risk models.

As Table 55-3 shows, even using these models, the risks of mesothelioma and lung cancer for building occupants and schoolchildren were estimated to be hundreds to thousands of times lower than estimated risks for workers exposed at the OSHA PEL.

Environmental Regulations

The EPA currently regulates the industrial use, environmental release, and disposal of asbestos-containing materials through a variety of environmental laws. Some commercial uses of asbestos, such as spray on ceilings or on fireproofing of steel beams in buildings, have been banned by the EPA. Stringent regulations have also led to a significant decrease in the use of asbestos in new manufactured products and new construction. Currently, the largest use of asbestos in the United States is in the production of asbestos cement pipes.

A much larger issue, in terms of both potential exposures and the cost to society, involves the regulation of asbestos currently in place in U.S. structures and products. In 1987, Congress passed the Asbestos Hazard Emergency Remediation Act (AHERA), which directed the EPA to require that all U.S. school buildings have surveys done to identify any asbestos-containing materials. However, AHERA did not specify what action should be taken if asbestos was found in a school.

In the first years after AHERA, a number of schools and public buildings carried out large-scale removal of asbestos

materials that were found, but this process was often extremely expensive and sometimes resulted in higher air concentrations of asbestos fibers in the building than before the removal.

Except for regulating environmental releases and disposal, there are no EPA regulations on what steps should be taken if asbestos is found in schools, public or commercial buildings, or private homes. However, in recent years, the EPA has issued recommended guidelines that asbestos-containing materials in good repair should be left in place or encapsulated, while asbestos materials that are damaged, deteriorating, or otherwise have the potential for releasing fibers into the air should be repaired or removed. The agency has also issued recommendations for homeowners who wish to remove or repair asbestos in their homes, although this is not directly regulated by either the EPA or OSHA.

Over the past decade, many public buildings have been surveyed for asbestos-containing materials, and disclosure of whether a building contains asbestos is now a common practice in real estate transactions.

Occupational Health Regulations

In 1995, OSHA issued updated standards regulating workplace exposures to asbestos in construction and general industry and a new standard regulating asbestos used in shipyards. These standards strictly regulate all activities that may involve exposure to asbestos by U.S. workers. These standards prescribe specific work practices that must be followed in manufacturing, installation, repair, removal, and disposal of all asbestos-containing products. The standards also include requirements for worker health and safety training and for medical surveillance for workers who may be exposed to asbestos in the course of their jobs.

Current OSHA permissible exposure limits. The current OSHA permissible exposure level (PEL) for workers exposed to airborne asbestos fibers is 0.1 fibers per cc as an 8-hour time weighed average (TWA), with a short term exposure limit (STEL) of 1.0 fibers per cc over a 30 minute exposure. This level was partly chosen because it represents the lowest practical limit of detection for asbestos fibers using phase contrast light microscopy (although lower concentration levels can be measured with electron microscopy). The OSHA standards are the same for all fiber types, and for all types of manufacturing processes, even though it is known from epidemiologic and animal data that some fibers are more pathogenic, and some industrial processes present either greater or lesser risks for asbestos-related diseases.

Medical surveillance programs for asbestos workers. Workers in areas where asbestos fiber levels are above the action level (regardless of whether respirators are used) or engaged in specific work activities (regardless of the results of air monitoring for asbestos) are required by OSHA to be entered in a medical surveillance program. The components of the exam, which are specified in the OSHA asbestos standard, include a standardized questionnaire, a physical exam, spirometry, and periodic chest x-rays. The purpose of this program appears to be case finding so that disability claims can be filed and further exposure prevented, since there are no effective treatments for asbestos-related diseases.

The OSHA standard requires only that medical surveillance be offered for workers currently exposed to asbestos. There are no provisions in the standard to require surveillance for workers with significant historical asbestos exposures, even though it is acknowledged that, because of the long latency periods for asbestos-related diseases, any asbestos-related diseases found on surveillance are likely to be due to exposures 20 to 40 years in the past, rather than recent exposures.

Since there are no effective treatments for asbestos-related disease, there are no significant health benefits from early detection of the disease. Some experts recommend that those with clinical asbestosis be restricted from further asbestos exposure, based on an assumption that further exposure may cause the asbestosis to progress faster, but this remains a controversial issue.

One important part of the asbestos medical surveillance is to assure that workers are medically qualified for industrial respirator use while performing the tasks of the job. The medical surveillance exams are seen by some physicians as an opportunity for worker education, and they use these exams to reinforce the importance of using proper protective equipment and good work practices to prevent inhalation of asbestos fibers. This interaction is also seen as an opportunity to encourage potentially asbestos-exposed workers to stop smoking, which increases their risk for asbestosis and lung cancer.

The Changing Demographics of Asbestos-Related Disease

The incidence of newly diagnosed cases of asbestos-related diseases appeared to peak in the United States in the 1970s and 1980s. A large proportion of these cases were workers with a history of heavy exposure to asbestos in U.S. shipyards and other industries 20 to 40 years earlier, in the decades during and just after World War II. This pattern is consistent with the known 20- to 40-year latency periods for all asbestos-related diseases.

Epidemiologic studies suggest that risk for asbestos-related disease is directly related to both cumulative asbestos exposure and the duration since first exposure. Individuals with lower cumulative exposures tend to have longer latency periods, with clinical disease appearing 40 or more years after the first exposure.

The incidence of newly diagnosed asbestos-related diseases in U.S. workers will probably continue to decline in the future because extensive regulation of workplace asbestos exposure was in place by the 1970s. Therefore, many experts predict that, after worker cohorts exposed before the 1970s die off sometime early in the next century, asbestos-related diseases will become rare in the United States.

However, in comparison to workers heavily exposed to asbestos in the 1940s and 1950s, cohorts of workers first exposed to asbestos in the 1960s and early 1970s are likely to have both lower cumulative doses of asbestos and longer latency periods for asbestos-related diseases. Therefore, asbestos-related diseases will probably still be diagnosed in U.S. workers for the first few decades of the twenty-first century.

Unfortunately, in many rapidly industrializing Third World nations, especially in Asia, the incidence of asbestos-related diseases is likely to increase rather than decline in coming years, due to extensive industrial use of asbestos-containing materials with little effective regulation to protect workers or the public.

REFERENCES

1. American Thoracic Society: The diagnosis of nonmalignant diseases related to asbestos, *Am Rev Respir Dis* 134:363, 1986.
2. *Annual report of the chief inspector of factories for the year 1899,* Part II, Reports, London, 1899, Her Majesty's Stationery Office.
3. Blot W et al: Lung cancer after employment in shipyards during WWII, *N Engl J Med* 299:620, 1978.
4. Bohlig H, Jacob G, Muller H: *Die Asbestose der Lunger,* Stuttgart, 1960, George Thieme Verlag.
5. Browne K: Asbestos related malignancy and the Cairns hypothesis, *Br J Ind Med* 48:73, 1991.
6. Browne K, Churg A: A threshold for asbestos-related lung cancer, *Br J Ind Med* 43:145, 1986.
7. Browne K, Smither WJ: Asbestos-related mesothelioma: factors discriminating between pleural and peritoneal sites, *Br J Ind Med* 40:145, 1983.
8. Carbone M et al: Simian virus 40-like DNA sequences in human pleural mesothelioma, *Oncogene* 9:781, 1994.
9. Churg A: Chrysotile, tremolite, and malignant mesothelioma in man, *Chest* 3:621, 1993.
10. Churg A: Current issues in the pathologic and mineralogic diagnosis of asbestos-induced disease, *Chest* 84:275, 1983.
11. Churg A: Fiber counting and analysis in the diagnosis of asbestos-related disease, *Hum Pathol* 13:381-382, 1982.
12. Churg A: Lung cancer cell type and asbestos exposure, *JAMA* 253:2984, 1985.
13. Churg A, Tron V, Wright JL: Effects of cigarette smoke exposure on retention of asbestos fibers in various morphologic compartments of the guinea pig lung, *Am J Pathol* 129:385, 1987.
14. Churg A et al: Mineralogic parameters related to amosite asbestos-induced fibrosis in humans, *Am Rev Respir Dis* 142:1331, 1990.
15. Cooke WE: Fibrosis of the lungs due to the inhalation of asbestos dust, *Br Med J* 2:147, 1924.
16. Cooke WE: Pulmonary asbestosis, *Br Med J* 2:1024, 1927.
17. Davis J et al: The pathogenicity of long versus short fibre samples of amosite asbestos administered to rats by inhalation and intraperitoneal injection, *Br J Exp Path* 67:415-430, 1986.
18. Davis JMG, Cowie HA: The relationship between fibrosis and cancer in experimental animals exposed to asbestos and other fibers, *Environ Health Perspect* 88:305, 1990.
19. Dement JM et al: Estimates of dose-response for respiratory cancer among chrysotile asbestos textile workers. In Walton WH, editor: *Inhaled particles V,* Oxford, 1982, Pergamon Press.

20. Doll R: Mortality from lung cancer in asbestos workers, *Br J Ind Med* 12:81, 1955.

21. Dreessen's public health bulletin 241: *A study of asbestosis in the asbestos textile industry,* Washington, DC, 1938, US Government Printing Office.

22. Epler GR, McLoud TC, Gaensler EA: Prevalence and incidence of benign asbestos pleural effusion in a working population, *JAMA* 247:617, 1982.

23. Finkelstein MM: A study of dose-response relationships for asbestos associated disease, *Br J Ind Med* 42:319, 1985.

24. Fleischer WE et al: A health survey of pipe covering operations in constructing naval vessels, *J Ind Hyg Toxicol* 28:9-16, 1946.

25. Frumkin H, Pransky G, Cosmatos I: Radiologic detection of pleural thickening, *Am Rev Respir Dis* 142:1325, 1990.

26. Gibbs AR: Role of asbestos and other fibres in the development of diffuse malignant mesothelioma, *Thorax* 649, 1990.

27. HEI-AR: *Asbestos in public and commercial buildings: A literature review and synthesis of current knowledge,* volume 45, Cambridge, Mass, 1991, HEI-AR.

28. Homa DM, Garabrant DH, Gillespie BW: A meta-analysis of colorectal cancer and asbestos exposure, *Am J Epidemiol* 139:1210, 1994.

29. Hughes JM, Weill H: Asbestosis as a precursor of asbestos-related lung cancer: results of a prospective mortality study, *Br J Ind Med* 48:229, 1991.

30. Hughes JM, Weill H: Asbestos exposure: quantitative assessment of risk, *Am Rev Respir Dis* 133:5, 1986.

31. Jones RD, Smith DM, Thomas PG: Mesothelioma in Great Britain in 1968-1983, *Scand J Work Environ Health* 14:145, 1988.

32. Kipen H et al: Pulmonary fibrosis in asbestos insulation workers with lung cancer, *Br J Ind Med* 44:96, 1987.

33. Lanphear BP, Buncher CR: Latent period for malignant mesothelioma of occupational origin, *J Occup Med* 34:718, 1992.

34. Lilis R et al: Asbestosis: interstitial pulmonary fibrosis and pleural fibrosis in a cohort of asbestos insulation workers: influence of cigarette smoking, *Am J Ind Med* 10:459, 1986.

35. Lippmann M: Deposition and retention of inhaled fibres: effects on incidence of lung cancer and mesothelioma, *Occup Environ Med* 51:793, 1994.

36. Merewether ERA, Price CW: *Report on effects of asbestos dust on the lungs and dust suppression in the asbestos industry,* London, 1934, His Majesty's Stationery Office.

37. Mossman BT, Gee JBL: Asbestos-related diseases, *N Engl J Med* 320:1721, 1989.

38. Murray H: *Montague-testimony. Report of departmental committee on compensation for industrial diseases, minutes of evidence,* London, 1907, His Majesty's Stationery Office.

39. Pelnar PV: Further evidence of nonasbestos-related mesothelioma, *Scand J Work Environ Health* 14:141, 1988.

40. Robinson BWS et al: Alveolitis of pulmonary asbestosis, *Chest* 90:396, 1986.

41. Rudd RM: New developments in asbestos-related pleural disease, *Thorax* 51:210, 1996.

42. Schwartz DA et al: The clinical utility and reliability of asbestos bodies in bronchoalveolar fluid, *Am Rev Respir Dis* 144:684, 1991.

43. Selikoff IJ: Constraints in estimating occupational contributions to current cancer mortality in the United States, *Cold Spring Harb Symp Quant Biol* 9:3, 1987.

44. Selikoff IJ: Mortality experience of insulation workers in the United States and Canada 1943-1976, *Ann N Y Acad Sci* 330:91, 1979.

45. Selikoff I, Lee D: In Lee D, Hewson E, Klun D, editors: *Asbestos and disease,* New York, 1978, Academic Press.

46. Selikoff IJ, Seidman H: Asbestos-associated deaths among insulation workers in the United States and Canada, 1967-1987, *Ann N Y Acad Sci* 643:1, 1991.

47. Sluis-Cremer GK, Bezuidenhart BN: Relation between asbestosis and bronchial cancer in amphibole asbestos miners, *Br J Ind Med* 46:537, 1989.

48. Smith DD: Asbestos-related pleural disease: questions in need of answers, *Clin Pulm Med* 1:289, 1994.

49. Smith DD: Plaques, cancer, and confusion, *Chest* 105:7, 1994.

50. Stanton M et al: Relation of particle dimension to carcinogenicity in amphibole asbestos and other fibrous minerals, *J Natl Cancer Inst* 67:965, 1981.

51. Voisin C et al: Asbestos-related rounded atelectasis, *Chest* 107:477, 1995.

52. Wagner JC, Pooley FD: Mineral fibres and mesothelioma, *Thorax* 41:161, 1985.

53. Weiss W: Cigarette smoke, asbestos, and small irregular opacities, *Am Rev Respir Dis* 130:293, 1984.

54. Yegles M et al: Role of fibre characteristics on cytotoxicity and induction of anaphase/telephase aberrations in rat pleural mesothelial cells in vitro: correlations with in vivo animal findings, *Carcinogenesis* 16:2751, 1995.

56

Chemical Carcinogenesis

Scott D. Phillips
Michael T. Parra

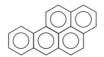

benzo(a)pyrene

- Cancer is a multistep process that includes induction, promotion, and progression

- The prevention of environmental and occupational cancers can best be accomplished by elimination of tobacco products and the use of sun blocking agents

Furth and Sobel[16] predicted more than 50 years ago that most cancers are the result of one or more genetic alterations at the level of the individual cell.

Tumors may be either benign or malignant. Benign tumors are derived from normally growing tissues; examples include neuromas, fibromas, and lipomas. Malignant tumors are derived from either the epidermis (ectoderm and endoderm) or the mesenchyma. Epithelial-derived malignant tumors are termed *carcinomas,* and malignant tumors of mesenchymal origin are called *sarcomas.* The latter are typically named after the tissue of their origin, such as rhabdomyosarcoma or leiomyosarcoma. As these altered cells reproduce, they become tumors, which may be either benign or malignant, depending on their pattern of growth: slow for benign tumors and more rapidly dividing for malignant tumors.

HISTORY

The first reports of chemical carcinogenesis have been attributed to Paracelsus. By the sixteenth century, it was recognized that miners of Europe developed a chronic wasting illness termed *Bergkrankheiten,* possibly due to exposure to the decay products of uranium that led to lung cancer. Following this was the identification of bladder tumors in dyestuff workers. The bladder cancer was thought to be due to the synthetic dyes, and not until 1938 was bladder cancer reproduced by the aromatic amines in experimental animals.

Percival Pott[30] in 1775 described cancer of the scrotum in English chimney sweeps. It was ultimately attributed to polycyclic aromatic hydrocarbons. These substances are

Environmental Protection Agency Carcinogen Designations

A. Human carcinogen: sufficient evidence from epidemiologic studies to support a causal association between exposure and cancer

B. Probable human carcinogen: weight of evidence of human carcinogenicity based on epidemiologic studies is limited; agents for which weight of evidence of carcinogenicity based on animal studies is sufficient
Two groups:
  B1: Limited evidence of carcinogenicity from epidemiologic studies
  B2: Sufficient evidence from animal studies; inadequate human and animal evidence of carcinogenicity

C. Possible human carcinogen; limited evidence of carcinogenicity in animals in the absence of human data

D. Not classifiable as to human carcinogenicity; inadequate human and animal evidence of carcinogenicity, or no data are available

E. Evidence of noncarcinogenicity for humans: no evidence for carcinogenicity in at least two adequate animal tests in different species or in both adequate epidemiologic and animal studies

International Agency for Research on Cancer Carcinogen Designations

1. Carcinogenic to humans: sufficient evidence of carcinogenicity

2A. Probably carcinogenic to humans: limited human evidence, sufficient evidence in experimental animals

2B. Possibly carcinogenic to humans: limited evidence in humans in the absence of sufficient evidence in experimental animals

3. Not classifiable as to carcinogenicity to humans

4. Probably not carcinogenic to humans

National Toxicology Program's Carcinogen Designation Scheme

1. Known to be a carcinogen. Sufficient evidence of carcinogenicity from studies in humans to indicate a causal relationship between the agent and human cancer

2. Reasonably anticipated to be a carcinogen
  2A: Limited evidence of carcinogenicity from studies in humans to indicate that causal relationship is credible
  2B: Sufficient evidence of carcinogenicity from studies in experimental animals

Table 56-1 Chemical agents that have been associated with cancer, not including chemotherapeutic agents

Chemical	Environmental Protection Agency	International Agency for Research on Cancer	National Toxicology Program
Aflatoxins	—	1	A
4-Aminobiphenol	—	1	A
Arsenic	A	1	A
Asbestos	A	1	A
Benzene	A	1	A
Benzidine	A	1	A
Bis (chloroethyl) ether	A	1	A
Coal tars	—	1	A
Coke production	—	1	A
Chromium (VI)	A	1	A
Diethylstilbestrol	A	1	A
Direct black 38	A	—	B
Direct blue 6	A	—	B
Direct brown 95	A	—	—
Estrogens	—	1	A
Methylhydrazine	A	—	—
2-Naphthylamine	—	1	A
Nickel	A	1	A
Tobacco (smoke)	—	1	—
Vinyl chloride	A	1	A

now recognized as human carcinogens by a variety of organizations throughout the world.

Chemical exposures have long been associated with cancer. Toxicologists are involved in the field of carcinogenesis from the etiologic and preventive standpoints. Mutagenesis and tumor formation are a type of end-organ response to chemicals in our environments and workplaces.

ORGANIZATIONS

Several organizations in the world are deeply involved in chemical carcinogenesis and the "rating" of substances according to their ability to induce cancers: the International Agency for Research on Cancer (IARC) of the World

Health Organization, the U.S. Environmental Protection Agency (EPA), and the National Toxicology Program (NTP) of the U.S. Public Health Service. Each of these agencies has categorized chemicals that have been tested into groups according to their ability to cause malignant transformation (see the above three boxes). Ratings of 1 or A signify ample evidence to include the chemical as a carcinogen in humans. Chemical carcinogenicity data are based on human and animal evidence. Benzene is recognized as a human carcinogen by all three organizations. Chemicals felt to be human carcinogens are listed in Table 56-1. Chemotherapeutic agents and ionizing radiation that may result in cancer are not listed. Certain environmental

Table 56-2 Common cancers that have been associated with certain occupations

Industry of material	Carcinogen	Site of associated cancer*
Asbestos	Asbestos	Lung
Brewing	Alcohol	Liver
Commercial fishing	Ultraviolet light	Skin
Demolition	Asbestos	Lung
Furniture manufacturing	Wood dusts	Nasal
Glue factories	Benzene	Leukemia
Insulation	Asbestos	Lung
Ion-exchange resin production	Bos (chloromethyl) ether	Lung
Isopropyl alcohol manufacturing	Isopropyl alcohol	Lung
Mineral oil	Polycyclic hydrocarbons	Lung
Nickel refining	Nickel	Respiratory
Ore manufacturing	Chromium	Lung
Outdoor occupations	Ultraviolet light	Skin
Pesticides—arsenic	Arsenic	Lung, skin
Petroleum production	Polycyclic hydrocarbons	Lung
Pigment manufacturing	Chromium	Lung
Rubber manufacturing	Aromatic amines	Bladder
Shipyards	Asbestos	Lung
Smelters	Arsenic	Lung, skin
Uranium mining	Ionizing radiation	Lung, others
Varnish	Benzene	Leukemia
Vinyl chloride	Vinyl chloride	Liver

From Costanza ME et al: *Cancer manual,* ed 8, Framingham, Mass, 1990, American Cancer Society, Massachusetts Division. Reproduced with permission.

scenarios or occupations are more likely to be associated with certain forms of cancer than others, as noted in Table 56-2.

The American Cancer Society is actively involved in supporting both patients and families in the prevention, diagnosis, and treatment of cancers.

OVERVIEW OF CANCER BIOLOGY

A multistep process in carcinogenesis has evolved during the last 80 years.[4,6,7,14] A two-stage model coining the terms *initiation* and *promotion* was originally proposed by Rous and Kidd in 1941.[33] This concept has been confirmed and supported by several other researchers.[15]

This initial model is generally believed to be a simplified approach. Many factors point to several steps within these two stages that may be required for a tumor to progress. Because of this, carcinogenesis is currently described as initiation, promotion, and progression.

MOLECULAR TARGETS AND CHEMICAL CARCINOGENESIS

Chemicals may cause genetic damage from either a single base pair substitution or gross chromosomal changes. These may lead to either altered expression of the gene or a change in the chemical function of the gene.[5]

Genes that are of particular importance include those involved in the proliferation and differentiation of cells. Many of these types of genes have recently come to be known as *protooncogenes* and *tumor suppressor genes.*

Protooncogenes are normal cellular genes that, when activated inappropriately as oncogenes, cause altered regulation of growth and differentiation pathways and enhance the probability of neoplastic transformation by the cell. Tumor suppressor genes are normal cellular genes that, when inactivated, may cause disregulation of growth and differentiation pathways and enhance the probability of neoplastic transformation. It is now becoming clear that the development of tumors common in adults (e.g., of the lung and breast) involves the loss or inactivation of multiple tumor suppressor genes or the activation of protooncogenes. The best-characterized example of this human tumor is that of the colon, in which three tumor suppressor genes (MCC, p53 DCC) and one protooncogene, K-*ras,* are frequently altered and specific genetic alterations are associated with progressive stages of tumor development.[13]

These findings support a multistage model of neoplastic development. Substances recognized currently as human carcinogens by most official organizations are shown in Tables 56-1 and 56-2. Chemicals have long been known or thought to be responsible for the cause of cancer. Molecular causes of human cancers have emerged in research into genetic and epigenetic changes from the interaction of a variety of environmental industrial compounds with DNA. It is commonly held that each tumor is descended from a single altered cell, referred to as *monoclonal* in origin. Cells must undergo multiple changes after modification to result in a tumor (Fig. 56-1). A cell may be attacked by an electrophilic chemical that can covalently bind to the cell's DNA. This forms a DNA-adduct, which may result in mutation. In the presence of a promoter, this process may lead to tumor initiation. Repair mechanisms are in place to combat the constant barrage of chemical attacks on the genome, such as free radical scavengers or tumor suppressor genes.

MECHANISMS OF CARCINOGENICITY

A variety of possible pathobiologic processes are implicated in carcinogenesis (see first box on p. 492). Attempts to categorize the carcinogens according to the mechanisms of action are not always possible because a single carcinogen may have multiple effects and, hence, may be perceived as operating as several different mechanisms.

Genetic changes induced by chemical carcinogens could include gene mutations, gene amplifications, chromosomal

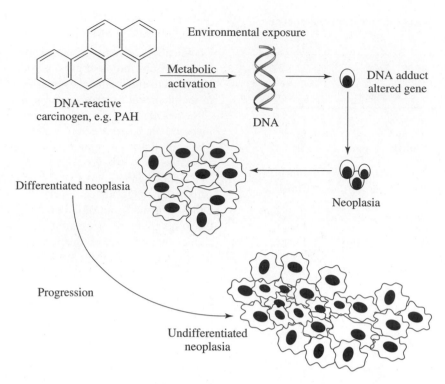

Fig. 56-1 Potential pathway by which environmental carcinogen exposure could produce tumor initiation, promotion, and progression.

Mechanisms of Carcinogenesis
1. Mutation
2. Receptor mediated
3. Mitogen
4. Cytotoxic
5. Others

Potential Genetic Mechanisms in Carcinogenesis
A. Distinguish whether direct or indirect receptor mediated
1. Proliferative—short-term or sustained
2. Altered differentiation. Question: transformation
B. Type
1. Hormones
a. Steroid E_{21}
b. Peptide
2. Growth factors (EGI, TPA, oncoproteins)
3. Cytotoxic-reparative, proliferative, (melamine) bladder stones/carbon tetrachloride, d-limioline
4. Inhibit apoptosis (phenobarbital)
5. H_2 antagonist, etc.
6. P450 inducers (PCBs), phenobarbital
7. Other spindle inhibition and reactive oxygen species

rearrangement, and aneuploidy (see box at right). Specific examples have been identified for each of these genetic changes. One such example is the observation of point mutations that activate protooncogenes and inactivate tumor suppressor genes in certain cancers. Chromosomal rearrangements that lead to activation of protooncogenes or inactivation of tumor suppressor genes are also documented.

Chemical carcinogen binding to DNA is easily found with radio-labeled carcinogens. Carcinogen-DNA adducts differ quantitatively and qualitatively in their mutagenic potential. Moreover, the adduct concentrations obtained with some carcinogens may vary widely among cell types of given tissues.[3]

The carcinogen-derived adducts and adducted bases in cells and tissues can be eliminated spontaneously by DNA repair processes.

Historically, carcinogenesis is divided into two to four phases, including initiation, promotion, and typically progression. The initial interaction of the chemical with DNA is termed *initiation*. Tumor promoters facilitate clonal expansion; those previously initiated allow them to form increased numbers of cancer cells. Progression is the process that allows the cells to become malignant cancers.

Carcinogenesis is a multistage process of induction followed by promotion and progression. The concept of a multistage process in carcinogenesis was first recognized during skin cancer experiments in mice. Polycyclic aromatic hydrocarbons (PAH) were applied (inducer) to the skin in extremely low doses. No skin tumors developed during the rodent's lifetime. This application was followed by weekly topical doses of croton oil (promoter), which resulted in multiple skin tumors. Significant delays of up to a year in the application of the promoter resulted in a similar number of tumors.[29] Initiaters alter the genetic material of the cell and do not result in cancer after a single exposure. These chemicals are genotoxic and bind to DNA. Multiple applications of an initiater may result in tumor formation. Promoters, by contrast, are not carcinogenic and do not bind to DNA as do initiaters; rather, they permit the initiated cell to develop into a neoplasia. Rarely, a chemical may be both an initiater and promoter; when both properties occur from one substance, the substance is referred to as a *complete* carcinogen.

Carcinogens may be termed either *primary* or *procarcinogens*. The former directly acts with DNA as a genotoxin; the latter requires metabolic activation before it can interact with the genome.

Most xenobiotics that result in cancer require some type of metabolic alteration, typically conversion to highly reactive electrophils,[25] as was discovered more than 20 years ago regarding the metabolism of azo dyes. It has been shown that the enzyme that most commonly results in activation of the substrate is of the P450 enzyme system. An interesting note is that distinct P450s are involved in the activation of different types of chemical carcinogens. For example, the metabolism of dichloromethane (methylene chloride) is oxidized by P450 IIE1 in various rodent models.[17] Others have shown that P450 ISF-G activates 2-naphthylamine to a carcinogen.[8]

Research shows that chemicals may be activated in one portion of the body, yet result in cancer in another area. For example, certain direct-acting chemicals such as *N*-methylnitrosourea (NMU) are activated in the liver and do not need metabolic activation, and similar agents can also show target organ specificity. An example of a chemical that requires metabolic activation to result in distant carcinogenesis is acrylonitrile (ACO). This is converted to cyanoethylene oxide in the liver and distributed throughout the body. After this distribution, cancer results in the brain without evidence of cancer at other sites.[18] Elimination routes are also important with regard to location of cancers in that some metabolites might be excreted in the urine and result in bladder cancer. It is apparent that carcinogenic compounds bind covalently to DNA or RNA to result in induction. This covalent binding to DNA results in a substrate-DNA adduct.[34] These may function either as inducers or as promoters. Certain genes, if they are targeted by chemical carcinogens, can result in disturbances of growth and differentiation. They are termed *protooncogenes* and are numerous. These may alter growth or differentiation by one of several mechanisms, including point mutations, chromosome translocations, or gene amplification. Also, inactivation of tumor suppressor genes may occur, which results in expression of tumorigenic processes.

Carcinogens may act on cellular constituents, including proteins, lipids, and nucleic acids, or directly with the genetic material within the cell. Certain carcinogens require "activation" whereas others may directly interact with those cellular components to result in the cascade of chemical carcinogenesis. Chemicals that require metabolic activation are termed *indirect acting*. They are generally stable in an environment and are more commonly encountered by the general population. Metabolic activity is affected by many factors, including species, gender, age, diet, and enzyme-inducing substances. Indirect-acting carcinogens are also known as precarcinogens or procarcinogens. Most indirect-acting xenobiotics, including those that are carcinogens, may be detoxified by oxidation to result in the ultimate carcinogen. Typically these reactions are through the P450 system. There are many forms of this enzyme system, and they have undergone a variety of nomenclature changes. The most recent seems to be a system of naming the subenzymes based on chromosomal location.[27]

Relatively few carcinogens are direct-acting, since by their nature are chemically unstable. Examples of "direct-acting" carcinogens are ethyleneimine, β-propiolactone, bis (chloromethyl) ether, bis (2-chlorol-ethyl) sulfide, diepoxybutane, ethylene oxide, methyl methane sulfonate, and nitrogen mustard (e.g., cyclophosphamide). Many of these compounds are alkylators of cellular macromolecules. Typically, they interact at the seven position of guanine and cytosine acids. They do not require metabolic activation for this interaction to occur. Some think that direct-acting carcinogens lack potency in that these species are so reactive because of the intervening metabolic processes that occur before they reach their final receptor. Compounds that have less reactivity may, in fact, be more potent. However, most direct-acting carcinogens do not represent an appreciable hazard to the general population, with the exception of those involved in the treatment of patients with chemotherapeutic agents.

Typically, we are rarely exposed to a single chemical; rather, mixtures tend to be the usual source of exposure. One substance may predominate. Examples include tobacco smoke and diesel exhaust fumes. The interactions of various mixtures may result in enhanced, reduced, or no significant effect on carcinogenesis. Mixtures may provide both inducers and promoters and result in an augmented effect. This chapter focuses on the effects of single exposures, with the understanding that this is seldom the case.

GENOTOXIC VERSUS EPIGENETIC CARCINOGENS

Genotoxic carcinogens are those that either react as such with genetic material or are converted by metabolism to react as intermediates and form adducts with genetic material, the cell. Direct- and indirect-acting carcinogens fall into the class of genotoxic carcinogens. The nongenotoxic or epigenetic carcinogens do not appear to bind to the DNA of the cell but may form adducts with other cellular constituents.

Host Factors That Can Modify a Carcinogenic Response

Species and strain
Route of exposure
Pharmacokinetics
DNA modification repair
Promotion
Specific target genes

Lung Carcinogens

Asbestos	Beryllium
Arsenic	Cadmium
Chloromethyl ethers	Vinyl chloride
Chromium	Formaldehyde
Mustard gas	Man-made mineral fiber
Nickel	Silica
Polyaromatic hydrocarbons	Wood dusts
Radon	Wood smoke
Acrylonitrile	Cutting oils

It is not known whether carcinogens act as initiators by causing point mutations activating oncogenes, by causing deletions in growth suppressor genes, or by acting on elements that regulate transcription or induce changes in DNA amplification. Because of these considerations, classifications of carcinogens are generally grouped into either genotoxic or epigenetic. However, this is complicated by the absence of clear-cut criteria for defining genotoxicity.

Material such as films and fibers may be considered as epigenetic carcinogens. Also, certain physiochemical factors such as osmolarity or abnormal pH induced by some nonphysiologic condition may lead to the development of cancer by epigenetic mechanisms. This may be especially true in the bladder. Certain conditions that allow the formation of crystals and calculi in the bladder, especially in male rats, have led to bladder tumors with lifetime high-level exposure. This is best seen with saccharine. Diverse types of compounds fall into this category.

Dong and Jeffrey[11] have reported that many chemical carcinogens cause tumors at specific sites or at limited sites; they term this *ganotrophy*. It includes a variety of tissue types and tissue sites including the following.

SITE AND SPECIES SPECIFICITY

It has long been known that specific chemicals cause tumors in specific organs. This is termed *organotropism*.[31] The organ specificity of chemicals has significant interspecies similarity. For example, vinyl chloride is known to induce angiosarcomas of the liver in rats, mice, and hamsters, as well as humans.[12]

Certain carcinogens are found to have species-dependent organ specificity. In dogs, monkeys, and humans, 2-naphthylamine causes bladder cancer, and it is known to produce hepatomas in mice; however, it has not been shown to be carcinogenic in cats or rabbits.[11] Factors that determine tissue specificity include species strain, route of exposure, pharmacokinetics, DNA modification repair, promotion, and specific target genes (see above box).

Lung carcinogens include many familiar agents. The most common that may result in lung cancer are smoking and radon (see box at top right). Hematopoietic malignancies including certain leukemias and lymphomas are associated with ionizing radiation and benzene; urinary tract cancers include benzedrine, 4-biphenylmeamine,

2-naphthylamine, NN bis (2-chloroethyl)-H-1,3,2-oxazak-phosphorine, 2-(bis) 2-chloroethyl (amino), tetrahydro-2-oxide, purine, 6-(1-methyl-4-nitroimadazol5-yl), thyo-/+, polycyclic aromatic hydrocarbons, asbestos, lead salts, cadmium, and petroleum products. Gastrointestinal cancers, colon and rectal cancer, and hepatocellular cancers are associated with aflatoxins, thiotrast (thorium dioxide), steroids (both antibiotic and estrogen types), vinyl chloride, and arsenic. Gall bladder cancer and pancreatic cancer are seen with cigarette smoking. Thyroid endocrine cancers can be seen with ionizing radiation. Breast cancer is seen with ionizing radiation, radium, and possibly asbestos. Germ cell (ovary and testis) cancers are associated with ionizing radiation, asbestos, dimethylformamide, chromates, and ionizing radiation. Prostate cancer can be associated with ionizing radiation and possibly cadmium, acrylonitrile, and dimethylformamide. Central nervous system chemicals such as astrocytomas can be seen with vinyl chloride, acrylonitrile, nitrosoureas, lead acetate, diethyl and dimethyl sulfate, ethylene oxide, 1,3-propane sulfone, and ionizing radiation. Dermatologic cancers such as melanomas, squamous cell, and basal cell carcinogens may result from ultraviolet radiation, arsenic, and polycyclic aromatic hydrocarbons.

INTERPRETATION OF ANIMAL CARCINOGENICITY TESTS

A long-term carcinogenicity study may be conducted on a variety of different agents thought to induce cancers. Commonly, this is done in rodent studies over a defined period of time, typically in two species in two sexes for 2 years in rats. Chemicals termed *carcinogens* are those that lead to a significant increase and instance of neoplasias of one or more tissue types in the exposed animals over an appropriate control group. To determine the appropriate dose for the long-term assay, information from short-term, 90-day exposure studies are used. Doses are then decreased from the 90-day dose, typically to a dose that does not alter the normal growth or survival patterns in these animals. Results obtained from these types of long-term assays do provide information regarding common and uncommon neoplasias. Evidence includes progression of tumors, latency of tumors, multiplicity, metastases, dose-response relationships, and structure-activity relationships.

A recent approach has been transgenic testing, which can be done either in vitro or in vivo. Transgenic cells are created when a specific gene is introduced, along with a promoter, into a cell to determine tumor induction upon exposure to a specific chemical or substrate. More recently, transgenic animals are used as a way of studying the consequences of introduction of various protooncogenes and activated oncogenes into specific tissue sites. This field is very exciting because transgenic mice have been shown to respond within weeks to months when exposed to a carcinogen, which allows for collection of a great deal of information in a relatively short period of time.

Short-term tests for mutagenicity typically are performed in vitro. The basis for these tests is the assumption that all carcinogens are mutagenic. Many agents known to be carcinogenic in humans are also mutagenic. A number of short-term tests are available. They all have in common the use of genetic damage as an end point. The most widely known is the mutagenicity assay developed by Bruce Ames and colleagues.[2] In this test, bacterial cells that are deficient in DNA repair lack the ability to grow without histidine. The bacterial cells are treated with several dose levels of the chemical compound. They revert to a histidine-positive phenotype. This results in the bacteria, typically *Salmonella typhimurium,* to mutate away from histidine. There are also several mammalian mutation assays, including the mouse lymphoma L5178Y (MOLY) assay, the Chinese hamster ovary (CHO) assay, and the V79 fibroblast assay. Tests can also be done indirectly, leading to the incorporation of radio-labeled thymidine into DNA as a repair mechanism.[1]

HUMAN BIOMARKERS

Human biomarker research has been exploding in recent years. For some time, markers of tumors have been measured in biologic fluids. Common biomarkers include prostate specific antigen (PSA), a serum test that is used in the diagnosis and screening of prostate cancer, and carcinoembryonic antigen (CEA), a protein used in the monitoring of patients during treatment for colon and breast cancer. Some commonly used tests are the CA-15-3 and CA-125, both used to monitor breast and ovarian cancer, respectively. Other serum markers include α-fetoprotein (α-FP), β-human choriogonodotropic hormone (β-HCG), and Ca19-9, which are used to assist in the diagnosis of carcinomas of the testes, liver, and pancreas, respectively. Many of these biomarkers are sensitive but lack specificity for certain types of cancers (e.g., CEA for cancer of the colon, breast, and lung). Because of this, other tumor markers such as the antimalign antibody (AMAS) in serum assay are in development to assist in the diagnosis and detection of cancer at earlier stages. A more complete listing of biomarkers can be found in Table 56-3.

Recently, genetic biomarkers have been studied. The most notable are the BRCA1 and BRCA2 cancer suscepti-

Table 56-3 Cancer biomarkers to detect established disease

Biomarker	Cancer site
Carcinoembryonic antigens (CEA)	Colorectal, breast
Cancer procoagulant (CP)	Colorectal
Carbohydrate antigens (CA)	Colorectal
CA-50	Colorectal, pancreatic
CA 15-3	Ovarian, colorectal, breast
CA 125	Breast
CA 549	Colorectal, breast
CA 19-9	Testicular, liver, pancreatic
CA 242	Pancreatic
CA M26	Colorectal, breast
CA M29	Colorectal, breast
Tissue polypeptide antigen (TPA)	Pancreatic
Tissue polypeptide specific antigen (TPS)	Pancreatic
Prostate specific antigen (PSA)	Prostate
Prostate acid phosphatase (PAP)	Prostate
α-Fetoprotein (AFP)	Testicular, liver, pancreatic
β-Human chorionic gonadotropin (β-HCG)	Testicular, liver, pancreatic
Mucinlike carcinoma associated antigen (MCA)	Breast
NCC-ST-439 (ST-439)	Breast
Nucleolar proliferation antigen (P120)	Breast
Cancer-associated serum antigen (CASA)	Ovarian
Protooncogene marker (C-erB-2)	Ovarian
α-Transforming growth factor (α-TGF)	Lung, pancreatic, colorectal
Plasma sialyl transferase (ST)	Lung, colorectal, ovarian, cervix, pancreatic
B-protein	Many
Disaccharide mucin marker (D-GAlNac or T-Ag)	Colorectal
Galactose oxidase mucin test (GO)	Colorectal
Gross cystic disease protein (GCDP)	Breast

Concerning many other markers that are available. Hee SQ, editor: *Biological monitoring: An introduction,* New York, 1993, Van Nostrand Reinhold.

bility genes. The BRCA1 gene was first localized in 1990 by Hall and associates at the University of California at Berkeley. Using linkage analysis, they mapped the area to the long arm of chromosome 17 (q12-q21).[20] The gene was identified in 1994 by Skolnick at the University of Utah. The BRCA1 codes for a protein of 1863 amino acids. Most mutations (± 70%) of the BRCA1 gene involve the truncation of the protein. Some authors suggested that women who are heterozygous for mutations of BRCA1 and BRCA2 genes may have up to a 90% lifetime risk for cancer of the breast, colon, ovary, and other sites with an early age of onset.[22,24,28] The prospect of having these cancer susceptibility genes raises important and difficult questions in the area of preemployment testing in industry.

MEDICAL MONITORING

In the past several years, screening populations for medical abnormalities has been proposed as a method of finding disease early. As these programs frequently occur in the realm of environmental toxicology and medicine, exposures generally are far less than in the occupational setting. There are several major concerns associated with programs such as these.[19,23] The potential benefits of screening would include the following:

1. Finding those who would have died from their disease without detection
2. Early detection may require less radical treatment in order to obtain a cure
3. The knowledge that one has a negative test
4. Reduction in costs due to potentially less therapy needed to cure an individual

The drawbacks of a shotgun-approach monitoring program include:

1. A longer period of morbidity, due to earlier detection of the disease process
2. Overtreatment of borderline abnormalities
3. Lack of reassurance for those with false-negative tests
4. Increased morbidity or mortality for those with a false-positive test
5. The potential hazard of the test procedure, such as open lung biopsy
6. The cost of a screening program

If a monitoring program is undertaken, the selected screening test(s) should have sufficient sensitivity and specificity to detect a disease process. The disease should be more likely in the population being screened than the general population. Patients should find the test(s) acceptable without undue discomfort. The consequences of a test result should be determined ahead of time. Appropriate follow-up and monitoring of results must be considered.

Because cancer is frequently an end point for screening programs, several organizations have evaluated the concept of screening programs for certain tumors. The International Union against Cancer, The American Cancer Society, and the Early Detection Working Guidelines of the National Cancer Institute (NCI) all have recommendations on screening for selected cancers. All of the organizations agree that physical examinations, breast self-examinations, pap smears, mammography, and fecal occult blood testing are important; the age of the person at screening varies. Screening for lung cancer and for stomach cancer, except in Japan, are not recommended. Prostate screening is recommended after the age of 40 by the NCI. Biomarkers are not universally recommended, though as tests become refined, recommendations in this area may change. Table 56-3 lists many current biomarkers that can be used in cancer screening.

CONCLUSION

Our knowledge of chemical-induced carcinogenesis is rapidly progressing. The genome has been mapped, and each year many new genes are identified that relate to cancer, such as the BRCA1 gene and breast cancer.

The prevention of environmentally and occupationally induced cancers can best be obtained by elimination of tobacco products. Reportedly, this accounts for up to 30% of all cases of newly diagnosed cancers in the United States. In fact, according to some, there has been no recent dramatic increased risk in cancers except for those due to asbestos and tobacco products. The control of well-known exposures such as tobacco, alcohol, and sun and knowledge of the age-specific variation in cancer could reduce rates by 80% to 90%.[10] Further research is needed into behavioral and other methods that could reduce exposure to environmental tobacco smoke and other preventable sources of carcinogens.

REFERENCES

1. Ames BM et al: Carcinogens are mutagens: a simple test system combining liver homogenates for activation in bacteria for detection, *Proc Natl Acad Sci U S A* 70:2281, 1973.
2. Ames BN, Shigenaga MK, Gold LS: DNA lesions, inducible DNA repair, and cell division: three key factors in mutagenesis and carcinogenesis, *Environ Health Perspect* 93:35, 1993.
3. Belinsky SA et al: Cell selective alkylation of DNA in rat lung following low dose exposure to the tobacco specific carcinogen 4-(N-methyl-N-nitrosamino)-1-(3-pyridyl)-1-butanone, *Cancer Res* 47:1143, 1987.
4. Berenblum I: The mechanism of carcinogenesis: the study of the significance of carcinogenic action related phenomena, *Cancer Res* 1:807, 1941.
5. Bishop JM: The molecular genetics of cancer, *Science* 235:305, 1987.
6. Bishop JM: Molecular themes in oncogenesis, *Cell* 64:235, 1991.
7. Case RAM et al: Tumours of the urinary bladder in workmen engaged in the manufacture and use of certain dyestuff intermediates in the British chemical industry. I. The role of aniline, benzidine alpha-naphthylamine and beta naphthylamine, *Br J Ind Med* 11:75, 1954.
8. Concelman GM Jr et al: Induction of transitional cell carcinomas of the urinary bladder in monkeys fed naphthylamine, *J Natl Cancer Inst* 42:825, 1969.
9. Costanza ME et al: *Cancer manual,* ed 8, Framingham, Mass, 1990, American Cancer Society, Massachusetts Division.
10. Doll R: Nature and nurture: possibilities for cancer control, *Carcinogenesis* 17:177, 1996.
11. Dong Z, Jeffrey AM: Mechanisms of organ specificity and chemical carcinogenesis, *Cancer Invest* 8:523, 1990.
12. Etoni C, Lefemine G: Carcinogenicity bioassay of vinyl chloride: current results, *Ann N Y Acad Sci* 246:185, 1975.
13. Fearon ER, Vogelstein B: The genetic model for colorectal tumorogenesis, *Cell* 61:759, 1990.
14. Foulds L: The experimental study of tumor progression: a review, *Cancer Res* 14:327, 1954.
15. Freidwald WF, Rous P: The initiating and promoting elements in tumor production, *J Exp Biol* 80:101, 1944.
16. Furth J, Sobel H: Neoplastic transformation of granulosa cells and graphs of normal ovaries into spleens of gonadectomized mice, *J Natl Cancer Inst* 8:7, 1947.
17. Guengerich FP, Kine D-H, Iwaski MI: Role of human cytochrome P-450IIE1 in the oxidation of many low molecular weight cancer suspects, *Chem Res Toxicol* 4:168, 1991.

18. Guengerich FP, Liebler DC: Enzymatic activation of chemicals to toxic metabolites, *Crit Rev Toxicol* 14:259, 1987.
19. *Guide to clinical preventive services. Part B. Neoplastic diseases. Report of the U S preventative task force,* ed 2, Baltimore, 1996, Williams & Wilkins.
20. Hall JM et al: Linkage of early-onset familial breast cancer to chromosome 17q21, *Science* 250:1684, 1990.
21. Hee SQ, editor: *Biological monitoring: an introduction,* New York, 1993, Van Nostrand Reinhold.
22. Hoskins KF et al: Assessment and counseling for women with family history of breast cancer. A guide for clinicians, *JAMA* 273:577, 1995.
23. MacLean CD: Principles of cancer screening, *Med Clin North Am* 80:1, 1996.
24. Marcus JN et al: Hereditary breast cancer: pathobiology, prognosis, and BRCA1 and BRCA2 gene linkage, *Cancer* 77:697, 1996.
25. Miller EC: Some current perspectives on chemical carcinogenesis in humans and experimental animals: presidential address, *Cancer Res* 38:1479, 1978.
26. Mottram JC: The origin of tar tumours in mice, whether from single cells or many cells, *J Pathol* 40:407, 1935.
27. Nebert DW et al: The P450 superfamily: updated listing on new sequences, gene mapping and recommended nomenclature, *DNA Cell Biol* 10:1, 1991.
28. Offit K, Brown K: Quantitating familial cancer risk: a resource for clinical oncologists, *J Clin Oncol* 12:1724, 1994.
29. Peraino C, Jones CA: The multistage concept of carcinogenesis. In: Sirca AE, editor: *The pathobiology of neoplasia,* New York, 1989, Plenum Press.
30. Pott P: Cancer scroti. In *The chirurgical works of Percival Pott,* London, 1775, Hawes, Clarke, Collins.
31. Rice JM, Frith CH: The nature of organo specificity chemical carcinogenesis. In Langebach R, Nes S, Rice JM, editors: New York, 1983, Plenum Press.
32. Rous P, Beard JW: The progression to carcinoma of virus-induced rabbit papillomas (shape), *J Exp Med* 62:523, 1935.
33. Rous P, Kidd JG: Conditional neoplasms and subthreshold neoplastic states, *J Exp Med* 73:299, 1941.
34. Weinstein IB: Chemical carcinogenesis. In Schien P, editor: *Medical oncology,* New York, 1985, Macmillan.

57

dioxin

environmental audits

- Environmental audits extend to all forms of property transfers

- The innocent purchaser defense may protect owners of property from liability if the government undertakes a cleanup project on their property

Environmental Audits and Property Transfers

Timothy R. Gablehouse
Scott D. Phillips

Before launching into a discussion of the risks from exposure to toxic materials presented to those conducting environmental assessments, a reminder of the reasons for environmental site assessments is in order. Environmental site assessments are today treated as routine activities, and the original point of conducting them has been lost. Today, people at financial institutions, attorneys, real estate agents, and the buyers and sellers of property refer to things like a "phase-1" environmental assessment as though everyone knows what it means.

Originally, the practice of conducting these environmental assessment studies, frequently called *environmental audits,* was to take advantage of the innocent purchaser defense to liability as an owner of property under the Comprehensive Environmental Response, Compensation, and Liability Act (CERCLA).[2] Very simply stated, the innocent purchaser defense may protect owners of property from liability if the government or a private party undertakes a cleanup project on their property.

In this very limited context, the standard that must be met to claim the innocent purchaser defense is that the purchaser had no reason to know that any hazardous substance had been released on the property. In order to demonstrate that they had "no reason to know," the purchaser must have undertaken, at the time of acquisition, all appropriate inquiry into the previous ownership and uses of the property consistent with good commercial or customary practice.

There has been little or no guidance regarding what level of effort was necessary to demonstrate good commercial or customary practice. An American Society for Testing and Material (ASTM) standard approach and checklist have been adopted;[5] however, there have been no cases or regulatory pronouncements that guarantee these standards really do establish the minimum level of activity necessary to preserve the innocent purchaser defense. Many financial institutions have reacted to the ASTM standard by requiring its use because their auditors typically look for such studies when they examine loan files.

Today, the point of conducting environmental assessments has expanded. Simply to mount a defense to CERCLA liability is no longer the driving point. It is clear to buyers and sellers of property that environmental liabilities extend well beyond the type of site that would be dealt with under CERCLA. In 1986, a federal district court ruling in Maryland set the stage for environmental audits to be liability driven rather than regulatory driven.[7] Thus, it is prudent for the buyer or seller of real property to conduct an environmental audit prior to the transfer of the property. Under the Superfund Amendments and Reauthorization Act,[6] there are purchasers' provisions with "due diligence" language that requires purchasers to have no prior knowledge or suspicion of hazardous material on the property in question. Only asbestos, lead, and PCBs are mandated in specific restricted environment for environmental assessments.[1,3,4]

The buyer and seller of today want to know about regulatory compliance costs. If the facility has been out of compliance, they want to know what it will cost to restore the facility to compliance. They want to know if neighboring property occupants have caused harm to the facility or if the facility has caused harm to them. Costs associated with nuisance and negligence cases are substantial, and the parties want to know if there is a potential for such suits. The environmental assessment of today is as focused on these other sorts of environmental compliance and liability issues as it is on the secured creditor defense.

SITE ASSESSMENTS

Some property owners conduct environmental site assessments of their own property for the purpose of determining regulatory compliance. Most of these assessments are, however, conducted when property or a business is being sold.

In a purchase transaction, the most important elements cover areas such as price and terms of the purchase. Typically, the parties have reached substantial agreement on these terms before they make the commitment to proceed with environmental assessment of the property. Unfortunately, this timing means that if the environmental assessment discovers compliance or contamination problems, the transaction has to be modified.

These modifications occur at the "eleventh hour," and there is extraordinary pressure on the consultant to quantify the costs of correcting the compliance or contamination problem. As the initial or "phase 1" environmental assessment is not designed to provide this level of detail, additional work is necessary. As the parties may have waited to the end of their negotiations to retain the consultant, the time available for additional work may be minimal. It is safe to say that the pressure on the consultant to provide concrete details in a very short period of time can be substantial.

The consultants must not allow this pressure to overwhelm their judgment on safe working conditions. All too often, work conditions are compromised to respond to the schedule demanded by the client. At this point, people get hurt and unnecessary exposure to toxics occurs.

ENVIRONMENTAL ASSESSMENT

The typical environmental assessment consists of the so-called phase 1 activity, which usually includes a search of public records and a site inspection. The search of public records is usually done by obtaining a report from a company that maintains a database of the public records. These records disclose the existence of information provided to the governmental agencies during the normal course of compliance activities. If the facility failed to properly report spills or tanks or anything that might normally be in these reports, the information is not present. The same thing is true of problems caused by the occupants of neighboring properties. This weakness in the public records is why "phase 1" activities are never limited to a public records search.

Phase 1 environmental assessments always include a site inspection (see first box on p. 501). The site inspection includes walking through the property and interviewing persons with knowledge concerning past or current uses of the property. During these inspections, the consultant is expected to note anything that suggests the presence of a compliance problem or contamination. These notes are not a guarantee that the problem exists. Instead, the process is intended to be a simple survey of possible problems.

With the exception of vacant and residential property, it is not unusual for the phase 1 report to find conditions that merit additional study in order to determine whether a compliance problem or contamination really is present. These so-called phase 2 studies typically include some sort of physical sampling of materials, soils, and water on the property.

Phase 2 activities may include sampling construction materials for asbestos, paints for lead, and soils and water for contamination (see second box on p. 501). Sampling techniques may involve hand tools and powered equipment such as large truck-mounted drilling equipment. Because many of the contaminants that can be anticipated at facilities can be toxic, personal protective equipment may be required.

Phase I: Evaluation of Existing Site Data, Property History, and Site Visit to Gather Information

Interviewing persons
Previous owners
Historical documents
Records of previous chemical use
Site maps
Underground storage tank (UST) records
Title reports
Hydrogeologic reports
Permits and licensures
Site visit
Adjacent geology
Building inspector reports
View of adjacent properties
Walk-through (depending on site)
Health department records

- What equipment will be necessary to take the samples?
- Will this equipment create hazardous conditions such as potential contact with overhead power lines?
- Does this equipment involve moving parts or other hazardous mechanical conditions so that untrained persons should be kept at a distance?
- Will the sampling produce hazardous materials that must be properly managed?
- Will the sampling produce trash such as protective equipment and gloves that need special handling?

- Will the sampling potentially liberate hazardous vapors or other materials to cause a potential exposure to hazardous materials?
- Is there a need for specialized equipment to avoid a risk of fire or explosion?
- Is there the potential for exposure to persons off the facility?
- Is the potential for exposure or accidents such that the local police and fire officials should be notified and briefed on response and avoidance?
- Is the potential for accidents such that specialized decontamination and medical treatment facilities are necessary?
- Will the use of protective equipment require specialized facilities for decontamination, changing, showers, breaks, and other types of support?
- Will workplace air or water sampling be required to detect releases?
- Will the employees of the facility feel threatened if they see consultant employees in their workplace who are wearing protective equipment they do not have?
- Should the phase 2 work be conducted in multiple stages so that risks can be better assessed and more refined work plans can be instituted?

Phase II: Evaluation of the Property is Done by Comprehensive Sampling

Soil sampling	Lead paint sampling
Water sampling	Radon sampling
Air monitoring	Hydrogeologic evaluation
Asbestos sampling	

Some people in the industry also refer to "phase 3" activities. This term is meant to include the work necessary to correct the compliance problem or remediate the contamination. In some regions, the term *phase 3* is meant to include additional site assessment and engineering activities leading to cleanup work. These activities are part of the process used to conduct cleanup projects and are beyond the scope of this chapter.

Both the Occupational Safety and Health Administration and the Environmental Protection Agency have regulations in place concerning the protection and training of employees who are working where hazardous substances may be present. Much of the focus of these regulations is on appropriate training, including the recognition and handling of hazardous substances. Proper handling includes the use of personal protective equipment.

These regulations do impose compliance burdens; however, their real importance is a recognition that, in dealing with unknown conditions, good employee training is the key to personal safety. Employees, with good plans, training, and experience, can recognize when conditions become unacceptable and then react appropriately.

PLANNING ASSUMPTIONS AND REALITIES

The consulting firms and others who are routinely hired to conduct site inspections need to live with the fundamental truth that environmental site assessments are intended to discover and quantify conditions of environmental contamination that are not known or are at least not fully understood by the current property owner or occupants. Employees of these firms are asked to discover these conditions without knowledge of the risks presented by whatever they may discover. These employees cannot rely upon what they have been told about the property, as the whole point of the investigation is to discover unknown conditions.

The consulting firm conducting these studies has usually been retained by counsel or the buyer. These clients are unlikely to have detailed information about the property and cannot provide the consultant with much, if any, meaningful information about the risks that may be present. Even in those cases where the property owner or occupant has retained the consultant, information provided by the client cannot be relied upon to guarantee that no risks are present.

In this setting, the consultant must create safe working conditions for its employees without complete information.

Specific Risks Typically Present at a Manufacturing Facility

- Unidentified containers of waste materials
- Unidentified containers of test products
- Storage areas where leftover materials may be kept
- Employee-used working containers of cleaners or other materials
- Chemicals or contamination in infrequently used areas within the facility
- Moving equipment such as belts, conveyors, fork trucks, elevators, and man lifts
- Dusts and other debris above ceilings
- In-process chemicals regardless of container
- Indoor air contamination
- Noise
- Contamination on equipment, floors or other building surfaces, and containers
- Equipment or materials that can cause eye injuries
- Slip and fall hazards due to slippery surfaces
- Burn hazards due to hot surfaces
- Hazards associated with the use of stepladders
- Rags contaminated with various materials

The consultant needs to develop standardized procedures and practices to anticipate, identify, and respond to potential exposures to toxic materials during environmental assessments. The practices and procedures must be specific enough so that the employees assigned to the project understand how they are to respond to anticipated conditions and to the unknown conditions they may encounter. The remainder of this chapter discusses the sorts of risks that may be present and the procedures and practices that may be useful to avoid these risks.

Phase 1 Risks

As discussed previously, phase 1 activities involve a site inspection. Depending upon the nature of the property or facility involved, the risks may be great or small (see box above).

The procedure used for this inspection is not typically a simple tour of the facility. Instead, the inspector is expected to look in corners, behind equipment, above ceilings, and around drug storage areas and, in general, to go into areas that the employees of the business occupying the facility do not normally go. The inspector is expected to look for contamination, in addition to understanding the more controlled practices the occupant of the property uses when handling chemical materials in the normal course of business.

Many companies have areas in the premises that they do not remember as containing old containers of materials or wastes. They may simply forget about old drums or containers of materials in the normal rush of daily operations. Many companies have tried new materials and then stored leftover quantities. Many companies allow employees

to use working containers of various cleaning and other materials that are unlabeled. The inspector in an environmental audit must identify all of these conditions to be thorough.

The inspector must also anticipate that any company operating on the property that is being inspected is not in compliance with occupational safety and health regulations. Just because the company does not require protective equipment in some areas does not mean the work environment is safe. In addition, the inspector has not had the benefit of whatever safety training has been provided to the employees. The inspector is likely not familiar with the workplace procedures and may well not recognize just the simple hazards present in the normal operations at the facility.

Environmental audits at vacant properties present their own special set of risks. There may typically be mechanical hazards associated with debris on the property. Unknown containers may be present. Even if containers are labeled, they are likely abandoned, and the labels most likely are not reflective of the actual contents.

Many times vacant property means farm or ranch land. Instead, the property may have been the home to various facilities that have subsequently been demolished. This demolition process may not have removed pipes, tanks, and other features. The property may have also been used for disposal of trash or toxic wastes or simply filled with dirt and construction debris.

As the inspector is supposed to be looking for signs of contamination, they may well encounter contamination in soils or water. This contamination may or may not be very obvious, depending upon the time of year and the contaminant present. Vapors or other ongoing releases from contaminated materials can be present and may also not be obvious.

Some types of facilities, such as facilities with laboratory operations, facilities engaged in research and development, and facilities that have been abandoned, present unusual risks.

Case example.   One of the most frightening environmental assessments we ever participated in involved an abandoned building. After some research, we made the decision to enter the building for an initial reconnaissance. After cutting the lock on the door, we entered the building, only to be confronted with floors and other surfaces that seemed to be coated with a very hard, rocklike substance. As we stood about 10 feet inside the door, we noticed that a pigeon had died in the building and fallen to the floor. This pigeon had mummified where it had fallen. There were no rodent tracks, no spider webs, and no evidence of insect activity. We recognized that we had entered an area that contained toxic materials and made a hasty retreat.

The role of planning.   In all of these cases, it is clear that the consultant needs to anticipate and plan so that the inspector is not exposed to potentially hazardous situations.

As many of the conditions that create risk are not known until the inspector arrives upon the scene, the plans must allow the inspector to exercise judgment and create guidelines within which that judgment is to be exercised.

Each environmental audit project should have a health and safety plan. This plan should be developed initially based upon the history of the site and the type of industry or facility currently present. If vacant land is involved, the plan should be based upon past uses of the land.

In every case, the consultant should make an effort to establish risks that may be present through phone calls or a scoping visit to the site prior to the inspection. This preinspection effort should include information on chemical materials present, types of operations, and necessary safety equipment.

Based upon the preinspection effort, health and safety data should be collected and reviewed for the chemicals present. This sort of data can be acquired either by material safety data sheets obtained from the facility to be visited or from various third-party published data sources. The inspectors visiting the site should review this data and make an independent decision on the sort of safety equipment for chemical exposure they believe should be taken on the site inspection.

The preinspection plan needs to anticipate the procedures by which the inspection will be conducted. Questions such as whether ladders or safety equipment like hard hats or special shoes are necessary need to be answered. Careful consideration should also be given to the number of people assigned to the inspection team.

When this review is complete, the site-specific health and safety plan can be prepared. This plan should indicate the types of chemicals and other risks anticipated. The plan should provide direction on the inspector's actions, should an unanticipated risk be encountered. The plan should describe the type of activities that may be included in the inspection, while also stating the sorts of activities that will be left to later phases. For example, guidelines such as the inspector is not to enter certain areas or is not to handle unknown containers must be stated and understood.

In some cases, the preinspection review notes areas of clear hazard to an inspector. For example, if areas with hazardous air conditions are known to exist in the facility, then a decision must be made on whether to include these areas in a phase 1 inspection. If zones of contamination are known to exist at the facility, then the same sort of decision must be made. If the consultant can already conclude that phase 2 work will be recommended for an area, then there is little point to performing a detailed phase 1 inspection in that same area.

The health and safety plan must also anticipate any risks that the inspection may present to other people in the facility. While these risks may not be great, it is distinctly possible for an inspector to cause the release of a hazardous chemical by, for example, accidentally dislodging a container. Simply

---

Some Specific Risks That May Be Present on Vacant Property

- Site debris such as nails and sharp objects
- Unconsolidated fill materials
- Unmarked physical hazards such as tank vaults and foundations
- Pipes and wires that are hidden by weeds or snow
- Contaminated soils
- Vapors from contaminated soils
- Contaminated water
- Vapors from contaminated water
- Unknown containers
- Explosion and fire hazards from unstable materials
- Snakes, spiders, and other unfriendly inhabitants of the property

---

having "extra" people moving through a workplace may create risks because of the disruption in the normal flow of activity.

Due consideration to alternative means of conducting the inspection should occur when operations at the facility present undue risks to the inspector or the inspection presents risks to the people normally present at the facility. It is frequently appropriate to conduct the inspection during off hours at the facility.

The final point to be considered are the qualifications of the people who will perform the inspection. Not only should they be adequately experienced in environmental regulations so that they can identify areas of noncompliance, but also they must be adequately trained to recognize and respond to the risks presented during inspections. Their training must include identification and handling of toxic or hazardous substances. Their training must also include general safety procedures necessary to being in an industrial or similar hazardous location.

Phase 2 Risks

It is appropriate to view phase 2 activities as specialized construction projects. As the sampling activities involved in phase 2 inspections typically require tools, drilling equipment, and other specialized equipment, the necessary health and safety plans must anticipate and include all of the risk presented by this equipment in addition to the risks of exposure to hazardous chemicals (see box above and boxes on p. 504).

Phase 2 activities typically involve intentional contact with areas having known or suspected contamination. The type and concentration of contamination are likely to be highly variable and may be unknown. In some areas, it is asbestos; in other areas, the material at issue is petroleum or solvent contamination. The material sampled varies from soil and water to construction materials. It is also frequently the case that containers of unknown materials are involved.

Specific Risks During Laboratory Operations

- Numerous containers of potentially reactive materials.
- Unlabeled containers.
- Containers of old materials that may be unstable.
- Surface contamination on tables and in reaction hoods.
- Experiments in progress may be unstable.
- Uncharacterized waste materials may be present.

Specific Risks in Research and Development Operations Beyond Those Mentioned For Labs

- Their experimental nature creates the potential for unpredictable events.
- Unintended byproducts may be present.
- Activities in progress may be unstable.
- Uncharacterized waste materials may be present.

Risks Involving Abandoned Properties Are Almost Innumerable

- Deterioration of the structure.
- The presence of animal and other biologic wastes.
- Microorganism action on abandoned materials can create toxic by-products.
- Unintended reactions of abandoned materials.
- Deterioration of tanks and vessels.
- The lack of ventilation may create an unsafe atmosphere in confined spaces.
- Unknown persons may abandon various materials at these locations.

The greatest risks are presented when phase 2 activities involve sampling of unknown materials and contaminated areas. In these situations, the materials may potentially be very hazardous and must be approached with the greatest caution. Sampling of unknown materials presents the greatest need for preplanning.

Preplanning activities for phase 2 work requires careful consideration of a number of factors in order to prepare an appropriate work plan and a health and safety plan.

As with phase 1 work, a detailed health and safety plan is necessary for all phase 2 work. This health and safety plan needs to be prepared in conjunction with the phase 2 work plan.

CONCLUSION

The objective for phase 2 work is to document whether contamination is present and provide enough information so that the other people interested in the transaction can assess the impact of the contamination. From this information, they can assess how to proceed. This assessment typically involves the use of escrows or the need for other work on the site. Because the information collected in phase 2 is critical, there is a great deal of pressure on the consultant to collect this information. Typically, this pressure includes a desire for the work to be conducted on an expedited basis.

The consultant must balance the client's desire for information with the need to create a safe workplace. The consultant needs to realistically assess how long the phase 2 work will take and provide the client with a clear indication of what steps are necessary to conduct the work in a safe manner while collecting the information desired. No client wants to require a consultant to work in an unsafe fashion; however, it is the consultant's obligation to inform the client about what schedule and work conditions are reasonable.

The consultant needs to be systematic in planning the work to be conducted. This systematic approach must anticipate potential risks to the inspector, other persons at the facility, and persons outside the facility. Work plans need to be established, and detailed health and safety plans should be prepared based upon the best information available. The inspectors need to be experienced and trained so that they can perform the work in compliance with plans as well as deal with unexpected conditions.

REFERENCES

1. Asbestos hazard emergency response act (AHERA). PL 15 USC 2641 et seq, 40 CFR 763, 1986.
2. Comprehensive environmental response, compensation, and liability act (CERCLA). PL 96-510, 42 USC 9601 et seq, 40 CFR 300, 1980.
3. Environmental Protection Agency polychlorinated biphenyl regulations. 15 USC 2605 et seq, 40 CFR 761, 1981.
4. Resource conservation and recovery act (RCRA). 42 USC 6991, 6992, and 6996 et seq, 40 CFR 280, 1985.
5. Standard practice for environmental site assessments: phase I environmental site assessment process, ASTM E 1527.
6. Superfund amendments and reauthorization act (SARA). PL 99-499, 1986.
7. *United States v Maryland Bank & Trust Co.*, 632 F Supp. 573, (D.Md. 1986).

58

benzene

- The physician's responsibility in environmental risk communication

- Understanding environmental risks

- Strengths and weaknesses of environmental epidemiology

- Personal vs. public risk: the critical difference

- Dealing with distressed patients or communities

Environmental Risks and the Clinician: Informing Worried Patients

Ronald E. Gots

In 1990, when Perrier, the natural sparkling water, was found to contain 15 ppb of benzene, three times the allowable drinking water limit of 5 ppb, the company promptly removed the product from the shelves. That satisfied an immediate concern but left unfinished business for the Perrier set. "What risks are in store for me from this contaminated drink?" they wondered. After all, if 5 ppb is the upper limit, then it stands to reason that 15 ppb must be dangerous.

The public views regulatory standards as sacrosanct. Below the number is safety; above it lies danger. The agencies are hard-pressed to dispel this inaccurate notion. How, after all, can they reassure the public that 15 ppb of benzene is all right to drink without undermining public confidence in their own standard of 5 ppb?

The notion that 5 ppb is the "safe" level—the level set by the regulatory agencies—but that 15 ppb is not harmful to an individual may seem incompatible, yet it is likely true. This seeming paradox highlights the line between the science of toxicology and the regulation of toxic substances. This important distinction must be understood by physicians, for they, after all, are the ones to whom frightened patients turn for answers.

Physicians routinely help their patients weigh risks for familiar clinical interactions. What are the chances that the radiation will cure my cancer? What are the risks of surgery? How likely is it that the medication will cause kidney failure? Answers to these and many other questions are routinely sought and generally given. Why, then, do physicians find it difficult to offer meaningful answers to patients worried about the effects of pesticides on their children or plant emissions in their neighborhood? The reason is partly rooted in uncertainties. Some of the answers are not clear.

More important, I believe, are two other factors. First is the unfamiliarity of most physicians with environmental toxicology and regulatory matters. Second is the popular pananxiety about environmental issues, to which physicians are not immune. However, absence of complete knowledge in these areas does not mean absence of any knowledge. Much is known about environmental toxicology, and knowledgeable physicians can provide meaningful insight for their worried patients.

The environmental risks discussed in this chapter are largely low-level chronic exposures. Other chapters in this book have considered acute toxicity and the more significant exposures, such as those in industrial settings. However, the arena of low-level exposures presents a great challenge to clinician-patient interaction because much of what patients "know" to be true has been influenced by popular writing and television programs, and much of that knowledge is either incorrect, unproven, or more relevant to the public at large than to a specific person.

I also provide to the reader some basic tools that can put environmental risks into an accurate scientific perspective that is intelligible to the layperson. Since most public information conveyed by the media is derived from two arenas, environmental epidemiology and regulatory risk assessment, the physician has to understand the inherent limitations of these two fields. Understanding these disciplines is essential to effective environmental risk communication.

REGULATORY TOXICOLOGY: A PRIMER FOR THE MEDICAL PRACTITIONER

Concern that low-level exposures "might" influence the overall public health is the central paradigm underlying environmental regulation. That, in turn, is interpreted by the individual as "this will hurt me." Common popular and regulatory beliefs about the environment are driven by such concepts as:

- If one can measure it, it must be eliminated.
- If animals respond to high doses, people will respond to low doses.

- There are no thresholds for carcinogens.
- If safety cannot be proven, risk must be assumed.
- Man-made is more dangerous than natural.
- Our health is worse or more precarious than it used to be.

To communicate what is known about environmental risks, the practitioner must understand the assumptions that underlie regulatory risk policy. Those assumptions lead to regulatory limits designed to protect against possible health effects in hundreds of millions of people. Thus, even if such a theoretical risk is trivial for an individual—say 1 in 100,000—it has a public health implication, for a 1 in 100,000 cancer risk means 2500 cases in a population of 250 million. Thus, although 15 ppb of benzene in Perrier poses no risk to the individual, it poses a theoretical risk to the public. Furthermore, the method by which these limits are set is both highly theoretical (there may be no risk at all) and quite conservative, with built-in margins of safety.

Mathematical risk assessment is the technique by which certain biologic data are converted into regulatory action. Often the data upon which such regulation is based consist solely of animal carcinogenicity studies. Invariably, these studies test large doses of the chemical, far higher than humans might ever experience from environmental exposures. To make judgments about low-dose human exposure from those high-dose animal data, mathematical formulae are used. These formulae are conservative, assuming, for example, that there is no threshold for a carcinogen. This mathematical extrapolation process is the field of quantitative risk assessment. Risk assessment is an instrument of social compromise, providing numeric answers in the face of vast scientific uncertainties. It is a necessary instrument, however, because the effects of low-level environmental exposures cannot be tested directly.

Examining the many assumptions inherent in risk assessment shows that the process does not reflect biologic behavior. In some cases, known human carcinogens are involved. In most chemical regulation, however, the agents are not known to produce cancer in people but only in experimental animals, and in a limited number of animal species, or even sexes or breeds, at that.

Rats, mice, and hamsters are not good predictors of each other; females and males respond differently; one genetic strain differs from the next. Clearly, such data cannot predict with any scientific solidity the response of human beings.

Where does this leave the Perrier drinkers? How do we communicate with them about the benzene risk? To answer this, let us explore the basis for the benzene standard.

We know scientifically that very high exposures to benzene can cause both disorders of blood production and at least one kind of leukemia. Initial recognition of benzene as a leukemogen came from observations in Turkey among shoemakers.[1] In their small, unventilated shops, they breathed an estimated 400 to 600 ppm of benzene, day in, day out for their working lifetimes. For comparison, 100 ppm is the same as 100,000 ppb; the Perrier contained 15 ppb. Leukemia rates in this group of workers appeared to be higher than expected, but leukemia was by no means common. The background rate of leukemia was 6 in 100,000. The exposed group's rate was 13 in 100,000. This twofold excess was seen consistently and was, therefore, a clear association, although the risk remained low. The overwhelming majority of workers did not develop leukemia, even with these extraordinary exposure levels.

Additional studies in American workers to evaluate the relationship of lower levels of benzene exposure to leukemias have suggested that some leukemias may occur even with exposures much lower than those in the Turkish workshop. However, no increased risk has been proven at levels less than approximately 10 ppm (10,000 ppb) when the substance is inhaled throughout a working lifetime.[26] Notice, we have not yet gotten to 15 ppb (the amount of benzene found in the Perrier) or begun to assess the effects of drinking 2 liters per day, in contrast to inhaling benzene day in, day out. At these extremely low levels, there may be a small theoretical or potential risk, but one that has not been established and that may or may not be real. It is this theoretical risk that drives the regulatory process and leads to the 5 ppb benzene standard.

As a tool of public policy, risk assessment has an important role. But its influence on society is now so great that the public must learn to understand what it is and what it is not. The physician communicating with a worried patient has a particular responsibility to understand these distinctions.

The fact that an agent is regulated and a permissible limit is set does not imply an actual risk to an exposed individual. Public health policy and personal risk are two separate issues.

ENVIRONMENTAL EPIDEMIOLOGY AS APPLIED TO RISK COMMUNICATION

If regulatory standards create popular perceptions of risk, so, too, do epidemiologic studies. Not infrequently, relationships identified in observational analytical studies (either case control or cohort) are picked up by the popular press and reported upon as if they had proven a causal connection. With every contradictory study comes a diminution in the public mind of the credibility of science: "How can they keep changing their minds?" Actually, it is a misinterpretation of the significance of such studies that leads to this misunderstanding. A single observational study, even a very good one, rarely establishes conclusively a causal relationship.

Epidemiologists have attempted to clarify the relevance of such studies. Realizing that a single study, or even a few, rarely proves causation, the question is, What does? In the mid-1960s, while the surgeon general was immersed in the issue of smoking and cancer causation, a set of

criteria was proposed by which the likelihood of a causal relationship (not a mere association) could be assessed. These have come to be known as the Hill criteria after Bradford Hill.

1. *Chronologic relationship.* The exposure must precede the disease if it is to be considered causal.
2. *Strength of the association.* The greater the magnitude of the association—relative risk of study cohort versus the control group—the more likely the significance.
3. *Intensity or duration of exposure.* If those with the greatest intensity and duration of exposure have the greatest chance of developing the disease, this supports causation.
4. *Specificity of association.* If the effect is a specific and unusual one, associated most commonly with the particular potential cause, then this supports causation.
5. *Consistency.* If many observers, in many experiments, find the same association, this supports causation.
6. *Coherence and biologic plausibility.* The connection between the potential cause and the possible effect must make biologic sense. It should also be found in other situations, such as experimental animals.[19,34]

The more of these criteria are met, the more likely it is that an observed outcome is causally connected to the studied potential cause. These criteria show that proving a causal connection between an exposure and a disease is no easy matter; such proof is rarely the result of a single observational epidemiologic study. In an editorial in the *New England Journal of Medicine*, Angell[2] noted the recent increase in epidemiologic research and cautioned against overinterpretation of the results. The number of studies has increased, the author explained, because many acute diseases have been addressed, and we are now facing chronic diseases with multifactorial etiologies: diet, lifestyle, environment, genetics, chronic infections, and other unknown causes. These potential causes can be studied only through epidemiologic research. The author warned how difficult the studies can be to interpret and how misleading the findings can be.

There is no question that epidemiologic studies of risk factors for disease are of growing interest and importance, both for individuals and for the public health. It is important, however, to remember the pitfalls in interpreting them and to be cautious in advising patients on the basis of single or conflicting studies. This is particularly true of studies purporting to show only weak associations between exposures and disease. These should be evaluated more critically, by researchers and clinicians alike.[2]

EXAMPLES OF POPULAR PERCEPTIONS IN ENVIRONMENTAL EPIDEMIOLOGY: USES AND OVERINTERPRETATIONS

Angell's warning about the interpretation of epidemiologic studies is particularly relevant in environmental toxicology. Here, popular perceptions and public pressures have pushed scientific investigations beyond the limits of scientific capabilities. The effects of small amounts of chemicals near waste sites, in indoor air, and in drinking water are not easily studied, yet the public wants answers. These societal concerns are placing greater and greater demands upon the scientific community, asking questions for which there are no answers and demanding answers to questions that defy scientifically valid studies. State departments of public health are in the middle of these issues and are central to this interface between science and policy. A group of citizens wants to know whether a variety of physical complaints came about because of their proximity to a nearby waste treatment facility. Their complaints are numerous, vague, widely varied, and subject to enormous reporting bias because of the pervasive perception that the waste site is causing a problem. The public health department, both a political creature and a scientific investigative organization, is caught in a dilemma. It is required politically to answer a question that may be scientifically impossible to investigate. One answer may be politically acceptable but scientifically inaccurate, and the other scientifically correct but politically dangerous. This tension between popular demand and scientific accuracy strains the public confidence in science and tests the power of scientists to maintain their integrity and to explain the limits of science to a hostile public.

Waste Site Epidemiology

The Pennsylvania Department of Environmental Resources and the U.S. Agency for Toxic Substances and Disease Registry (ATSDR) recently studied a group of citizens in central Pennsylvania who complained of a variety of symptoms they attributed to a nearby waste treatment facility.[3] By the time the study took place, the residents had formed an active citizens' group and had filed lawsuits. Their story appeared in *Family Circle Magazine* under the title "Cluster Diseases: Is Your Family at Risk?"[17]

The epidemiologic study consisted of a symptom survey carried out in the study population and a nearby control population. This cross-sectional survey asked the participants about their symptoms and whether they had ever had cancer. Importantly, and to their credit, the researchers went to the actual medical records to check the validity of the answers to the cancer question. The findings were quite revealing. The symptom questionnaire revealed more symptoms in the study group than in the control group. This finding is typical in communities involved in real or perceived chemical threats. It has no causal meaning because symptoms would be expected to follow both perceived and real chemical poisoning. The study group also had a 30% higher reported incidence of cancer, but when medical records were actually reviewed, their medically proven cancer rates were no different from the control group's.[3] Thus, the study group had overreported cancer by 30%. Whether they truly believed that they had cancers when they did not or whether this difference represented intentional

overreporting is not known. It does illustrate, however, the unreliability of questionnaires that ask for the self-reporting of ailments. If even cancer is misreported, how accurate are the reports of symptoms such as fatigue, headaches, itchy eyes, and insomnia?

More recently, a similar survey was performed in Tucson, Arizona, where the drinking water of a number of residents had been contaminated with trichloroethylene (TCE) from approximately 1944 to 1981.[4] Once again, symptom questionnaires were used. The ATSDR cautioned that the results of this cross-sectional survey could not establish a causal connection to TCE, since reporter bias was extreme, actual amounts of contaminated water in control and target populations were unknown, and diseases and symptoms were not verified. Notwithstanding this disclaimer, it is clear that the public views excess reports of symptoms and diseases in the target population as proof that people's health was adversely affected by the water.

This self-reporting of symptoms is merely one of the experimental design impediments in the study of health effects of waste sites.[16] This dependent variable (the effect or outcome) is unreliable. Frequently, equally unreliable is the independent variable (potential cause): the characterization of the actual exposure.

Other popular areas of environmental epidemiology are based upon variable, often shaky scientific data.

Electric and Magnetic Fields

Much attention has been focused on the potential health effects of electromagnetic fields. The question commonly posed is, Do high power lines that produce electric and magnetic fields cause adverse health effects in people? When Wertheimer and Leeper, in 1979, described a correlation between childhood leukemia and proximity to power lines, the public concern began.[35] In fact, the study was merely a cross-sectional survey in which the independent variable (field strength) had never been measured but was assumed based upon wiring configurations. Since then, many other studies have been performed, some finding weak associations between fields and outcomes, such as childhood leukemias, and others finding none.* In these studies, outcomes are objective: Cancer is a clear end point, for example. The independent variable, field strength (either magnetic or electric), is far harder to fix, however. It varies widely from time to time and place to place, even in the same room of the same house. Other variables are impossible to control fully. Studies have not shown a dose-response relationship between believed field intensities and adverse outcomes. There is no animal model connecting such fields to cancer. The biology of this phenomenon is unclear and is not explained by any current understanding of how cancers are produced. Thus, to date, Hill's criteria are not satisfied. Electric and magnetic fields have not been shown to cause cancer. The perception

*References 9, 13, 21, 23, 29, 30, 33.

Table 58-1 Experimental inaccuracies

Issue	Independent variable	Dependent variable	Biases	Confounders
Waste site effects	Rarely	Rarely	Rarely	Rarely
Low-level water contamination	Rarely	Sometimes	Rarely	Rarely
Electric and magnetic fields	Sometimes	Usually	Sometimes	Sometimes
"Sick buildings"	Rarely	Rarely	Rarely	Rarely
Occupational cancer	Usually	Usually	Sometimes	Sometimes

From Gots RE: *Toxic risks: science, regulation, and perception,* Boca Raton, Fla, 1993, Lewis Publishers.

of the public is otherwise. Books such as *Currents of Death: Power Lines, Computer Terminals and the Attempt to Cover Up Their Threat to Your Health* and *Cross Currents* have taken the preliminary and inconclusive data in the literature and concluded that the causal relationship is well established. Moreover, this literature asserts that our government has plotted to withhold the truth from the American public.[6,7]

Summary of Environmental Epidemiology

Environmental epidemiologists are searching intensely for two important tools: outcome measures that enable subtle and specific objective assessments of chemical effects and exposure end points that permit an objective assessment of, rather than conjecture about, a subject's actual exposure. Studies of enzyme systems, immunologic parameters, and neurologic and neurophysiologic function are all part of this research landscape. The critical goal is to find more effective, specific, objective, and reproducible ways of measuring independent (exposure) and dependent (outcomes) variables. Until that is accomplished, environmental epidemiology will be plagued by lack of reproducibility, biases, and enormous uncertainties. Table 58-1 identifies and rates qualitatively the experimental inaccuracies that plague these areas of research. The quality of the studies with regard to the control of dependent variables, independent variables, and biases are qualitatively rated as "usually," "sometimes," and "rarely." The greater the number of "rarelys," the less reliable the study. Studies investigating community health effects associated with waste sites and sick buildings are the most unreliable.

PERSONAL VERSUS PUBLIC RISK

The fact that a carcinogen is regulated or that it is given a not-to-exceed number tells nothing about the effect of that substance upon an exposed individual. Substances are regulated because of potential for harm, and numbers are chosen according to presumed margins of safety. But how do we explain this to a worried public? What do we tell people living near a hazardous waste site or a mother worried about the effect of Alar-contaminated apples on her toddler?

Weighing Emotional Distress Versus Health Concerns

Because environmental worries play such a large role in perceptions of risk, it may not be possible to dispel fears with cold logic and science. Effective risk communication requires the communicator to know whether the patient or the community group is motivated primarily by health concerns or by emotional distress.

Social scientists argue that health concerns play a minor role in public distress and that communicators who ignore the emotional impact of environmental dangers do so at their peril.* Sandman has called these emotional aspects "outrage" and has done, I believe, an effective job of raising our consciousness regarding this public motivator.[28] While emotional aspects of an environmental concern can be important or even paramount, they are by no means always central. Situations exist in which health concerns predominate, while emotional distress (Sandman's "outrage") is minor. For example, a nuclear power facility or a hazardous waste site in the neighborhood provokes emotional distress; here, health concerns are, indeed, secondary. By contrast, electric power lines overhead, a sudden release of a chemical from a plant, or benzene contamination of Perrier water generate health concerns primarily. In these instances, the consuming public was (or is) more worried about health than outraged at the situation. Understanding these distinctions—whether emotional concerns or health concerns form the central core of public distress—is essential to the institution of an effective dialogue. Bringing health data into a forum dominated by emotional hostility can be counterproductive. In such situations, dealing with the distress factors must come first.[11,18,28] However, when health worries form the nidus of community concerns, those must be addressed.[14,15] Table 58-2 provides a tool for the communicator to balance these public motivators—health or emotional distress.

Health concerns shown on the X axis range in severity from "none" to "panic." Emotional distress (Y axis) moves along a continuum from none to severe, responses I call "none," "annoyance," "anger," and "outrage." The most severe degree of emotional distress is what Sandman refers to as "outrage." Since the context of environmental risks and perceptions varies greatly, it is important to categorize public perceptions in this fashion and to attempt to find the matrix block that best represents the situation at hand.

A few examples will illustrate this approach. Benzene in the Perrier water generated health concerns but little emotional distress. Health concerns resulted from the fact

*References 5, 8, 10, 11, 18, 20, 22, 24, 25, 27, 31.

Table 58-2 Health concern versus indignation matrix

		Health concerns			
		None 1	Worry 2	Fear 3	Panic 4
I N D I G N A T I O N	None A	1A	2A	3A	4A
	Annoyance B	1B	2B	3B	4B
	Anger C	1C	2C	3C	4C
	Outrage D	1D	2D	3D	4D

From Gots RE: Public versus personal risk: the challenge in environmental risk communication, *Technology: Journal of the Franklin Institute* 331A:59, 1994.

Table 58-3 Rating on health concern versus indignation matrix for various environmental risk situations

Situation	Health concern versus indignation matrix
Toxic gas release (immediately following)	3A, 4A 3B, 4B
Toxic gas release (week later)	2A 2B 2C
Fire and explosion at a chemical plant (immediately following)	3A, 4A 3B, 4B
Benzene in perrier	2A, 3A, 4A
Hazardous waste site in neighborhood	2C, 3C, 2D, 3D
Plant stack emissions	2B, 2C, 2D
Dioxin in fishing lake	2C, 2D
Solvent contaminated school	3A, 4A, 3B, 4B
Firemen exposed to PCBs	3A, 4A
Compost facility in neighborhood	1C, 2C, 1D, 2D
Tank farm in neighborhood	1C, 2C, 1D, 2D
Electric power line (in place)	2A, 3A
Hazardous waste incinerator to be constructed in neighborhood	2D, 3D
Waste treatment facility in neighborhood	2D, 3D

From Gots RE: Public versus personal risk: the challenge in environmental risk communication, *Technology: Journal of the Franklin Institute* 331A:59, 1994.

that levels exceeded federal drinking water standards by threefold, a fact that many would view with alarm. However, because this was seen as an accident and because the Perrier company responded promptly with information and a recall, most people were not overly distressed at the company. Thus, health concerns ranged (depending upon the indi-

vidual) from worry to panic; emotional distress was low. Blocks 2 to 4 on the matrix can be used to characterize the public perceptions.

By contrast, a compost facility in a neighborhood (a situation in which I communicated with the neighbors) generated a great deal of emotional distress because of the odors and unsightliness. Health issues were raised to get the attention of regulators, but, in actuality, they were not of primary concern. In this instance, the community fell into blocks 9, 10, 13, and 14, with few or no health concerns but significant emotional distress. Examples of health risk situations with their primary matrix locations are provided in Table 58-3.

In recent years, the emotional distress issue has become so central to discussions of environmental risk communication that health concerns have been given short shrift. In fact, there has developed a tension between social scientists and technical people engaged in communication activities. The social scientists focus exclusively upon community distress, while the technical experts focus upon numbers. Moreover, each accuses the other of doing the wrong thing. The fact is that there is a place for both disciplines, the relative balance of each determined by the balance of concerns identified by the matrix.

When Health Concerns Predominate

In the normal course of practice, physicians provide health risk information. It is called "informed consent." They routinely convert statistics and probabilities to individual, personal information. When a child develops meningitis, the physician lets the concerned family know the prognosis. The physician does not know what will actually happen to that child but knows what the chances (probabilities) are based on statistical data and can use these data to communicate. The risks of surgery, the dangers and benefits of medications, and the likelihood that cancer chemotherapy will be beneficial all require the physician to convert probabilities to personal risk messages. The patient demands it, the law demands it, and physicians comply.

Environmental risk communication is no different. Probabilistic analyses must be converted into the kind of personal health information that doctors routinely provide.

Consider the electric power issue brought to the fore by environmental alarmists.[6,12] The public has now become concerned about this uncertain and likely marginal health risk. Factual, personal health information might go something like this: even if we accept (from the variable and inconsistent epidemiologic data) the worst case risk seen thus far, the chances of any child developing leukemia from such exposures is trivial. It changes from 1 in 10,000 to 4 in 10,000. From the public health standpoint, that difference may be important in arguing for public protection. From the standpoint of the individual, however, the increased risk is lost in the noise of background risks.

Perhaps two specific examples may further illustrate the contextual issues in risk communication. Assume a neighborhood discovers that its drinking water was contaminated with 10 ppb of a chlorinated aliphatic chemical. Assume further the following facts:

1. There is one positive animal carcinogenicity study in female rats of one strain when given the maximally tolerated dose of this agent.
2. Fifty other animal studies have been negative for cancer.
3. Twenty human epidemiologic studies in exposed workers have all been negative.
4. Quantitative risk assessment has indicated that the lifetime cancer risk engendered by 70 years of drinking this water is 4×10^{-6}.

Given these facts, the following personal health messages regarding the cancer-causing potential of this exposure would all be accurate.

1. We just don't know.
2. Science is uncertain.
3. This is a cancer causer/carcinogen.
4. This is probably not a human carcinogen.
5. This is possibly a carcinogen, but likely a weak one.
6. The studies have shown the following [a complete description].
7. Considering the nature of the chemical and the amount of your exposure, there is almost no risk to you.

Assume now that we have to pick only one of these messages. We do not have the time to educate fully or an audience with the scientific background to understand the nuances of the studies and the risk assessment. The question, then, is which of these messages is most helpful. If the purpose of the communication is to assist the concerned public in understanding how this contaminated water may affect them, I believe that the last message best serves that purpose. It is truthful, accurate, and reassuring at the same time.

Consider a second example, this time involving a more potent carcinogen. A neighborhood is found to contain soil contaminated with a potent carcinogen. The following facts are true.

1. At extraordinarily low doses of this carcinogen, every species of animal develops cancer.
2. Three of 20 human epidemiologic studies have found a positive association between exposures and malignancies.
3. Risk assessment in this community has suggested a 5×10^{-5} potential lifetime risk considering 70 years of exposure to the soil.

Given these facts, the following personal health messages regarding the cancer-causing potential of this exposure would all be accurate:

1. This is the most potent carcinogen known to man.
2. Science is uncertain.

3. This is probably a human carcinogen.
4. The studies have shown the following [a complete description].
5. Considering the amount of your exposure, there is almost no risk to you.

Assume as before that we have to pick only one of these messages. Again, we do not have the time to educate fully or an audience with the scientific background to understand the nuances of the studies and the risk assessment. If the purpose of the communication is to assist the concerned public in understanding how this contaminated soil may affect them, I believe that, once again, the last message best serves that purpose.

While the general wisdom seems to be the more information, the better, it may seem a radical suggestion that we minimize offering information about carcinogenicity in these situations. What I am suggesting, categorically, is that providing such information, without a frame of reference, is more misleading than excluding it would be.

Providing a Context for Risk Information

Let us assume that an environmental exposure poses, according to quantitative risk assessment, a 1-in-100,000 theoretical risk to a person. How do we provide a frame of reference? One way I have found useful is to use words associated with a more familiar example. For example, we might ask a group of concerned citizens to attach a word to the risk of dying during a coronary bypass operation: severe, moderate, minimal, or trivial. Next, we offer numbers: a 50% chance of dying; a 1% chance; a 1-in-1000 chance; a 1-in-10,000 chance; or a 1-in-100,000 chance. Audiences with whom I have used this risk quiz invariably describe a 50% chance of dying as severe and a 1-in-100,000 chance as trivial. Most describe 1-in-1000 and 1-in-10,000 chances as minimal or trivial. One can then use those very same descriptive terms to qualify an environmentally induced risk of 1 in 10,000 or 1 in 100,000. This method, then, provides a frame of reference for such risks.

Another useful method is comparative risks, for example, the risk of dying in an automobile crash. Risk communicators steeped in the social sciences tell us that the use of such comparative risks is generally inappropriate and inflammatory. One cannot and should not compare voluntary with involuntary risks. I agree that such comparisons must be used carefully. It must be explicitly stated that these are not being used to trivialize concerns but purely and solely to offer a perspective, a context. After all, 1 in a million has little meaning, but a vivid example, such as the chance of being hit by lightning or of being struck by a falling airplane while on the ground, brings significance to those numbers.

Finally, a useful cancer risk communication tool is to compare background risks with the theoretical, incremental risk created by an environmental exposure. The background risk of contracting cancer is between 25% and 30%, approximately 0.30. An incremental additional risk of 1 in 10,000 converts that risk to 0.3001, a small, incremental change. Most low-level environmental risks are at that level or lower, essentially lost in the expected background.

THE DANGERS OF MISCOMMUNICATION OF ENVIRONMENTAL RISKS

"Fifty thousand children will get cancer from eating alar contaminated apples," read a headline in the *New York Times*. That number, derived from risk assessment modeling, was the product of an environmental group's effort to draw instant national attention to pesticide residues in foods—an effort that did, indeed, grab the attention of Americans.

It was clearly a misrepresentation of risk assessment data to present this as a truism to the American public. It was not fact, and the public was consequently misled. The result, however, was tens of thousands of worried parents, whose distress continues to this day.

It is often easier for physicians to simply go along with their patients' firm beliefs that something in the environment has produced an illness or is posing a risk. There are, however, dangers in supporting false perceptions. People can lose their jobs or be uprooted from their communities. Children may be removed from schools. Some particularly vulnerable people may become environmental hermits, removing themselves and their children from all societal encounters.

I evaluated a family from a medium-sized town in Mississippi. By the time I saw their records, the family had moved to a log cabin in the woods. The children, ages 9 and 7, had been pulled out of school and were being taught at home. Their mother, having read about chemicals and their widespread health effects, related pest extermination of their home to her flulike symptoms (probably viral). She subsequently viewed every childhood illness as chemically induced. A physician confirmed her belief that she and her entire family had been poisoned.

Ultimately, these young children were removed from school and friends, told they were abnormal (suffering from multiple chemical sensitivities [MCS]), and consigned to a life of invalidism and isolation.

Thus, misperceptions about environmental risks are not benign. They carry grave consequences. Physicians, exercising their Hippocratic oath to do no harm, have the responsibility to warn and evaluate when those approaches are warranted and to reassure when circumstances demand it.

Labels and Warnings

Health warnings and labels are a form of risk communication, a regular feature of consumer products. These expressions of the public's "right to know" have, at times, produced health warnings both bizarre and misleading. An example appeared on page 1 of the *Wall Street Journal* in March 1993.[32] California's peculiar cancer warning requirements, it seems, necessitated a label on ordinary beach sand destined for children's sandboxes. That prompted a worried father to return the sand and abandon the sandbox. This issue raises a fundamental question about risk communication: What is it that the public has the "right to know"? About what, when, and in what manner should the public be informed? Information too simplified, too separated from its context, can mislead rather than instruct. Absent qualifiers and context, overly simplified information becomes more hazardous than helpful. Whether it is a child who cannot have her sandbox because of a remote risk, a woman who has an unnecessary abortion for fear of a chemical described as a "reproductive hazard," or a man who abandons his house because he is notified of a cancer hazard from a nearby plant, limiting the "right to know" can produce poor choices and distress.

How dangerous is sandbox sand, really? How does it compare with other cancer causers? Sand, asbestos, and cigarettes have, under some circumstances, caused cancer. Both rhinovirus (common cold) and HIV are viruses that can make people sick. They are, in one respect, the same, yet in others, they are entirely different. These are the differences that are the casualties of generic labeling. The "nuances" of cancer labels are lost in the oversimplification. Such nuances are not merely scientific complications; they are central to the understanding and decision making of the consuming public. Does this substance cause cancer in people, animals, or both? How much does it take to cause cancer? Will my child get cancer if I let her play in the sand? How does this activity compare with other risks of cancer? In other words, what do I do about this and how seriously am I to consider this risk? That is, after all, what most people really want to learn from a label. The father who bought the sand for his daughter's playbox would understandably return it having read the label ". . . causes cancer." What if he had been given more complete and scientifically accurate information? For example, "This is ordinary beach sand. A few animal studies have been positive for cancer at high exposure levels. Human studies have all been negative, despite years of investigation in heavily exposed workers. The likelihood of getting cancer from playing in a sandbox is infinitesimally small." Obviously, this does not readily lend itself to a label. But, I would ask, which better serves the truth? If one must simplify, given these scientific realities, which is more accurate: not mentioning cancer at all or labeling the sand as a cancer causer?

Community Right to Know

AB2588 is a California air toxics law that, among other things, requires companies to notify the community if chemical pollutants exceed certain arbitrary state or regional air board guidelines. In California, companies are explicitly enjoined from placing exposures into context.

They are, in effect, required to tell people that they are at risk without any meaningful and informative discussion of the extent of the risk, comparison of risks, or severity of risk, all of which are essential underpinnings of a true "right to know." They are, in fact, required to mislead the public and to frighten unnecessarily. Thus, if a chemical exceeds a guideline for a reproductive toxin by threefold, a pregnant woman so informed is understandably concerned about the fate of her offspring. To her, the risk to her fetus may seem just as likely and extreme as if she had taken thalidomide or suffered from German measles, even though the facts of her exposure represent a vanishingly small risk to her baby and, by comparison to those other risks, almost no risk at all.

Typically, medical and surgical informed consent tends to qualify and quantify the numbers. By contrast, environmental warnings and labels never do that. As a result, the public does not know what to be afraid of or how afraid to be. The labels on the sand and on the asbestos both say "causes cancer." That would be like a label on both a full-sized Ford and a Tonka toy truck that says, "Warning: Four-wheeled vehicles kill people." The right to know has, in the words of Lewis Carroll, made our world more and more curious, but it has not made it better informed. Those risks that create real and significant hazards for individuals should be identified and discussed. Those that pose small public health risks should be kept in their proper perspective. The alternative is a confused public that cannot distinguish between major and trivial risks and views every environmental hazard, minor or serious, as potentially catastrophic. The physician plays a central role in placing personal environmental risks in their proper perspective.

SUGGESTED READINGS

1. Abramson JG: The Cornell Medical Index as an epidemiologic tool, *Am J Public Health* 56:287, 1966.
2. Andelman JB, Underhill DW: *Health effects of hazardous waste sites,* Chelsea, Mich, 1987, Lewis Publishers.
3. Baker DB et al: A health survey of two communities near the Stringfellow waste disposal site, *Arch Environ Health* 43:325, 1988.
4. Bond SS et al: Epidemiologic problems related to medical coverage of new diseases. In American Public Health Association: *111th annual meeting of the American Public Health Association, Dallas, Texas, November 1983,* Washington, DC, 1983, American Public Health Association.
5. Dawber TR: *The Framingham study: the epidemiology of atherosclerotic disease,* Cambridge, Mass, 1980, Harvard University Press.
6. Dunne MP et al: The health effects of chemical waste in an urban community, *Med J Aust* 152:392, 1990.
7. Grisham JW, editor: *Health aspects of the disposal of waste chemicals,* New York, 1986, Pergamon Press.
8. Hance BJ, Chess C, Sandman PM: *Industry risk communication,* Boca Raton, Fla, 1990, Lewis Publishers.
9. Hennekens CH, Buring JE: In SL Mayrent, editor: *Epidemiology in medicine,* Boston, 1987, Little, Brown.
10. Hertzman C et al: Upper Ottowa Street landfill site health study, *Environ Health Perspect* 75:173, 1987.
11. Hopwood DG, Guidotti TL: Recall bias in exposed subjects following a toxic exposure incident, *Arch Environ Health* 43:234, 1988.

12. Janerich DT et al: Cancer incidence in the Love Canal area, *Science* 212:1404, 1981.
13. Landrigan PJ: Epidemiologic approaches to persons with exposures to waste chemicals, *Environ Health Perspect* 18:93, 1983.
14. Last JM, editor: *A dictionary of epidemiology,* New York, 1983, Oxford University Press.
15. Last JM, Wallace RB, editors: *Public health and preventive medicine,* ed 13, Norwalk, Conn, 1992, Appleton and Lange.
16. Lewis HW: *Technological risk,* New York, 1990, Norton.
17. McGrew RE: *Encyclopedia of medical history,* New York, 1985, McGraw-Hill.
18. Morgenstern H: Uses of ecologic analysis in epidemiologic research, *Am J Public Health* 72:1336, 1982.
19. New Jersey Department of Health, Environmental Health Hazard Evaluation Program: *Health survey of the population living near the Price Landfill, Egg Harbor Township, Atlantic County,* Trenton, NJ, 1983, New Jersey Department of Health.
20. Ozonoff D et al: Health problems reported by residents of a neighborhood contaminated by a hazardous waste facility, *Am J Ind Med* 11:581, 1987.
21. Roht LR et al: Community exposure to hazardous waste disposal sites: assessing reporter bias, *Am J Epidemiol* 122:418, 1985.

REFERENCES

1. Aksoy M, Erdem S, Dincol G: Leukemia in shoe-workers exposed chronically to benzene, *Blood* 44:837, 1974.
2. Angell M: The interpretation of epidemiologic studies, *N Engl J Med* 323:823, 1990.
3. ATSDR (Agency for Toxic Substances and Disease Registry), Division of Health Studies: *Study of disease and symptom prevalence in residents of Yukon and Cokeburg, Pennsylvania,* Atlanta, 1990, ATSDR.
4. ATSDR (Agency for Toxic Substances and Disease Registry): *Disease and symptom prevalence survey, Tucson International Airport site, Tucson, Arizona,* Atlanta, 1995, ATSDR.
5. Baker F: Risk communication about environmental hazards, *J Public Health Policy* 11:341, 1990.
6. Becker RO: *Cross currents,* Los Angeles, 1990, Tarcher.
7. Brodeur P: *Currents of death: power lines, computer terminals and the attempt to cover up their threat to your health,* New York, 1989, Simon and Schuster.
8. Chess C, Hance BJ, Sandman PM: *Improving dialogue with communities: a short guide for government risk communication,* Trenton, NJ, 1988, New Jersey Department of Environmental Protection.
9. Coleman MP et al: Leukaemia and residence near electricity transmission equipment: a case-control study, *Br J Cancer* 60:793, 1989.
10. Covello VT: Social and behavioral research on risk: its use in policy formulation and decision-making. In Homburger F, editor: *Safety evaluation and regulation of chemicals,* Basel, 1985, Karger.
11. Covello VT, Sandman PM, Slovic P: *Risk communication, risk statistics, and risk comparisons: a manual for plant managers,* Washington, DC, 1988, Chemical Manufacturers Association.
12. Fitzgerald FT: Sounding board: decisions about life-threatening risks, *N Engl J Med* 331:193, 1994.
13. Fulton JP et al: Electrical wiring configurations and childhood leukemia in Rhode Island, *Am J Epidemiol* 111:292, 1980.
14. Gots RE: Risk communication: a few observations from a physician/toxicologist/communicator, *Hazardous Substances and Public Health* 4:6, 1994.
15. Gots RE: *Toxic risks: science, regulation, and perception,* Boca Raton, Fla, 1993, Lewis Publishers.
16. Gots RE, Gots BA, Spencer J: Proving causes of illness in environmental toxicology: "sick buildings" as an example, *Fresenius Envir Bull* 1:135, 1992.

17. Hales D: Cluster diseases: is your family at risk? *Family Circle Magazine,* March 1990.
18. Hance BJ, Chess C, Sandman PM: *Improving dialogue with communities: a risk communication manual for government,* Trenton, NJ, 1988, Division of Science and Research Risk Communication Unit, New Jersey Department of Environmental Protection.
19. Hill AB: The environment and disease: association or causation? *Proc R Soc Med* 58:295, 1965.
20. Konheim CS: Risk communication in the real world, *Risk Anal* 8:367, 1988.
21. McDowell ME: Mortality of persons resident in the vicinity of electricity transmission facilities, *Br J Cancer* 53:271, 1986.
22. McGuire WJ: Public communication as a strategy for inducing health-promoting behavioral change, *Prev Med* 3:299, 1984.
23. Michaelson SM: Influence of power frequency electric and magnetic fields on human health, *Ann N Y Acad Sci* 502:55, 1987.
24. NRC (National Research Council): *Improving risk communication,* Washington, DC, 1989, National Academy Press.
25. Otway H: Experts, risk communication, and democracy, *Risk Anal* 7:125, 1987.
26. Rinsky RA et al: Benzene and leukemia: an epidemiologic risk assessment, *N Engl J Med* 316:1044, 1987.
27. Sandman PM: *Explaining environmental risk,* Washington, DC, 1986, U S Environmental Protection Agency, Office of Toxic Substances.

28. Sandman PM: *Responding to community outrage: strategies for effective risk communication,* Fairfax, Va, 1993, American Industrial Hygiene Association.

29. Savitz DA: Case-control study of childhood cancer and exposure to 60-Hz magnetic fields, *Am J Epidemiol* 128:21, 1988.

30. Savitz DA: Power lines and cancer risk, *JAMA* 265:1458, 1991.

31. Starr C: Social benefit versus technological risk, *Science* 165:1232, 1969.

32. Stipp D: Cancer scare: how sand in a beach came to be defined as human carcinogen, *Wall Street Journal,* March 22, 1993, A1.

33. Tomenius L: 50-Hz electromagnetic environment and the incidence of childhood tumors in Stockholm County, *Bioelectromagnetics* 7:191, 1986.

34. United States Department of Health, Education, and Welfare: *Smoking and health: a report of the surgeon general,* Washington, DC, 1964, U S Government Printing Office.

35. Wertheimer N, Leeper E: Electrical wiring configurations and childhood cancer, *Am J Epidemiol* 109:273, 1979.

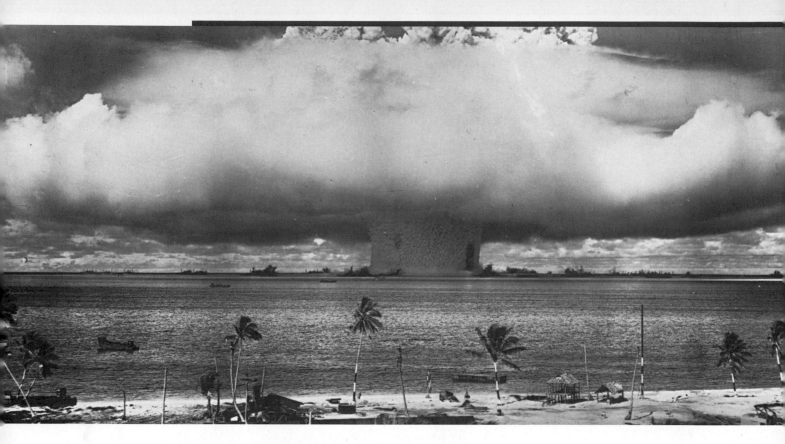

*Gigantic Water Column which reached 5000 feet rises
into the first phase of the characteristic mushroom
following the first underwater atom bomb explosion at
Bikini, July 25th. At the 2000 feet base of the column
in left foreground is the cruiser USS Salt Lake City. In
the right foreground, the Japanese battleship Nagato.
July 25, 1946.*

(Courtesy UPI/Corbis-Bettmann)

59

Ionizing Radiation

Rudi H. Nussbaum
Wolfgang Köhnlein

Cs^{137}

cesium 137

ionizing radiation

- The relative biological damage from ionizing radiation varies with the type, energy, and target

- External sources of radiation affect the body very differently from internal sources

In assessing why radioactivity ought to be considered among globally distributed toxicants we must realize that large populations all over the globe live in an environment contaminated by man-made ionizing radiation. To name some major sources, nuclear weapons production has severely contaminated the atmosphere, ground and surface waters, seas, and oceans. Several billion (10^9) curies of radioactive waste is stored on large, permanently contaminated areas of our globe, partly in corroded storage vessels, in leaking tanks, or in dilapidated production facilities. This mixed radioactive and chemical waste exists in a variety of mostly poorly known physical and chemical conditions, including potentially highly explosive toxic mixtures (e.g., at Hanford, Washington). It includes long-lived radioisotopes with half-lives from decades to several tens of thousands of years (Table 59-1). For example, global contamination includes more than 10^8 curies of radioactive krypton-85 released into the atmosphere from reprocessing of nuclear fuel, as well as worldwide radioactive fallout from atmospheric nuclear weapons tests, including about 3×10^7 curies of strontium-90 and cesium-137 combined, together with 10^7 curies of carbon-14. Immense quantities of radioactivity have been left in caverns and atoll formations after underground and underwater tests, the long-term isolation of which from the biosphere remains rather uncertain.[35]

In terms of human suffering,

- Many thousands of excess lung cancers can be associated with uranium mining, with a disproportionate share of the burden falling on indigenous or colonized people.

Table 59-1 Some characteristics of environmentally important radionuclides

Radionuclide	Critical organ	Physical half-life	Biologic half-life (approximate)
Americium-241	Bone, kidneys	458 years	60-140 years
Arsenic-76	Whole body	27 hours	11 days
Carbon-14	Whole body, genes	5730 years	12-40 days
Cerium-144	Bone, liver	284 days	0.5-4 years
Cesium-137	Muscle, whole body	31 years	70-140 days
Chromium-51	Bone, lung	28 days	1.7 years
Iodine-129	Thyroid, breast	16 million years	138 days
Iodine-131	Thyroid, breast	8 days	12-138 days
Krypton-85	Lung, fatty tissue	11 years	—
Manganese-54	Lung, liver	310 days	25-40 days
Neptunium-239	Bone	2.3 days	>40 years
Phosphorus-32	Bone, blood	14 days	3.2 years
Plutonium-238	Bone, liver	86 years	>40 years
Plutonium-239	Bone, liver	24,390 years	>40 years
Plutonium-241 → Americium-241	Bone, liver	13 years	>40 years
Ruthenium-103	Lung, kidney	39.5 days	3-30 days
Ruthenium-106	Lung, kidney	368 days	3-130 days
Sodium-24	Whole body	15 hours	11 days
Strontium-90 → Yttrium-90	Bone, lung	27.7 years	18-50 years
Tritium (H-3)	Whole body, genes	12.3 years	4-18 days
Xenon-133	Lung	5.3 days	—
Zinc-65	Whole body, ovaries, prostate	245 days	200 days-2.5 years

Data from Healy JW: *Los Alamos handbook of radiation monitoring* (LA 4400), Washington, DC, 1970; and Brodine V: *Radioactive contamination,* New York, 1975, Harcourt, Brace, Jovanovich.

- Considering only long-term contamination from known atmospheric tests, conservative estimates by independent scientists predict at least an additional 430,000 radiogenic cancer fatalities until the year 2000, increasing eventually to more than 2 million.[34,35] These estimates do not include an uncertain number of genetic effects passed on to future generations or thousands of reported cases of nonneoplastic disease among large populations residing within the areas affected by fallout from nuclear installations, such as Hanford, Washington, Savannah River, South Carolina, Fernald, Ohio, or the Nevada test site.

IONIZING RADIATION AND ITS BIOLOGIC EFFECTS

Ionizing radiation comprises emissions from the radioactive decay of naturally occurring radioisotopes, from those produced in nuclear reactors and accelerators, or from direct radiation released by these installations. The biologic damage caused by ionizing radiation is due to high-speed particles (usually electrons) traveling through cells and depositing concentrated amounts of energy, knocking out electrons from biomolecules (ionization), breaking chemical bonds, and causing a variety of other biochemical changes. The path of primary disturbances is described as an "ionization track." The amount of energy transferred to nearby biomolecules is usually many times larger than the energies involved in normal cell chemistry and metabolism.

Radiogenic health hazards are associated with a variety of complex lesions such as single- or double-strand breaks in the DNA helix of cell nuclei, severance of chemical bonds in essential proteins, and induction of oxidative or structural damage to cell membranes that control intercellular communication and defensive mechanisms, even at very low dose levels where there is little or no genomic DNA damage.

Given this complexity of interactions, it is not surprising that relative biologic effectiveness varies with type, energy, and target of the radiation.[74]

- α-Particles: ionized helium atoms, very short range, densely ionizing along very short track; if originating externally, they can be stopped by the skin; highly damaging if emitted internally
- β-Particles: high-energy electrons, considerably less densely ionizing along medium-range path; require thin material barriers for stoppage
- γ-Rays or x-rays (electromagnetic radiation with energies varying from a few thousand electron-Volt (keV) to several million electron-Volt (MeV), highly penetrating: ionization density varies inversely with energy; require thick layers of heavy material for shielding at high energies
- Neutrons: electrically neutral constituent particles of atomic nuclei, similar in mass to electrically charged protons; highly penetrating, dense indirect ionizations by collisions with light atoms, primarily hydrogen in human tissue; shielding requires thick layers of material

External and Internal Radiation Exposure

Physical and biologic half-life. External sources of radiation affect the body very differently from internal sources. Erecting shielding (such as in remote-control handling of radioactivity in nuclear weapons production or in handling radioactive sources in nuclear medicine) or distancing oneself from a localized external source greatly reduces the health hazard. However, large populations have been involuntarily subject to both external exposure (from dispersed environmental contamination due to fallout from weapons tests, reactor accidents, wastes leaking into the groundwater, and the like) and internal exposure, as a consequence of inhalation and ingestion. In addition to posing a radiation hazard, many of these radioactive contaminants are chemical toxicants as well.

Tissue exposure from radioactivity lodged inside the body diminishes only by physically decreasing emissions (radioactive decay) or by physiologic elimination of the contaminant. The decrease in rate of radioactive emissions from radioactive materials is determined by the physical half-life of the radioisotopes involved. Emissions decrease exponentially with time. The half-life describes the elapsed time for the initial rate of emission to fall by 50%. It takes a time period of nearly 7 half-lives before the original activity of any radioactive source has fallen below 1% of its initial value ($[\frac{1}{2}]^7 = 0.08$). Physical half-lives are specific to a particular radioisotope, and, for those most important for environmental contamination, half-lives vary from hours to geological time periods. They are physical constants, unalterable by human intervention. For radioactivity lodged inside the body, however, total tissue exposure (dose) is determined by a combination of physical half-life and the body's ability to eliminate radioactive contaminants by excretion. Time scales for bodily excretion vary with chemical and physical properties of the radioactive deposit, with its location in the body and with individual differences in metabolic rates. In contrast to radioactive decay, physiologic elimination of radioactivity does, in general, not follow an exponential trend with time. Often, there is a steep initial loss from the body or a contaminated organ, followed by elimination at a much lower rate. Therefore, tabulated biologic half-lives represent approximate values only, obtained under specific conditions. In some favorable cases, the retention time can be shortened by intervention in body chemistry (decontamination treatment). Representative physical and biologic half-lives of some environmentally important radioisotopes are listed in Table 59-1, together with organs in which these radioisotopes tend to concentrate.

Units of radioactivity and radiation dose. Radiation hazard is related to both the strength of the source (activity) and the total radioactive energy absorbed per unit volume of tissue (dose).

Activity is measured in number of radioactive disintegrations per second (Becquerel or Bq) or the larger traditional unit curie (1 Ci = 3.7×10^{10} Bq). Often larger or smaller units are defined by metric prefixes such as *mega* (M), *milli* (m), *micro* (μ), or *pico* (p):(1 MBq = 10^6 Bq = 2.7×10^{-5} Ci = 27 μCi; 1 mCi = 10^{-3} Ci = 3.7×10^7 Bq; 1 μCi = 10^{-6}Ci; 1 pCi = 10^{-12} Ci). Daily gaseous emissions from an exhaust stack may be recorded in thousands of curies, and soil and water contamination may be expressed in Bq/km^2 or Bq/kg and pCi/liter, respectively.

Relative biological effectiveness for different radiation exposures. Biologic injury from a given type of ionizing radiation depends on the amount of radioactive energy deposited into a physiologically critical volume of tissue or a specific organ (quantified by units of absorbed dose).

For the purpose of radiation protection, we must compare the same biologic effect resulting from exposures to different types of radiation. It is convenient to define an *effective dose* or *dose equivalent* (resulting in a certain biologic effect), related to the physically absorbed dose by a multiplying factor, relative biologic effectiveness (RBE) in the relation:

$$\text{Effective dose} = \text{RBE} \times \text{Absorbed dose}$$

Metric and traditional units for effective dose have been used in the literature (with metric prefixes), such as:

$$1 \text{ Sievert (Sv)} = 100 \text{ rem or } 10 \text{ mSv} = 1 \text{ cSv} = 1 \text{ rem}$$

For absorbed dose:

$$1 \text{ Gray (Gy)} = 100 \text{ rad or } 10 \text{ mGy} = 1 \text{ cGy} = 1 \text{ rad}$$

The RBE varies with type and energy of radiation, with the biologic effect studied (end point), and with dose and dose rate.

Influenced by concerns of industry and radiologists,[15] the International Commission on Radiological Protection (ICRP) has defined RBE for x-rays, γ- and β-radiation of all energies to be unity (i.e., 1 Gy = 1 Sv for these types of radiation).[33] Such a definition is inconsistent with radiobiologic experiments and reports by other international expert commissions. Specifically, if the RBE for medical and industrial x-ray exposures is actually significantly greater than unity, compared to γ-radiation, it has important ramifications for assessing radiation risks for the public, since radiation protection standards are based on risk factors derived from high-energy γ-exposures.[56]

In a recent study, using the frequency of induced chromosome aberrations in human blood lymphocytes in vitro as the indicator (end point) and comparing 250 kVp x-rays at varying doses with Co-60 γ-rays (mean energy of about 1.5 MeV, with RBE defined as unity), x-rays showed an inverse dose-effect relation with an RBE of 2.7 at doses below 1 mGy, diminishing to a value of 1.6 at a dose of about 10 mGy. In this comparison, the dose rate was held at a constant 1 Gy/min.[20]

The rate at which radiation is absorbed appears to be important. There is growing epidemiologic evidence that long-term protracted accumulation of low doses is more injurious to human health than the same dose applied all at once.[56,57,87]

Stochastic and deterministic health effects: threshold doses. Radiogenic induction of cancer or of genetically transmitted damage is an example of stochastic effects. Such damage is the result of ionizing tracks traversing a cell nucleus that result in critical mutations. For stochastic effects, higher doses result in higher probability that more cells in a given volume will be hit or that more than one track will traverse any one cell, translating into higher risk for mutations. There is no threshold dose below which there is zero risk.

For deterministic radiation effects, however, often a minimum dose (threshold) must be exceeded before radiogenic damage can be observed, and its severity is related to the dose. Acute radiation sickness, such as nausea, hair loss, diarrhea, radiation burns, or leukopenia, is considered a deterministic effect.

No threshold dose for cancer or genetic effects of radiation. The lowest radiation dose a cell nucleus can receive is one ionization track. The latter usually results in a large number of broken bonds and other biomolecular lesions, including possible genetic mutations. Cells have effective repair mechanisms in place for many lesions, but *not all damage, even from a single track, can be repaired with 100% efficiency.* This conclusion is based on epidemiologic studies that have shown excess cancer induction at very low doses and at very low dose rates.[56,57] Under those exposure conditions, not a single ionizing track has traversed the nucleus of a large fraction of the cells of exposed individuals, while for a small fraction of cells, the nuclei were hit by a single ionizing track only. In a carefully documented microdosimetric argument, based on many published studies, Gofman has shown that there exists no threshold dose or dose rate below which there is zero risk for stochastic radiogenic damage.[30]

Effects of Natural Background Radiation

Life on earth has evolved under continuous and gradually diminishing exposures to cosmic radiation by neutrons and charged high-energy particles, as well as to terrestrial α-, β-, and γ-rays. The origins of these various types of radiation are solar emissions of nuclear particles, nuclear reactions of these particles with the earth's atmosphere, and the radioactive decay of very long-lived radioisotopes, distributed throughout the earth's crust (e.g., potassium-40, uranium, and the noble gas radon, including its decay products). This biologic fact in no way supports, however, a conjecture that, therefore, exposures to low doses of naturally present or man-made ionizing radiation must have beneficial effects on human health (hormesis hypothesis).[46] There exists no credible epidemiologic evidence for this conjecture. On the contrary, a large study in Great Britain (confirmed by others in the United States) concluded that a major fraction of childhood cancer deaths are associated with natural background radiation (as discussed later). Also, extrapolating

from a study of 65,000 underground miners among whom more than 2700 died of lung cancer, an international team of scientists concluded that in the general U.S. population about 11% of lung cancer deaths among smokers and 30% among never-smokers might be due to exposure to naturally occurring radon gas and its radioactive daughter isotopes in homes.[47]

Useful data about activities and estimated annual effective doses from natural radionuclides and from those dumped into the environment by nuclear weapons production and tests have been collected from a variety of sources by a public research group.[32]

HEALTH HAZARDS FROM IONIZING RADIATION

High doses of ionizing radiation from nuclear explosions result in many serious health effects within hours, weeks, or months.[44,66] For those who were spared from or survived acute radiation injuries, a lifespan study of about 100,000 Hiroshima-Nagasaki survivors, alive in 1950, has shown dose-dependent long-term risks for induction of radiogenic cancers of virtually all known types with latency periods that can span many decades. Although the statistical risk analysis has been weighted toward medium to high-dose effects, excess cancers have been observed down to very low doses.[7,56,57] Thus, while some tissue seems to be more radiosensitive than others, no cancer is known to be specific to radiation exposure.

Similarly, most noncancerous health effects that have been found to be associated with radioactivity are also known to be associated with other toxicants, such as chemical pollutants.

Protracted Low-Dose Exposures

The literature on radiation-related health effects from low-dose exposures is vast and beset with contradictions and open questions.[56] Practically all pertinent health research has been funded by government agencies whose primary mission has been nuclear weapons production and promotion of nuclear technologies. Such activities are often accompanied by unavoidable or accidental releases of radioactivity into the environment. There exist conflicts of interest between the efficient production of weapons or electricity and the responsibility for radiation protection of workers and the general public. Effective protection of employees has been monitored by contracted epidemiologic studies. An assessment of the "state of knowledge" in this area of science must, therefore, include a recognition of the politicoeconomic force field in which radiation researchers have been operating, lest the reader of mainstream medical literature be misled into concluding that most of what we need to know about the health impacts of low-level radiation has been firmly established and that deviating findings have no credible scientific foundation. Collated conclusions from several extensive reviews, a discussion of their respective merits, and a collection of essential references permit a more differentiated evaluation.* Here, only a limited selection of essential or very recent references can be listed.

Somatic, Genetic, and Congenital Health Effects of Ionizing Radiation

In a large number of epidemiologic studies, among A-bomb survivors or nuclear worker populations, cancer cases in excess of "normal" background rate have been ascribed to the individuals' exposures, a so-called somatic effect of radiation. The designation *radiogenic* cancers has statistical meaning only (i.e., it refers to populations) and can never be applied to an individual case. This greatly complicates the establishment of fair standards of liability for occupational safety on employers or government agencies. As a practical matter, agencies and contractors operating nuclear installations have largely been indemnified against claims of liability.[60]

In contrast to a vast literature on somatic effects of radiation,[7,56,88] few studies link risks to offspring and parental radiation exposure at low doses (*genetic* effects). Yet, there is no doubt that low doses of ionizing radiation do induce unrepaired or unrepairable mutations in cell nuclei (see later in this chapter), which makes the induction of genetic effects at low doses biologically rather likely, even if it is difficult to ascertain them unambiguously from a second-generation statistical study. The BEIR V report by the National Research Council reviews various past estimates of excess genetic effects per rem exposure per generation (Table 59-2).[7] Gofman[29,31] has reviewed the literature about chromosome aberrations, such as deletions and translocations, that are associated with serious birth defects and mental handicaps, such as the Wolf-Hirschhorn syndrome or trisomy 21 (usually known as Down syndrome), respectively.[1] Mutagenic research suggests that a large part of congenital defects and genetic diseases of unknown origin are consequences of deletions and translocations at the submicroscopic level. Such lesions can be induced by very low doses of ionizing radiation (and at low dose-rates).

A study of leukemia clusters among young people born in the vicinity of the Sellafield nuclear installation in Great Britain suggested a genetic component via radiation exposure of their fathers. References to the important debate over this interpretation and to subsequent studies—some corroborating, some refuting it—as well as other relevant studies can be found elsewhere.[56,57,73]

Another class of health effects are those following exposure before birth, manifest at or after birth (*congenital* effects). One of the most comprehensive studies was started about 40 years ago in Great Britain (Oxford Survey of Childhood Cancers; OSCC). It unambiguously linked increased cancer risks (including leukemia) in children under 15 years to obstetric x-ray studies of their mothers during pregnancy. The risk coefficients per unit dose derived from the OSCC survey[10,41,54] are considerably larger than those

*References 10, 15, 28, 56, 57, 87.

that were obtained from the A-bomb study.[7,87] This discrepancy has been explained as a consequence of natural selection among the Japanese survivor population, which raises doubt about transferring radiogenic risks derived from this rather special group of people to predict exposure hazards among ordinary populations.[82,83]

The vast collection of data for all British childhood cancer cases allowed the Birmingham team to make several concomitant discoveries, such as a threefold higher risk for first than for third trimester exposures during pregnancy, the greatly increased susceptibility of prenatally exposed children to infections during cancer latency periods (associated with immune depression), and an association of juvenile cancer mortality rates with variations in natural terrestrial background doses.[40] The last finding led the researchers to conclude that a major fraction of all juvenile cancers are associated with natural background radiation.

Among children of A-bomb survivors, nonmalignant congenital defects, such as abnormal brain development and small head size, have also been related to a single prenatal exposure, down to doses less than 20 mGy.[92]

ESTABLISHING LEVELS OF EXPOSURE OR DOSE

By law, radiation workers must wear individual dosimeters (monitors or badges containing thermoluminescent or x-ray films) during working hours. These badges are read out at regular intervals, and the workers' exposure records form the basis for long-term occupational health studies. At low external doses, dosimeter readings become uncertain. Also, health effects from exposures can easily be masked by a variety of other factors also associated with the frequency of the disease under investigation. If sufficient information is available about the workforce and their work environment, ingenuity, medical insight, and astute observations of trends can inform the researchers' choices of controlling or modifying factors to be included in the analysis. These choices, in turn, determine the sensitivity of a particular statistical methodology to detect relatively small but significant excess radiogenic risks.[39]

For other populations, such as Hiroshima-Nagasaki survivors, external doses had to be estimated from complex computer models, simulating the intensity of the radiation flash from the two bombs.[7] Additional doses due to fallout, an important contribution to exposures for survivors at great distances from the epicenter (low-dose cohorts), were, however, not included in the dose estimates.[56]

Where exposures to internal radioactivity are likely to have played a major role in observed health effects, such as among some nuclear workers and among populations in environmentally contaminated regions, dosimetry models are beset with many uncertainties. For exposures to environmental contamination, their accuracy depends on reliable estimates of deposition rates, subject to highly variable microclimatic conditions, to variations in topography, and to uncertain transfer factors to pastures, vegetables, dust, and the like, as well as to dietary habits of individuals.[86]

Biologic Dosimetry

Ionizing radiation, even at low doses, induces observable chromosome aberrations, such as dicentrics in T-lymphocytes of the human peripheral blood. With suitable methods for dose-effect calibration, a sensitivity of 100 mSv and possibly 50 mSv can be achieved for determining single acute radiation exposures.[45,91] One drawback of this method is a loss of dicentrics during normal processes of cell division in vivo. In adults, a half-life of about 1.5 years has been found.[6] For protracted and relatively constant exposures, such as those of most nuclear workers or airline personnel, the assumption can be made that an equilibrium concentration of dicentrics will be established such that the number of newly induced aberrations equals those eliminated by normal metabolic processes of the body. Under these circumstances, a much higher sensitivity of about 10 mSv can be achieved.[69,70]

Depression in monocyte count appears to be associated with internal exposure to radiation from bone-seeking radioactive particulates.[8,9] Monocytes are part of the im-

Table 59-2 Selected radiogenic cancer risk estimates for exposures at low doses, acute or protracted

| | Exposure conditions | | | | Excess cancer risk per 10^4 p-cGy* | |
Reference	Dose range cGy	Dose rate	Applicable population	Applicable follow-up	Observed risk	Lifetime risk (estim.)
Nussbaum-Köhnlein[56,57]	1-11	acute bomb γ	~90,000 A-bomb survivors	1950-1985	9.1	33
Same	11-69	acute bomb γ	Same	1950-1985	2.8	9.3
Gofman[30]	0-5	acute bomb γ	Same	1950-1985	5	30
Same	0-5	acute bomb γ	Recalculated for U.S. population	1950-1985	—	26
Knox et al,[41] Muirhead, Kneale[54]	<0.5	acute x-ray prenatal	~24,000 British children who died of cancer	age 0-15 years	13 (mortality)	n.a.
Bithell, Stiller[10]	<0.5	acute x-ray prenatal	Same as above	age 0-15 years	17.5 (incidence)	n.a.
Modan et al[52]	1.6 mean to breast	acute x-rays	~11,000 Israeli children, age 5-9 years	23-37 years after exposure	relative risk >12 for breast cancer†	n.a..
Mancuso, Stewart, Kneale[56,57]	2.2 mean (~equal to background)	low rate	~28,000 nuclear workers Hanford (WA)	1944-1986 deaths	*Working life risk* 85 for all workers >440 for exposures after age 58	
Wing et al[56,57]	1.7 mean <5 for 68%	low rate	~8,000 nuclear workers Oak Ridge (TN)	1943-1984 deaths	*Working life risk* ~110 average for all workers, all ages	
Beral et al[56]	0.8 mean	low rate	~23,000 British nuclear workers	1951-1982 ~19 years mean follow-up	*Working life risk* ~165 average for all workers, all ages	

*For example, for a lifetime excess cancer risk for 30 per 10^4 person-cGy: exposing 15,000 people to an average accumulated dose of 10 cGy (100 mGy) will on average lead to [(30 cancers)/10^4 p-cGy] $(1.5 \times 10^4 \times 10$ p-cGy) = 450 extra radiogenic cancer deaths over the lifetime of these 15,000 people.
†This means that exposed children have a twelve-fold higher risk for developing breast cancer as adults than unexposed controls.

Range of estimated lifetime risk values for protracted low-dose exposures of normal populations by international radiation commissions‡

UNSCEAR (1988)[87]	2-5	Fatal cancers per 10^4 p-cGy
BEIR V (1990)[7]	4	Fatal cancers per 10^4 p-cGy
ICRP (1990)[33]	5	Fatal cancers per 10^4 p-cGy

‡Including recommended dose rate effectiveness factor (2), not supported by human studies.[30,56]

mune defense system; they are formed in bone marrow, and they migrate out of the bloodstream into tissue and engulf foreign matter such as particles of uranium or plutonium. Monocyte count, if it can be calibrated, could probably be developed for biologic dosimetry, especially for radioactivity lodged in the body.[58]

EPIDEMIOLOGIC METHODS FOR ASCERTAINING HEALTH EFFECTS

Cohort and Case-Control Studies

In an epidemiologic cohort study, an exposed population is compared with an unexposed or less exposed one. It is important that the compared populations are similar in age and sex distribution, socioeconomic conditions, and a variety of other factors with known influences on disease rates. Cohort studies yield relative risks, a comparison of risk with and without exposure. If individual doses are known, relative risks can be related to dose. Selection effects must be taken into account. For example, nuclear workers as a group have been selected for good health, and high pay is an important factor in maintaining good health. This is illustrated by the fact that mortality for all causes among nuclear workers in the United States and in Great Britain has been found to be about 25% lower than national averages (health worker effect). Therefore, reliable estimates of radiation risks must derive from comparisons between subcohorts of the same workforce, ranked according to levels of exposure. In addition, internal selection associated with job categories must be accounted for.[39]

In a case-control study, the level of exposure of individuals with a certain disease (or for whom the disease was the primary cause of death) is compared with that of matched controls from the same population who, except for being free of the studied disease, are otherwise as similar as possible. The British study of childhood cancers is an example of a case-control study.[41]

Ecological and Clinical Studies

For populations exposed to radioactive fallout, only average doses or (as a substitute) air, surface soil, or water contamination in different geographic areas can be estimated. In such ecologic studies, disease or mortality rates among populations from more exposed geographic areas are compared with those from less contaminated ones. Several ecologic studies have found excess cancers and other diseases among populations exposed to environmental contamination as a consequence of radioactive fallout from weapons tests or accidental nuclear explosions, such as the Chernobyl catastrophe (see pp. 526-527).[35,56,57] For example, an elevated incidence of leukemia was found among residents of Utah who had been affected by fallout from nuclear tests at the Nevada site.[83]

Epidemiologic studies can also be used to formulate new hypotheses of disease-exposure relationships. For example, Gofman analyzed a large number of clinical studies to establish the association of breast cancer incidence with previous exposures to diagnostic x-ray films.[28]

Two recently published ecologic studies spawned intense debate about the legitimacy of such studies in suggesting (as opposed to proving) an association of radioactive contamination of the environment with cancer mortality near the Oak Ridge, Tennessee, nuclear installation and with breast cancer incidence in four U.S. geographic areas.[49,55] Examples of other ecologic studies are presented in the section on population exposures.

RADIATION PROTECTION STANDARDS AND OCCUPATIONAL HEALTH STUDIES

Shortly after the end of World War II, when various nations took the political decision that nuclear weapons production was a matter of highest national priority, it became necessary to establish standards for "allowable" exposures of both nuclear workers and the public that would not seriously impede the operation of production facilities.[15] Most Western governments adopted recommendations by the International Commission on Radiological Protection (ICRP), a self-appointing commission of 13 scientists and radiologists, for their legal norms. These recommendations by the ICRP have been derived primarily from extrapolations from high-dose risks among the A-bomb survivors, combined with radiobiologic data. Table 59-3 reviews the history of "allowable" exposures, a reflection of gradual revisions of previously underestimated health risks from low-dose exposures.

Given the early recognition that medium to high doses of ionizing radiation are effective in the induction of cancers, a preoccupation with carcinogenesis has persisted in radioepidemiologic studies at the expense of attention to excess numbers of nonneoplastic diseases associated with exposures.

Table 59-3 Whole body dose limits as recommended by the International Commission on Radiological Protection

	Allowable dose	
	Occupational	**General public**
1951-1954	0.5 rad/week	0.5 rad/year
1955-1959	0.3 rem/week 200 rem/lifetime averaging 5 rem/year	0.5 rem/year
1959-1977	5 (age 18) rem/year or 3 rem/13 weeks	0.5 rem/year
1977-1989	50 mSv (5 rem)/year	1.7 mSv (0.17 rem)/year
1990-	*20 mSv/year* averaged over 5 years, not to exceed 50 mSv in any 1 year	*1 mSv/year* in special circumstances 1 mSv averaged over 5 years

From Barish RJ: Health physics concerns in commercial aviation, *Health Phys* 59:199, 1990.

Health Studies among Workers in Nuclear Installations

As reflected in Table 59-3, radiogenic risk estimates by the ICRP have continued to support the expectation that exposures to occupational doses well below official permissible levels would not induce any observable excess cancers or other diseases (the "null hypothesis"). Thus, the focus of most epidemiologic studies among workers in weapons production plants has been a test of this hypothesis. This emphasis might have misled the researchers of a large number of studies of radiation health effects toward inconclusive results. A critical review of 124 government-sponsored occupational studies, most of them showing negative findings, found serious flaws in their research design.[27]

In many reported investigations, the methodology used is not sensitive enough to detect an association at low doses. In order to improve statistical power, several worker studies can be pooled (meta-analysis).[91] However, this methodology may lead to other problems: Recently, a very large set of data from diverse worker populations in different countries was combined. The investigators claimed highest accuracy for their values of radiogenic cancer risks under protracted low-dose exposures. Unfortunately, heterogeneities among various components of the data sets led to averaging of trends, which reduced the study's sensitivity such that the result remained inconclusive.[14,39] To posit a "safe" threshold dose on the strength of this and other inconclusive findings[46] is, however, unwarranted when lack of sensitivity is a much more probable reason for negative findings.

Several occupational studies involving smaller but more homogeneous groups of workers and employment conditions have established statistically significant association of low-dose radiation exposure with excess malignancies. While none of these findings have been refuted on scientific grounds, they have been attacked and dismissed by critics as "aberrant" or "accidental."[63] These unwelcome results have been routinely ignored when downward revisions in radiation protection standards were contemplated.[7,33,56,57] The presumption that radiation poses a particularly low risk for genetically transmitted effects at low-dose exposures has recently been challenged by the following findings of leukemia clusters near a British nuclear installation.

Among young people whose fathers worked at the Sellafield (West Cumbria) nuclear plant, a high correlation of excess leukemia was found with parental doses received prior to conception. A sixfold to sevenfold increase in risk was found for external doses above 10 mSv, received within 6 months prior to conception.[26] The broad ramifications of this finding for genetic transmission of malignancies have led to vigorous debate. Additional studies around other nuclear installations provided both corroborative and nonsupportive evidence for Gardner's hypothesis. Inhaled or ingested radioisotopes may also have played an important role, even though internal dose estimates were not available.

For additional references to the ongoing debate about Gardner's hypothesis, see reviews elsewhere.[56,57]

The enhanced hazards due to exposures from internal isotopes have recently been investigated in another study of nuclear workers.[55,65]

Official estimates of somatic radiogenic cancer risk at low and protracted exposures, based on extrapolations from the A-bomb survivor study and some animal studies, have been about an order of magnitude lower than those obtained from mortalities at the lowest dose levels of the Japanese survivors, as well as from several occupational studies, as illustrated in Table 59-2. Such inconsistencies and open questions have been discussed in previous reviews.[56,57]

Military Personnel (Atomic Soldiers)

About 250,000 members of the U.S. armed forces participated in the nuclear weapons testing program. Numbers for other nuclear nations, foremost the former Soviet Union and China, are not known but can be expected to be very large as well. Only a few follow-up health studies have been published. Some found excess cancers among the exposed,[13] while another government-commissioned study claimed negative findings,[62] followed by much controversy about the scientific credibility of this study.[76] A reanalysis of the data used by the scientists of the National Academy of Sciences, corrected for the neglected healthy soldier bias, came to quite opposite conclusions.[12] Atomic veterans are still battling for appropriate medical care as a minimal recognition for their sacrifices in support of their country's nuclear policies.[48]

A study of cancer mortality among military personnel stationed at the Hanford, Washington, Nuclear Installation during periods of high radioactive releases has been initiated. It has been delayed by a lack of cooperation from the Department of Veterans Affairs.

Nuclear Emergency Workers (Chernobyl Liquidators)

Elsewhere, government authorities are not forthcoming, either, with reliable health studies after radioactive releases.

Recent unofficial reports from medical officers of the republics of the former Soviet Union state that about 25,000 of several hundred thousand liquidators (emergency workers who attempted to bury the melting reactor core) have already died, many of them by their own hands. There exists to date no confirmation of these disturbing numbers in the Western scientific literature.

Uranium Miners

Many hundreds of thousands of miners in various countries have been employed to bring forth the basic ore for nuclear weapons production.[35] The former Soviet Union, together with East Germany, had organized the Wismut Company, a contractor that employed workers in the rich uranium mines in the German Ore Mountains. After the collapse of both regimes, the secret records of 450,000 workers were discovered, indicating that at least 15,000 workers had already died of silicosis and about 10,000 to 15,000 of lung cancers.[36] Epidemiologic studies of uranium miners have uncovered only the tip of the iceberg in terms of lung cancer deaths and other diseases.[47,71,72,75] Some of these studies also showed that mortality risk factors for α-radiation are inversely related to the average yearly exposure rate of miners, a finding that has important ramifications for the protracted low-dose exposures of residents to α-emitting radon gas in homes.[18]

Cancers Among Commercial Airline Personnel

Airline crews are subject to cosmic irradiation, consisting mainly of neutrons and high-energy γ-rays.[5,24,43,59,68] Mean annual dose equivalents can be estimated from physical[67] and biologic dosimetry.[68] Accumulated doses depend on flight altitude and routes, as well as on fluctuating solar activity. Mean annual effective doses between 10 mSv and 25 mSv have been reported, which for a working life may add up to 300 mSv.

A cancer mortality and incidence study among Canadian male pilots showed significant excess rates for several cancers, including Hodgkin's disease and nonmelanoma skin cancer.[4] By using the population of British Columbia as the control group, the positive findings represent an underestimation of true excess incidence and mortality rates, considering the reported reduced mortality for all causes (80% of that for the general population). No correction was applied for this obvious healthy worker effect. The findings suggest an association of cancer with exposure to low doses of ionizing radiation, possibly in synergism with a range of electromagnetic frequencies and, for rectal cancer, with a high-fat diet.

High-altitude exposure, aviator status, and both also correlate significantly with cancerous conditions of the skin, testicles, bladder, and thyroid in a study of U.S. pilots.[5] An investigation of cancer incidence among Finnish airline cabin attendants found a significant excess risk for breast cancer (about double) and for bone cancer (about fifteenfold) among female workers, compared to the Finnish population.[61]

A study of chromosome aberrations induced in lymphocytes of pilots and stewardesses also confirms effects of very-low-dose exposures in this occupation.[69]

Mutational Effects among Radiotherapy Technicians

Messing and colleagues[50] investigated whether mutant frequency in peripheral T-lymphocytes of radiotherapy technicians, exposed on the average to 0.3 cGy per month of Co-60 γ-radiation, can be associated with recently absorbed dose. The study cohort consisted of 13 exposed technicians wearing dosimeters. The matched controls were 12 physiotherapy technicians working in the same hospital with no radiation exposure. The analysis revealed that the mutation frequency is linearly correlated with dose in the range from 0 to 0.7 cGy. In radiotherapy patients (treated for breast cancer), the Messing group observed after much higher doses (4 Gy) mutation frequencies of only 1% of those at the very low doses and dose-rates. This would suggest that at higher doses multiple damage and cell killing become prominent, reducing the mutation yield. The findings are consistent with earlier observations among nuclear medicine technicians.[51] Significantly elevated risks for leukemia and various cancers were also found among Chinese x-ray workers.[88]

CONSEQUENCES OF EXPOSURES TO THE GENERAL POPULATION

Exposures from Natural and Medical Background Radiation

Averaged over the U.S. population, about 55% of background radiation dose originates from radon and its radioactive decay products; 27% from cosmic, terrestrial, and internal exposure; and about 18% from man-made sources, including medical exposures.[7]

Useful estimates of concentrations of naturally occurring and man-made radioisotopes (including those from weapons tests), as found in seawater, continental waters, surface soils, and rocks, and effective doses from these sources have been summarized in a recent publication.[32]

On the basis of his cancer risk estimates, Gofman suggested that background and medical radiation induce about 25% of all "spontaneous" cancers in the U.S. population,[30] while Stewart and her team determined that natural background radiation accounts for a major fraction of all childhood cancers.[40] A recent comprehensive analysis of the radiologic literature led Gofman to conclude that medical x-ray exposures over past decades can account for at least 75% of all female breast cancers.[28]

Congenital effects of low doses of prenatal x-ray exposures have already been discussed.[41,54] They showed the particularly high susceptibility of the fetus for radiation injury. Combining these findings with those among the A-bomb survivors, which concluded that tissue of the female breast is about 2.5 times as sensitive to cancer induction as all other tissue taken together,[21] we might expect that young female children would be particularly sensitive to breast cancer induction from x-ray exposures. Modan and associates[52] found an increased risk of cancer for the most recent 5-year period of a long-term follow-up study of Israeli children who had scalp irradiation for tinea capitis between 1949 and 1959. The original cohort included 10,834 irradiated children. Estimated mean doses were 9 cGy to the thyroid, 4.8 to 6.6 cGy to the pituitary, and 1.6 cGy to the breast. Until 1982, there were no indications of more cancer risk than matched controls. Since then, however, incidence of breast cancer in girls increased significantly, showing a long latency period for induction in childhood. A very high relative risk of about 12 (with a large uncertainty) was found in women who had been exposed to a mean breast dose of 1.6 cGy at age 5 to 9 years. Thyroid cancers eventually became also more frequent in the exposed population.

Contamination from Nuclear Weapons Tests

Clinical reports and unofficial health surveys by citizen groups, independent scientists, and investigative reporters have found consistent patterns of unexplained increases in various health problems among exposed populations and their children.[15,19,17,25] These groups include residents of areas contaminated by deliberate or accidental radioactive releases[8,9] or by fallout from nuclear test sites,[38] as well as tens of thousands of military personnel from various nuclear nations, who had been involved in exercises or cleanup operations.[48] The global environmental and health consequences of nuclear weapons production, including miners, workers in weapons production plants, military personnel, and civilian populations, have recently been surveyed in detail by a team of researchers in the fields of environmental and occupational medicine, epidemiology, environmental engineering, and ecology.[35] This volume brings together extensive, hitherto scattered or unavailable data about the human toll of the nuclear arms race.

In the epidemiologic literature, there exist considerably fewer comprehensive studies of health effects among populations affected by internal exposures from radioactive fallout than among those subjected to external exposures. One of the major reasons is that estimates of effective doses from contamination by internal radioisotopes are beset with unavoidable uncertainties.[57,74] Yet, there is little doubt that a large number of people all over the globe have suffered ill health as a consequence of partly external, partly internal contamination from atmospheric nuclear weapons testing.[35] We review here a few examples from an emerging consistent pattern among reports from various sources that suggest that—depending on levels of exposure—various types of cancers, depressed immune response, miscarriages, stillbirths, first-through sixth-day infant mortality, deformities, and an increase of neuroblastoma and Down syndrome in newborns are probably associated with contamination from radioactive fallout.

Increases in leukemia rates among U.S. children have been linked to deposition of low concentrations of strontium-90 in food, milk, and human bone, originating from atmospheric testing. The strongest association was found with acute and myeloid leukemia rates among 5- to 9-year-olds about 5.5 years after the peaks in fallout. Regional differences in leukemia rates corresponded to different levels of strontium-90 deposition. An additional indicator for a causal relation was the drop in leukemia rates several years after cessation of atmospheric tests.[2]

Near the nuclear test sites in Nevada, a case-control study was conducted involving 1177 individuals (cases) who died of leukemia between 1952 and 1981 and 5330 persons who died of other causes (controls). The authors estimated active bone marrow dose from external exposure to radioactive deposition on the soil from fallout to range from 0 to 3 cGy. The median bone marrow dose from fallout was 0.32 cGy for all cases and controls, to be compared to a dose of 0.49 cGy from terrestrial and cosmic background radiation accumulated over the period of fallout (7 years). A significant association with external marrow dose was found for acute leukemias discovered from 1952 to 1963 among those individuals who were younger than 20 years at exposure. The corresponding risk values at these very low external exposures are about double those predicted by the BEIR V report.[7] While the difference was formally not statistically significant, the consistency of the results with several previous studies of populations exposed to fallout from the Nevada atmospheric bomb tests suggests a causal relation.[81]

While positive associations were observed between leukemia and external exposure, internal exposures from inhaled or ingested fission products are likely to have played a dominant role if tissue concentrations of radioisotopes were correlated with levels of external contamination.

Similarly, a statistically significant excess of thyroid neoplasms was found among schoolchildren who were exposed to fallout between 1951 and 1958 in communities of Southwestern Utah, Southeastern Nevada, and Southeastern Arizona. Estimated doses from radioactive iodine isotopes to the thyroid ranged from 0 to 460 cGy (17 cGy average for Utah).[38]

The Chernobyl Nuclear Disaster

Since 1986, contamination from the reactor explosion at Chernobyl devastated the health of many people in the Ukraine and in Belarus, with an unexpected and particularly invasive form of thyroid cancer affecting many children of the area.[3,37,84] Even at rather low levels of radioactive deposition in Germany, far from the source of the radioactive emissions, increased incidence of neonatal and infant mortality, as well as trisomy 21 (Down syndrome), was observed.[77-79] The evidence for serious health detriment among the exposed population, far above and beyond official reports by government agencies and industry officials, has been reviewed more extensively elsewhere.[56,57]

Recently, a clinical health study was conducted in Israel among a group of 1560 new immigrants from the former Soviet Union, including reactor "liquidators" and two groups of former residents from areas of higher and lower contamination of the soil with cesium-137. Their classification according to internal contamination was validated by measurements of cesium-137 body burden.[42] Among the highly irradiated liquidators, there was considerably higher incidence of acute radiation effects than among the residents of the most contaminated areas. There were about 2.5 times as many cases of bronchial asthma among children from the more exposed areas. Respiratory, central nervous system, and cardiovascular disorders were significantly more prevalent in liquidators than in the two other groups. Among adolescents, cardiovascular disease and, among children, respiratory and central nervous system disorders were significantly elevated among those from the more exposed communities. Asthma prevalence among children potentially exposed in utero appeared to be increased eightfold. The authors interpret this large increase to be a manifestation of depressed immune function, consistent with blood plasma studies among members of the affected population.[23]

Summarizing their findings, the authors conclude that a preoccupation with carcinogenesis as the principal consequence of radioactive contamination has led to a distorted view of health effects of low-level radiation. Mutagenesis may also result in nonneoplastic abnormalities.

However, based on their own research as well as on other studies published in Russian journals, the authors emphasize that the observed occurrences of exposure-related stress disorders in persons exposed to radiation from the Chernobyl accident (e.g., hypertension among older adults[23]) is not a valid argument against the etiologic role of food contamination by cesium-137, possibly in synergism with other pollutants.[22]

Leukemia Clusters Near Civilian Nuclear Power Plants

Leukemia is a very rare disease, especially childhood leukemia. From the time in the mid-1950s when Alice Stewart first showed that prenatal x-ray examinations could nearly double the risk of a child to die of leukemia (or other cancers),[41] it took the U.S. Food and Drug Administration almost 30 years to issue warnings about x-raying pregnant women. It is now generally accepted that an increased incidence rate of childhood leukemia is an early indication of past radiation exposure. Such increases have been reported around nuclear installations in the United States, Great Britain, and Germany.

United States. After the near-meltdown of the core of one of the Three Mild Island (TMI) nuclear reactors near Harrisburg, Pennsylvania, in March 1979, a federally supported study claimed that no more than 15 curies of I-131 were released from the stricken plant. This number was admittedly an estimate, obtained from an environmental dosimetric model, involving a great number of assumptions and unknown parameters.[15] On the basis of that amount of radioactivity, the official reports predicted that the accident should not have resulted in any observable health effects. When concerned citizens started to receive reports of increases in leukemia and lung cancers in the areas downwind of the plant, a community health survey was initiated with assistance by some independent scientists that compared areas with higher and lower radioactive exposure. The results are still tied up in court proceedings.

An increased risk of leukemia was found in a five-town area of Massachusetts near Plymouth, location of the Pilgrim I nuclear plant. This plant is known to have released various radioisotopes during the years 1974 and 1975. Here, the excess was found primarily among adults and the elderly. The authors suspect the source of radioactive contamination

to be atmospheric trapping of radioactive effluents into a coastal wind flow pattern.[16] Sparked by public concern, the U.S. National Cancer Institute sponsored a subsequent study that could not confirm excess leukemia cases. This negative finding could, however, be shown to be due to a lack of sensitivity of the applied methodology.[56]

Great Britain. A study of childhood leukemia in the vicinity of two reprocessing plants, four power plants, and two weapons production sites, extending over 20 years, revealed enhanced rates compared to national averages with relative risks ranging from 1.2 to 3.2.[64]

Germany. In the neighborhood of the nuclear power plant Krümmel alongside the Elbe River, 8 cases of leukemia were reported within a 7-year period (1989 to 1995). During a 10-year period 1980 to 1990, only 0.7 cases would have been expected. The power reactor started operating in 1983. External doses calculated on the basis of environmental monitoring records provided by the operator, combined with official risk estimates are insufficient to account for such an effect. However, families with leukemia cases have preferentially consumed food grown in the area, where microclimatic conditions favor concentrations of deposits. Chromosomal analyses of blood samples taken from members of affected families showed a more than sixfold increase in dicentric aberrations over the standard rate. Competing risk factors such as medical x-rays, parental occupational exposures, chemicals, previous diseases, and radon could be excluded. All cases of leukemia were diagnosed 5 to 11 years after the plant had been started. A detailed account on the Krümmel cluster was presented at the Tenth International Congress of Radiation Research held at Würzburg, Germany, the city where C. W. Roentgen discovered x-rays 100 years ago.[70]

THE DILEMMA OF NUCLEAR WASTE
Temporary Storage and Radioactive Contamination

Residue from weapons production. Most U.S. nuclear weapons plants, such as Rocky Flats, Colorado, Savannah River, South Carolina, Fernald, Ohio, and Hanford, Washington, have released large amounts of radioactive materials into the environment, both on-site and off-site, as a consequence of cold war production pressures. The 570-square-mile Hanford site is probably the most contaminated area of them all. Makhijani and colleagues[35] (Table 6.4) present estimates of radioactive and chemical hazardous substances released into the air and the soil, as well as into the Columbia River and into underground aquifers. Massive unavoidable and intentional releases of airborne radioactive materials such as iodine-131 and other radioisotopes have long been suspected by Hanford "downwinders" to be associated with clusters of serious illness, including thyroid disease, cancers, miscarriages, impaired immune response, and long-term illnesses of the central nervous system.[15,17,19,25] This spectrum of ailments shows remarkable similarity to that suspected to be associated with contamination by fallout from atmospheric nuclear explosions, as described earlier.

Radioactivity, released into the Columbia River and at first diluted by its large volume of flow, was found to be unexpectedly reconcentrated in fish and shellfish, a primary staple for many people living along the river, particularly for Native Americans. By 1947, radioisotope concentrations in fish tissue and in oysters harvested hundreds of miles down river, past the mouth of the Columbia in Willapa Bay, had reached values more than 100,000 times those in river water.[80] Yet, all aquatic studies by Hanford biologists had been classified as secret, and until very recently, the public has never been informed about possible health hazards from these releases.

At Hanford alone, about 68 million gallons of high-level radioactive waste, containing 374 million curies, is stored in 177 tanks, of which 68 have been identified as leaking or potentially leaking into the ground, with some radioactive plumes seeping steadily toward the Columbia River. About 40 of the tanks present a risk of fire or explosion due to incomplete knowledge of the mix of organic and inorganic chemicals, including hydrogen gas.[35]

Spent fuel from civilian nuclear power plants. A nuclear reactor that generates 1000 MW electric power requires about 30 tons of nuclear fuel (uranium enriched to about 3% U-235, packaged in 12-foot by ½-inch steel alloy rods) each year. For the production of this fuel, more than 200 tons of relatively low-level radioactive waste (tailings, retaining about 85% of its original radioactivity) were generated during mining and enrichment operations.[35] This waste must be kept isolated from people and their water supplies. At the power plant, after a normal "burnup" cycle (fissioning of U-235), about 30 tons of spent fuel, containing about 18 million curies of radioactivity, must be removed each year from the reactor. At that level of specific activity (300 Ci/b), heat production remains so high that the spent fuel rods must be cooled for decades to prevent rupture. Since even after decades of planning and the expenditure of many billions of dollars in public funds, there is no permanent repository for high-level waste in place, power companies had to build large storage pools next to the reactors on their terrain for temporary storage. At several plants, these pools are already filled to capacity, and some present an environmental hazard since they are vulnerable to earthquake damage, corrosion, or both.

Decommissioning and transportation After about 25 to 30 years of operation, nuclear power reactors must be decommissioned. Besides the spent fuel, highly radioactive parts of the plant such as reactor vessels, steam generators, and tons of other heavily contaminated equipment must be safely stored. There are grave concerns about safety in transportation over public roads or waterways across hundreds of miles. Permanent disposition of these wastes and the spent fuel remains an unsolved problem of public safety.

Permanent Radioactive Waste Repository

The U.S. Department of Energy, guided by political expediency rather than sound scientific evaluation, has focused its attention for a permanent repository of high-level nuclear wastes on a controversial site in a politically weak state, Nevada.[86] The site is known as Yucca Mountain, not very far from the nuclear test site. High-level waste, much of it with very long half-lives (see Table 59-1), must be kept isolated from the biosphere for near-geologic time periods. If geologic stability would have been given top priority over other concerns for site selection, the granite deposits along the Atlantic coast of the United States would have had to be considered as serious alternatives. In the area of Yucca Mountain, however, geologists have identified 32 active faults at the repository site and concluded that volcanic and tectonic activity could endanger the integrity of the repository long before its radioactivity would have decayed.[11]

The bottom line of the nuclear waste dilemma is that there is no proven solution for the safe, long-term management of vast amounts of long-lived radioactive waste.[35]

FOOD IRRADIATION

In a text on toxicology, it is appropriate to include one particular industrial application of relatively small quantities of nuclear waste materials for the purpose of increasing the shelf life of food by sterilization from very-high-dose irradiation. High doses of radiation, used to kill microorganisms, also affect various vitamins. Moreover, with very high doses of ionizing radiation, complex radiolytic processes take place, such as the production of highly reactive oxygen free radicals, together with the formation of toxic hydrogen peroxide in all foods that contain water. Neither the overall nutritional quality of irradiated food nor the possible toxicity of even small concentrations of radiolytic contaminants has been sufficiently investigated to support claims of safety.[89]

CONCLUSION

While the nuclear nations have taken great pains to do most of their aboveground and underground nuclear testing far away from their own population centers—usually at the expense of indigenous or "low use" populations elsewhere—this chapter shows clearly that the health risks to both nuclear workers and to the general public at home are much larger than most official publications have led the medical profession and guardians of public health to believe.

Future generations will undoubtedly ask, "What did the experts at the end of the twentieth century know about the toxicity of ionizing radiation and, especially, of the health risks from low-level radioactive contamination of the environment?" Future historians may look into this handbook for answers. If health authorities do not step in energetically to educate the public and the lawmakers, these historians will have cause to wonder out loud, "That much was known and so little was done to protect the people and to preserve a healthy environment for posterity?"

REFERENCES

1. Altherr MR et al: Molecular confirmation of Wolf-Hirschhorn syndrome with a subtle translocation of chromosome 4, *Am J Hum Genet* 49:1235, 1991.

2. Archer VE: Association of nuclear fallout with leukemia in the United States, *Arch Environ Health* 42:263, 1987.

3. Averkin JI, Abelin T, Bleuer JP: Thyroid cancer in children in Belarus: ascertainment bias? *Lancet* 346:1223, 1995.

4. Band PR et al: Mortality and cancer incidence in a cohort of commercial airline pilots, *Aviat Space Environ Med* 61:299, 1990.

5. Barish RJ: Health physics concerns in commercial aviation, *Health Phys* 59:199, 1990.

6. Bauchinger M et al: Time-effect relationship of chromosome aberrations in peripheral lymphocytes after radiation therapy for seminoma, *Mutat Res* 211:265, 1989.

7. BEIR V, National Research Council: *Health effects of exposure to low levels of ionizing radiation,* Washington, DC, 1990, National Academy Press.

8. Bertell R: Internal bone-seeking radionuclides and monocyte counts, *Int Perspect Publ Health* 9:21, 1993.

9. Bertell R, Calloyannis B: *Health problems of Rongelap people. A report to Congress,* Toronto, 1989, International Institute of Concern for Public Health.

10. Bithell JF, Stiller CA: A new calculation of the radiogenic risk of obstetric X-raying, *Stat Med* 7:857, 1988.

11. Broad WJ: A mountain of trouble, *New York Times Magazine* November 18, 1990.

12. Bross ID, Bross NS: Do atomic veterans have excess cancer? New results correcting for the healthy soldier bias, *Am J Epidemiol* 126:1042, 1986.

13. Caldwell GG, Kelley DB, Heath CW: Leukemia among participants in military maneuvers at a nuclear bomb test, *JAMA* 244:1575, 1980.

14. Cardis E et al: Direct estimates of cancer mortality due to low doses of ionising radiation; an international study, *Lancet* 344: 1039, 1994.

15. Caufield C: *Multiple exposures,* Chicago, 1990, University of Chicago Press.

16. Clapp RW et al: Leukaemia near Massachusetts nuclear power plant, *Lancet* 5:1324-1325, 1987.

17. D'Antonio M: *Atomic harvest,* New York, 1993, Crown.

18. Darby SC, Doll R: Radiation and exposure rate, *Nature* 344:824, 1990.

19. Del Tredici R: *At work in the fields of the bomb,* New York, 1987, Harper & Row.

20. Dobson RL et al: Biological effectiveness of neutrons from Hiroshima bomb replica: results of a collaborative cytogenetic study, *Radiat Res* 128:143, 1991.

21. Dohy H et al: Cancer incidence in atomic bomb survivors, *Radiat Res* 137(2 suppl):1, 1994.

22. Edwards M: Chernobyl, *National Geographic* 186:70, 1994.

23. Emerit I et al: Transferable clastogenic activity in plasma from persons exposed as salvage personnel of the Chernobyl reactor, *J Cancer Res Clin Oncol* 120:558, 1994.

24. Friedberg W et al: Galactic cosmic radiation exposure and associated health risk for air carrier crew members, *Aviat Space Environ Med* 60:1004, 1989.

25. Gallagher C: *American ground zero,* Cambridge, Mass, 1993, MIT Press.

26. Gardner MJ: Father's occupational exposure to radiation and the raised level of childhood leukemia near Sellafield nuclear plant, *Environ Health Perspect* 94:5, 1991.

27. Geiger HJ et al: *Dead reckoning: a critical review of the Department of Energy's epidemiological research,* Washington, DC, 1992, Physicians for Social Responsibility.

28. Gofman JW: *Preventing breast cancer: the story of a major, proven, preventable cause of this disease,* ed 2, San Francisco, 1996, Committee for Nuclear Responsibility.

29. Gofman JW: *Radiation and human health,* New York, 1983, Pantheon Books.

30. Gofman JW: Radiation-induced cancer from low-dose exposure: an independent analysis, San Francisco, 1990, Committee for Nuclear Responsibility.

31. Gofman JW: *Radiation-inducible chromosome injuries,* San Francisco, 1992, Committee for Nuclear Responsibility.

32. Institute for Energy and Environmental Research: *Science for democratic action* 4:7, 1995.

33. International Commission on Radiological Protection: *Recommendations of the ICRP,* Oxford, 1991, Pergamon.

34. International Physicians for the Prevention of Nuclear War (IPPNW): *Radioactive heaven and earth,* New York, 1991, Apex Press.

35. International Physicians for the Prevention of Nuclear War and Institute for Energy and Environmental Research; Makhijani A, Hu H, Yih K, editors: *Nuclear wastelands: nuclear weapons production worldwide and its environmental and health consequences,* Cambridge, Mass, 1995, MIT Press.

36. Kahn P: A grisly archive of key cancer data, *Science* 259: 448, 1993.

37. Kazakov VS, Demidchik EP, Astakhova LN: Thyroid cancer after Chernobyl, *Nature* 359:21, 1992.

38. Kerber R: A cohort study of thyroid disease in relation to fallout from nuclear weapons testing, *JAMA* 270:2076, 1993.

39. Kneale GW, Stewart AM: Factors affecting recognition of cancer risks of nuclear workers, *Occup Environ Med* 52:515, 1995.

40. Knox EG et al: Background radiation and childhood cancer, *J Soc Radiol Prot (GB)* 8:9, 1988.

41. Knox EG et al: Prenatal irradiation and childhood cancer, *J Soc Radiol Prot (GB)* 7:3, 1987.

42. Kordysh EA et al: Health effects in a casual sample of immigrants to Israel from areas contaminated by the Chernobyl explosion, *Environ Health Perspect* 103:936, 1995.

43. Krain LS: Aviation, high altitude, cumulative radiation exposure and their association with cancer, *Med Hypotheses* 34:33, 1991.

44. Kusano N: *Atomic bomb injuries,* Tokyo, 1995, Tsukiji Shokan.

45. Lloyd DC et al: Chromosomal aberrations in human lymphocytes induced *in vitro* by very low doses of X-rays, *Int J Radiat Oncol Biol Phys* 61:335, 1992.

46. Loken MK: Physician's obligations in radiation issues, *JAMA* 258:673, 1987.

47. Lubin JH et al: Lung cancer in radon-exposed miners and estimation of risk from indoor exposure, *J Natl Cancer Inst* 87:817, 1995.

48. Manning M: Atomic vets battle time, *Bull Atomic Scientists* 51:54, 1995.

49. McRae C: Comments on "Cancer mortality near Oak Ridge, TN" and response (Mangano JJ), *Int J Health Serv* 25:333, 1995.

50. Messing K et al: Mutant frequency of radiotherapy technicians appears to be associated with recent dose of ionizing radiation, *Health Phys* 57:537, 1989.

51. Messing K, Seifert AM, Bradley WEC: In vivo mutant frequency among technicians professionally exposed to ionizing radiation. In Sorsa M, Norppa H, editors: *Monitoring of occupational genotoxicants,* New York, 1986, Alan R Liss.

52. Modan B et al: Increased risk of breast cancer after low-dose irradiation, *Lancet* 8639:629, 1989.

53. Morgan KZ: ICRP risk estimates: an alternative view. In Jones RR, Southwood R, editors: *Radiation and health: the biological effects of low-level exposure to ionizing radiation,* Chichester, Engl, 1987, John Wiley.

54. Muirhead CR, Kneale GW: Prenatal irradiation and childhood cancer, *J Radiol Prot* 9:209, 1989.

55. Musolino SV et al: Comments on "Breast cancer: evidence for a relation to fission products in the diet" and response (Sternglass EJ, Gould JM), *Int J Health Serv* 25:475, 1995.

56. Nussbaum RH, Köhnlein W: Inconsistencies and open questions regarding low-dose health effects of ionizing radiation, *Environ Health Perspect* 102:656, 1994.

57. Nussbaum RH, Köhnlein W: Health consequences of exposures to ionizing radiation from external and internal sources: challenges to

radiation protection standards and biomedical research, *Medicine & Global Survival* 2:158, 1995.

58. Ogunranti JO: Haematological indices in Nigerians exposed to radioactive waste, *Lancet* 1:667, 1989.

59. Paretzke HG, Heinrich W: Radiation exposure and radiation risk in civil aircraft, *Radiat Prot Dosim* 48:33, 1993.

60. Pritikin TT: Hanford: where traditional common law fails, *Gonzaga Law Rev* 30:523, 1994/95.

61. Pukkala E, Auvinen A, Wahlberg G: Incidence of cancer among Finnish airline cabin attendants, 1967-92, *BMJ* 311:649, 1995.

62. Robinette C, Jablon S, Preston T: *Mortality of nuclear weapons test participants. National Research Council,* Washington, DC, 1985, National Academy Press.

63. Rojas-Burke J: Oak Ridge cancer findings hotly debated, *J Nucl Med* 32:11N, 1991.

64. Roman E et al: Childhood leukemia in West-Berkshire, Basingstoke and North Hampshire district health authorities in relation to nuclear establishments in the vicinity, *BMJ* 294:597, 1987.

65. Rooney C et al: Case-control study of prostatic cancer in employees of the United Kingdom Atomic Energy Authority, *BMJ* 307:1391, 1993.

66. Salomon F, Marston RQ: *The medical consequences of nuclear war,* Washington, DC, 1986, National Academy Press.

67. Schalch D, Scharmann A: Strahlenexposition in Verkehrsflugzeugen, *Naturwissenschaftliche Rundschau* 46:348, 1993.

68. Scheid W et al: Biological and physical dosimetry after chronic occupational exposure to ionizing radiation: a comparative study, *Stud Biophys* 138:205, 1990.

69. Scheid W, Weber J, Traut H: Chromosome aberrations induced in the lymphocytes of pilots and stewardesses, *Naturwissenschaften* 80:528, 1993.

70. Schmitz-Feuerhake I et al: *Leukemia in the proximity of a German boiling water reactor.* Proceedings of the 10th International Congress of Radiation Research, Würzburg, 1995.

71. Schneider K: A valley of death for the Navajo uranium miners, *New York Times,* May 3, 1993.

72. Sevc J et al: A survey of the Czechoslovak follow-up of lung cancer mortality in uranium miners, *Health Phys* 64:355, 1993.

73. Sever LE: Parental radiation exposure and children's health: are there effects on the second generation? *Occup Med* 6:613, 1991.

74. Shapiro J: *Radiation protection,* Cambridge, Mass, 1990, Harvard University Press.

75. Shields LM et al: Navajo birth outcomes in the shiprock uranium mining areas, *Health Phys* 63:542, 1992.

76. Smith RJ: Study of atomic veterans fuels controversy, *Science* 221:733, 1983.

77. Sperling K et al: Bewertung eines Trisomie 21 Clusters, *Med Genetik* 6:378, 1994.

78. Sperling K et al: Frequency of Trisomy-21 in Germany before and after the Chernobyl accident, *Biomed Pharmacother* 45:255, 1991.

79. Sperling K et al: Significant increase in trisomy-21 in Berlin nine months after the Chernobyl reactor accident: temporal or causal relation? *BMJ* 309:158, 1994.

80. Stenehjem M: Indecent exposure, *Natural History* 9:6, 1990.

81. Stevens W et al: Leukemia in Utah and radioactive fallout from the Nevada test site: a case-control study, *JAMA* 264:585, 1990.

82. Stewart AM, Kneale GW: A-bomb survivors: further evidence of late effects of early deaths, *Health Phys* 64:467, 1993.

83. Stewart AM, Kneale GW: Acute injuries of A-bomb survivors: their epidemiological importance (in press).

84. Stsjazhko VA et al: Childhood thyroid cancer since accident at Chernobyl, *BMJ* 310:801, 1995.

85. Technical Steering Panel: *Summary: radiation dose estimates from Hanford radioactive material releases to the air and the Columbia River,* Olympia, Wash, 1994, 98504-7651: Nuclear Waste Program, Department of Ecology.

86. U S Department of Energy: *Closing the circle on the splitting of the atom,* Washington, DC, 1995, Office of Environmental Management, Department of Energy.

87. United Nations Scientific Committee on the Effects of Atomic Radiation: *Sources, effects and risks of ionizing radiation,* New York, 1994, United Nations.

88. Wang JX et al: Cancer incidence among medical diagnostic x-ray workers in China, 1950 to 1985, *Int J Cancer* 45:889, 1990.

89. Webb T, Lang T, Tucker K: Food irradiation: who wants it? Rochester, Vt, 1987, Thorsons Publishers.

90. Weber J, Scheid W, Traut H: Biological dosimetry after extensive diagnostic x-ray exposure, *Health Phys* 68:266, 1995.

91. Wilkinson GS, Dreyer NA: Leukemia among nuclear workers with protracted exposure to low-dose ionizing radiation, *Epidemiology* 2:305, 1991.

92. Yoshimaru H et al: Further observations on abnormal brain development caused by prenatal A-bomb exposure to ionizing radiation, *Int J Radiat Biol* 67:359, 1995.

60

nonionizing radiation wave

- The dose of nonionizing radiation is not cumulative, in contrast to that of ionizing radiation

- Ultraviolet radiation exposure results in skin cancer, which is largely preventable

- Snowblindness can result from exposure to a combination of VLR and UVR radiation

- Inhalational exposure to the laser "plume" can pose a health hazard to health care personnel who work with lasers

Nonionizing Radiation

Scott D. Phillips

Nonionizing forms of radiation are those with wavelengths longer than ionizing radiation. There is an inverse relationship between wavelength and energy value. The longer the radiation wavelength, the less the energy emitted. The order of decreasing energy is ultraviolet radiation (UV), visible light, infrared radiation, microwave radiation, and radiofrequency radiation (Table 60-1). The term *ionization* refers to the energetic removal or addition of electrons from the outer shells of atoms that could lead to the production of ions. In the past, nonionizing radiation (NIR) was considered too weak to result in the formation of ions that could induce adverse health effects, unless physical heating occurred. The ability to produce ionization in tissues requires approximately 10 to 12 electron volts (eV). This may result in alterations of nucleic acids, which is responsible for radiation sickness. The energy of radiofrequencies in the 1 MHz range is approximately 3 billion times too weak to result in tissue ionization. As one ascends on the energy scale of NIR, microwave radiation (MWR) is only about one ten-thousandth of the energy needed to cause ionization in tissues. The biologic effect of NIR is a function of type of radiation, dose (duration and intensity), and absorption. The dose of NIR is not cumulative, in contrast to that of ionizing radiation.

The environment may alter many forms of NIR. For example, as ultraviolet light enters the upper atmosphere and is absorbed by ozone. Infrared radiation (IFR) and MWR are absorbed by water vapor. Particulates and gases in the atmosphere may also affect the availability of a particular type of radiation on an organism.

Table 60-1 Nonionizing radiation characteristics

Type of radiation	Energy range	Frequency range	Wavelength range
Ionizing	>12.4 eV	>3000 THz	<100 nm
Ultraviolet	6.2-3.1 eV	1500-750 THz	200-400 nm
Visible	3.1-1.8 eV	750-429 THz	400-700 nm
Violet			400-424
Blue			424-491
Green			491-575
Yellow			575-585
Orange			585-647
Red			647-700
Infrared	1.8 eV-1.2 meV	429 THz-300 GHz	700 nm-1 mm
Microwave	1.2 meV-1.2 μeV	300 GHz-300 MHz	1 mm-1 m
Radiofrequency	1.2 μeV-1.2 neV	300 MHz-300 kHz	1 m-1 km

Modified from NIOSH Technical Report: *Ionizing radiation,* NIOSH Publ No 78-142, Washington, DC, 1978, National Institute of Occupational Safety and Health.

MICROWAVE RADIATION

The biologic effect of MWR on organisms is a function of the water content, vascularity, and dielectric properties of tissues. Microwave energy converts into thermal energy during absorption by the tissues. It is the production of heat that results in tissue damage. There is nonuniform heat production following significant exposures. This is due to the density differences between tissues, such as bone versus muscle. The rate at which energy absorbs is the specific absorption rate (SAR). The unit of measure for the SAR is watts per kilogram. With these units, different substances and tissues can be categorized. Ten mW/cm^2 of energy increase body temperature 1°C. The body absorbs approximately 60 watts of energy. This is an acceptable temperature elevation. The normal resting basal metabolism results in 1 to 1.3 watts/kg.[7] Two factors determine thermal dose: the peak tissue temperature and the duration that temperature is maintained.[4] The body's own thermoregulatory mechanisms modulate the increase.

The penetration of MWRs increases with the length of microwave (Table 60-2). There are four general MWR bands (Table 60-3). These wavelengths range from television to cloud detection radar frequencies. There is overlap between these long wave forms of MWR and radiofrequency radiation (RFR) energy. The health effects tend to be similar. There are several known bioeffects reported from MWR[1,9,10] (see box on p. 533).

INFRARED RADIATION

Any source of heat yields infrared radiation (IRR). Sources of industrial production include power generation plants, foundries, and traffic. Certain occupations, including users of industrial or medical lasers, steelworkers, steam generation plant workers, and bakers, place people at risk to greater amounts of IRR.

Table 60-2 Microwave penetration into tissues

Band	Wavelength	Penetration
Super high frequency	<0.03 m	Epidermis
Super high frequency and ultra high frequency	0.03-0.1 m	Subcutaneous
Ultra high frequency and very high frequency	0.25-2 m	Through body

Table 60-3 Common uses of typical microwave frequencies

Uses	Wavelength	Frequency	Band
Television	10-1 m	30-300 MHz	Very high frequency (VHF)
Microwave ovens	1-0.1 m	0.3-3 GHz	Ultra high frequency (UHF)
Communications	10-0.01 m	3-30 GHz	Super high frequency (SHF)
Weather radar	0.01-0.001 m	30-300 GHz	Extra high frequency (EHF)

Infrared radiation is in the wavelength between 700 nm and 1 mm. This form of energy does not penetrate beneath the epidermis. It can result in acute thermal skin burns and alter pigmentation. Infrared radiation has three wavelength spectra. Infrared-C has the longest wavelength, and IR-A has the shortest (Table 60-4).

Some of the shorter forms of IRR are implicated in "glass blowers' cataract." In this instance, heat transfers from the

Animal and Human Physiologic Effects of Microwave Radiation	
Behavioral	Developmental
Cardiovascular	Environmental
Cataracts (human)	Genotoxic
Central nervous system	Hematologic
Circadian rhythms	Metabolic

Table 60-4 Infrared wavelengths; IR-A is nearest to the visible spectrum

Radiation form	Wavelength
Infrared	700 nm-1 mm
IR-A	1.4 μm-760 nm
IR-B	3-1.4 μm
IR-C	1 mm-3 μm
Ultraviolet	200-400 nm
UV-A	315-400 nm
UV-B	280-315 nm
UV-C	<280 nm

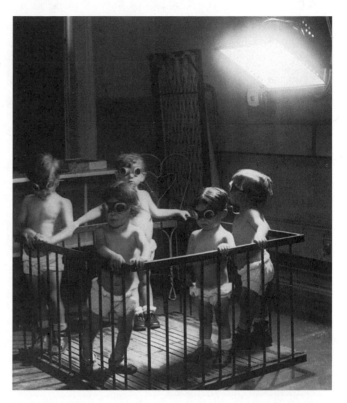

Fig. 60-1. Ultraviolet light treatment. (From Bettman Archive, New York City.)

iris to the lens. This may result in opacification if the amount and duration are sufficient.[8] Other ocular effects include drying of the cornea and potential retinal damage from protein denaturation. Arc welders are another occupation with increased risk of NIR ocular damage. In welders, both IRR and ultraviolet radiation (UVR) may result in ophthalmologic toxicity. Protective goggles prevent these adverse effects. Studies on "incandescent hot bodies" in industry suggest a threshold effect below 8 W-sec/cm^2. Therefore, it is important to limit exposures at or below this area with engineering controls or protective glasses.[12]

VISIBLE LIGHT RADIATION

The human eye is able to detect light between the red and violet spectra (see Table 60-1). The peak sensitivity of the retina is at 555 nm in the green band. Besides environmental sources, pulsed lasers and electronic flashes are sources of visible light radiation (VLR) that may induce retinal injury. Normal exposures to VLR do not result in ocular pathology. However, prolonged exposure by purposeful staring at the sun or "snowblindness" causes ocular injury. The latter is evidenced by scotoma, keratitis, iritis, and photophobia. Snowblindness results from a combination of VLR and UVR.

Overillumination in the visual field (glare), if severe, can cause iritis. This is an important area of concern with the widespread use of video display terminals (VDT). Nuisance glare is economically and socially important because of VDTs. Glare-reducing screen devices are now available to combat this problem. Shielding with screens or appropriate sunglasses is the best preventive measure.

ULTRAVIOLET LIGHT RADIATION

Ultraviolet light radiation exposure is mostly from sunlight but can be from man-made sources. Indoor fluorescent lights emit UV-C inside the tube that then stimulates phosphors to emit white light. Very little UV-C is detectable beyond the bulb. Some industrial processes, including welding, foundry work, and lasers, create UVR.

Nonionizing radiation ranges from 200 nm to 400 nm (see Table 60-1). Within the UVR spectrum, there are three regions, A, B, and C (see Table 60-4). Ultraviolet-A is an important contributor in the formation of cataracts and less with skin effects, while UV-B is responsible for the majority of adverse effects. Ultraviolet-C radiation is germicidal (Fig. 60-1). The use of UV-C as a method of food sterilization is an area of significant social controversy, though scientifically based health risks are lacking.

The major health risk from exposure to UVR is sunburn and carcinogenesis. Other health effects include photosensitization reactions, solar keratosis, wrinkling, and cataracts. The use of tanning beds and increased outdoor activities have led to an epidemic of skin cancers in North America. Ultraviolet exposure increases with closeness to the equator and higher elevation. Squamous cell carcinoma

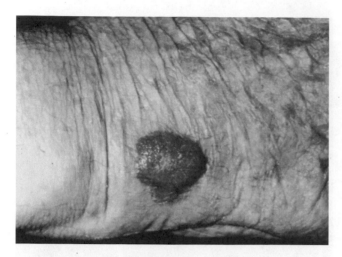

Fig. 60-2. Squamous cell carcinoma arising within sun-damaged skin on the dorsal hand of a farmer. (From Zenz C, Dickerson OB, Horvath EP: *Occupational medicine,* ed 3, St Louis, 1994, Mosby.)

Table 60-5 Health risks of lasers by class: Embedded laser is a class II, III, or IV laser or system that is contained in a protective housing and operated at a lower classification

Laser class	Health risk
I	Cannot emit laser radiation at known hazard levels, typically 0.4 microwatts (μW) at visible wavelengths
II	Low-power visible lasers that emit above class I levels but at radiant power not above 1 mW; the concept is that the human aversion reaction to bright light will protect a person above that
IIIa	Intermediate power lasers (1-5 mW); hazardous only for intrabeam viewing; some limited controls are recommended
IIIb	Moderate-power lasers (5-500 mW, pulsed 10K/cm^2 or diffuse reflection limit, whichever is lower)
IV	High-power lasers (500 mW) are hazardous to view under any conditions

is most closely associated with sun exposure (Fig. 60-2). The association between sun exposure and melanoma is more complex but is increased in those who have had severe sunburns at young ages.

Occupations that result in significant sun exposure include highway workers, agricultural workers, and fishers.

Most adverse effects of UVR on the skin are preventable. Though most of the damage is due to the effects of UV-B, protection against UV-A is probably also important. Several sunscreens with sun protective factors (SPFs) greater than 15 block both UV-A and UV-B. The use of tanning beds or salons should be discouraged by physicians. The avoidance of midday sun helps to prevent the damaging effects of UV-A on the eye. Many glasses have the ability to allow VLR to pass while blocking UVR. Sunglasses should have this same UVR blocking property.

LASERS

The term *laser* stands for *l*ight *a*mplification by *s*timulated *e*missions of *r*adiation. Uses are typically commercial, including medical, welding, photolysis, fiber optics, communications, antipersonnel, range finding, and other military applications. The laser process utilizes the release of photons from atoms whose electrons move to a lower energy level. This results in light scattered emissions. Laser light is the same wavelength in phase (coherence) and plane (collimation). By this "focusing" a single-watt laser can produce 100 million times more irradiance than a 100-watt light bulb.[6]

Lasers are classified into four major groups based on potential health hazards. This classification scheme (Table 60-5) ranges from class I, essentially harmless, to class IV, which is very dangerous and a fire hazard. Laser radiation (LR) may involve several different spectra. Infrared radiation–emitting lasers include neodymium:yttrium and carbon dioxide. Visible light emitters include helium-neon,

dye, and krypton lasers. Excimer lasers emit radiation in the UV range.

The health risks of lasers are mainly to the skin and eye, depending on the type and power of the emitter. Tissue damage that occurs is principally due to thermal injury related to the beam power emitted. In the eye, this focused beam results in retinal photocoagulation and ocular damage. Depending on the intensity of the dose exposure, a variety of ocular injuries occur, including blindness. Lasers used in medicine vaporize tissue, creating smoke that may carry contagious organisms. Papillomavirus in laser smoke may be transmitted to medical caregivers. Protection of workers' and patients' eyes from exposure to certain laser beams is important. With lasers that may vaporize tissue, masks that filter viral and other particles should be worn.

The use of LR as weaponry is typically with very-high-power beam class IV lasers. These can reflect on impact to within several meters of the target. Military uses of lasers include range finders, designators, antimaterial (Star Wars program), and antipersonnel lasers (APL). The latter blind opposing troops. Examples of APLs include the Daser,[3] Cobra,[11] and Dazzle Gun.[2] These weapons result in blindness that is either temporary, to immobilize opposing forces, or permanent.

Eye shielding and appropriate eyewear for caregivers must be available and worn to avoid accidental ocular injury. The recommended use of protective eyeware in medical applications was available since their introduction.[5] Medical laser manufacturers typically supply eyeware. However, buyers must rely on manufacturers to supply the appropriate type. Absorptive types of eyewear are better than reflective protection. Each type of laser has a particular type of protective lens. In some medical applications, eye shields are used to allow the user to align the laser and have unobstructed views during the procedure while being adequately protected. The American National Standards Institute has established guidelines for eye protection (ANSI Z136.1-1986).

REFERENCES

1. Aldrich TE, Easterly CE: Electromagnetic fields and public health, *Environ Health Perspect* 75:159, 1987.
2. Anderberg B, Wolbarsht M: Blinding lasers: the nastiest weapon? *Mil Techn* 1990; 3:58-623.
3. Anderberg B, Wolbarsht M: Hand-held lasers are waiting in the wings, *Armed Forces J Int* 60-1, 1992.
4. Dewhirst MW: Animal modeling and thermal dose, *Radiol Clin North Am* 27:509, 518 1989.
5. Dixon J: *Surgical application of lasers,* Chicago, 1983, Year Book.
6. Elkington AR, Frank HJ: *Clinical optics,* Oxford, 1991, Blackwell Scientific.
7. Gandhi OP: Dosimetry: the absorption properties of man and experimental animals, *Bull N Y Acad Med* 55:1016, 1979.
8. National Institute for Occupational Safety and Health: *Criteria for a recommended standard: occupational exposure to ultraviolet radiation,* Cincinnati, 1972, U S Department of Health, Education, and Welfare, National Institute for Occupational Safety and Health.
9. Peterson RC: Bioeffects of microwaves: a review of current knowledge, *J Occup Med* 25:103, 1983.
10. Polk C, Postow E: *CRC handbook of biological effects of electromagnetic fields, Boca Raton, Fla, 1987, CRC Press.*
11. Tapscott M, Atwal K: New weapons that win without killing on DoD's horizon, *Defense Electron* 41-6, 1993.
12. U S Department of Health, Education, and Welfare: *Research report, determination of ocular threshold levels for infrared radiation cataractogenesis,* DHHS Publ 80-121, Rockville, Md, 1980, National Institute for Occupational Safety and Health.

61

Residential Radon and Lung Cancer

Mark J. Upfal

Christine Johnson

$$Ra^{226} \longrightarrow Rn^{222}$$

radon daughters

- While the pulmonary carcinogenicity of radon is well established in mining studies, there remains scientific uncertainty and public debate about the magnitude of the cancer risk associated with residential exposure

- Many scientists believe that radon may be second only to cigarette smoke as a cause of lung cancer

- Primary prevention through environmental control is believed to be highly effective in reducing ambient exposure to ambient radon

- Radon is associated with lung cancer in underground uranium miners in a dose-dependent fashion

- Radon is derived from the radioactive decay of uranium

Indoor air quality has received considerable public attention in recent years, as the trend toward energy efficiency with "tighter" buildings and lower air exchange rates has contributed to higher levels of indoor air pollution. Among the various air contaminants found in the residential environment, radon may be among the most hazardous as well as the most controversial. While the pulmonary carcinogenicity of radon is well established in mining studies, there remains scientific uncertainty and public debate about the magnitude of the cancer risk associated with residential exposure. Based upon the mining data, many scientists believe that radon may be second only to cigarette smoke as a cause of lung cancer. Primary prevention through environmental control is believed to be highly effective in reducing ambient exposure to ambient radon. The technology for detection and mitigation of elevated radon levels in homes is available and practical, and many scientists believe it to be a cost-effective public health effort. Nonetheless, there is confusion about what level of exposure should require action. This chapter provides a perspective on radon exposure, hazard assessment, health effects, and management.

Radon gas is derived from the radioactive decay of radium, a ubiquitous element found in rock and soil. The decay series begins with uranium-238 and goes through four intermediates to form radium-226, with a half-life of 1600 years. Radium-226 then decays to form radon-222 gas. Radon's half-life, 3.8 days, provides sufficient time for it to diffuse through soil and into homes, where further disintegration produces the more chemically and radiologically active radon progeny (or radon daughters). These include isotopes of lead, polonium, and bismuth with half-lives of less than 30 minutes[3,26]; they are the major source of human exposure to α-radiation (high-energy, high-mass particles, each consisting of two protons and two neutrons). This α-radiation can transform cells in the respiratory tract, resulting in the putative mechanism for the development of radon-induced lung cancer.[58]

HISTORIC PERSPECTIVE

Chronic pulmonary disease among miners has been recognized since at least the beginning of the sixteenth century. In the rich central European ore mines of Schneeberg, Germany and Joachimsthal, Czechoslovakia, middle-aged men wasted away from a lung condition then known as *bergkrankheit* (mountain disease) as these miners extracted copper, iron, silver, cobalt, arsenic, bismuth, nickel, radium, and uranium. By the end of the nineteenth century, and before radon had been discovered by Rutherford, Härting and Hesse reported this condition to be cancer of the lung with an onset after approximately 20 years of mining.[25] In 1913, Arnstein reported on 665 deaths among miners between 1875 and 1912. Of these, 276 (42%) were due to lung cancer, 64 (9.6%) due to tuberculosis, 119 (18%) due to other pulmonary disorders, and 206 (31%) from nonpulmonary etiologies.[6] Later in the twentieth century, radon was associated in a dose-dependent fashion as a cause of lung cancer among these and other underground miners,[34,40] working in a wide variety of settings, including iron, tin, fluorspar, uranium, and gold mines. As various epidemiologic investigations of miners began to demonstrate consistent reports of a dose-dependent association between radon exposure and lung cancer, the National Academy of Sciences examined these studies and issued its BEIR IV Report,[44] which established radon as a cause of lung cancer in the mines and a concern for exposure in the home. Animal investigations provided additional evidence substantiating the carcinogenicity of radon.[13] Most recently, a pooled analysis of 11 underground mining cohort studies confirmed the prior conclusions of the BEIR IV report.[36,37] This analysis of 65,000 men and more than 2700 lung cancer deaths established a consistently linear relative risk of lung cancer associated with radon exposure. The exposure-response trend for miners who never smoked was triple that of the smokers.

Awareness about radon as a potential hazard in the home was heightened in the mid-1980s, when the home of Stanley Watras, a worker at the Limerick nuclear power plant in Pennsylvania, was found to have extraordinarily high levels of radon (2700 pCi/l).[71] Subsequently, studies of the geographic distribution of radon demonstrated levels in many homes that were as high as those known to be carcinogenic from the mining studies.[11,49] On the basis of miner epidemiology and geographic distribution of exposure, the U.S. Environmental Protection Agency initially estimated that 5000 to 20,000 annual lung cancer deaths could be attributed to radon. This has been updated to a point estimate of approximately 14,000 annual radon-induced deaths and is consistent with the recent National Cancer Institute estimate of 10,000 annual lung cancer deaths due to radon among smokers (11% of all lung cancer deaths among smokers) and 5000 among never-smokers (30% of lung cancer deaths among never-smokers).[36]

SOURCES OF RESIDENTIAL RADON EXPOSURE

Imperceptible by odor, taste, and color, radon causes no symptoms of irritation or discomfort. Exposure can be detected only by empirical measurement. Radon seeps from the soil into buildings primarily through sump holes, dirt floors, floor drains, cinder-block walls, and cracks in foundations and concrete floors[70] (Fig. 61-1). When trapped indoors, radon can become concentrated to hazardous levels. However, outdoors, it is diluted to levels that pose relatively little or no health risk.

Radon gas can enter a building by diffusion, but pressure-driven flow is a more important mechanism.[71] Negative pressure in the home relative to the soil may be caused by exhaust fans and by rising warm air created by fireplaces, clothes dryers, and forced-air heating systems. In addition to pressure differences, the type of building foundation (basement versus slab-on-grade) can affect radon entry.

There is considerable regional and local variation in the amount of radon emanating from the earth and concentrating inside homes, with residential levels varying by orders of magnitude. Surveys performed by the U.S. Environmental Protection Agency (EPA) and state programs have found elevated radon levels throughout the United States. In the recent EPA National Residential Radon Survey,[46] the mean household radon level detected was 1.25, with about 6% of American homes exceeding 4 pCi/L. This survey was based upon year-long α-track measurements averaged over several locations in the home. It has been estimated that more than 600,000 homes exceed 10 pCi/L[54] and more than 100,000 homes exceed 20 pCi/L.[21] In Clinton, New Jersey, near a geologic formation high in radium called the Reading Prong, all 105 homes tested were above the action level, and 40 had levels exceeding 200 pCi/L.[71] In the Stanley Watras basement discussed previously, also located on the Reading Prong, levels as high as 2700 pCi/L were detected.[22]

Although the most important determinant is likely to be source strength from the soil,[48] there are many other determinants of indoor radon levels. However, factors such as local geology, building structure, and meteorology alone are inadequate predictors of risk. Currently, the only way to determine indoor radon concentration is by actual measure-

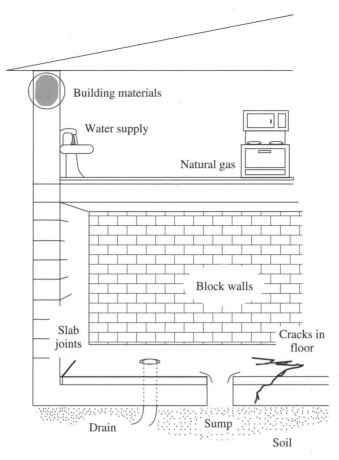

Fig. 61-1 Sources of radon and common entry points. (From Samet JM, editor: *TSDR case studies in environmental medicine,* Atlanta, 1992, US Department of Health and Human Service.)

ment. In a home located nearby the Watras home, measured radon concentrations were at levels considered safe, yet both houses are located on the same geologic formation. Other factors that can affect radon levels include soil porosity, atmospheric pressure, foundation type, building materials used, entry points for soil gas, building ventilation rates, and source of water supply. Ambient levels tend to be highest during the heating season (in temperate climates) and in the basement and lower levels of buildings. Levels above the second floor are generally unlikely to have high levels of radon.

RESPIRATORY DOSE AND UNITS OF MEASURE

Because of their charged state and solid nature, radon progeny rapidly attach to most surfaces they encounter, including walls, floors, and airborne particulates. They can be inhaled either as free, unattached particles or attached to airborne dust. The smaller dust particles can deposit the radon progeny deep in the lungs. The ionized progeny tend to attach to the respiratory epithelium.[19] During subsequent decay, α-emissions may cause respiratory epithelial stem cells to undergo malignant transformation. It is estimated that a lung cancer would result from, on the average, 4×10^9 hits of such cells by α-emissions.

Because radon exposure is imperceptible, and levels cannot be accurately predicted on the basis of geologic, climatic, or architectural factors, measurement is important. However, the ambient radon and radon daughter levels are not the only factors affecting the exposure of an individual. The relationship between measured ambient radon and the dose of α-emissions that reaches target cells in the respiratory tract is complex. Some factors that may influence pulmonary radiation dosimetry include characteristics of the ambient air, the breathing pattern, the volume and flow characteristics of inhalation, lung architecture, and the histobiology of the respiratory tract. Free or unattached radon progeny deposit on the respiratory epithelium more efficiently than progeny attached to dust or other airborne particles and may be more hazardous.[19,23,58] Thus, theoretically, a dusty environment (e.g., a mine) might result in a lower degree of radon dosimetric exposure than a cleaner environment (e.g., a home) with the same ambient radon level. Whether someone is a nasal breather or a mouth breather may affect the proximal filtration of particulates and hence the quantity of radioactive particles depositing on the respiratory tract. The quantity and deposition of inhaled radon decay products vary with the flow rate in each airway segment. Thus, lung architecture, which may be influenced

---

Factors Affecting Respiratory Tract Dose

- Ambient radon gas level
- Characteristics of the inhaled air
- Volume and flow rate of air inhaled
- Breathing pattern
- Architecture of the lungs
- Biologic characteristics of the respiratory tract

---

by age, sex, race, and other determinants of anatomy, can affect dosimetry in ways that are not well understood. Finally, histobiologic characteristics can impact the exposure dose through mechanisms such as mucociliary clearance removing particles from the lower respiratory tract and the mucus layer acting as a shield.

Consequently, two settings with the same measured radon level may result in quite different levels of ambient α-radiation. Likewise, two individuals in the same environment may also experience different exposure doses to the target cells in their respiratory epithelium. Factors affecting respiratory tract dose are highlighted in the box above.

While the concentration of radon progeny may more directly relate to the risk of lung injury, the readily available technology for indoor air measurements usually detects radon gas itself. These measurements are expressed in picocuries per liter (pCi/L) of air, where a picocurie is equivalent to 0.037 becquerels (disintegrations per second).

HEALTH EFFECTS OF RADON

Considerable epidemiologic evidence establishes radon as an occupational lung carcinogen. Although questions remain about the extrapolation of mining data to the general population and about the exact nature of the exposure-response relationship, there is little controversy about whether radon is a carcinogenic agent. An increasing risk of lung cancer with radon dose has been demonstrated repeatedly in a variety of types of underground mines (e.g., gold, tin, uranium, fluorspar) scattered across the globe (including the United States, Canada, South Africa, China, eastern Europe). Despite great differences in these studies, including varying mining conditions with concomitant exposures and the use of various analytic methods and control populations, risk estimates are remarkably consistent. Although most of the miners studied were smokers, radon is considered to have an independent effect. The association between lung cancer and radon exposure among underground miners has even been observed among nonsmoking and light-smoking miners.[56]

At lower exposures, the exposure-risk curve appears linear, but then seems to flatten out at the higher levels of mining exposure.[10] There is limited evidence that, in addition to lung cancer, the frequency of bronchial dysplasia, detectable with sputum cytology, may also be associated with radon exposure in a dose-dependent fashion.[42] The role of genetic susceptibility factors as they interact with radon

exposure is currently of interest but poorly understood. Genetic polymorphisms of susceptibility genes such as glutathione S-transferase (GST) M1 and M3 are currently being examined among lung cancer patients with exposure to pulmonary carcinogens such as tobacco smoke, occupational carcinogens, and radon.[4] Mutations in the p53 tumor suppressor gene have also sparked interest among radon investigators.[64]

The histology of lung cancer has been known to differ between smokers and nonsmokers, with a higher proportion of adenocarcinomas among nonsmokers and increasing proportions among former smokers, rising with the number of years of smoking cessation.[43] Most lung cancers associated with radon are bronchogenic, with all histologic types represented.[24] However, small-cell carcinoma may occur at a higher frequency among both smoking and nonsmoking populations of underground miners than in the general population.[5,14,20]

The effect of risk modifiers such as age, race, sex, exposure duration, latency period, dose rate, and smoking history (discussed later in this chapter) is not well understood. Studies suggest a decreasing relative risk with time since last exposure, as well as an inverse dose-rate effect (lower exposures for a long period of time may be more hazardous than higher but briefer exposures, with cumulative exposure dose being comparable).[29]

Although there have been hypotheses generated regarding an association between radon and cancers other than those of the respiratory tract (e.g., myeloid leukemia,[28] renal cancer, melanoma, and others[7]), there is currently little evidence to establish such a relationship, and there is evidence to suggest the absence of such associations.[15,67] No acute health effects or other chronic health effects, malignant or otherwise, have been established for exposure to radon under usual exposure conditions. Ingestion of radon in contaminated water appears to be of relatively less concern than inhalation exposure.[12,72]

Smoking and Radon as Risk Factors for Lung Cancer

Smoking has been shown to be the predominant cause of lung cancer. In combination with smoking, the risk of radon-induced lung cancer appears to be somewhat higher, and the overall risk of lung cancer (whether radon- or smoking-induced) may be considerably higher. The joint effect based upon recent data analyses is estimated to be more than additive but less than multiplicative. This suggests that prior risk estimates based upon a multiplicative model may have overestimated the risk among smokers and underestimated the risk among nonsmokers.[39] Still, if the joint effect is more than additive, radon would have a more deleterious effect in smokers than in nonsmokers. However, given a joint effect that is less than multiplicative, the carcinogenic effect of radon would be far more difficult to detect in an epidemiologic study that includes smokers than in a study of pure never-smokers (see pp. 543-544).

Age and the sequence of exposure may also influence the joint effect relationship. The multiplicative joint effect model seems to overestimate risk most for middle-aged miners, while it seems to offer a better fit for the youngest and oldest age categories.[60] Recent evidence suggests that exposure to radon that precedes smoking may enhance the joint effect (supramultiplicative), while smoking prior to radon exposure may result in a reduced joint effect (significantly less than multiplicative). This would be consistent with radon acting as the initiator, with cigarette smoking promoting the carcinogenic effect.[66]

Risk Estimates

While risk estimation is an imperfect science, it provides the best method to quantify concerns about radon. Most of what we currently know about the human carcinogenicity and the risk of radon exposure is from mining studies.[37] However, uncertainty regarding the application of this mining data to residential populations results from the many differences between mines and homes, as well as differences between miners and the general public. Despite this uncertainty, the evidence for the carcinogenicity of radon may be stronger than that for many other agents that are accepted as important public health concerns. Levels of radon found in many American homes are as high as those in some of the mines determined to have elevated lung cancer rates. If current estimates are correct, radon may be second only to cigarette smoke as a cause of lung cancer, resulting in an estimated 14,000 (7000 to 30,000) annual deaths in the United States[65] and about 2000 annual deaths in West Germany.[61] While there is some epidemiologic evidence from residential studies to suggest the association of radon with lung cancer, the studies to date have been conflicting and inadequate to accurately quantify risk.* Nonetheless, on the basis of current knowledge, radon has been ranked by the EPA as one of our top priority environmental health problems. The National Cancer Institute,[36] the National Academy of Science (BEIR IV),[44] the National Council on Radiation Protection,[45] and others have independently derived risk estimates similar to those of the EPA. Recent estimates suggest that approximately 11% of all U.S. lung cancer cases among smokers and 30% of cases among never-smokers may be attributed to radon.[36] According to the EPA, the lifetime risk of death to the average American due to radon-induced lung cancer may approximate 1 in 300 (0.3%). At the 4 pCi/L action level, the risk may exceed 1%.[55,70]

Because the prevalence of exposure to radon is so high and because lung cancer mortality is so common (approximately 153,000 annual deaths[18]), even a very small relative risk level (as low as 1.1 to 1.3) would make radon an extremely important public health risk factor (with an attributable risk comparable to a weekly major airliner

crash). However, in addition to the prodigious challenges of detecting small relative risks, the presence of smoking as the primary cause of lung cancer makes the carcinogenic effect of radon remarkably elusive to epidemiologic detection.[69] Unfortunately, negative or conflicting outcomes of studies with inadequate power or design limitations are often misinterpreted by the lay public, the popular media,[32] and even by radon investigators and other scientists as evidence that risk may be minimal or absent, even in the face of human epidemiologic data to the contrary.

Many factors influence the risk of lung cancer due to radon exposure; among these are age, duration of exposure, time since initiation of exposure, and cigarette smoking. In assessing the risk of radon in a home, one must consider not only the level of radon but also the occupants and their lifestyles. Are there any smokers? Are there children? How much time is spent in the home? Where do occupants sleep? The highest radon levels are typically found in basements, where levels may be double or triple the level in the rest of the home. In colder climates, radon levels are often higher in the winter and lower in the summer.

RESIDENTIAL EPIDEMIOLOGY OF RADON AND LUNG CANCER

The establishment of a dose-response relationship between radon in the mines and the recognition of high levels of radon in many homes led to a search for direct evidence linking radon to lung cancer in the residential environment. In consideration of many important differences between exposure in mines and homes (presence of dust and occupational carcinogens such as arsenic and diesel exhaust, activity level of miners, demographic differences, magnitude and duration of radon exposure, and so on), such direct evidence would help reduce uncertainties associated with risk extrapolation. Initially, a number of ecologic investigations were performed with variable results.[50] A review of these studies and an analysis of the limitations of this approach have led to the conclusion that ecologic studies would not have the power to detect the carcinogenic effect of domestic radon and that well-designed case-referent investigations would be required.[38,62,63] Further, even case-control studies may be unenlightening unless they are limited to never-smokers, with large numbers of subjects, or are limited to populations with relatively high levels of exposure.[68]

Recently, a number of case-control investigations have been undertaken, seven of which have been completed to date. However, due to inadequate power and other practical and theoretical limitations, the completed studies do not, individually or in combination, alter existing estimates of the magnitude of the residential carcinogenic effect based on data from mining studies. Regarding those studies currently underway and pending completion, it is unclear whether, alone or in combination, they will have adequate power to detect the estimated carcinogenic effect of radon in the residential environment.

---

* References 1, 9, 33, 52, 59, 69.

To date, approximately 20 studies of domestic radon and lung cancer risk have been initiated; they include more than 12,000 lung cancer cases and 19,000 referents.[51] While these studies may have improved on the earlier ecologically based studies, there is still a paucity of subjects who are neither current nor former smokers (see discussion to follow). Further, accurate assessment of historic exposure remains a major challenge for all investigators. Several retrospective investigations of residential radon exposure among lung cancer cases and referents have been published, with variable outcomes. This section will briefly describe those completed investigations from Shenyang, China[9]; New Jersey[59]; Sweden[52,53]; Winnipeg, Manitoba[33]; and Missouri.[1,2]

The Chinese study[9] examined 308 female cancer registry cases (185 smokers) and 362 controls in an area of China with "exceptionally high rates of lung cancer among women." Radon was measured with year-long α-track detectors. Radon levels, however, were not particularly elevated, with a median exposure of 2.3 pCi/l and only 20.1% of the levels above 4 pCi/l. One might predict that the predominance of background cases of lung cancer would not likely be due to radon in an area with such a high rate of disease and without unusually high levels of exposure. Indoor benzo[a]pyrene and particulate levels were found to be very high in this community, due to the prevalent use of woodburning stoves. Background cases of lung cancer that might have been caused by such pollutants or other risk factors in this community would obscure the ability of a case-control study to detect a carcinogenic effect of radon (unless the joint effect of radon and these factors is multiplicative). Not surprisingly, no association was found between radon and lung cancer, and there were no significant trends within subcategories of smoking or histologic type.

A positive trend was detected by the New Jersey investigation of 433 female lung cancer cases and 402 controls.[59] However, this was driven by very small numbers in the highest exposure category. This trend was strongest for light smokers. There was no trend for nonsmokers, although few nonsmokers were represented. Exposure covered an average of 21 years during the prior 5 to 30 years and was detected by 1-year α-track measurements. Radon exposure was generally low in this population, with a median of 0.6 pCi/L, and only 1% of the measurements above 4 pCi/L.

The Swedish National study of 1360 cases and 2847 controls detected a positive trend in its overall analysis, with a similar trend within smoking and histologic subcategories.[52] Compared with exposures below 1.4 pCi/L, a relative risk of 1.3 was found for exposures between 3.8 and 10.8 pCi/L, and a relative risk of 1.8 was determined for higher exposures. These results were considered to be consistent with the risk projections of the mining studies. Two separate control groups were used and yielded similar results. Only 10% of the cases were alive at the time of interview, with the remainder of the survey data collected by proxy. Two control groups were used, one matched on age and the other matched on both age and vital status. Radon was measured with α-track detectors for 3 months during the heating season, representing an average of 23 years of exposure, with a mean level of 2.9 pCi/L and 25% of the measurements exceeding 3.1 pCi/L. Theoretically, the impact of using 3-month heating season measurements would be to overestimate radon exposures (and thus underestimate the carcinogenic effect of radon).

A positive trend was also detected in the Stockholm, Sweden, study of 210 cases and 400 controls, but this trend did not persist when exposure was weighted.[53] The greatest effect was seen in nonsmokers and for small-cell and squamous cell carcinoma. One year α-track measurements covered an average of 26 years of exposure, with mean radon levels of 3.5 pCi/L and 28% of the measurements above 4.1 pCi/L.

No association between radon exposure and lung cancer was found in the Winnipeg, Manitoba, study, either in the overall analysis or in the subcategory analyses.[33,35] Histologically confirmed incident cases ($n = 738$) from the Winnipeg cancer registry were 1:1 matched on age and sex with controls randomly selected from the telephone directory. Cases and controls differed significantly in education, ethnicity, and smoking status. Interviews were performed by proxy for 35% of the cases and 11% of the controls. Mobility was relatively high, with an average of 9 homes per subject, 5 of which were in Winnipeg. Only about 61% of eligible homes and 34% of occupied homes were measured with 1 year of α-track detection. The mean radon level in the occupied areas of the homes was 3.2 pCi/L, with 25% of the measurements above 4 pCi/L. An increase in relative risk for lung cancer due to exposure was not detected for any histologic type of lung cancer after adjusting for smoking and education. The odds ratio for ever versus never smoking was 12.8 in this study.

The Missouri study examined 538 nonsmoking white women and 1183 controls, but the definition of nonsmoker included ex-smokers.[1,2] The mean of the exposures assessed with year-long α-track devices was 1.8 pCi/L, with under 7% of the measurements above 4 pCi/L. An average of about 20 years of residence during the period of 5 to 30 years prior to diagnosis or enrollment was accounted for by the measurements. Due to mortality of the cases, about two thirds were interviewed by proxy, while controls were all alive and personally interviewed. About half of the lung cancer cases were histologically confirmed. There was little evidence of an association between radon and lung cancer for all of the data combined, although there was a suggestive trend for adenocarcinoma among women personally interviewed. Those with "in person" interviews demonstrated increased risk in the highest exposure category, a significant dose-response trend with categoric analysis, and a near-significant dose-response trend with continuous analysis. The most potent risk factor in this study, as expected, was prior history of smoking. Additionally, saturated fat intake, nonmalignant lung disease, environmental tobacco smoke (ETS), and occupational exposure were identified as risk factors associated with lung cancer. Adjustment for ETS exposure did not significantly alter the risk estimates for radon.

A combined analysis of three of the completed studies (Stockholm, New Jersey, and Shenyang) was unrevealing, consistent both with the risk projections of the mining studies and with the null hypothesis. Additional case-control investigations of residential radon and lung cancer are currently underway worldwide, with results expected in the next few years. Attempts are being made to standardize some of the data collection methodology and to organize combined analyses of the data generated. Despite the large numbers of subjects that such combined analyses would provide, however, it remains unclear whether these studies will have the power to add to our knowledge of radon and lung cancer beyond what we already know based upon the mining studies. Some of the major challenges faced by all such investigations include problems associated with tracking and full participation of subjects and current occupants of residences, accurate recreation of historic exposure profiles, the inclusion of smokers or former smokers, selection of a region with relatively high radon exposures, and choice of an adequate control group.

Although the sample size is quite small, a recent observation from Ulmhausen, Austria, may be of interest.[16] This town is divided between east and west, with a heavily fractured granite gneiss geologic formation causing high radon levels (up to 7400 pCi/L) on the east side. During a recent 10-year period, the east side, with a median indoor radon concentration of 50.5 pCi/L and a population of 1000, experienced 24 cases of lung cancer, while there were only 5 cases in the west side of town, with a median radon concentration of 4.9 and a population of 1600. This results in an odds ratio of 7.7 for those who live in the east side of town.

Recreating Historic Exposure Profiles

Currently, the gold standard for exposure assessment is a year-long α-track measurement performed in all of the homes inhabited by the subject during a period 5 to 30 years prior to lung cancer diagnosis or enrollment as a control. Inherent is the assumption that the homes have not changed significantly over the years and that radon exposure measurements performed at the time of the study and in the location that the samplers are placed would represent the subject's actual exposure history. However, such assumptions are somewhat tenuous. Architectural changes in homes; settling and cracking of foundations; changes in home occupancy and use patterns; differences in the current occupants' use of heating and air conditioning systems, windows, and doors; the trend toward energy-efficient tightening of homes in recent years; and many other factors may affect radon levels. Limited subject recall of their prior

residences and where they spent their time compounds these problems of exposure assessment. Even if there were no measurement error and results were actually representative of exposure in the locations where the α-track devices were installed, it would be nearly impossible for the investigator to adequately account for radon exposure levels when the subject was not present in these specific locations. Even with full identification of prior residences, with 100% participation and measurement of these prior homes, the best any investigator could hope for is a relative and crude assessment of exposure.

In addition to using α-track measurements, some investigators are currently experimenting with biologic monitoring of subjects[31] and the use of heirloom glass or porcelain objects that may act as dosimeters of exposure during the life of the object.[41] Biologic monitoring is based on the formation of lead-210 as radon decays. This radioisotope deposits in bone, with a half-time on the order of 10 or 20 years. Gamma emissions from this isotope can then be detected with extremely sensitive detectors surrounding the subject's head. While this method may account for complete time-weighted-average exposures independent of where the subject spent his or her time and would remedy the problems associated with current measurements in homes, the method has its own limitations. Sensitivity of the technique for residential subjects with average or lower than average radon exposures may need to be further developed prior to broader epidemiologic application of the method. Due to the characteristics of logarithmic decay, high-level exposure in the distant past may not be adequately distinguished from lower-level exposure in the recent past. The investigator must be careful to consider and account for other sources of lead-210 (including diet).

Heirloom objects, such as a picture frame kept in the subject's bedroom for the prior 30 years, provide the potential for serving as integrated sampling devices, accumulating long half-time α-emitting radon decay products, which become embedded into the glass. However, the inconsistent availability of such objects among subjects, combined with technical challenges in using them for measurement limits their utility. Further, the problem of using a stationary sampling device as a surrogate for a mobile human's exposure is similar to the α-track device.

Including Smokers and Former Smokers in Case-Control Studies of Radon

Because of the prevalence of both radon exposure and lung cancer, a very small relative risk (on the order of 1.1 to 1.3) results in a very high attributable risk, posing a major epidemiologic dilemma. Compounding this problem is that of the currently unknown joint effect of radon and smoking. The best evidence suggests that the joint effect lies somewhere between additive and multiplicative. While the carcinogenicity of radon would thus be greater among smokers, detecting it would be much more difficult. As a simplistic example, suppose radon has a relative risk of 1.2 among nonsmokers, and smoking has a relative risk of 10. If the joint effect of the two risk factors were multiplicative, then the overall relative risk of an exposed smoker (compared with the unexposed nonsmoker) would be 12. In a case-control study of smokers alone, the relative risk to be detected would be the risk of the exposed smoker compared with that of the unexposed smoker (12 vs. 10). This would be the same as the relative risk one would need to detect in a case control study limited to nonsmokers (1.2).

Then again, if the joint effect were additive, the exposed smoker would have a risk of 10.2 compared with the unexposed nonsmoker. A study limited to smokers would need to detect a relative risk of 10.2 to 10, or 1.02. One can readily appreciate that if the joint effect is much below multiplicative, it may be extremely difficult to detect the effect of radon in a case-control study that is predominantly composed of smokers. Further, because the cancer risk of a former smoker may be closer to that of a smoker than a nonsmoker, including ex-smokers in a case-control study would create the same difficulty. As noted previously, detecting the effect of radon epidemiologically would be difficult enough without this added complexity. Because most studies are heavily represented by smokers, it is currently unclear that we will ever answer the controversy about residential radon with our current investigations.

Conclusions About the Carcinogenicity of Radon

Although there are uncertainties associated with extrapolating from mines to homes, the data are currently stronger for associating residential radon with cancer than most other well-established human environmental hazards. There is extensive human epidemiologic evidence, as well as animal studies that corroborate the findings. Risk is demonstrated in a linear dose-dependent fashion fairly consistently in a wide variety of studies scattered across the globe. Residential exposures are not much lower than those that are carcinogenic in occupational studies, and in many homes exposures are as high. However, asbestos has generated considerable controversy and concern for exposure at levels that are many orders of magnitude below those known to be carcinogenic in occupational cohorts. Dioxin, an agent for which most putative risks are currently speculative, generates even greater public concern. Even if the risk estimates are imprecise or inaccurate, the magnitude of estimated risk to the public of radon exceeds that of these other agents by many orders of magnitude. Perhaps the difference in public reaction to these carcinogens relates to the fact that asbestos and dioxin are man-made and in commercial use, while radon is a natural pollutant.

Residential radon investigations to date, and perhaps into the future, remain relatively noncontributory to our knowledge about the agent's carcinogenicity. Because the studies lack statistical power, the inconclusive results must not be interpreted as evidence contrary to the conclusions of the mining studies. Perhaps the greatest error made in interpretation of radon investigation results by radon investigators, journalists, and the lay public alike is considering an inconclusive study to be evidence of the lack of carcinogenicity of residential radon or evidence that the magnitude of the risk is low.

PREVENTION

Currently, no effective methods are available for the early diagnosis and treatment of lung cancer (radon-induced or otherwise).[27] The most effective methods of prevention are the detection and mitigation of high radon levels and the modification of other simultaneous risk factors such as smoking. Several studies have noted optimistic biases in the public's assessment of residential radon risk that may discourage testing and subsequent implementation of control measures.[30,73,74] While the general public tends to be somewhat apathetic about radon, the lay press sometimes paints a picture of overreaction. The diversity of perspectives on the issue presented by the lay press may be more confusing than enlightening for the public. Thus, physicians and public health professionals should promote public awareness so that the radon problem is seen in perspective, leading to radon detection and appropriate mitigation action when indicated.

Radon Detection

Because radon levels cannot be accurately predicted solely on the basis of factors such as location, geology, home construction, and ventilation, measurement is the key to identifying the problem. Detection is inexpensive and very easy for the homeowner to perform. Previously, the EPA had recommended a two-step strategy, with an initial 2- to 7-day charcoal canister screening measurement followed by a 3- to 12-month integrated α-track confirmation measurement. This approach had the benefit of more accurate assessment prior to mitigation but suffered from the problem of compliance due to the multiple steps in the process. Many homeowners would take the first measurement but then fail to follow through the process of confirmatory measurement and mitigation. Thus, current recommendations are for a simpler single screening step, followed by mitigation if indicated. Screening measurements using charcoal canister kits should be made under "closed house measurement conditions,"[71] preferably in the basement or lowest livable area in the house. Such measurements are "worst case" and do not represent actual exposure conditions. Nonetheless, charcoal canister measurements provide reasonable guidance for a public mitigation strategy. The charcoal canister is an inexpensive ($10 to $20) small can containing charcoal behind a filter permeable to radon gas but impermeable to radon progeny.

If screening levels exceed 4 pCi/L, the EPA recommends action to reduce radon levels in the home, although this "action level" does remain somewhat controversial. Some individuals may choose to perform the more definitive measurements over a longer period of time in the occupied areas of the home (e.g., bedrooms) using an α-track device. This would be more representative of actual exposure conditions. The α-track device contains a small piece of plastic in a filtered container. As the radon gas that has entered the container decays, the α-particles etch tracks on the plastic piece that can be counted by a special technique. The cost of the α-track device is roughly twice that of the charcoal canister, and it may be used to measure cumulative exposure over a longer period (several months to a year).[47]

Radon Mitigation

In general, if detection and mitigation methods are applied rationally and if current risk estimates are correct, the costs of protection from radon exposure may compare favorably with other measures initiated to lower the risk of death from other hazards (e.g., highway and other transportation hazards, occupational exposure hazards, other environmental hazards). Because of the likely synergy between radon and cigarette smoking, however, the most important and most cost-effective method for reducing radon-induced lung cancer among smokers would be smoking cessation. Unfortunately, smoking cessation may be more difficult for most individuals than radon mitigation. Further, even after smoking cessation, radon mitigation would provide additional risk reduction benefit.

Radon mitigation methods include sealing the foundation, creating negative pressure in the soil and pressurizing the home,[27] and increasing ventilation, including installing heat exchangers, ventilating basements and crawl spaces, and ventilating sump holes and floor drains to the outside of the house. Enhancement of ventilation, however, should be carefully designed to avoid negative pressure changes that could increase radon entry to the home. Preventing soil gas entry is more important than increasing whole-house ventilation.[8] This involves sealing the foundation or depressurizing the soil. Using vapor barriers around the foundation, sealing cracks and holes with epoxies and caulks, and sealing the crawl space from the rest of the house are all methods with some application. However, sealing the foundation tends to be far less effective than depressurizing the soil. Subslab suction is a technique of soil depressurization that can reduce radon levels by as much as 99%.[27] Suction puts the soil at a lower pressure than the home and prevents inward migration of soil gas. It requires sinking ventilation pipes below the foundation to continuously pump out soil gas (Fig. 61-2). Capped pipes can be installed during the construction of a home to terminate in a space under the foundation, to allow for the installation of subslab suction at a later date, if indicated (see Fig. 61-2). This and other very simple construction techniques can reduce the subsequent cost of reducing radon levels.[27] Mitigation contractors should be carefully

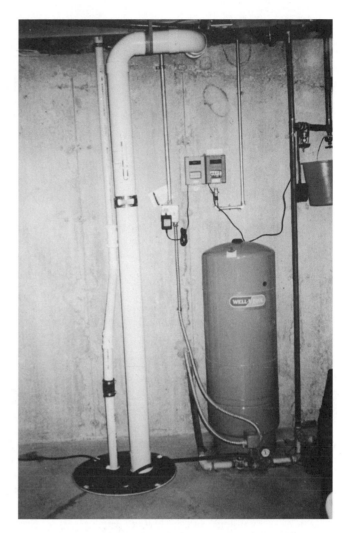

Fig. 61-2 Ventilation pipes below the foundation continuously pump out soil gas. Typical residential subslab ventilation system.

chosen to avoid unnecessary or inappropriate installations; that is, buyer beware.

The EPA recommends mitigation whenever the annual average concentration of radon exceeds their action level in the occupied areas of the home. Recognizing that reducing exposures below 4 pCi/L may be difficult, the agency has recommended that homes at lower levels of exposure consider mitigation on a case-by-case basis. As previously noted, a variety of factors affect exposure dose and risk in addition to ambient exposure level. These and other factors may be considered by families or individuals contemplating mitigation. Such factors may include the number and ages of the occupants, their patterns of occupancy, simultaneous exposure to other lung carcinogens (e.g., smoking), their expected duration of residence in the home, the cost of mitigation, and their available financial resources. An elderly couple on a modest fixed income exposed to 6 pCi/L and contemplating moving to an apartment in several years may not find radon mitigation to be a reasonable investment; a

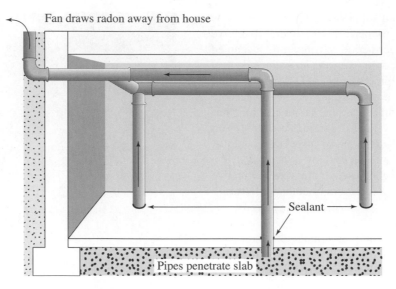

Fan draws radon away from house

Sealant

Pipes penetrate slab

Fig. 61-3 Subslab depressurization. (From Samet JM, editor: *TSDR case studies in environmental medicine,* Atlanta, 1992, US Department of Health and Human Services.)

financially secure family that spends a lot of time indoors and intends to live in the home for decades may consider the decision from a very different perspective.

A recent examination of mitigation methods in homes with very high radon levels found that, while basement sealing was not effective, soil depressurization, properly installed mechanical ventilation with heat exchange technology, and multilayer floor construction with evacuation of air between the floor and bottom slab all achieved significant reduction of ambient radon levels (Fig. 61-3).[17] Soil depressurization, the most effective method, reduced winter basement levels about 200-fold, and ground floor levels about 400-fold. When using mechanical ventilation with heat exchange, improper installation with the development of negative pressure in the basement could actually raise radon levels. With this technique, the basement must be maintained under positive pressure with respect to the outdoors.

SUMMARY

Among the various air contaminants found in the residential environment, radon may be among the most hazardous as well as the most controversial. While the pulmonary carcinogenicity of radon is well established in mining studies, scientific uncertainty and public debate remains about the magnitude of the cancer risk associated with residential exposure. Based upon the mining data, many scientists believe that radon may be second only to smoking as a cause of lung cancer. Primary prevention through environmental control is believed to be highly effective in reducing ambient exposure to radon. The technology for detection and mitigation of elevated radon levels in homes

is available, practical, and may be cost-effective compared with other public health efforts.

REFERENCES

1. Alavanja CRM et al: Attributable risk of lung cancer in lifetime nonsmokers and long-term ex-smokers (Missouri, United States), *Cancer Causes Control* 6:209, 1995.
2. Alavanja CRM et al: Residential radon exposure and lung cancer among nonsmoking women, *J Natl Cancer Inst* 86:1829, 1994.
3. American Medical Association Council on Scientific Affairs: Radon in homes, *JAMA* 258:668, 1987.
4. Anttila S et al: Pulmonary expression of glutathione S-transferase M3 in lung cancer patients: association with GSTM1 polymorphism, smoking and asbestos exposure, *Cancer Res* 55:3305, 1995.
5. Archer VE: Lung cancer risks of underground miners: cohort and case-control studies, *Yale J Biol Med* 61:183, 1988.
6. Arnstein A: Sozialhygienische Untersuchungen über die Bergleute in den Schneeberger Kobalt-Gruben, insbesodere über das Borkommen des sogenannten Schneeberger Lungenkrebses, *Osterreich. Sanitätswesen* 38:64, 1913.
7. Axelson O: Cancer risks from exposure to radon in homes, *Environ Health Perspect* 103(Suppl):37, 1995.
8. Bierma TJ: Radon risk factors: evaluating the health implications of home exposure, *J Environ Health* 51:277, 1989.
9. Blot WJ et al: Indoor radon and lung cancer in China, *J Natl Cancer Inst* 82:1025, 1990.
10. Brill AB et al: Radon update: facts concerning environmental radon: levels, mitigation strategies, dosimetry, effects and guidelines, *J Nucl Med* 35:368, 1994.
11. Cohen BL: Radon levels in United States homes by states and counties, *Health Phys* 60:243, 1991.
12. Collman GW et al: Radon222 concentration in groundwater and cancer mortality in North Carolina, *Int Arch Occup Environ Health* 61:13, 1988.
13. Cross FT: *Radon inhalation studies in animals,* Publ No DOE-ER-0396, Springfield, Va, 1988, National Technical Information Service.

14. Damber L, Larsson LG: Combined effects of mining and smoking in the causation of lung carcinoma, *Acta Radiol* 21:305, 1982.

15. Darby SC et al: Radon and cancers other than lung cancer in underground miners: a collaborative analysis of 11 studies, *J Natl Cancer Inst* 87:378, 1995.

16. Ennemoser O et al: Exposure to unusually high indoor radon levels, *Lancet* 341:828, 1993.

17. Ennemoser O et al: Mitigation of indoor radon in an area with unusually high radon concentrations, *Health Phys* 69:227, 1995.

18. Gloeckler Ries LA et al: *SEER cancer statistics review, 1973-1991,* NIH Publ No 94-2789, Washington, DC, 1994, National Institutes of Health, National Cancer Institute.

19. Gofman JW: *Radiation & Human Health,* San Francisco, 1981, Sierra Club Books.

20. Gottlieb LS, Husen LA: Lung cancer among Navajo uranium miners, *Chest* 81:449, 1982.

21. Guimond RJ: Radon risk and EPA, *Science* 251:724, 1991.

22. Hanson DJ: Radon tagged as cancer hazard by most studies, researchers, *C&EN,* Feb 6, 1989.

23. Harley NH: Interaction of alpha particles with bronchial cells, *Health Phys* 55:665, 1988.

24. Harley N et al: Contribution of radon and radon daughters to respiratory cancer, *Environ Health Perspect* 70:17, 1986.

25. Härting FH, Hesse W: Der Lungenkrebs, die Bergkrankheit in den Schneeberger Gruben, *Vierteljahrsschr f gerichtl Med u öffentl Gesundheitswesen* (N F) 30:296; 31:102, 1879.

26. Hendee WR, Doege TC: Origin and health risks of indoor radon, *Semin Nucl Med* 18:3, 1987.

27. Henschel DB: *Radon reduction techniques for detached homes,* ed 2, EPA Publ No 625/5-87/019, Washington, DC, 1988, US Environmental Protection Agency.

28. Henshaw DL, Eatough JP, Richardson RB: Radon as a causative factor in induction of myeloid leukemia and other cancers, *Lancet* 335:1008, 1990.

29. Hornung RW, Deddens J, Roscoe R: Modifiers of exposure-response estimates for lung cancer among miners exposed to radon progeny, *Environ Health Perspect* 103(Suppl 2):49, 1995.

30. Johnson FR, Luken RA: Radon risk information and voluntary protection: evidence from a natural experiment, *Risk Anal* 7:97, 1987.

31. Laurer GR, Qui TG, Lubin FH: Skeletal lead-210 levels and lung cancer among radon-exposed tin miners in Southern China, *Health Phys* 64:253, 1993.

32. Leary WE: Studies raise doubts about need to lower home radon levels, *New York Times,* September 6, 1994, p B7.

33. Létourneau EG et al: Case-control study of residential radon and lung cancer in Winnipeg, Manitoba, Canada, *Am J Epidemiol* 40:310, 1994.

34. Lorenz E: Radioactivity and lung cancer: a critical review of lung cancer in the miners of Schneeberg and Joachimsthal, *J Natl Cancer Inst* 5:1, 1944.

35. Lubin JH: Invited commentary: lung cancer and exposure to residential radon, *Am J Epidemiol* 140:323, 1994.

36. Lubin JH et al: Lung cancer in radon-exposed miners and estimation of risk from indoor exposure, *J Natl Cancer Inst* 87:817, 1995.

37. Lubin JH et al: *Radon and lung cancer risk: a joint analysis of 11 underground miners studies,* Publ No 94-3644, Washington, DC, 1994, National Cancer Institute, National Institutes of Health.

38. Lubin JH, Samet JM, Weinberg C: Design issues in epidemiologic studies of indoor exposure to radon and risk of lung cancer, *Health Phys* 59:807, 1990.

39. Lubin JH, Steindorf K: Cigarette use and the estimation of lung cancer attributable to radon in the United States, *Radiat Res* 141:79, 1995.

40. Ludewig P, Lorenser E: Untersuchung der Grubenluft in den Schneeberger Gruben auf den Gehalt an Radiumemanation, *Z f Phys* 22:178, 1924.

41. Mahaffy JA, Parkhurst MA, James AC: Estimating past exposure to indoor radon from household glass, *Health Phys* 64:381, 1993.

42. Michaylov MA, Presssyanov DS, Kalinov KB: Bronchial dysplasia induced by radiation in miners exposed to 222Rn progeny, *Occup Environ Med* 52: 82, 1995.

43. Muscat JE, Wynder EL: Lung cancer pathology in smokers, ex-smokers and never smokers, *Cancer Lett* 88:1, 1995.

44. National Academy of Science Committee on the Biological Effects of Ionizing Radiation, National Research Council: *Health risks of radon and other internally deposited alpha-emitters: BEIR IV,* Washington, DC, 1988, National Academy Press.

45. National Council on Radiation Protection: *Evaluation of occupational and environmental exposures to radon and radon daughters in the United States,* NCRP Report No 78, Bethesda, Md, 1984, NCRP.

46. National Radon Database: *The national residential radon survey,* Washington, DC, 1993, U S Environmental Protection Agency.

47. *National radon measurement proficiency (RMP) program, proficiency report:* Tennessee, Washington, DC, 1988, US Environmental Protection Agency.

48. Nero AV: Radon and its decay products in indoor air: an overview. In Nazaroff WW, Nero AV, editors: *Radon and its decay products in indoor air,* New York, 1988, John Wiley.

49. Nero AV et al: Distribution of airborne radon-222 concentrations in US homes, *Science* 234:992, 1986.

50. Neuberger JS: Residential radon exposure and lung cancer: an overview of published studies, *Cancer Detect Prev* 15:435, 1991.

51. Neuberger JS: Residential radon exposure and lung cancer: an overview of ongoing studies, *Health Phys* 63:503, 1992.

52. Pershagen G et al: Residential radon exposure and lung cancer in Sweden, *New Engl J Med* 330:159, 1994.

53. Pershagen G et al: Residential radon exposure and lung cancer in Swedish women, *Health Phys* 63:179, 1992.

54. Puskin JS, Nelson CB: EPA's perspective on risks from residential radon exposure, *JAPCA* 39:915, 1989.

55. Puskin JS, Yang Y: A retrospective look at Rn-induced lung cancer mortality from the viewpoint of a relative risk model, *Health Phys* 54:635, 1988.

56. Roscoe RJ et al: Mortality among Navajo uranium miners, *Am J Public Health* 85:535, 1995.

57. Samet JM: Radon and lung cancer, *J Natl Cancer Inst* 81:745, 1989.

58. Schoenberg JB et al: Case-control study of residential radon and lung cancer among New Jersey women, *Cancer Res* 50:6520, 1990.

59. Schoenberg JB et al: Lung cancer and exposure to radon in women—New Jersey, *MMWR Morb Mortal Wkly Rep* 38:715, 1989.

60. Steenland K: Age specific interactions between smoking and radon among United States uranium miners, *Occup Environ Med* 51:192, 1994.

61. Steindorf K et al: Lung cancer deaths attributable to indoor radon exposure in West Germany, *Int J Epidemiol* 24:485, 1995.

62. Stidley CA, Samet JM: Assessment of ecologic regression in the study of lung cancer and indoor radon, *Am J Epidemiol* 139:312, 1994.

63. Stidley CA, Samet JM: A review of ecologic studies of lung cancer and indoor radon, *Health Phys* 65:234, 1993.

64. Taylor JA et al: p53 Mutation hotspot in radon-associated lung cancer, *Lancet* 343:86, 1994.

65. *Technical support document for the 1992 citizen's guide to radon,* Document No400-R-92-011, Washington, DC, 1992, US Environmental Protection Agency.

66. Thomas D et al: Temporal modifiers of the radon-smoking interaction, *Health Phys* 66:257, 1994.

67. Tomasek L et al: Radon exposure and cancers other than lung cancer among uranium miners in West Bohemia, *Lancet* 341:919, 1993.

68. Upfal M, Divine G, Siemiatycki J: Design issues in studies of radon and lung cancer: implications of the joint effect of smoking and radon, *Environ Health Perspect* 103:58, 1995.

69. Upfal MJ et al: Indoor radon and lung cancer in China, *J Natl Cancer Inst* 82:1722, 1990 (letter).

70. US Environmental Protection Agency: *A citizen's guide to radon: what it is and what to do about it,* EPA Publ No OPA-86-004, Washington, DC, 1986, EPA.

71. US Environmental Protection Agency: *Radon reference manual,* EPA Publ No 520/1-87-20, Washington, DC, 1987, EPA.

72. US Environmental Protection Agency: *Removal of radon from household water,* EPA Publ No OPA-87-011, Washington, DC, 1987, EPA.

73. Weinstein ND et al: Optimistic biases in public perceptions of the risk from radon, *Am J Public Health* 78:796, 1988.

74. Weinstein ND, Sandman PM, Roberts NE: Perceived susceptibility and self-protective behavior: a field experiment to encourage home radon testing, *Health Psychol* 10:25, 1991.

Appendix I

Cybertoxicology

Jerry V. Glowniak

- The Internet is a worldwide system of computers that individuals can access to obtain information in many different areas

- There are multiple ways of getting information from the Internet through services such as the World Wide Web

- There are various methods for locating toxicologic information on the Internet

- There are many medical resources on the Internet, including toxicologic resources that provide useful information

The early 1990s witnessed an explosive growth in telecommunications eagerly embraced by the scientific and medical communities. One of the most salient features in this growth was the development of computer networks and electronic bulletin boards. Computers can be connected together by means of special cabling and communication software to form networks that permit the sharing of resources and information. Computers connected together at a single organization or institution form a local area network (LAN). Another method of linking computers is through electronic bulletin boards. Using standard telephone lines and a modem,* an individual with a personal computer can connect to a central computer that provides various services such as electronic mail, teleconferencing, and access to databases and computer files. Two problems limit the widespread use of these technologies: Different computer networks use different communication standards that make it difficult or impossible to exchange information, and long-distance communication using a modem is expensive. These two problems were solved in an unexpected way by the development of the Internet. This chapter describes the Internet, the largest computer network in the world, and methods for using it to access medical resources, with a special emphasis on toxocologic information.

*Modem is an acronym for *mo*dulator *dem*odulator. A modem sends messages by converting a computer's digital signals into analog signals that can be transmitted on telephone lines. A receiving modem converts the signals back into digital form.

HISTORY OF THE INTERNET

In the late 1960s, the Department of Defense (DoD) became interested in long-distance computer communications. In 1969, the Advanced Research Projects Agency (ARPA, also at various times called DARPA, the Defense Advanced Research Projects Agency) of the DoD funded a networking experiment between computers at the University of Utah, the University of California at Santa Barbara, Stanford, and the University of California at Los Angeles. The purpose of the experiment was to develop methods of sharing information and resources between computers by using communication standards that were highly reliable and capable of functioning with any type of computer or operating system. High reliability was required so that the network could continue to function when some of the communication links became inoperative or signals were degraded, as might occur during a war. The communication links and associated hardware for transferring information between these centers was referred to as the "backbone" network and was called the ARPANET. The success of this experiment attracted other academic and research centers that connected their LANs to ARPANET. By the early 1980s, approximately 20 universities and 1000 computers were connected to ARPANET. During this time, a series of communication standards was developed that described all aspects of computer communication from application programs to methods for routing information through the network. In 1978, the DoD declared that any computer that used the ARPANET had to use these standards for communication. This group of standards, or protocols, was formally defined in a set of approximately 50 documents. The entire set became known as the TCP/IP protocol suite, named after its two most important protocols: TCP (the transmission control protocol) and IP (the Internet protocol). These protocols were made freely available so that any institution or commercial organization could use them to write communication software.

In the 1980s, all military computers and networks were split off from ARPANET to form a distinct but connected network, MILNET. Then ARPANET, along with its connected networks and their computers, began to be referred to as the Internet. By 1985, ARPA, which had neither the funds nor the interest in developing or running a civilian network, decided to withdraw funding from ARPANET. At this point, the Internet nearly came to an end. Fortunately, the National Science Foundation (NSF), which had been developing its own networking projects for supercomputers, decided to fund an expanded version of ARPANET that interconnected major academic, scientific, and research centers across the United States. It funded the creation of a new backbone

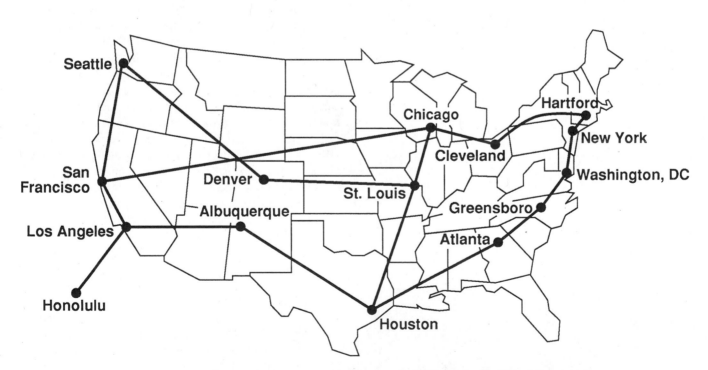

Fig. I-1 Structure of the major Internet backbone network, NSFNET, in the United States at the beginning of 1995. The 15 nodes indicated by city names are the points at which the regional networks connected to NSFNET. Links between the nodes are fiber optic cables leased from MCI. By the middle of 1995, the U.S. government stopped funding for the backbone network, and large telecommunication companies began carrying most of the Internet traffic. (From Glowniak JV: Medical resources on the Internet, *Annals of Internal Medicine* 123:123-129, 1995.)

network, NSFNET, that became operational in 1988 and consisted of leased, high-speed telephone lines that interconnected all portions of the United States through hubs at 14 major sites. The NSF also funded the creation of regional networks that connected the LANs of institutions together. Thus the Internet was a three-tiered structure: LANs at local institutions connected together to form regional networks, which connected to the NSFNET backbone. All the links on NSFNET were capable of transmitting up to 1.5 million bits of information per second (1.5 Mbps), equivalent to transmitting 30 to 40 pages of text per second. The NSFNET was markedly successful. Many more institutions connected to the regional networks, and the capacity of NSFNET was becoming saturated. In 1992, NSFNET created a new, higher-speed network capable of transmitting 45 Mbps, equivalent to 1000 pages of text per second. Figures I-1 and I-2 show the structure of NSFNET and one of the regional networks in early 1995.

By 1993, it was clear that the Internet had appeal to many commercial organizations who were willing to pay for connections to the Internet. Thus, the U.S. government terminated funding for NSFNET in 1995 except for networking projects in restricted areas. Long-distance Internet traffic was then handled primarily by the major telecommunication carriers, MCI, Sprint, and AT&T, and by an assortment of smaller telecommunication companies that created a much more complex backbone structure than NSFNET. At the local level, a marked demand for access to the Internet sparked the creation of commercial Internet service providers (ISPs) who sold connectivity to institutions and individuals. In this scheme, an individual purchased access to an ISP, who then supplied the high-speed links to the Internet backbone.

Although the Internet originated in the United States, the backbone network was connected to computer networks in other countries from its earliest days: ARPANET had

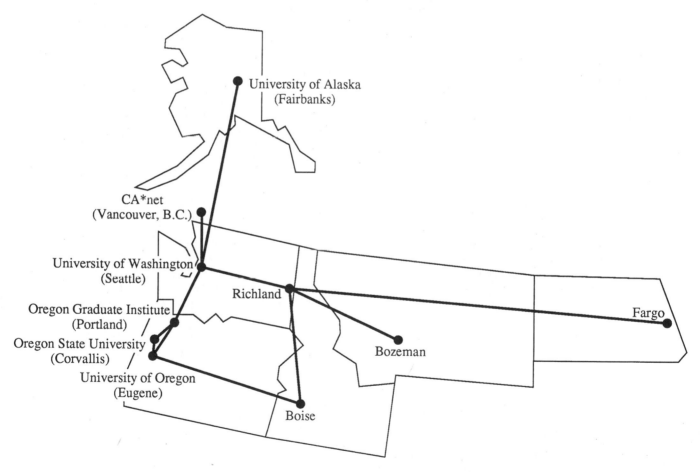

Fig. I-2 NorthWestNet, one of the regional networks sponsored by NSF. Only the major connecting links and hubs are shown. Over 200 academic, research, and commercial networks, primarily in the Portland and Seattle areas, are connected to NorthWestNet. NorthWestNet connects to the United States backbone network, previously NSFNET, at Seattle. CA*net is the national Canadian backbone network on the Internet. It connects to the U.S. backbone network in western Canada through NorthWestNet. (From Glowniak JV: An introduction to the Internet, part 1: history, organization and function, *J Nucl Med Technol* 23:56, 1995.)

connections to Europe, Canada, and Japan. The only requirements for connecting to the Internet were that these networks had to use the TCP/IP protocols and conform to the naming conventions adopted for computers and networks on the Internet (discussed later). The types of organizations that can connect to the Internet, the structure of the national backbone networks, and the type of traffic allowed are all determined individually by each country. Thus, in a manner similar to the telephone system, there is no central organization that controls the Internet. The Internet is growing rapidly and becoming more international in scope. As of January 1997, the Internet was composed of more than 16 million computers on 800,000 networks in 92 countries.

ORGANIZATION OF THE INTERNET

The basic organizational unit on the Internet is the network. All computers on the Internet belong to a network. A network

may consist of one to thousands of computers. In order to facilitate communications, each computer on the Internet is assigned a unique number called its IP number or IP address. An IP address is represented by a string of numbers separated by periods. Part of this string identifies the network and another part a specific computer on the network (see box below). All computer communication on the Internet takes place using IP addresses. Since IP addresses are difficult for humans to remember, a parallel system of computer and network identification was developed called the *domain name system* (DNS). It employs a naming scheme that is similar to that for IP addresses in that computers are identified by names consisting of strings of characters separated by periods. A portion of the name identifies the network and a portion identifies a single computer on the network (see box below). The character strings are words or character combinations that ideally are easy to remember

---

IP Addresses and Computer Names on the Internet

Every computer on the Internet must have an IP address that uniquely identifies that computer. An IP address is a 32 bit* string:

10011101 01100010 00001000 00001001

(Spaces are added for convenience in reading; they are not part of the address.) This string is usually written as 8-bit segments. Each segment is represented by its equivalent decimal integer, which lies in the range 0-255 with the integers separated by periods. Each IP address consists of two parts: The leftmost one to three numbers form the network portion of the address. The remaining numbers form the host, or computer, portion of the address. If the leftmost number in an IP address is in the range 1-127, this number is the network portion of the IP address. If the leftmost number is in the range 128-191, the leftmost two numbers are the network address. If the leftmost number is in the range 192-223, the leftmost three numbers form the network address. Thus, the above IP address written in decimal form is:

```
        host address portion
                 |
                ___
               |   |
          157.98.8.9
          |       |
         _____
              |
        network address portion
```

which is a computer at the National Institute for Environmental Health Sciences at the National Institutes of Health. As explained in the text, a Network Information Center assigns the network portion of the address to a network. The network then assigns the host portion of the address to its computers. Since this network can assign the rightmost two numbers, this network could contain $256 \times 256 = 65,536$ computers.

A parallel system of identifying computers is the domain name system (DNS). While every computer on the Internet must have an IP address, DNS names are optional, though the vast majority of computers have these names. Portions of a DNS name are written in hierarchical order from left to right, with the most specific portion on the left (the host name) and the most general portion on the right (the top level domain name). As an example, the DNS name for the above IP address is

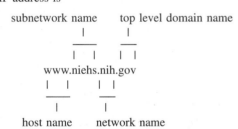

The host name of this computer, www, indicates that this is a World Wide Web server. Every named computer must have a host name, a network name, and a top level domain name. Subnetwork names are optional. In some instances, primarily with email, only the network and top level domain names are required for contacting remote computers. The domain name system is case insensitive, and computer names can be entered in upper or lower case in commands or as part of email addresses and URLs.

---

*A bit is a *binary digit*, either 0 or 1.

and describe the system is some way. The DNS also imposes a hierarchy of networks that is reflected in the computer names. Originally, all networks were divided into seven main categories called *top level domains* that described the primary activity of each of the categories (Table I-1). Since the Internet was at first composed of computers only in the United States, there was no system to identify foreign networks. As other countries joined the Internet, new top level domains were created for foreign networks. These domains were designated by two letter codes assigned to each country. Thus, the top level domain for computers in the United Kingdom is "uk." This naming scheme is not universally applied. Some networks outside the United States use the three-letter codes com, int, org, and net in Table I-1 as top level domains while some networks in the United States use "us," the country code for the United States, as the top level domain.

As mentioned previously, computers communicate using IP addresses, not domain names. The domain name of a remote computer must be converted to its IP address before the remote computer can be contacted. Since there are no logical connections between IP addresses and domain names, conversions occur by consulting lists of IP addresses and their corresponding domain names. It would be difficult, however, for most computers to handle a complete list of IP addresses and impossible to keep it up-to-date. Instead, portions of the list are kept on several thousand computers around the Internet known as *name servers*. Each name server contains an up-to-date list of IP addresses and domain names for a defined network or group of networks. When a domain name is entered on a computer, the computer's DNS software automatically contacts its name server and asks for an IP address. If the local name server does not have the IP address, other name servers are contacted until one with a

Table I-1 Top level domains

Code	Meaning
edu	educational
com	commercial
gov	government
mil	military
net	network
org	organization
int	international
us	United States
uk	United Kingdom
de	Germany
ch	Switzerland

The top level domains for computer networks in the United States are represented by the three-letter codes shown above and the country code "us." Top level domains for foreign networks are com, int, org, and net two-letter codes that identify the country where the network resides. There are over 100 such codes, which are often derived from the country name as it is spelled or used in the particular country (*de* for Deutschland, *ch* for Cantons of Helvetia—the Latin name for the region that includes Switzerland).

listing for the domain name is found. The IP address is then returned to the local computer and substituted for the domain name.

The Internet can be thought of as a network of networks or, perhaps, a hierarchy of networks. Each component network is an independent entity entirely under the control of the organization that owns the network. Each organization decides whether to connect to the Internet, which computers will have Internet access, and the type of services available. Nevertheless, some central organization is required to coordinate assignment of DNS names and IP addresses to assure these assignments are unique. In the early days of the Internet, a central registry assigned domain names and IP addresses to all computers and networks. When the size of the Internet increased to hundreds of thousands of computers, this scheme became unworkable. In its place, a system of network information centers (NICs) was created. The NICs, the most important of which is the InterNIC (Internet network information center), coordinate their activities and are responsible for registering networks and assigning top level domain names, network names, and the network portion of IP addresses to individual networks. Networks are assigned blocks of IP addresses. It is the responsibility of the networks to assign the host portion of domain names and IP addresses to their computers. Since a network can use some, none, or all of the IP addresses assigned to it, it is impossible to know how many computers there are on the Internet, though various counting methods have been developed.

THE CLIENT-SERVER MODEL

All Internet communications involve a local computer accessing resources on a remote computer. The remote computer may be on the same network or anywhere on the Internet. The method of accessing the remote computer depends upon the resources desired: electronic mail, downloading of files, or an interactive session. Access methods are referred to as *Internet services,* each of which is governed by protocols that describe how the interactions are to occur. The protocols are implemented by software or application programs. There are a large number of software programs for the Internet services, particularly for the World Wide Web and E-mail.

The software for an Internet service is split into two parts: a client that resides on the local computer and a server on the remote computer. The user interacts with the client, which accepts user input, formats it according to the particular protocol, and sends the request to the server. The server accepts the request, performs whatever function is required, and sends the results back to the client. The client then displays the results to the user. In general, a client for a particular service can interact only with a server for the same service, although exceptions exist. Clients and servers are software programs, though the terms are often used interchangeably for the computers on which the programs

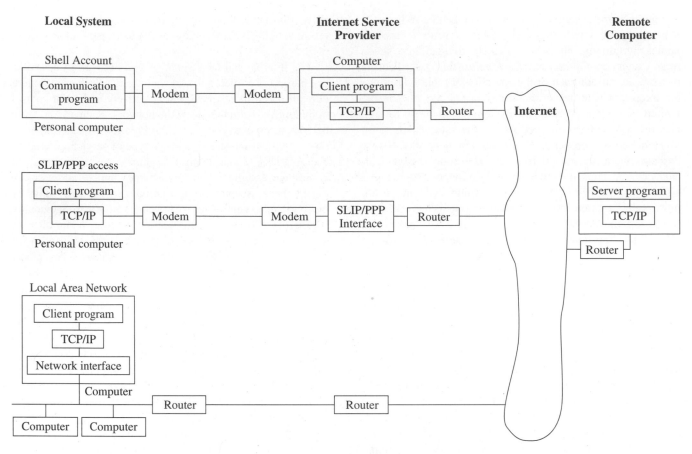

Fig. I-3 Methods of Internet access. Personal computers can connect to the Internet by standard telephone lines and modems. With a shell account, the client programs for the Internet services and the networking (TCP/IP) software are on the Internet service provider's (ISP) computer. SLIP or PPP access allows a user's computer to become a full-fledged computer on the Internet. The user's personal computer runs the Internet client programs and networking software. Computers on a local area network (LAN) are connected together by special cabling and can communicate with each other or pass messages beyond the LAN through a router. A router is a device that directs traffic between networks. All connections between the ISP and the remote computer through the Internet are represented as a cloud whose structure is unimportant to the user.

reside. In practice, the terms *client* and *server* are often not used, the meaning being derived from context. The actual sending and receiving of information are not performed by the application program itself, but rather by the TCP/IP software that handles all aspects of the connection between the two computers (Fig. I-3). The TCP/IP software creates connections and passes information from the application programs between computers in a manner that is independent of both the types of computers and their operating systems.

INTERNET ACCESS

There are several different ways of accessing the Internet. Most large medical, academic, and research institutions in the United States provide some form of access to their members. Since these institutions typically can afford high-speed connections to the Internet, they often provide the best access. The most common method for connecting to the Internet is by means of a personal computer using a modem and standard telephone lines to connect to an ISP. There are three requirements for Internet access: application programs for the Internet services, networking software (TCP/IP software), and an ISP that supplies the physical link to the Internet (see Fig. I-3). In the discussion that follows, Internet access is described for a personal computer connecting to an ISP through a modem.

One of the driving forces that made the Internet so popular has been the emergence of proprietary ISPs that sell access to individuals. There are hundreds of such providers, competition among whom has markedly reduced the price of Internet access. They range from large international vendors to local providers who service a small geographic area. There are ISPs in all large and medium-size metropolitan areas within the United States. These vendors advertise widely in computer-oriented magazines and publications. A major new development that began in 1994 is the availability of Internet access through traditional computer online services such as America Online, Prodigy, CompuServe, Delphi, and GEnie. A more recent addition has been the Microsoft Network. Vendors offer different levels of service and various pricing schemes.

For the individual user, one of the major decisions about connecting to the Internet is the type of access. There are two major access methods: text-based interfaces and graphic user interfaces. As the name implies, text-based interfaces display text on the computer screen, and commands or options are typed on a keyboard. An example of a text-based system is DOS. Graphic user interfaces such as Macintosh and Windows-based systems use text and graphic elements to display information and allow user input with a mouse.

The simplest way to connect to the Internet is through a "shell" account. With this method, all that is required is a computer with a communication program and a modem. All the Internet application programs and the TCP/IP software are on the ISP's computer. The user logs onto this system in a manner similar to accessing an electronic bulletin board. After logging in, the user must enter commands understood by the ISP's computer operating system. The most common operating system on the Internet is UNIX,* a system preferred for its superior networking and multiuser capabilities. It is beyond the scope of this chapter to describe UNIX, but it has a command and file structure similar to DOS. Most sites, however, offer a menu format in addition to a UNIX interface so no knowledge of UNIX is required to use the system. The main disadvantage of a shell account is that a user cannot access the graphic capabilities of the World Wide Web, and files downloaded from the Internet are stored on the ISP's computer. A separate transfer from the ISP's computer to the individual's personal computer is required if a user wishes to have a copy of a file or program on his or her own computer. With a shell account, the individual's personal computer is used as an input-output device and is not a computer on the Internet.

The second type of access is called SLIP (serial line Internet protocol) or PPP (point to point protocol) access and allows a user's computer to become a full-fledged computer on the Internet. With this type of access, the user's personal computer is assigned, temporarily, its own IP address, which permits direct downloading of files from the Internet. The SLIP or PPP connection allows a user to access all the graphic and multimedia capabilities of the World Wide Web. (The user's computer must have the hardware and software for capabilities for displaying multimedia data to be able to do this.) Unlike a shell account, a user must install and run

* As used here, *UNIX* refers to a family of closely related, mostly proprietary operating systems. The most common systems are SunOS, Solaris, Ultrix, AIX, HP-UX, and Linux.

Table I-2 World Wide Web access methods

Service	Access method	Port number
Electronic mail	email	25
File transfer	ftp	21
Gopher	gopher.	70
Remote login	telnet	23
USENET	news	119
World Wide Web	http	80

Web browsers can connect to multiple Internet services. Each service is identified by an access method, which is the first part of a URL. Servers for Internet services are assigned standard port numbers, which are shown in the third column.

all the Internet application and TCP/IP programs on her or his own computer. In addition, more computer memory, higher processing speeds, and faster modems are required than for a shell account.

INTERNET SERVICES

The resources on the Internet are accessed by Internet services, each of which has its own distinctive features and is defined by one or more protocols. All these services function in the client-server mode. To access a service, a user activates a client program on the local computer and supplies it with the IP address or domain name of a remote computer that is running a corresponding server. There are dozens of Internet services, but most users need to be familiar with only a few of them to access most of the information on the Internet (Table I-2). The major services are described here, and a few examples in UNIX format are given. For these examples, user input is given in bold text and is followed by a carriage return. Computer prompts and messages are displayed as ordinary text. Client software for all the Internet services is available for both text-based and graphic systems.

Electronic Mail

Electronic mail, or E-mail, is probably the most widely used service on the Internet. There is a wide diversity of mail programs, but all of them allow a user to create, edit, and send messages and store received mail. Mail addressing on the Internet uses the following format:

username@computername

where *username* is the way an individual is identified by the mail program on the local system (on UNIX systems, this is often the same as the user's login name), and *computername* is the domain name of the computer that handles mail for a given network. No spaces are allowed anywhere within the address. The vast majority of mail systems allow addresses to be in either upper or lower case. To simplify mail addressing, many networks use "aliases" for the computer that sends and receives mail. An *alias* is an alternative name for a computer that is usually shorter than the full domain name. A common practice is to use only the network portion of a domain name as an alias for the computer that handles mail.

Originally, mail programs could send and receive only ordinary text. An extension of the standard Internet mail protocol called MIME (multipurpose Internet mail extensions) allows a user with a MIME-compatible mailer to send and receive messages that contain graphics, video or audio clips, or computer programs. Depending on how the mailer is configured, these elements can be displayed or run when the mail message is read, or they can be sent as attached files that can be displayed or run independently of the text in the message.

A useful extension of simple E-mail is the mailing list. A *mailing list* is a group of individuals who communicate through a mail program called a *mailing list manager* (MLM), which accepts E-mail messages and sends copies of the message to all members on the list. Mailing lists are organized around specific subjects and may function as an interactive discussion group or as a means of disseminating information from some source. Anyone with access to E-mail can join a mailing list. There are thousands of mailing lists on the Internet, several hundred of which are devoted to medical topics. A mailing list has two E-mail addresses. One address is used for administrative functions. A user sends messages to this address for subscribing and unsubscribing to the list and as means of getting information about the list. The other address is for posting messages to all members on the list.

USENET

USENET (a contraction of *users' network*), or network news, is a service that consists of thousands of discussion groups on every imaginable topic. Unlike a mailing list that resides on a single computer, a USENET discussion group can exist on thousands of computers worldwide. Messages to a USENET newsgroups are stored in special files on a computer and are not forwarded to individuals. A user reads these messages with a newsreader program. Through the newsreader, an individual can read, reply to, and save messages of interest. The system administrator decides whether to install USENET on the local computer and what newsgroups will be available. One unique feature of USENET is that sites offering this service are connected to other USENET sites with which they exchange messages. There are tens of thousands of USENET sites worldwide, and a message posted at one site can be delivered to many other sites. A user who posts a message to a USENET group specifies how far the message is to be distributed—to local, regional, national, or international sites. Strictly speaking, USENET is not part of the Internet. In the early days, USENET postings were passed between computers using standard telephone lines and modems. This method was rather slow. Using the Internet as a transport medium markedly increased the speed at which

posting could be exchanged, and the majority of USENET sites now use the Internet. There are a few dozen USENET newsgroups related to medicine, and some of these such as sci.med.pharmacy deal in issues related to toxicology.

Telnet

Telnet, a text-based service, is used to log on to remote computers. Telnet is the most versatile service on the Internet and potentially gives the greatest possible access to a computer's resources. A user with unrestricted telnet access to a computer appears to be logging in directly to the remote computer. System administrators, however, usually limit the resources available to a user, especially at telnet sites that are freely accessible by the general public. A telnet session allows a user to run any program on a remote computer, including Internet application programs such as ftp, E-mail, and text-based versions of the World Wide Web (assuming, of course, these services are available on the remote computer, and an individual has permission to use them). Most public telnet sites present the user with a menu, and the user can access only the files and services on the menu. Some computers offer publicly available gopher clients and text-based clients for the World Wide Web. For private accounts, access requires both a login name and a password. At public sites, a password is usually not required, and occasionally a login name is also dispensed with. An example of a public telnet site that offers a text-based client for the World Wide Web, called *lynx,* is at the University of North Carolina. On a UNIX system, a user types:

> **telnet public.sunsite.unc.edu**
> login:**lynx**
> TERM=(unknown)**vt100**

Gopher

The gopher program appears superficially similar to telnet except that a login or password is never required. A user accesses gopher by activating a gopher client and supplying it with the name of a computer running a gopher server. After connecting to the remote computer, a menu is downloaded. A user chooses a menu item that may return another menu, display a text file, or provide some service such as searching a database. The major difference between gopher and telnet is that resources reached by telnet reside on or are activated by a single remote computer. While menu items displayed by gopher may reside on the remote computer, they may also be linked to resources on other computers (primarily gopher servers) anywhere on the Internet. With each menu item, there is an associated location of the resource. When a user chooses a menu item, the gopher client connects to the computer where the resource is located and downloads the information. Thus, a single gopher server can be used to access multiple sites on the Internet. Some servers have links to thousands of other gopher servers on the Internet. The gopher server at the University of Minnesota, where the original gopher program was written, has links to most of the publicly available gopher servers on the Internet. It can be reached by typing:

gopher gopher.tc.umn.edu

FTP

Thousands of computers on the Internet serve as archives for computer files that are freely available to the general public. These files can include anything from simple text files to complete books and a large variety of computer programs for all types of computers. In particular, nearly every type of client program used on the Internet can be found in some of these archives. A user can download these files using an ftp (file transfer protocol) client. As with telnet, a user login name and password are required. At public sites, the login name is "anonymous," and the password is the user's E-mail address. After connecting to the remote site, a user moves between directories and selects files for downloading. As an example, Mosaic, a program for accessing the World Wide Web, can be found at the National Center for Supercomputing Applications at the University of Illinois at Urbana-Champaign. To access this site, a user types:

ftp ftp.ncsa.uiuc.edu
Name:**anonymous**
Password:**glowniak@ohsu.edu**

The author's E-mail address is used as a password. After logging in, a message may be presented to the user, followed by a prompt, commonly "ftp>" on UNIX and other text-based systems. Initially, the program is in the root directory. The "dir" or "ls" command can be used to obtain a directory listing. The user changes directories by using the "cd" command, followed by a directory name or directory path. When a file of interest is found, a user types "get" followed by the file name, and the file is downloaded to the user's computer. On graphical systems, these functions are performed by clicking on corresponding items with a mouse.

The World Wide Web

The service that has caused the explosive growth of the Internet is the World Wide Web (WWW). Unlike gopher or telnet, where documents are simple text files, WWW documents can contain hypertext. *Hypertext* is any word, phrase, or image that is linked to another resource. In a displayed WWW document, the hypertext element is highlighted in some manner. When a user selects the element, typically by clicking on it with a mouse, the linked resource is retrieved and displayed. Like gopher, the linked resource can reside anywhere on the Internet. The resource can be another hypertext document, an image, an audio or video clip, or a program that performs some specific function such as searching a database.

A WWW document is a text file that can be associated with other types of files such as image, audio, or video files that are collectively referred to as *multimedia* files. The WWW documents and their associated files are called *Web*

pages. The primary or introductory Web page on a WWW server is called the *home page.* The home page for the library of the National Institute of Environmental Health Sciences is shown in Figure I-4. The methods by which a Web client and server interact are described in the hypertext transfer protocol (http).

The reason Web pages can contain such diverse elements is that WWW documents contain special formatting codes that describe how the Web page is to be rendered. The set of formatting codes and the rules for using them are called the *hypertext markup language* (html), and WWW documents are often referred to as *html files.* These codes describe how text is to be displayed, what resources hypertext is linked to, and what multimedia elements are to be included in the Web page. The multimedia elements are not part of the WWW document itself. Rather, they are distinct files on the Web server that are referenced in the WWW document. A WWW client, more commonly called a *Web browser,* downloads WWW documents, reads the formatting codes, and creates a Web page. If the WWW document contains references to multimedia (which are usually images), the browser retrieves these files and incorporates them into the Web page.

A Web browser is more than a WWW client program. Browsers include software that allows them to connect to ftp, gopher, and other types of servers. In order to access information on the WWW and other types of servers, browsers use a special notation called uniform resource locators (URLs) for designating files on the Internet. A URL is a string of characters that contains several elements, most commonly an access method, a computer name, a directory path to a file, and a file name (Fig. I-5).

There are dozens of different Web browsers. Several are available free on the Internet, such as Mosaic, the original graphic Web browser from the University of Illinois at Urbana-Champaign. The most popular Web browser is the Mosaic-based program, Netscape, from Netscape Corporation (http://home.netscape.com). As with several browsers available from proprietary sources, a free version of Netscape is available, as well as a version with more extensive features that can be purchased. Another commonly used browser is Internet Explorer from Microsoft.

LOCATING RESOURCES ON THE INTERNET

While the Internet consists of millions of computers, only a small fraction of them, perhaps less than 1%, allow public access. Nevertheless, this amounts to tens of thousands of computers. Since the Internet has no central organization, there is no logical pattern to where resources are located, and there is no official registry of what resources are available. By the early 1990s, it became clear that some method of cataloging information was required. Various organizations and individuals have independently developed a number of methods for indexing Internet computers and their resources as well as means for searching and retrieving information from these indices. Because so much of the information is on the World Wide Web or can be accessed through it, most of the indices and their search programs (also called *search engines*) are on the World Wide Web. New indices and search programs are continuously being developed. Most are available free on the Internet, while others are proprietary, available either as software or as online services. A few of the more useful search methods are described here.

Archie (derived from *archive*) is a program for locating files at FTP sites. An archie server consists of a database of a large number of public FTP sites and a list of all the files they contain. The server has a search program that can be accessed by an archie client. There are several commercial archie clients, and others are available free on the Internet. There are also several dozen public archie clients that can be

Welcome to the National Institute of Environmental Health Sciences Library

The NIEHS Library primarily serves the scientific and administrative staff of <u>NIEHS</u>. Secondarily, the Library provides limited services to the public. The public may use the collection as a reference collection 8:30-5:00 Monday-Friday, and may borrow books from the NIEHS Library by going through standard interlibrary loan channels at their own business, public, or academic library.

 ## <u>NIEHS Library and Information Services</u>

Including details on New Arrivals in the library, photocopy services, interlibrary loan, book ordering and journal subscriptions, reference services, and CD-ROM and LAN support.

 ## <u>Web Sites</u> selected for NIEHS users

These include scientific research, government information and organizations, libraries, news sources, and reference tools.

 ## <u>NIEHS Library Gopher</u>, including the NIEHS bibliography.

The resources available through the gopher include biomedical databases, electronic journals, and more.

<u>NIEHS Home Page</u>   <u>Enviro-Health Clearinghouse</u>

<u>Search the WEB!</u>   <u>Comments on our Web page?</u>

Fig. I-4 The home page for the library of the National Institute for Environmental Health Sciences (http://library.niehs.nih.gov/home.htm). This figure demonstrates the main elements of a typical Web page. Home.htm is an html file (a WWW document) that contains the text and instructions for creating the Web page. This Web page incorporates nine separate images: the two horizontal patterned lines and the seven square images. The images are downloaded from the Web server as separate files distinct from the home.html file. There are eight hypertext links on this page indicated by the underlined words. Clicking on a link retrieves another Web page or a gopher menu.

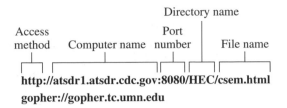

http://atsdr1.atsdr.cdc.gov:8080/HEC/csem.html

gopher://gopher.tc.umn.edu

Fig. I-5 Uniform resources locators. The World Wide Web utilizes uniform resource locators (URLs) to locate resources on the Internet. A URL has five main components: (1) an access method followed by a colon and two forward slashes, (2) the name or IP address of a computer on the Internet, (3) a colon followed by a port number, (4) a forward slash followed by a directory path to a file with directory and subdirectory names each followed by a forward slash, and (5) a file name. Additional elements, such as user input to a search program, are added to the right end of a URL. A port number identifies the location of a particular Internet service on a remote computer. All connections to remote computers occur through ports, numbered 1 through 65,535. Servers for commonly used Internet services operate through standard ports, such as World Wide Web, port 80; gopher, port 70; and E-mail, port 25. If a user does not specify a port on the remote computer, the standard port number is used. If a server uses a nonstandard port for a service, as in this illustration, the port number must be explicitly stated. See Table I-2 for a list of the access methods used in URLs and the standard port numbers of these services. The minimum information required in a URL is an access method and a computer name or IP address. If no directory or file names are given, the home page is usually displayed for a Web site; for gopher or ftp URLs, the main menu and the root directory, respectively, are displayed.

accessed by telnet. After connecting to an archie server, the user enters a search term. The server returns a list of file and directory names that contain the search term along with the sites at which they are located. It is important to understand that archie searches for file and directory names, not file contents. As an example, a public archie client at Rutgers University can be used to locate file names that contain the word *dioxin*. A user types:

>**telnet archie.rutgers.edu**
>login:**archie**
>archie>**prog dioxin**

The "prog" command is used to perform a search for a keyword, in this case, dioxin.

Of the many search programs on the WWW, Yahoo is one of the easiest to use. Yahoo lists sites by categories and subcategories. A user can search by choosing successive subcategories until a list of sites on a specific topic is found. Yahoo also permits keyword searching. Unlike archie, Yahoo can do limited searches of Web pages and returns a list of sites and documents that can be accessed by clicking on their names. The URL for Yahoo is http://www.yahoo.com.

Two programs that perform more exhaustive searches are the Webcrawler at http://www.webcrawler.com and Lycos at http://www.lycos.com. These sites do keyword searching and allow users to customize a search by setting various parameters. As with Yahoo, a list of sites is returned with

links to these sites. There are Web sites that contain lists of search engines with links to their home pages. One of these is the Meta-Index at CERN—the European Laboratory of Particle Physics at the University of Geneva in Switzerland. Its URL is http://cuiwww.unige.ch/meta-index.html. The MetaCrawler at the University of Washington (http://metacrawler.cs.washington.edu:8080) keeps a database of search engines and sends queries to all the engines when a user enters a search term. The MetaCrawler organizes the results and presents them to the user in a uniform format.

MEDICAL RESOURCES ON THE INTERNET

Several sites on the Internet catalog medical resources and can be used as starting points for searching for specific information. A few sites that have extensive references to general medical resources are discussed here, and more are listed in the Internet Resources and Suggested Reading sections. Most of these are on the World Wide Web, but some of the more important sites, such as the National Institutes of Health, can also be reached by gopher or occasionally telnet.

An important resource for many types of medical information is the National Institutes of Health, whose home page is located at http://www.nih.gov (gopher access at gopher.nih.gov). Web pages are available for all the institutes from this site. One of its many resources is CANCERNET at the National Cancer Institute (http://www.nci.nih.gov), which has information on all types of cancer arranged by organ system and cancer type under its Physician Data Query system (PDQ). Another resource is CANCERLIT (CANCER LITerature), a listing of citations and abstracts from the current cancer literature. The NIH home page has a link to the Guide to Grants and Contracts that details grants and program announcements at the NIH. Publications from several institutes are available, such as the Center for Disease Control and Prevention's CDC daily summaries and *Morbidity and Mortality Weekly Report*.

The National Library of Medicine can be reached by gopher (gopher.nlm.nih.gov) or the World Wide Web (http://www.nlm.nih.gov). There are numerous databases that can be accessed at this site. Some databases are free to the general public, such as CANCERLIT, AIDSLINE, and HSTAT (Health Services/Technology Assessment Texts), while others such as MEDLINE and TOXNET (*tox*icology *net*work) require personal accounts.

The University of Michigan sponsors the Clearinghouse for Subject Oriented Internet Resource Guides. This is one of the major projects for cataloging Internet resources and can be reached by gopher at una.hh.lib.umich.edu. The major feature at this site is a list of approximately 200 guides on multiple subjects, each of which is a more or less exhaustive listing of Internet resources on specific topics. About a dozen guides are related to health and medical subjects. The most comprehensive listing of general medical resources is the *Medical Resources—Clinical Guide* by Gary Malet and Lee

Hancock. A Web site that contains most of this material and is more easily accessed is the Medical Matrix at http://www.slackinc.com/matrix. There are several other lists of medical resources on the Internet. A compendium of these lists can be found at the American Medical Association's Web site, http://www.ama-assn.org/med_link/links.htm; the American College of Physicians, http://www.acponline.org is another high quality source of medical Web sites.

TOXICOLOGY RESOURCES

A large number of Internet sites offer toxicology and environmental health resources. An exhaustive review of these sites is not possible, but the major resources are described here, along with others of particular interest. As with all sites on the Internet, information changes rapidly. Individual Web pages, gopher documents, and occasionally entire Web sites may be changed or removed from the Internet. If a user has trouble locating a particular resource, the various search programs mentioned earlier can be used to find information. In addition, many sites have search functions for locating resources locally. Nearly all the sites described have a number of links to other toxicology sites which facilitates finding resources.

Government Agencies

The National Institutes of Health has a great deal of material on toxicology at the National Institute for Environmental Health Sciences (http://www.niehs.nih.gov). The home page has a bulletin board that lists meetings and events, postdoctoral fellowships, and grants and awards. Of the NIEHS publications that can be accessed from this page, the most important is *Environmental Health Perspectives,* the journal of the National Institute of Environmental Health Sciences. As with many other medical and scientific journals, abstracts of articles are available, along with other material such as indexes and editorials. A search program is available for finding information in the abstracts. There are online methods for subscribing to the printed version of the journal. A link to a mail program allows individuals to send comments and questions to the staff. Another Web server at the National Institute of Environmental Health Sciences is for the National Toxicology Program (NTP, http://ntp-server.niehs.nih.gov). Information on this server includes the complete biennial report on carcinogens, the NTP annual plan, and the NTP liaison office announcements. A bibliography of NTP publications is available with instructions for requesting reprints by email, fax, or telephone. A link on the home page lists other NTP participating agencies.

The National Center for Toxicological Research (NCTR), a branch of the Food and Drug Administration (FDA), has a gopher site at gopher.nctr.fda.gov. The mission of NTCR is to conduct peer-reviewed scientific research on the toxicity of products regulated by the FDA; to evaluate genetic aberrations, birth defects, cancer, and/or biochemical alterations in animals; and to develop methods to improve the FDA's assessment of human risk and exposure to hazardous substances. Research is organized under nine different program areas, such as the quantitative risk assessment program and the neurotoxicology program.

A Web site with extensive material is the Agency for Toxic Substances and Disease Registry (ATSDR) located at http://atsdr1.atsdr.cdc.gov:8080. A user-configurable search program for documents at this site is available on the home page. The ATSDR, an agency of the Public Health Service, performs specific functions relating to the effects on public health of hazardous substances in the environment. This site has a hazardous materials database that includes a map of the United States. Clicking on a state returns a list of sites in that state that are contaminated with hazardous materials along with ancillary information, such as health assessments and consultations for a site. A toxicologic profile database contains over 200 chemicals with online information about their toxicities. A useful document is ToxFAQ (toxicology frequently asked questions) that allows a quick search for information on common toxic chemicals. There is a separate list for the ATDSR/EPA's top 20 hazardous substances. Another link describes medical management guidelines for acute chemical exposures. Some of the chemical listed include ammonia, benzene, formaldehyde, phenol, and xylene. One interesting link at this site is the Case Studies in Environmental Medicine page (http://atsdr1.atsdr.cdc.gov:8080/HEC/csem.html), a self-instruction publication designed to increase a physician's knowledge about hazardous substances and to aid in the evaluation and treatment of patients. A user chooses a topic, such as lead or radon, and is presented information on the substance. A posttest can be taken that allows a physician to receive category I continuing medical education (CME) credits. Congressional testimony on toxicology and public health issues for the 103rd and later Congresses is also available.

Perhaps the most comprehensive source of toxicology information on the Internet is at the National Library of Medicine (NLM, http://www.nlm.nih.gov). Access to most of the information at NLM requires a personal account. Instructions for obtaining an account are available on the home page. There are two especially useful resources for toxicologic information at NLM: MEDLARS (*med*ical *l*iterature *a*nalysis and *r*etrieval *s*ystem) is a computerized system of databases oriented to biomedical research and patient care, such as MEDLINE and TOXLINE (a bibliographic database on the toxicity of drugs); TOXNET is similar to MEDLARS, offering files and databases on toxicology and related areas. A user can get a description of TOXNET at http://tamas.nlm.nih.gov/~boyda/htdocs/TOXNET/factsheets/toxnet.html. Eleven separate databases can be accessed through TOXNET, such as

HSDB (Hazardous Substances Data Bank), a databank of more than 4300 potentially hazardous chemicals with toxicity data, detection methods, and regulatory requirements cosponsored by ATSDR

RTECS (Registry of Toxic Effects of Chemical Substances), which contains descriptions of acute and chronic toxic effects on over 100,000 chemicals; the database is maintained by the National Institute for Occupational Safety and Health (NIOSH)

DART (Development and Reproductive Toxicology), a bibliographic database incorporating more than 14,000 literature citations on teratology published since 1989

Division of Specialized Information Services (sis.nlm.nih. gov), which gives a description of the Toxicology Information Outreach Project, a program for disseminating toxicologic and environmental information to historically black and minority universities

In addition to these services, several experimental Web pages are under development that provide an even greater range of references and services.

Universities

Major sources of medical and scientific information are Web sites at universities and research institutions. Many of the resources at these organizations are the work of one or a few individuals, rather than a dedicated staff such as at the NIH. For this reason, the quality of information is more variable. Several sites with interesting material are presented here. There are many other such sites on the Internet, often describing local programs and resources, that can be located with the search programs described previously.

Toxikon is a multimedia project from the emergency medicine department of the University of Illinois at Chicago developed by Mark Crockett (http://toxikon.uih.uic.edu/toxikon). Links at this site allow users to look up antidotes to common toxins and to access toxicology teaching cases. An interesting feature is *The Poison Review,* a bimonthly newsletter that critically analyzes articles in the current medical literature pertaining to toxicology. Articles relevant to clinical practice are reviewed and abstracts prepared. A selection of these articles is available at Toxikon, along with subscription information for the newsletter.

The University of Pittsburgh has a catalog of Internet toxicology resources listed on a Web page (http://www.pitt.edu/~martint) maintained by Thomas Martin. One set of links provides information on toxicology mailing lists such as ACMT-NET, Occ-Env-Med-L, Poison-Net, and ToxList (see the Internet resources section). Another link leads to a Web page devoted to poison information resources that contains, among other topics, a database of poison control centers.

Oregon State University hosts EXTOXNET—the Extension Toxicology Network, which can be reached by gopher (gopher://sulaco.oes.orst.edu/70/1/ext/extoxnet) or the WWW (http://ace.orst.edu/info/extoxnet). It is a toxicology information base and forum that is a cooperative undertaking of the University California at Davis, Michigan State University, Oregon State University, and Cornell. This site also has an automatic information mail server called ALMANAC that sends requests for toxicologic information by E-mail to individuals. Some of the resources at this site are toxicology fact sheets, pesticide information profiles (PIPs), and toxicology information briefs (TIBs), which are short descriptions of issues that pertain to pesticides such as health and environmental effects. The TIBs are intended to assist in the understanding and interpretation of PIPs.

Commercial Organizations

There are commercial organizations that deal with toxicology or have related material, primarily information sources, although other activities such as consulting firms advertising on the WWW are also represented. A few of the informational resources are described here. The Environmental Journalists Web page lists many of the previously mentioned Web sites and many others related to the environment. The Web page (http://www.sej.org) classifies environmental resources by topic and has a page devoted to chemicals and toxicology. The Chemical Industry Institute of Toxicology (CIIT) is located in Research Triangle Park, North Carolina (http://www.ciit.org). The home page describes CIIT as a not-for-profit toxicology research institute dedicated to providing an improved scientific basis for understanding and assessing the potential adverse effects of chemicals, pharmaceuticals, and consumer products on human health. It is supported by approximately 50 industrial organizations. Cambridge Scientific Abstracts (http://www.csa.com) provides access to a large database of scientific and medical information. A personal account is required to use this service. One service available at this site is Environmental RouteNet, which accesses both public and proprietary resources such as TOXLINE.

CONCLUDING REMARKS

The Internet opens a new vista of communication that allows individuals to access information around the world. A variety of medical resources are available through the Internet, and, undoubtedly, more will become available in the future. The Internet and telecommunications in general are rapidly growing areas. In the future, new technologies will allow faster communications that permit high speed applications such as real-time audio and video services to be offered over the Internet. These advances in telecommunications have implications for the medical field that are just beginning to be realized.

SUGGESTED READING

There are many articles in the medical literature on the Internet, but better sources of information are books on the Internet. There are hundreds of books about the Internet, ranging from general introductions to specific topics such as the World Wide Web, E-mail, USENET, and Netscape. The books and articles listed here are introductory material on the Internet, as well as a few sources for general medical information.

INTERNET-RELATED MATERIAL

Duntemann J, Pronk R, Vincent P: *Web explorer pocket companion,* Foster City, Calif, 1995, IDG Books Worldwide.

Flynn P: *The World Wide Web handbook: an HTML guide for users, authors, and publishers,* London, 1995, International Thompson Computer Press.

Glowniak JV: An introduction to the Internet, part III: Internet services, *J Nucl Med Technol* 23:231, 1995.

Kehoe BP: *Zen and the art of the Internet. A beginner's guide,* Englewood Cliffs, NJ, 1994, PTR Prentice Hall.

Krol E: *The whole Internet: user's guide & catalog,* ed 2, Sebastopol, Calif, 1994, O'Reilly & Associates.

Levine J: *Internet for dummies quick reference,* Foster City, Calif, 1994, IDG Books Worldwide.

Manger J: *Netscape navigator,* London, 1995, McGraw-Hill.

Schatz BR, Hardin JB: NCSA Mosaic and World Wide Web: global hypermedia protocols for the Internet, *Science* 265:895, 1994.

GENERAL MEDICAL RESOURCES

Glowniak JV: Medical resources on the Internet, *Ann Intern Med* 123:123, 1995.

Hancock L: *Physicians' guide to the Internet,* Philadelphia, 1995, Lippincott-Raven Publishers.

McKinney WP et al: A guide to Mosaic and the World Wide Web for physicians, *M D Computing* 12:109, 1995.

INTERNET RESOURCES

All references except for E-mail addresses are given as uniform resource locators (URLs), the format required for Web browsers. To access telnet, ftp, and gopher sites with text-based, nonbrowser programs, use the appropriate access command followed by the site name. For example, to connect to the InterNIC by telnet with a Web browser, a user enters **telnet://rs.internic.net.** On a UNIX system, the command **telnet rs.internic.net** would be used.

General Internet Resources

University of North Carolina	Public text-based Web browser telnet://public.sunsite. unc.edu. Login:lynx
University of Minnesota	Gopher server with multiple links gopher://gopher.tc.umn.edu
University of Illinois, Urbana-Champaign	FTP access to Internet application programs ftp://ftp.ncsa.uiuc.edu. Mosaic programs are found in the Web/Mosaic directory
Netscape Corporation	Information on how to obtain Netscape http://home.netscape.com
Rutgers University	Public archie client program telnet://archie.rutgers.edu. Login: archie

University of Michigan	Clearinghouse for Subject Oriented Internet Resource Guides gopher:// una.hh.lib.umich.edu
Internet Network Information Center (InterNIC)	Internet information source and databases telnet://rs.internic.net. Login: whois http://www.internic.net

World Wide Web Search Programs

AltaVista	http://altavista.digital.com
The Webcrawler	http://www.webcrawler.com
Lycos	http://www.lycos.com
Yahoo	http://www.yahoo.com
CERN—European Laboratory of Particle Physics	http://cuiwww.unige.ch/meta-index.html
MetaCrawler, University of Washington	http://metacrawler.cs.washington.edu:8080

Medical Resources

National Institutes of Health	http://www.nih.gov gopher://gopher.nih.gov
National Cancer Institute	http://www.nci.nih.gov
National Library of Medicine	http://www.nlm.nih.gov
Virtual Hospital, University of Iowa	http://vh.radiology.uiowa.edu
World Health Organization	http://www.who.ch
American Medical Association	http://www.ama-assn.org
British Medical Journal	http://www.bmj.com/bmj
American College of Physicians	http://www.acponline.org
Medical Matrix	http://www.slackinc.com/matrix
American Medical Association	http://www.ama-assn.org/med_link/links.htm
MEDWEB at Emory University	http://www.gen.emory.edu/MEDWEB/keyword.html

Toxicology Resources

Mailing lists

ALMANAC, E-mail server: for catalog of resources, send message for general information, send message	Almanac@sulaco.oes.orst.edu send extoxnet catalog send guide

ACMT-NET—For members of the American College of Medical Toxicology. For information, send E-mail to Paul Pentel, pente001@maroon.tc.umn.edu or Steve Curry, stevec@samaritan.edu

Occ-Env-Med-L—Occupational and Environmental Medicine Mailing List at Duke University. To subscribe, send message "subscribe occ-env-med-1" or "subscribe occ-env-med-1-digest" (for a digest) to majordomo@list.mc.duke.edu. For more information, consult http://dmi-www.mc.duke.edu/oem or send E-mail to the above address with the message "info occ-env-med-1".

Poison-Net—For information, contact http://www1.pitt.edu/~martint/pages/poisonet.htm or send message "info poison-net" to listproc@ucdavis.edu.

ToxList—For information contact Geoff Rule at gsr1@cornell.edu

Government agencies

National Institute of Environmental Health Sciences — http://www.niehs.nih.gov

Agency for Toxic Substances and Disease Registry — http://atsdr1.atsdr.cdc.gov:8080

National Center for Toxicological Research, FDA — gopher://gopher.nctr.fda.gov

National Toxicology Program, NIEHS — http://ntp-server.niehs.nih.gov

TOXNET, National Library of Medicine — http://tamas.nlm.nih.gov/~boyda/htdocs/TOXNET/factsheets/toxnet.html

Specialized Information Services, NLM — http://sis.nlm.nih.gov

Tri-Service Toxicology Consortium — Military toxicology information http://www.navy.al.wpafb.af.mil

Environmental Protection Agency — http://www.epa.gov

Universities

University of Illinois at Chicago — Toxikon project http://toxikon.uih.uic.edu/toxikon

University of Pittsburgh — http://www.pitt.edu/~martint

University of Oregon — EXTOXNET gopher://sulaco.oes.orst.edu/70/1/ext/extoxnet
http://ace.orst.edu/info/extoxnet

Kansas University Medical Center, Dept. of Pharmacology, Toxicity, and Therapeutics — http://www.kumc.edu/research/medicine/pharmacology/dhp.html

University of Oklahoma, Toxicology Program — http://www.cpb.uokhsc.edu/cop/tox/outox.html

Johns Hopkins Community of Science, Genome Database — A database of NIH funded toxicology research http://cos.gdb.org/best/fedfund/nih-select/toxicology.html

University of Utah — Material Safety Data Sheets gopher://atlas.chem.utah.edu/70/11/MSDS

National University of Singapore — Poisons Information Database http://vhp.nus.sg/PID

Commercial and other organizations

Cambridge Scientific Abstracts — http://www.csa.com

Environmental journalism — http://www.sej.org

Chemical Industry Institute of Toxicology — http://www.ciit.org

Appendix II

Review Questions

CHAPTER 1 A BRIEF HISTORY OF OCCUPATIONAL, INDUSTRIAL, AND ENVIRONMENTAL TOXICOLOGY

Match the following environmental release with the appropriate location.

Principal toxin		Location/year
1. ___ Methyl isocyanate	**A**	Minimata Bay, Japan, 1950s
2. ___ Aldicarb	**B**	Serveso, Italy, 1976
3. ___ HCN gas	**C**	Turkey, 1956
4. ___ Methylmercury	**D**	Texas, 1990
5. ___ Dioxin	**E**	Staffordshire, England, 1900s
6. ___ TOCP (ginger jake)	**F**	Louisville, Kentucky, 1960–1970
7. ___ Hexachlorobenzene	**G**	Ann Arbor, Michigan, 1975
8. ___ Hydrofluoric acid	**H**	Bhopal, India, 1984
9. ___ Carbon dioxide	**I**	United States, 1930
10. ___ Cadmium	**J**	Cleveland Clinic, Cleveland, Ohio, 1928
11. ___ PAHs	**K**	Ypres, Belgium, 1915
12. ___ Arsenic	**L**	California, 1985
13. ___ Mustard gas	**M**	Lake Nyos, Cameroon, 1986
14. ___ Vinyl chloride	**N**	Epping, England, 1965
15. ___ Cyanide	**O**	Japan, 1939
16. ___ Pancuronium	**P**	Manchester, England, 1910
17. ___ Chlordecone	**Q**	Donora, Pennsylvania, 1948
18. ___ Methylene dianiline	**R**	James River, Virginia, 1973
19. ___ Photochemical air pollution	**S**	Guyana, 1978

CHAPTER 2 ARTISTS AND ARTISANS

1. Glazes are dangerous to the artist during all of the following phases of production except
   a. initial powder form
   b. application to ceramics
   c. during firing
   d. after firing
2. An artist presents to your office asking you to develop a safety program for his busy silk screen shop in his garage. You explain why this will be difficult for him but inadvertently give him one piece of bad advice. Which is it?
   a. Adhering to PELs assures artists a wide margin of safety.
   b. He cannot rely on labeling to identify potential problem toxins.
   c. The design of their workshop, especially with ventilation, is important.
   d. Training in safe practices is essential.
3. A young ceramicist complains of fatigue, back pain, disequilibrium, and leg pain. Which one of the following would be least likely to cause these problems?
   a. Mercury
   b. Cadmium
   c. Lead
   d. Solvents
   e. Carbon Monoxide

CHAPTER 3 ATHLETES

1. Significant nitrogen dioxide exposures can produce all of the following except
   a. methemoglobinemia
   b. bronchiolitis fibrosa obliterans
   c. noncardiogenic pulmonary edema
   d. nonlactate metabolic acidosis
   e. aplastic anemia
2. Risks to swimmers competing in indoor swimming pools include all of the following except
   a. contact dermatitis
   b. erosion of dental enamel termed *swimmers' erosion*
   c. hepatitis
   d. increased alveolar chloroform concentrations
3. Which of the following would be consistent with androgenic anabolic steroid abuse?
   a. Delayed closure of epiphyseal growth plates
   b. Increased serum high-density lipoproteins (HDL)
   c. Peliosis hepatis
   d. Hypoglycemia
   e. Decreased libido

4. Which presentation would *not* be consistent with hypervitaminosis A?
   a. Desquamating erythematous rash
   b. Sensory peripheral neuropathy
   c. Hair loss
   d. Hepatotoxicity
   e. Pseudotumor cerebri
5. A 32-year-old, otherwise healthy male bodybuilder presents to the emergency department comatose with new-onset seizures. He has a history of ingesting nutritional supplements. This presentation would be most consistent with which nutritional supplement?
   a. γ-hydroxybutyrate
   b. Tryptophan
   c. Arginine
   d. Vitamin D
   e. Ornithine
6. A few days prior to an international athletic competition, a soccer player develops signs of an upper respiratory tract infection with fever, cough, nasal congestion, and sinus pressure. As the patient's physician, what is the best treatment advice?
   a. Instruct the athlete to take an over-the-counter cold preparation, since nonprescription medications are not restricted.
   b. Give the athlete a written prescription for a decongestant, instruct him to declare all medications prior to competition, and send written notification to the head physician responsible for the athletic event.
   c. Prescribe pseudoephedrine, a decongestant whose use is not restricted by the International Olympic Committee.
   d. Consult the athletic governing body under which the athlete is competing as to the status of a particular medication.
7. Based upon chlorine's high water solubility, the major toxicologic effects would be expected to be exerted on
   a. upper airway
   b. lower airway
   c. kidneys
   d. liver
8. In which occupation would an exposure to nitrogen dioxide be uncommon?
   a. Missile site personnel
   b. Silo filler
   c. Indoor ice skating rink personnel
   d. Manufacturer of lacquers and jet fuel
   e. Manufacturer of rubber and plastics

CHAPTER 4 AVIATION PERSONNEL

1. The liquid phase of gasoline
   a. contains a greater percentage of aromatic hydrocarbons than the vapor phase
   b. contains no benzene
   c. is mostly aromatics
   d. consists of long-chain (c_{18} and greater) hydrocarbons
2. JP-4
   a. is pure napthene hydrocarbons
   b. produces no carbon monoxide in a fire
   c. is a blend of AVGAS and kerosene
   d. contains no lead

3. AVGAS
   a. always has a higher lead content than U.S. auto fuel
   b. never has a lower octane rating than auto fuel
   c. contains 30% benzene
   d. is soluble in water
4. Hydraulic fluids
   a. cause dermatitis
   b. have large amounts of tri-ortho cresyl phosphate
   c. are in aircraft systems but no more than a few quarts
   d. have no petroleum distillates

CHAPTER 5 CARPENTERS AND LOGGERS

1. A characteristic of hypersensitivity pneumonitis that differentiates it from organic toxic dust syndrome is that
   a. it requires repetitive exposure to the inciting agent
   b. patients may present very ill-appearing with an acute flulike illness, respiratory distress, and a fever as high as 41° C
   c. it may occur after exposure to more than one type of organic dust of 1 to 5 microns in size
   d. avoidance of the inciting agent is the key to treatment and management
   e. bronchial hyperactivity may be found on methacholine challenge
2. Nasal carcinoma in woodworkers has definitively been linked to all of the following except
   a. phenol
   b. turpenes
   c. formaldehyde
   d. coal tar pitch volatiles
   e. alcohol consumption
3. All of the following are true of pulmonary symptoms in woodworkers except
   a. decline in FEV_1 across the workweek has been shown to be correlated with long-term pulmonary dysfunction
   b. pulp and papermill workers showed an inverse relation between length of employment and pulmonary function
   c. asthma due to occupational exposure to western red cedar is mediated by plicatic acid–specific immunoglobulins
   d. methyl mercaptan, hydrogen sulfide, and chlorine are commonly encountered pulmonary toxins in pulp and paper mills
4. The dermatoses listed below have been linked to these causal agents except
   a. mahogany and irritant dermatitis
   b. pentachlorophenol and chloracne
   c. nickel in tools and contact dermatitis
   d. benzene and toxic vitiligo
   e. TCMBT and dry, peeling skin
5. The use of the fungicide pentachlorophenol has been linked to all of the following toxic effects except
   a. excessive release of heat
   b. gastrointestinal complaints
   c. non-Hodgkin's lymphoma
   d. blindness
   e. interference with oxidative phosphorylation

6. Of this list of compounds to which carpenters and loggers may be exposed, there is evidence to support the role of each as a human carcinogen except
   a. toluene
   b. benzene
   c. coal tar pitch volatiles
   d. epoxy resins
   e. phenol
7. Which one of the following is true regarding hypersensitivity pneumonitis?
   a. Granulomatous lesions are not found on lung biopsy.
   b. Endotoxin's role in the etiology accounts for all symptoms in the studies reported to date.
   c. There is evidence to support the role of inhaled hexachlorobenzene in the development of hypersensitivity pneumonitis in pigeon breeders.
   d. The IgE levels are often elevated.
   e. Bronchospasm excludes the diagnosis.
8. Which of the following statements regarding respiratory problems in carpenters and loggers is true?
   a. Woodworkers exposed to medium-density fiberboard have been shown to have decreased mucociliary function compared with workers using traditional fiberboard.
   b. The rotten egg odor of hydrogen sulfide warns a victim of exposure at all concentrations above 100 to 150 ppm.
   c. Sulfur dioxide is a colorless gas that is more readily deposited in the lower airways.
   d. Only inhaled substances can induce hypersensitivity pneumonitis.
9. All of the following appear to have some role in the development of hypersensitivity pneumonitis except
   a. endotoxin
   b. histamine
   c. concomitant pulmonary infection
   d. immune regulation via suppressor T cells
   e. serum precipitating antibodies

CHAPTER 6 CONCRETE WORKERS AND MASONS

1. The most common cause of cement-induced dermatitis is
   a. chromium
   b. zinc
   c. cobalt
   d. nickel
2. All of the following have been shown to decrease the incidence of cement-induced dermatitis except
   a. addition of ferrous sulfate to cement
   b. addition of lime to cement
   c. rapid decontamination
   d. protective gloves
3. The treatment of cement-induced skin disease includes all of the following except
   a. prevention
   b. topical steroids
   c. increase exposure to allow acclimation
   d. antibiotics for superinfections

4. The most common cement-induced respiratory disease is?
   a. Asbestoses
   b. Silicosis
   c. Chronic obstructive pulmonary disease
   d. Oat cell carcinoma
5. Which of the following are false concerning chromium?
   a. It causes mutation when reduction occurs in close proximity to the nucleus.
   b. It is added to cement to improve its strength.
   c. The trivalent form is carcinogenic.
   d. Chromium content in U.S. cement is less than 0.2%.
6. To decrease the potential pulmonary irritation, NIOSH has recommended all of the following except
   a. periodic air sampling
   b. water application to the cutting blade
   c. respiratory protection for 50 mg/m^3 parts cement dust or more
   d. yearly chest radiographs

CHAPTER 7 DIVERS

1. The biologic effects of a gas are determined by
   a. relative concentration in the total breathing gas
   b. percent of the total gas mixture
   c. partial pressure of the gas
   d. valence of the gas
2. Oxygen
   a. was first recognized to have toxicity in patients requiring prolonged mechanical ventilation
   b. is a CNS, pulmonary, and retinal toxin primarily
   c. is detoxified by free radicals
   d. never should be a cause for a seizure in a patient who has been taken off oxygen in a HBO chamber
3. Nitrogen narcosis
   a. is rarely encountered in amateur diving
   b. can be lessened if the diver is a regular drinker of alcohol
   c. can be lessened if the diver has a small amount of alcohol before the dive
   d. is exacerbated by carbon dioxide
4. The so-called high-pressure neurologic syndrome
   a. was first identified by Behnke in the mid 1930s
   b. is seen in patients who require long-term ventilator care
   c. can be life-threatening
   d. is associated with cardiac conduction disturbances
5. Which of the following have been known to contaminate the breathing supply of divers?
   a. CO
   b. CO_2
   c. Oil vapors
   d. Any gas or vapor
   e. All of the above
6. Sources of CO_2 to which divers are exposed include all of the following except
   a. excess production due to work and elevated metabolism
   b. microorganisms
   c. inadequate ventilation systems
   d. diver's own air supply
   e. exhausted CO_2 absorbent

7. Which of the following represents the symptom triad associated with CO_2 intoxication?
   a. Ataxia, aphasia, dysphonia
   b. Asterixis, diarrhea, seizures
   c. Clonus, nystagmus, dysphonia
   d. Dyspnea, somnolence, headache
8. The most common form of visual disturbance associated with oxygen toxicity is
   a. blurred vision
   b. double vision
   c. impaired ability to accommodate
   d. tunnel vision
   e. rotatory nystagmus
9. The primary enzyme responsible for degradation of superoxides is
   a. alcohol dehydrogenase
   b. aldehyde dehydrogenase
   c. SOD
   d. epoxide dysmutase
10. Oxygen exerts its toxicity primarily on which two systems?
    a. GI and hematologic
    b. CNS and skin
    c. CNS and cardiac
    d. GU and CNS
    e. CNS and pulmonary

CHAPTER 8 DOCTORS, NURSES, AND DENTISTS

1. The most significant route of exposure for elemental mercury is
   a. dermal
   b. enteral (GI)
   c. inhalation of vapors
2. Severe, large exposures of inhaled mercury vapor resulting in acute bronchiolitis may be treated with
   a. intubation and oxygenation
   b. chelation with BAL (British anti-lewisite)
   c. chelation with DMSA (Succimer)
   d. all of the above
3. Ethylene oxide is classified as a probable human carcinogen based on
   a. animal studies demonstrating malignancy
   b. several cohort studies demonstrating increased incidence of leukemia
   c. evidence of sister chromatid exchanges and DNA morphology alterations in humans
   d. all of the above
4. Chronic exposure in humans to nitrous oxide in poorly ventilated settings or with repeated recreational abuse has been associated with
   a. leukemia
   b. lung cancer
   c. peripheral neuropathy
   d. colon cancer
5. Formaldehyde inhalation has been most closely associated with which of the following malignancies in animals?
   a. Bladder cancer
   b. Hepatoma
   c. Testicular cancer
   d. Nasopharyngeal cancer

6. Which of the following have been associated with occupational exposure to the general anaesthetic halothane?
   a. Diarrhea
   b. Peripheral neuropathy
   c. Hepatitis
   d. Lung cancer

CHAPTER 9 DOMESTIC AND BUILDING MAINTENANCE WORKERS

1. All of the following combinations of cleaning agents result in liberation of irritant or toxic gas except
   a. ammonia and sodium hypochlorite
   b. bleach, urine, and HCl
   c. HCl and sodium hypochlorite
   d. water and bleach
2. Decontamination of phenol burns is best accomplished by
   a. water
   b. polyethyleneglycol solutions
   c. creosol
   d. ammonia
3. HF dermal exposures
   a. should be treated as if they were thermal burns
   b. generally appear like normal skin after exposure
   c. respond to cortisone cream application
   d. are painless
4. All of the following are true of calcium therapy for HF exposures except
   a. topical application of calcium gluconate is the preferred initial therapy after decontamination
   b. injections of calcium chloride are necessary for severe burns
   c. intraarterial calcium gluconate is indicated for extensive burns of the hand which do not respond to topical application
   d. nebulized calcium gluconate is useful for pulmonary exposures

CHAPTER 10 DRY CLEANERS

1. The chemical characteristics that give perc its particular toxicity include all of the following except
   a. affinity for lipid tissues
   b. chlorinated hydrocarbon
   c. water solubility
   d. volatile
2. Pulmonary absorption of perc
   a. is not the main route of occupational exposure
   b. is followed by rapid, near-total pulmonary elimination
   c. is decreased by high tidal volumes
   d. is minimal
3. Hepatotoxicity from perc
   a. is common and usually results in mild elevation of LFTs
   b. is probably from an epoxide intermediate
   c. is uncommon because perc is 90% eliminated by the kidneys
   d. occurs only with large acute exposures

4. All of the following are useful acutely and the days following after perc exposure except
   a. breath concentration of perc
   b. serum concentration of perc
   c. LFTs
   d. bun/creatinine

5. Tetrachlorethylene is also known as which of the following?
   a. PCE
   b. Perc
   c. Perchloroethylene
   d. All of the above

6. The most commonly used solvent in the dry cleaning industry is
   a. TCE
   b. F-113
   c. 1,1,1-trichloroethylene
   d. perc
   e. TIDE

7. Stoddard solvent contains of all of the following except
   a. paraffins
   b. naphthalene
   c. aromatic hydrocarbons
   d. benzene
   e. petroleum

8. Perc is eliminated primarily by
   a. kidneys
   b. lungs
   c. enterohepatic circulation
   d. skin and hair
   e. stool

9. Intravascular hemolysis has been reported following acute exposure to
   a. benzene
   b. TCE
   c. chloroform
   d. Perchloroethylene
   e. CCl_4

10. The treatment for acute exposure to perc is
    a. mainly supportive
    b. naloxone
    c. chelation
    d. DMSA

CHAPTER 11 ELECTRICIANS

1. Toxicity from PCBs is determined by
   a. the viscosity of the fluid
   b. the percentage of furans, dioxins, and PCQs
   c. the pH of the fluid
   d. the age of the fluid

2. Furans and dioxins are produced when
   a. acids react with PCBs
   b. chlorinated gases are used in production processes
   c. PCBs are heated
   d. PCBs are exposed to sunlight

3. The typical manifestations of PCB toxicity are
   a. nonspecific complaints such as headache and fatigue
   b. chloracne and laboratory hepatitis
   c. retinal depigmentation
   d. chronic muscle wasting

CHAPTER 12 ELECTROPLATERS

1. What are the manifestations of renal toxicity from cadmium?
2. What are the manifestations of the effects of cadmium on bone metabolism?
3. Where are nonoccupational sources of cadmium found?
4. What is the significance of the low-molecular-weight proteins in cadmium toxicity?
5. What is the role of metallothionein in cadmium toxicity?
6. What is the difference in toxicity between trivalent chromium (Cr^{+3}) and hexavalent chromium (Cr^{+6})?

CHAPTER 13 EXTERMINATORS

1. Muscarinic effects of organophosphate poisoning include
   a. respiratory muscle weakness
   b. tachycardia
   c. bronchorrhea
   d. fasciculations

2. Delayed effects of organophosphate toxicity
   a. are possible only if the patient had an acute toxicity requiring 2-PAM
   b. may actually be patients with ongoing absorption of OP without sufficient 2-PAM and atropine
   c. usually manifest as incontinence and cranial nerve pathology
   d. are seen only with carbamates

3. Pyrethrums and synthetic pyrethroids
   a. are rapid acting
   b. are extremely toxic to humans when mixed with piperonyl butoxide
   c. can "age" to the sodium channel
   d. are stored in adipose tissue

4. Atropine
   a. is contraindicated in organophosphate poisoned patients who are tachycardic
   b. should be given in small doses
   c. decreases the effectiveness of 2-PAM when treating carbamates
   d. should always be used when 2-PAM is used

5. Pyrethrin toxicity is characterized by
   a. rash, atrial fibrillation, hepatic carcinoma
   b. rash, wheeze, agitation
   c. bronchorrhea, lethargy, vomiting
   d. pulmonary fibrosis, peripheral neurologic symptoms, prolonged QT syndrome

CHAPTER 14 FARMERS AND FARM PERSONNEL

1. Anhydrous ammonia
   a. is a liquid at atmospheric pressure
   b. is non-toxic in its gaseous form
   c. has an odor threshold below its irritant threshold
   d. burns should not be decontaminated with copious water

2. Manure pits
   a. generate simple asphyxiants and metabolic toxins, but have high ambient oxygen concentrations
   b. are not associated with hazards unless skin contact with waste occurs
   c. do not require self contained breathing apparatus for safe entrance
   d. have potentially explosive levels of methane

3. All of the following are true of silos except
   a. Oxygen limited silos produce oxides of nitrogen.
   b. Conventional silos capture carbon dioxide.
   c. Trench silos are relatively safe from respiratory hazards.
   d. The danger from toxic gases is limited to the silo itself.

CHAPTER 15 FIREFIGHTERS

1. The thermal degradation of organic material in oxygen poor environments is
   a. combustion
   b. pyrolysis
   c. smoke
   d. products of combustion
2. Smoke inhalation as an independent variable increases mortality because of cutaneous burns by
   a. 10%
   b. 20%
   c. 50%
   d. 95%
3. Acrolein has been associated with all of the following except
   a. pulmonary edema
   b. skin burns
   c. ciliastasis
   d. decreased respiratory rate
4. Hydrogen cyanide is produced by the combustion of which of the following except
   a. wool
   b. silk
   c. nylon
   d. asphalt
   e. all of the above
5. The bronchospasm caused by inhalation of irritant gases is best treated with
   a. hyperbaric oxygen
   b. epinephrine
   c. inhaled B_2 agonists
   d. inhaled steroids
6. The generally accepted criteria for treating fire victims with hyperbaric oxygen include all of the following except
   a. carboxyhemoglobin greater than 30
   b. pregnant females
   c. persistent neurologic findings
   d. soot stained sputum

CHAPTER 16 FLOOR AND CARPET LAYERS

1. Methacrylate metabolism
   a. is carried out by cytochrome P-450
   b. occurs for only a small percentage of methacrylate, as it is largely eliminated unchanged in the kidney
   c. occurs in many tissues but especially the kidney
   d. results in hippuric acid formation
2. Methacrylate can be classified as a
   a. potent teratogen
   b. potent carcinogen
   c. potent embryotoxin
   d. weak mitogen

3. The following chemical changes increase the sensitizer effect of acrylates:
   a. α-methylation
   b. increased acrylic double bonds
   c. polymerization
   d. UV curing
4. The following method of hand protection is the minimum requirement for successful prevention of dermatitis:
   a. latex gloves
   b. vinyl gloves
   c. double gloving with latex gloves
   d. 0.48-mm butyl rubber gloves
   e. 0.07-mm-thick 4-H gloves
5. Acrylic acids and esters have been demonstrated to cause
   a. Raynaud's phenomenon
   b. wrist drop
   c. axonopathy
   d. demylenating neuropathy

CHAPTER 17 FLORISTS AND GROUNDSKEEPERS

1. Dithiocarbamates have all of the following properties except
   a. disulfiram reaction with alcohol
   b. potent skin and mucous membrane sensitizers
   c. multiple carbon-sulfur bonds
   d. inhibition of cholinesterase
2. Plant dermatitis occurs by all of the following mechanisms except
   a. mechanical irritation
   b. allergic sensitization
   c. photosensitization
   d. pseudophytodermatitis
3. Pentachlorophenol cannot
   a. uncouple oxidative phosphorylation
   b. induce myocardial sensitization
   c. cause thyroid cancer
   d. produce chloracne
4. A patient occupationally exposed to an organotin compound would be expected to have which one of the following?
   a. Gastric carcinoma
   b. Peripheral neuropathy
   c. Blue discoloration of the skin
   d. Cardiac arrest
5. Concerning poison ivy:
   a. It is an insignificant problem in occupational medicine.
   b. Urushiol is considered the toxic component.
   c. The rash develops about a week after exposure in previously exposed workers.
   d. Hyposensitization should be considered if the patient may be reexposed.
6. Which group contains the common phytophotosensitizers?
   a. Sesquiterpene lactones
   b. Alkylcatechols
   c. Quinones
   d. Furocoumarins

CHAPTER 18 FOOD PREPARATION PERSONNEL

1. The respiratory symptoms of meat-wrapper's asthma are exacerbated by all of the following except
   a. types of additives to the plastic
   b. the amount of phthalic anhydride in the fumes created by heating
   c. history of cigarette smoking
   d. temperature to which the plastic is heated
   e. use of a self-adhesive glue when applying the product label
2. Individuals in the food industry may be exposed to furocoumarins (psoralens) and develop a phytophotodermatitis. This is most commonly seen in those handling which of the following?
   a. Kale
   b. Artichoke hearts
   c. Leeks
   d. Celery
   e. Squash
3. Individuals handling fish may acquire which of the following problems as a result of direct contact with the fish slime?
   a. Erysipeloid
   b. Grain itch
   c. Paronychia
   d. Deep space infection of the hand
4. Which of the following substances is responsible for the development of meat wrapper's asthma?
   a. Zinc
   b. Mellitic anhydride
   c. Phthalic anhydride
   d. Plicatic acid
5. All of the following statements regarding meat wrapper's asthma are true except
   a. Most of the symptomatology is related to the respiratory system.
   b. Any worker who uses a hot wire to cut plastic or uses heat to attach labels is at risk.
   c. Prevalence rates range from 12% to 80%.
   d. Cardiac arrythmias are commonly associated with meat wrapper's asthma.

CHAPTER 19 HAIRDRESSERS AND COSMETOLOGISTS

1. The most common allergen to induce allergic contact dermatitis in hairdressers is
   a. glyceryl monothioglycolate (GMTG)
   b. nickel
   c. phenylenediamine
   d. hydrogen peroxide
2. Which of the following statements is true?
   a. Dermatitis of the palms of the hands is characteristic of hairdresser's dermatitis.
   b. Hairdressers with allergic contact dermatitis to glyceryl monothioglycolate can work with ammonium thioglycolate.
   c. Positive patch tests aid in the diagnosis of thesaurosis.
   d. Hairdressers with a history of atopy should not be patch tested.

3. Thesaurosis is a lung storage disease believed to be linked to exposure to
   a. polyvinylpyrrolidone
   b. formaldehyde
   c. dimethylhydantoin
   d. lanolin
4. Which of the following statements is true?
   a. There exists no animal model for thesaurosis.
   b. Multiple epidemiologic studies have linked thesaurosis and exposure to aerosol cosmetics.
   c. The presence of PAS-positive lesions confirms the diagnosis of thesaurosis.
   d. Thesaurosis should be treated with sodium cromolyn.
5. Which one of these statements is false?
   a. Exposure to brilliantine is linked to bladder cancer.
   b. Most case-control studies suffer from recall biases.
   c. Exposure to aerosols is linked to lung cancer.
   d. Exposure to bromates is linked to cardiac failure.

CHAPTER 20 JEWELERS

1. Which of the following dermal conditions is least likely to occur in a jeweler?
   a. Skin abrasions and burns
   b. Allergic contact dermatitis
   c. Black dermographism
   d. Argyria
   e. Chloracne
2. A jeweler whose task is electroplating complains of dyspnea. Which of these chemicals is least likely to be a cause of this complaint?
   a. Gold potassium cyanide
   b. Copper cyanide
   c. Potassium cyanide
   d. Nickel sulfate
   e. Phenol (carbolic acid)
3. Which of the following metals is associated with black dermographism?
   a. Silver
   b. Gold
   c. Antimony
   d. Zinc
   e. Iron
4. Which of the following alloys, which is often a component of pierced earrings, is commonly associated with cutaneous hypersensitivity and atopic eczema?
   a. Nickel
   b. Silver
   c. Brass
   d. Aluminum
   e. Cobalt

5. From the following histories of present illness, which symptom complex represents the most common type of systemic illness encountered in jewelers?
   a. A 50-year-old man who drills metal settings presents with numbness, tingling, and erythema of his fingertips of several years' duration. The symptoms appear to be worse when the weather is cold.
   b. A 49-year-old man with tremor and rigidity of his extremities and progressive, occasional confusion that has developed over the past year. His job involves the application of gold and silver finishes to soldered items.
   c. A 46-year-old woman who files gem stones presents with episodic sneezing, rhinorrhea, and dry cough. She has had two episodes of wheezing that required β-agonist inhalational therapy at the local emergency department within the past 8 months.
   d. A 30-year-old male solderer with a complaint of persistent headache and periodic sleeplessness for 2 weeks.
   e. A 29-year-old man responsible for pickling plate metals presents with colicky abdominal pain, flatulence, and three episodes of explosive diarrhea.

CHAPTER 21 MECHANICS

1. Describe the "degreaser flush" phenomenon.
2. What are the most common types of chemicals mechanics encounter and their route of exposure?
3. What is the role of determining hydrocarbon concentrations in biologic samples? Why are they a better indicator of worker exposure than workplace air samples?
4. What special considerations must be taken into account in interpreting biologic samples?
5. What is the most important health aspect to monitor in solvent-exposed workers?

CHAPTER 22 MILITARY PERSONNEL

1. You are coming out of the military clinic where you work, when you are pinned down by a news crew about your reaction to a recent article that appeared in the *New York Times*. Diligent reports there made a careful comparison between cancer rates of Persian Gulf war veterans and comparable figures from a national cancer registry and concluded that the veterans were twice as likely to develop cancer as the national average. Discuss the strengths or weaknesses of such a study and how you would tend to view the results.
2. Background: You are tasked to determine the likelihood that a patient's symptoms result from an occupational exposure. The patient is a 35-year-old male F-16 crew chief complaining of dyspnea and headache. He is just getting over a case of bronchitis and has been sleep-deprived due to a new baby at home plus exams he has been studying for in night school. The patient responded 2 days ago to an F-16 "hot-foot" by dousing the front landing gear of the aircraft with a fire extinguisher, which he tells you contained "1211." He tells you that the brake pads, which contain a high level of magnesium, were so hot they were about to "flash."

Question: What is the chemical formula of halon 1211?
Question: What is the likelihood that his symptoms are occupationally related, and what (if any) is the mechanism of action?
   a. Symptoms are *not* occupationally related, continue treatment for bronchitis, refer to family-practice clinic.
   b. Symptoms are *not* occupational related, recommend the patient catch up on sleep, refer to family-practice clinic.
   c. Symptoms *are* occupationally related, symptoms are due to CNS and cardiac dysrhythmias caused by Halon 1211 reacting at high temperatures. Document occupational exposure, and recommend follow-up exams of cardiopulmonary function.
   d. Symptoms *are* occupationally related, symptoms are "metal fume fever" due to exposure to magnesium metal fumes. Document occupational exposure, and recommend chelation treatment.
3. Using the description in the NBC propagation section of this chapter about the Soviet agent FT and your knowledge of basic metabolic pathways, describe the mechanism of FT toxicity and the metabolic pathway(s) affected. What other signs or symptoms would you expect to see with FT toxicity? How would you treat a patient suffering from exposure to an agent similar to FT?
4. You are at home watching a local drama unfold on cable TV when you are paged by the chief resident from the emergency room. Being flown into the hospital from a farm is a National Guardsman who has been involved in a standoff there with a separatist group that was operating a methamphetamine lab to purchase arms and spread their propaganda. You're aware that the compound just burned to the ground and that the National Guard has been firing CS gas canisters into the compound. The patient started hyperventilating at the scene, complained of headache, nausea, and vomiting, and passed out while en route to the hospital. He is very pale, and his nailbeds and lips are blue. The resident has available a CD-ROM database containing treatment recommendations for different agents. You tell the resident to query the CD-ROM database for treatment recommendations for
   a. CS gas
   b. smoke inhalation from the fire
   c. exposure to chemicals in the methamphetamine lab
   d. HCN gas

CHAPTER 23 MORTICIANS

1. What factors increase the airborne exposure of formaldehyde?
2. List other potent skin and respiratory toxins that morticians use.
3. Formaldehyde exposure increases the bronchospastic and irritant effects of other irritant substances that were previously tolerated by the worker: true or false?
4. Formaldehyde causes squamous metaplasia and chromosomal alterations, and thus it is known to be definitely carcinogenic: true or false?

CHAPTER 24 OFFICE PERSONNEL

1. Health complaints by office workers thought to be related to the workplace invariably
   a. are caused by mass hysteria
   b. involve the skin, respiratory system, nose, throat, and eyes
   c. are explained by physical and chemical factors alone
   d. are independent of the type of work being performed at the site

CHAPTER 25 PAINTERS AND FURNITURE REFINISHERS

1. All of the following chemicals can cause a peripheral neuropathy except
   a. hexane
   b. carbon disulfide
   c. methyl butyl ketone
   d. methylene chloride
   e. benzo(a)pyrene
2. Toluene 2,4-diisocyanate causes bronchospasm by
   a. Ig E-mediated mechanism only
   b. indirect pharmacologic blockade of the β-adrenergic receptors
   c. reacting with the amino groups of proteins to form haptens, resulting in a hypersensitivity reaction
   d. suppressing the cough reflex
3. Acute isocyanate exposure
   a. results in the sensation of numbness in the throat
   b. causes rhinitis, cough, and dyspnea
   c. is not associated with bronchospasm
   d. results in a severe lactic acidosis
4. Methacholine and other pharmacologic challenges
   a. are safe tests with few consequential side effects
   b. are most helpful when they do not result in bronchospasm
   c. cannot confirm the diagnosis when they are positive
   d. are most helpful when they are negative and the patient has ongoing exposures and symptoms
5. Solvent-induced hepatotoxicity
   a. is a common consequence of aromatic and aliphatic hydrocarbon exposure
   b. have never been reported after toluene and xylene exposures
   c. should be considered after the diagnosis of alcohol-induced hepatotoxicity has been excluded
   d. is idiosyncratic

CHAPTER 26 PEDIATRIC LABORERS

1. Green tobacco sickness
   a. is caused by inhalation of burning tobacco
   b. is most often seen in adult smokers
   c. is common in tobacco stringers
   d. is seen primarily in adolescent croppers
2. Children can receive significant lead exposure as a result of which of the following exposures?
   a. Home-going lead on parental clothing, skin, hair, or shoes
   b. Home-based cottage industries
   c. Living near industrial sites employing lead in processes.
   d. As a result of home renovations
   e. All of the above

CHAPTER 27 PHOTOGRAPHERS AND FILM DEVELOPERS

1. All of the following might be used as toners except
   a. selenium
   b. gold
   c. uranium
   d. glacial acetic acid
2. Which of the following statement best describes a "fixative"?
   a. Stabilization of the developed image
   b. Oxidizing dye couplers that make images visible
   c. Digitized image processing
   d. A chemical process attaching silver nitrate crystals to plastic film
3. All of the following agents are used in developing, except
   a. hydroquinone
   b. metol
   c. alkalis
   d. dichromate
4. Which agent is a depigmenting chemical?
   a. Selenium
   b. Gold salts
   c. Hydroquinone
   d. Sulfur dioxide
5. Dark room developing in open trays may result in which of the following?
   a. Lichen planus
   b. Hyperpigmentation
   c. Cardiac arrhythmias
   d. Splenomegaly

CHAPTER 28 PLUMBERS

1. Colophony
   a. is an acid derivative
   b. is a pine resin derivative
   c. causes asthma but not dermatitis
   d. helps keep the solder melting point low
2. PVC adhesives
   a. should be cleaned immediately if accidently spilled on the skin
   b. form carbon monoxide when metabolized
   c. are generally nontoxic
   d. can cause porphyria cutanea tarda
3. Freon
   a. should not be considered cardiotoxic
   b. is a halogenated hydrocarbon
   c. accumulates in fatty tissue
   d. causes nummular eczema
4. Trifluorochloromethane
   a. has been shown to induce hepatic carcinoma
   b. is a liquid at room temperature
   c. can cause asystole at high concentrations
   d. is the active metabolite of Freon 11

CHAPTER 29 POLICE AND LAW ENFORCEMENT PERSONNEL

1. Which of the following agencies does not support a law enforcement function?
   a. FBI
   b. CIA
   c. DEA
   d. ATF
2. The most toxic selenium compound is
   a. metallic selenium
   b. selenites
   c. selenates
   d. hydrogen selenide
3. Which of the following has been shown to increase the excretion of selenium?
   a. Bromobenzene
   b. Methylbenzene
   c. Trichloroethylene
   d. Pentachlorophenol
4. Smokers may demonstrate "normal" levels of carboxyhemoglobin as high as
   a. 1%
   b. 10%
   c. 0%
   d. 0.75%
5. Which of the following indicates surgical bullet removal in order to prevent lead intoxication?
   a. Bullet fragments retained in soft tissue
   b. Bullet in the hip joint space
   c. Bullet fragments in subcutaneous tissue
   d. Removal is not indicated for that purpose
6. Which of the following statements is true?
   a. Testicular cancer is common in men over 50.
   b. Testicular cancer is very common in police officers.
   c. Testicular cancer has been reported in microwave radar operators but the statistical significance is not proven.
   d. Testicular cancer is clearly caused by handheld radar devices.
7. One acute hazard in "clean labs" is
   a. methane gas
   b. hydrogen sulfide
   c. carbon monoxide
   d. explosion
8. Handling large amounts of cocaine for long periods of time will
   a. not alter a urine drug screen
   b. could possibly alter a urine drug screen
   c. definitely will alter a urine drug screen

CHAPTER 30 PRINTERS

1. Toluene is metabolized to all of the following except
   a. benzoic acid
   b. hippuric acid
   c. ortho-cresol
   d. phenol
2. Toluene
   a. has been demonstrated to be largely expired unchanged in the lungs
   b. can cause symptoms below the TLV-TWA
   c. is lipophobic
   d. is rarely used as a solvent
3. Toluene
   a. exposure can be documented by a positive qualitative assay for urine hippuric acid
   b. can be measured in the urine but does not correlate to toxicity
   c. does not induce the cytochrome P-450
   d. is a CNS stimulant

CHAPTER 31 ROOFERS AND ROADBUILDERS

1. What are the main toxic exposures in roofers and road builders?
2. What are the most important acute toxic effects of coal tar and asphalt fumes?
3. What is the most significant long-term health hazard associated with exposure to coal tar fumes?
4. What are tar warts, and how should they be managed?
5. What is the importance of a "bay region" in a PAH?
6. How can the exposure of a worker to PAHs be estimated?
7. What are some important nonoccupational sources of PAHs?

CHAPTER 32 SANDBLASTERS

1. What are the differences in exposure history and radiographic appearance between acute and chronic silicosis?
2. Name some of the methods used to control silica exposure in sandblasting.
3. A 35-year-old man who has worked as a sandblaster for 10 years has a chest x-ray showing nodular opacities in the upper zones of his lungs. He is asymptomatic. What is indicated diagnostically and therapeutically?
4. What is the pathologic appearance of chronic silicosis?
5. What are the clinical and radiographic differences between PMF and simple silicosis?
6. What should you suspect in your patient with PMF who develops a sudden decline in respiratory function?
7. Name two extrapulmonic manifestations of disease associated with silica exposure.

CHAPTER 33 SEWER AND SANITATION PERSONNEL

1. The highly water-soluble gases include all of the following except
   a. ammonia
   b. sulfur dioxide
   c. hydrogen chloride
   d. nitrogen dioxide
2. The gradual decrease in the rotten egg odor during a hydrogen sulfide spill is a reliable indicator that ambient concentrations of hydrogen sulfide are decreasing. True or false?
3. Hydrogen sulfide
   a. is virtually undetectable below 15 ppm
   b. has a TWA/TLV of 10 ppm
   c. has no chronic ocular effects
   d. is lighter than air and rapidly dissipates from an enclosed space
4. Examples of simple asphyxiants include all of the following except
   a. carbon dioxide
   b. methane
   c. carbon monoxide
   d. helium

CHAPTER 34 SHIP AND DOCKYARD PERSONNEL

1. What is the approximate latent period for the development of lung cancer following heavy asbestos exposure?
   a. 5 years
   b. 10 years
   c. 15 years
   d. 20 years
2. All of the following toxicants are found in shipbuilding except
   a. lead
   b. chromium
   c. asbestos
   d. phosgene
3. Welders in the shipbuilding trade are exposed to all of the following except
   a. lead
   b. halogenated biphenyls
   c. asbestos
   d. manufactured mineral fibers
4. A shipping manifest details cargo and must be located where on the loaded ship that is transporting the cargo?
   a. Bulkhead
   b. Captain's quarters
   c. Bridge
   d. Shipwright's office
5. Red lead is used as a rust retardant. What is the chemical nature of red lead?
   a. Pb_2O_6
   b. Pb_4Cr_6
   c. $Pb_3poison4$
   d. Pb_3O_4
   e. Pb_2SO_4
6. What compound is commonly found in the building of small crafts?
   a. Styrene
   b. Asbestos
   c. methyl lMethyl methacrylate
   d. Benzene
7. Shipfitters perform which of the following functions?
   a. Plumbing
   b. Woodworking
   c. Material moving
   d. Electricians
8. At what level of blood lead do persons have measurable inhibition of pyrimidine-5′-nucleotidase
   a. 15 µg/dl
   b. 30 µg/dl
   c. 60 µg/dl
   d. 90 µg/dl
9. For laborers with a last measured blood lead level of 35 µg/dl, when should the next biomonitoring be done?
   a. 6 months
   b. 1 year
   c. 2 years
   d. 5 years
10. With an airborne lead level of 75 mg/m^2, what type of respiratory protection is required by OSHA?
   a. Half-mask, with HEPA filters
   b. Full facepiece, air-purifying
   c. Full facepiece supplied-air
   d. SCBA

CHAPTER 35 SHOEMAKERS

1. Which of the following hematologic abnormalities has been associated with occupational exposure to benzene in the shoe industry?
   a. Multiple myeloma
   b. Aplastic anemia
   c. Acute myelogenous leukemia
   d. All of the above
2. Hydrocarbon neuropathy most likely results from exposure to which of the following compounds?
   a. n-hexane
   b. n-pentane
   c. methyl-ethyl ketone
   d. cyclohexane
3. Which of the following tumors has been associated with the footwear industry?
   a. Hepatoma
   b. Adenocarcinoma of the nose
   c. Seminoma
   d. Renal adenoma
4. Chronic exposure to toluene is likely to cause which of the following effects?
   a. Peripheral neuropathy
   b. Bone marrow failure
   c. Organic brain syndrome
   d. Infertility
5. Women in the footwear industry are most likely to have
   a. a high incidence of congenital malformations in their children
   b. a high incidence of twins
   c. a high risk of ovarian carcinoma
   d. a high spontaneous abortion rate

CHAPTER 36 SMELTERS AND METAL RECLAIMERS

1. Which of the following statements about occupational lead exposure is correct?
   a. Lead enters the body primarily via the gastrointestinal tract.
   b. Initially, the majority of the lead is found within the soft tissues.
   c. Of all the body tissues, bone has the highest affinity for lead.
   d. Lead is actively eliminated via the biliary tract.
   e. All of the above.
2. Lead poisoning has been associated with which of the following disease states?
   a. Microcytic anemia
   b. Seizures
   c. Gout
   d. Impotence
   e. All of the above
3. Which of the following physical examination findings is consistent with lead exposure?
   a. Irritability
   b. Wrist weakness
   c. Bluish gum discoloration
   d. Pallor
   e. All of the above

4. Chelation therapy is indicated in which of the following workers?
   a. A symptomatic patient with a BPb of 50 μg/dl
   b. A symptomatic patient with a BPb of 80 μg/dl
   c. An asymptomatic patient with a BPb of 70 μg/dl
   d. An asymptomatic worker prior to routine BPb screening
   e. a, b, and c
5. Which of the following is a potential exposure in a smelter associated with a foundry?
   a. Lead fumes and dust
   b. Sulfur dioxide
   c. Arsenic trioxide
   d. Silica dust
   e. All of the above

CHAPTER 37 WELDERS

1. Polymer fume fever
   a. is characterized by an immediate urticarial reaction
   b. severity corresponds to urine fluoride level
   c. occurs after ingestion of Teflon
   d. may be mistaken for pneumonia
2. A persistent febrile pulmonary illness after welding fume exposure may be
   a. siderosis
   b. welder's asthma
   c. chemical pneumonitis
   d. polymer fume fever
3. Acute metal fume fever
   a. is rarely caused by ZnO
   b. correlates with the predilection for asthma or bronchospasm
   c. may be cytokine mediated
   d. is irreversible
4. A 56-year-old welder is being evaluated for chronic cough. Which would be the least helpful diagnostically?
   a. Smoking/tobacco history
   b. Detailed history of welding practices
   c. PFTs
   d. Sputum culture

CHAPTER 38 ZOOKEEPERS AND VETERINARIANS

1. The primary cause for a veterinarian's exposure to anesthetic gases is
   a. frequent endotracheal tube disconnections during surgery
   b. excretion by the animals
   c. leaking gas canisters
   d. drug-drug interactions
2. Charcoal filters used to absorb waste gases are ineffective for all of the following reasons except
   a. they are not frequently changed
   b. they do not absorb nitrous oxide
   c. charcoal filters are never used for this purpose
   d. all of the above

3. Which of the following birth defects have been linked to maternal exposure to waste anesthetic gas exposure?
   a. Hypospadias
   b. Spina bifida
   c. Multiple digits
   d. Club foot
   e. Supernumerary nipples
4. Mortality rates for veterinarians are increased for all of the following reasons except
   a. suicide
   b. malignant melanoma
   c. colon cancer
   d. lymphoma
   e. lung cancer
5. Ethylene oxide has been associated with which of the following?
   a. Mesothelioma
   b. Gastric carcinoma
   c. Myelofibrosis
   d. Retroperitoneal fibrosis
   e. Nasal carcinoma

CHAPTER 39 DYNAMITE AND EXPLOSIVES

1. The primary components of dynamite include all of the following except
   a. ammonium nitrate
   b. sodium nitrate
   c. ethylene glycol dinitrate (EGDN)
   d. polyethylene glycol
   e. dinitrotoluene (DNT)
2. Dinitrotoluene replaced which of the following components of dynamite in the early 1960s?
   a. EGDN
   b. TNT
   c. DMSO
   d. CCl_4
   e. PEG
3. What is the primary hazard involved during the manufacturing of dynamite?
   a. Methemoglobinemia formation
   b. Hemolysis
   c. Marrow aplasia
   d. Anemia
   e. Explosion
4. The nitrate esters used in the explosives industry do which of the following?
   a. Immediate arterial vasodilation of variable duration
   b. Delayed arterial vasodilation of variable duration
   c. Coronary artery effects only
   d. No vascular effect
   e. Cerebral vascular effects only
5. The toxin-related headaches suffered by workers in the dynamite industry are typically described as
   a. mild and transient
   b. throbbing with a sensation of facial heat
   c. well localized to the occipital region
   d. relieved by acetaminophen
   e. almost never occurring in these workers

6. Workers in the explosives industry may suffer angina or myocardial infarction as the result of which of the following phenomena?
   a. Constant exposure to ethylene glycols
   b. Rebound coronary vasospasm upon withdrawal of nitrates
   c. Hypoxia secondary to poor work space ventilation
   d. Elevated levels of carboxyhemoglobin
   e. Sulfhemoglobin formation

7. Which of the following is not an effect of prolonged exposure to trinitrotoluene?
   a. Cataract formation
   b. Joint pain
   c. Dermatitis
   d. Cardiomyopathy
   e. Peripheral sensory neuropathy

8. The diagnosis of nitrate compound toxicity is suggested by which of the following triads?
   a. Nausea, vomiting, diarrhea
   b. Muscle fasiculations, syncope, seizures
   c. Headache, hypotension, tachycardia
   d. Salivation, lacrimation, bronchorrhea
   e. Wide gait, foot drop, dermatitis

9. Early dynamite workers prevented nitrate withdrawal symptoms from developing during off hours by
   a. reducing work load on Fridays
   b. increasing work load on Fridays
   c. keeping a piece of dynamite in their hatbands
   d. using nitroglycerine spray
   e. doing nothing special to prevent these symptoms

10. Biologic monitoring for explosives workers
   a. is highly effective
   b. has not been adequately studied
   c. involves serial methemoglobin determinations
   d. involves urinary nitrate levels daily
   e. is best done with serum EGDN levels

CHAPTER 40 FERTILIZER

1. Which of the following are possible sources of nitrate exposure?
   a. Contaminated well water
   b. Fertilizers
   c. Meat preservatives
   d. Vegetable-carrot juice, spinach
   e. All of the above

2. Methemoglobinemia may be induced by which of the following?
   a. Aniline/aminophenols
   b. Nitrobenzene
   c. Chlorates
   d. Copper sulfate
   e. All of the above

3. The following treatments may be used for patients with nitrate toxicity except
   a. 100% oxygen
   b. methylene blue
   c. HBO
   d. exchange transfusion
   e. amyl nitrite

4. The following diagnosis are causes of direct cellular hypoxia except
   a. carbon monoxide
   b. inert gases
   c. cyanide
   d. H_2S

5. Which of the following treatments may be used for patients whose eyes have been exposed to anhydrous ammonia?
   a. Chemical neutralizing solution
   b. Allow patients to rub their eyes
   c. Maintain contact lenses in place to minimize chemical penetration
   d. Immediate copious amounts of tap water or saline irrigation

6. In patients who develop methemoglobinemia, which of the following coexisting disorders is most likely to result in hemolysis?
   a. G-6-PD deficiency
   b. Iron deficiency
   c. Porphyria
   d. Iron overload
   e. Sickle cell trait

7. The "blue baby syndrome" has been associated with methemoglobin formation from what source?
   a. Local anesthetics
   b. Parental occupational exposure
   c. Antibiotics
   d. Well water
   e. Zinc ingestion

8. What is the most important treatment that can be rendered to patients who have developed methemoglobinemia while preparing to administer methylene blue?
   a. Packed red blood cells
   b. Atropine
   c. 100% oxygen
   d. Intravenous fluids
   e. Hyperbaric oxygen

9. The intermediate syndrome occurs in which of the following settings?
   a. Immediately after organophosphate exposure
   b. 24 to 96 hours after an acute cholinergic crisis
   c. In conjunction with methemoglobinemia
   d. 6 to 8 hours after a cholinergic crisis
   e. 2 to 3 weeks after a cholinergic crisis

10. Sewage application as fertilizer results in all of the following problems except
   a. accumulation of organic compounds that can enter the human food chain
   b. accumulation of pathogens that can pose a public health problem
   c. accumulation of heavy metals that can enter the human food chain
   d. accumulation of organic compounds that can enter the human food chain
   e. accumulation of methane gas that can pose a public health problem

CHAPTER 41 GLASS MANUFACTURE

1. Which of the following is not generally suffered by glass-blowers?
   a. Bronchitis
   b. Methemoglobinemia
   c. COPD
   d. Chronic cough
   e. Airway hyperresponsiveness
2. Pain caused by hydrofluoric acid burns that does not respond to topical therapy may respond to which of the following modalities?
   a. Hyperbaric oxygen
   b. Nitrous oxide
   c. Sulfadiazine
   d. Intraarterial calcium chloride
   e. Intraarterial calcium gluconate
3. Which of the following is associated with an increased incidence of lung cancer?
   a. Copper
   b. Lead
   c. Antimony
   d. Arsenic
   e. Nickel
4. The best workplace prevention for UV keratitis is
   a. topical ocular anesthetics
   b. engineering control
   c. protective lenses
   d. NIOSH-approved respirators
5. For glass blowers, which of the following has the greatest effect on the development of increased mouth pressures?
   a. Poor dental hygiene
   b. The size of the glass piece being blown
   c. The amount of heat utilized
   d. Preexisting pulmonary disease in the blower
6. Which of the following is not considered to be a significant health problem for workers in the glass manufacturing industry?
   a. Lung cancer
   b. Stomach cancer
   c. Colon cancer
   d. Heat-related illness
   e. Cardiomyopathy
7. Which of the following toxins could potentially affect both gunsmiths and glass manufacture workers?
   a. Chlorine
   b. Hydrofloric acid
   c. Selenium
   d. Ytrium
   e. Vanadium
8. The hallmark of heat stroke is
   a. hypotension
   b. CNS involvement
   c. cardiac arrhythmias
   d. GI involvement
   e. visual disturbances
9. Inhaled hydrofluoric acid fumes can be treated with
   a. aerosolized steroids
   b. PEEP
   c. aerosolized calcium gluconate
   d. aerosolized sodium bicarbonate
   e. aerosolized antibiotics
10. Hydrofluoric acid burns can result in clinically significant
   a. hyperkalemia
   b. hypermagnesemia
   c. hypercalcemia
   d. systemic florosis
   e. hypocalcemia

CHAPTER 42 HEALTH CARE

1. Glutaraldehye is used in hospitals as a sterilizing agent. It is also found in high concentrations in
   a. x-ray film processing chemicals
   b. bathroom cleaning chemicals
   c. the emergency department as an instrument sterilizer
   d. animal area disinfectants
2. In 1928, the Cleveland Clinic was the site of what significant hospital environmental disaster that resulted in the death of more than 100 people, including health care workers?
   a. Chlorine gas release
   b. Xylene contamination of the water supply
   c. X-ray department fire
   d. Cryptosporidiosis
   e. Nitrous oxide contamination of oxygen lines
3. Regarding the previous question, what was the cause of the deaths?
   a. Cyanide produced by the burning of nitromethylcellulose in the x-ray film
   b. Hydrogen sulfate produced by the burning of nitromethylcellulose in the x-ray film
   c. Aerosolized silver produced by the burning of nitromethylcellulose in the x-ray film
   d. Chlorine produced by the burning of nitromethylcellulose in the x-ray film
   e. Carbon dioxide produced by the burning of nitromethylcellulose in the x-ray film
4. Acute exposure to methyl methacralate has been reported to cause all of the following adverse health effects except
   a. respiratory tract irritation
   b. peripheral neuritis
   c. allergic contact dermatitis
   d. irritant contact dermatitis
   e. occupational asthma
5. Phenol is used as a disinfectant on glassware, instruments, and floors in hospitals. Differing exposures to phenol can cause all of the following except
   a. pancreatitis
   b. skin burns
   c. hypopigmentation of the skin
   d. seizures
   e. death

6. A toxic substance found in hospitals that is similar to formaldehyde and used to sterilize heat-sensitive equipment such as endoscopes is
   a. methyl paraben
   b. chloramine
   c. hexachlorophene
   d. glutaraldehyde
   e. paraldehyde

7. Laboratory animal allergy (LAA)
   a. is due to IgA mediated reactions
   b. is due to IgM mediated reactions
   c. was first identified in the early 1990s
   d. is not necessarily more prevalent in those with an atopic history

8. Measurable urine levels of which drug have been demonstrated in health care workers working with AIDS patients?
   a. DDI
   b. AZT
   c. DDA
   d. Acyclovir
   e. Pentamidine

9. Which of the following represents a good biologic monitor for formaldehyde exposure in health care workers?
   a. Blood formaldehyde levels
   b. Urine formaldehyde levels
   c. Serum formate levels
   d. Urine formate levels
   e. There is no good biologic monitor for formaldehyde

10. The primary route for toxic exposure to mercury for health care workers is
    a. oral
    b. bloodborne
    c. inhalational
    d. skin
    e. none; health care workers are not exposed to mercury

11. Which of the following causes sensitization leading to occupational asthma in health care workers employed specifically in nursing homes?
    a. Talc
    b. Arsine
    c. Psyllium
    d. Lead
    e. Latex

CHAPTER 43 MATCH PRODUCTION

1. Phossy jaw from match production was due to
   a. yellow phosphorus
   b. green phosphorus
   c. red phosphorus
   d. manganese trisulfide

2. Most safety matches contain
   a. ammonium phosphate
   b. potassium chlorate
   c. boric acid
   d. yellow phosphorus

3. A facial eczematous rash has been reported in match makers that is thought to be the result of
   a. yellow phosphorus
   b. potassium chlorate
   c. phosphorus-sesquisulfide bichromates
   d. carbon monoxide

4. Though yellow phosphorus is no longer used in the manufacture of matches in the United States, it is found in all of the following industries except
   a. munitions
   b. food processing
   c. semiconductor
   d. rodenticides

5. Ingestion of white phosphorus can result in all of the following except
   a. GI symptoms
   b. garlic breath
   c. smoking luminescent stool
   d. pulmonary edema

6. Chronic industrial exposure has resulted in all of the following except
   a. Lucifer's jaw
   b. Osteomyelitis
   c. Japanese match workers
   d. Nephritis

7. Sudden death in acute phosphorus poisoning may be related to a direct cardiac effect or
   a. hypocalcemia
   b. hypokalemia
   c. hypernatremia
   d. hypoxia

8. Red phosphorus has all of the following properties, except
   a. nonvolatile
   b. nonabsorbable
   c. faster burning than yellow phosphorus
   d. insoluble

9. A book of modern-day paper matches contains how much potassium chlorate?
   a. 110 mg
   b. 220 mg
   c. 500 mg
   d. 750 mg

10. All of the following can be found in matches except
    a. antimony trisulfide
    b. potassium bichromate
    c. potassium chlorate
    d. potassium chloride

CHAPTER 44 NATURAL GAS

1. Natural gas is the gaseous form of petroleum. During its processing all of the following are removed except
   a. sulfur compounds
   b. water
   c. ozone
   d. liquid hydrocarbons

2. Natural gas is primarily a mixture of
   a. C1 to C4 hydrocarbon gases
   b. C5 to C10 hydrocarbon gases
   c. C12 to C20 hydrocarbon gases
   d. C5 to C10 hydrocarbon liquids
3. All of the following may be trace contaminates in natural gas, except
   a. mercaptans
   b. carbonyl sulfide (COS)
   c. helium
   d. carbon monoxide
   e. methylene chloride
4. Natural gas is classified based on the hydrogen sulfide content. Dry natural gas typically contains what percent of hydrogen sulfide?
   a. 7 to 40%
   b. 1 to 5%
   c. 0%
   d. not more than 2%
5. Natural gas may have the following hazardous effects except
   a. fire hazard
   b. explosion hazard
   c. asphyxiation
   d. endogenous metabolism to CO
6. Formaldehyde can be found as a contaminate in natural gas from which one of the following sources?
   a. Landfill gas
   b. Naturally occurring
   c. Hydrogen sulfide treatment
   d. Compressor lubricants
7. Asphyxiation, the major health concern, occurs at what level?
   a. 10 ppm
   b. 100 ppm
   c. 1,000 ppm
   d. >100,000 ppm
8. Natural gas has which odor warning properties?
   a. Excellent
   b. Good
   c. Poor
   d. None
9. Which one of the following is both a natural contaminate and is reintroduced to natural gas prior to delivery for home use as an odorant?
   a. Mercaptans
   b. Benzene
   c. Hydrogen sulfide
   d. Vinyl chloride
10. Which of the following is the primary toxic agent in the sour gas segment of the natural gas industry?
    a. Nitric oxide
    b. Hydrogen sulfide
    c. Methane
    d. Octane
11. Prolonged H_2S exposure has been associated with all of the following except
    a. knockdown
    b. pulmonary edema
    c. olfactory fatigue
    d. death
    e. visual hallucinations

CHAPTER 45 PHARMACEUTICAL

1. Among the antibiotics, which is the most common agent causing occupational asthma?
   a. Penicillin
   b. Ciprofloxacin
   c. Vancomycin
   d. Clindamycin
   e. Bacitracin
2. Which of these statements are true?
   a. The allergen causing allergic contact dermatitis is usually less than 500 daltons.
   b. Barrier creams have been proven effective in preventing contact dermatitis.
   c. The initial approaches to the treatment of contact urticaria and contact dermatitis differ.
   d. Dry and cold environments usually increase the dermal absorption of compounds.
   e. The most common site of contact allergy is the face.
3. Compared to the general public, workers in the pharmaceutical industry
   a. have increased risks of committing suicide
   b. have increased rates of colon and breast cancers
   c. have decreased rates of leukemias and melanomas
   d. have increased rates of mortality
   e. have decreased rates of spontaneous abortions
4. Which is a true statement concerning psyllium?
   a. It expands exponentially in water.
   b. Psyllium dust is usually 2 to 3 mm in diameter.
   c. Psyllium is inert in the lung.
   d. Psyllium is lipophilic.
5. Which statement is true for workers involved in manufacturing birth control pills?
   a. There is an increased risk for spontaneous abortions.
   b. Symptoms of occupational exposure include increased libido in males and decreased intermenstrual bleeding in females.
   c. Incidences of hyperestrogenism have been reported only in Third World countries where there are limited governmental regulations on the pharmaceutical industry.
   d. They have increased rates of breast cancer.

CHAPTER 46 PLASTICS

1. All of the following are thermoplastics except
   a. polyethylene
   b. polyvinyl chloride
   c. polypropylene
   d. polyurethanes
2. Fillers are added to plastics for all of the following reasons except
   a. opacity
   b. color
   c. improved electrical properties
   d. reinforcement
3. Polymethyl methacrylate is used for what in the plastic industry?
   a. Bone cement
   b. Filler
   c. Fire retardant
   d. Colorant

4. All of the following are latex rubbers except
   a. acrylate-butadiene
   b. acrylonitrile-butadiene
   c. latex
   d. styrene-butadiene

5. Chloroprene monomer is used in the production of which substance?
   a. Neoprene
   b. Acrylate
   c. Butadiene
   d. PVC pipe

6. Ethylene thiourea is a rubber accelerator that may cause what clinical findings?
   a. Hepatocellular cancer
   b. Disulfiram-like reaction
   c. Acryosteolysis
   d. Stomach cancer

7. TDI is used in the production of what compound?
   a. Polyurethane
   b. ABR rubber
   c. SBR rubber
   d. Dimethyl fromamide

8. Studies report sensitization rates in TDI workers to be
   a. 1%
   b. 15%
   c. 32%
   d. 65%

9. Plasticizers are compounds that have what toxicity?
   a. Irritate mucous membranes
   b. Hepatocellular cancer
   c. Allergic asthma
   d. Neuropsychiatric injury

10. Styrene is metabolized to what biomarker?
   a. Toluene
   b. Xylene
   c. Phenylglyoxlic acid
   d. Butadiene

CHAPTER 47 RAILROAD

1. Which of the following is the most important component of DEF with regard to carcinogenicity?
   a. Adsorbed hydrocarbons
   b. Particulates
   c. Moisture
   d. Carbon content
   e. Chlorine

2. Which of the following are not important diagnostic criteria for RADS?
   a. Age of the patient
   b. Abrupt symptom onset
   c. Significant hyperactivity to methacholine
   d. Absence of preexisting pulmonary disease
   e. Symptoms that require medical care within 24 hours of onset

3. Which of the following individuals would be most likely to develop RADS after an inciting exposure?
   a. A 22-year-old male with a history of asthma since childhood
   b. A 40-year-old female schoolteacher
   c. A 28-year-old male, previously healthy
   d. A 65-year-old male smoker
   e. None of the above

4. A 32-year-old, healthy, nonsmoking male firefighter runs into a burning building with no respiratory protection and emerges several minutes later carrying an unconscious elderly woman. Two hours later, the firefighter is taken to the emergency department with the complaint of shortness of breath, wheezing, and chest tightness. All lab results are normal, and his carboxyhemoglobin is reported to be 4%. He is observed for several hours and discharged to home, but his wheezing persists over the subsequent weeks. The most likely diagnosis for this patient is
   a. carbon monoxide poisoning
   b. carbon dioxide poisoning
   c. cyanide poisoning
   d. reactive airways dysfunction syndrome
   e. nitrogen oxide poisoning

5. Phosphine intoxication can cause which of the following?
   a. Hemolysis
   b. Pancreatitis
   c. Choreoathetosis
   d. Neurobehavioral changes
   e. Delayed-onset pulmonary edema

6. Which of the following have been responsible for deaths of personnel entering sealed railcars?
   a. Electric shock
   b. Fumigants
   c. Organophosphates
   d. Carbamates
   e. Polychlorinated hydrocarbons

7. The appropriate biologic marker to assess occupational exposure to creosote is
   a. 1-HP
   b. mandelic acid
   c. TTCA
   d. TCA
   e. hippuric acid

8. The most significant intoxicant related to the acute exposure to DEF is
   a. PAH
   b. CS_2
   c. carbon monoxide
   d. carbon black
   e. paradichlorobenzene

9. Which of the following agencies published guidelines for the placement of warning signs on fumigated rail cars?
   a. EPA
   b. NIOSH
   c. OSHA
   d. FDA
   e. ATSDR

10. Which of the following is a significant machine shop hazard for railyard workers?
    a. Salicylates
    b. Camphor
    c. Phosphorus
    d. Direct black 38
    e. Lead

CHAPTER 48 SEMICONDUCTOR

1. The state-of-the-art clean room design uses which type of ventilation?
   a. Airtight rooms where air is continuously filtered
   b. Clean work stations with individual exhaust hoods
   c. Vertical laminar flow rooms
   d. All of the above
   e. None of the above
2. The management of severe glycol ether exposure may include all of the following except
   a. removal from exposure
   b. intravenous naloxone
   c. intravenous ethanol
   d. hemodialysis
   e. intravenous calcium
3. The severity of hydrofluoric acid exposure is dependent upon all of the following except
   a. concentration
   b. effects of hydrogen ion
   c. contact time
   d. prior state of affected tissue
   e. effects of fluoride ion
4. Gallium arsenide
   a. is biologically inert
   b. is a poor substance to use for semiconductors because of slow electron movement
   c. dissociates in vivo with liberated inorganic arsenic, exerting toxic effect
   d. all of the above
   e. none of the above
5. The semiconductor industry
   a. has a well-delineated toxicologic history, and very little is unknown about the effects of substances used
   b. has recently lost its lead ahead of Japan in the world market and will have difficulty regaining it
   c. has a large labor force with approximately 70% involved in direct product handling
   d. none of the above
   e. all of the above
6. Which of the following toxins is not generally considered a hazard in the semi-conductor industry?
   a. Diborane
   b. Arsine
   c. Phosphine
   d. Silicon
   e. Ozone

7. Which of the following materials is capable of causing hemolysis?
   a. TCE
   b. Phosphorus
   c. Lithium
   d. Ozone
   e. Arsine
8. Which of the following substances causes arsenic toxicity?
   a. Arsine
   b. Gallium arsenide
   c. Gallium
   d. Aluminum phosphide
   e. TOCP
9. Which of the following semiconductor industry toxins is capable of causing noncardiogenic pulmonary edema?
   a. Gallium arsenide
   b. Diborane
   c. Arsine
   d. HF
   e. Silicon
10. Which of the following is never used to treat HF toxicity?
    a. Topical calcium gluconate
    b. Intraartertial calcium gluconate
    c. Topical magnesium sulfate
    d. Intravenous magnesium citrate
    e. Copious amounts of H_2O

CHAPTER 49 TEXTILE MANUFACTURE

1. Which of the following characterizes the toxicity of carbon disulfide?
   a. Pancreatitis
   b. Axonopathy
   c. Cardiomyopathy
   d. Macular degeneration
   e. Osteoarthritis
2. Which of the following dyes have been used in the textile industry as well as in hair dyes?
   a. Direct blue 6 and direct brown 95
   b. Mordant green and brilliant red
   c. Direct brown 95 and direct blue 6
   d. Direct black 38 and direct blue 6
3. Which of the following has not been specifically associated with work-related toxins in the textile industry?
   a. Pernicious anemia
   b. Byssinosis
   c. Bladder cancer
   d. Sporotrichosis
4. Crease resistance is imparted to fabric by the use of which of the following chemicals?
   a. CS_2
   b. Direct brown 38
   c. Formaldehyde
   d. Hydrogen fluoride
   e. 2,5 Hexandione

5. The OSHA permissible exposure limit (PEL) for formaldehyde is
   a. 1 ppm
   b. 0.5 ppm
   c. 2 ppm
   d. 10 ppm
   e. 0.75 ppm
6. Which of the following carcinogenic chemicals was used in the manufacture of children's pajamas in the 1970s?
   a. Tris (2,3dibromopropyl) phosphate
   b. Triortho-cresophosphate (TOCP)
   c. Azo-benzidine
   d. N,N diethyldithicarbamate
7. Which of the following is characterized by symptoms that occur on days other than Monday?
   a. Grade V byssinosis
   b. Grade II byssinosis
   c. Metal fume fever
   d. Grade IV byssinosis
   e. Mill fever
8. Aliphatic hydrocarbons are often used to clean parts and equipment in textile mills and plants. All of the following chemicals are used for this purpose except
   a. Stoddard's solvent
   b. 2,5 hexandione
   c. kerosene
   d. mineral spirits
9. Which of the following represents a significant pathologic effect of long-term exposure to low levels of carbon disulfide?
   a. Glomerulonephritis
   b. Deep venous thrombosis
   c. Accelerated atherogenesis
   d. Pulmonary fibrosis
   e. Cortical blindness
10. Which of the following can be used as a marker to monitor worker exposure to carbon disulfide?
   a. Urinary retinol binding protein
   b. Urinary β-2 microglobulin
   c. Urinary trichloracetic acid (TCA)
   d. Urinary 2-thiothiazolidine-4-carboxylic acid
   e. Plasma CS_2 levels

CHAPTER 50 TOOL AND DIE AND MACHINISTS

1. A trade journeyman of the tool and die industry could perform the following except
   a. welding
   b. superfinishing
   c. engraving
   d. smelting
   e. milling

2. Common potential toxic exposures for workers within the tool and die industry include all of the following except
   a. metal operation exposures to carbonaceous products, machining fluids, acids and alkalis, and cyanide
   b. foundry-type molding exposures to sulfur dioxide, silica, carbon monoxide, and hydrogen cyanide
   c. plastic products manufacturing exposures to polymers, additives, isocyanates, and formaldehyde
   d. rubber products manufacturing exposures to dusts, vulcanizing agents, activators, and reinforcing agents
   e. All of the above are potential toxic exposures.
3. Which statement is correct?
   a. Machining fluids have five basic functions.
   b. Mineral oil forms of machining fluids always contain 100% paraffin or naphtherine.
   c. Synthetic machining fluids have been in use since the 1930s.
   d. Irritant contact dermatitis (ICD) is the most common cause of contact dermatitis in the occupational setting.
   e. A job site with workstation evaluation concerning machining fluid exposure and dermal and/or respiratory effects can usually be bypassed.
4. Which of the following statements is true?
   a. Silicosis requires the inhalation of any silica particle with favorable alveolar space deposition characteristics.
   b. Most cases of classic silicosis cause non–activity-related respiratory symptoms in the early years of the disease process.
   c. The chest radiograph correlates well with the exposure duration for silicosis.
   d. Treatment of silicosis is causative in nature.
   e. None of the above are true.
5. Which statement is true?
   a. The American Cancer Society in its 1995 publication identified particular cancer types to be associated with tool and die workers.
   b. The three most common target organs of known occupational carcinogens, according to the American Cancer Society, are the lung, gastrointestinal tract, and bladder.
   c. There appears to be an association between bladder cancer and the tool and die industry.
   d. There is overwhelming evidence for multiple myeloma association with tool and die workers.
6. Which of the following pulmonary effects have not been noted to occur after working with this alloy?
   a. Asterixis
   b. Asthma
   c. Pulmonary fibrosis
   d. Noncardiogenic pulmonary edema
7. Which of the following symptoms occur in nonallergic, irritant-type contact dermatitis?
   a. Sensation of "skin stiffness"
   b. Hives
   c. Multiple verrucae
   d. Pustules
8. Classic silicosis chest x-rays involve
   a. up to 10-mm-diameter rounded opacities
   b. up to 8-mm nonrounded opacities
   c. 15-mm or larger rounded opacities
   d. no rounded opacities

9. Which of the following malignancies has been associated with work in the tool and dyemaking industry?
   a. AML
   b. ALL
   c. CML
   d. Multiple myeloma
10. Carcinogenicity of cutting oils is dependent upon
   a. the chlorine content
   b. the pH of the solution
   c. viscosity
   d. the concentration of PAHs

CHAPTER 51 OUTDOOR AIR POLLUTION AND ISSUES OF QUALITY

1. All of the following are "criteria pollutants" except
   a. CO
   b. lead
   c. NO_x
   d. SO_2
   e. CO_2
2. All of the following may affect lung function, except
   a. CO
   b. ozone
   c. NO_x
   d. SO_2
   e. CO_2
3. Particulates may include
   a. sulfates
   b. acid aerosols
   c. latex
   d. silica
   e. all of the above
4. Regulation of particulates to the PM_{10} level is adequate to prevent adverse health effects.
   a. True
   b. False
   c. No relation
5. Which of the following is a secondary pollutant?
   a. Carbon monoxide
   b. Ozone
   c. Oxides of nitrogen
   d. Oxides of sulfur
   e. Lead
6. Air pollution is associated with excess health effects in all except
   a. respiratory diseases
   b. asthma
   c. bronchitis
   d. leukemia
   e. increased physician visits
7. Which of the following is responsible for the majority of SO_2 emissions?
   a. Automobile exhaust
   b. Atmospheric generation
   c. Power plants
   d. Agriculture
   e. Forest fires

8. Regarding filtering of particulates, what characteristic does not favor deep penetration into the respiratory tract?
   a. High water solubility
   b. Particles > 100 μm
   c. High environmental concentration
   d. Mouth breathing
   e. Pulmonary hypertension
9. Thermal inversions result in
   a. confining air pollution over a specific area
   b. increased turnover of particulates
   c. decreased production of ozone
   d. decreased emergency department visits
   e. cleaner air
10. Confounding variables in studying the health effects of air pollution include all except
   a. aeroallergens
   b. cigarette smoking
   c. socioeconomic factors
   d. industrial contributors
   e. chronic liver disease

CHAPTER 52 INDOOR AIR QUALITY

1. "New carpet" odor arises from a substance formed in situ by means of a ring-closure reaction.
   a. True
   b. False
2. Environmental tobacco smoke has both vapor and particulate components.
   a. True
   b. False
3. Operating electronic devices (computers, video terminals, printers) may emit significant quantities of volatile organics.
   a. True
   b. False
4. Untreated hypersensitivity pneumonitis seldom results in permanent lung damage.
   a. True
   b. False
5. Rhinitis can be triggered by complexes formed between isocyanates and immunoglobulin E (IgE).
   a. True
   b. False
6. Mass psychogenic illness and sick-building syndrome result from volatile organic compounds.
   a. True
   b. False
7. Tricyclic antidepressants are effective in treating multiple chemical sensitivity syndrome (MCS).
   a. True
   b. False
8. Measurement of ambient volatile organic compounds (VOC) is an essential part of any IAQ investigation.
   a. True
   b. False
9. Indoor carbon dioxide levels above 1000 ppm indicate insufficient outdoor air makeup to the area.
   a. True
   b. False

10. Pontiac fever is caused by *Legionella pontiacensis.*
    a. True
    b. False

CHAPTER 53 WATER POLLUTION

1. The "hydrologic cycle" refers to
    a. the cycle of water molecules from large salt-containing bodies of water such as oceans and seas, to freshwater lakes and streams
    b. the circulation of water among the ocean, atmosphere, and land
    c. the dilution of potential toxins threatening an ecosystem
    d. progress made in controlling pollution through federal legislation
    e. suitable (potable) groundwater obtained via collection from springs that flow to the surface in accessible geologic formations

2. Which of the following are considered to be "nonpoint" sources of water pollution?
    a. Discharge of pollutants from drainpipes of factories into bodies of water
    b. Pollution resulting from personal uses of water such as drinking, cooking, bathing, and laundering
    c. Surface runoffs that may occur in chemically treated agricultural areas
    d. Decaying matter resulting in increased oxygen consumption by aerobic bacteria
    e. Coagulating agents such as lime, aluminum, ferric salts, or synthetic polyelectrolytes

3. The etiology of "acid rain" is thought to be
    a. the combination of rain and sulfur oxides emissions from the combustion of fossil fuels
    b. the evaporation of low-pH water from lakes undergoing eutrophication
    c. wastewater from syrup-storage-tank drains used in the soft drink industry
    d. a direct result of HR 961 (Clean Water Act Reauthorization)
    e. the movement and final evaporation of water through subsurface soil layers found underneath unregulated nuclear power plants

4. Which class of chemical compounds is responsible for the eutrophication of lakes?
    a. Heavy metals
    b. Organochlorines
    c. Dioxins
    d. Phosphates
    e. Aromatic hydrocarbons

5. Which of the following accurately describes the biochemical oxygen demand test?
    a. A measure of the oxygen used by microorganisms (which oxidize organic matter biochemically)
    b. A screening test used to indirectly measure the lime content of distilled beverages
    c. An assay developed by the pulp industry to measure limiting nutrients for freshwater flora
    d. The earliest known objective measurement of coliforms (used by ancient Romans monitoring the Cloaca Maxima)
    e. A measurement of oxidizing microorganisms contaminating municipal wastewater treatment plants

6. All of the following are protected runoff sources of water except
    a. New York
    b. Boston
    c. Lisbon
    d. Boulder

7. Groundwater in the United States is
    a. high in minerals, high in turbidity
    b. low in minerals, high in turbidity
    c. low in minerals, low in turbidity
    d. high in minerals, low in turbidity

8. All of the following are water pollutants except
    a. infectious matter
    b. radioactive matter
    c. organic chemicals
    d. oxides of nitrogen

9. What is the principal form of arsenic in drinking water?
    a. Arsenate
    b. Arsenite
    c. Cacodylic Acid
    d. As^{+3}

10. Nonpoint sources of pollution include all of the following except
    a. polychlorinated dibenzofurans
    b. sediment
    c. organic nutrients
    d. nitrogenous fertilizer

CHAPTER 54 NOISE POLLUTION

Please answer questions 1 through 9 as true or false.
1. Noise has the following properties:
    a. Sound power is a property of the noise source and is independent of the observer.
    b. Sound intensity experienced by an observer depends on the sound power of the noise and the distance between the source and the observer.
    c. Sound power level, sound intensity level, and sound pressure level are all quoted in dB.
    d. Noises of the same sound pressure levels (in dBA) pose the same risk to human hearing.

2. The noise level measured by an observer is 80 dB when machine 1 is in operation. The noise level when machine 2 is in operation is 83 dB.
    a. The noise level will be 163 dB when both machines are in operation.
    b. The noise level will be 85 dB when both machines are in operation.
    c. When the distance between the observer and machine 1 is doubled, the noise level experienced by the observer when machine 1 is in operation will be 40 dB.
    d. When the distance between the observer and machine 1 is doubled, the noise level experienced by the observer when machine 1 is in operation will be 77 dB.

3. A machine placed in the center of a large workroom with a high ceiling produced a noise level of 83 dBA for the operator.
   a. If the machine is relocated to the side of the room close to a wall, but away from any corner, the operator will be exposed to a noise level of 86 dBA.
   b. If the machine is relocated to a corner of the room, the operator will be exposed to a noise level of 92 dBA.
   c. If the machine is relocated to a corner of the room, and the walls are lined with noise-absorptive materials, the operator will be exposed to a noise level of 83 dBA.
   d. If the machine and the operator are placed on a raised platform in the center of the room, the noise exposure level will be 80 dBA.

4. Regarding noise as a health hazard,
   a. what you cannot hear will not harm you, so noise at frequencies inaudible to human hearing is not hazardous to health
   b. the ACGIH threshold limit value for long-term noise exposure is a time-weighted noise level of 85 dBA for an 8-hour day and 5-day workweek
   c. long-term listening to a person's favorite music at high sound levels (> 100 dBA) will not have any adverse effect of hearing
   d. if a worker accrues a noise dose of 55% in the morning and 60% in the afternoon, he would have exceeded the noise exposure limit if that day was his normal working day

5. Acute acoustic trauma
   a. can be treated medically (e.g., with dextran), unlike noise-induced hearing loss (NIHL)
   b. usually presents as a bilateral conductive hearing loss affecting all frequencies
   c. would almost always occur if a person is exposed to 145 dBA without hearing protection
   d. can present with symptoms of hyperacusis, sound distortion, and pain

6. Noise-induced hearing loss (NIHL)
   a. usually presents initially as a bilateral high-frequency sensorineural hearing loss
   b. over 90% of sufferers complain of tinnitus
   c. is an unlikely diagnosis in a right-handed hunter with a profound unilateral sensorineural hearing loss in the right ear and normal hearing in the other ear
   d. is more likely to occur in a noise-exposed person concurrently exposed to toluene as compared to a similarly noise-exposed worker without toluene exposure

7. A proper audiometric assessment of the noise-exposed worker should comply with the following guidelines:
   a. The worker should not work for a 16-hour period prior to the test, even with the use of hearing protection
   b. A qualified audiologist or medical practitioner has to perform the assessment
   c. Pregnant workers in the third trimester should not be tested because of a health risk to the fetus
   d. Reporting of the results to the worker should be both verbal and in writing

8. Besides noise and presbyacusis, other causes of bilateral high-frequency sensorineural hearing loss are
   a. smoking
   b. ampicillin
   c. otitis media
   d. upper respiratory tract viral infection

9. A hearing conservation program (HCP)
   a. has the objectives of control of the noise hazard and prevention of noise-induced hearing loss (NIHL)
   b. is required when workers are exposed to an environmental noise level of 87 dBA
   c. should have audiometric assessments of exposed workers as an integral component
   d. may reduce the incidence of accidents at the workplace

10. All of the following chemicals have ototoxicity characteristics except
    a. solvents
    b. smoking
    c. vancomycin
    d. ozone

CHAPTER 55 ASBESTOS

1. All of the following are associated with asbestos exposure except
   a. lung cancer
   b. asbestosis
   c. mesothelioma
   d. hypercalcemia

2. The only serpentine asbestos is
   a. chrysotile
   b. crocidolite
   c. amosite
   d. actinolite

3. Asbestos fibers range from
   a. 0.001 to 0.3 microns
   b. 0.001 to 3.0 microns
   c. 0.1 to 3 microns
   d. 1 to 3 microns

4. The most important route of exposure is
   a. oral
   b. dermal
   c. inhalation
   d. a and b

5. Which type of asbestos is least toxic in causing asbestosis?
   a. Crocidolite
   b. Amosite
   c. Amphibole
   d. Chrysotile

6. Inflammation in asbestosis begins within what time period following first exposure?
   a. Days
   b. Weeks
   c. Months
   d. Years

7. Asbestos-related pleural changes represent
   a. early mesothelioma
   b. early lung cancer
   c. asbestosis
   d. previous asbestos exposure

8. What percent of pleural plaques that are found on autopsy were visible on x-ray?
    a. 5%
    b. 15%
    c. 35%
    d. 75%
9. How does asbestos function in carcinogenesis?
    a. Initiator
    b. Promotor
    c. Progressers
    d. Producers
10. According to a survey study, what percent of public and private buildings contain asbestos?
    a. 5% to 10%
    b. 10% to 20%
    c. 20% to 40%
    d. 40% to 75%

CHAPTER 56 CHEMICAL CARCINOGENESIS

1. Malignant tumors of epithelial origin are termed
    a. sarcomas
    b. carcinomas
    c. fibromas
    d. ectodermomas
2. One of the earliest identified occupational cancers was caused by
    a. radon
    b. fuller's earth
    c. CA 19-9
    d. beryllium
3. All of the following are recognized as human carcinogens except
    a. arsenic
    b. chromium (VI)
    c. nickel
    d. dieldrin
4. All of the following are tumor suppressor genes except
    a. MCC
    b. p53
    c. DCC
    d. K-ras
5. Protooncogenes, when inappropriately activated, cause
    a. altered growth and differentiation
    b. opsonization of the carcinogen
    c. expression of suppressor genes
    d. benign cancers
6. Each of the following may be a step in carcinogenesis except
    a. promotion
    b. deletion
    c. initiation
    d. progression
7. Persons in the furniture manufacturing industry may be at increased risk of nasal cancer from what compound?
    a. Aromatic amines
    b. Wood dusts
    c. Vinyl chloride
    d. PCBs

8. All of the following may alter gene expression that may contribute to cancer except
    a. Oncoproteins
    b. Phenobarbital
    c. Cimetidine
    d. Estrogen-like steroid compounds
    e. PAHs
9. All of the following are lung carcinogens except
    a. radon
    b. arsenic
    c. nickel
    d. methyl mercury
10. All of the following are good biomarkers of ovarian cancer except
    a. CA 15-3
    b. CA 125
    c. CASA
    d. C-erB-2

CHAPTER 57 ENVIRONMENTAL AUDITS AND PROPERTY TRANSFERS

1. Which of the following is not part of a phase 1 assessment?
    a. Air monitoring
    b. Geological records
    c. Permits and licensing
    d. Title search
2. Which of the following is not part of a phase 2 assessment?
    a. Water sampling
    b. Soil sampling
    c. Laboratory testing
    d. UST records
3. Radon sampling is an example of what type of assessment?
    a. Phase 1
    b. Phase 2
    c. Phase 3
    d. Hydrogeological
4. What risks are encountered when assessing abandoned properties?
    a. Structure deterioration
    b. Unknown deposited chemicals
    c. Vapors from contaminated water or soil
    d. Burn hazards due to hot surfaces
5. All of the following are mandated by law for evaluations except
    a. asbestos
    b. polychlorinated biphenyls (PCBs) in transformers and capacitors
    c. underground storage tanks (USTs)
    d. cadmium
6. Under SARA, the innocent purchaser provisions implies the following except
    a. prior knowledge of property contamination
    b. a suspicion of hazardous waste associated with the property
    c. the purchaser is required by law to remediate the property after purchase
    d. the principal responsible parties may be financially responsible for remediation of the property

CHAPTER 58 ENVIRONMENTAL RISKS AND THE CLINICIAN: INFORMING WORRIED PATIENTS

1. What year was the alleged scare from benzene in Perrier?
   a. 1980
   b. 1985
   c. 1990
   d. 1993
2. All of the following are false except
   a. If it can be measured, it must be eliminated.
   b. There is no threshold for carcinogens.
   c. Man-made is more hazardous than natural.
   d. The general health of the public is improving.
3. What is the background rate for leukemia?
   a. 1 per 100,000
   b. 6 per 100,000
   c. 10 per 100,000
   d. 50 per 100,000
4. At what level of benzene is there no increased risk of leukemia?
   a. 1 ppm
   b. < 10 ppm
   c. 100 ppm
   d. 500 ppm
5. All of the following are part of the "Hill Criteria" except
   a. temporality
   b. intensity
   c. consistency
   d. $p = .05$
6. The response of the public to potential exposure sources includes all these reactions except
   a. annoyance
   b. anger
   c. outrage
   d. reason
7. Are odors a frequent or rare cause for concern by the public?
   a. Frequent
   b. Rare
8. The physician is viewed by the public as
   a. an effective communicator
   b. usually on the side of insurance companies
   c. generally trusted
   d. well trained in risk communication
9. The public usually keeps public health risks in their proper perspectives, true or false?
10. Mathematical risk assessment is a technique in which
    a. biologic data is converted into regulatory action
    b. the public uses it to understand risk
    c. low doses of chemicals are tested
    d. few uncertainties are used

CHAPTER 59 IONIZING RADIATION

1. What is the estimated global amount of krypton-85 that has been released into the atmosphere?
   a. 10^3 curies
   b. 10^5 curies
   c. 10^8 curies
   d. 10^9 curies

2. It has been estimated that until the year 2000, there will be an additional excess of lung cancer. What is the excess?
   a. 50,000
   b. 100,000
   c. 250,000
   d. 430,000
3. Alpha particles have all of the following characteristics except
   a. high-energy electrons
   b. ionized helium atoms
   c. short track
   d. stopped by the skin
4. Gamma rays have all of the following characteristics except
   a. highly penetrating
   b. neurons
   c. long track
   d. electromagnetic energy
5. The lowest radiation dose a cell can receive is
   a. One ionization track
   b. One Sievert
   c. REM
   d. RBE

CHAPTER 60 NONIONIZING RADIATION

1. Infrared radiation has a wavelength that ranges from
   a. 700 nm to 1 mm
   b. 400 to 700 nm
   c. 3 MHz to 300 GHz
   d. 200 to 280 nm
2. The unit of frequency for microwave radiation is
   a. nanometer
   b. megahertz
   c. hertz
   d. gray
3. Which ultraviolet spectrum is felt to be responsible for ocular injury?
   a. UV-A
   b. UV-B
   c. UV-C
   d. UV-D
4. Skin cancer is associated with which form of nonionizing radiation?
   a. Infrared radiation
   b. Visible radiation
   c. Ultraviolet radiation
   d. Radiofrequency radiation
5. Which type of nonionizing radiation is most important for the production of heat?
   a. Microwave radiation
   b. Ultraviolet radiation
   c. Infrared radiation
   d. Visible radiation
6. Damage to tissues from nonionizing radiation is generally due to
   a. genotoxicity
   b. thermal injury
   c. opening of ion channel
   d. coherence

7. Lasers may emit all of the following except
   a. ultraviolet radiation
   b. visible radiation
   c. infrared radiation
   d. radiofrequency radiation
8. The human body is essentially transparent to microwaves that are
   a. < 0.03 meters
   b. 0.03 to 0.1 meters
   c. 0.1 to 1 meters
   d. > 2 meters
9. The best established human bioeffect of microwave radiation is
   a. chromosomal damage
   b. lymphocyte transformation
   c. calcium efflux
   d. cataract formation
10. All of the following health effects have been noted from laser use except
    a. retinal photocoagulation
    b. thermal burns
    c. neuropsychiatric effects
    d. viral exposure

CHAPTER 61 RESIDENTIAL RADON AND LUNG CANCER

1. Radon is the result of
   a. radioactive decay of uranium
   b. radioactive decay of plutonium
   c. atomic bomb fallout
   d. decay of beryllium
2. Radon has a half-life of
   a. 3.8 days
   b. 1 year
   c. 25 years
   d. 1600 years
3. The EPA has set an "acceptable" level of radon of
   a. < 4 pCi/L
   b. 6 pCi/L
   c. 10 pCi/L
   d. 35 pCi/L

4. The National Residential Radon Survey found that the mean level of radon was
   a. 1.25 pCi/L
   b. 4.25 pCi/L
   c. 10.5 pCi/L
   d. 15 pCi/L
5. Radon emits what type of particle?
   a. Alpha
   b. Beta
   c. Gamma
   d. Delta
6. How many homes are estimated to exceed 20 pCi/L?
   a. 10,000
   b. 25,000
   c. 100,000
   d. 750,000
7. One home on the Reading Prong was found to have radon levels of
   a. 150 pCi/L
   b. 2700 pCi/L
   c. 3000 pCi/L
   d. 4500 pCi/L
8. It is estimated that a lung cancer results from how many alpha hits?
   a. 1×10^5
   b. 4×10^9
   c. 6×10^5
   d. 8×10^9
9. All of the following affect respiratory tract dose except
   a. breathing pattern
   b. characteristics of inhaled air
   c. humidity
   d. ambient CO_2 level
10. All of the following mining types have been found to have elevated radon levels, except
    a. gold
    b. tin
    c. uranium
    d. coal

Review Answers

CHAPTER 1 A BRIEF HISTORY OF OCCUPATIONAL, INDUSTRIAL, AND ENVIRONMENTAL TOXICOLOGY

1. H		11. P	
2. L		12. E	
3. J		13. K	
4. A		14. F	
5. B		15. S	
6. I		16. G	
7. C		17. R	
8. D		18. N	
9. M		19. Q	
10. O			

CHAPTER 2 ARTISTS AND ARTISANS

1. d
2. a
3. e

CHAPTER 3 ATHLETES

1. e	5. a
2. c	6. d
3. c	7. a
4. b	8. e

CHAPTER 4 AVIATION PERSONNEL

1. a
2. c
3. a
4. a

CHAPTER 5 CARPENTERS AND LOGGERS

1. a	6. d
2. e	7. c
3. c	8. d
4. d	9. c
5. d	

CHAPTER 6 CONCRETE WORKERS AND MASONS

1. a	4. c
2. b	5. b
3. c	6. d

CHAPTER 7 DIVERS

1. c	6. b
2. b	7. d
3. d	8. d
4. c	9. c
5. e	10. e

CHAPTER 8 DOCTORS, NURSES, AND DENTISTS

1. c
2. d
3. d
4. c
5. d
6. c

CHAPTER 9 DOMESTIC AND BUILDING MAINTENANCE WORKERS

1. d
2. b
3. b
4. b

CHAPTER 10 DRY CLEANERS

1. c
2. b
3. b
4. b
5. d

6. d
7. d
8. b
9. d
10. a

CHAPTER 11 ELECTRICIANS

1. b
2. c
3. b

CHAPTER 12 ELECTROPLATERS

1. Proteinuria is an early manifestation of cadmium-induced renal toxicity. This results from proximal renal tubular and glomerular damage. The progression of disease leads to elevation of the serum creatinine. An increase in incidence of renal calculi has been reported among these workers.

2. Osteomalacia, osteoporosis, and pathologic fractures result from increased urinary loss of calcium and phosphorus, inhibition of renal hydroxylation of vitamin D, and inhibition of gut absorption of calcium.

3. Some of the nonoccupational sources of cadmium are from industrial by-products (e.g., plastics, batteries, machinery) that enter the food chain, certain foods (e.g., seafood, meat by-products, fruits, grains), acidic beverages that leech cadmium from glaze, tobacco, and recreational hobbies (e.g., soldering, welding, smelting, grinding).

4. Early cadmium-induced renal tubule damage results in the diminished resorption of low-molecular-weight proteins, namely, β-2-microglobulin, lysozyme, and retinol-binding protein. Since the presence of these proteins in the urine is one of the first signs of chronic cadmium toxicity, workers should have their urine routinely screened and occupational exposure discontinued if this abnormality is identified.

5. Metallothionein is a transport protein that binds to cadmium to form a nontoxic complex. When cadmium exists in the "free" or "unbound" state, cellular toxicity occurs. Such conditions can result from either the saturation of available protein-binding sites by excess cadmium or the dissociation of cadmium from metallothionein upon renal tubular resorption. Metallothionein also serves as a carrier for other essential trace metals. This function can be impaired in cadmium toxicity to contribute to cellular derangement.

6. The reduced form of chromium (Cr^{+6}) is more hazardous than its trivalent form because of its increased tissue and cellular permeability. Hexavalent chromium can cause localized burns and inhibit nucleic acid function when it is oxidized to its trivalent state upon entry into cells. Owing to the diminished solubility of the trivalent chromium compounds, they are less likely to cause tissue injury and are not considered cancer risks.

CHAPTER 13 EXTERMINATORS

1. c
2. b
3. a
4. d
5. b

CHAPTER 14 FARMERS AND FARM PERSONNEL

1. c
2. d
3. b

CHAPTER 15 FIREFIGHTERS

1. b
2. b
3. b

4. e
5. c
6. d

CHAPTER 16 FLOOR AND CARPET LAYERS

1. c
2. d
3. b
4. e
5. c

CHAPTER 17 FLORISTS AND GROUNDSKEEPERS

1. d
2. d
3. c

4. b
5. b
6. d

CHAPTER 18 FOOD PREPARATION PERSONNEL

1. e
2. d
3. a
4. c
5. d

CHAPTER 19 HAIRDRESSERS AND COSMETOLOGISTS

1. c
2. b
3. a
4. a
5. c

CHAPTER 20 JEWELERS

1. e
2. e
3. b
4. a
5. c

CHAPTER 21 MECHANICS

1. "Degreaser flush" is the result of vasodilatation of the superficial cutaneous blood vessels of the face and neck. This reaction occurs in some individuals who are exposed to trichloroethylene (TCE) vapors and consume alcohol. It appears that repeated exposure to TCE vapors must first occur before this reaction happens. It starts approximately 30 minutes after consumption of alcohol, peaks within an hour, and gradually fades over the next hour. No other physiologic changes are recorded during this reaction. The response can still be triggered with alcohol consumption 3 weeks after the last vapor exposure to TCE.
2. Chemicals used as degreasers and solvents represent the chief exposure mechanics encounter. These complex solutions contain varying amounts of aliphatic and aromatic hydrocarbons as well as oxygenated and halogenated hydrocarbons. The major routes of exposure are dermal contact and vapor inhalation.
3. Biologic samples assess the degree of exposure in workers as a preventive measure. They determine if the workers' exposure to potentially harmful agents is kept below a level not believed to cause toxic effects. Biologic samples are a better indicator of a worker's exposure than workplace air sampling because they include the workload of the worker and the physical properties of the solvents. Labored activity increases a worker's minute ventilation and exposure to inhaled toxins.
4. The worker must be assessed for other sources of contamination. Tobacco smokers have higher blood benzene levels than nonsmokers. Phenol is a urinary metabolite of benzene and is also used to measure a worker's exposure to benzene. Certain cosmetics and medications can lead to elevated urinary phenol levels and must be considered in evaluating a worker's exposure to benzene. Another consideration is the type of laboratory method used in the analysis of biologic samples. The Fujiwara test can qualitatively measure urinary metabolites of trichloroethylene, but this test can yield false positives if other halogens are present.
5. Chronic exposure to hydrocarbon solvents can lead to neurobehavioral and intellectual impairment. It is important to monitor solvent-exposed workers for neurologic symptoms. Assessment can be made through neurophysiologic screening questionnaires. The questionnaires can ascertain disorders in affect, memory, and personality. The questionnaires are highly sensitive but have a high degree of false positives. It should be noted that a number of other processes (e.g., alcoholism, Alzheimer's disease, electroconvulsive therapy) may cause these same symptoms.

CHAPTER 22 MILITARY PERSONNEL

1. Healthy worker effect. The healthy worker effect can be seen when proportionate mortality studies are used to describe disease risk. Because the incidence of one kind of disease may be low (heart), deaths occur more often from other disease (cancer).
2. Difluorochlorobromomethane; c.
3. As a fluoroacetate, FT is related to the rodenticide sodium fluoroacetate in that it blocks the action of cis-aconitase. This results in a buildup of citrate in the tricarboxylic acid cycle, which allosterically inhibits the action of phosphofructokinase (PFK). Blocked energy metabolism results in reduced oxygen consumption. Because of the resulting delay in metabolic depression, onset of symptoms is not immediate. Depression and convulsions may result, followed by death from cardiac arrest or ventricular fibrillation. Treatment involves removal of the exposure source, supportive care, and administration of glycerol monoacetate.
4. d.

CHAPTER 23 MORTICIANS

1. Embalming autopsied body, paraformaldehyde powders, spills, inadequate room ventilation.
2. Glutaraldehyde, methanol, isopropanol, phenol.
3. True. This is the definition of *sensitizer*.
4. False. Although formaldehyde causes these precancerous changes, it is suspect as a carcinogen and requires further study.

CHAPTER 24 OFFICE PERSONNEL

1. b

CHAPTER 25 PAINTERS AND FURNITURE REFINISHERS

1. d
2. c
3. b
4. d
5. c

CHAPTER 26 PEDIATRIC LABORERS

1. d
2. e

CHAPTER 27 PHOTOGRAPHERS AND FILM DEVELOPERS

1. d
2. a
3. d
4. c
5. a

CHAPTER 28 PLUMBERS

1. b
2. a
3. b
4. c

CHAPTER 29 POLICE AND LAW ENFORCEMENT PERSONNEL

1. b   5. b
2. d   6. c
3. a   7. d
4. b   8. b

CHAPTER 30 PRINTERS

1. d
2. b
3. c

CHAPTER 31 ROOFERS AND ROADBUILDERS

1. The primary toxic exposures in these occupations are fumes from heated coal tar pitch and asphalt. Asphalt fumes are less toxic than coal tar fumes. Solar radiation may exacerbate the toxicity of asphalt and coal tar fumes. Other exposures include dust, hydrogen sulfide, and solvents. Roofers may, on occasion, come in contact with sawdust, if using wood shingles, or fiberglass, if laying insulation. Road builders may be exposed to exhaust fumes and may be at risk for carbon monoxide toxicity if working in enclosed spaces.

2. Fumes from coal tar and, to a lesser extent, asphalt fumes are skin and eye irritants and photosensitizing agents. Workers complain of burning skin and pruritus and develop erythema and blistering after exposure to these fumes. These symptoms are referred to as the *burns* or the *smarts* and are worsened by exposure to solar radiation and cold wind. Ocular burning and erythema are also common and also worsened by solar radiation. Dark skin color is protective against the skin but not the ocular symptoms.

3. Coal tar is a human carcinogen. Workers chronically exposed to coal tar are at increased risk of developing skin, lung, gastric, and hematologic cancers. Asphalt fumes are carcinogenic in animals but to a lesser extent than coal tar fumes. It is not certain that asphalt fumes are human carcinogens.

4. *Tar wart* is the slang name for a keratoacanthoma in workers using coal tar or pitch. These are benign, dome-shaped skin tumors that most often develop on the face after decades of exposure to pitch. Because they resemble squamous cell cancer and have the potential to progress to cancer, they should all be removed and sent for pathologic examination.

5. A PAH that contains a bay region (see Fig. 20-1) is likely to be carcinogenic. Bay regions allow the PAH to be metabolized to a diol epoxide. Diol epoxides are very reactive and can bind to and damage DNA. Repetitive DNA damage can result in cancer. Important PAHs that contain bay regions include benzo(*a*)pyrene, chrysene, and dibenz(*a,h*)anthracene.

6. The simplest way to estimate PAH exposure is to measure the concentration of coal tar or asphalt fumes in the workplace air. Total fumes correlate only roughly with PAH exposure, so a more accurate method would be to measure total PAH concentration or to measure the concentration of specific PAHs, such as benzo(*a*)pyrene. This is technically more difficult than the first option and is rarely used. An experimental method to estimate exposure to harmful PAHs is to measure adducts between PAHs and white blood cells, DNA, or serum albumin.

7. Cigarette smoke is perhaps the most important source of PAHs in smokers. Coal tar–containing psoriasis remedies contain PAHs, as do numerous food products, including smoked or barbecued meats, roasted nuts and coffee, and vegetable oil. Polluted water, soil, and air often contains PAHs.

CHAPTER 32 SANDBLASTERS

1. Chronic silicosis is much more common than acute silicosis; it occurs after decades of exposure to moderate levels of free crystalline silica. Acute silicosis occurs after just a few years of enormous silica exposure. Radiographically, chronic silicosis is characterized by upper-zone rounded opacities, which may coalesce into large areas of fibrosis, with basilar emphysema. "Eggshell" lymph node calcification may also be seen. Acute silicosis, by contrast, presents a ground-glass radiographic appearance, and what fibrosis is present is linear and occurs in the lower lung zones.

2. Methods used to control silica exposure in sandblasting include measurement of exposure and identification of the sources of exposure, replacing silica-containing materials with silica-free materials, isolation and enclosure of work processes, limiting the amount of time a sandblaster may spend in the blasting chamber, personal protective equipment, and special ventilation in blasting areas.

3. Your 35-year-old patient has presumptive chronic simple silicosis, which is currently asymptomatic. If he is a smoker, he will likely develop disabling chronic obstructive pulmonary disease before he would be disabled by his silicosis. He should cease his exposure to silica immediately, as he has developed these radiographic changes after only 10 years of exposure; if he smokes, he should quit. A PPD should be placed to test for tuberculosis exposure. If his PPD is positive, he may require empiric isoniazid therapy. Should his diagnosis be in doubt (he may have sarcoidosis or histoplasmosis or tuberculosis), he should have a bronchoscopy with bronchial alveolar lavage to look for acid-fast bacilli. He may progress to lung biopsy, should his disease become symptomatic, or should the diagnosis of tuberculosis be seriously entertained (tuberculosis is a treatable illness and silicosis at this time is not). Pulmonary function tests may show a restrictive pattern (or obstructive, if he is a smoker) and may help serve as baseline for future evaluations of disability. Chest CT may reveal confluent disease (evidence of PMF) which would change your patient's prognosis. At this time, however, there would be little reason to perform lung CT on this asymptomatic patient.

4. On pathologic section, the lung affected by chronic silicosis contains silicotic nodules: whorled collagen around a hyalin center, with an inflammatory margin. The nodules expand to fibrose the structures of the lung: parenchyma, vessels, airways, pleura. Steelworkers with silicosis tend to have stellate lesions of reticulin and collagen, instead of the classic silicotic nodule. Acute silicosis is pathologically quite different: silicotic nodules are not seen; instead, the alveoli are filled with proteinaceous material.

5. Progressive massive fibrosis is distinguished radiographically and pathologically from simple silicosis by the degree of fibrosis and the appearance of coalescent lesions. The radiographic findings are associated with end-stage silicosis and show marked emphysematous changes with diffuse small nodular lesions. Patients are hypoxic at rest and advance to respiratory failure, cor pulmonale, or both.

6. Any patient with silicosis who develops a sudden decline in respiratory function must be evaluated for pneumothorax (caused by spontaneous rupture of the basilar bullae associated with advanced silicosis) and mycobacterial infection.

7. Numerous autoimmune diseases (rheumatoid arthritis, scleroderma, and progressive systemic sclerosis) have been linked with silica exposure, even in the absence of pulmonary disease. Renal disease (nephrotic syndrome and even end-stage renal disease) has also been associated with exposure to silica.

CHAPTER 33 SEWER AND SANITATION PERSONNEL

1. d
2. false
3. b
4. c

CHAPTER 34 SHIP AND DOCKYARD PERSONNEL

1. d   6. a
2. d   7. a
3. b   8. a
4. c   9. a
5. d   10. c

CHAPTER 35 SHOEMAKERS

1. d
2. a
3. b
4. c
5. d

CHAPTER 36 SMELTERS AND METAL RECLAIMERS

1. c
2. e
3. e
4. e
5. e

CHAPTER 37 WELDERS

1. d
2. c
3. c
4. d

CHAPTER 38 ZOOKEEPERS AND VETERINARIANS

1. a
2. c
3. a
4. e
5. b

CHAPTER 39 DYNAMITE AND EXPLOSIVES

1. d   6. b
2. b   7. d
3. e   8. c
4. a   9. c
5. b   10. b

CHAPTER 40 FERTILIZER

1. e   6. a
2. e   7. d
3. e   8. c
4. b   9. b
5. d   10. e

CHAPTER 41 GLASS MANUFACTURE

1. b   6. e
2. e   7. c
3. d   8. b
4. c   9. c
5. b   10. e

CHAPTER 42 HEALTH CARE

1. a   7. d
2. c   8. e
3. a   9. e
4. b   10. c
5. a   11. c
6. d

CHAPTER 43 MATCH PRODUCTION

1. a   6. d
2. b   7. a
3. c   8. c
4. b   9. a
5. d   10. d

CHAPTER 44 NATURAL GAS

1. c	7. d
2. a	8. c
3. e	9. a
4. c	10. b
5. d	11. e
6. c	

CHAPTER 45 PHARMACEUTICAL

1. a
2. a
3. a, b
4. a
5. a

CHAPTER 46 PLASTICS

1. d	6. b
2. b	7. a
3. a	8. b
4. c	9. a
5. a	10. c

CHAPTER 47 RAILROAD

1. b	6. b
2. a	7. a
3. c	8. c
4. d	9. a
5. e	10. e

CHAPTER 48 SEMICONDUCTOR

1. c	6. c
2. b	7. e
3. b	8. b
4. c	9. b
5. d	10. d

CHAPTER 49 TEXTILE MANUFACTURE

1. b	6. a
2. d	7. b
3. d	8. b
4. c	9. c
5. e	10. d

CHAPTER 50 TOOL AND DIE AND MACHINISTS

1. d	6. a
2. e	7. a
3. d	8. a
4. e	9. d
5. c	10. d

CHAPTER 51 OUTDOOR AIR POLLUTION AND ISSUES OF QUALITY

1. e	6. d
2. a	7. c
3. e	8. b
4. b	9. a
5. b	10. e

CHAPTER 52 INDOOR AIR QUALITY

1. a	6. b
2. a	7. b
3. a	8. b
4. b	9. a
5. a	10. b

CHAPTER 53 WATER POLLUTION

1. b	6. d
2. c	7. c
3. a	8. d
4. d	9. a
5. a	10. a

CHAPTER 54 NOISE POLLUTION

1. a. T	6. a. T
b. T	b. F
c. T	c. T
d. T	d. T
2. a. F	7. a. F
b. T	b. F
c. F	c. F
d. T	d. T
3. a. T	8. a. F
b. F	b. F
c. T	c. F
d. T	d. T
4. a. F	9. a. T
b. T	b. T
c. F	c. T
d. T	d. T
5. a. T	10. d
b. F	
c. T	
d. T	

CHAPTER 55 ASBESTOS

1. d	6. a
2. a	7. d
3. b	8. b
4. c	9. b
5. a	10. c

CHAPTER 56 CHEMICAL CARCINOGENESIS

1. b	6. b
2. a	7. b
3. d	8. e
4. d	9. d
5. a	10. b

CHAPTER 57 ENVIRONMENTAL AUDITS AND PROPERTY TRANSFERS

1. a	4. all
2. d	5. d
3. b	6. c

CHAPTER 58 ENVIRONMENTAL RISKS AND THE CLINICIAN: INFORMING WORRIED PATIENTS

1. c	6. d
2. d	7. a
3. b	8. c
4. b	9. false
5. d	10. a

CHAPTER 59 IONIZING RADIATION

1. c
2. d
3. a
4. b
5. a

CHAPTER 60 NONIONIZING RADIATION

1. a	6. b
2. c	7. d
3. a	8. d
4. c	9. d
5. c	10. c

CHAPTER 61 RESIDENTIAL RADON AND LUNG CANCER

1. a	6. c
2. a	7. b
3. a	8. b
4. a	9. d
5. a	10. d

Review Answers

Appendix IV

Toxin Guide

Chapter number	Chapter title	Subject/toxin discussed	Other chapters discussing the subject/toxin	Chapter location
2	**Artists and artisans**	Lead (glazes)	26, 28, 29, 34, 36, 41, 47, 51, 57	p. 9
		Manganese	34	
		Cadmium	12, 37	
		Chromium	6, 12, 20	
		Gold	4, 20, 22, 61	
		Silver cyanate	—	
		Hydrofluoric acid	9, 25, 41, 48	
		Dyes	19, 25, 30, 49, 56	
3	**Athletes**	Oxides of nitrogen	14, 39, 44, 51	p. 19
		Anabolic steroids	—	
		Chlorine	5, 9, 44	
		Supplements	—	
		Antihistamines	—	
		Erythropoietin	—	
4	**Aviation personnel**	Jet fuels	22	p. 29
		Lubricants	21, 47, 50	
		Gasoline	21, 22	
		JP-4	—	
		JP-5	—	
		JP-7	—	
		Triorthocresyl phosphate	—	
		Avgas	2, 20, 22, 61	
5	**Carpenters and loggers**	Plicatic acid	—	p. 33
		Exotic woods	—	
		Chlorine	3, 9, 44	
		Hydrogen sulfide	33, 40, 44	
		Methylmercaptan	—	
		Pentachlorophenol	—	
		Copper	—	
		Nickel	20	
6	**Concrete workers and masons**	Chromium	2, 12, 20	p. 41
		Cement	—	
		Cobalt	41	
		Calcium hydroxide	—	
		Silica	32, 36, 41	
		Asbestos	26, 28, 34, 42, 53, 55, 56, 57	
		Lime	—	
7	**Divers**	Oxygen	—	p. 49
		Nitrogen	—	
		Carbon dioxide	14, 15, 33, 44	
		Carbon monoxide	15, 29, 33, 36, 47, 51	

Continued.

Chapter number	Chapter title	Subject/toxin discussed	Other chapters discussing the subject/toxin	Chapter location
8	Doctors, nurses, and dentists	Glutaraldehyde	42	p. 61
		Mercury	20, 25	
		Methylmethacrylate	42, 46	
		Ethylene oxide	38, 42, 56	
		Nitrous oxide	—	
		Antineoplastic drugs	—	
		Chemotherapeutic drugs	—	
9	Domestic and building maintenance workers	Chlorine	3, 5, 44	p. 67
		Ammonia	14, 15, 40	
		Chloramine	—	
		Hydrofluoric acid	2, 25, 41, 48	
		Phenol	—	
		Sodium hypochlorite	—	
		Dettol	—	
10	Dry cleaners	Perchloroethylene	—	p. 73
		Carbon tetrachloride	—	
		Trichloroethylene	53, 58	
		Stoddard solvent	21	
		Naphtha	30	
		F-113	—	
		Trichloroethane	—	
11	Electricians	Polychlorinated biphenyl (PCB)	—	p. 83
		Furans	—	
		Polychloroquaterphenyl (PCQ)	—	
		Dioxins	58	
		Polychlorinated dibenzofuran (PCDF)	—	
12	Electroplaters	Solvents	22, 25, 33, 34, 35, 41, 45, 48, 49, 53, 54	p. 89
		Cyanide	15, 20, 50	
		Cadmium	2, 37	
		Chromium	2, 6, 20	
		Acids	2, 9, 25, 29, 41, 42, 48	
		Alkalis	42	
		Heavy metals	40	
		Electricity	—	
13	Exterminators	Organophosphates	26, 40	p. 101
		Pyrethrin	—	
		Pyrethroids	—	
		Arsenic	53, 56	
14	Farmers and farm personnel	Ammonia	9, 15, 40	p. 105
		Oxides of nitrogen	3, 39, 44, 51	
		Methane	33, 44	
		Carbon dioxide	7, 15, 33, 44	
		Carbon	—	
		Nonionizing radiation	17, 29, 60	
		Mycotoxins	—	
		Pesticides	17, 38	

Chapter number	Chapter title	Subject/toxin discussed	Other chapters discussing the subject/toxin	Chapter location
15	**Firefighters**	Carbon monoxide	7, 29, 33, 36, 47, 51	p. 113
		Cyanide	12, 20, 50	
		Acrolein	—	
		Carbon dioxide	7, 14, 33, 44	
		Particulates	51	
		Ammonia	9, 14, 40	
		HCl	—	
		Isocyanates	—	
		Phosgene	—	
		Sulfur dioxide	51	
16	**Floor and carpet layers**	Methylmethacrylate	—	p. 123
		Glues	—	
		Adhesives	—	
		Acrylates	—	
		Epoxies	—	
		Polyesters	—	
		Ethyl acrylates	—	
17	**Florists and groundskeepers**	Tetramethylthiuram	—	p. 135
		Fungicides	—	
		Pesticides	14, 38	
		Dithiocarbamates	—	
		Nonionizing radiation	14, 29, 60	
		Ultraviolet light	34, 50, 60	
		Tuppalin-A	—	
18	**Food preparation workers**	Psoralens	—	p. 143
		Meat wrappers' asthma	—	
19	**Hairdressers and cosmetologists**	Phenylenediamine	—	p. 147
		Glycerol monothioglycolate	—	
		Polyvinylpyrrolidone	—	
		Lauryl sulfates	—	
		Hydrogen peroxide	—	
		Thioglycolate	—	
		Lanolin	—	
		Dyes	2, 25, 30, 49, 56	
		Detergents	—	
		Brilliantine	—	
		Bromates		
20	**Jewelers**	Cyanide	12, 15, 50	p. 153
		Gold	2, 4, 22, 61	
		Silver	—	
		Platinum	—	
		Nickel	5	
		Mercury	8, 25	
		Chromium-6	2, 6, 12	
21	**Mechanics**	Diesel	22, 47	p. 171
		Gasoline	4, 22	
		Degreaser	47, 50	
		Stoddard solvent	10	
		Lubricants	4, 47, 50	
		Benzene	26, 56, 58	
		Methylethylketone (MEK)	35	

Continued.

Chapter number	Chapter title	Subject/toxin discussed	Other chapters discussing the subject/toxin	Chapter location
22	Military personnel	Trimethyl propane phosphate	—	p. 182
		Jet fuels	4	
		Gasoline	4, 21	
		Avgas	2, 4, 20, 61	
		Diesel	21	
		Magnesium thorium	—	
		Solvents	12, 25, 33, 34, 35, 42, 45, 48, 49, 53, 54	
		Hypergallic propellants	—	
		Halon	—	
23	Morticians	Formaldehyde	26, 38, 42, 49, 50	p. 195
		Glutaraldehyde	—	
24	Office personnel	Volatile organic chemicals (VOCs)	—	p. 203
		Environmental tobacco smoke	26, 52, 56, 58, 61	
		Carbonless paper	—	
		Multiple chemical sensitivity (MCS)	—	
		Sick building syndrome	52, 58	
25	Painters and furniture refinishers	Hydrofluoric acid	2, 9, 41, 48	p. 211
		Dyes	2, 19, 30, 49, 56	
		Solvents	12, 22, 33, 34, 35, 42, 45, 48, 49, 53, 54	
		Varnish	—	
		Lacquers	—	
		Methylene chloride	45	
		Toluene diisocyanate (TDI)	—	
		Isophorone diisocyanate (IPDI)	—	
		Hexamethylene diisocyanate (HDI)	—	
		Benzo[a]pyrene	31	
		Mercury	8, 20	
26	Pediatric laborers	Green tobacco	—	p. 219
		Lead	2, 28, 29, 34, 36, 41, 47, 51, 57	
		Organophosphates	13, 40	
		Environmental tobacco smoke	24, 52, 56, 58, 61	
		Benzene	21, 56, 58	
		Formaldehyde	23, 38, 42, 49, 50	
		Asbestos	6, 28, 34, 42, 53, 55, 56, 57	
27	Photographers and film developers	Potassium ferrocyanide	—	p. 227
		Hydroquinone	—	
		Aminophenol	—	
		α-naphthol	—	
		Selenium	—	
		Ammonium thiosulfate	—	
		Hypochlorites	—	
28	Plumbers	Lead	2, 26, 29, 34, 36, 41, 47, 51, 57	p. 231
		Asbestos	6, 26, 34, 42, 53, 55, 56, 57	
		Solder flux	—	
		Zinc	37	
		Tetrahydrofuran	—	
		Cyclohexanone	—	
		Fluorocarbons	—	

Chapter number	Chapter title	Subject/toxin discussed	Other chapters discussing the subject/toxin	Chapter location
29	Police and law enforcement personnel	Lead	2, 26, 28, 34, 36, 41, 47, 53, 57	p. 233
		Carbon monoxide	7, 15, 33, 36, 47, 51	
		Selenious acid	12	
		Cocaine	—	
		Tetrahydrocannabinol (THC)	—	
		Nonionizing radiation	14, 17, 60	
30	Printers	Toluene	—	p. 243
		Azoridine	—	
		Carbon black	—	
		Pigments	2, 19, 25, 49, 56	
		Naphtha	10	
		n-hexane		
		Isopropyl alcohol	—	
31	Roofers and roadbuilders	Coal tar	—	p. 247
		Benzo[a]pyrene	25	
		Asphalt	—	
		Polycyclic aromatic hydro-carbon (PAHs)	36, 44, 56	
		Fiberglass	—	
32	Sandblasters	Silica	6, 36, 41	p. 255
33	Sewer and sanitation personnel	Hydrogen sulfide	5, 40, 44	p. 265
		Methane	14, 44	
		Carbon dioxide	7, 14, 15, 44	
		Hydrogen cyanide	—	
		Carbon monoxide	7, 15, 29, 36, 47, 51	
		Endotoxin	—	
		Solvents	12, 22, 25, 34, 35, 42, 45, 48, 49, 53, 54	
34	Ship and dockyard personnel	Asbestos	6, 26, 28, 42, 53, 55, 56, 57	p. 275
		Lead	2, 26, 28, 29, 36, 41, 47, 51, 57	
		Manganese	2	
		Ultraviolet light	17, 50, 60	
		Styrene	46	
		Solvents	12, 22, 25, 33, 35, 42, 45, 48, 49, 53, 54	
35	Shoemakers	2.5-Hexandione	—	p. 282
		Benzene oxide	—	
		Tri-orthocresylphosphate (TOCP)	—	
		Methylethylketone (MEK)	21	
		Toluene	—	
		Solvents	12, 22, 25, 33, 34, 42, 45, 48, 49, 53, 54	
		Vinyl chloride	46, 56	
		Leather dust	—	
36	Smelters and metal reclaimers	Lead	2, 26, 28, 29, 34, 41, 47, 51, 57	p. 291
		Carbon monoxide	7, 15, 29, 33, 47, 51	
		Silica	6, 32, 41	
		PAHs	31, 44, 56	
37	Welders	Metal fumes	47	p. 303
		Polymer fumes	—	
		Siderosis	—	
		Colophony	—	
		Iron	—	

Continued.

Chapter number	Chapter title	Subject/toxin discussed	Other chapters discussing the subject/toxin	Chapter location
37	**Welders—cont'd**	Zinc	28	
		Cadmium	2, 12	
		Aluminum	—	
38	**Zookeepers and veterinarians**	Ethylene oxide	8, 42, 56	p. 311
		Anesthetic gases	—	
		Ionizing radiation	42, 59	
		Pesticides	14, 17	
		Formaldehyde	23, 26, 42, 49, 50	
39	**Dynamite and explosives**	Nitrates	40	p. 321
		Oxides of nitrogen	3, 14, 44, 51	
40	**Fertilizer**	Ammonia	9, 14, 15	p. 327
		Heavy metals	12	
		Hydrogen sulfide	5, 33, 44	
		Organophosphates	13, 26	
		Nitrates	39	
		Methemoglobin formation	—	
		Sewage study	—	
41	**Glass manufacturer**	Hydrofluoric acid	2, 9, 12, 25, 48	p. 337
		Heat	—	
		Silica	6, 32, 36	
		Lead	2, 26, 28, 29, 34, 36, 47, 51, 57	
		Cobalt	6	
		Zirconium dioxide	—	
42	**Health care**	Glutaraldehyde	8	p. 345
		Ethylene oxide	8, 38, 56	
		Formaldehyde	23, 26, 38, 49, 50	
		Methyl methacrylate	8, 46	
		Pentamidine	—	
		Organic solvents	12, 22, 25, 33, 34, 35, 45, 48, 49, 54	
		Ionizing radiation	38, 59	
		Asbestos	6, 26, 28, 34, 53, 55, 56, 57	
		Acids	2, 9, 25, 29, 41, 48	
		Alkalis	12	
		Latex	—	
43	**Match production**	Chromates	—	p. 351
		Phosphates	—	
		Antimony	—	
44	**Natural gas**	Methane	14, 33	p. 359
		Hydrogen sulfide	5, 33, 40	
		Chlorine	3, 5, 9	
		Chlorine dioxide	7, 14, 15, 33	
		Bromine	—	
		Carbonyl sulfide	—	
		Mercaptans	—	
		PAHs	31, 36, 56	
		PAH-nitrogenated	31, 36, 56	
		Oxides of nitrogen	3, 14, 39, 51	
45	**Pharmaceutical**	Methylene chloride	25	p. 367
		Estrogen	—	
		Solvents	12, 22, 25, 33, 34, 35, 42, 48, 49, 53, 54	
		Psyllium dust	—	
		Antibiotics	—	
		Chloroquine	—	

Chapter number	Chapter title	Subject/toxin discussed	Other chapters discussing the subject/toxin	Chapter location
46	Plastics	Styrene	34	p. 373
		Butadiene	—	
		Toluene diisocyanate (TDI)	—	
		Toluene diamine (TDA)	—	
		Polyurethane	—	
		Polyvinyl chloride	35, 56	
		Methyl methacrylate	8, 42	
47	Railroad	Diesel exhaust	21, 22	p. 379
		Carbon monoxide	7, 15, 29, 33, 36, 51	
		Lead	2, 26, 28, 29, 34, 36, 41, 51, 57	
		Reactive Airway Dysfunction Syndrome (RADs)	—	
		Cutting oils	50	
		Lubricants	4, 21, 50	
		Degreasers	21, 50	
		Metal fumes	37	
48	Semiconductor	Arsine	—	p. 387
		Phosphine	—	
		Ozone	51	
		Silicon	—	
		Diborane		
		Solvents	12, 22, 25, 33, 34, 35, 42, 45, 49, 53, 54	
		Gallium arsenide	—	
		Hydrofluoric acid	2, 9, 12, 25, 41	
49	Textile manufacture	Azo-dyes	2, 19, 25, 30, 56	p. 395
		Byssinosis/dust	—	
		Benzidine	—	
		Solvents	12, 22, 25, 33, 34, 35, 42, 45, 48, 53, 54	
		Formaldehyde	23, 26, 38, 42, 50	
		Carbon disulfide	—	
50	Tool and die and machinists	Cutting oils	47	p. 403
		Formaldehyde	23, 26, 38, 42, 49	
		Cyanide	12, 15, 20	
		Ultraviolet light	17, 34, 60	
		Lubricants	4, 21, 47	
		Degreasers	21, 47	
51	Outdoor air pollution and issues of quality	Oxides of nitrogen	3, 14, 39, 44	p. 419
		Sulfur dioxide	15	
		Ozone	48	
		Carbon monoxide	7, 15, 20, 33, 36, 47	
		Lead	2, 26, 28, 29, 34, 36, 41, 47, 57	
		Particulates	15	
52	Indoor air quality	4-Phenylcyclohexene (4-PC)	—	p. 427
		Environmental tobacco smoke	24, 26, 56, 61	
		Sick building syndrome	24, 58	
		Multiple chemical sensitivity	58	
		Bioaerosols	—	
		Volatile organics	—	
53	Water pollution	Radon	56, 57, 59, 61	p. 437
		Asbestos	6, 26, 28, 34, 42, 55, 56, 57	
		Arsenic	13, 56	

Continued.

Chapter number	Chapter title	Subject/toxin discussed	Other chapters discussing the subject/toxin	Chapter location
53	Water pollution—cont'd	Solvents	12, 22, 25, 33, 34, 35, 42, 45, 48, 49, 54	
		Trichloroethylene	10, 58	
54	Noise pollution	Solvents	12, 22, 25, 33, 34, 35, 42, 45, 48, 49, 53	p. 451
		Smoke	—	
55	Asbestos	Asbestos	6, 26, 28, 34, 42, 53, 56, 57	p. 471
56	Chemical carcinogenesis	Radon	53, 57, 59, 61	p. 489
		Dyes	2, 19, 25, 30, 49	
		Benzene	21, 26, 58	
		PAHs	31, 36, 44	
		Acrylonitrile	—	
		Ethylene oxide	8, 38, 42	
		Environmental tobacco smoke	24, 26, 52, 58, 61	
		Vinyl chloride	35, 46	
		Arsenic	13, 53	
		Asbestos	6, 26, 28, 34, 42, 53, 55, 57	
57	Environmental audits and property transfers	Air	—	p. 499
		Asbestos	6, 26, 28, 34, 42, 53, 55, 56	
		Lead	2, 26, 28, 29, 34, 36, 41, 47, 51	
		Radon	53, 56, 59, 61	
58	Environmental risks and the clinician: informing worried patients	Benzene	21, 26, 56	p. 505
		Trichloroethylene	10, 53	
		Sick building syndrome	24, 52	
		Multiple chemical sensitivity	51	
		Dioxins	11	
		Environmental tobacco smoke	24, 26, 52, 56, 61	
		Magnetic fields	—	
59	Ionizing radiation	Ionizing radiation	38, 42	p. 517
		Strontium	—	
		Cesium	—	
		Radon	53, 56, 57, 61	
		Uranium	61	
		Potassium-40	—	
		Plutonium	—	
		Chernobyl	—	
60	Nonionizing radiation	Nonionizing radiation	14, 17, 29	p. 531
		Ultraviolet light	17, 34, 50	
		Visual	—	
		Infrared	—	
		Radio frequency	—	
		Microwaves	—	
		Lasers	—	
61	Residential radon and lung cancer	Radon	53, 56, 57, 59	p. 537
		Uranium	59	
		Radium	—	
		Gold	2, 4, 20, 22	
		Tin	—	
		Fluospar	—	
		Environmental tobacco smoke	24, 26, 52, 56, 58	

Index